Handbook of human intelligence

Handbook of human intelligence

Edited by ROBERT J. STERNBERG

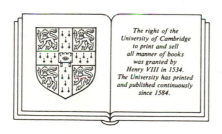

The right of the
University of Cambridge
to print and sell
all manner of books
was granted by
Henry VIII in 1534.
The University has printed
and published continuously
since 1584.

CAMBRIDGE UNIVERSITY PRESS

Cambridge
New York New Rochelle
Melbourne Sydney

Published by the Press Syndicate of the University of Cambridge
The Pitt Building, Trumpington Street, Cambridge CB2 1RP
32 East 57th Street, New York, NY 10022, USA
10 Stamford Road, Oakleigh, Melbourne 3166, Australia

First published 1982
Reprinted 1984, 1985, 1986, 1988

Printed in the United States of America

Library of Congress Cataloging in Publication Data
Main entry under title:
Handbook of human intelligence.
Includes indexes.
1. Intellect. 2. Intellect – Research.
I. *Sternberg, Robert J.*
BF431.H3186   153.9   82–1160   AACR2
ISBN 0 521 22870 0 hard covers
ISBN 0 521 29687 0 paperback

Contents

v

Contributors

Jonathan Baron
Department of Psychology
University of Pennsylvania

Ann L. Brown
Center for the Study of Reading
University of Illinois

Joseph C. Campione
Center for the Study of Reading
University of Illinois

John B. Carroll
L. L. Thurstone Psychometric
Laboratory
University of North Carolina

Louise Carter-Saltzman
Department of Psychology
University of Washington

Lynn A. Cooper
Learning Research
and Development Center
University of Pittsburgh

Natalie Dehn
Department of Computer Science
Yale University

William K. Estes
Department of Psychology
and Social Relations
Harvard University

Roberta A. Ferrara
Center for the Study of Reading
University of Illinois

Harry J. Jerison
Department of Psychiatry
University of California
Los Angeles

Laboratory of Comparative
Human Cognition
Communications Program D-003
University of California
San Diego

Janet S. Powell
Department of Psychology
Yale University

Dennis T. Regan
Department of Psychology
Cornell University

D. Dean Richards
Department of Psychology
University of California
Los Angeles

William Salter
Department of Psychology
Yale University

Sandra Scarr
Department of Psychology
Yale University

Roger Schank
Department of Computer Science
Yale University

Victoria Seitz
Department of Psychology
Yale University

Robert S. Siegler
Department of Psychology
Carnegie-Mellon University

Richard E. Snow
School of Education
Stanford University

Robert J. Sternberg
Department of Psychology
Yale University

Elanna Yalow
School of Education
Stanford University

Edward Zigler
Department of Psychology
Yale University

Preface

The investigation of intelligence is rapidly becoming central to psychology as a discipline, and to all disciplines involved in the scientific study of the mind. The reburgeoning of interest in the field of intelligence that we have witnessed in recent years could result in a healthy and thriving subdiscipline of psychology (which would crosscut a number of other disciplines as well). But fields of psychology (and other sciences) in these early stages of growth (or regrowth) can also develop into stunted and quickly moribund endeavors, especially if they become task- or method-centered rather than problem-centered.

In view of these considerations, the time seemed to be ripe for a *Handbook of Human Intelligence* – a volume that would help guide research in intelligence at this critical juncture and that would point out directions for research during at least the 1980s. Each chapter in the handbook (a) poses the critical questions and issues that need to be addressed by research in the given subfield, (b) reviews and evaluates recent contributions to the subfield to assess the importance of the questions the contributions address and how well the contributions address them, and (c) indicates lines of inquiry that have been and are likely to continue to be valuable (and valueless) to pursue. The chapters are written for psychologists and others who have a general background in psychology, but not necessarily any specialized knowledge about the various subfields covered. Thus each chapter can serve as an introduction to a given subfield of intelligence to novices in the area and as an evaluative review of the subfield to experts.

This book does not provide the kinds of literature reviews found in *Psychological Bulletin* articles or *Annual Review of Psychology* chapters. In fact, contributors were told to avoid detailed literature reviews of these kinds. Nor is this a sourcebook of techniques for the study of intelligence. I hope readers will find the present chapters more lively and provocative than pieces of that sort usually are. The idea in soliciting authors for these chapters was to find people who could both provide direction to the field and characterize the directions the field has taken so far.

The handbook covers a wide range of topics in intelligence. Indeed, in constructing a table of contents, I tried to include all of what I believed to be the areas in which major contributions to research on intelligence are being and will continue to be made. Unfortunately, contributors of two chapters and their replacements – "Neuropsychology of intelligence" and "Psychophysiology of intelligence" – failed to come through with their promised chapters. As a result, the general area of the physiology of intelligence failed to receive the representation it deserved in this compendium.

The book is divided into five major parts. The first part, "The nature of intelligence and its measurement," contains two chapters intended to serve as introductions to

xi

the remainder of the volume. The first, "Conceptions of intelligence," attempts to provide an organizing and integrating framework for the chapters in the remaining parts. The second, "The measurement of intelligence," provides a rather comprehensive history of the general field of intelligence and its measurement. Thus the first chapter is an overview of the field as it stands today; the second is an overview of how the field got to be the way it is today. The second part, "Cognition, personality, and intelligence," contains three chapters relating various aspects of cognition and intelligence, ranging from the lower "levels" of processing to the higher ones: "Attention, perception, and intelligence," "Learning, memory, and intelligence," and "Reasoning, problem solving, and intelligence." Part II also includes one chapter relating personality and intelligence, one on artificial and human intelligence, and one on mental retardation and intelligence. These chapters are all largely concerned with delineating the nature of intelligence as it exists within the individual. In contrast, the chapters in the third part of the book, "Society, culture, and intelligence," focus on delineating the nature of intelligence as it relates to and is defined by society and culture. This part contains chapters on education and intelligence, social policy and intelligence, and culture and intelligence. The chapters in Part IV, "The phylogeny and ontogeny of intelligence," relate intelligence to even broader contexts – the life span of the individual, the human ancestors of the individual, and the ancestors of the species as a whole. The fifth part, "Metatheory of intelligence," consists of just a single chapter, "Theories of intelligence," which raises epistemological issues concerning theorizing about intelligence as it has been done both in this handbook and elsewhere.

I am grateful to the Office of Naval Research, the National Institute of Education, and the Army Research Institute, which jointly funded a conference of handbook contributors in San Diego in January 1980. Dr. Marshall Farr of the Office of Naval Research was particularly helpful in putting together the funding that made this conference possible. I am also grateful to Susan Milmoe, Behavioral Science Editor of Cambridge University Press in New York, for her tremendous support of the project in all its phases. Finally, I thank the contributors for their willingness to undertake a difficult and challenging task.

R.J.S.

PART I

The nature of intelligence and its measurement

1 *Conceptions of intelligence*

ROBERT J. STERNBERG AND WILLIAM SALTER

We seek here to distill from the chapters of this handbook ideas that unify what otherwise might appear to be a series of unintegrated and possibly unintegrable conceptions of the nature of intelligence and the circumstances surrounding the manifestation of intelligence. We shall organize our overview by the main headings of the book (excluding only the introductory and concluding parts): "Cognition, personality, and intelligence," "Society, culture, and intelligence," and "The phylogeny and ontogeny of intelligence." We shall conclude with a discussion of those themes that seem to run throughout the handbook. Obviously, this scheme is only one of the many possible schemes that might be used to organize the chapters; but then, our choice of unifying ideas also represents only one of the innumerable partitionings of ideas that might have been selected. We freely admit that our overview is a subjective one that derives from and is guided by some interaction between the content of the chapters and the content that was in our minds before we ever read the chapters. We hope the interaction is a fruitful one in conveying some of the unities that we think tie together the various chapters.

The term *intelligence* is used in many different ways by many different authors of the chapters of this book. As integrators, we face the difficult task of trying to decide whether to "impose" a single definition of intelligence on all of these contributors, and thereby risk being untrue to some of the authors' conceptions of what intelligence is, or whether instead to try to find no common definition at all, and thereby risk writing an "integration" with no integrating theme. Because we believe that there is a definition of intelligence, at a very general level, that would be acceptable to most, if not all, the contributors to this book, as well as to many others who have studied intelligence, we shall attempt to define intelligence, as have others before us, as "goal-directed adaptive behavior." At the end of the chapter, we will argue that this definition does indeed fit the body of ideas and research presented in this book.

1.1. COGNITION, PERSONALITY, AND INTELLIGENCE

The chapters in this section of the handbook are all heavily influenced by the "information-processing" viewpoint. From this point of view, human cognition can be understood largely in terms of the ways in which people process information mentally. This viewpoint is very much a reaction to stimulus-response (S-R) theorizing (cf. Miller, Galanter, & Pribram, 1960): Whereas S-R theorists were interested primarily in the antecedents and consequents of intelligent behavior, information-processing psychologists are interested primarily in the mental phenomena that intervene between stimulus and response. The contributors to this part of the book focus on a great diversity of issues pertinent to these mental phenomena; but some

3

issues seem to form a common core in at least several of the chapters: (a) the processes underlying intelligent behavior, (b) the strategies into which these processes combine, and (c) knowledge and its representation.

PROCESSES UNDERLYING INTELLIGENT BEHAVIOR

All of the authors seem to agree that a necessary condition for understanding intelligence is the identification of the processes that in combination constitute intelligent behavior. The authors do not all agree just what processes should serve as the focus of research; how, if at all, these processes should be classified; or how the processes should be identified. We shall discuss each of these issues in turn.

The processes that constitute the core of intelligent behavior.   Although all of the chapters deal with processes of intelligent behavior, they by no means all deal with the same processes. Sternberg and Powell (Chapter 15) view various theories of intelligence as being distinguished in part by the "level of processing" at which they deal, and argue that a substantial portion of the difference in focus among investigators is due to differences in emphasis on various levels of processing. For example, "encoding" seems to be an important process in many information-processing theories, from theories describing perceptual performance to theories describing complex problem-solving performance. But encoding can occur at many different levels, depending upon the information contained in the stimulus to be encoded, the ability of the individual to encode the information contained in the stimulus, and the individual's perception of the use to which the encoded information will be put. Thus the level of encoding required in letter-matching tasks of the kind studied by Hunt, Lunneborg, and Lewis (1975; see Cooper & Regan, Chapter 3) might be quite different from that required by the insight tasks that have been studied by Maier (1970; see Sternberg, Chapter 5).

Because levels of processing represent a continuum, or even possibly a number of continua embedded in a multidimensional space, any cut points chosen for discussion will of necessity be arbitrary. For convenience, we will discuss processes used in perception, learning and memory, reasoning, and complex problem solving. It should be noted, however, that these psychological functions do not necessarily represent different or even discrete levels of processing: Complex "perceptual" processes may be every bit as deep in the processing required as are simple "reasoning" processes.

In the literature on attention, perception, and intelligence, reviewed by Cooper and Regan (Chapter 3), the single process that has probably received the most study is that of access to overlearned codes stored in long-term memory. The task most often used for studying this process is the Posner and Mitchell (1967) letter-comparison task. In this task, subjects are asked to decide whether two letters, for example, *A,a,* are either identical in physical appearance (which they obviously are not) or identical in name (which they are, in that they are both the same letter). Hunt et al. (1975) found a modest but significant relationship between name-match time minus physical-match time, on the one hand, and measured verbal ability, on the other; since this initial discovery, the reported level of relationship (r equal to about $-.3$) has been replicated a number of times by several different investigators. Because the name- minus physical-match time difference score seems to represent a relatively pure measure of lexical access time unconfounded by sheer physical recognition time, some investigators (including Hunt et al., 1975) have concluded that lexical access time is in some sense a precursor of, and possibly even a causal agent in, complex verbal processing of the kind measured by standard verbal scholastic aptitude tests.

We believe that this interpretation of the obtained correlation may overstate the degree of dependence of complex verbal processing on very simple processes. We further believe that the relatively modest correlations obtained from the study of very simple processes from laboratory-type perceptual tasks has often led to overestimation of the role of simple processes in the kinds of performance most of us would call intelligent. An alternative explanation of the correlation utilizes the levels-of-processing framework. According to this view, the mental "comparison" process can occur at many different levels of processing, ranging from very low-level physical matching through name matching up to complex semantic matching, as when an individual is asked whether two words represent members of the same semantic category (e.g., both *poodle* and *collie* are kinds of dogs). The higher the level of processing at which the comparison is executed, the higher will be the magnitude of the correlation between comparison time and measured verbal ability. In fact, Goldberg, Schwartz, and Stewart (1977) have found evidence of just such a pattern of correlations for matches of successively higher "levels," and Jackson (1978) has shown that the match need not even be verbal for the correlation to occur. According to this view, the correlation represents not a causal relationship between simple lexical access time and verbal ability, but rather the closeness of the level of comparison required to that required in verbal aptitude tests, as, for example, when a person has to compare the meanings of two words and decide whether they are antonyms (or synonyms). In this levels-of-processing view, a table of intercorrelations for successively higher levels of comparison would form a Guttman simplex, with tasks requiring comparisons at nearer levels showing higher correlations, and tasks requiring comparisons at more distant levels showing lower correlations. The idea of a continuum of complexity, of course, has been used in interpreting performance in a number of intellectual tasks (Guttman, 1965; Jensen, 1970; Marshalek, 1977). We believe, then, that the particular level of comparison required by the Posner Mitchell name-matching task represents only one point along a continuum of complexity of comparisons, and that the particular level of processing required has been accorded more importance than it deserves in the study of individual differences because this level just happens to be that which is required in a well-known and well-respected laboratory paradigm. The obtained correlation between the lexical-access-level comparison parameter and measured verbal ability is fairly modest because there is a fairly large discrepancy in levels of processing between pure name matching and complex semantic matching. The correlation becomes stronger as the level of processing of the laboratory-type task gets closer to the level of processing required by the verbal ability test. The relationship is not a direct causal one, however, but rather one derived indirectly from shared *type* of processing (i.e., comparison) and from not altogether discrepant *levels* of processing for the given type of processing in the two kinds of activities. Thus the level of this and other intertask relationships is jointly determined by type and level of processing.

The literature on learning, memory, and intelligence, reviewed by Estes (Chapter 4) and discussed in the context of retarded performance by Campione, Brown, and Ferrara (Chapter 8), has been a disappointment for many. On the one hand, ability to learn has seemed to many to be one important aspect of intelligence (see, e.g.,

"Intelligence and Its Measurement," 1921; R. Sternberg, Conway, Ketron, & Bernstein, 1981); on the other hand, correlations between parameters (indexes estimating aspects of performance) of learning tasks and scores on intelligence tests have generally been weak. We believe, again, that discrepancies in levels of processing are at least partly to blame for many of the low correlations. There exists an extensive literature on levels of processing in learning (see, e.g., Cermak & Craik, 1979; Craik & Lockhart, 1972), and the literature suggests that learning, like perception, can take place at many different levels. The kinds of learning required by ability tests such as synonyms – where a person may be asked to choose between two possible meanings of a word that differ from each other only in subtle ways – or arithmetic problem solving – where fairly sophisticated algorithms may have to be brought to bear on the problems at hand – were probably at fairly deep levels of processing when these kinds of learning occurred. The kinds of learning that have been studied in many laboratory investigations of individual differences in learning, on the other hand, have been quite simple, requiring what may well have been fairly superficial processing with little opportunity or reason to process the new information in a way that would result in truly long-term retention.

In this view, then, we would not expect much correlation between scores on basic learning tasks and scores on intelligence tests. Instead, we would want to investigate learning situations closer to those that were required for acquisition of the information needed for high performance on intelligence tests or, ideally, situations comparable to those found in everyday life. An example of such learning is that studied by Werner and Kaplan (1952) and by Powell and Sternberg (1981), in which subjects were required to learn meanings of new words presented in everyday reading contexts (see also Sternberg, Powell, & Kaye, in press). When learning scores from the vocabulary-in-context task were correlated with ability scores, Powell and Sternberg obtained correlations that were moderate to high (about .6); this finding suggests that if the level of learning in the experimental task is matched to that which is required for the information needed for the ability tests (IQ, reading, and vocabulary), high correlations can be obtained. Again, we attribute these correlations at least in part to shared kinds and levels of processing.

Correlations of IQ-test scores with parameters estimated from reasoning tasks (e.g., analogies, linear syllogisms, series completions, categorical syllogisms, and the like) of the kind studied in the literature reviewed by Sternberg (Chapter 5)have generally been moderate, often in the .40 – 60 range. Because the tasks studied by investigators of reasoning have often been similar or identical to those found on IQ tests, what is perhaps surprising is that the correlations have not been even higher. Given the high degree of overlap in both the kinds and the levels of processing of the laboratory and ability-test items, one might expect correlations approaching levels of reliability for the tests and tasks. We believe that there are at least three reasons why such high correlations have generally not been obtained. First, whereas ability-test scores tend to be accuracy scores obtained under moderately speeded conditions, reasoning-task scores tend to be latency scores obtained under heavily speeded conditions. Several lines of work have converged to suggest that the abilities involved in speed and accuracy of processing may be distinct and distinguishable (e.g., Carroll, 1980; Egan, 1976; Lohman, 1979a, 1979b; R. Sternberg, 1977, 1980a). Indeed, the issue of just how speed and power are related is a time-honored one in psychometric testing (Cronbach, 1970). Second, when test items are adapted to laboratory use, they are frequently simplified, for example, by reducing the number of alternative answer options (R. Sternberg, 1977) or by using item stems that are just not as difficult as those found on most ability tests (R. Sternberg, 1977, 1981a). Thus the level of processing required in the performance of the laboratory task may, in fact, be reduced below that required in the performance of the standardized test. Third, we believe that the degree of repetition of item types required for reasonably precise individual measurement of parameters in laboratory tasks may result in a degree of routinization that does not appear in IQ-test performance, where items solved are often of multiple types or at least of differing character within a given type. In effect, in the laboratory, the novelty wears off, and the ability to deal with novelty may be an essential part of the intelligence that the tests measure (although only in part) (see Snow, 1980, 1981; R. Sternberg, 1980b, 1981a). In sum, then, the laboratory tasks used in the study of reasoning, and the circumstances surrounding the administration of these tasks, may bear less resemblance to ability tests and the circumstances surrounding their administration than initially may appear to be the case.

Finally, we turn to the complex tasks studied in the problem-solving literature, and especially the insight tasks reviewed by Sternberg (Chapter 5). There is not much literature relating performance on complex problems to performance on intelligence tests, although what literature there is generally suggests, somewhat surprisingly, that the correlations are not very high at all and, indeed, that performance on various insight tasks is not even highly intercorrelated. There is good reason to believe, however, that the weak correlations that have been obtained in studies by the Gestalt psychologists, such as Maier (1970), may have been due to unreliability of measurements; a very recent study (Jacobs & Dominowski, 1981) suggests that with more reliable measurements, ability to solve insight problems does emerge as a stable individual-differences variable. At present, there just is not enough literature to draw firm conclusions about relations between problem solving and intelligence (but see Raaheim, 1974, for an interesting discussion of this relationship).

Categorization of the processes of intelligent behavior. Several taxonomic principles are offered by the various chapter writers, either explicitly or implicitly, for the categorization of the processes of intelligent behavior. The ontological status of these classification schemes is not entirely clear at the present time. All of the chapter authors appear to believe that classification schemes can be at least heuristically useful. Some think that different kinds of processes actually differ functionally in a qualitative way. But none of the authors commit themselves to saying whether the distinctions go beyond function to the representation of differences in the ways various kinds of processes are generated or executed.

One distinction that is common in the cognitive literature is that between executive and nonexecutive processes, or between metacognitive and cognitive processes (see Campione et al., Chapter 8; Sternberg, Chapter 5; and Sternberg & Powell, Chapter 15). Whereas some theorists believe that executive processes, which are postulated to control or activate nonexecutive ones, are different in kind from nonexecutive ones, others view this distinction as superfluous or even deceptive. Whether or not the distinction is needed seems to depend in part upon the form of the theory underlying the account of information processing. For example, production-system theories do not need two kinds of processes; flow chart theories seem to need the two kinds, or at least some way of getting the flow charts built, the processes in them started, and the execution of the strategies continuing. Whether the human processing system requires the distinction is simply unknown at the present time.

A second distinction is that between processes involved in learning, on the one hand, and processes involved in performing what has already been learned, on the other (see Campione et al., Chapter 8; Dehn & Schank, Chapter 7; Estes, Chapter 4; Sternberg, Chapter 5). Campione et al. further distinguish between rehearsal and organizational processes, whereas Sternberg further distinguishes among acquisition, retention, and transfer processes. The view of learning and executive processes as distinct is not shared by everyone. Butterfield (1980) has argued that the distinction between executive and nonexecutive processes is sufficient to account for the difference between performance and learning, so that the present distinction is unnecessary. Other authors do not take a position on whether the two distinctions are both required (e.g., Estes; Dehn & Schank), and still others seem to argue that both distinctions are needed to account for the range of processes individuals use in task performance (e.g., Campione et al.; Sternberg).

A third distinction is that between controlled processes, on the one hand, and automatic ones, on the other (see Estes, Chapter 4). Controlled processes (or, more generally, controlled processing) are capacity-limited, usually serial in combination, and under subject control; automatic processes (or, more generally, automatic processing) are capacity-unlimited, usually parallel in combination, and not under subject control. It seems likely that a given "process" can be controlled or automatic, depending upon the circumstances of its execution. For example, a process may become automatized through practice. Thus it appears likely that this distinction is orthogonal to the others, and can apply within as well as between processes.

A fourth distinction, which we introduced earlier, is that between levels in the execution of a given process. This distinction, like the controlled–automatic one, seems to apply within as well as between processes. A process, such as encoding, can be executed at a number of levels, depending upon the requirements of a given task, the subject's abilities, and the interaction between the two. This distinction is crossed with the ones just discussed, in that we would propose that any process can be executed at multiple levels.

We believe that at this stage of psychological investigation, process taxonomies serve a useful heuristic function in highlighting ways in which processes are similar to and different from each other. We also believe that there exist valid functional distinctions among processes, and that at least one source of individual differences in human intelligence derives from differential availability, accessibility, and efficiency in execution of various kinds of processes (as well as in execution of multiple processes of a given kind). We would not seek to press the distinction among kinds of processes beyond the functional level, however, because at the present time there exist no good ways of validating any one taxonomy in comparison to others. Indeed, the search for such a means of validation would seem to be a useful direction for present pursuit.

Identification of the processes of intelligent behavior. The chapters of this handbook discuss a number of ways by which processes of intelligent behavior can be identified. We shall describe some of these methods, emphasizing that our list is neither exhaustive nor even mutually exclusive, and attempting to evaluate the strengths and weaknesses of the various methods.[1]

A first approach to the identification of the processes of intelligent behavior is what might be referred to as a *cognitive-correlates approach* (Pellegrino & Glaser, 1979; R. Sternberg, 1981b). In this approach, subjects are tested in their ability to perform

tasks that contemporary cognitive psychologists believe measure basic human information processes. Such tasks include, among others, the Posner and Mitchell (1967)
letter-matching task and the S. Sternberg (1969) memory-scanning task. Subjects
are usually tested via either tachistoscope or a computer terminal, and the principal
dependent measure of interest is response time (see Cooper & Regan, Chapter 3).

The proximal goal in this research is to estimate parameters representing durations of execution for the information processes constituting intelligent behavior in
each task, and then to investigate the extent to which these processes correlate
across subjects with each other and with scores on measures commonly believed to
assess intelligence (e.g., the Raven Progressive Matrices test). The distal goal of
cognitive-correlates research is to bring about some kind of integration between
individual-differences research and mainstream cognitive psychological research, in
particular, by providing a theoretical grounding from cognitive psychology for differential research (Hunt, Frost, & Lunneborg, 1973). Thus, instead of trying to draw
theoretical conclusions from correlating scores on one empirically derived test (e.g.,
reasoning) with scores on another empirically derived test (e.g., vocabulary), the
cognitive-correlates researcher draws theoretical conclusions from correlating
scores on an empirically derived test with parameters generated by a cognitive model
of some aspect of mental information processing.

On the one hand, cognitive-correlates researchers like Hunt (1978), Jensen
(1979), Keating and Bobbitt (1978), and Jackson and McClelland (1979) (see
Cooper & Regan, Chapter 3; Estes, Chapter 4) must be given credit for providing a
cognitive-theoretical base for individual-differences research to supplement the psy-
chometric-theoretical base that had existed earlier. On the other hand, one might
question, and we do, whether these researchers are providing the optimal cognitive-
theoretical base. As we stated earlier, we believe that the relatively low correlations
attained between task parameters and psychometric test scores might be the result
of psychometric tests' drawing upon lower-level abilities of the kinds studied by
cognitive-correlates researchers only in the most peripheral way. In the terminology
we prefer, the level of processing studied by these investigators tends to be too low.
But whether or not this is the case, these investigators deserve considerable credit
for reawakening interest among cognitive psychologists in individual differences in
mental information processing.

A second approach to the identification of the processes of intelligent behavior is
what might be referred to as a *cognitive-components approach* (Pellegrino & Glaser,
1979; R. Sternberg, 1977, 1981b). In the cognitive-components approach to understanding mental abilities, subjects are tested in their ability to perform tasks of the
kinds actually found on standard psychometric tests of mental abilities, such as
analogies, series completions, mental rotations, and the like (see Campione et al.,
Chapter 8; Cooper & Regan, Chapter 3; Sternberg, Chapter 5). Subjects are usually
tested via a tachistoscope or a computer terminal; response time is ordinarily the
principal dependent variable, but error rate and pattern of response choices can be
secondary dependent variables. These latter variables are of more interest in this
approach than in the cognitive-correlates approach because the tasks tend to be
more difficult, and thus more susceptible to erroneous responses.

The proximal goal in this research is, first, to formulate a model of information
processing in performance on IQ-test types of tasks; second, to test the model while
estimating parameters for the model; and finally, to investigate the extent to which
these processes correlate across subjects with each other and with scores on stan-

dard psychometric tests. Because the tasks that are analyzed are usually taken directly from IQ tests, or are very similar to tasks found on IQ tests, the major issue in this kind of research is not whether there is any correlation at all between cognitive task and psychometric test scores. Rather, the issue is one of isolating the locus or loci of the correlation that is obtained. In other words, one seeks to discover what processes of task performance are the critical ones from the standpoint of the theory of intelligence.

The distinction between cognitive-correlates and cognitive-components research is not a wholly clear-cut one. The differences between the two approaches are almost certainly matters of emphasis rather than kind. There appear to be at least two major differences in emphasis. First, if one were willing to accept our proposal of a continuum of levels of information processing, extending from perception in very simple identification tasks to problem solving in very complex inferential tasks, one would find cognitive-correlates researchers tending to study tasks measuring processes at the lower end of the continuum and cognitive-components researchers tending to study tasks measuring processes at the higher end of the continuum. Second, there seems to be more emphasis in cognitive-components research on the formulation, fitting, and testing of formal information-processing models.

As in many kinds of research, there have been some pleasant and some unpleasant surprises in cognitive-components research. One of the more agreeable surprises has been the ability of formal componential models to account for large amounts of both task and person variance in response times and response choices (see Cooper & Regan, Chapter 3; Sternberg, Chapter 5). One of the less pleasant surprises has been that the magnitudes of correlations between information-processing latencies and psychometric test scores have often been only moderate (often in the .4–.6 range). Recent efforts have attempted to raise these correlations by studying executive functioning separately from nonexecutive functioning, and by studying performance in nonentrenched tasks (see Bethell-Fox, Lohman, & Snow, 1981; Kyllonen, Lohman, & Snow, 1981; R. Sternberg, 1980b, 1981a). We believe that a major contribution of this approach will be judged to be its demonstration that IQ-test tasks can be decomposed into sets of processes accessible to cognitive-experimental methods of analysis.

A third approach to the identification of the processes of intelligent behavior can be used in conjunction with either of the preceding approaches, or in conjunction with some other approach. This is the *cognitive-training approach,* which is aptly described in Campione et al. (Chapter 8). The approach begins with an analysis of some kind of task performance. The analysis is then tested by training subjects to perform the given task according to the processes specified by the task analysis. The task analysis is viewed as supported if the subjects can be instructed in the set of processes, and as unsupported if the subjects cannot be instructed.

At a practical level, the cognitive-training approach can be helpful in telling us what processes of cognitive functioning are and are not trainable with reasonable amounts of effort, and in actually effecting improvement in cognitive functioning. We are somewhat less impressed with the utility of the approach for drawing theoretical conclusions about the processes of intelligent task performance. First, whereas successful training of a cognitive strategy for performing a particular task does imply that people might use the given set of processes in spontaneous performance of the task, it does not imply that people necessarily use that set of processes if untrained, or even that they are likely to use them. Second, if training fails, it is not at all clear what conclusions one can draw, because the relation between process use and process trainability is unclear. Finally, we would note that a training program based on a given theory can succeed even if the theory is incorrect, and fail even if the theory is correct. Thus we believe that the cognitive-training approach provides an excellent supplement to other approaches, but is not a replacement for them.

A fourth approach to the identification of the processes of intelligent behavior, and the last we shall describe, is a *computer-based approach* (see especially Dehn & Schank, Chapter 7), in which the proposed processes of intelligent behavior are simulated on a computer. The basic idea is to program a computer to perform certain intelligent functions, and then to determine whether its output simulates human behavior. This approach is unique among the ones we have considered in that it results not only in analysis of output, but in actual production of output. And if a given computer program is executed successfully, it is possible to use quantitative as well as qualitative tests to compare the output of the computer to the output of human beings. Although the point has been made many times before, it is worth repeating that no one is claiming that the anatomy (hardware) of the computer, or the language (software) used by the computer, is analogous to that of a human being. The only claim made is that the executing program functionally simulates human performance.

We have very high regard for the computer-based approach, and high hopes for its future. Some problems with this approach in the past have been the difficulty of communicating a given process theory to the scientific public; ambiguity in what is being claimed as being analogous to human behavior and what is simply a bookkeeping aspect of program behavior that is needed to make a computer program run; and limitations in the range of information processing to which the approach can be applied. But we view computer-oriented psychologists as having come a long way over the last few years in dealing with all of these problems, and we see no reason to believe that, insofar as any of these problems remain, they are inherent in the method. Rather, they seem to be glitches that will be ironed out with time. Hence we believe that this approach will be useful, in conjunction with other procedures, in future investigations of intelligent behavior.

In concluding this section, we wish to emphasize our view that there is no one right approach to identifying the processes of intelligent behavior, although some approaches may turn out to be more productive than others. The optimal strategy for identifying the processes of intelligent behavior is almost certainly one employing a variety of approaches, all of which (it is hoped) will converge upon a countable set of processes. To the extent that the approaches converge in their conclusions – and we believe that to some extent they already do – our confidence in their outcomes is appreciably increased.

STRATEGIES UNDERLYING INTELLIGENT BEHAVIOR

All of the contributors to Part II of the handbook seem to agree that strategy choice and execution represent key manifestations of intelligent behavior. If their claim went no further than this, it might be of no great interest, because strategies are, after all, essentially collections of component processes. But the claim does seem to go beyond the minimal one that processes are important in combination as well as in isolation. The contributors seem to believe that there are emergent properties of strategies that go beyond their merely being collections of processes – that the whole

is greater than the sum of its parts, and that part of the locus of intelligent functioning resides in this augmented whole. We concur with this belief. In discussing the
role of strategy in intelligent behavior, we will describe and evaluate the roles of what
seem to come out of the chapters as emergent properties of strategies. (We shall
considerably reduce the length of our discussion by dealing *only* with emergent
properties.)

Differential accessibility and availability of various strategies.   Some strategies
may work much better for a given task than others. For example, in learning lists of
words, subjects will almost always do better if they rehearse than if they do not. A
major distinction between the performance of retarded and normal subjects appears
to be in their differential use of rehearsal, with normal subjects using it regularly and
retarded subjects using it only rarely. Retarded subjects can be trained to rehearse,
in which case their performance on episodic learning tasks can approach or even
reach that of normal subjects. But the training proves not to be easily transferable,
and often not even durable (see Campione et al., Chapter 8; Estes, Chapter 4).
Whereas training may have rendered the rehearsal strategy available, it for some
reason remains relatively inaccessible to the retarded subjects. In Flavell's (1970)
terms, subjects may continue to show a production deficit even when they are
known not to have a mediation deficit.

Although the rehearsal deficit in learning by retarded subjects is one of the most
striking examples of differential accessibility of strategies, the difference can be seen
in other kinds and levels of processing as well, and in different gradations of normal
subjects as well as in normal versus subnormal levels of functioning. Cooper (1982),
for example, has found that under limited circumstances, it is possible to train
holistic or analytic strategies for perceptual performance; but subjects seem to have
strong preferences for one or the other in their performance of such tasks. In the
reasoning domain, Mathews, Hunt, and MacLeod (1980) and R. Sternberg and Weil
(1980) have found preferences for linguistic, spatial, or mixed linguistic–spatial
strategies that can also be resistant, although not necessarily immune, to training
attempts (see Cooper & Regan, Chapter 3; Sternberg, Chapter 5). Snow (1980) has
also found strategy differences in spatial ability tasks such as paper folding.

We conclude that an important area for future investigation is what it is that
makes certain strategies more or less accessible to persons performing tasks requiring intelligence. In the great bulk of research done to date, the issue of availability
versus accessibility has been ignored; and even in research that has considered the
issue, little progress has been made in eliciting the factors that contribute to differential accessibility of strategies. One area of research that may be fruitful in this
regard is that of styles, which is considered next.

Effect of style on strategy.   The effectiveness of a strategy in performing a task can
be influenced by the way in which the strategy is executed. In particular, individuals
can approach tasks with varying "styles" of performance. Differences in style are
reflected particularly by varying degrees of metacognitive reflection by individuals
upon their cognitive performance – before and after that performance as well as
while it is taking place (see Baron, Chapter 6; Campione et al., Chapter 8; Sternberg,
Chapter 5). A given strategy executed in an impulsive way can result in quality of
performance much lower than would have been attained had the strategy been
executed in a reflective way. At the opposite extreme, excessive reflection on task

performance can paralyze the individual, causing him or her to have difficulty in completing tasks. As Baron has pointed out, proclivities seem to differ from abilities in that they manifest themselves in an optimal way when exercised in moderation: One seeks some kind of happy medium, say, between extreme reflectivity and impulsivity.

We find the case made by Baron for the further study of cognitive styles of strategy execution to be an appealing one. We particularly agree that training in proclivities may provide a useful entrée into the training of intellectual performance in general (see Feuerstein, 1979, 1980, for a similar point of view). On the other hand, we have found the literature on cognitive styles generally disappointing, and prior to reading Baron's chapter, we would not have been inclined to endorse further research on styles with anything but lukewarm enthusiasm. From our former vantage point, cognitive-styles research had been tried but had succeeded only in moderate degree: First, the style constructs were often only barely distinguishable from standard cognitive abilities; second, and largely as a result of the preceding problem, their incremental validity in external prediction, over and above that of cognitive tests, seemed to be marginal at best; third, they seemed often to rest only upon a weak theoretical foundation; fourth, they seemed to elude reliable measurement, so that even alternative tests of the same style (e.g., rod-and-frame test and embedded-figures test for psychological differentiation) did not seem very highly correlated with each other; and fifth, research on styles just did not seem to be yielding exciting new insights. We are now inclined to believe that the seemingly slow progress of research on cognitive styles may have resulted from overreliance on psychometric technology for investigation of styles. Such techniques of investigation may need supplementation by the more cognitive techniques that have been brought to bear upon the study of mental abilities such as inductive reasoning, verbal comprehension, and the like (see Cooper & Regan, Chapter 3; Estes, Chapter 4; Sternberg, Chapter 5). It would be useful, for example, to demonstrate directly the effect of two alternate styles – say, impulsivity and reflectivity – on individual components of information processing in an intellectual task. To our knowledge, this kind of investigation has not yet been attempted.

Aptitude–strategy interactions. During the 1960s and 1970s, there was a large volume of work on aptitude–treatment interactions. The goal of much of the work was to demonstrate that the suitability of an instructional treatment often depends upon learner characteristics. The results were generally disappointing, with remarkably few replicable aptitude–treatment interactions turning up (see Cronbach & Snow, 1977). Many of the failures in this area seem to be attributable to lack of statistical power (Cronbach & Snow, 1977), to the need for process analysis and explicit consideration of strategies (Cronbach & Snow, 1977), and to inadequate operationalization of psychological conceptualizations (Bond & Glaser, 1979; Roth-kopf, 1978). We believe that a primary limitation was the absence of explicit formulations of either the aptitude processes measured by the tests or the processes of learning that resulted from the instructional treatments.

There now exists a small, but, we believe, significant, literature that suggests that when explicit information-processing models are used to study task performance, it is possible to demonstrate clearly one form of aptitude–treatment interaction, an "aptitude–strategy" interaction, by which the efficacy of a strategy for learning how to perform a task or for solving a task is seen to depend upon a person's pattern of cognitive abilities (Gavurin, 1967; MacLeod, Hunt, & Mathews, 1978; Mathews et al., 1980; R. Sternberg & Weil, 1980; see Cooper & Regan, Chapter 3; Sternberg, Chapter 5). This literature, of course, deals only with a tiny fraction of the aptitude–treatment interaction domain. But what is interesting about this group of studies as a whole is their demonstration of interactions between task performance, on the one hand, and patterns of spatial versus verbal abilities, on the other. These clear demonstrations are in contrast to most of the aptitude–treatment literature on the verbal–spatial distinction, which has been quite confusing, at best (see Cronbach & Snow, 1977). Like Cronbach and Snow, we are concerned that the aptitude–treatment approach, like the cognitive-styles approach, might be abandoned prematurely out of desperation from a lack of exciting results. We view the use of explicit information-processing models and methods of data analysis as providing the potential for new life in what otherwise might be viewed by some, ourselves included, as dying areas of research. In the present case, we believe that as we learn more about main effects of strategy optimality, it will prove to be important to investigate as well interactions between strategy optimality and individuals' ability patterns. We would hope that the next few years will see a considerable increase in research in this area, and especially an increase in research from an information-processing point of view.

KNOWLEDGE AND ITS REPRESENTATION

A repeated theme in the chapters of Part II is that intelligence cannot be well understood without reference to knowledge and its internal representation. There are a number of streams of research in cognitive psychology that converge on this conclusion, for example, research on propositional and analogue representations (see Cooper & Regan, Chapter 3; Estes, Chapter 4), research on representation of complex knowledge bases (see Dehn & Schank, Chapter 7; Estes; Sternberg, Chapter 5), and research on the representation of information in reasoning tasks such as linear syllogisms (see Sternberg).

Historically, the research by Chase and Simon (1973) on expertise in chess playing may be seen as something of a turning point for thinking about the importance of knowledge and its representation. These investigators found that what seemed to distinguish experts from novices was not differences in processes of playing chess, but rather differences in the knowledge base upon which experts could successfully draw. In Chapter 7, Dehn and Schank present the evolution of some of these views. Efforts to improve artificial intelligence programs by improving their processing systems eventually seemed to reach a dead end. These investigators and others have concluded that an essential ingredient in intelligent performance is the organization of knowledge in a way that makes it highly accessible and conveniently usable. In particular, intelligent individuals can use their knowledge bases to decide effectively what information is relevant, and what information is irrelevant, to a task at hand. This point can be illustrated by an analysis of the insight problems discussed in Sternberg (Chapter 5). Almost all individuals have the necessary knowledge base to solve the problems: What is difficult is figuring out what information is relevant.

When the information-processing movement got started, there was so much excitement about the possibility of identifying the processes people used in performing tasks that questions of knowledge and its representation came to take a distant second place to questions of process. Recent research by investigators such as

Anderson (1978), Cooper (1975), Kosslyn (1978), and Shepard (1975) has gone a long way toward reinstating an interest in representation, and the work of Chase and Simon (1973) and Chi, Glaser, and Rees (1982), among others, has helped reawaken an interest in the role of knowledge in intelligent performance. Nevertheless, we share the concern of Campione et al. (Chapter 8) that there would be little gain in replacing an overemphasis on process with an overemphasis on knowledge and its representation. If there is a message to be learned from the recent history of information-processing psychology, it would seem to be that process, knowledge, and representation ought to be understood in their interactions with one another. Isolation of any subset of these is useful, but only as a temporary expedient for experimental investigation. Knowledge is acquired by learning processes acting upon some kind of stimulus material in a way that results in successful encoding of the new information in some form in the mind. Problems are then solved by retrieving this information and applying it to the problem at hand. Whether or not the information will be retrieved will depend in large part upon how the information is stored, and in large part upon the efficacy of the retrieval processes themselves. Inevitably, process, knowledge, and representation are closely intertwined; they need to be understood in interaction if we are to understand how intelligence is acquired and, later, how it operates in various kinds of tasks and situations.

1.2.   SOCIETY, CULTURE, AND INTELLIGENCE

The chapters in Part III of the handbook examine intelligence in various social contexts. The contexts examined here are rather different, and the chapters take quite different orientations to the relationships between social context and intelligence. Nevertheless, several common themes run throughout: (a) that all intelligent behavior occurs in a social context that includes goals, expectations, demands, and a history of prior experience; (b) that the common element in intelligent behavior across situations and across individuals is goal-directed activity; (c) that the distinction between competence and performance is a critical one in conceptualizing intelligence; (d) that detailed task analyses, including analysis of the relationship of the task to the individual, are necessary for the development of a complete conceptualization of intelligence; (e) that differences in knowledge are an important source of individual differences in performance, and that such knowledge differences may be in large part the result of contextual differences; and (f) that conceptualizations of intelligence are not, and cannot be, value-free.

INTELLIGENCE AND SOCIAL CONTEXT

The contributors to Part III agree that all intelligent behavior occurs in a social context that includes goals, expectations, demands, and a history of prior experiences. Snow and Yalow (Chapter 9) maintain: "Our concept of intelligence is, to a significant extent, an emergent property of education. Education exercises native faculties of intelligence already in place, or education produces intelligence, or both." And education is conducted via social institutions – schools – that are essentially sources of goals, expectations, and demands presented through an organized sequence of educational experiences. Zigler and Seitz (Chapter 10) view intelligence largely in terms of social competence, which depends crucially upon social environment; in a similar vein, they see family support systems as particularly important targets for intervention, because the family is an important interpreter of social context for the developing individual. By focusing on the family, these authors are, of course, focusing upon one virtually universal source as well as interpreter of social context. Finally, the authors from the Laboratory of Comparative Human Cognition (Chapter 11) claim that "cultural differences reside more in the situations to which particular cognitive processes are applied than in the existence of a process in one group and its absence in another." The idea of a situation, in this context, seems implicitly to contain embedded within it the goals, expectations, demands, and history that are so important in shaping intellectual performance.

This relativistic, contextual approach to intelligence suggests an underlying multidimensional conception of intelligence, a conception consistent in spirit with that of the more "cognitively oriented" contributors to this handbook. In such a conception, intelligence is composed of a number of (at least theoretically) distinct abilities. But the contextual approach adds an important new element: The same abilities or dimensions can be manifested in quite different ways, depending upon the demands made by the cultural or social groups to which a given individual belongs. Moreover, in various social or cultural groups, the relative importances of particular abilities may vary widely, suggesting that quite different bundles of abilities might characterize the "most intelligent" members of various groups, and hence intelligence itself.

We certainly concur with the necessity of a multidimensional conception of intelligence. We also concur with the notion that contextual factors affect the expression and perhaps even the levels of various abilities. However, we believe that some "contextualists" may tend to overstate the extent to which contextual effects on intelligence should affect the tasks cognitive psychologists study. First, we believe it is the weights of the abilities, rather than the abilities themselves, that change from one cultural or societal context to another (see R. Sternberg, 1980b). Hence the tasks cognitive psychologists study may be more or less important in various contexts, depending upon the importance of what these tasks measure in the various contexts; but we believe that the abilities measured by these tasks are of at least nontrivial importance in many cultures, and probably in most of them. We are not precluding at all the possibility that cross-cultural researchers may be able to tell us, at some future time, what other tasks we ought to be studying in order better to understand the nature and manifestation of intelligence in other cultures. In the meantime, though, the tasks we are studying (see Part II) seem like a reasonable start toward understanding intelligence in some variety of environmental contexts. Second, we would emphasize that the rather microscopic analyses cognitive psychologists have tended to do complement, rather than contradict, the more macroscopic analyses that contextualists seem to prefer. We see no inconsistency in the two positions. Instead, researchers relating society to the nature of intelligence provide the opportunity to take cognitive methods of analysis and place them in the broader context they need to be fully meaningful. If they do not fit in this context, then we, as cognitive psychologists, are as eager to know this as are cross-cultural psychologists.

In sum, the contextualist approach, in combination with the more microscopic approach of cognitive psychologists, helps clarify the range of issues that a complete theory of intelligence must address (see also Sternberg & Powell, Chapter 15). Such a theory, according to this view, must consider the ways in which the social environment sets the problems that intelligence is used to solve. In the same spirit, from a developmental point of view, a theory must deal with the ways in which social environment fosters the development of some, and hinders the development of other, ways of solving the problems it sets.

INTELLIGENCE AS GOAL-DIRECTED

A common element in the manifestations of intelligence in diverse situations within an individual's life and across individuals and social groups is the goal-directed, even practical, character of intelligent performance. This commonality is in the spirit of definitions and conceptions of intelligence that focus upon the adaptive value of intelligence, although it should be noted that *adaptive* here is not meant in its strictly biological sense. The basic idea is that a social context (be it a classroom, a tribe, a family, a profession, or whatever) sets up a variety of problems, and intelligence consists in large part of the ability to solve these problems. Clearly, there is considerable overlap in the problems that are posed in a variety of environments, and considerable overlap in the abilities used to solve different problems. But the importance of social factors in defining intelligence means precisely that there is not perfect overlap in either problems or mixes of abilities across social settings.

What remains invariant across settings is the idea of the individual functioning intelligently in response to demands set from the outside. A crucial aspect of such intelligent functioning is understanding that there is a problem to be solved ("problem finding"), defining it rather precisely, and attempting to solve it. This conception has a fundamentally pragmatic character to it: Solving the problems of life is placed at the center of the conception of intelligence. It should be noted that this conception is compatible with information-processing models of intelligence, factor models of intelligence, or any other models that allow for multiple dimensions of intelligence that have their most important manifestations in real-world adaptation. What is added to models of these kinds is the notion of purposiveness underlying intelligent activity, as well as the notion that intelligence fundamentally has to do with responses to external demands (which may be internalized within the individual!). But intelligence does not reside exclusively within the individual, but rather in the individual's responses to the demands of his or her societal, cultural, or other context.

The three chapters in this section characterize the purposive aspect of intelligence quite differently, but all share an emphasis on the importance of goal-based, practical conceptualizations of intelligence. Snow and Yalow, who deal with intelligence in school settings in Chapter 9, make clear their belief that intelligence is knowable in part through success on school tasks. Zigler and Seitz (Chapter 10), with their emphasis on social competence and their concern with the social-policy utility of research on intelligence, argue that a conceptualization based on "pure" mental abilities considered outside their social context is of little use. The contributors from the Laboratory of Comparative Human Cognition (Chapter 11) make explicit the idea that intelligence must be conceptualized with reference to quite specific social demands, and that more general mental abilities – though useful theoretical entities – must always be explicitly connected to their roles in meeting such demands.

Within cognitive psychology, the idea that goals are important goes back, in recent times, to Miller et al. (1960). Whereas cognitive psychologists such as Miller et al. have been concerned primarily with the ways in which goals affect cognitive processing, contextual psychologists have been concerned primarily with where the goals come from, how they are transmitted, and how they manifest themselves in human behavior. Again, then, we see the cognitive and contextualist positions as consistent and complementary. The two positions may be perceived as dealing with two sides of the same coin, both of which must be seen fully if we are to understand the phenomenon under consideration.

THE COMPETENCE–PERFORMANCE DISTINCTION

All of the chapters in the "Society and intelligence" section stress the distinction between competence and performance. The visible expression of competence – performance – is viewed as depending in part upon the context in which behavior occurs. Zigler and Seitz (Chapter 10) provide an example of a retarded person who could operate a complicated piece of machinery quite competently; but when the machine was rotated 30°, the person was confused and unable to operate it. One could obviously argue that this operator was less competent than a skilled machine operator; more to the point, however, is the fact that, in a very well specified context, the person *was* able to exhibit skilled performance. As noted earlier in discussing Campione et al. (Chapter 8), part of what made this person's performance "retarded" was its unfortunate lack of cross-situational transfer. The members of the Laboratory of Comparative Human Cognition (Chapter 11) discuss a Mexican tribe in which the children are involved in pottery making from an early age; these children exhibit conservation of quantity at an earlier age than do Swiss or American children, but only in very specific contexts.

The sensitivity of performance to context suggests that methods to assess competence – that is, ways of attempting to elicit performance – must be designed with consideration of contextual factors, and must have considerable diversity in order to reflect the diversity of possible contexts in which performance may occur. This observation obviously has implications for testing and measurement. It also seems to require that a full theory of intelligence address the ways in which various contexts may affect the expression of a given competence.

We applaud the stated distinction between competence and performance, which arises out of a cognitive framework as well, although for different reasons. We believe that the contextual rationale is every bit as important as the cognitive one: Whether a given competence will or will not be expressed in performance depends upon external contextual, as well as upon internal, factors.

TASK ANALYSIS

All of the chapters in Part III stress the importance of detailed task analysis. To some extent, the tasks on an intelligence test, or in life, can be seen as part of the context of performance. Moreover, familiarity with both the nature and the content of tasks will vary, depending upon past experiences. From a contextual perspective, then, a detailed task analysis must include a detailed examination of the past and present environments in which a person has found and continues to find him- or herself.

Different environments pose different problems, and these problems can be represented by different types of tasks. The contextual perspective would see the need for varying tasks in the measurement of mental abilities as driven largely by the various types of contexts people experience; indeed, the multidimensional nature of intelligence can only be seen as being due to the multidimensional kinds of demands the environment places on individuals. A multifaceted notion of intelligence has no meaning outside of task demands. To the extent that the multiple dimensions of psychometric or cognitive analysis are the result of contrived tasks that have no representation in the external environment, these dimensions do not represent intelligence in any meaningful sense at all.

Both the psychometric and cognitive conceptualizations, on the one hand, and the contextualist one, on the other, advocate sampling of a wide and surprisingly similar range of tasks; but the interpretations accorded to differences in performance vary. From the psychometric or cognitive (or other "internally oriented") perspective, such ranges in measurement derive from the need to sample different underlying abilities of which people possess different amounts. In the contextualist view, the sampling is needed because of the range of environmental demands one meets; tasks are of value only to the extent they represent real demands of environments people do or might plausibly encounter. On the average, internally oriented psychologists seem inclined to interpret differences in test or task performance as differences in amounts of underlying abilities, whereas contextually oriented psychologists seem more inclined to attribute differences in performance to differences in the preparation for the test materials the subject has encountered as a result of previous interactions with the environment. In fact, these two perspectives may, in the limiting case, say the same thing in different ways, because all but the strictest hereditarians would agree that experience is largely responsible for shaping the development of abilities.

An important distinction in the contextualist perspective is that between the form of a task and its content – the actual terms in which a problem is instantiated, as opposed to the formal problem itself. Because different cultures work with very different contents in the everyday problems and activities of life, a given form of problem may appear quite difficult when presented with one kind of content, but quite easy when presented with another. Internally oriented psychologists also vary content, but it often seems that they do so more to add dimensions of stimulus variation than to attain representation of the kinds of contents people encounter in their transactions with real environments of everyday life.

THE ROLE OF KNOWLEDGE IN INTELLIGENCE

The contextualists emphasize differences in knowledge as important sources of individual differences in intelligent performance. Knowledge is accumulated as a function of experience. Not only do differences in knowledge derive from contextual sources; knowledge itself comes to form a part of a person's context of problem solving. The contextual perspective maintains that knowledge must be fully considered in a complete conception of intelligence, where knowledge is seen on the one hand as a product of context, and on the other as a creator of context.

The stress on knowledge in the contextualist view is quite consistent with the contextualist stress on the role of content in task analysis. It is also consistent with recent cognitive views of intelligence, which are again beginning to emphasize the role of knowledge in intelligence (see Campione et al., Chapter 8; Siegler & Richards, Chapter 14; see also Chi, Feltovich, & Glaser, 1981; R. Sternberg, 1981b). One of the most striking examples of the role of knowledge on intelligent performance actually arises from the cognitive literature. Hayes and Simon (1976) have shown that a given formal problem structure can vary widely in difficulty, depending solely upon the content used to express that form (see also Polson & Jeffries, 1982; Sternberg, Chapter 5).

Although recent cognitive and contextualist perspectives have both emphasized the important role of knowledge in intelligent performance, it is probably worth pointing out one difference as well. In the contextualist perspective, knowledge is of interest largely because of its derivation from and contribution to the creation of cultural and societal contexts. In the cognitive perspective, knowledge structures are seen as of interest in their own right and as distinct from the processes that operate upon them; but the roles of society and culture are barely considered. Thus the cognitive view is essentially internal; the contextualist view is essentially external. The two views are again complementary, but little work seems to have been done to date on their interface, with aptitude–treatment interaction research one of a few notable research areas that are at the interface.

VALUES IN THE CONCEPTUALIZATION OF INTELLIGENCE

The contextualist approach to intelligence implies that conceptions of intelligence are not and cannot be value-free. Basically, this is because the definition of intelligence is itself a social and cultural product, and will inevitably reflect social and cultural values. The definers of intelligence and the designers of intelligence tests cannot transcend their culture. Science is a part of culture, and cultural values are always incorporated into science in some degree. As long as that fact is understood and accepted by people who study and measure intelligence, by those who administer and use intelligence tests, and by those whose futures are affected by performance on such tests, the dangers of confusion and miscommunication are minimized. It is only when the importance of values is minimized or even denied, or when the value bases of such tests are deemed an inappropriate topic of discussion, that serious problems arise.

Much of the appeal of the contextualist framework is in its usefulness in developing a broad intellectual stance from which research and theory on intelligence may be viewed. Intelligence and research on intelligence occur in a cultural context and only in a cultural context. Internally oriented psychologists must avoid the hubris of absolutism: Psychometric, cognitive, and other paradigmatically based theories of intelligence may be supplanted as our knowledge of the role of intelligence in everyday contexts increases. Or they may be found to be increasingly useful: It is too early to tell. The contextualist position would maintain, not without a trace of irony, that even a contextualist conception of intelligence is a social and cultural product, and thus should be viewed in relative terms. There is an appealing modesty in this position that we might all be well-advised to adopt.

One might argue, as some have (e.g., Jonathan Baron, personal communication), that the contextualist position is too relativistic, in that it implies that in some sense intelligence will be indicated by different mental and behavioral events at different times and in different places. But we would argue that, in fact, what counts as goal-directed adaptive behavior may well change with time and place. The definition of intelligence does not change, but the mental and behavioral events that give content to the formal definition do. In a rapidly developing society, who is *intelligent* may actually change over the course of people's lifetimes, and for sociocultural rather than biological reasons. The behavior that might have been ideally adaptive – ideally intelligent – in a hunting culture may not even have a place in an industrial culture. What is intelligent in one culture may be irrelevant in the next, or actually unintelligent, as, for example, when mechanization makes certain routine hand-done operations an extravagant waste of time.

I.3.   THE PHYLOGENY AND ONTOGENY OF INTELLIGENCE

The chapters in Part IV of the handbook all deal with the development of intelligence, but in very different chronological frameworks. "The evolution of biological intelligence" deals with development over evolutionary time; "Genetics and intelligence" deals with development over the life-span of an individual and his or her recent ancestors; "The development of intelligence" deals with development over a single individual's life-span. A common theme in all three chapters seems to be the respective roles of environmental and nonenvironmental factors in the development of intelligence. (We have selected the term *nonenvironmental* to contrast with *environmental* because it seems to be the most neutral term available for what we intend to convey: We hope its neutrality and scope compensate for its lack of euphony and precision.) Naturally, what is seen as environmental differs in each of the chapters, with the meaning determined in part by the time scale and level of analysis under consideration.

The three chapters deal with somewhat different senses of *intelligence, environmental factors,* and *nonenvironmental factors,* and we will begin our discussion by outlining what these senses seem to be. For Jerison (Chapter 12), intelligence is defined as the total information-processing capacity of the organism, measured via an "index of encephalization," which represents the size of the brain in excess of that needed to control routine bodily functions. Using this definition, one can compare various species without concern for the particular cognitive and behavioral activities they engage in. It is a gross capacity measure, and thus can be thought of as indexing a crude form of competence, although a competence different in level of analysis from the more fine-grained competences isolated by cognitive psychologists. For Jerison, the environment consists of inanimate factors – the geological, topographical, and climatological setting in which species live – and animate factors – the range and types of living species with which an individual interacts either directly or indirectly – that influence adaptation. Nonenvironmental factors consist primarily of the genetic material in species-specific aggregates.

For Scarr and Carter-Saltzman (Chapter 13), intelligence is defined implicitly via the dependent measures used in research on the transmission of intelligence from one generation to the next. These measures are typically the Stanford–Binet, the Wechsler, or roughly comparable intelligence tests. The environment consists of the family, school, and general social milieu in which the person lives. These factors are defined operationally by various measures such as family size, social class level, and the like. Nonenvironmental factors affecting levels of measured intelligence are genetic; but the genesis dealt with by Scarr and Carter-Saltzman is on a scale much smaller than that dealt with by Jerison.

Siegler and Richards (Chapter 14) view intelligence as a prototype (along the lines suggested by Neisser, 1979). Thus to them, intelligence is a concept with no defining features but with a number of prototypical instances. Lay assessments of intelligence are made by comparing individuals to one or more prototypes of the "intelligent person." In this view, intelligence can mean different things in different societies, cultures, or even subcultures. Moreover, it can mean different things for people of different ages. Siegler and Richards note that intelligence is perceived as comprising different kinds of abilities at different ages in the life span. The environment with which Siegler and Richards deal in their presentation consists largely of the range of learning tasks and problems encountered by the individual; the nonenvironmental factors consist largely of the individual's internal mental state, which is determined in part by knowledge and skills previously acquired through interactions with the environment.

For Jerison, then, intelligence may differ between species, but is treated as essentially invariant within species (for the kinds of analyses Jerison conducts, which is not to say that Jerison denies the existence of within-species differences). For Scarr and Carter-Saltzman and for Siegler and Richards, intelligence is analyzed as a uniquely human phenomenon: Scarr and Carter-Saltzman focus particularly on variation across individuals, whereas Siegler and Richards focus especially on developmental variation within individuals over the course of the life-span.

In the evolution of intelligence – the subject of Jerison's chapter – both environmental and nonenvironmental factors are important. Evolution is a product of two basic forces: changes in the environment and random mutations in genetic material, which either allow or do not allow adaptation to the environment and its changing character. Different environments make different phenotypes differentially successful in reproducing, and random mutations result in varying genotypes that, in turn, may lead to varying phenotypes.

In this formulation, the environment defines what are called *niches*, which can be thought of as representing constellations of biological and behavioral attributes that are tailored to the environment. The set of niches is often referred to as *niche space*. Some niches in niche space may be unoccupied, in the sense that there are no species with particular constellations of attributes. Other niches in niche space may be potentially occupied by multiple species, in which case competition between species may arise.

There are at least three ways in which this large-scale evolutionary perspective is helpful in understanding the interplay between environmental and nonenvironmental factors in intelligence. First, the range of possible environmental factors constrains the range of possible nonenvironmental factors that can be relevant to intelligent behavior. That is, the only possible genetic differences that can matter in the long-term life of a species are those that might lead to differential reproductive efficacy in an actual or possible niche space and location in that space. The reverse is also true: The only possible environmental differences that might matter in the long term are those that do or could result in differential reproductive results for some species. Thus environmental and nonenvironmental factors and their interactions must be considered together, with all deserving careful attention.

Second, there are a great many niches that do not require a high degree of intelligence, as measured by encephalization. In Jerison's view, then, intelligence can be seen as just another biological characteristic, more important in some niches than in others. Species of monkeys, for example, vary widely in their encephalization; this variation makes some species far more suitable than others for language experiments, say, but does not appear to contribute to differential success in the wild, even though there are clearly varying adaptive strategies followed and varying niches occupied by the species. Niche space is multidimensional, and intelligence is differentially important in different regions of the niche space. This relativistic perspective is helpful in avoiding excessive anthropomorphism: Our preoccupation with intelligence is *ours*. It is not clear that intelligence, except when defined so broadly as to lose much of its meaning, is really of such great importance as we might make it out to be when we look at its functioning across species.

Third, niche space can provide a heuristically useful metaphor for the nature of intelligence itself: If intelligence is conceptualized multidimensionally, particular niches would require, and metaphorically correspond to, particular combinations of the constituents of intelligence. This metaphor suggests that different human "intelligences" might be differentially useful in the rich niche space of human society. Furthermore, the metaphorical extension of niche space suggests that various constellations of the constituents of intelligence might combine with differential effectiveness with various bundles of other, noncognitive attributes.

The importance of environmental, nonenvironmental, and interactive forces also emerges from Scarr and Carter-Saltzman's chapter, although their concerns are not the same as Jerison's. Scarr and Carter-Saltzman are especially interested in accounting for observed variation in human intelligence, and in partitioning that variance among genetic, environmental, and interactive sources. As mentioned previously, the major dependent variable in most of the studies they review is a score on a standard intelligence test. The relatively few studies that attempt more fine-grained analyses – for example, by using subtest scores – generally show weak or null differential results. It is difficult to know exactly what to make of these null results, because most workers in the field of intelligence accept a multidimensional definition of intelligence, and hence might expect at least some differential heritability for the multiple dimensions. Our own view is that there may be measurement problems of two kinds. First, the subscores may be quite a bit less reliable than total scores, so that it is more difficult to obtain meaningful results, especially with small effects. Second, the subscores may not represent an optimal partitioning of abilities. In particular, we would like to see studies done in which subscores represent processing components rather than structural factors. Although we believe that differential hereditary patterns might be more likely to be found with this partitioning, given perfect measurement, we recognize that process component scores tend, if anything, to be even less reliable than structural factor scores.

A basic idea in the analysis by Siegler and Richards (Chapter 14) is that intelligence develops through the acquisition of successively more complex and ecologically valid rules for dealing with problems presented by the environment. The child brings some current state of knowledge (nonenvironmental factors), both declarative and procedural, to bear on a problem presented by his or her encounters with the world (environmental factors). In order for the child to learn, two criteria must be satisfied. First, the child must encounter problem situations that permit differentiation between the child's current rule and the correct rule (i.e., problems to which the child's current rule will give an incorrect response, whereas the correct rule will, of course, give the correct response). Second, the attributes of the problem situation that differentiate the correct rule from the child's incorrect one must be salient to the child. Whether the difference will be salient will depend in large part upon the child's internal state.

We find the Siegler–Richards approach (see also Siegler, 1981, for a more detailed description of the approach) highly inventive, insightful, and useful for distinguishing cognitive rules in the problems that these investigators have studied. One concern we have, which might equally well apply to other approaches to the investigation of intelligence, is that the "rules" for dealing with most of the consequential problems life throws one's way are not nearly so well defined as are the rules in the constrained problems Siegler and Richards have studied. The extent to which rule learning for very well defined problems resembles rule learning for fuzzily defined problems (with fuzzily defined rules) is unknown, but if the concept-formation and concept-attainment literatures are any indication, the resemblance may not be great. The kinds of psychological processes relevant to the learning of well-defined concepts, such as those studied by Bruner, Goodnow, and Austin (1965), have not seemed very relevant to the learning of ill-defined concepts such as those studied by Rosch (1978) and her associates. Thus we cannot help but have some concerns about the ecological validity of this approach as it has been used so far. In saying this, we emphasize again that the same criticism could easily be directed at most of the cognitively oriented approaches we considered earlier.

To summarize, the chapters in this part of the handbook describe how environmental and nonenvironmental factors operate, individually and in interaction, to influence intelligent behavior. The chapters deal with somewhat different senses of the various terms (*intelligence, environmental factors, nonenvironmental factors*), but are in consensus that both kinds of factors do affect intelligent performance at all the levels at which intelligence might be investigated. In this respect, we find the chapter authors of Part IV in agreement with those of the other parts. We now turn to a consideration of what we perceive as the overall themes of the book.

I.4.   CONCLUSION

We believe that if there is a common theme in the highly diverse viewpoints presented in this handbook, it is that intelligence is expressed in terms of adaptive, goal-directed behavior. The subset of such behavior that is labeled "intelligent" seems to be determined in large part by cultural or societal norms. Each of the terms – *adaptive* and *goal-directed* – needs some elaboration.

Adaptive behavior is behavior that confronts and meets successfully the challenges that are encountered. These challenges can be either internal ones set by the organism itself, or external ones presented by the outside world. Because the challenges of varying internal and external environments will differ from one organism to the next (and a fortiori, from one species to the next), it is impossible to specify any one set of behaviors that constitute "intelligent behaviors." What is adaptive in one individual or species may be maladaptive in another. Yet we doubt that those who wish to assess intelligence need despair entirely: There are commonalities in the environments of members of a species, and the greater the extent of these commonalities, the greater the extent to which intelligent assessment of intelligence is possible. Similarly, the more restricted the range of organisms and environments one studies, the greater the extent to which it is possible to conduct fine-grained analyses of intelligent performance. We believe that differences in level of analysis are due in large part to the range of organisms and environments studied. (Compare, for example, the range reviewed by Jerison in his chapter on evolution to the range reviewed by Cooper & Regan, Estes, and Sternberg in their chapters on cognition.) What we must remember, however, is that not only do levels and kinds of intelligence differ from one organism to the next, but the extent to which any one test tests intelligence also differs from one organism to the next. For this reason it is essential that any test purporting to measure intelligence be shown to have both construct validity and predictive validity for the particular environments in which it is used. In the mad scramble to rank order individuals for purposes of selection, placement, and diagnosis, we must not forget that tests of intelligence are proxies for consequential intelligent behaviors, not the consequential intelligent behaviors themselves. What constitutes an appropriate proxy depends upon the challenges that the individual and the society in which he or she lives set for that individual.

Goal-directed behavior is behavior that is ultimately purposive. It is not enough for behavior merely to be adaptive: It is possible to adapt to the demands in an environment so as to do nothing more than minimally "get by." We believe that intelligent behavior must be understood in terms of the short- and long-term goals to which it contributes. The meeting of challenges cannot be termed "intelligent" if the performance involved in meeting these challenges is aimless. What constitutes an aim or a purpose can vary greatly across individuals and species, and must be construed very broadly, but we believe it a consensus of the authors that some purpose, however remote or otherwise far-removed, must motivate intelligent acts.

The study of adaptive, goal-directed behavior requires detailed analysis of carefully selected tasks. First, the tasks must be carefully selected to assure that they do measure what constitutes intelligent behavior for a given individual or set of individuals. Second, the tasks must be carefully analyzed if we are to understand the constituents of intelligent behavior. Although the contributors' emphases are different, they seem to agree that at least two kinds of analysis are necessary – internal and external. Internal analysis views the constituents of task performance in relation to task performance as a whole. It seeks to understand these constituents without losing sight of the whole that constitutes the performance. The contributors to Part II emphasize task analysis of this kind. External analysis views the whole of task performance or its constituents in relation to the environment in which task performance takes place. It seeks to understand how task performance fits into the world in which the individual lives. The contributors to Part III emphasize task analysis of this kind. The contributors to part IV seem to split in their emphases, with Jerison stressing external and Siegler and Richards internal analyses; Scarr and Carter-Saltzman emphasize each about equally.

It is doubtful that there exists any best approach to studying intelligence, because intelligence can mean such diverse things in different settings, and because each method has its regions of strength and weakness when applied to the particular problems that confront a theorist of intelligence. But we are encouraged by what we believe are broad areas of agreement among theorists about what constitute important problems to study, and about viable ways in which they can be studied. This agreement is shown, we believe, by the fact that common themes do run through each of the parts of the book, with converging views on many of these themes, and by the higher-order agreements we have discussed in this concluding section. We believe that, however modest they may be, the contributions of scientists such as the ones represented in this book provide an important affirmation of the possibility, and, we hope, the probability, of understanding intelligent behavior, and eventually of being able to guide behavior in a direction that is at the same time intelligent for individuals and for the collectivities into which they enter.

NOTES

Preparation of this chapter was supported by Contract Noo01478C0025 from the Office of Naval Research to Robert J. Sternberg.
1 For a more detailed description and discussion of these various approaches, see R. Sternberg (1981b).

REFERENCES

Anderson, J. R. Arguments concerning representations for mental imagery. *Psychological Review*, 1978, *85*, 249–177.

Bethell-Fox, C. E., Lohman, D. F., & Snow, R. E. *Componential and eye movement analysis of geometric analogy performance* (Tech. Rep. No. 16). Stanford, Calif.: Stanford University, School of Education, Aptitude Research Project, 1981.

Bond, L., & Glaser, R. ATI, but mostly A and T with not much I. *Applied Psychological Measurement*, 1979, *3*, 137–140.

Bruner, J. S., Goodnow, J. J., & Austin, G. A. *A study of thinking.* New York: Wiley, 1956.

Butterfield, E. C. On Sternberg's translation of *g* into metacomponents and on questions of parsimony. *Behavioral and Brain Sciences*, 1980, *3*, 573–614.

Carroll, J. B. *Individual difference relations in psychometric and experimental cognitive tasks.* (NR 150–406 ONR Final Report). Chapel Hill, N.C.: L. L. Thurstone Psychometric Laboratory, 1980. (NTIS No. ADA-086057; ERIC Document Reproduction Service No. ED 191-891)

Cermak, L. S., & Craik, F. I. M. (Eds.). *Levels of processing in human memory.* Hillsdale, N.J.: Erlbaum, 1979.

Chase, W. G., & Simon, H. A. Perception in chess. *Cognitive Psychology*, 1973, *4*, 55–81.

Chi, M. T. H., Feltovich, P. J., & Glaser, R. Representation of physics knowledge by experts and novices. *Cognitive Science*, 1981, *5*, 121–152.

Chi, M. T. H., Glaser, R., & Rees, E. Expertise in problem solving. In R. J. Sternberg (Ed.), *Advances in the psychology of human intelligence* (Vol. 1). Hillsdale, N.J.: Erlbaum, 1982.

Cooper, L. A. Mental rotation of random two-dimensional shapes. *Cognitive Psychology*, 1975, *7*, 20–43.

Cooper, L. A. Strategies for visual comparison and representation: Individual differences. In R. J. Sternberg (Ed.), *Advances in the psychology of human intelligence* (Vol. 1). Hillsdale, N.J.: Erlbaum, 1982.

Craik, F. I. M., & Lockhart, R. S. Levels of processing: A framework for memory research. *Journal of Verbal Learning and Verbal Behavior*, 1972, *11*, 671–684.

Cronbach, L. J. *Essentials of psychological testing* (3rd ed.). New York: Harper & Row, 1970.

Cronbach, L. J., & Snow, R. E. *Aptitudes and instructional methods.* New York: Irvington, 1977.

Feuerstein, R. *The dynamic assessment of retarded performers: The learning potential assessment device, theory, instruments, and techniques.* Baltimore: University Park Press, 1979.

Feuerstein, R. *Instrumental enrichment: An intervention program for cognitive modifiability.* Baltimore: University Park Press, 1980.

Flavell, J. H. Developmental studies of mediated memory. In H. W. Reese & L. P. Lipsitt (Eds.), *Advances in child development and behavior* (Vol. 5). New York: Academic Press, 1970.

Gavurin, E. I. Anagram solving and spatial ability. *Journal of Psychology*, 1967, *65*, 65–68.

Goldberg, R. A., Schwartz, S., & Stewart, M. Individual differences in cognitive processes. *Journal of Educational Psychology*, 1977, *69*, 9–14.

Guttman, L. The structure of relations among intelligence tests. In *Proceedings, 1964 Invitational Conference on Testing Problems.* Princeton, N.J.: Educational Testing Service, 1965.

Hayes, J. R., & Simon, H. A. The understanding process: Problem isomorphs. *Cognitive Psychology*, 1976, *8*, 165–190.

Hunt, E. B. Mechanics of verbal ability. *Psychological Review*, 1978, *85*, 109–130.

Hunt, E. B., Frost, N., & Lunneborg, C. Individual differences in cognition: A new approach to intelligence. In G. H. Bower (Ed.), *The psychology of learning and motivation* (Vol. 7). New York: Academic Press, 1973.

Hunt, E., Lunneborg, C., & Lewis, J. What does it mean to be high verbal? *Cognitive Psychology*, 1975, *7*, 194–227.

"Intelligence and its measurement: A symposium." *Journal of Educational Psychology*, 1921, *12*, 123–147; 195–216; 271–275.

Jackson, M. D. *Memory access and reading ability.* Unpublished doctoral dissertation, University of California, San Diego, 1978.

Jackson, M. D., & McClelland, J. L. Processing determinants of reading speed. *Journal of Experimental Psychology: General*, 1979, *108*, 151–181.

Jacobs, M. K., & Dominowski, R. L. Learning to solve insight problems. *Bulletin of the Psychonomic Society,* 1981, *17,* 171–174.

Jensen, A. R. Hierarchical theories of mental ability. In W. B. Dockrell (Ed.), *On intelligence: Contemporary theories and educational implications.* Toronto: Ontario Institute for Studies in Education, 1970.

Jensen, A. R. *g:* Outmoded theory or unconquered frontier? *Creative Science and Technology,* 1979, 2(3), 16–29.

Keating, D. P., & Bobbitt, B. L. Individual and developmental differences in cognitive-processing components of mental ability. *Child Development,* 1978, *49,* 155–167.

Kosslyn, S. M. Measuring the visual angle of the mind's eye. *Cognitive Psychology,* 1978, *10,* 356–389.

Kyllonen, P. C., Lohman, D. F., & Snow, R. E. *Effects of item facets and strategy training on spatial task performance* (Tech. Rep. No. 14). Stanford, Calif.: Stanford University, School of Education, Aptitude Research Project, 1981.

Lohman, D. F. *Spatial ability: A review and reanalysis of the correlational literature* (Tech. Rep. No. 8). Stanford, Calif.: Stanford University, School of Education, Aptitude Research Project, 1979. (a)

Lohman, D. F. *Spatial ability: Individual differences in speed and level* (Tech. Rep. No. 9). Stanford, Calif.: Stanford University, School of Education, Aptitude Research Project, 1979. (b)

MacLeod, C. M., Hunt, E. B., & Mathews, N. N. Individual differences in the verification of sentence–picture relationships. *Journal of Verbal Learning and Verbal Behavior,* 1978, *17,* 493–507.

Maier, N. R. F. *Problem solving and creativity in individuals and groups.* Belmont, Calif.: Brooks/Cole, 1970.

Marshalek, B. *The complexity dimension in the radex and hierarchical models of intelligence.* Paper presented at the annual meeting of the American Psychological Association, San Francisco, 1977.

Mathews, N. N., Hunt, E. B., & MacLeod, C. M. Strategy choice and strategy training in sentence–picture verification. *Journal of Verbal Learning and Verbal Behavior,* 1980, *19,* 531–548.

Miller, G. A., Galanter, E., & Pribram, K. H. *Plans and the structure of behavior.* New York: Holt, Rinehart, & Winston, 1960.

Neisser, U. The concept of intelligence. In R. J. Sternberg & D. K. Detterman (Eds.), *Human intelligence: Perspectives on its theory and measurement.* Norwood, N.J.: Ablex, 1979.

Pellegrino, J. W., & Glaser, R. Cognitive correlates and components in the analysis of individual differences. In R. J. Sternberg & D. K. Detterman (Eds.), *Human intelligence: Perspectives on its theory and measurement.* Norwood, N.J.: Ablex, 1979.

Polson, P., & Jeffries, R. Problem solving as search and understanding. In R. J. Sternberg (Ed.), *Advances in the psychology of human intelligence* (Vol. 1). Hillsdale, N.J.: Erlbaum, 1982.

Posner, M. I., & Mitchell, R. Chronometric analysis of classification. *Psychological Review,* 1967, 74, 392–409.

Powell, J. S., & Sternberg, R. J. *Acquisition of vocabulary from context.* Paper presented at the annual meeting of the American Psychological Association, Los Angeles, August 1981.

Raaheim, K. *Problem solving and intelligence.* Oslo: Universitetsforlaget, 1974.

Rosch, E. Principles of categorization. In E. Rosch & B. B. Lloyd (Eds.), *Cognition and categorization.* Hillsdale, N.J.: Erlbaum, 1978.

Rothkopf, E. Z. The sound of one hand plowing. *Contemporary Psychology,* 1978, 23, 707–708.

Shepard, R. N. Form, formation, and transformation of internal representations. In R. L. Solso (Ed.), *Information processing and cognition: The Loyola Symposium.* Hillsdale, N.J.: Erlbaum, 1975.

Siegler, R. S. Developmental sequences within and between concepts. *Monographs of the Society for Research in Child Development,* 1981, 46, Serial No. 189.

Snow, R. E. Aptitude processes. In R. E. Snow, P.-A. Federico, & W. E. Montague (Eds.), *Aptitude, learning, and instruction: Cognitive process analyses of aptitude* (Vol. 1). Hillsdale, N.J.: Erlbaum, 1980.

Snow, R. E. Toward a theory of aptitude for learning: I. Fluid and crystallized abilities and their correlates. In M. P. Friedman, J. P. Das, & N. O'Connor (Eds.), *Intelligence and learning*. New York: Plenum, 1981.

Sternberg, R. J. *Intelligence, information processing, and analogical reasoning: The componential analysis of human abilities*. Hillsdale, N.J.: Erlbaum, 1977.

Sternberg, R. J. Developmental patterns in the encoding and combination of logical connectives. *Journal of Experimental Child Psychology*, 1979, *28*, 469–498.

Sternberg, R. J. A proposed resolution of curious conflicts in the literature on linear syllogisms. In R. Nickerson (Ed.), *Attention and performance VIII*. Hillsdale, N.J.: Erlbaum, 1980. (a)

Sternberg, R. J. Sketch of a componential subtheory of human intelligence. *Behavioral and Brain Sciences*, 1980, *3*, 573–584. (b)

Sternberg, R. J. Intelligence and nonentrenchment. *Journal of Educational Psychology*, 1981, *73*, 1–16. (a)

Sternberg, R. J. Testing and cognitive psychology. *American Psychologist*, 1981, *36*, 1181–1189. (b)

Sternberg, R. J., Conway, B. E., Ketron, J. L., & Bernstein, M. People's conceptions of intelligence. *Journal of Personality and Social Psychology: Attitudes and Social Cognition*, 1981, *41*, 37–55.

Sternberg, R. J., Powell, J. S., & Kaye, D. B. The nature of verbal comprehension. *Poetics*, in press.

Sternberg, R. J., & Weil, E. M. An aptitude × strategy interaction in linear syllogistic reasoning. *Journal of Educational Psychology*, 1980, *72*, 226–239.

Sternberg, S. The discovery of processing stages: Extensions of Donders' method. *Acta Psychologica*, 1969, *30*, 276–315.

Werner, H., & Kaplan, E. The acquisition of word meanings: A developmental study. *Monographs of the Society for Research in Child Development*, 1952, No. 51.

2   *The measurement of intelligence*

JOHN B. CARROLL

A prime goal of scientific discovery and technological development is the production of new knowledge – knowledge that can be disseminated through communications in scientific journals, monographs, books, and the like. This knowledge can be taken advantage of, generally, only at the cost of some special attention and study by the user. Much of the output of psychological and educational research is of this character; that is, the fruits of this research are mainly writings intended to provide educators with guidance on how various aspects of schooling should be conducted.

Often, however, particularly in the physical and biological sciences, scientific knowledge can become embodied in some kind of physical object or substance – a "long-lasting" razor blade, a color television set, or a new drug or vaccine. Most of the time, a razor blade, a color television set or an over-the-counter drug can be employed quite successfully by the ordinary lay person who has not the faintest idea of the technology in metallurgy, electronics, biochemistry, or whatever, that went into its development and production. There are, of course, many technological products, such as supersonic airplanes, electron microscopes, or radiation therapy machines, whose use requires a high degree of specialized training.

At least some of the products of educational research are concrete physical things. One of these products – insofar as it may consist of a set of one or more physical objects like test stimulus arrays, response devices, or scoring keys – is the mental test. The mental test is a concrete product of the subdiscipline and technology known as psychometrics, which is somewhat analogous to the knowledge-embodying products of technology in the physical and biological sciences.

As in the case of a new drug, it would not ordinarily take much skill for a person without specialized training to administer the test to him- or herself or to others. Without a knowledge of the circumstances it would be difficult to predict whether such an action would have beneficial or adverse consequences. Certain it is, however, that a lay person (or, particularly, a person who undergoes a "psychological test") would ordinarily be unaware of the technology that produced the test, just as he or she would be unaware of the technology involved in the discovery, development, and production of the drug. And just as a lay person might be inclined to have reasonable doubts about the usefulness or efficacy of a prescribed drug, so a lay person (or a test subject) might entertain reasonable doubts about the value and precision of a psychological test. A mental test usually *looks* like a rather simple object, consisting, perhaps, of a series of tasks based on visual or auditorily presented verbal, mathematical, or symbolic materials. The scientific knowledge that may have gone into the selection and construction of these tasks, or that would be employed in the analysis of performances on these tasks, would hardly be evident from superficial examination of a mental test.

29

The intention of this chapter is to give a view of the development and present status of the scientific knowledge that lies at the base of psychological tests, with special reference to tests of "intelligence" or intellectual capacity. It suggests that no matter how simple (or apparently simpleminded) the test content may appear to be, the selection or devising of this content, and the analysis of people's performances on these tests, is undergirded with a substantial amount of knowledge and technology, and that although the present theory and technology are highly sophisticated, there are reasonable grounds for questioning at least some of it and for thinking that new and profitable directions for research can be found.

The focus is on tests of so-called intelligence, IQ, or mental ability, partly because of space limitations, but more because this is currently (and has been since its beginnings) one of the most controversial fields of testing. Psychological and educational tests exist in great variety and profusion, as can be verified by consulting O. K. Buros's latest compilation, *Tests in Print II* (1974). Much of the basic psychometric technology to be discussed here pertains to all types of tests. Problems of reliability, validity, scaling, standardization, and the like have to be considered in connection not only with tests of mental abilities but also with tests of educational achievement, personality, interests, attitudes, motor skills, and the rest. But there are somewhat special considerations – linked to basic psychological issues about the nature of human capacities – that apply with particular force in the domain of tests of intellectual abilities; these will be discussed here in due course. Little attention will be paid to the measurement of educational achievement except insofar as tests of intellectual ability may be said to be, or can be shown to be, tests of educational attainment.

Even in considering the field of mental ability testing, I must limit the scope considerably. Except to outline historical antecedents in other countries (particularly England, France, and Germany), I focus on developments in the United States. Little consideration is given to the use of IQ tests in clinical practice to diagnose mental retardation and so-called learning disabilities. The emphasis is on "group" tests – that is, tests given to fairly large groups of people at a time, and usually of the "paper-and-pencil" variety. Starting roughly in the 1920s, such tests have often been used in schools to yield measures of intellectual capacity to serve as a partial basis for ability grouping, selection for special classes, and so on, and tests of this type have increasingly been used in connection with admission to higher education.

The approach is descriptive and historical. I trace the history of the mental testing movement, with special attention to its technological aspects, through two somewhat arbitarily defined periods: (a) an "early" or "developmental" period beginning in the late 19th century, during which the foundations of theory and practice in psychometrics were laid down; and (b) a "modern" period starting around 1935 with the founding of the Psychometric Society and its journal *Psychometrika,* during which many refinements were made in the technology of testing and during which testing became a major enterprise.

Each period is introduced with an overview of its major developments and achievements. This introduction is followed by a detailed discussion of particular topics that are regarded as essential to the scientific study of tests of intellectual ability and to the orderly development of their applications in educational settings. These topics, which are closely interrelated, are as follows:

1. *Theories and doctrines concerning the nature of what is to be measured.* All measurement has to do with (at least) the ordering (placing in an ordinal series) of a defined class of objects with respect to some attribute or attributes. In the case of

in the army work. Notable examples of such tests were the National Intelligence Test (designed for Grades 3–8), the Terman Group Test of Mental Ability (designed for Grades 7–12), and Thurstone's Psychological Examination for College Freshmen. Notions of "standardization" (the derivation of norms for representative samples of the population for which a test was designed) and "validation" (establishment of substantial correlation of test scores with independent measures of the attributes being tested or predicted) were developed during this period. Some of the tests recognized somewhat independent dimensions of ability; for example, beginning in about 1925, Thurstone's American Council on Education Psychological Examination for College Freshmen yielded two scores, a "linguistic" and a "quantitative"; similar scores ("verbal" and "mathematical") were produced by the Scholastic Aptitude Examinations constructed by C. C. Brigham for the College Entrance Examination Board (CEEB), starting in 1926. The culmination of this trend, for the period under consideration here, was represented by E. L. Thorndike's development in 1927 of his CAVD test, which contained four quite different parts (completion, arithmetic, vocabulary, and directions) and yielded scores on "altitude," "width," and "area."

These and many other tests became widely used in schools and colleges, and the publication and distribution of tests grew into a large, and often highly lucrative, enterprise. The concept of "intelligence" or "scholastic aptitude" came into general acceptance, but the notion that intelligence or scholastic aptitude reflected largely the effects of native endowment in interaction with schooling was, apparently, slow in coming. Writing in 1925, Joseph Peterson had this to say:

The popular mind today ... neglects innate individual differences. Many of the weaknesses of our present educational system are directly due to the view, now disappearing, that we are born "free and equal" in the sense that all alike can learn what the schools teach. Failures, according to this view, are attributed to stubbornness, laziness, etc., rather than to inability or to innate differences in the structure and organization of individuals. [P. 15]

This sketchy overview of the development of group tests of mental ability has omitted many details, and even some major developments. Some of these details will be filled in during consideration of specific aspects of the testing movement as it developed during the period now in view.

NOTIONS OF MENTAL ABILITY

What does one seek to measure in developing a test of "mental ability"? One can interpret the efforts of Galton, Cattell, Binet, and many others in the developmental period of mental testing as oriented toward the diagnosis and verification of an "ordinary language" concept of intelligence whereby it is recognized that human beings exhibit, somewhat independently of the amount of education to which they have been exposed, grades of intelligence ranging from idiocy or feeblemindedness, through average, up to genius. Galton was most interested in the characteristics of genius; Binet, at least in his earlier practical work, was concerned with distinguishing grades of mental deficiency and contrasting them with the abilities of the average child. Galton was unsuccessful in discovering tests that would exhibit the mental powers of a genius; he must have been surprised to find that recognized geniuses had no greater prowess in sensory acuity and speed of reaction than the average person. By focusing his attention on relatively complex mental tasks, Binet was successful in devising a scale that distinguished grades of mental deficiency. The psychologists who developed the Army Alpha and Beta examinations were evidently attempting to take seriously the advice offered by Galton, namely, that one should "obtain a general knowledge of the capacities of a man by sinking shafts, as it were, at a few critical points" (Galton, in a letter appended to Cattell, 1890). For these army psychologists, the critical points were abilities to understand language to perform reasoning with semantic and quantitative relationships, to make "practical judgments," to infer rules and regularities from data, and to recall general information. Operationally, every one of the more successful tests of intelligence, whether of an "individual" or "group" type, employed a rather wide array and variety of tasks involving the understanding and manipulation of verbal and nonverbal materials and problems. Although some of these tasks intersected those specifically taught in school, the emphasis was on tasks that reflected the individual's ability to profit from his total experiential history.

The general view of the nature of intelligence implied here was later expounded in considerable detail by E. L. Thorndike (Thorndike, Bregman, Cobb, & Woodyard, 1927). Thorndike saw intelligence as a general capacity that manifests itself in a large variety of tasks; it is, in effect, a capacity for forming bonds or connections among ideas, concepts, and so on. Persons of high intelligence are those who have the capacity to form a large number of bonds and have had the opportunity (through experience, education, etc.) to do so. Insofar as the capacity to form bonds might be regarded as innate, and the actual formation of these bonds is thought to be a result of appropriate opportunities to form them, Thorndike viewed intelligence as having both hereditary and environmental components.

A somewhat similar theory, the "sampling theory" of intelligence, was proposed by a Scottish psychologist (and chief author of a series of "Moray House" intelligence tests used widely in schools in the United Kingdom), Godfrey Thomson (Brown & Thomson, 1921). According to this view, any mental task "samples" a wide variety of mental operations; the correlation between two tests is therefore a function of the amount of overlap between the sets of operations thus sampled. (In a sense, Thomson foreshadowed the "information-processing" approach that is in favor in contemporary psychology; Thomson, however, never attempted to specify the details of how mental operations enter into tasks.)

Nevertheless, a satisfactory *definition* of intelligence or mental ability was always elusive. The few definitions that were enunciated by leaders in mental testing seldom corresponded very well with the actual measurement procedures embodied in their tests. For example, one definition of intelligence offered by Binet (1890) would hardly yield suggestions about how to operationalize the concept: "What we call intelligence, in the narrow sense of the term, consists of two chief processes: First, to perceive the external world, and then to reinstate the perceptions in memory, to rework them, and to think about them" (p. 582, my translation). At another point, Binet (Binet & Simon, 1909, 128 ff.) laid down three criteria for intelligent thought: (a) *la direction,* the taking and maintaining of a given mental set; (b) *l'adaptation,* the adaptation of thought for the purpose of obtaining a given end; and (c) *la critique,* the taking of a critical attitude toward one's thought, and correcting it where necessary.

We have seen that, in the early years of the period we are considering, use was made of relatively simple tasks, usually involving powers of sensory acuity and judgment (e.g., detecting small differences in the weights of two visually similar objects) or speed of reaction time in responding to stimuli (e.g., naming colors). Selection of these tests was based on the apparently plausible hypothesis that intelligence resides in the individual's power to respond sensitively and quickly. Of these early types of tests, perhaps only one has survived in current measures of intelligence – the memory-span test – and even this is recognized to be a measure of a rather special dimension of intelligence. It was only when Binet developed tests of more "complex" processes that he could feel that he was measuring something that revealed mental ability differences. It may be noted, however, that Binet's approach was *developmental:* He was essentially the first to trace the development of certain abilities over the age range of childhood and early adolescence. A criterion for the acceptance of a task into his series was that it show not only progressive increase in performance over these ages but also consistent relationships with degrees of mental deficiency over these ages. (Otherwise, a test of a motor skill like walking might have been included.)

A symposium on the meaning of intelligence published in 1921 (E. Thorndike et al., 1921) produced a tremendous profusion of definitions and opinions. Intelligence was variously described as "ability to learn" (Buckingham, p. 273), as "the power of good responses from the point of view of truth or fact" (Thorndike, p. 124), as "the ability to carry on abstract thinking" (Terman, p. 128), as "the ability of the individual to adapt himself adequately to relatively new situations in life" (Pintner, p, 139), as "involving two factors – the capacity for knowledge and the knowledge possessed" (Henmon, p. 195), or as "the capacity to acquire capacity" (Woodrow, p. 207). Beardsley Ruml, who later, as an economist, introduced the idea of the withholding tax, declined to enter the debate because there was insufficient precision in the terms and concepts to form a basis for discussion, and because of "an absence of factual material on so many essential points" (p. 143). Henmon added the caution that "the so-called general intelligence tests are not general intelligence tests at all but tests of the special intelligence upon which the school puts a premium" (p. 197).

Perhaps it was truly premature to expect any consensus on the meaning of intelligence at this early date.[1] Yet the tests must have been measuring *something,* and to a degree their reliability as measurements, and their validity in predicting school and other kinds of performances, had been established. Despite the fact that Binet's definitions of intelligence differed considerably from those espoused by the authors of group tests of intelligence, there was evidence from the work with the army that scores from the Army Alpha Examination correlated rather highly with ratings derived from tests of the Binet type (Yerkes, 1921).

So far unmentioned in our overview of this developmental period is the work of the British psychologist Spearman, who very early in the century published a strikingly original interpretation of some data[2] that he had collected in a village school in Hampshire, England (Spearman, 1904b). Setting up a matrix of correlations among the test scores and academic ranks, Spearman noticed that they could be arranged and analyzed in a special way, "hierarchically," to show that all the variables measured just one "factor" in common, but to different degrees. From this discovery, Spearman developed what he called (somewhat misleadingly) the "two-factor" theory of intelligence, whereby each test of a set is regarded as measuring one "general" factor in common with all the other tests and, in addition, a "specific" factor that is unique to that test. Spearman devoted the major part of his professional life to attempting to establish the universality of this two-factor theory and, in addition, to explicating the psychological nature of the general (G or g) factor. His major writings that bear on this subject are the books *The Nature of "Intelligence" and the Principles of Cognition* (1923), *The Abilities of Man* (1927), and (with L. Wynn Jones) *Human Ability* (1950). This work embroiled Spearman in many controversies, for he was often accused by his critics of "selecting" his data – that is, selecting tests in such a way as to cause the data to fit the two-factor theory. Eventually, Spearman conceded that not all tests could be interpreted solely in terms of a two-factor theory; his later writings recognize the appearance of "group" factors (and even two other specialized "general factors" – perseveration and oscillation) alongside the original g factor. What Spearman's original g factor seems to correspond to, in current interpretations, is the fact that almost any set of mental tests, no matter how different, will *tend* to exhibit *positive* intercorrelations (assuming that the test scores are all oriented in the same way, i.e., that numerically "high" scores represent the more desirable, competent behaviors). What really interested Spearman was the psychological nature and interpretation of whatever it is that tends to produce positive correlations among all mental tests. To this end, he held that the "general" factor is central and supreme in all tests of intelligence. He even thought it had identifiable physiological correlates.

Spearman's *Nature of "Intelligence" and the Principles of Cognition* (1923) may be thought of as the result of a detour he took out of statistical psychology into cognitive psychology. Virtually unknown to today's cognitive psychologists, but potentially highly rewarding, it was a thoroughgoing analysis of reasoning processes as they are exhibited in solving syllogisms, making inferences from propositions, solving mathematical problems, and the like. From this work, and from the empirical data (much of it from group intelligence tests) amassed in *The Abilities of Man* (1927), he arrived at the notion that the "general" factor represents the power of reasoning, or the "noegenesis" of abstract entities. To the extent that a test measures a general factor, Spearman saw in it operations of the "education of relations" and the "education of correlates." A vocabulary test, for example, often requires the subject to notice similarities or differences in meaning, whereas a verbal analogies test ("Father is to mother as son is to _____ ") requires the noticing of correlative or analogous relationships. According to this theory, an intelligence test (to the extent that it is "loaded" with g) measures the extent to which an individual can perform such mental operations.

At about the time that Spearman published his *Nature of "Intelligence"* Thurstone (1924) published a book with a similar title, but it was concerned more with the nature of perceptual processes in intelligence, and for various reasons it failed to have the impact that Spearman's work did. Indeed, it was all but ignored by Thurstone himself in his later work.

Out of the controversies surrounding Spearman's two-factor theory and the attempts to put it to empirical test, there gradually emerged a somewhat different, and perhaps better-articulated, view of mental abilities. Spearman himself, but even more his co-workers and students, sought to explain the fact that matrices of correlations among test variables did not always conform well to the two-factor theory. It was noticed that specific groups of intelligence tests – by virtue of special similarities in content, format, or the response processes involved – tended to exhibit intercorrelations that were greater than would be predicted by the two-factor theory. Already in 1927, Spearman recognized the existence of group factors of intelligence apart from *g*. In cooperation with the American educational psychologist Karl Holzinger, Spearman and his associates initiated a "Unitary Trait Study" in the early 1930s to seek information on what kinds of "group factors" could be established empirically and interpreted psychologically in useful ways.

In the meantime, Thurstone, who had early been involved in the army examining program and who had been one of the most creative test developers, was seeking improved mathematical formulations of the problem of identifying "factors" of intelligence. The story of these efforts by Spearman, Holzinger, Thurstone, and others to delineate the factors of intelligence belongs more properly, however, to the discussion of the "modern period."

THEORIES OF MEASUREMENT AND SCALING

Psychological measurement involves difficult problems concerning the nature of the scales on which measurements are taken, the units of measurement, the existence of an origin or zero point, and the numerical operations that can legitimately be performed with the measurements. No indications have come to my attention that early developers of intelligence tests concerned themselves with such problems. To be sure, in his *Grammar of Science* (1892), Karl Pearson (who is discussed later as a collaborator of Galton in the development of the correlation coefficient) recognized the need for a science or theory of measurement, but he did not discuss any peculiarly psychological problems of measurement. Galton, Spearman, Binet, and other early workers in the measurement of intelligence apparently relied on traditional concepts of measurement as they had come down from Euclid and Newton. Modern doctrines of the foundations of measurement took shape only in the work of the philosopher-physicist von Helmholtz (1885) and the mathematician Hölder (1901), but this work was not to influence psychological measurement until much later, for example, in the writings of B. O. Smith (1938) and S. S. Stevens (1951).

It is, nevertheless, instructive to examine the assumptions about measurement that were made by early developers of intelligence tests. It is convenient to depart somewhat from a strictly chronological treatment in order to begin with a look at the rather special measurement characteristics of Binet's mental age scale. Subsequently attention will be given to the tradition that began with Galton and other British psychologists and was carried on by group intelligence testers in the United States.

Implicitly, the first problem that confronted Binet was whether mental ability varies continuously (i.e., exists in different gradations that can be as small as one likes) or exists in some set of discrete steps or classifications. He was, after all, set the task of distinguishing "abnormal" or mentally retarded children (as a group) from "normal" children (as a group). As a result of his empirical work, he apparently came to realize quite early that mental ability or intelligence can best be thought of as varying continuously and that different degrees of intelligence can be ranged along a scale. (In Binet's time, the dominant theories of individual differences, especially in personality, were essentially typologies. Thus Binet's achievement in recognizing the continuous variation of intelligence was perhaps more significant than it seems today.)

A quotation from Binet suggests still other implications about measurement theory:

The basic idea of this method is the establishment of what we shall call a metric scale of intelligence [*échelle métrique de l'intelligence*]; this scale is composed of a series of tests, of increasing difficulty, starting at the lowest intellectual level that one can observe, and ending at an average and normal level of intelligence, wherein to each test there corresponds a different mental level. [Binet & Simon, 1905, p. 194, my translation]

What is striking here is the idea of a scale composed of tasks of increasing difficulty where, in addition, each task corresponds to a different level of ability or "mental age" (a concept Binet originated). There was nothing like this in the previous history of mental testing, and, in fact, there are few parallels to such a scale in ordinary experience (except perhaps the erection of bars at increasing heights to test jumping ability, or the testing of minerals for hardness by finding which ones of a graded series of substances – from soapstone to diamond – could produce scratches in them). One other idea that is implicit here was perhaps not so new – the idea that the outcome of each task would be binary, that is, would consist of either passing or failing.

Binet was, of course, a little too optimistic in seeming to suggest that each task would correspond exactly and reliably to a particular mental level. As the Binet scale developed, it was found necessary to use a number of tasks at each level of mental age. From this point on, the task of determining a person's mental age was reminiscent of one of the psychophysical methods devised by Fechner, Wundt, and others to determine the level of a person's sensitivity to faint stimuli or to a small physical difference in stimuli. In fact, it is in the psychometric analysis of a Binet-type scale that we see the strong resemblance of psychometric methods to those of psychophysics, a resemblance that was capitalized on in later developments in "test theory" (of which more will be said subsequently). That is, just as one tests hearing ability by presenting sounds of increasing loudness or softness, and determines the limen (threshold) at which the individual hears a sound half the time, so one determines mental age by presenting different tasks in order to find the level on the mental age scale where the individual can pass half (or some other fraction) of the tasks. Such testing is readily done when the examination is conducted for one child at a time; it is much more difficult to accomplish under group testing conditions.

Later developments of Binet-type tests, particularly at the hands of Terman (1916) in his Stanford–Binet test, led to an elaborate technology for this type of scale, involving the careful selection and placement of tasks on the scale in such a way as to produce approximately constant means and standard deviations of intelligence quotients over different ages. (This implied, of course, that the scale was conceived to apply not only to normal and mentally retarded children but also to children at the upper ranges of ability.) The idea of an intelligence quotient came from the German psychologist Stern (1912), who had noticed that as chronological age increased, variation in mental ages increased proportionally; thus he saw that it would be possible to obtain a ratio whose standard deviation would be approximately constant over chronological age if mental age was divided by chronological age.

Despite the interesting psychometric characteristics of the Binet-type scale, neither Binet nor any of his followers gave much thought to the question whether such a scale would be homogeneous in the sense that every task or item would measure the "same" kind of mental ability. One can perceive that this would not necessarily be the case. Binet's scale depended mainly on the fact that nearly all human functions, whether cognitive or not, tend to mature at some specified rate, and more or less in a fixed order. But different mental functions could mature at different rates. Intelligence as derived from Binet-type tests is therefore essentially a measure of average rate of growth of various mental functions – a measure not of *momentary* mental growth (in the sense of a first derivative), but of rate of mental growth as estimated from the cumulative performance or achievement up to the time of testing. It can easily be shown that as a consequence it has an element of constancy automatically built into it, if one assumes that competencies once achieved are not forgotten or lost. Amid the discussions of the "constancy of the IQ," the implications of this fact were not clearly seen until a later phase of the history of mental tests.

Let us turn now to the measurement assumptions underlying the group testing tradition. The kinds of tests employed by Galton and Cattell in the early "experimental laboratory" phase of the testing movement most often yielded scores based on direct physical measurements – speeds of reaction expressed in fractions of a second or the physical magnitudes of stimuli or stimulus differences that could be apprehended by the subject. As such, they had the properties of other kinds of physical measurement. Very few of these tests, therefore, had "binary score" characteristics. It seems to have been assumed that any mental abilities measured by these tests were in direct relation to the score levels attained – an assumption that probably was justified.

When Binet-type items began to be applied in group tests of intelligence, shortly after the turn of the century, the measurement assumptions changed rather radically, although it is probable that few psychologists gave much thought to this change. A "test" became an assemblage of items; generally each item or task yielded a binary score (pass or fail). The test score became the number of such items that were passed, and the resulting scale was called a "point scale." When the test was given under a time limit, the score became the number of items that the examinee was able to attempt *and pass* within that time limit. Test constructors recognized that the items might differ in difficulty; in fact, the usual practice (as it still is today) was to arrange the items in approximate order of difficulty, starting with the easier ones, apparently under the assumption that this made for a better adjustment of the examinee to the demands of the task as a whole. Also, it meant that the slower examinees were likely to attempt a greater number of items than otherwise, if difficulty of an item entailed a greater amount of time. As in the case of Galton's and Cattell's tests, it was assumed that whatever mental ability was being measured by the test would be in direct monotonic relation to the total score, that is, to the number of items passed. Such an assumption was somewhat more questionable in this case than in the case of the simple tests employed by Galton and Cattell, for several reasons. First, there was an inadequate guarantee that the separate tasks were homogeneous with respect to what they measured; two persons might obtain precisely the same score, yet pass completely different items and thus exhibit quite different mental abilities. Imagine an analogous situation of a test with half the items in English, half in French; if a person scored 50% correct, it might be that he passed only the items in English, or only the items in French, depending on which language he knew. In the group intelligence tests that were constructed in the early days, the only guarantee of item or task homogeneity was the judgment of the test constructor. Second, scores could depend upon either the level of the examinee's abilities (which could be thought of as the probability that he could pass any item picked at random) or the speed with which he could attempt them, or upon some combination of the two. Third, the difficulty levels of items were assessed according to the average performance of a group and would not necessarily correspond to their difficulty levels for a given individual.

The seriousness of these problems of scaling was seldom perceived in the developmental phases of the mental testing movement. We find only hints of it in the writings of E. L. Thorndike. Perhaps the earliest clear recognition of the relation between the patterns of scores on individual items and individuals' total scores is to be found in the work of David A. Walker (1931, 1936, 1940), a Scottish psychologist working with educational achievement measurements. Walker pointed out that this relation could range from what he called "hig" (from "higgledy-piggledy-ness") to its converse, "unig." The "unig" situation would exist when "a given answer-pattern completely determines the score-scatter" (1931, p. 75) (that is, each score x is composed of correct answers to the x easiest items), whereas maximum "hig" would occur when all the scores with value x might be composed of a random selection of the possible combinations of answers on the individual items of varying difficulty. It is interesting to note that Walker's concept of "unig" anticipated by some years the notion of what later came to be called a "Guttman scale" (Guttman, 1941); also, Walker's continuum from "hig" to "unig" corresponds to Loevinger's (1947) continuum from maximum "heterogeneity" to maximum "homogeneity." Nevertheless, Walker's concerns did not extend to the question whether the units of measurement represented by point scores are equal, nor to the question whether the "unig" condition he described would necessarily reflect true homogeneity of the items with respect to the functions they measured.

A test score obtained as the number of items correctly answered (with possibly an adjustment for "guessing" made by subtracting a fraction of the number of incorrect answers) is called a "raw score." Such raw scores have quite arbitrary meanings. Their direct interpretation has to depend upon a knowledge of the characteristics of the total assemblage of items – for example, on a knowledge of whether they are generally easy or difficult. Even a conversion of a raw score to a *percentage correct* score would help very little. This fact was recognized by early mental testers, with the consequence that elaborate techniques (foreshadowed by Galton, 1885, with his concept of the percentile) were worked out for interpreting scores with respect to the performances of stated groups, for example, ninth graders, 14-year-olds, or representative groups of college students. Thus was developed the "normative" interpretation of test scores. The more reputable and responsible publishers of group intelligence tests provided extensive tables of "norms," that is, correspondences between scores and the percentile ranks of those scores in typical groups. Scores could also be interpreted normatively by means of "standard scores" or "T-scores," that is, values that expressed how far above or below an average a score would be, measured by the standard deviation of the scores of representative groups.

All these normative interpretations of test scores were useful but left something to be desired. A normative interpretation does not really characterize the performance of an individual, for it tells little about the absolute level of that person's abilities. The problem of relating mental test scores to absolute, or quasi-absolute, levels of abilities was never satisfactorily solved in the developmental period of mental testing; in fact, it is a problem even today, although (as will be pointed out) the technology for solving it is now much more advanced.

STATISTICAL METHODS AND MENTAL TEST THEORY

Quantitative and statistical methods have played a large and necessary role in the development of mental tests. It is convenient to organize the discussion of these methods from the perspective of the present day, which would treat them under a number of somewhat separate topics:

1.   *Univariate descriptive statistics:* methods for characterizing the distribution of the measurements of a given variable over a sample of things (objects, persons, events, etc.) measured.
2.   *Inferential statistics:* statistical methods for making inferences concerning populations from the statistics obtained from samples of those populations.
3.   *Bivariate and multivariate descriptive statistics:* methods for characterizing the joint distributions of two or more measurements over a sample of things measured and for predicting measurements on a given variable from one or more other variables.
4.   *"Mental test theory"*: a collection of special statistical methods and theorems that have to do with the reliability and validity of measurements, particularly the kinds of measurements derived from mental tests.
5.   *"Factor analysis"*: a collection of special mathematical and statistical methods that provide models for the identification of fundamental dimensions underlying the observed measurements from mental tests or other sources.

The beginnings of the work in univariate descriptive statistics, and to some extent that in inferential statistics, occurred well before the start of the developmental period of mental ability testing that is in view here. Most of the major developments in the other topics mentioned in this list had their beginnings during this period, however. In fact, many of the advances, even in "pure" statistics, were occasioned by the technological requirements of the mental ability testing movement. A detailed account of developments up through about 1928, with emphasis on origins in the 19th century, is to be found in Helen Walker's *Studies in the History of Statistical Method* (1929), actually a revision of her doctoral thesis at Teachers College, Columbia University.

By the time of Galton and Cattell, the theory of the Gaussian law of error – what is now conventionally called the normal probability distribution – had been worked out, and early in the 19th century, Quetelet, the astronomer royal of Belgium, had shown how it could be applied to the analysis of various kinds of vital and social statistics. Concepts of central tendency (indicated, for example, by the arithmetic mean of a series of observations) and of variation (as measured by the "probable error" or the standard deviation) were known. It fell to Galton (1885), however, to make the first wide use of the normal probability distribution in psychological and educational contexts. He made frequency distributions of his mental test results and suggested the use of the normal curve in assigning class grades. He can be regarded as the inventor of what is now called the percentile rank. Univariate statistical methods continued to be developed and applied throughout the period under review here, particularly by Karl Pearson in a series of publications starting in 1894, G. Udny Yule (1911), Ronald Fisher (1925), and many others, principally in England, and often in fairly close contact with psychologists concerned with the development of mental tests.

Because of their close conceptual relationships with probability distributions, the methods of inferential statistics received much early development in the period under consideration here. In connection with mental tests, they were used mainly in research on the application of tests – for example, in deciding whether there were significant differences between test scores of different sexes, social classes, races, and so on. However, even as late as 1935, the "small sample" statistical methods developed by Fisher (1925), "Student" (the pseudonym of one of Fisher's students), and others were practically unknown in the United States (Rucci & Tweney, 1980). Fortunately, American psychologists in the early days tended to employ such a conservative standard in testing statistical differences (a "critical ratio" of four times the probable error, corresponding to $p < .007$) that they only infrequently made "Type I errors" – rejecting the hypothesis of no difference when it was in fact true.

It is in the domain of bivariate and multivariate descriptive statistics that the development of statistical methods had a particularly close association with the development of mental tests, for fundamental to the methodologies surrounding mental tests is the statistical concept of *correlation* or *association*. Reading Helen Walker's (1929, chap. 5) account of its development, one may be surprised to discover that the technical concept of correlation is hardly a hundred years old, having first arisen in the mind of Galton around 1875, in connection with his studies of the inheritance of traits such as the sizes of peas, and yet not appearing in published form until 1886 (Galton, 1886, 1889). (The nontechnical concept of correlation is embedded in ordinary language, as in expressions of the form "The more intelligent, the more (or less) rich." The technical concept provides a measure of the degree of relationship between the variables X and Y.) Actually, Galton conceived correlation in terms of *regression,* a term deriving from the fact that the mean heights of sons, for example, tend to "regress" toward the mean height of the fathers. The first exact formula for computing what is today the most prevalent correlation measure, the Pearson product-moment correlation coefficient, was not published by Karl Pearson until 1896, even though, as Walker points out, many earlier mathematical statisticians (e.g., Laplace, Plana, Gauss, Bravais) had been "on the verge" of formulating it. Nevertheless, after the publication of Pearson's work, there was a period of intense activity for about 10 years during which most of the basic correlation methodologies were developed, including, for example, the standard deviations and correlations of weighted sums, multiple correlation and regression theory, and theorems on the probable errors of estimates. Practically all this work was accomplished by Pearson and his students and associates in England.

Strangely, it appears that Galton, the discoverer of the technical concept of correlation, did not recognize its usefulness in the analysis of mental test results; at least, I have found no indication of his having applied it to the mental test data that he collected at his Anthropometric Laboratory in the years 1884–1890. Instead, Galton applied his correlation and regression concepts to the problem of measuring the role of inheritance in passing traits from generation to generation.

Correlation theory has continued to play an important role in genetics (and in the applications of genetics in psychology), but one of the first applications and refinements of correlation theory in connection with mental tests is that of Spearman in his *American Journal of Psychology* paper "The Proof and Measurement of Association between Two Things" (1904a). In this and a further paper (Spearman, 1904b), he not only showed how correlation theory could be applied to establish dimensions of mental ability, but also developed several formulas for dealing with the role of error in test results. Spearman saw the correlation coefficient as a measurement of the extent to which two variables may be taken to measure one underlying variable in common. He was the first to apply the correlation coefficient as a measure of the reliability of measurements; these reliability coefficients (though he did not at that time call them that) played a role in his famous formula for "correction for attenuation," a formula for estimating the amount of correlation that would exist between two series of measurements if they could be freed of all error. However, it was not until 1910 that a further derivation of reliability theory was made, independently by Spearman and by William Brown, the so-called Spearman–Brown prophecy formula for predicting the effect of the length of a test (or the number of replicate measurements) on its reliability. (Derivation of this formula is a trivial exercise for present-day students of test theory.)

The work of Spearman and Brown generated what may be regarded as two rather independent subfields in quantitative psychology: one, the specialty known as "factor analysis" and the other, what has come to be called "mental test theory." Factor analysis is concerned mainly with the identification of the "dimensions" of mental ability, whereas test theory is concerned with making reliable measurements of mental abilities. (Both factor analysis and test theory can, of course, be applied to other types of measurements.) Actually, there are intimate relations between factor analysis and test theory, but particularly today the specialties tend to be quite separate: they are usually treated in different university courses and taught by different specialists, who tend to publish in different sets of journals. And, somewhat surprising to state, factor analysis and test theory are usually treated quite separately from the basic statistical methodology that encompasses the further refinements of correlation theory that ensued from the work of Pearson.

In the United States, the person most instrumental in disseminating the new discoveries in correlational methods and mental test theory was E. L. Thorndike. His book, *Introduction to the Theory of Mental and Social Measurements* (1904), contained detailed discussions of statistical methods, including correlation, appropriate for the construction and application of mental tests. Thorndike was even able to take some advantage of Spearman's then recent contributions to reliability theory. The result was a flurry of activity in applying the new methods to a variety of test data in psychology and education. It is rather amusing to note the frequency with which new correlation formulas were "discovered" by American educational statisticians – often these formulas were mere mathematical variants of those already presented by British workers.

By the time of the establishment of the army testing program in World War I, the principles of basic statistical methods, including correlation, were fairly well understood, and they played a large role in the selection, refinement, and analysis of the army tests. In fact, Yerkes's (1921) statistical report of the army testing program contains one of the early applications of multiple correlation in psychological testing, used to discover the optimal weighting of two or more tests in predicting an independent criterion. Correlations among the separate tests in test batteries were computed in order to see which tests best contributed to the aggregate score and which were more independent of the others. By this time, also, simple item-analysis techniques had been developed and were used to arrange items in order of difficulty and to select items that best discriminated individuals on the total score scale.

Probably the person most responsible for the dissemination of psychological measurement statistics in the 1920s was Truman L. Kelley, who for a number of years (1920–1931) was associated with Terman's activities at Stanford University in the further development of the Stanford–Binet scale and a variety of other tests. Kelley's book *Statistical Method* (1923) "marked an important milestone in the application of rigorous statistical methodology to problems in psychology, education, and other social science fields" (Flanagan, 1961, p. 343). It summarized nearly all the previous relevant work in statistical method and presented many new contributions from Kelley himself. The book was the basic text for a generation of workers in psychological and educational measurement. Another classic work by Kelley was *The Interpretation of Educational Measurements* (1927), which presented a unified account of mental test theory as it had developed up to that time. Kelley was also a contributor to the development of factor analysis; his monograph *Crossroads in the Mind of Man* (1928) contained some important new derivations.

Statistical methods, test theory, and factor analysis in the 1920s had still not become so highly specialized that they could not be easily encompassed within the expertise of a single individual. One other figure who started to become prominent at this time was L. L. Thurstone (1887–1955). Whereas Kelley had been identified principally with educational measurement, Thurstone was identified primarily with psychology. Early on, he was a contributor to the field of psychophysics, being responsible for several famous "laws" of comparative judgment (Thurstone, 1927). The author of a theoretical work on the nature of intelligence (Thurstone, 1924) and a brief text on statistics (1925a), he was one of the most creative workers in the development of psychological tests. His work in the construction of psychological examinations for college admissions has already been mentioned. All of this work impelled Thurstone's quantitatively oriented mind to seek the elevation of psychological testing to the status of a truly "quantitative, rational" science. Although Thurstone made few fundamental contributions to mental test theory, save perhaps for his so-called absolute scaling methods (Thurstone, 1925b, 1928), he systematically summarized the major parts of test theory for his students in a small monograph, *The Reliability and Validity of Tests* (1931a). This monograph was the inspiration for many later developments in test theory among his students and co-workers, of which we will say more in our survey of the "modern" period of mental testing.

Thurstone's major contributions were in the field of factor analysis, a field heavily dominated between 1904 and about 1931 by Spearman, who was mainly concerned to establish and validate the two-factor theory he had announced in 1904. From the standpoint of today's theory and technology, Spearman's methodology was quite unsophisticated. It used relatively simple algebraic procedures in order to "factor" a matrix of intercorrelations. Because of the unavailability of efficient computing procedures, Spearman and his students generally used small sets of variables – rarely more than 20 or 25, and more commonly 10 or 12.

Progress was relatively slow. Techniques for establishing new group factors were primitive. A major part of Spearman's scientific output was of a polemical nature, arguing against critics of his rather narrow two-factor theory. It may be said that scientific progress in the analysis of mental abilities was held back by the lack of adequately refined mathematical and statistical methods for such an analysis. Nevertheless, Spearman was sufficiently optimistic in the early 1930s about the prospects of new findings to establish, with Karl Holzinger at the University of Chicago, a large "Spearman–Holzinger Unitary Trait Study" to search for "group factors" of mental ability.

By this time, Thurstone was literally just down the street from Holzinger at the University of Chicago, yet the two never collaborated directly. Thurstone's major contributions came through his recognition that the factor analysis of correlation matrices required sophisticated methods of determinants and matrix algebra, and although the basic theorems had long been known to mathematicians (e.g., Bôcher, 1907), they were known to few psychologists. Thurstone set about learning them, under tutelage, and by 1931 he was able to sketch a new model for factor analysis that was, in effect, a generalization of Spearman's model to multiple factors (Thurstone, 1931b). A more complete version of this model was published several years later, as *The Vectors of the Mind* (Thurstone, 1935), and within a year or so, Thurstone and his wife, Thelma, and their students were starting to assemble a major data base to test out these new formulations. The results of this study were published as a monograph, *Primary Mental Abilities* (Thurstone, 1938a), setting the stage for an entirely new phase in the development of theories of mental abilities, discussion of which is reserved for my treatment of the modern period of mental ability test development.

Advances in computational technology have had a large role in the development of mental ability test methodology. The computational methods available to people like Galton and Cattell were primitive in the extreme; aside from the slide rule, there were practically no aids to hand computation. The period after Thorndike's introduction of statistical methods to American psychologists saw the production of numerous "worksheets" for computing correlation coefficients – many of them exceedingly clever – that facilitated computations but that still relied essentially on hand tabulations and mental arithmetic (Otis, 1923); Toops, 1921). Tests had to be scored by hand, although fairly efficient methods utilizing "scoring keys" were devised early in the century. Mechanical aids such as machines for basic arithmetic operations were introduced only gradually, and their use was cumbersome and error prone. Hollerith machines using punched cards had been introduced by the U.S. Census Bureau early in the century and received some use in the army examining program of World War I, but their use was limited to providing data for simple hand tabulations. Even as late as 1935, their uses in performing any elaborate statistical calculations were extremely limited, although Warren and Mendenhall (1929) had developed a method for computing correlations partly by tabulating machine. From the late 1920s until well into the 1950s, the mechanical desk calculator was the essential tool of the statistician. It is a practical certainty that many published research results contained egregious errors that were the fault of the investigators, not the printers. Of course, errors occur even with present-day electronic facilities, but these errors are rarely of a primitive computational kind. The more basic point that should be made here is that the lack of efficient methods for collecting, tabulating, and analyzing statistical data seriously impeded progress during the developmental phases of the mental ability test movement.

Previous sections have outlined the theoretical and methodological developments that occurred in the early phase of the mental ability test movement. To examine the actual impact of these developments on the construction and use of tests, it may be helpful to take a look at several group tests that were in wide use at the end of the period: a form of the Henmon–Nelson Tests of Mental Ability that was designed for use with elementary-school children, a form of the California Tests of Mental Maturity that was designed for use with secondary-school students, and one of the annual editions of the American Council on Education Psychological Examination, designed for use with college students. All three tests were constructed and published around 1935.

The Henmon–Nelson Test of Mental Ability, Elementary School Examination (Henmon & Nelson, 1932–1935), is a group test designed for students in elementary school, Grades 3–8. It was first published in the years 1932–1935 and early achieved wide popularity because of the simplicity of its format and scoring (from the standpoint of the test user), the small amount of time required to administer it (30 min), and its low cost. Actually, this test is one of a set of three, each test in the set being designed for a different range of grade levels. (The other two levels are a High School Examination for Grades 7–12 and an Intelligence Test for College Students, by the same authors.) The test has been revised several times; one revision was published in 1957–1958 by Tom A. Lamke and M. J. Nelson, and a further revision was published by Joseph L. French in 1973.

The test itself consists of a series of 90 items printed in a booklet. At the outset of the test, the examinee is given examples and practice exercises for the several types of items he or she will encounter in the test, such as vocabulary, sentence completion, "classification" (finding which one of a set of stimuli cannot logically be grouped with the others), series completion, analogies, and arithmetic problems. All items in the test proper are in multiple-choice format; the student has to find the one correct or "best" answer from the five choices offered, indicating the choice by marking in a particular space. The marks are registered through carbon onto a grid underneath; the test can then be scored relatively easily (though manually) by counting the number of marks that fall in designated positions on the grid. (In this way, the test makes use of the Clapp–Young Self-Marking Device, patented in 1929.) The items are arranged in order of "difficulty"; at the same time, the several types of items appear in more or less random order, it being assumed that the student has been adequately instructed at the outset of the test in how to do each type.

Many of the item types require the student to be able to read printed English; others employ numerical or geometrical ("spatial") material. After the introduction to the test, the student is given 30 min to do as many items as possible – 90 items in 30 min, or 3 items per min on the average. It is a rare student who does all the items in this time. The raw score is the number of items answered correctly within the time limit.

There are three forms of the test, and according to the test manual they may be regarded as equivalent – that is, as yielding scores that could be expected to be approximately the same regardless of which form is administered. Tables are supplied whereby the test user can easily convert the raw scores to mental ages and thence to IQs. Normative data, based on a total of about 5,000 cases sampled from various elementary schools around the country, are given for each grade for which the test is designed. Separate reliability coefficients, found by the odd–even technique and the Spearman–Brown formula, are reported for each age and each grade. These reliabilities are all high, being consistently in the upper .80s or in the .90s. It should be remarked, however, that such reliabilities may well be inflated by the fact that there is a speed element in the test. When a test is "speeded," there will be variation in the numbers of items attempted by the examinees, and when scores on the odd items are correlated with those on the even items, a consequence of such variation in numbers of items attempted is that a rather high degree of correlation is inevitable. The use of odd–even reliability coefficients may therefore give a falsely favorable impression of the actual accuracy of the test scores. The authors failed to recognize this fact; they also failed to report equivalent-form reliabilities, something that they could easily have provided.

The "validity" of the test as a measure of intelligence or mental ability was ascertained by correlating scores of the test with other measures presumed to reflect intelligence. Correlations of the scores with results of other widely known group intelligence tests are reported as ranging from .54 to .92. Such values are regarded as being generally satisfactory, particularly the upper range of these values (9 of the 19 correlations reported were above .80). The authors also imply that the scores should correlate well with scholastic performance, because they report that in the process of selecting items for the test, they retained only those items that "proved to differentiate between pupils of known superior and known inferior mental ability" (Henmon & Nelson, 1932–1935, manual). They fail to say exactly how pupils' superior or inferior abilities were "known," but presumably the criterion was scholastic success as reflected in teachers' grades.

In their manual Henmon and Nelson make various suggestions concerning use of the test results. They state their belief that the test measures "those aspects of mental ability which are important for success in academic work." The scores are to be interpreted as measures of general mental ability but not as indexes of school achievement specifically taught in a common curriculum:

Although knowledge is required to answer the items, they were selected to reflect ability to profit from exposure to learning in a variety of situations. High performance on the test requires the efficient utilization of verbal and numerical symbols and the ability to acquire and retain information in common symbol form for use at later times in the solution of verbal, quantitative and abstract reasoning problems. [Manual]

They believe that the results will be most valuable to teachers when pupils' performances on the test are compared to their performances in school work; in this way teachers can arrive at a judgment about whether students are working up to capacity. The implication is that students with low scores on the test *and* with low scholastic performances are probably working up to their rather limited capacities. Students with high scores on the test and *low* academic achievements are ones who need help and special attention. If a student makes low scores on the test, but still does quite well academically, it is recommended that the scores on the test be "checked" through the administration of individually administered tests such as the Stanford–Binet.

Several experts in psychological measurement commented upon the test in a kind of "consumer's report" compiled by Buros (1941). Anne Anastasi, who later became one of the nation's leading authorities on individual differences (see Anastasi, 1958), remarked that "the use of a single score based on a hodgepodge of different types of items could be questioned, if one wanted a particularly fine or discriminative measure. But like other tests of its kind, this scale serves the practical purposes of (a) preliminary rapid exploration, and (b) rough classification of broad groups" (in Buros, 1941, p. 221). Howard Easley stated: "The content and standardization of these three tests seem as satisfactory as those of the better group tests of intelligence, but not strikingly more so" (in Buros, 1941, p. 222). J. P. Guilford, later to become the originator of a widely known theory of intelligence (Guilford, 1967), proclaimed: "An examination of these group tests and the manuals and scoring keys that accompany them impresses one immediately with the kind of care and expertness with which one wishes all tests were constructed" (in Buros, 1941, p. 222). Although they had certain reservations about details, all these experts were willing to accept the test as a well-constructed, highly useful measure of mental ability.

The test can be appraised as the natural resultant of trends that had been initiated by Binet and other early developers of mental tests. The kinds of items included can be regarded as group test derivatives of the sorts of tasks included in the Binet scale – simple problems involving the understanding of words and verbal expression, the manipulation of numerical and spatial information, and the recognition of logical distinctions and classifications. It could be argued that the materials in the test items were not specifically taught in the school curriculum, but that successful school learning would require the student's ability to perform problems with such materials. (A few items obviously require certain kinds of specific information, but this information is of such a general and widely disseminated character that it would be only the less "able" students who might have failed to acquire it.)

The construction and standardization of the Henmon–Nelson Test of Mental Ability obviously involved various technologies that had been fashioned throughout the early days of the testing movement. The items had been selected from pools of items that had been submitted to teachers, tried out on a number of occasions, and evaluated for their overall "difficulty" (as reflected in the proportions of students in different grades able to pass them) and for their power of "discriminating" among groups of students of "known" mental ability. Reliability and validity coefficients had been duly computed according to Pearson and Spearman's formulas, and norms had been compiled on the basis of fairly representative samples. The format was carefully devised in the light of experience with printed tests of this type, and the scoring and administration of the test had been honed and refined to a point of high efficiency – as much efficiency, that is, as could be achieved prior to the development of test-scoring machines.

Another example of a group intelligence test developed during the early period is the California Test of Mental Maturity, Advanced Series, 1937 edition (Sullivan, Clark, & Tiegs, 1936–1939). This test was designed for pupils from Grades 7–14. According to the authors' manual, its "primary purpose is to make for each pupil a diagnostic evaluation of those mental abilities which are related to, or determine, his success in various types of school activity in order that the teacher may utilize this information directly in aiding students who have learning difficulties." In contrast to the test just considered, it yields not a single score but a whole series of scores that can be plotted on a "diagnostic profile." It is

based on the philosophy, researches and important inferences of outstanding leaders in this field, as well as the work of the authors. The analytical comparison of the various sections of the test indicates a definite central factor, yet the same analysis reveals a specificity for each test sufficient to justify its inclusion as a measure of a more or less unique factor.... This series of tests is unique in that each battery is preceded by tests of visual acuity, auditory acuity, and motor coordination, the purpose of which is to detect those pupils with defects sufficiently serious to prevent obtaining a valid diagnosis of mental maturity with the remainder of the test. In general, the mental maturity test proper samples memory (immediate and delayed); maturity of apperceptive processes; spatial relationships; and logical and mathematical aspects of reasoning. Certain tests are presented in both verbal and non-language form in order to obtain a separate evaluation of each.... The authors of these tests believe that the multiple-factory [*sic*] theory of intelligence comes nearer to explaining observable phenomena than does the strong central-factor theory alone... [and] believe that progress in determining the nature of mentality and the value of tests of mental maturity is dependent largely upon further studies in factor analysis which employ analytical and statistical techniques. [Manual]

The battery consists of 16 tests and takes a total of 1½ hours to administer. (Generally, it would have been administered in a series of class sessions on different days.) The first 3 tests, presumably measuring visual acuity, auditory acuity, and motor coordination, are not to be counted in the total scores, but their results are to be examined by the teacher for insight into whether the remainder of the test is to be regarded as valid for the individual pupil. The 13 remaining tests are generally quite short but exhibit considerable ingenuity in their construction. Only some of them utilize a multiple-choice format. The scoring is to be done by hand, using a series of answer keys. (Later editions of the battery were converted to machine-scoring formats.) In general, the subtests represent extensions of Stanford–Binet tasks to a group testing situation. For example, Test 4, of "immediate memory," represents an ingenious procedure for testing digit memory span in a classroom test. Test 5 involves delayed recall of paragraph meaning: A story is read near the beginning of the test, and memory for its contents is tested at the end of the test. Three tests of "spatial relationships" require the student to "sense right and left" (determining whether pictured hands and similar items are "right" or "left"), to detect whether pairs of geometric figures are rotated or "flipped over," or to find the shortest path through a maze (thus exhibiting "foresight in spatial situations"). Various "reasoning" items are presented mainly in pictured form; for example, in a test of "opposites," the student has to find the "opposite" of a picture of a cake (it turns out to be a picture of a lemon, because while a cake is sweet, a lemon is sour). Even analogies are presented in pictorial form: a *speedometer* is to a *car* as a *thermometer* is to a (*rose, sun, turnip, airplane*), where all the italicized words are pictured. Other reasoning items include number series and various types of numerical problems (e.g., how to make up $5.51 with exactly 15 coins). The last 3 tests are tests deliberately using verbal presentation, arithmetic problems, syllogistic inferences, and vocabulary.

The test manual gives a variety of data on the statistical characteristics of the results, chiefly split-half reliabilities and tables of norms. The authors do not seem to be aware that the split-half reliabilities given for each grade, all quite high in magnitude, are probably inflated because of the speededness of the tests. (They insist, however, that "this is a power rather than a speed test" [manual]). Intercorrelations among the tests are not reported, although their inclusion would have enabled the user to assess the extent to which the separate tests measure distinct abilities.

The manual presents much advice to teachers on interpreting results. For example,

A student who reveals high ability in Tests 9–13 inclusive, and who rates low in Tests 14–15, may lack reading ability.... Where disability is not due to some remediable cause, a student who cannot detect differences and similarities or sense relationships is simply missing important elements of his environment; if in addition he fails to sense quantitative relationships and fails in manipulating both quantitative and non-mathematical ideas, he is destined to live on a low plane intellectually. Such students tend to remain in a simple concrete world; they do not generalize easily, must often be given their principles and generalizations as facts, and must depend upon memory rather than ability to deal with ideas. Notwithstanding these disabilities, some students do well in situations involving common sense (because of experience) while more brilliant inexperienced students will fail. Students who do poorly on these tests cannot go far beyond limits set in general by their mental ages. While this is true of the types of activities which constitute the ordinary school program, many students who do poorly on these tests nevertheless have talent in music, art, or some other special field. It is well to follow this general test with tests of specific aptitude.

Maturity of the apperceptive processes with reference to ideas and growth of meaning is revealed by Test 16 [of vocabulary]. The verbal factor is recognized as an important and more or less independent element of mental maturity. Meaning is added gradually and skill in using verbal symbols is primarily a matter of training.... A high rating in this test is evidence of the capacity to profit by experience, resulting in a high degree of development of the verbal factor. However, a low or even an average rating is not a definite proof of native limitation of the verbal factor; favoring circumstances and specific training in language may have been lacking.

After the total test scores have been recorded and the relative rating in language and non-language factors obtained, the teacher will have revealed to her whether or not the student will probably learn best through language or non-language activities. [Sullivan, Clark, & Tiegs, 1936–1939, manual]

The important influence of Binet, Terman, and others on the development of this test is evident. In fact, its chief author, Elizabeth Sullivan, had worked with Terman and published her research on applications of the Stanford–Binet scale (Sullivan, 1926). The test already shows, however, evidence of the then new indications that mental ability was to be described not in terms of a single "general factor" but also, or instead, in terms of a series of differentiated traits. Just how much of the technology of mental testing is incorporated into the test is unclear; there is no indication in the manual about the use of item analysis or other test-refinement procedures.

Nevertheless, one commentator (Raymond B. Cattell) in Buros's (1941) compilation was able to say:

These tests are exceedingly well designed from the point of view of adaptation to school needs and the convenience of the teacher. All the data regarding consistencies, standardization, correlation with school progress, etc., that one could reasonably demand, are clearly presented in the handbook of instructions.... An admirable feature of this test is the courageous manner in which the authors come out into the open regarding the purpose, principles, and theory of test design. [P. 208]

A little later, he comments:

They offer a profile which "analyzes and summarizes the various factors which are measured by the test situations," and claim that this "reduces the mystery which has surrounded the meaning of mental age and intelligence quotient." This attempt to produce for special consumption a "psychology without mystery" ends by appearing to the psychologist to be "mystery without psychology." No proof is offered that these subtests do, in fact, test independent factors or that one is justified in generalizing from them to performances in everyday life which happen to have the same verbal label. [P. 208]

Another commentator (F. Kuhlmann) is more critical:

We do not believe there is much merit in labeling tests as regards functions measured, as the authors have done; first, because it cannot be done correctly by inspection; and second, because these labels are not of much value until we know also how these functions enter into school achievement in different school subjects. Also, when a battery is divided into several different measures the tests assigned to measure any particular function tend to become inadequate in number and range to do so reliably. It would be hazardous, indeed, to conclude from the score on two brief tests that a child has a poor memory, for example. It seems to be implied also that the child mind is simply the adult mind in miniature, so that all tests should measure the same function at all ages. . . . The authors' distinction between language factor and nonlanguage factor tests is also somewhat misleading. Language enters both, the real distinction being that in the former the child has to read test material, while in the latter he is told what to do with picture material and, with a few exceptions, no reading is involved. [Buros, 1941, p. 209]

What Kuhlmann is complaining about is a problem that has persisted up to the present day: Though total scores on mental ability tests can be shown to be rather highly correlated with total progress in school, it is very difficult to prove detailed relationships between separate kinds of mental ability and particular activities in school learning. He also points to a difficulty that has cropped up in all "multifactor" batteries of mental ability: It is hard to obtain reliable measures of different kinds of mental ability within very short time limits.

One more widely used group intelligence test deserves to be examined, this one issued by the prestigious American Council on Education (ACE). A "psychological examination" constructed by L. L. Thurstone and Thelma Gwinn Thurstone was issued annually by ACE from 1924 to 1954; for present purposes we select the one published for 1935, the 12th edition of the test. According to Thurstone and Thurstone (1936), it was ordered by 493 institutions, testing a total of 189,506 students. The article by the Thurstones reports data on the distributions of scores for 58,402 students from 266 colleges, but, in a change from former years, "in order to discourage the use of test results as the basis for comparative ranking of institutions, this year the names of the colleges have been deleted" (p. 296).

The test was issued in both hand-scored and machine-scored editions; although the test contents of these editions were slightly different, the authors claim that scores on them had been shown to be equivalent. The hand-scored edition, at any rate, had five parts:

1.   *Completion* (40 items, 10 min). The examinee has to write answers to items such as "Burnt sugar, used for coloring and flavoring, is called (7 letters)." [Answer: caramel]
2.   *Arithmetic* (20 items, 20 min). The examinee has to supply the answers to arithmetic reasoning problems such as "A freight train travelling at the rate of 15 miles per hour requires 80 minutes between two stations. What time does an express train going 48 miles per hour require for the trip: ——hrs. ——min. ——sec."
3.   *Artificial Language* (30 items, 13 min). After vocabulary, grammar rules, and examples for an artificial language are given, the examinee has to evaluate the correctness of translations of sentences like "Slupup girdigro paresba."

4.   *Analogies* (29 items, 10 min). In each item, the examinee has to detect a relationship
            exemplified in two geometric figures and find which of several other figures
            exemplifies this same relationship to a third figure.
5.   *Opposites* (33 items, 7 min). Each item presents four words; the examinee has to
            find which two are either the same or opposite in meaning; for example, in the
            group (many, ill, few, down) *many* and *few* are opposite in meaning. Many of the
            words used in the test are relatively infrequent and unfamiliar.

No data are presented on the reliability of this instrument or on the manner in
which it was constructed. Buros's (1941) compilation contains, however, a long
series of citations of research articles by several authors reporting on correlations
between the various annual editions of this test and scholastic success in college.
It would appear that many of these correlations were sufficiently high to justify
continued use of the examinations for placement and other purposes in colleges.
Only in a later article by the Thurstones do we find validity coefficients reported.
For data collected in 1933 and 1934, correlations of the ACE Psychological Examination Score with average scores in introductory courses in various subjects were
about .50. Furthermore, the Thurstones had started to recommend the computation of separate L ("linguistic") and Q ("quantitative") scores. The L score was to
be computed by adding scores on the completion, opposites, and artificial language subtests, whereas the Q score was to come from the arithmetic and analogies subtests. According to the Thurstones, "the two constellations are correlated
(.55) but do not represent primary factors. Both of these composites are complex
as to their primary factorial composition" (Thurstone, Thurstone, & Adkins, 1939,
p. 298).

Our examination of these three tests bears out the statement already made that
during the early developmental period, up to about 1935, the science of mental
testing progressed from its crudest beginnings to a stage of high development.
The procedures developed by Binet for gauging mental growth by individually
administered tests had been adapted for use in group intelligence tests. Theories
of intelligence had been formulated, and technologies for constructing, standardizing, and validating mental tests had been developed, utilizing advances in statistical methods that occurred during this period. There was widespread acceptance
of the notion that mental ability as measured by intelligence tests played an
important role in students' school success. By 1935 there were the beginnings of
interest in the differentiation of mental abilities, but there were as yet few indications of the role of such differential mental abilities in school performances.

PRACTICES IN THE USE OF TESTS

As we have seen, by 1935 intelligence tests of various sorts had been widely
applied in a variety of settings. These uses were reviewed in a number of textbooks designed for psychologists, teachers, and other practitioners. One example
is a work by Pintner (1931), a professor of education at Teachers College, Columbia University, and an author of intelligence tests. Pintner points out that the
development of psychological tests was in the beginning "closely bound up with
the study of mental deficiency and abnormality" and shortly afterward with the
study of juvenile delinquency and of the dependent child. "The next striking
phenomenon," he says, "was the appearance of the very bright or superior
child.... It is doubtful whether the very decided superiority of some children was

really appreciated before the advent of the psychological examination." With the coming of the group test method,

it became possible to test large numbers of school children. This brought in the period of school surveys on a large scale with their direct and important influence for the purpose of instruction. At the same time the group method was extended to other groups of individuals, soldiers in the army, prisoners, college students, and the like.... We note also the extension of the use of tests to special groups of individuals... the blind and the deaf. [P. 226]

Later he continues:

During all this development the use of intelligence tests in the study of racial differences has been going on. The most thoroughgoing studies have been made on the negro in America.... The possibilities in this line of work are very great, although there are certain inherent difficulties that have not yet been fully overcome.... The field of industry and commerce is one of the latest fields in which intelligence tests have been adopted. [P. 227]

Devoting separate chapters to uses of tests in different situations, Pintner notes that, in the elementary school,

the chief practical uses of tests up to the present time have centered around their value for the purpose of classifying children into more or less homogeneous intelligence groups, and also for predicting their future success in school work. These two purposes are intimately bound up with each other. Classification in homogeneous groups is justifiable because intelligence correlates highly with school success, and therefore, the more homogeneous the group the more likely are the children in the group to advance together at about the same rate, be that rate relatively fast, normal, or slow. [P. 239]

McClure (1930) had in fact found, through a questionnaire sent to a number of large city school systems, that the most important use of psychological tests was for sectioning classes into homogeneous groups. Nevertheless, evidence that homogeneous grouping of children with respect to intelligence actually made for more effective educational programs was very scarce. Most of the reports, according to a review by Rankin (1931), were negative. The failure of homogeneous grouping, Rankin thought, might be attributed to the probability that this practice was not ordinarily accompanied by appropriate modifications of curriculum materials and instructional practices for different classifications of learners. Keliher (1931) had attacked the whole practice of homogeneous grouping on the ground that it did not square with an educational theory that conceives education as growth and takes the whole child into account. Further, Keliher pointed out, as did many others, that children are so specific in their abilities that it is difficult if not impossible to achieve true homogeneity of grouping. Despite all this, it appears that homogeneous grouping was widely practiced by 1930. (In a later section of this chapter, we shall see that the practice continued for many years.) Pintner (1931) confirms this in his summary statement:

It is evident from the survey in this chapter of the use of intelligence tests with school children that such tests are at present being used very widely and for many different purposes. They have not come to be considered an integral part of every school system, but the time is not far distant when they will be considered as essential for the health, happiness and advance of every child.

   At present tests are being used for the purpose of classifying children into more or less homogeneous groups.... Most reports of such classifications are favorable, and justice is being done to all types of children by this procedure.... A natural corollary to this movement of sectioning according to ability will be the gradual differentiation of the course of study in terms of capacities of the various groups of pupils. Little has been done in this respect, but the indications are that attempts in this direction will be made now that the individual differences have been so clearly demonstrated. [Pp. 268–269]

At the high-school level, Pintner was able, at the time he was writing, to point to the fact that selection for admission to the high school "was, and still is, partly on the basis of intelligence," even though the percentage of the population of high-school age children enrolled in school had increased from about 12 in 1910 to about 47 in 1926. He seemed to express concern in his statement that "as the proportion of children going to high school increases the average intelligence decreases" (p. 275). Mort and Featherstone (1932), in a review of the uses of psychological tests in schools, note that use of such tests for admission to high school "doubtless underlies much of the investigation that has been carried on" concerning the predictive value of intelligence-test scores for success in high school, but they remark that, as compared to the question of admission requirements for colleges, "there is less significance in the question of initial estimate before admission [to high school], for it is coming to be generally conceded that the high school should be available for all who choose to come. Therefore, at the high-school level, psychological tests are of value, for the most part, in guidance after admission" (p. 302). Pintner (1931) was nevertheless able to point to many studies showing substantial correlations between intelligence-test scores and high-school success, both in particular courses and as reflected in overall averages. He also noted that the average intelligence-test scores of students in different types of curricula varied, students in "classical" or "academic" courses having higher average scores than those in "general," "vocational," or "commercial" curricula. "The general picture resulting from these various studies is that of a decrease in intelligence as the course becomes less abstract or more practical in nature" (p. 284).

At the college level, the use of intelligence tests for admissions purposes appears to have begun shortly after World War I. Pintner states, "During the war, and for several years thereafter, Army Alpha was used widely in colleges and universities" (p. 295). He cites a 1923 report by Wood, who stated:

In 1919 the Office of Admissions at Columbia University inaugurated an experiment for the purpose of discovering the value of the Thorndike College Entrance Intelligence Examination for High School Graduates as a criterion for admission to Columbia College. From an attitude of healthy if not severe skepticism toward the use of intelligence tests for this purpose, the whole college administration came, within the space of two years, to consider the intelligence tests as an indispensable part, not only of the admission machinery, but also of the administration of the college in the Dean's Office. [Quoted in Pintner, 1931, p. 295]

Presumably, the favorable attitudes toward intelligence as a selection criterion resulted from findings concerning the correlations between mental ability scores and scholarship records. Wood reported, for example, a correlation of .67 for 111 students who remained in college for two years. (This correlation is, it should be noted, somewhat higher than those usually obtained for students already selected partly on the basis of scholastic aptitude tests; it appears that Wood's group was largely an *unselected* group.) Summarizing coefficients of correlation found between intelligence scores and college academic records, Toops (1926) reported a median coefficient of .46 based on reports from 43 colleges; Pintner reported later data with a similar magnitude of coefficients. It will be recalled that Thurstone, Thurstone, and Adkins (1939) reported even higher coefficients. In any case, from 1919 to 1935 there was increasing use of intelligence or scholastic aptitude tests in connection with college admission, based on the finding that there were very substantial relationships between scores on these tests and performance in various types of academic college courses. Because records of scholastic aptitude scores were for the most part maintained only in college admissions offices, it is probable that there was little "contamination of the criterion" involved in these findings; that is, it is improbable that professors giving academic grades were informed of the aptitude-test scores, and thus the correlations are not spuriously biased toward the high side.

Apparently intelligence-test scores were rarely used in colleges and universities for purposes other than admissions. There are few reports of their further use in sectioning, failing, or counseling students. Nevertheless, some interesting correlates of intelligence were found: Younger students were found to have higher intelligence-test scores (a finding that can also be observed in elementary and secondary schools, particularly when students are promoted partly on the basis of performance); also, the more intelligent students reported spending somewhat less time in study (A. Crawford, 1929).

Throughout the school system, from elementary school to the university, the use of intelligence tests seems to have been predicated on the assumption that their scores reflected mainly innate or at least relatively unalterable characteristics of students having to do with their capacity to do school work. Although it was noted that average scores were correlated with demographic variables such as socioeconomic class, race, urban–rural environment, and so on, there does not seem to have been any serious consideration whether children's home backgrounds, or even their schooling, would have had any important influence on their performances in mental tests. E. L. Thorndike et al. (1927) had, to be sure, recognized the difficulty of distinguishing between types of tests that measure mental "maturity" and those that measure the effects of training. But the question whether test scores were "biased" by cultural factors, for example, was hardly ever raised during the developmental period of the mental testing movement. The general attitude among educators and the public toward intelligence tests during this period seems to be well reflected in the following quotation from Pintner's (1931) text:

Intelligence tests have done much to show that all children are not created free and equal with respect to their mental abilities. A child's abilities are determined by his ancestors, and all that environment can do is to give opportunities for the development of his potentialities. It cannot create new powers or additional abilities. This, then, is the main function of education, to measure the inherited capacities of the child and to so arrange the environment as to give full opportunities for all these capacities to develop to the uttermost. [Pp. 520–521]

An overall appraisal of the developmental period of the mental testing movement would have to observe that although major technological advances had occurred to produce a new type of social instrument that in the climate of the times received wide acceptance, the exact nature of this instrument, and its true significance, was largely unexplored. It is evident that by 1935 educators and psychologists were rather well satisfied with what had been created, but at the same time they were highly optimistic about the possibilities of its future development.

2.2.   THE MODERN PERIOD

OVERVIEW

"The pioneering stage in psychometrics may be considered to have ended in the 1930s," says Philip DuBois (1970, p. 112) in his history of psychological testing. Or, as Walter Monroe (1945) put it, it was in this period that measurement moved from "adolescence to maturity." The beginning of the modern period, as we are calling it, may with some justification be placed in the year 1935, the date of the founding of the Psychometric Society by a group of scholars who had been called together by Louis Leon Thurstone and some of his colleagues at the University of Chicago (for details, see Dunlap, 1942). It was Thurstone and the leaders of the Psychometric Society, notably Paul Horst, who were primarily responsible for the origination and dissemination of theoretical and technological developments that had a major impact on mental testing during this period.

We have seen that, by 1935, group mental testing had become widely adopted throughout all levels of education. By this time, also, it was beginning to be utilized in business and industry. (It had, of course, been used extensively in the military during World War I, but by 1935 mental testing in the military had become dormant.) Mental ability testing had become an established subject matter for research and teaching in nearly all the major universities, both in departments of psychology and in departments of education. Among the university centers of research in mental ability testing that were particularly prominent at the time were those at Columbia (especially at Teachers College), Stanford, Harvard, Minnesota, Ohio State, Iowa, California, and Chicago. (Centers of research in England and Scotland were also still very active.) Thousands, or more like millions, of intelligence tests were administered every year in elementary and secondary schools, often with a kind of blind faith in the scores. Increasingly, colleges and universities were using mental ability test results in their admissions and placement processes, although it was not until 1937 that the CEEB established scholastic aptitude tests as a regular part of its admissions testing program.

Most of the mental testing that was being done in 1935 was based on the view that "intelligence" was a more or less unitary trait. Most tests of intelligence yielded a single score for an individual – expressed usually as an "intelligence quotient" or some derivative of the intelligence quotient. The common view – even at most of the university research centers just named – was that intelligence-test scores reflected some largely innate capacity of the individual to think in abstract terms, to learn in school, and to adapt to the requirements of an increasingly complex technological society. Intelligence tests were valued as scientific measurements to the extent that they showed high degrees of reliability and validity as indicated by the techniques developed by Spearman, Kelley, and other early scholars in mental testing.

Presaged in the later years of the testing movement's early period, but taking full form only in the 1940s and 1950s, two striking technological developments were initiated around 1935, chiefly by Thurstone and his colleagues at the University of Chicago: (a) multiple-factor analysis, a mathematical technique whereby it was clearly shown that "intelligence" is not a simple unitary trait; and (b) the refinement of the statistical theory of mental tests, leading to new ways of constructing mental tests and studying their measurement characteristics. Both of these developments had a substantial impact upon the development and construction of mental tests during the modern period.

The history of testing throughout the modern period can be traced through the publications of a remarkable husband-and-wife team based at Rutgers University in New Jersey. It was shortly before 1935 that Oscar K. Buros, then an assistant professor who had been trained at Teachers College, became disturbed with the laxity of the standards by which mental tests were being published and distributed. He decided to initiate a series of publications that would constitute a kind of "consumer's report" on mental and educational tests. The first two of these compilations were published by the School of Education at Rutgers, but by 1941 Buros and his wife Luella were able to establish their own independent nonprofit publishing house (which they later called the Gryphon Press). Increasingly weighty tomes were issued in 1941, 1949, 1953, 1959, 1965, and 1972, with reviews of literally thousands of mental and educational tests; the *Eighth Mental Measurements Yearbook* appeared shortly after Buros's death in March of 1978.

The objectives of the Buros series, as described in the introduction to the *Seventh Yearbook* (Buros, 1972), were

(a) to provide information about tests published as separates throughout the English-speaking world; (b) to present frankly critical reviews written by testing and subject specialists representing various viewpoints; (c) to provide extensive bibliographies of verified references on the construction, use, and validity of specific tests; (d) to make readily available the critical portions of test reviews appearing in professional journals; and (e) to present fairly exhaustive listings of new and revised books on testing, along with evaluative excerpts from representative reviews which these books receive in professional journals.

But the Buroses attached much importance to other objectives of a "crusading nature":

(f) to impel test authors and publishers to publish better tests and to provide test users with detailed information on the validity and limitations of their tests; (g) to inculcate test users with a keener awareness of the values and limitations of standardized tests; (h) to stimulate contributing reviewers to think through more carefully their own beliefs and values relevant to testing; (i) to suggest to test users better methods of appraising tests in light of their own particular needs; and (j) to impress test users with the need to suspect all tests unaccompanied by detailed data on their construction, validity, uses, and limitations – even when products of distinguished authors and reputable publishers.

Nevertheless, they concluded:

Our success in attaining the last five missionary objectives has been disappointingly modest. Test publishers continue to market tests which do not begin to meet the standards of the rank and file of MMY and journal reviewers. At least half of the tests currently on the market should never have been published. Exaggerated, false, or unsubstantial claims are the rule rather than the exception. Test users are becoming more discriminating, but not nearly fast enough. [Pp. xxvii–xxviii]

These quotations suggest that although the modern period saw the introduction of many innovations and refinements in the theory and practice of mental testing, these innovations and refinements were not utilized and applied as widely and as uniformly as they might have been. In fact, many tests published and circulated during the modern period did not even meet the criteria of excellence that had been established by 1935. The Buroses may be given credit for helping the field to police its own activities, but even the efforts of special committees of professional organizations such as the American Psychological Association (APA) and the American Educational Research Association (AERA) in publishing quasi-official technical standards for tests (APA, 1954, 1966, 1974) were not sufficient to ensure that all test-development activities conformed to these standards. Still less did the run-of-the-mill intelligence tests of the time take advantage of the technological refinements introduced during the period.

We can, however, discern the influence of Thurstone and other leaders in psychometrics in many published tests and in a variety of research and testing programs that appeared or occurred during the modern period. The prototype of the many "multifactor batteries" developed during the period was the Thurstones' own Primary Mental Abilities (PMA) battery, an experimental edition of which was published as early as 1938 (Thurstone, 1938b). This battery was based on the findings of Thurstone's (1938a) first major study of mental tests employing the multiple-factor analysis method, a study in which at least seven somewhat independent "factors" of mental ability had been identified. The PMA battery offered tests of seven factors, designated by capital letters and described as follows: P, perceptual ability; N, numerical ability; V, verbal ability; S, spatial-visualizing ability: M, memory; I, induction or generalizing ability; and D, deductive or reasoning ability. More formal versions of the PMA battery were published subsequently (Thurstone & Thurstone, 1946–1965), for several age levels, but it may be remarked that these tests were never subjected to as much careful refinement, standardization, and validation as they might have been. Reviewers of these tests in the Buros *Yearbooks,* at least, expressed considerable dissatisfaction with their measurement characteristics. The importance of the PMA battery was that it first brought into general awareness the concept of differentiable mental ability factors.

Mental testing took new strides in the personnel programs of World War II. As had been the case in World War I, many well-known psychologists contributed their talents and energies to the speedy development and validation of tests suitable for use in the selection and training of millions of armed forces personnel for their varied tasks. At the foundation of the testing programs of the several armed forces components were one or more "general classification" tests that resembled the group intelligence tests of earlier periods. For example, there were developed, for the army, the Army General Classification Test (AGCT) and the Officer Qualifying Test (OQT), and for the army air force, an Army Air Force Qualifying Test. These tests were fashioned along familiar lines, and generally yielded single scores, although in its later versions the AGCT had separate scores for reading and vocabulary, arithmetic computations, arithmetic reasoning, and spatial relations. Some of the armed services developed and validated tests to measure special aptitudes. Especially in the army air force, under the direction of Flanagan (1948), Thurstone's ideas about primary mental abilities, and his methods of factor analysis, were utilized to develop batteries of special tests for the selection of pilots, navigators, bombardiers, and other classes of personnel. Many of these tests were "printed classification tests" (Guilford, 1947); others were tests involving various kinds of apparatus, motion picture films, and the like to measure perceptual and psychomotor skills. In this and other testing programs much was learned about improved and more efficient techniques of constructing tests, analyzing results, and using those results in personnel decisions (R. Thorndike, 1949). R. L. Thorndike and Hagen (1959) followed up the subsequent careers of over 10,000 men who had taken air force tests during the war, finding that although a factor of general ability differentiated the average scores of people going into different occupations, the predictive value of test profiles for success in those occupations was not impressive.

After the war, J. P. Guilford, who had been in charge of much of the factor-analytic investigation done in the army air forces, built upon this work to conduct, with the support of the Office of Naval Research, a 20-year "high level aptitudes" project to study the full range of mental abilities that might be measured (Guilford & Hoepfner, 1971). In the course of this work he conceived a new model of the structure of mental abilities, which he called the structure of intellect (SI) (Guilford, 1956, 1967). He and one of his students also published a multifactor battery called the Guilford–Zimmerman Aptitude Survey (Guilford & Zimmerman, 1947–1956).

Another important testing and research program that stemmed from work done during the war was Project Talent (Flanagan, Dailey, Shaycoft, Gorham, Orr, & Goldberg, 1962). Inspired by the promising results of factor-analytic investigations he had supervised in his wartime work, Flanagan (1951–1960) had constructed a multifactor test battery called the Flanagan Aptitude Classification Tests (FACT). This battery was offered for general use through a commercial publisher, but Flanagan also felt that a parallel battery should be constructed and placed in the public domain so that long-range studies of the identification and utilization of human abilities could be conducted. He initiated the first major steps for the undertaking in what he called Project Talent. Some 23 aptitude and achievement tests, as well as several questionnaires and interest inventories, were administered to about 140,000 high-school students around the country in March 1960. There have already been several long-term follow-ups of the students in this sample, disclosing important new information about the growth of mental abilities and the way in which they interact with students' educational and occupational choices (Flanagan & Cooley, 1966; Flanagan & Jung, 1971; Jencks, Smith, Acland, Bane, Cohen, Gintis, Heyns, & Michelson, 1972).

Multiple-factor analysis theory was also brought to bear in the construction by the United States Employment Service (USES) of an extensive series of tests to measure a number of special mental and other abilities thought to be important in different occupations (Dvorak, 1947). The USES published reports about the validity of these tests for predicting success in numerous occupations.

Commercial publishers were alert to the possibilities of developing multifactor batteries for wide use in secondary schools. One of the most highly regarded of such batteries is the so-called DAT, Differential Aptitude Tests, published by the Psychological Corporation (Bennett, Seashore, & Wesman, 1947–1975). This battery offers separate scores on verbal reasoning, numerical ability, abstract reasoning, space relations, mechanical reasoning, clerical speed and accuracy, and language usage (with separate scores on spelling and "correct" English usage).

Little attempt was made to make the subtests "pure" measures of primary mental abilities; the goal was to develop tests that would have the greatest practical use in educational and vocational counseling in high schools. Some of the tests emphasize generalized mental abilities; others stress mastery of skills and knowledges taught in schools. Much labor was expended in item analysis, standardization, and validation of the tests; voluminous data are presented in accompanying manuals concerning correlations of test scores with success in various subjects, with college grades, and with educational and vocational placement after graduation from high school. The "differential" aspect of this battery implies that differences among scores on the several subtests are intended to be useful in counseling; the publishers have provided a casebook that illustrates how counselors can employ profiles of test scores. (Later in this section, the DAT is examined in more detail.)

Many other multifactor batteries were published during the period, and continuing interest in and demand for them is suggested by the fact that several entirely new batteries of this type have recently come to my attention, for example, the International Primary Factors Battery (W. Horn, 1973) and the Comprehensive Abilities Battery (Hakstian & Cattell, 1976), based on the continuing research (reviewed by J. Horn, 1976) that has been done in the identification of factors of mental ability.

In the meantime, there was movement toward the much greater use of mental ability tests in the college admissions process, and there was more extensive research into the refinement of such tests. I have already given brief mention, in the overview of the early period of the test movement, to the work of Carl C. Brigham in the experimental development of a so-called scholastic aptitude examination. It is appropriate at this point to describe Brigham's work in more detail, because its effects were felt mainly in the modern period of mental testing. Brigham's early experiences, as described in an interesting biographical memoir by Downey (1961), included writing a doctoral dissertation on the Binet intelligence tests and service under Yerkes in the development of the army psychological examinations in World War I. At Princeton in the 1920s, Brigham developed a test that was used as early as 1925 in connection with admission to the university. Shortly thereafter, the CEEB turned to him to construct a similar examination for experimental use in a small number of "Ivy League" colleges. One of Brigham's innovations at that time was the use of "experimental sections" in the tests of successive years to explore the usefulness of new items and item types and to serve as a basis for making successive forms relatively equivalent in their derived scales. The intensive study that Brigham devoted to each new item of his tests involved tabulations of answers to each alternative of every multiple-choice item and the use of a mechanical apparatus for timing students' responses to items. Brigham was evidently the first to develop systematic item-analysis procedures using large samples. He was also the first to emphasize the importance of "test security" (accounting for the return of all examination materials) in the administration of admissions tests.

Brigham carefully avoided calling his test an "intelligence test." Although he had earlier believed that tests like the Army Alpha measured intelligence and that the low average scores of certain immigrant populations indicated poor prospects for their success in America, he retracted these views in a famous article published in 1930. Downey (1961) gives this quotation from one of Brigham's private memoranda:

The testing movement came to this country some twenty-five years ago accompanied by one of the most serious fallacies in the history of science, namely, that the tests measured *native intelligence* purely and simply without regard to training or schooling. I hope nobody believes that now. The test scores very definitely are a composite including schooling, family background, familiarity with English, and everything else, relevant and irrelevant. The *"native intelligence"* hypothesis is dead. [P. 27]

Brigham also recognized the important difference between verbal and mathematical aptitudes (as revealed in the relatively low intercorrelations between tests of these aptitudes). The Scholastic Aptitude Examinations (SAT), first adopted by the CEEB as a regular part of its admissions examination program in 1937, have to this day included separate verbal and mathematical sections, each yielding a score on a scale that Brigham himself introduced – a scale with a mean of 500 and a standard deviation of 100 and with a range of 200–800, in a defined population of college admissions candidates.

Under Brigham's direction, the CEEB built a staff in Princeton, near the university, to construct the successive editions of the SAT (and later other objective-type CEEB examinations). This staff carried on after Brigham's death in 1943, continuing to meet his high standards of test construction. For various reasons that need not be gone into here, this staff was merged in 1947 into a new organization, the Educational Testing Service (ETS), that had been proposed by James B. Conant, then president of Harvard University. This organization undertook the further development and administration of the CEEB examinations, including the SAT, as well as the construction and administration of many other testing programs, many of which have involved tests of general intellectual development (e.g., the aptitude tests of the Graduate Record Examination and the National Teacher Examination). The ETS also became a major center of research on the theory of mental tests, with the addition of persons such as Harold Gulliksen, Ledyard Tucker, Frederic Lord, and William Angoff to its staff. Gulliksen and Tucker, it may be noted, had been close associates of Thurstone's at Chicago. Through the research of these specialists in mental test theory, the measurement characteristics of tests produced by ETS have been of particular excellence, although it cannot be said that *all* their research has yet been reflected in the actual development of tests.

Throughout the years of the modern period, the SAT gained wide acceptance not only among the Ivy League colleges that constituted the original membership of the CEEB, but also among numerous state universities, engineering schools, and public and private colleges in different parts of the country. Whereas, for purposes of studying candidates' qualifications, the early constituents of the CEEB were more interested in the results of essay achievement examinations in various subjects, these and other CEEB constituents increasingly found more usefulness in the SAT scores. (The essay examinations of the earlier days were for the most part abandoned after 1942.) SAT scores, many admissions officers concluded, were better indicators of the true promise of many capable students from unknown high schools who might not have been as well prepared (or coached) as their preparatory-school competitors. In this way, use of SAT scores in the college admissions process tended to even out the disparities in educational advantages between candidates from the wealthier, upper-class families and those from more plebeian backgrounds.

The SAT did not continue to be alone in its field. In 1959, E. F. Lindquist of the University of Iowa, having resigned from his associations with the CEEB (he had been a member of the board's Committee of Aptitude Examiners, which monitored the construction and administration of the SAT), established the American College Testing Program (ACT), which quickly grew to serve large numbers of colleges and universities, particularly in the Midwest and West. In contrast to the SAT, the ACT battery of examinations is much more heavily loaded with materials measuring generalized educational achievements in English usage, mathematics, social studies, and natural science. Above all, it seems to stress *reading* comprehension ability. According to a reviewer, "ACT suffers by comparison with the SAT in psychometric care and sophistication, is about equal in validity for predicting collegiate success, and excels somewhat in the variety and extent of ancillary services offered" (W. L. Wallace, in Buros, 1972, p. 615).

PSYCHOMETRICS AND THEORIES OF INTELLECTUAL ABILITIES

To provide a perspective from which we can view modern developments in psychometrics, it seems desirable at this point to examine the logical foundations of a viable theory of intellectual abilities. To do so, it is necessary, unfortunately, to couch the discussion in rather general and abstract terms. Also, brevity demands that many essential details be omitted and many terms be left inadequately defined.

Mental tests typically consist of collections of tasks that examinees can be asked to perform in some given (relatively short) period of time. These tasks, or at least some components of them, may be considered to be a sample of the almost infinite domain of tasks that an individual might be required to perform in some conceivable context in the course of real life, but the samples of tasks appearing in mental tests are constrained in at least two important ways.

First, from a practical point of view, only certain kinds of tasks can conveniently be included in a psychological test. They must be tasks that are small enough to be completed successfully by at least some examinees in a relatively short period of time, and normally they must not involve any complicated apparatus for stimulus presentation or for the examinee's performance of his response. This constraint may appear to make the tasks somewhat artificial; for example, it is not normal in real life for a person to be confronted with the task (one that often appears in mental tests) of identifying which of a group of words does not fall into the same semantic classification as the others. Nevertheless, it might be argued that such "artificial" tasks represent or contain elements of larger tasks that might be encountered in real life.

Second, the tasks in a mental test are selected in such a way that it is reasonable to suppose that (except for lucky guesses) successful performance of a task requires some one or more kinds of intellectual competence or potential and that any other kinds of competence that might be required are not critical, in the sense that all examinees may be assumed to possess these noncritical competences in a sufficient degree. (For example, it is normally assumed that all examinees taking a "paper-and-pencil" test can in fact hold a pencil and make certain required kinds of marks with it.) Initially, the selection of tasks for a mental test is a matter that is up to the judgment of the test constructor, but there are, as we shall see, empirical operations whereby the test constructor's judgments become less critical.

Given the characteristics of mental tests as we have described them, we now attempt to state the requirements of an adequate theory of such tests, that is, a theory of what such tests measure and how well they measure whatever that may be. An adequate theory, it would seem, ought to give a satisfactory account of at least the following:

1.   *The extent to which the tasks, singly or in groups, can or do yield reliable measures of the characteristic behaviors of individuals performing such tasks.* To the extent that the measures derived from the tasks are in fact reliable (and we will leave this term undefined for the moment), it may be inferred that individuals may be arranged or ordered on a scale or continuum reflecting different degrees of competence with respect to the class or classes of tasks represented by those for which their performance has been observed.

2.   *The extent to which successful performance on each task, or group of tasks, reflects some particular kind of cognitive competence or potential.* The theory must therefore offer a satisfactory classification of the various kinds of cognitive competences that might be observed. To each kind of competence it may be assumed that there corresponds a scale or continuum containing different degrees of competence.

3.   *The source or cause of the individual differences observed with respect to any scale of cognitive competence so identified.*

These three requirements of a theory of intellectual abilities constitute problems to be solved empirically. Psychometric theory is concerned primarily with the first two of these problems. What is conventionally termed "test theory" is addressed to the first problem, and what has come to be known as "factor analysis" is devoted to the second problem. The third of these problems can in principle be approached only by appeal to more general methodologies of investigation in the behavioral sciences, for example, by observational and experimental studies, and will not be dealt with here except in passing. Psychometric techniques, nevertheless, play a critical role in this third class of studies because they are essential in establishing reliable and distinguishable variables for use in such studies.

TEST THEORY IN THE MODERN PERIOD

As we have seen, the foundations of test theory were laid in the early period of the mental test movement, initially by Spearman, Brown, Thorndike, Kelley and others. Test theory in the early period, however, was concerned chiefly with the "reliability" of measurements that were *already quantified* (e.g., "number correct" scores on mental tests, and "intelligence quotients"); concern for exactly how this quantification took place was expressed only in the development of various "item-analysis" techniques that would ensure that all items or tasks involved in obtaining a given measurement would tend, on the average, to be consistent with one another and thus contribute effectively to the reliability of the measurement. Reliability was defined as the extent to which observed measurements reflected a "true" underlying score as opposed to "error." This approach has come to be known as "classical" test theory (Novick, 1966; Stanley, 1971).

In the modern period, there have been many elaborations of test-analysis techniques arising from classical test theory. Gulliksen's (1950) text, Lord and Novick's (1968) treatise, and Stanley's (1971) chapter summarize many of these. Kuder and Richardson's (1937) formulation of a class of procedures for estimating reliability from the "internal consistency" of the items or tasks composing a test and Cronbach's (1951) derivation of a so-called coefficient alpha, a generalization of some of the Kuder–Richardson results, led to determinations of reliability that were in some ways more accurate (because they took more data into account) and more convenient (because they could at the same time be based on the administration of a single test). Test theorists began to look more closely at the effects of different distributions of item difficulties on the measurement characteristics of total test scores. Over a considerable period, attention was devoted to the so-called attenuation paradox (Loevinger, 1954; Lord, 1955; Tucker, 1946), whereby it seemed that maximum reliability, but reduced validity for measurement of an underlying ability, was attained when the distribution of item difficulties was "peaked," that is, when all item difficulties were near 50% difficulty. The paradox was resolved when it was shown that it depended on misapplication of correlation coefficient formulas and that in many circumstances the distribution of item difficulties should not be peaked at all. (The issue has, in fact, led to a great many misunderstandings among test analysts, misunderstandings that prevail even now in some quarters.) A related issue that has been studied extensively is that of how item scores can be weighted to produce optimal measurement characteristics of total scores (Stanley & Wang, 1970). In general, special weighting schemes have little advantage over simple counts of items with unit weights.

A current concern of test theorists that is essentially an outgrowth of classical test theory is the development of what Lord (1971) has called "tailored testing," that is, a procedure for optimizing the efficiency of a mental test by the sequential administration of items. In early stages of such testing, a brief test composed of items of a wide range of difficulty is administered to make a rough determination of the examinee's level of ability; the subsequent items are selected in such a way as to "zero in" on the level of ability so established. The motivation for developing these procedures seems to have arisen from the possibility of administering tests by an interactive computer terminal; extensive efforts by the CEEB to adapt such procedures to group testing resulted in the finding that they resulted in very little significant improvement in the accuracy of measurement and were rather impractical besides. It is ironic that tailored testing is in a sense a modern adaptation of procedures that have long been used in connection with individual tests such as the Stanford–Binet.

Other modern developments from classical test theory have included consideration of the implications of unreliability for the measurement of change or test gains (Cronbach & Furby, 1970), the development of optimal methods for establishing equivalent scales on different tests of the same trait (Angoff, 1971b), and studies of various sources of unreliability such as sampling of items, and the effects of practice, fatigue, and chance guessing.

Contrasting with the "classical" approach to reliability is one that emphasizes problems of statistical estimation and that is derived from the work of R. A. Fisher (1925) in statistical inference. Seminal papers by Baker (1939) and Hoyt (1941) got this "ANOVA" (analysis-of-variance) approach off the ground; later developments by Stanley (1961) and others have made it possible to determine the relative effects of different sources of variation underlying ability as opposed to variation owing to "test form," task difficulty, and so on and their interactions. Stanley (1971) believes that this ANOVA or "components-of-variance" approach makes for much greater precision and flexibility in the estimation of reliability. A still further development of this approach, called "generalizability theory," is due mainly to Cronbach and his associates (Cronbach, Gleser, Nanda, & Rajaratnam, 1972; Cronbach, Rajaratnam, & Gleser, 1963); it provides procedures for estimating the reliability of a test according to degree to which the scores represent those that would be derived from a "universe" of measurements (items, raters, or the like).

A persistent theme in the development of mental tests is a concern with the way in which successful versus unsuccessful performance on a given item or task relates to an underlying "latent trait" continuum of ability. Binet (Binet & Simon, 1905) assumed that a one-to-one correspondence could be established between graded tasks and mental ages, but experience with Binet-type scales revealed that the correspondence was far from exact. What is needed, either in connection with Binet-type scales or in connection with the "point scales" associated with group mental ability tests that are scored in terms of number correct, is a model for the probability of an examinee's successfully passing an item or task as a function of (among other things) the characteristics of the task (principally, its "difficulty" and "discriminating power") and the examinee's position on an underlying continuum of ability. Such a function has been called the item-characteristic function (Lord & Novick, 1968). A satisfactory model of the item-characteristic function should enable one to establish units of measurement for the ability scale, demonstrate the extent to which two or more items measure this continuum to known degrees, and derive information on the examinee's placement on the ability scale from his or her performances on the set of items thus selected.

Progress in developing satisfactory models of this type has been relatively slow; for example, Ferguson's (1942) and Finney's (1944) contributions, in which they assumed that item success is related to the ability scale by a cumulative normal distribution function, represented only a slight advance over that of Thurstone (1925b) 17 years earlier. Modern developments are the work primarily of Lord (1952; cf. Lord & Novick, 1968), Birnbaum (1968), and Rasch (1960), but these developments are really only elaborations of the earlier models, taking more parameters into account or resorting to the use of somewhat more tractable mathematical expressions. Their models do, however, provide reasonably satisfactory solutions to some of the problems of test construction, except that they are limited to circumstances in which one can assume that every item measures the same ability (or composite of abilities).

Satisfactory models for determining whether two or more items measure the same ability (or composite of abilities) and for relating performances on such items to underlying scales of ability have been elusive and controversial. Loevinger (1947) took the tack of contrasting a model of a "perfectly homogeneous test" (in which all items measure an underlying scale perfectly) with that of a completely "heterogeneous" test (in which all items measure different abilities – each perfectly, however.) Her "perfectly homogeneous" test actually followed the model described earlier by Walker (1931), Guttman (1941), and Carroll (1945), in which, if an examinee passes an item of a given level of difficulty, he or she passes all items of lower levels of difficulty, and, conversely, if an examinee fails an item of a given level of difficulty, he or she also fails all items of greater difficulty, difficulty being defined by the proportion of examinees failing an item. Loevinger's contribution was to suggest a measure of the extent to which a test approximates perfect homogeneity, in her sense of the term. There are, however, a number of still unresolved difficulties in Loevinger's approach, because it does not take systematic account of sources of unreliability; consequently, most tests show relatively low degrees of homogeneity – probably spuriously low.

It would seem that the question whether sets of items can be regarded as measuring the same abilities could be answered by techniques of correlational or factor analysis, but these techniques present difficulties stemming from the inappropriateness of the usual methods of computing correlations (Carroll, 1961). Some of these difficulties are overcome by methods proposed by Wherry and Winer (1953) and Loevinger, Gleser, and DuBois (1953), among others. Few improvements have been made in these methods, however, and they have not been widely applied in test construction. In this connection, it should be noted that Wherry and Gaylord (1943) were the first to point out that the interpretation of reliability coefficients determined by Kuder–Richardson, or similar methods, required the (often false) assumption that all the items measure a single ability (or composite of abilities). This fact has often been ignored; Lord and Novick (1968, p. 95) dodge the issue by observing that there is no general agreement about the meaning of homogeneity. They nevertheless offer reasons for concluding that a perfectly homogeneous test is one in which Cronbach's coefficient alpha is equal to the theoretical reliability of the test; the problem here is that there is no way of confidently determining the theoretical reliability of the test.

In the state of current knowledge, there is no satisfactory way of guaranteeing the construction of tests that are completely "homogeneous" in the sense that all items measure the same ability despite the presence of unreliability of measurement.

Several recent discussions have expressed considerable dissatisfaction with the present status of mental test theory. Lumsden (1976), for example, has this to say:

Test theory has had few major ideas. I can list only five.
1.   the decomposition of obtained scores into true and error components;
2.   the duality of psychophysics and psychometrics;
3.   the notion of unidimensionality;
4.   the conception of test validity as theoretical equivalence, usually called construct validity;
5.   the scaling ideas derived from various item characteristic curve models.
Apart from the first, these ideas have been hesitatingly and unconfidently applied. [P. 251]

Lumsden gives less credence to Bock and Wood's (1971) suggestion that test theorists are discouraged by the uncritical use of tests than to his own belief that "the shreds of theory that have been developed and the timeworn true score models are not rich sources of ideas about testing, and the ideas that are generated seem to relate mainly to the internal workings of the models" (p. 251). Likewise, Levy (1973) comments that "the holy cows of item analysis, standardization and indices of reliability appear to receive more attention from test constructors than elucidation of meaning" and urges that we need "tests constructed to test hypotheses, and fewer hypotheses about tests" (p. 36). Despite their acid criticisms, both of these writers strike a somewhat optimistic note by giving examples of promising test-development activities, or prescriptions for them, like Lumsden's (1976):

The new test theorists ... will be primarily test constructors and validity people who attempt to realize their dreams. ... They will not test a new model with a few items from the SAT files (or from a computer), find a mediocre fit to some dubiously relevant criterion, and then go on to the next. Rather, they will set out the requirements for the application of the model against a user-for-blood standard of efficiency. [P. 277]

Although mental test theory has made considerable progress toward establishing a satisfactory theory of mental test *scores,* it appears that it has made little progress toward a theory of the abilities that those scores presumably measure. Let us now consider whether any progress toward such a theory has been made by a different and by now quite separate branch of psychometrics, factor analysis.

FACTOR ANALYSIS IN THE MODERN PERIOD

Introducing his review of "factor analysis to 1940," Dael Wolfle (1940) remarked:

A single correlation coefficient is relatively easy to interpret. If the correlation is high, it may be assumed that there is considerable overlap between the determiners of the goodness of performance; if the correlation is low, it may be assumed that there is little overlap between the two sets of determiners. But if one is faced with a large table of correlations, the task of explaining all the complex interrelations is almost hopeless. Factor analysis provides one method of summarizing these relations, thereby making it easier for the psychologist to interpret and explain them. [P. 1]

Wolfle went on to state two important goals of all factor analysis investigations: simplification – explaining the correlations by means of a small set of values that can be regarded as having generated the correlations, and the association of these values with a small set of "factors" that will be "more fundamental in nature than the original tests" (p. 1).

Considerable progress in factor analysis had been made in the early period; the main achievement had been Spearman's elaboration of a theory claiming that correlations among mental tests could be explained chiefly by one common or "general" factor and that any residuals were to be attributed to the influence of "specific" factors. It proved impossible to support this claim in all cases, however. Various mathematical techniques were advanced, chiefly in Great Britain, to show that correlation matrices often contained evidence of the influence of "group" factors in certain sets of tests, but the methods developed to analyze correlation matrices for group factors were somewhat subjective and cumbersome.

During the 1930s, L. L. Thurstone, at the University of Chicago, developed methods of factor analysis that made no initial assumptions concerning a "general" factor or "group factors"; they were intended to arrive at the most parsimonious and psychologically meaningful description of the data to which they were applied, whether the data contained one, two, or any number of factors. Some of the important ideas advanced by Thurstone (1931b, 1935, 1940, 1947) in an extensive series of publications were the following: the notion of *common-factor variance,* and the associated *communalities* of particular tests, representing the variance that exists in common among the tests in a particular set and thus the variance that can be analyzed into common factors; the notion of *rotation to simple structure,* whereby a purely mathematical description of a set of data was transformed to a psychologically meaningful and (in some ways) more parsimonious description; and the notion of *correlated factors* and *oblique-factor structure,* whereby underlying entities or "factors" could themselves be correlated and explained by a further factoring at a higher order of analysis. Thurstone also introduced several mathematical techniques of factoring that were computationally simpler, though less elegant, than some of those advanced by Hotelling (1933), Burt (1938), and others; chief of these was the so-called centroid method.

(Nowadays the more elegant methods are usually used, because the high-speed electronic computer has made them practicable and convenient.)

The fundamental model underlying any method of factor analysis, as Thurstone saw it, is one whereby any observed test score of any examinee is to be explained or interpreted as a weighted sum of the examinee's scores on a set of underlying hypothetical entities called factors or, sometimes, latent traits. Generally there is interest only in so-called common factors, that is, factors that can be shown to manifest themselves significantly in performance on more than one test variable. (Any factors that remain specific to given test variables are attributed to error or to the idiosyncrasies of the particular test variables.) The model whereby a test score is a weighted sum of scores on underlying factors is, in statistical terms, a "linear" model similar to the kind of model used in many other branches of statistics. Such a model implies, incidentally, that high values on one underlying factor can compensate for low values on another underlying factor. Two people having the same observed score on a given test variable could therefore be assumed to arrive at that score in quite different ways, one by being very good in one ability and poor in another, the other by having the converse pattern of abilities. Although nonlinear models of factor analysis are now available (McDonald, 1962), there is as yet no evidence of serious difficulties in accepting the implications of the purely linear model for the usual types of ability tests.

Because one has no way of knowing in advance what the underlying entities or factors are, or how they operate to generate observed data, one must try to solve for the parameters of a factor analysis model by applying one of various approaches to the analysis of empirical data from a set of variables. Usually the data analyzed are in the form of a matrix of correlations among the variables. The problem of factor analysis, therefore, may be thought of as one of determining how many common factors are needed to explain the correlations among a set of variables and then determining an appropriate and psychologically meaningful set of weights for these variables. Thurstone's methods provided, by the mid-1930s, what was widely regarded as a more satisfactory and reasonable group of procedures for solving this problem than had been previously available, and these methods were adopted in most of the factor-analytic research in the United States.

From today's perspective, Thurstone's methods yield results that are generally quite similar to those yielded by procedures developed elsewhere. Perhaps a principal reason for the acceptance of his methods was the fact that the first major application of his procedures produced strikingly interesting results. Thurstone's skill in test construction also contributed to his success. His monograph *Primary Mental Abilities* (1938a) was a factor analysis of 57 assorted mental test variables, yielding 13 centroid factors that were rotated to a "simple structure." Nine of the factors were interpreted psychologically (some quite definitively, others somewhat tentatively) as representing distinct types of mental abilities:

    S – Space
    V – Verbal Comprehension
    W – Word Fluency
    N – Number Facility
    I – Induction
    P – Perceptual Speed
    D – Deduction
    M – Rote Memory
    R – Reasoning

Subsequent analyses (e.g., Kaiser, 1960) of these same data, using more advanced methodologies, have shown that most of the original factors stand, although there have been slight reinterpretations of their meanings. In the framework of the factor model, each of these factors was thought of as a distinct underlying ability that would manifest itself in any test that called for its use. Individuals who had a low level of a particular ability would be handicapped in their performance on any test involving it, particularly if the test were a "pure" test of that ability in the sense that it called on no other abilities.

Thurstone's results lent support to a rather different concept of intelligence from the one that had dominated the earlier period of the test movement; that is, they supported the concept that there is not *one* kind of intelligence, but *many*. Most of the tests that Thurstone used in his PMA study were expanded forms of tasks or items that had been used in the conventional group intelligence tests of the period. From the factor-analytic viewpoint, group intelligence tests were "hodgepodges" of mental tasks; the single scores derived from such tests were seen as masking the true pattern of abilities that the examinee might have. If a person received a high score on one of these "omnibus" intelligence tests, it could mean simply that he or she happened to have a high standing on all or nearly all of the abilities tapped by such a test. An average score could reflect any one of many different patterns of abilities – either average standings on a number of abilities or some combination of high and low standings on different abilities.

Further, the new results opened the way to the idea that in the realm of the intellect, people could have a wide variety of strengths as well as weaknesses. This fitted in with the notion that people might differ widely in their aptitudes for different educational programs, occupations, and avocations. Children with relatively low standings on general intelligence were not thereby doomed to failure in everything of an intellectual nature that they might undertake; rather, it was thought, their low scores on the composite test might conceal some particular kind of talent.

In the early years of factor analysis investigations, there had not been time to assemble evidence on whether the underlying factors were of genetic or of environmental origin, or of some combination of these origins. The common opinion, however (possibly influenced by the intellectual climate of the time), seems to have been that the "factors" identified in factor-analytic investigations were largely genetic in origin.

From the standpoint of the requirements for an adequate theory of intelligence tests, the significance of multiple-factor analysis methodology was that it seemed to offer an objective way of identifying and classifying the kinds of competence that might be found in test performances.

In the modern period up to the present, factor-analytic research has proceeded along two relatively independent lines. On the one hand, efforts have been directed toward the improvement and refinement of the methodology itself; on the other hand, the available methodology has been widely applied in the search for new factors of ability and more satisfactory psychological interpretations of the factors identified.

Progress in methodology. Despite his extensive contributions to factor-analytic methodology, Thurstone was able to offer only partial or approximate solutions for several difficult mathematical and theoretical problems. Mainly, these are problems of indeterminacy. One of these concerns how many factors one should accept as being significantly in the "common-factor space." A related problem is how best to estimate the "communalities" of the variables, that is, what proportion of variance in each variable is to be identified as being in the common-factor space. These problems arise principally because empirical data always contain at least some error variance, and thus it is difficult to decide where to draw the line between true common-factor variance and error variance (C. Crawford, 1975).

A second major problem has to do with the notion of "simple structure" and the rotation of the coordinate framework to yield a structural description of the data that is regarded as psychologically meaningful and interpretable. This problem arises from the mathematical fact that there is an infinity of factor matrices that can generate a given correlation matrix, a fact analogous to the familiar truth that there is an infinity of pairs of numbers whose product is equal to some given number. Thus there is a problem of selecting the matrix that is most readily interpretable.

A third major problem has to do with the kinds of models that one tries to fit to factor-analytic data – either models that are maximally parsimonious in terms of the number of underlying factors hypothesized or models that, although they are less parsimonious, may provide a more reasonable description of the data from a psychological point of view.

Considerable progress has been made toward solving all these problems, which are interrelated in complex ways.

Among major contributions to the first problem (estimating the number of significant common factors and thereby estimating the communalities of test variables) have been Guttman's (1940) proof of a lower bound to the communalities and his (1953) development of image factor analysis; Kaiser and Caffrey's (1965) development of "alpha factor analysis," relating factor analysis to the reliability and generalizability concepts of test theory; and Jöreskog and Lawley's (1968) further development of methodologies that permit significance tests. These last authors introduced a distinction between "exploratory" factor analysis, in which one simply seeks statistically sound factorial descriptions of data, and "confirmatory" factor analysis, in which one tests statistical hypotheses about the structure of the data.

The second major problem – that of rotation to simple structure – has been approached by so-called analytical methods that rely on some type of mathematical criterion of good fit, replacing the subjectively determined graphical rotation methods employed by Thurstone and others. Analytical methods of rotation were first introduced in 1953 (Carroll, 1953; Saunders, 1953), but the currently most widely used and generally satisfactory procedure is that developed by Kaiser (1958), the so-called varimax method for orthogonal factors. There now exist at least a half-dozen analytic methods from which a researcher can select according to his taste; in general, these methods yield highly similar results for a well-designed study. The problem of indeterminacy in rotation of factor axes is seen to lie essentially in the adequacy or inadequacy of the data subjected to factor analysis. The essential purpose of rotation to simple structure is to achieve the simplest possible description of variables, that is, by making as many as possible of their weights or loadings close to zero. By the same token, it clarifies the description of factors, by revealing which variables have substantial loadings on each factor, as contrasted to loadings near zero. Factors are interpreted by inferring what psychological (or other) attributes of variables with high or substantial loadings distinguish them from variables with near-zero loadings.

There has been interest in the investigation of various models of factor analysis. One of the major contributions falling in this category is Schmid and Leiman's (1957) development of a largely objective method of determining, from Thurstone-type results, a hierarchical factor structure that is not as parsimonious as Thurstone's but conforms more closely to the factor models preferred by such workers in the British tradition as Vernon (1961). Vernon's model specifies a general factor, two broad group factors (*v:ed*, a verbal–numerical–educational factor, and *k:m*, a practical–mechanical–spatial–physical factor), and narrower factors that would correspond to Thurstone's primary factors, all these factors being orthogonal and independent. Any covariance found among obliquely rotated primary factors by Thurstone's methods can be, in effect, redistributed to the general and broad group factors of Vernon's model by the Schmidt–Leiman technique. Thus the Thurstone and Vernon models are interconvertible. The interconvertibility of models was recognized as early as 1938 by Holzinger and Harman, who provided an alternative, "bifactor" solution for the data analyzed by Thurstone (1938a) and already described here. A procedure similar to the Schmid–Leiman orthogonalization was devised by Cattell and White (R. Cattell, 1965); a study by Hakstian and Cattell (1978) exemplifies its application.

Other methodological developments include McDonald's (1962) nonlinear factor analysis model and Tucker's (1963) three-mode factor model, through which one can study factor-analytic data with an added data dimension, such as different testing occasions, different testing methods, or different observers. The utility of these methods has not as yet been sufficiently explored.

A general comment on the present state of the art of factor analysis is that even if there is still room for further refinement, methodologies are now available to do about anything one might like to do with factor analysis. The advent of high-speed computers, beginning around 1954 (as far as psychometricians were concerned), was particularly critical for the development of factor analysis because of the large and complex computations required. Computations that would have taken months in 1940, if they were thought practicable at all, can now be performed in a matter of seconds. Perhaps the only aspect of factor analysis that is in great need of further development is the factor analysis of large numbers of binary test items according to appropriate scaling models.

FACTOR-ANALYTIC STUDIES IN COGNITIVE ABILITIES

Thurstone himself, together with his colleagues and students, followed up the findings of his PMA study (1938a) with an extensive series of investigations of various factor "domains," such as those of perception (Thurstone, 1944), language (Carroll, 1941; C. Taylor, 1947), and number (Coombs, 1941). The object was to confirm or to refine the interpretations of the factors discovered in the PMA study and to see whether further factors could be disclosed. Systematic variations were introduced into the variables in order to test hypotheses suggested by ambiguities in the interpretation of previous results. For example, it was found that facility in numerical computations was best tested when the computations were extremely simple and speeded, as in the addition or multiplication of pairs of single-digit numbers; Coombs also obtained results that suggested that the Number factor was not limited to numerical material but could also operate in the manipulation of other well-learned symbolic rule systems.

The difficult and ambitious enterprise of studying cognitive abilities by factor-analytic methods has been carried on since Thurstone's day by numerous investigators, not only throughout the United States, but also in such countries as Sweden (Werdelin, 1961), Switzerland (Meili, 1964), and Germany (Jäger, 1967). By 1951, J. W. French compiled a summary of factorial investigations in which he listed 59 different factors of ability and scholastic achievement that had been "identified with sufficient certainty to receive a name" (p. 200). French and his colleagues at ETS assembled two successive "kits" of tests of confirmed factors of mental ability (J. French, 1954; J. French, Ekstrom, & Price, 1963). In preparation for making a third such kit, Ekstrom (1973; see also Ekstrom, French, & Harman, 1979) published a review of the existing literature on cognitive factors, concluding that there was sound evidence for at least 20 different factors of mental ability; the resulting kit (Harman, Ekstrom, & French, 1976) has tests of 23 factors.

One of the most active investigators has been Guilford, who directed a 20-year "high-level aptitudes" project and who by 1971 (Guilford & Hoepfner, 1971) claimed the confirmation of some 98 factors of cognitive ability. Other active investigators include R. B. Cattell (1971) and J. L. Horn (1968), whose concern with the relations of cognitive ability factors to personality traits set them somewhat apart from other groups of investigators.

The proliferation of mental factors beyond the small number – about seven – identified with reasonable confidence by Thurstone up to the large numbers reported by Guilford and his colleagues has been puzzling to many psychologists. Does this proliferation result somehow from artifacts of the methodology, or does it correspond to an actual complexity of "mental life"? Questions have also been raised about the number of factors that are of substantial importance in the conduct of everyday life, education, and other activities; it had been observed (Ellison & Edgerton, 1941) that relatively few of Thurstone's primary mental abilities had significant correlations with any kind of scholastic success. (Chiefly, only verbal and reasoning abilities were found to have more or less reliable correlations with school grades.)

Responses to the "proliferation" problem took several different directions. Methodologists (e.g., Linn, 1968), of course, retreated to their studies and computer terminals to reexamine the statistical bases for establishing factors. Guilford, however, saw the proliferation of factors as an indication that mental life is so structured that it is entirely reasonable to expect the existence of a large number of factors. During the course of his 20-year aptitude project, he developed a three-dimensional taxonomic model for classifying the large number of factors he claimed to have discovered. This model, which he called the structure-of-intellect (SI) model, postulated that a given factor could be classified in terms of the Contents that were involved, the mental Operations that were required in tests of the factor, and the types of Products that resulted from these operations. The model set forth four types of Contents, five types of Operations, and six types of Products. On the assumption that a factor could be defined in terms of exactly one type of Content, one type of Operation, and one type of Product, and that any combination of Content, Operation, and Product could generate a factor, Guilford predicted that continued research would eventually be able to identify 120 different factors. Having found factors representing a great many of these combinations, he directed his efforts toward discovering factors that represented all of the remaining combinations in his taxonomic model. Guilford's SI model has been criticized on various grounds, partly methodological (J. Horn, 1967) and partly logical (Carroll, 1972). The methodological criticism was that Guilford was too ready to accept factors on the basis of subjective judgments and fits to his data that might actually be due to the operation of chance. The criticism from the standpoint of logic was that there was nothing in Guilford's data that *required* or even positively indicated the classificatory constructs that he postulated, because all the factors are, in any event, claimed to be orthogonal and independent.

A different approach to the problem was implicit in the work of R. B. Cattell (1971). Some years ago, Cattell (1943) called attention to a possible distinction between what he called "fluid" intelligence and "crystallized" intelligence, the former representing basic capacity and the latter representing abilities acquired through learning, practice, and exposure to education. These were viewed as group factors standing beside a *g* or general factor. Both fluid and crystallized intelligence could be regarded as having associated with them a larger number of factors representing rather narrow abilities at the level of Thurstone's Primary Mental Abilities. In effect, Cattell espouses a hierarchical model of intellectual abilities; in a hierarchy, it is more or less inevitable that the terminal branches of the tree will proliferate. The hierarchical analysis by Hakstian and Cattell (1978), mentioned previously, of correlations among 20 primary factors revealed 6 oblique second-stratum factors: Fluid Intelligence, Crystallized Intelligence, Visualization Capacity, General Retrieval Capacity, General Perceptual Speed, and General Memory Capacity. These in turn were shown to be accounted for by three oblique factors at a third stratum: Original Fluid Intelligence, Capacity to Concentrate, and School Culture. This study represents an expansion of the hierarchical model of intellectual abilities. Similar developments at the hands of J. L. Horn (1978) and his colleagues present evidence of still further broad factors of ability standing alongside narrower "primary" factors that represent specialized abilities.

Most researchers in factor analysis, it would appear, assume that factors correspond to rather permanent constitutional traits or attributes of individuals – possibly arising in part from genetic sources. The tests measuring such factors are assumed to elicit the operations of these traits – somewhat in the way that a weight-lifting task calls on the individual's muscular powers. But factors can also be looked upon as manifestations of learned competencies. It can be easily demonstrated that if two types of content tend to be learned or practiced together (as opposed to *not* being learned together), tests of those contents will tend to have a positive correlation, giving rise to an underlying factor. The Canadian psychologist George Ferguson (1956) has put forward an interpretation of factor-analytic results relying on the notion that learning leads to the acquisition of abilities that can generalize and transfer to various performances. A factor, therefore, reflects the set of performances to which an ability can generalize and transfer. The full consequences of Ferguson's position have never been worked out in application to the variety of factor-analytic results that are now available, although a sketch of such an application to results in the verbal ability domain has been offered by Carroll (1962). Ferguson's theory does not exclude the possibility that individual differences in genetic and constitutional traits set differential limits on individuals' development of their abilities, but it draws attention to the way in which learning processes can be used to account for factor-analytic findings. Further discussions of a "learning-theoretic" interpretation of factors may be found in *Intelligence and Experience* by J. M. Hunt (1961, 297 ff.).

The latest developments in the theory of the abilities measured by mental tests have arisen from the information-processing approach that has been widely adopted in contemporary cognitive psychology. The performance of any mental task is conceived as involving the simultaneous (parallel) or sequential operation of mental processes upon inputs from external stimuli or from internal "memory stores," governed by learned "executive" routines, and resulting in further operations or responses involving either peripheral motor systems or internal memory stores. For example, the response to a multiple-choice vocabulary item appearing on a mental test would involve (among other things) reading the words shown in the item, recognizing templates for these words in an internal memory store, retrieving semantic information for these words, comparing different pieces of semantic information, and selecting a response on the basis of these meaning comparisons. E. Hunt, Frost, and Lunneborg (1973) assume that such mental processes have individual-difference parameters like speed, probability of transfer between different memory stores, capacity of memory stores, and the like, and have attempted to correlate subjects' performances on mental tests with their performances on experimental tasks that are specially designed to permit the derivation of these parameters. They have turned up some interesting and suggestive correlations, and there is now much activity, not only at Hunt's own laboratory at the University of Washington but elsewhere, seeking to extend and confirm these results (see Carroll & Maxwell, 1979). In a frankly speculative article, Carroll (1976) has tried to interpret the 24 factors measured by the ETS Kit of Factor Reference Tests (J. W. French, Ekstrom, & Price, 1963) in terms of Hunt's information-processing model, drawing attention to the kinds of mental operations, strategies, and memory stores that may be involved and to the way in which individual differences in underlying parameters may be revealed in factor test scores. A related development is Sternberg's (1977) procedure for the "componential analysis" of mental tasks like the solution of syllogisms and analogical reasoning problems.

This line of work is too recent for confident evaluation, but it promises to permit much more rigorous statements about the nature of the cognitive abilities measured by standardized mental tasks. Even then, it will be necessary to investigate in detail the influences giving rise to individual differences in the parameters of mental tasks. (A more detailed discussion of some of this work is to be found in Cooper & Regan, Chapter 3.)

THEORIES OF MEASUREMENT AND SCALING

Serious attention to providing a theoretical basis for psychological measurement came only in the modern period of the testing movement. Foundations had been laid in mathematics (Hölder, 1901) and in the physical sciences (Bridgman, 1927; Campbell, 1928). Bridgman had stressed the definition of physical measurements (of length, mass, etc.) in terms of the operations employed in obtaining them, and Campbell had set out the requirements for what he called fundamental measurement, the assignment of numerals in terms of equality of additive units, as opposed to measurements derived from them. Building on these foundations, B. O. Smith (1938), an educator, was one of the first to examine the nature of the scales underlying psychological and educational measurements; Smith suggested that most such measurements are of a derived rather than a fundamental type, in

Campbell's sense. (This suggestion was probably misguided, however: Psychological measurements are neither fundamental nor derived.)

The system of scale types proposed by Stevens (1946, 1951) has been most influential in current discussions of measurement theory in psychology. Stevens viewed measurement as the assignment of numerals to objects or events according to rules. He recognized four basic types of measurement scales, in increasing order of "strength": nominal, ordinal, interval, and ratio. (Some writers, like Jones, 1971, object to regarding nominal scales as measurements.) Stevens's scale types are differentiated by the properties of the number system that are used in defining them; for example, ordinal scales use only the transitive asymmetric relationships of the number system (e.g., 1 is less than 2, 2 is less than 3, thus 1 is less than 3), whereas ratio scales imply equality of units, equality of ratios (thus, e.g., the ratio of 4 to 2 is the same as the ratio of 8 to 4), and an absolute zero. Stevens claimed that psychological measurements are only rarely on ratio or even interval scales; the scales underlying psychological tests of ability, he believed, are no more than ordinal because they provide only a ranking of the individuals measured. If this claim is taken seriously, it has been argued, it implies that many types of statistics that are ordinarily applied to test-score data (e.g., arithmetic averages, standard deviations, and correlation coefficients) are not strictly appropriate; more valid would be "nonparametric" statistics such as medians, percentiles, and rank-order correlation coefficients. This claim does not, however, make necessary the use of nonparametric methods in testing hypotheses in inferential statistics (Gaito, 1980).

In recent years, work on the theory of psychological measurement has focused on providing a more rigorous axiomatic formulation (Krantz, Luce, Suppes, & Tversky, 1971; Suppes & Zinnes, 1963), but there has as yet been little use of such formulations to consider the conditions under which psychological measurements could have stronger than ordinal properties. Most test theorists have continued to rely on the assumption, widely made by early workers in the field, that abilities tend to be distributed normally, that is, according to the Gaussian normal probability function; they point out that many traits that are measured in fundamental units (e.g., adult height) tend to follow this distribution. Under this assumption it is asserted that if psychological measurements follow approximately normal distributions, or can be transformed to scales that do so, they may be presumed to be measured on scales with at least interval properties. There are difficulties entailed in this assumption, however, stemming from the fact that an approximately normal distribution can be generated simply from the aggregation of a large number of equiprobable events. Observed normal distributions of mental abilities, therefore, may represent mathematical artifacts, and the inference that their scales have interval properties may be invalid, if only for this reason.

It seems obvious that further work is desirable to provide an adequate theoretical basis for the scales on which mental abilities are measured, or, if necessary, to show that it is impossible to provide such a basis. One direction to explore is the attempt to relate item characteristics or test scores more directly to measurements that have clearly interval or even ratio scale properties, such as time, information-theoretic values (bits of information), or logarithmic word-probabilities. Such measurements could be obtained through the administration of individual items at computer terminals and through the analysis of the item tasks themselves in terms of the psychophysical and other dimensions of the stimuli and in terms of the number and characteristics of the operations involved in their performance. Sternberg's (1977) componential analysis techniques would be of use in this. Related techniques are illustrated in studies by Pellegrino and Glaser (1979, 1980) of inductive reasoning tasks and by Egan (1979) and Lohman (1979) of spatial ability items.

STATISTICAL AND COMPUTATIONAL TECHNOLOGY

While test theorists and factor analysts devoted themselves to the specific statistical problems that arose in the construction of tests and the identification of factors underlying them, statisticians continued to refine procedures of general utility in behavioral science investigations. These procedures were used (and sometimes misused) in studies that were designed to evaluate applications of mental ability tests or to identify the probable causal antecedents of individual differences revealed by such tests.

The modern period saw a great expansion in the technology of the correlational method, used in general to describe relationships among variables. A problem that often arises in connection with mental ability tests, and indeed in many other circumstances, is that of finding the best way of combining a set of independent variables – such as the subscores of a test battery – to predict the values of one or more dependent or criterion variables. The simplest way of combining variables is to add them up, each with some definite weight or coefficient, but the question arises: What are the best weights? A solution to this problem was reached around the turn of the century by Pearson (1896) and Yule (1897), through what is known as the multiple correlation, or multiple regression, technique. An early application of the technique occurred in Yerkes's (1921) report on army testing in World War I; extensive use of the method was delayed, however, until efficient algorithms for manual computations were adapted by Wherry (1932) from mathematical work of Doolittle (1878). It was not until the advent of electronic computers in the 1950s that computation of multiple correlations and associated parameters became really practicable for large numbers of variables. An extension of this technique for predicting optimal combinations of criterion variables, known as canonical correlation, was developed by Hotelling (1935) but did not come into even moderate use until the days of the electronic computer. A further generalization to any number of sets of variables was provided by Horst (1961).

All these methods concern merely the identification and description of relationships among variables, without necessary implication of causality. When measurements of variables are taken at different times, however, some inferences about causal relations may be attempted, as was shown by Wright (1921); this technique of path analysis, so called, has only recently been applied to any substantial extent in the analysis of psychological data (Werts & Linn, 1970; see also Bentler, 1980; Maruyama & McGarvey, 1980; L. Wolfle, 1980). A closely related technique, the cross-lagged panel correlation, has been applied, for example, in a study of whether intelligence "causes" achievement (Crano, Kenny, & Campbell, 1972). These and other techniques have greatly increased behavioral scientists' ability to identify and interpret relationships between mental ability tests and other variables (Tatsuoka, 1973). They help in studying performance on mental ability tests from a developmental point of view, that is, as the resultant of basic, fundamentally biological capacities in interaction with environmental influences such as home background and learning experiences at school and elsewhere. Studies using causal analysis might give encouragement to the proposition that many of the so-called primary abilities arise because certain groups of skills and knowledges tend to be learned together as the result of fairly specific and identifiable learning experiences. For example, the abilities represented by the spatial visualization factor may be enhanced by early experience with toys and games that involve perception and mental manipulation of visual patterns. Similarly, the verbal factor may appear in factor-analytic studies because children (and older people) differ in the amount of early and continued exposure to complex oral and written language patterns – vocabulary, syntax, discourse, and so on – that they receive at home and at school.

Much progress has been made in refining other aspects of statistical technology, such as sampling theory and experimental design. Sampling theory can be important in the design of large-scale surveys in which mental test data are involved. The theory of experimental design can be called into play in the design and analysis of mental testing procedures conducted under very carefully controlled conditions, as in an experimental laboratory.

The great advances in computer technology that began to be made in the late 1940s not only facilitated the development of new procedures in the statistical analysis of psychometric data (Cooley & Lohnes, 1962; B. Green, 1966) but also were accompanied by corresponding advances in the technology of scoring tests and manipulating test-score data. It became possible to score test answer sheets very rapidly and accurately by optical scanning devices, and to produce elaborate test-score reports by computer. In a number of schools and universities, facilities became available whereby students could take tests at a computer terminal. The possibility of having such tests "tailored" for the particular ability level of the examinees has been under investigation (Lord, 1971), but as yet the practice of giving such tailored tests has not become widespread. Most group tests of intelligence and scholastic aptitude are still administered in traditional ways; that is, examinees, seated at desks, make their answers by marking in test booklets or on answer sheets, and (typically) are given a uniform time limit to complete their work. In this respect, the process of administering group tests has changed very little in the last 50 years. Nevertheless, the kind of research being explored by E. Hunt, Frost, and Lunneborg (1973; E. Hunt, 1976) and Sternberg (1977) may suggest new procedures in test administration, involving the extensive use of computer terminals (Cory, Rimland, & Bryson, 1977).

PRACTICES IN TEST CONSTRUCTION, STANDARDIZATION, AND
VALIDATION

Practices in test construction, standardization, and validation in the modern period can be illustrated through an examination of several widely used group intelligence and scholastic aptitude tests.

The 1973 Henmon–Nelson Tests of Mental Ability. Earlier we examined the 1932–1935 edition of these tests. Except for a few refinements in format, the 1973 edition (J. L. French, 1973) is highly similar to earlier versions. The number of items, the arrangement of the items in "cycle-omnibus" form, and the time limits are the same as they were 40 years before. The test format and printing are somewhat modernized, and the examinee can make his responses either with the Clapp–Young Self-Marking Device used earlier or on an "MRC" card (the same size as a standard Hollerith/IBM card, but printed with spaces for answers) so that the test answers can be scored at a central point (i.e., the Measurement Research Center at the University of Iowa). The technology of test construction has been brought to bear on the test only with respect to the selection of items and the procedures of norming and validation. Actually, the *types* of items are very much the same as in earlier editions. The test manual (J. L. French, 1973) does not attempt to describe the processes by which new items were generated, but it states:

In selecting items for all levels of the 1973 revision, great care was taken to insure that each item had both a statistically significant biserial correlation with the total test score of which the item was a part and a progressively higher percent of pupils passing the item from one grade to the next in the level for which it was designed. Items with biserials of less than .30 were eliminated. Typical correlations ran in the mid to upper .40's with some running as high as the .50s and .60's.

The item types are described in the manual as being tests of "word knowledge, verbal analogies, verbal classification, sentence completion, numerical problem solving, number series, pictorial analogies, and pictorial classification"; it is remarked that such items

have stood well the test of time and a large proportion of them survived item analysis in the 70's.... By providing an opportunity to solve problems involving these symbol systems, the tests are avowedly measures of general abstract reasoning ability – the type of ability involved in the successful solution of most school-oriented tasks.... Such concepts as "social," "practical," or "mechanical" intelligence are not tapped by the Henmon–Nelson tests.

The general purpose and philosophy of the tests are much the same as before:

Like their predecessors, [these tests are] designed to measure those aspects of mental ability which are important for success in academic work and in similar endeavors outside the classroom. Scores may be interpreted as measures of general mental ability, or academic aptitude, but not as indices of school achievement specifically taught in a common curriculum. Although knowledge is required to answer the items, they were selected to reflect ability to profit from exposure to learning in a variety of situations. High performance on the test requires the efficient utilization of verbal and numerical symbols and the ability to acquire and retain information in common symbol form for use at later times in the solution of verbal, quantitative and abstract reasoning problems.

A test of general mental ability... is built upon the premise that the separable factors contributing to this ability are themselves substantially intercorrelated. Long-standing research has established that varying degrees of competence in the types of mental operations measured by the Henmon–Nelson tests are in fact significantly related to success in school work. As with any test, however, the results from a single administration should be interpreted as representing the individual's *current level of developed ability* and, as such, are more useful for short than long range prediction. Repeated testings at intervals of two or three years are recommended to establish more stable patterns of performance and bring predictive information up to date.

In attempting to persuade the user that the tests are reliable measures, the manual gives a series of stepped-up odd–even reliability coefficients, generally in the .80s and low .90s, but cautions that this procedure of determining reliability "leaves something to be desired for tests in which speed may be a factor in determining an individual's score. Because there is a definite time limit, the Henmon–Nelson tests do have, for some pupils, an element of speededness." Thus the test reviser made no attempt to obtain reliabilities of speeded tests by equivalent-form methods, as he might easily have done, or to take advantage of various methods of determining these reliabilities by statistical procedures suggested by Gulliksen (1950) and others (e.g., Guttman, 1955).

The manual proposes to establish the validity of the test by citing correlations between test scores (or IQs derived from the test) and scores on standardized achievement tests. A table (table 10 in the 1973 manual) shows such correlations ranging from a high of.86 with the reading subtest of the Iowa Test of Basic Skills, down to.60 with the arithmetic score on the same test. It is not stated whether these correlations are based on data obtained from testings done at closely similar times (giving concurrent validity) or at widely spaced times, the Henmon–Nelson test being given earlier (giving predictive validity). In any case, the rather high correlation coefficients tend to suggest that the Henmon–Nelson test, with its large complement of printed verbal materials, measures the cumulative effect of school achievement – regardless of how well it measures "general abstract reasoning ability."

A brief but generally favorable review of the 1973 revision of the Henmon–Nelson test appeared in the *Eighth Mental Measurements Yearbook* (Buros, 1978). If we turn back to the *Fifth Mental Measurements Yearbook* (Buros, 1959), however, we find reviews of a very similar previous revision (Lamke & Nelson, 1957–1958). Here we find Leona Tyler (widely known for textbooks on testing and individual differences) praising the revision as exemplifying "the application of the newest technology of mental measurement to one of our oldest testing problems" (in Buros, 1959, p. 472). Similarly, D. Welty Lefever, a professor of education at the University of Southern California, seems highly favorable to the revision. Both Lefever and Tyler, however, are concerned that the test produces only a single score. As Lefever puts it,

Will a relatively short test (90 items in 30 minutes) carrying a heavy verbal emphasis and yielding a single score serve the purposes for which an intelligence test is being administered?... According to the authors, research findings support the position that "factor" tests or multiscore tests have not predicted scholastic success any better than tests producing a single global score. Subtests in multiscore batteries which apparently have little to do with success in a given subject matter field often yield higher correlations with grades in that field than do the subtests which, because of the nature of their content, ought to be the best predictors.... If a single predictor of school success is needed which can be given in less than a class period and scored with a minimum of time and effort, serious consideration should be given the Henmon–Nelson test. On the other hand, if guidance involving some differentiation among aptitudes is required and if a profile showing the strengths and weaknesses of each counselee is desired, a more complex test battery will be more appropriate. [In Buros, 1959, pp. 470–471]

The Differential Aptitude Tests (DAT). This multiscore aptitude battery, developed by Bennett, Seashore, and Wesman (1947–1975) at the Psychological Corporation, is intended primarily for use in educational and vocational guidance at the secondary-school level. It contains not only tests of several "mental abilities" identified in factor-analytic researches but also several tests that are avowedly measures of certain types of school achievements – English language usage and spelling – on the assumption that these are particularly relevant for guidance decisions. Among test batteries of its type, it is exemplary in the thoroughness with which its standardization and validation have been conducted.

Each of the two equivalent forms of the battery published in 1947 contained eight subtests, taking about 4 hours to administer: verbal reasoning, numerical ability, abstract reasoning, clerical speed and accuracy, mechanical reasoning, space relations, spelling, and grammar. A revised pair of forms published in 1961–1962 had these same subtests, with the same items, but with a reduction of the number of response options in one of the tests, and elimination of the correction-for-guessing scoring for four of the tests. Thus the presently available forms are practically identical to those copyrighted in 1947, but the changes in scoring necessitated a revised set of norms. Although the battery is not intended to contain a test of "intelligence," certain combinations of scores will yield high correlations with group intelligence test scores. The battery is accompanied by a manual containing voluminous data concerning test characteristics, norms, and validity coefficients, and by other aids – for example, a casebook – to help high-school counselors learn how to use the test results.

In the manual, the battery is described as a compromise "between the desire to measure 'pure' mental abilities that emerge from factor analysis and the practical necessities continually encountered by personnel and guidance workers through the years." Many of the tests resemble those investigated in factor-analytic studies such as those of Thurstone and others. The manual gives no information, however, about how test items were generated or selected, nor does it give any information about whether item-analysis procedures were employed in constructing the tests. Nevertheless, the reliability data given for the tests provide assurance that the subscores are satisfactorily reliable for individual guidance purposes.

The DAT battery has received extensive reviews, generally highly laudatory, in Buros's *Mental Measurements Yearbooks* (Buros, 1953, 1959, 1965, 1972, 1978). A sample of general comments is as follows: "One of the more valuable tools for sound vocational and educational guidance available today is represented by the Differential Aptitude Tests" (Bechtoldt, in Buros, 1953, pp. 676–677). "The test items show signs of rare ingenuity.... In summary, the DAT have been carefully developed and standardized by competent authors who have done an exceptionally good job in making information about these tests available to the public" (Berdie, in Buros, 1953, pp. 679, 680). "[The DAT] constitutes the best available foundation battery for measuring the chief intellectual abilities and learned skills which one needs to take account of in high school counseling" (Carroll, in Buros, 1959, p. 673). "Reviewers in the past have justifiably dubbed the DAT as the 'best' available instrument of its kind" (Quereshi, in Buros, 1972, p. 1049).

Nevertheless, reviewers have pointed to certain deficiencies. Several complained about the lack of information on test-construction procedures. Keats asserted that "it is the responsibility of the test constructor to investigate the question [of test homogeneity] and so to be able to assure users that the test scores have an unambiguous meaning – at least in this sense.... The research," he went on (writing in the 1965 *Yearbook*), "is certainly not beyond present methods of analysis, either theoretically or computationally" (p. 1004). Carroll, writing in the 1959 *Yearbook,* complained about the out-of-date standards of English usage that seem to have been observed in the "grammar" test, and Keats, in the 1965 *Yearbook*, pointed out that the 1961–1962 revision took no cognizance of this complaint. Considerable discussion centered on the "differential aptitude" aspects of the battery. As Humphreys noted, "For efficiency in differential prediction, it is desirable to have a battery with low intercorrelations. While the intercorrelations among the tests in the present battery are low enough to make the battery useful, they are not as low as possible. Purer tests than several of those used here are available" (in Buros, 1953, p. 681). Frederiksen wrote: "The question might be legitimately raised as to how 'differential' the tests are, especially for predicting academic criteria" (in Buros, 1959, p. 675). Schutz concluded: "Thus, despite the extensive predictive validity coefficients for the separate DAT subtests, the *differential* validity of the tests in predicting various criteria is still without substantiation" (in Buros, 1965, p. 1006).

The redundancy of the tests and the inefficiency of using separate subscores have also been criticized. As Carroll noted in the 1959 *Yearbook:*

The authors make much of the fact that the DAT battery is a group of tests, each of which is valid and useful in itself; they appear to advise against the combination of weighted scores. In the notable controversy about clinical versus "statistical" prediction they are on the side of "clinical" prediction. Paradoxically, this position prevents them from displaying some of the undoubted powers of the test in affording statistical prediction from weighted combinations of scores. [In Buros, 1959, p. 673]

But Keats pointed out that the latest manual, published in 1966, contains little information on the possibilities of using multiple correlations and weighted combinations of scores. On the basis of a factor analysis, Quereshi concluded that "three factors generally account for about 90 per cent of the reliable variance, indicating that the battery probably encompasses three factors, but definitely no more than four." He asserted, therefore, that "the DAT, despite its technical superiority over its competitors, represents a substantial degree of inessential duplication of time, effort, and expense." Quereshi also pointed out that the extensive norms, based on more than 50,000 cases, were still not as representative as they might have been. He summarized his feelings in the following words: "It [the DAT battery] has not so far lived up to the promise of a differential instrument, but no other instrument for the given age range has yet succeeded in this respect. However, the DAT, if certain steps are taken, has better chances of attaining an acceptable level of differential efficiency than any other comparative [*sic*] battery" (in Buros, 1972, p. 1052).

Quereshi did not report interpretations of the factors he found, nor did he state whether they were correlated in such a way as to suggest that a general factor underlay them. In an article entitled "Lost: Our intelligence? Why?" McNemar (1964) noted that developers of multifactor batteries like the DAT seem deliberately to have avoided conceding any role of a general intelligence factor in such tests. Citing data from the DAT and five other multifactor batteries, he drew attention to what he called "a very disturbing aspect of the situation":

Those who have constructed and marketed multiple aptitude batteries, and advocated that they be used instead of tests of general intelligence seem never to have bothered to demonstrate whether or not multitest batteries provide better predictions than the old-fashioned scale of general intelligence.... Indeed, one can use the vast accumulation of data on the validity of the Psychological Corporation's DAT to show that better predictions are possible via old-fashioned general intelligence tests. [P. 875]

It would be my speculation, supported by a variety of evidence that cannot be given here in detail, that a large part of whatever predictive validity the DAT and other multiple aptitude batteries have is attributable to an underlying general factor that enters into the various subtests, such as those purporting to measure verbal ability, numerical ability, reasoning, spatial ability, and so on; possibly the speededness of many such subtests could account for some part of this general-factor variance, but certainly not all of it. At the same time, the "multifactor" aspect of these batteries reflects the fact that some skills tend to become specialized, on account of either genetic or environmental factors (or both). Some examinees are shown to have verbal, numerical, clerical, or other skills that are above or below what would be expected on the basis of their general intelligence. Some of the validation information from the tests suggests that account has to be taken of these special skills or traits in the predictive, selective, and guidance uses of the tests. But McNemar's point that the role of a general factor of intelligence cannot be overlooked should be taken seriously, in connection not only with the DAT but also with the other tests described here, and ones similar to them. Available multifactor batteries do not provide sufficiently clear measures of general and special skills factors to support accurate determinations of the role of these factors in predicting school grades, professional and job training, or occupational success.

The college board scholastic aptitude test (SAT). The work of C. C. Brigham in developing for the CEEB a test of "scholastic aptitude" to be used for general prediction of success in college and university studies has already been mentioned. Various putatively equivalent forms of this test, known widely to college applicants and their parents as the SAT, are constructed periodically at the ETS in Princeton, New Jersey, and administered to more than a million college applicants every year at numerous testing centers throughout the country and even abroad. It represents, or at least potentially represents, the highest standard of test-construction technology now available.

The SAT is a "secure" test; that is, the forms (or even the items, except for a few that have been released) are not open to public inspection, and copies of the test that are actually used are carefully guarded and accounted for. A publication edited by Angoff (1971a) constitutes, in effect, a "manual" for the test and presents voluminous details about the test itself and the procedures by which test items are developed and selected for inclusion in successive forms, successive test components are equated to one another, and norms are established. It also contains much information (even though it is only a sample of the information actually available) about the predictive validity of the SAT and the various factors that affect scores (coaching, practice and growth, fatigue and anxiety, etc.). (It also contains information pertinent to the Achievement Tests that are offered by the CEEB, but I will leave aside consideration of these tests here.)

For a general description of the test, I could do little better than to offer excerpts from P. H. DuBois's review in the *Seventh Mental Measurements Yearbook* (Buros, 1972):

Like many developments in measurement, the SAT is a direct descendant of the Army Alpha. The original plan was formulated by Robert M. Yerkes, Henry T. Moore, and Carl C. Brigham. Later Brigham became responsible for its development. A conscious effort was made to develop an instrument that would measure neither school achievement nor general mental alertness. With the passage of time, resemblance to its prototype lessened: subtests became fewer; speededness was reduced; and emphasis was placed upon two relatively homogeneous item types – verbal and mathematical. Currently the two subscores are referred to as SAT-V and SAT-M.

Even today, nearly three decades after Brigham's untimely death, the SAT continues a number of features which he initiated: (a) an attempt to measure "aptitude for college studies" rather than intelligence; (b) equating of numerous forms so that the predictive scores are stable irrespective of the time and place the student takes the test; (c) extensive and systematic use of item analysis; and (d) tryout of all new material before items are used operationally.

Items with known statistical characteristics are organized in sections requiring 30 or 45 minutes each for a total testing time of three hours. Within each block of items, arrangement is in terms of increasing difficulty, with "the mean difficulty of each block ... equal to that of the test as a whole."

Test content is selected to avoid as far as possible any inequities to any subclass of the intended population. The SAT-M requires as background only the mathematics taught in grades 1–9, while the SAT-V is related to social, political, scientific, artistic, philosophical, and literary areas. The earlier literary focus of the verbal items has been abandoned for a broader orientation, while the mathematical material now depends less on formal knowledge and more on "logical reasoning and ... the perception of mathematical relationships."

As is well known, SAT scores are reported with a mean 500 and standard deviation 100. It is not so well known that the standardization group consists of 10,654 students who took the test in April, 1941. Through somewhat involved methods, the various forms are equated accurately to one another and to the form yielding the initial norms.

Ask for any conventional statistic about the SAT and one can be practically certain that it will be available: reliabilities, validity coefficients, and item data.... The internal consistency reliability estimates for 12 recent forms cluster closely around .91 and .90 for the verbal and mathematical scores, respectively; the parallel-form reliabilities average two points lower. In the 1950's the average correlation between the two parts was in the middle .50's; more recently, it has been in the high .60's, possibly reflecting a decreasing emphasis on specific knowledge in the two areas. [It may also reflect an increasing verbal load in the mathematical part, however.]

From the beginning, the SAT has been found to have reasonably good validities for predicting college achievement. Also it has been found consistently that the SAT increases the validity of the high school average or rank. Studies made in 1927 showed a median validity of the school record of .52, a median validity of the SAT of .34, and of the combination of both, .55. . . . Currently, typical validities are .39 for SAT-V, .33 for SAT-M, .55 for the high school record, with a multiple correlation of the order of .62. The picture today is not greatly changed from that in 1927 except that both SAT validities and school grade validities have increased, and the increment of the SAT over the high school record is a little greater than it was. [Pp. 646–647]

A few notable details are absent from this account. For example, the SAT test is completely "objective," all items being of the multiple-choice type with five options per item. The exact composition of the sections is not quite as homogeneous as DuBois implies. A typical verbal section, for example, will contain antonym items, sentence completion items, analogies items, and reading comprehension items. From a factor-analytic viewpoint, such a section would tap both the V (verbal knowledge) factor and a verbal reasoning factor. The mathematical sections consist of two "formally distinct item types: general mathematics items common in form to many other tests, and data sufficiency items" (Angoff, 1971a, p. 17). In one factor-analytic study of the mathematical section, 6 mathematics factors and 10 *verbal* factors were tentatively identified (Pruzek & Coffman, 1966). The matter of the validity of the SAT in predicting college success is, of course, much more complex than could be conveyed in DuBois's account. It is necessary to emphasize that validity coefficients vary widely depending on various circumstances – the type of college, the selectivity of the college, and so forth. According to Fincher (1974), "Analysis of data over a thirteen-year period [in the university system of Georgia] gives firm evidence of the SAT's incremental effectiveness in supplementing the high school record as a predictor of college grades"

(p. 304). The validity of the test in predicting grades in particular institutions, however, is not the whole story. Colleges and universities differ markedly in the average intellectual quality of their student bodies. From the standpoint of the prospective applicant, the SAT score gives some guidance about the range of institutions, on this dimension, in which he or she is likely to be accepted and find an appropriate match for his or her level of academic ability. If it were possible to assign students to higher-education institutions randomly, the correlation of the SAT with college success would very probably be much higher than the figures usually reported.

Reviewers of this test in Buros's *Mental Measurement Yearbooks* generally approach it with what almost appears to be reverence and awe. DuBois, whose review (in Buros, 1972) has already been extensively quoted, finds little if any fault with the test, and defends it:

The SAT is not without its detractors, some of whom regard it as a "tool of the academic establishment." Of course it is! But it is a good tool, perhaps the best that can be devised with present psychometric technology. No attempt is made to adjust SAT scores for sex, socioeconomic status, race, or educational background. In this reviewer's opinion, such attempts would be difficult to justify. Adding substantially to the prediction of academic achievement as contrasted with the use of high school grades alone, the SAT has repeatedly proved its usefulness to colleges. It helps to pick those who fit in best in the program of a particular institution, and, of course, it can be supplemented with any other information that admissions officials may wish to use.

The question has arisen of whether or not it fits the needs of the students as well as those of the colleges and universities. No good end would be served by blunting this instrument. Certainly there are many aptitudes other than verbal and mathematical that some colleges might like to know about, such as musical, spatial, mechanical, and clerical abilities. College entrance examining could be broadened so that a profile of testable characteristics adequate for educational and vocational counseling would become available. . . . Obviously the CEEB program could be broadened further. But even in a broadened program the present SAT measures would be important. [P. 648]

In the same volume of the *Yearbooks*, Wimburn Wallace concludes his review with a comparison of the SAT with its nearest competitor, the ACT – a comparison that, he says, "favors the SAT overall. . . . Although validities against college achievement criteria are not strikingly different, the content mix, psychometric quality, and pertinent research efforts appear to be superior in the SAT." His only significant complaint would seem to be that "the content and format of the test have been essentially the same for a very long time. . . . The investigation of, or experimentation with, various and new test types for the SAT has been sporadic. . . . There should be sustained, regular effort toward new test development" (pp. 648–649). Actually, Angoff's compilation (1971a, 156 ff.) reports numerous studies designed to find new and valid content for the SAT; little of use, however, could be found. Various recommendations about possible new types of test content were made by a Commission on Tests appointed by the CEEB in 1967 to "undertake a thorough and critical review of the Board's testing function in American education and to consider possibilities for fundamental changes in the present tests and their use in schools, colleges, and universities" (CEEB, 1970, p. xiii), but thus far these recommendations have not been followed up, possibly because they have been seen to be unfeasible.

In earlier *Yearbooks*, we find little criticism of the SAT. In the 1965 issue,

Wayne Zimmerman raises the question why it should take as long as a half day to obtain accurate measurements of just two abilities. In the 1953 issue, Frederick B. Davis (author of well-known reading comprehension tests), complains that the items

lack originality and interest. The passages on which the reading items are based seem dull and, in general, poorly written. The difficulty of the items based on them often seems to derive from the muddiness of the passages rather than from the necessity for close reasoning or sensitiveness to implications on the part of the examinee.... As in the case of most tests, some faulty items can be found.... The validity data indicate that this test is about as useful for predicting academic success as a test of its limited scope can be. Tests that have been commercially available for twenty years are about equally useful. Any unique merit in using the *Scholastic Aptitude Test* lies in the fact that one can be reasonably sure that the examinees will not have had access to it beforehand and that it be administered and scored with scrupulous care and accuracy. [Pp. 383–384]

It is a matter of opinion whether the current forms of the SAT show any improvement over those criticized by Davis in 1953.

The truth-in-testing laws now in place or proposed in many states seem to be based, in part, on public misunderstanding of the theory and rationale of intellectual and scholastic aptitude testing. To the extent that these laws require testing agencies to publish their tests after their use in particular administrations, and to disclose answers, they are based on the assumption that the tests are nothing more than tests of achievement of learned skills and knowledges. In a sense, of course, the tests do reflect learned skills and knowledges, but these are intended to be skills and knowledges that have been acquired, and that have matured, over the long course of an individual's child and adolescent life, not those that can be readily learned and markedly improved over a short period. The tests are intended to sample long-acquired skills, not to focus on particular items of content that could somehow be described in advance and prepared for by the examinee. It is probably true (Slack & Porter, 1980) that certain test-taking skills and, to a limited extent, content knowledge in vocabulary and mathematics, can be improved somewhat through well-designed coaching programs sufficiently to affect favorably some small proportion of admissions decisions that are made partly on the basis of test scores. It is debatable, however, whether the cost–benefit ratio for the examinees is sufficient to justify attendance at coaching schools and similar programs.

The recommendation made by agencies like the CEEB that examinees not place undue confidence in the effects of coaching on their scores is a sound one if it is assumed (as appears to be the case) that well-motivated examinees can acquire test-taking skills either in their schooling or on their own, by working through published samples of tests. Unfortunately, thorough studies of this assumption are lacking, although Powers and Alderman (1979) found that students reported some benefits from studying a test-familiarization booklet published by the CEEB. An even better recommendation to prospective examinees would be to attend seriously to their schooling over the period of years necessary to acquire mastery of the intellectual skills measured by the SAT and other admissions tests (for advice to school administrators on this point, see Thomson & DeLeonibus, 1978). If some of the vocabulary items, reading passages, and mathematical problems placed in scholastic aptitude tests seem obscure, arcane, or contrived, it is because only in this way can the higher reaches of verbal and mathematical skills be effectively sampled and measured. Actually, it can be shown (see Carroll, 1980b) that average SAT scores (e.g., 416 on the SAT-V and 455 on SAT-M) reflect levels of verbal and mathematical skills far lower than those one might desire a student to attain from a secondary-school education.

THE USE AND MISUSE OF INTELLIGENCE TESTS IN SCHOOLS

By the opening of what we are calling the "modern" period of the mental test movement, the practice of using intelligence tests in schools, particularly the primary schools, for general diagnosis of pupils' presumed learning capabilities had become well established. Many schools used scores on such tests, along with records of actual school achievement, as a basis for "ability grouping," that is, placement of pupils in groups of "fast," "average," and "slow" learners, apparently with the conviction that pupils' needs could be better served in this way. Bright pupils would presumably be given instruction that allowed them to progress faster through the assigned curriculum units, with appropriate "enrichment" through the introduction of additional material. At the high-school level, such pupils would be more likely to be assigned to college-preparatory courses in mathematics, science, social studies, language, and the humanities. The less able students were given instruction with simpler content and at a slower pace; at the high-school level they were encouraged to take courses in business, shop, and other vocational subjects. The rationale for these procedures was the notion that mental ability scores were indicators of learning capacities that were at least to a large extent permanently fixed in students; the evidence cited as supporting this notion consisted of the many substantial correlation coefficients found between mental ability test scores and school grades. If students made low scores on mental ability tests, it could be rather confidently predicted that they would do poorly in the more difficult and advanced aspects of school work. Therefore, it was reasoned, they would be better off, in their general adjustment to school and in their school progress, if they were assigned to relatively easy tasks and easy subject matter.

Research on the efficacy and usefulness of ability grouping had up to 1935 yielded no clear conclusions, and the findings continued to have a negative tone even throughout the modern period (see reviews by Findley & Bryan, 1971, 1975; Svensson, 1962). Most of the research on ability grouping, however, pertained to differentiated streams of learners within a narrowly defined curriculum area, for example, groups of fast and slow learners in a particular social studies course. Findings regarded as negative consisted of observations that a slow group made no greater progress as a segregated group than they would have made had they been taught along with the fast group. It was rare that researchers in ability grouping had an opportunity to study situations in which instruction was appropriately differentiated for groups of varying abilities.

This research on ability grouping was probably irrelevant to the question whether students should be guided into different high-school curricula – academic curricula for the intellectually superior, and nonacademic, "general" curricula for those regarded as having mediocre intellectual abilities. Because of tradition and the weight of school administrators' experience in student assignments, it was practically impossible to conduct an adequately designed experiment. Such an experiment would have required something like random assignment of representative groups of students to courses of different types of content and difficulty levels.

Actually, if such an experiment had been done, it is highly likely that the usefulness of ability grouping would appear to have been justified to a much greater degree than it was by the usual study with a single subject matter. That is, we may confidently predict (and school administrators would also have predicted) that most low test scorers would fail in the more difficult courses, and most high test scorers would be bored and unchallenged in the less difficult courses. In the 1940s and perhaps in the 1950s, such an experiment (if it could have been conducted at all, in view of practical and ethical considerations) would have been regarded as a supreme vindication of the usefulness of mental test scores as a basis for student guidance and assignment. In fact, as late as 1959, James B. Conant suggested that only about 15–20% of the high-school student population possessed the talents fitting them for college-preparatory courses and eventual entrance to college. In Conant's own terms of reference, he may have been approximately correct. The difficulty comes in defining the proper terms of reference. That is, if by "possessing talents" it is meant that students have acquired *developed* general abilities, knowledges, and skills needed for success in academic work, one may agree with Conant, but if it was also implied that no other students in the age cohort could have developed those same abilities if they had been exposed to suitable learning and educational experiences from their earliest years, there is a reasonable doubt about the soundness of Conant's assertion. At least, we shall have to say that the evidence for thinking that only some small proportion of the population has an inherent potential *at birth* for developing "academic talent" is totally inadequate. It is beyond the scope of this chapter, however, to consider the problem in any detail; it is discussed in Scarr and Carter-Saltzman, Chapter 13.

It is of interest and relevance, however, to note the impact of research into mental abilities on the British educational system in the early days of the modern period, and the subsequent course of events. The post–World War I years in Britain were marked by an often bitter struggle between those who desired to maintain the traditionally highly selective school system (and defend the "public-school" system represented by Eton, Winchester, and the rest) and those who sought to reform the system by raising the school-leaving age and making secondary education widely and freely available to children of the working classes (Simon, 1974). There were problems of both economics and ideology. The Education Act of 1902 had already laid the foundation for a system of publicly maintained secondary schools, but the number of places allotted to non-fee-paying students continued to be very small. Whereas in the early years of the century selection for free places in secondary schools was based mainly on teachers' reports, from about 1924 on, mental tests played an increasingly important role. As Simon notes:

From the outset tests were integrally related to the selection of a few children from among many at the age of 11, on the grounds of capacity to profit from the academic secondary course. Accordingly the relevant curriculum was taken as given and as the yardstick for diagnosing "intelligence"; the children who could "take it" were intelligent, those who could not lacked ability. There could hardly be a better recipe for crystallising school practice at the secondary stage, and the influence stretched down to crystallise primary schools into a selective pattern. [Pp. 239–240]

Intelligence testing in school selection was sold to the public as a scientifically justified procedure (Simon, 1974):

In a popular exposition of the new "science" of mental testing in 1933, to a radio audience, Cyril Burt [psychological consultant to the London County Council] outlined the conclusions arrived at about the functioning of the human mind. It was a simple, clear, straight-forward statement admitting no doubts, inviting no argument. "By intelligence the psychologist understands inborn, all-round intellectual ability. It is inherited, or at least innate, not due to teaching or training; it is intellectual, not emotional or moral, and remains uninfluenced by industry or zeal; it is general, not specific, i.e., it is not limited to any particular kind of work, but enters into all we do or say or think. Of all our mental qualities, it is the most far-reaching." The exposition closed with an affirmation with ominous overtones for the educational system: "Fortunately it can be measured with accuracy and ease."

Even within the small world of mental testing, or psychometry, there were differences on this question which might have been cited; notably disagreement with the claim that the *ad hoc* tests, produced to meet urgent administrative needs, measured an innate and unchangeable power of the human mind. One of the most distinguished investigators in the field, Godfrey Thomson, held that there were no grounds to say that the "intelligence" measured by tests was a given quantity transmitted by inheritance; in his view environmental factors accounted for as much as 50 per cent of the variance in test scores. But, once again, so far as the school system was concerned the categoric Burt interpretation was both relevant and requisite, provisos an unnecessary complication. According to this, it was only necessary to take a child's I.Q., or intelligence quotient, when he entered school, allocate him to the relevant stream or differentiated course, and see him through at the given level until he left. This was to plan education in accordance with the child's needs, it was asserted, since it was now known that the I.Q. accurately represented a quota of innate "intelligence" which would not, indeed could not, change. [Pp. 241–242; in a footnote, p. 242, Simon points out that Burt expressed similar views in a broadcast talk in 1950.]

Because even by the late 1930s the publicly maintained secondary-school system continued to stress an academic curriculum, increasing pressure built up in the general public, particularly in the Labour Party, to establish a system that would better serve the needs of the great bulk of the students from middle and working classes. To be sure, there were various kinds of vocational and technical schools available, but progressives were of the opinion that the existing secondary schools should have a more diversified and widely appealing curriculum, with a more democratically composited student body. The upshot was the establishment, by the Board of Education, of a Committee on Curriculum and Examinations in Secondary Schools. It was perhaps characteristic of the educational politics of the time that the chairman was a former headmaster of a public school, Sir Cyril Norwood, who could not have been expected to be especially sympathetic to progressive ideas. The committee's report was released in 1943. Simon (1974) terms it "the most discreditable of official reports" and remarks that "directed to justifying the Board doctrine of securing a hierarchy of maintained schools in traditional terms, it justified the unjustifiable in the richest of rhetoric" (p. 283).

The report made little mention of intelligence tests ("the major prop of the Board policy on the scientific front," Simon notes, p. 283), but from the evidence and witnesses listed as being considered or heard by the committee, it is plain that its conclusions were strongly influenced by then current factorial theories of intelligence.[3] In a section concerned with "Variety of Capacity," the report (Norwood, 1943) asserts:

The evolution of education has in fact thrown up certain groups, each of which can and must be treated in a way appropriate to itself. Whether such groupings are distinct on strictly psychological grounds, whether they represent types of mind, whether the differences are differences in kind or in degree, these are questions which it is not necessary to pursue. [P. 2]

The report goes on to describe three "types" of students: (1) "the pupil who is interested in learning for its own sake, who can grasp an argument or follow a piece of connected reasoning"; (2) "the pupil whose interests and abilities lie markedly in the field of applied science or applied art"; and (3) "the pupil [who] deals more easily with concrete things than with ideas" (pp. 2–3). On this basis the report recommended that a tripartite school system be maintained: a "grammar school" for pupils in Category 1, a "technical school" for pupils in Category 2, and a "modern" school for pupils in Category 3. Evidently this tripartite school system was proposed to accommodate the notion of a "general" factor of intelligence, along with the notion of a "practical" factor (probably similar to what would be called a "spatial" factor today) as identified by Alexander (1935) and others: Grammar schools would be designed for those high in g and verbal skills; technical schools would be appropriate for those high in practical and spatial factors; modern schools would be suitable for pupils with lesser abilities in g and the practical factor.

It would appear that many local authorities in Britain actually went ahead with implementing the recommendations of the Norwood report, although in recent years the trend in Britain has been toward comprehensive secondary schools somewhat similar to those in the United States, Sweden, and other countries. It is not our purpose here to review later developments; we merely note this rather remarkable instance in which research on mental abilities seemed to have had signal influence on the formulation of educational policy, however misguidedly.

In defense of British psychometrists, however, we may note that they, "however firmly (if erroneously) they claimed to measure levels of intelligence accurately, were affronted at the crudities of the Norwood typology" (Simon, 1974, p. 327). Burt (1943) attacked the Norwood report vigorously, and numerous subsequent researches had the effect of weakening the validity of Norwood's claims. For example, Lambert (1949) was unable to find clear separations between the presumed types and suggested that "for the whole distribution a bilateral school in which alternative curricula differing slightly in bias would be provided would appear to be more suitable than separate grammar and technical schools" (p. 79). She also found that interests were not fixed at age 11 and that consequently a decision about the type of school a child might be suited for might be premature at that age.

Simon comments on the regressiveness of this whole period in Great Britain in the following words:

In sum, throughout the late 1940s and the 1950s, when so much might have been accomplished, the development of secondary education for all was restricted and distorted by the dead hand of a doctrine brought to a point during the depressed 1930s – the doctrine that secondary education is not for all, that only the selected qualify for a complete form of it.... In the end it was the breakdown of the supportive ideology of "intelligence" testing, through sheer over-use of tests and exposure of all their inherent weaknesses, upsurge in the secondary modern schools comparable to earlier outbreaks in the 1890s and 1920s, and growing parental revolt that broke open the closed circle. [Pp. 331–332]

This is not to say that either "intelligence" tests or selective grammar schools were completely eliminated. There are still today, in Britain, secondary schools for which one of the criteria for selection is passing of a verbal reasoning test, along with achievement tests in English and mathematics. On the basis of research in one such school, Richardson (1956) asserted that "an intelligence test seems to be necessary" (p. 23), because such a test had significantly higher validity against school grades than any other single test. If one assumes that the test measured some of the generalized developed abilities prerequisite for success in a selective school, its use may have been justified as a practical matter, but it would be wrong to assume that pupils selected by such a test were thereby shown to be innately different from pupils failing the test; it could be that the latter had simply not had the early advantages enjoyed by those passing the test. Furthermore, recent evidence in Britain (e.g., Christie & Griffin, 1970) suggests, again, that there is no particular advantage in setting up selective schools as opposed to nonselective, comprehensive schools.

In the United States, of course, public secondary schools have been of a comprehensive type for decades, and all vestiges of selection for such schools have long since disappeared. Mental ability tests are used in secondary schools mainly for guidance purposes, if at all – for example, in helping students decide upon choice of courses and curricula.

Test publishers offering group intelligence tests for use in elementary schools have noted a marked decline in sales, because many school systems have followed the lead of the New York City schools in abandoning the use of such tests altogether (Loretan, 1965). Many reasons have been given for their abandonment. For one thing, educators feel that teachers are liable to be unduly influenced by the results; that is, test scores are too likely to be used to "type" a child as a slow learner and thereby to inhibit proper instruction. Second, it is felt that group intelligence tests are not sufficiently accurate in view of their speededness and in view of the conditions under which they are usually given. Third, it is thought that the tests yield little information that cannot be gained from well-designed achievement tests in various school subjects. Fourth, it has been recognized, increasingly, that group intelligence tests of the conventional sort tend to measure the kinds of verbal and reasoning skills that, on the average, are more likely to be acquired by middle-class, majority-group children than by children from various types of "disadvantaged" backgrounds; thus it is said that the tests are "biased" against the latter groups of children, in the sense that these children have had meager opportunities to learn the verbal and reasoning skills measured by the tests. In the past, there were flagrant misuses of intelligence tests, for example, in using English-language intelligence tests to classify children who had little or no knowledge of English.

Granting all these objections to the use of group intelligence tests in elementary schools, one may nevertheless feel that some losses have been entailed in their abandonment. It is not completely certain, for example, that intelligence tests measure nothing beyond what can be measured by achievement tests. The fact that scores on intelligence tests and on achievement tests are generally highly correlated does not necessarily mean that they are measuring the same thing; it may signify only that whatever is measured by intelligence tests *tends* to be learned to the same or much the same degree as the skills and knowledges that are specific to a particular subject matter. If group intelligence tests measure certain skills (e.g., general vocabulary and language comprehension, general reasoning power, ability to manipulate symbol systems, etc.) that are not directly taught in schools, an intelligence test – wisely used and interpreted – may yield information that will not become apparent through teacher observations, achievement tests, and the like. Considering that group intelligence tests have changed little in the last 30 or 40 years and have been inadequately reflective of newer developments in test theory, the factor-analytic investigation of human ability, and the study of cognitive growth, it is conceivable that mental tests could now be developed that would have some real value in the process of education. What this writer has in mind would be a series of tests of intellectual skills – language production and comprehension in both their spoken and written aspects, reasoning abilities of different types with both verbal and mathematical content, ability to visualize and manipulate visual forms, ability to register and remember arbitrary content, ability to make rapid and accurate comparisons of series of printed symbols, and so forth – that would be specially devised to provide meaningful scales of ability and mastery in these skills. The tests would be criterion-referenced rather than norm-referenced, so that a score would concretely point to the types and levels of intellectual tasks of which the student had or had not attained mastery. Special techniques of test construction – departing from conventional test-theoretic procedures – might be required to prepare such tests. Test constructors would need to address themselves to the psychological attributes of the test stimulus materials and the components of the intellectual process required to respond to them appropriately. In tracing the course of students' intellectual development, teachers could use these tests not only to gauge progress but also as a guide to instructional procedures designed to promote such progress.

Mental ability tests in college admissions. Successive generations of college-bound students have been, many would say, all too familiar with the role of scholastic aptitude tests – those of the CEEB, those of the ACT, or those of still other agencies – in college admissions. The evidence assembled by Angoff (1971a) shows moderate to substantial validity of the CEEB's SAT, given prior to college entrance, in predicting academic success in selective colleges (in terms of grades, retention, and other criteria). If there is any test upon which all feasible applications of test theory have been made, it must be the SAT. It is agreed among test experts that even with all the refinements that test theory, factor analysis, and other psychometric developments can offer, tests of the SAT type can never attain a validity beyond a certain point – represented by a correlation coefficient of about .6 after "correction" for test and criterion unreliabilities and for restriction of range. Much more seems to be involved in college "success" than whatever is measured by the SAT; the SAT is not claimed to be a measure of motivation, personality, creativity, or other traits that might be relevant. The CEEB, and the ETS (which prepares and administers the test), has repeatedly cautioned college admissions officers against the exclusive use of test scores in the admissions process. Even when test scores are used judiciously, however, it cannot be denied that they play a considerable role, although the actual extent of this role is difficult to measure or state precisely because SAT scores tend to be correlated with other types of information. Thus it is likely that the rank order of applicants determined by a selection board *with* the use of SAT scores would be substantially the same as the rank order determined *without* the availability of SAT scores. Nevertheless, it seems that the primary case for using SAT scores rests on the fact that they contribute a significant amount of information over and above the high-school record (Fincher, 1974).

This is not the place to consider the large and controversial literature on the pros and cons of using scholastic aptitude tests in college or university admissions, at either the undergraduate or the graduate level. Nor can we comment on the experience of some institutions, like Bowdoin College, that have abandoned the use of such tests in the admissions process. We cannot go into the knotty problems of restriction of range, criterion contamination, cultural bias, the effects of coaching, and other factors affecting the validity of predictive tests. Many of these matters are treated quite thoroughly in the technical manual for the SAT compiled by Angoff (1971a). It may be pointed out here, however, that the scientific examination of all these problems is a challenge that draws upon the full resources of statistical methodologies and theories of measurement that have been developed over the years.

From the standpoint of the theory of mental abilities, furthermore, several comments are appropriate:

1. To the extent that tests of the SAT type are valid in predicting college or graduate-school success, it is undoubtedly because they provide a good indication of the extent to which applicants *at the time of testing* have developed or acquired, and are able to exhibit through their performance on a test, certain general intellectual skills in handling verbal, quantitative, and symbolic information that are contributory or even necessary to high-level success in academic studies, and, in addition, to intellectual pursuits in postcollege years.

2. A low score on such a test is no guarantee that the individual cannot acquire, during a subsequent period, the skills and abilities that are tested, but it is an indication, at least, of the probability that the individual could acquire these skills and abilities, if at all, only with much expense of time and effort and with careful instruction. This statement is an inference from at least two types of evidence: First, it has been repeatedly shown that coaching in short courses aimed at increasing SAT scores has meager effects, if any; second, the increases in mean SAT scores that occur from the third to the fourth year of the secondary school are very small. Furthermore, I can find little evidence that special compensatory or remedial courses for low-scoring students conducted for a period of a year or two in colleges have any major effects in increasing the level of the students' academic abilities, although they may indeed increase their abilities to cope with the demands of academic studies (Gordon & Wilkerson, 1966; Rayburn & Hayes, 1975).

3. Nevertheless, there is actually relatively little knowledge about the extent to which the aptitudes and abilities measured by scholastic aptitude tests can be improved by special training and guidance. The fact that previous efforts to improve them have been generally disappointing does not demonstrate that no such efforts can be successful.

2.3.   REVIEW AND ASSESSMENT: THE CURRENT SCENE

In the preceding sections I have been concerned with presenting the rather checkered history of theory and practice in group mental ability testing. Obviously, an enormous amount of effort has been devoted to the development, analysis, and application of measures of mental ability. But has all this effort been properly oriented to achieve socially useful results? Has it been based on a correct set of assumptions about the nature of the human organism – its biological substrate and its capacities for learning and adaptation? Has the testing movement been founded on acceptable presuppositions about the nature and goals of education in relation to the goals of human society?

These are very difficult questions. In part this is because they involve individual and societal values which appear to have changed significantly over the period reviewed here and about which there can be much discussion and debate among different sectors of the public. In part the difficulty of these questions is due to the incompleteness of our knowledge about individual behavior and the workings of education and society. A complete discussion of them would take us far beyond the scope of this chapter, which is limited to considering the contributions the theory and technology of testing might make to the resolution of current issues and problems. Nevertheless, they are questions that must be faced in thinking about the future of the mental testing movement and the kind of public support that it may or may not deserve.

In arriving at some tentative conclusions and recommendations, it may help to consider some of the issues raised by the controversies that have surrounded the testing movement.

PUBLIC CONTROVERSIES ABOUT MENTAL TESTING

Public controversy about mental testing and its consequences is not new; it goes back at least five decades, as Cronbach's (1975) thoughtful essay recounts. In the 1920s, debate was centered around questions of invidious ethnic comparisons, with overtones of doubt about the supposed immutability ("constancy") of intelligence and the elitist implication that education could not erase or even reduce intellectual inequality. One senses that during the whole period from the 1920s to the 1960s, when debate became extremely public and acrimonious, there was a latent, seldom-expressed concern over the use of intelligence tests in schools to sort children into ability groups, to bar students from the more selective schools and colleges, or, to put it bluntly, to determine young people's careers and eventual fates.

In England, the use of the so-called 11+ examinations for grammar-school selection increasingly disturbed the more liberal-minded sectors of the population, even though the tests were sometimes praised because they did, at least, provide a basis for admitting to grammar schools some working-class children who might otherwise have been turned away. Young's (1958) satiric essay on an eventual "meritocracy" of the intellect was in part a response to the great emphasis on intelligence testing in British education.

In the United States, an analogous phenomenon occurred, but at the college level, as many colleges found themselves forced to be more selective than previously (Hills, 1971, p. 681) and increasingly emphasized scholastic aptitude test results in the selection process. Chauncey and Dobbin's (1963) book on mental testing, addressed to the general public, probably did little to allay concern about testing in education, even though these authors asserted that "intelligence tests... measure only the individual's capacity for learning" (p. 21), that they "measure not innate ability but a developed ability in which innate ability and learned behavior are mixed in unknown proportions" (p. 22), and that "scholastic aptitude tests include verbal and numerical content but omit the non-academic tasks... [and] have all of their content devoted to skills taught in schools" (p. 32). Public concern about mental ability testing has been at least partly responsible for the abandonment of the use of intelligence tests in many public school systems throughout the country, and the use of ability grouping in schools has recently been put under severe restrictions by court decisions asserting that ability grouping limits educational opportunities. Currently, there is considerable feeling in some quarters that the use of scholastic aptitude tests in college admissions should be sharply curtailed or at least put under certain controls that are felt to be necessary.

Though there seems to have been general public acceptance of the need and utility of mental ability and aptitude testing in the armed forces during World War II, criticism of the overuse, misuse, and possible discriminatory effects of such tests in business and industry became frequent in the 1950s and 1960s, leading eventually to legislation and government regulations that had the effect of mandating demonstrated validity of any employment selection tests, including mental ability tests, that might be used (Ash, 1966; Baxter, 1969; U.S. Office of Personnel Management and ETS, 1980).

Much of the debate during this period stemmed from the civil rights movement and criticized the possible "cultural bias" of mental tests. It was asserted that the tests were oriented to tapping abilities and achievements valued in white, middle-class education and culture, and that persons in various minority groups, with different cultures, or even different dialects and language backgrounds (Labov, 1969), were put under a great handicap by the tests. At the 1968 meeting of the APA, a group of black psychologists presented a manifesto calling for a moratorium on the use of psychological and educational tests in schools with students having disadvantaged backgrounds, presumably until further research could be done to correct defects in tests and testing procedures.

During the 1960s, the Russell Sage Foundation initiated studies of the social effects of testing. As Orville Brim notes in his preface to the first volume (Goslin, 1963) of a series of reports,

the increasing use of tests in the United States constitutes a change in emphasis from traditional bases for the determination of status, such as race, sex, religion, and order of birth, to a greater reliance on this new criterion, performance on a standardized test of ability.... The source of this change can be traced to a number of factors, including the growing concern for education in America and the greater technological complexity of the society which makes it of increased importance that individuals occupy positions for which they are well suited. It is notable that the growth of standardized testing has come about as a direct result of the application of social science techniques to the solution of a problem; that is, how to select the best-qualified individuals for the various educational and occupational positions in society.

At present virtually nothing is known about what effects the testing movement is having on our society, and on the individuals who are directly affected by test results. The social consequences of standardized testing have not been considered systematically by testers or by social scientists, despite the expanding importance of the movement and the number of decisions being made on the basis of test results. [P. 3]

Goslin's volume set the stage for the social-effects studies by reviewing evidence available at the outset, discussing the possible favorable and unfavorable effects of mental testing on the individual and on the society. Echoing Young's (1958) forecast of a meritocracy of intellect, he stated: "One conceivable consequence of a greater reliance on tested ability as a criterion for the assignment of educational or occupational status is a more rigid class structure based on ability" (p. 191) – an idea that was to be further expanded by Herrnstein (1973). On the basis of extensive interviews, Brim, Neulinger, and Glass (1965) found that adults' estimates of their intelligence were more frequently based on "success in work" than on intelligence test scores; the tests were seen to measure mostly learned knowledge, and to be accurate. These findings, at least, were reassuring in some ways, as were also those of Holmen and Docter (1972), who in a study of the "testing industry and its practices" reported that, "generally, improvement of the instruments has met with more success than improvement of processes at the user level. . . . The good practices at the test-research and development level are not sufficient at this time to offset testing system inadequacies at the test user level" (p. 171). Holmen and Docter were thus more concerned about the uses and misuses of testing than about the theoretical foundations of such testing; nevertheless, they presented a thoughtful account of criticisms of testing that bear on its theoretical aspects.

Public debate grew to orchestral proportions chiefly as a result of a famous (or, some would say, notorious) article by Jensen (1969), which among other things asserted that (a) compensatory education for disadvantaged groups had "apparently" been a failure, (b) various lines of evidence "make it a not unreasonable hypothesis that genetic factors are strongly implicated in the average Negro–white intelligence difference" (p. 82), and (c) the race differences were evident chiefly in "Level II," "conceptual ability," and not in "Level I," "associative ability." In the public outcry against the allegedly racist connotations of these statements, the extensive and generally defensible scholarly review that Jensen offered of the theory of intelligence and its measurement was ignored. Jensen (1972, 1973a, 1973b) has, however, shown remarkable persistence in defending his views on the heredity–environment issue that he almost unwittingly brought to public attention. He has been joined by others who lean to genetic explanations, like Eysenck (1973); the antihereditarian forces have been led by Kamin (1974), an experimental psychologist with no previous involvement in the testing movement, who asserts that "there exist no data which should lead a prudent man to accept the hypothesis that I.Q. test scores are in any degree heritable" (p. 1). The debate at this writing seems to have run its course, although the CBS television program on the "IQ Myth" hosted by Dan Rather (Ravitch, 1975) and the statements made by geneticist Richard Lewontin on a PBS "Nova" program, sponsored by the American Association for the Advancement of Science, to the effect that Jensen's conclusions were racist and scientifically invalid, have certainly added fuel to it; the latest "flap" has been the allegation that widely cited twin data assembled by Sir Cyril Burt were fraudulent (Wade, 1976).[4]

Almost paradoxically, the most recent public concern about mental ability testing has been over the decline, noted by the ETS and the CEEB, of the average SAT scores made by college admissions applicants over the past decade. This concern has expressed itself, in my opinion correctly, not in alarm over a decline in the nation's supply of innate intelligence but in distress about declining standards in schools, decreasing student motivation and effort, and other possible factors in the test-score decline. There is as yet no convincing evidence about the causes of the decline, although a study by Harnischfeger and Wiley (1976) points the finger to curricular changes in schools, among other things.

A comment, written by a younger-generation philosopher of science with a

Marxist orientation, encapsulates some of the issues at the center of attention in present-day debate. Here Putnam (1973) is discussing aspects of psychology that cannot, he feels, be interpreted in a reductionist framework but, rather, must be examined in terms of social organization and societal beliefs:

As an example, let us take a look at the concept of "intelligence" – a concept in vogue with racist social scientists these days. The concept of intelligence is both an ordinary language concept and a technical concept (under the name "IQ"). But the technical concept has been shaped at every point to conform to the politically loaded uses of the ordinary language concept.

The three main features of the ordinary language notion of intelligence are (1) intelligence is hard or impossible to change. When one ascribes an excellent or poor performance to high or low skill there is no implication that this was not acquired or could not be changed; but when one ascribes the same performance to "high intelligence" or "low intelligence" there is the definite implication of something innate, something belonging to the very *essence* of the person involved. (2) Intelligence aids one to succeed, where the criterion of "success" is the criterion of *individual* success, success in *competition*. It is built into the notion that only a few people can have a lot of intelligence. (3) Intelligence aids one no matter what the task. Intelligence is thought of as a single ability which may aid one in doing anything from fixing a car or peeling a banana to solving a differential equation.

These three assumptions together amount to a certain social theory: The theory of elitism. The theory says that there are a few "superior" people who have this one mysterious factor – "intelligence" – and who are good at everything, and a lot of slobs who are not much good at anything.

The IQ test was constructed to preserve the elitist features of the concept in the following way. (1) The IQ test was standardized so that IQ scores would not change much with age, thus preserving the illusion of a measure of something unchanging.... (2) the IQ test was "validated" by selecting the items so that they would predict "success" in college – [and this] is 100% a statistical artifact of this method of validation. (3) The third feature of the ordinary language concept – that IQ is a *single* factor – was harder to ensure. All of the statistical evidence turned out to be against this hypothesis. In fact it turns out that over a hundred different factors contribute to one's score on IQ tests. So one just takes an average, weighting the factors so that they predict success in school, and *calls* the result "*Intelligence* Quotient." And... lo and behold! One has people with "high IQ" and people with "low IQ," "gifted people"... and "dull people."... In short, one recovers the full ordinary language use of the concept – but now with the appearance of "scientific objectivity." [Pp. 141–142]

Along with the misunderstandings and misinterpretations to be found in this excerpt there are points that need serious discussion. One hopes that Putnam does not mean to imply that *all* social scientists who study intelligence are elitist or racist, if indeed definitions of those terms could be agreed upon. One must question his assumption that the validation of intelligence tests is "100% a statistical artifact," as well as his statement that "over a hundred different factors" contribute to one's score on an IQ test. Not even Guilford (1967), whose work Putnam seems to be referring to, would agree with that statement. Also, one finds it hard to square Putnam's idea that the ordinary language concept of intelligence includes whatever it takes to peel a banana with his complaint that intelligence gets defined in terms of scholastic success in college. Nevertheless, central issues raised or implied in Putnam's discussion are the following:

1.   the question whether intelligence is a valid concept, and, if so, whether it corresponds to a "single ability" that generalizes to all kinds of activities, or to a multiplicity of abilities;
2.   the possible genetic bias of intelligence, and its modifiability; and
3.   the relevance of intelligence to scholastic success.

These have in fact been the predominant issues in the history of criticism of the testing movement. There have of course been many others, such as the allegation that the testing "industry" is a sort of cartel that exerts undue control over people's lives, but discussion of such issues is beyond my present scope.

What lessons are to be learned by specialists in mental measurement from public controversies on their subject matter? Cronbach (1975) has written:

Inquiry is best left unrestricted. But the person publishing or popularizing a study does have responsibility for anticipating what his words will suggest to the rightists and leftists, the exploiters and the *descamisados*. He is not irresponsible when his conclusions sway public decisions; he is irresponsible if his careless writing does so.

Our greatest difficulty is our innocence. To spotlight one question, pleased that social science can answer it, often casts closely related questions into a deeper shadow.

The testers of the 1920s could conceive of no risk or error save that of failure to take the tests seriously. The spokesmen for tests, then and recently, were convinced that they were improving social efficiency, not making choices about social philosophy. Their soberly interpreted research did place test interpretation on a more substantial basis. But they did not study the consequences of testing for the social structure – a sociological problem that psychologists do not readily perceive.

The social scientist is trained to think that he does not know all the answers. The social scientist is not trained to realize that he does not know all the questions. And that is why his social influence is not unfailingly constructive. [P. 13]

Let us be a little more specific. The social scientist has the responsibility not only to conduct his research according to the most advanced methodological canons and in the light of the most advanced knowledge that has accumulated in his field, but also to view his work in the broadest possible context of psychological and social theory. Factor analysts and test theorists have not always been mindful of this latter responsibility. There has been a tendency among them, for example, to hypostatize *ability* as something to be taken for granted, and defined merely by the carrying out of certain measurement and statistical operations. They sometimes fail to remind themselves that the concept of ability must be defined in terms of process rather than structure, and that ability is a manifestation or characterization of behavior that must be described and explicated in terms of its antecedents, not only those of a biological character but also those that stem from environmental experiences. Although factor analysts and test theorists need not be specialists in psychological theory, they should be thoroughly grounded in it.

More immediately, what should be the response of measurement specialists to public controversy? Many, of course, will choose to continue doing the things they want to do and are competent to do, and they have a right to do so, in the interests of scientific endeavor. But the interests and competences of others may be such as to allow them to shape their work to provide knowledge or technology that will be responsive to issues raised in current controversies, along lines that I shall suggest shortly.

NEW DIRECTIONS FOR MENTAL TEST RESEARCH

Possibly in part as a result of public controversies, the interest within psychology in the study of mental abilities is today as strong as it ever has been. New texts and treatises, edited volumes, symposia, and other writings on the subject abound (Brody & Brody, 1976; Buss & Poley, 1976; Cancro, 1971; Eysenck, 1973, 1979;

D. Green, 1974; D. Green, Ford, & Flamer, 1971; Humphreys, 1979; Husén, 1975; Jensen, 1980; Resnick, 1976; Royce, 1973; L. Tyler, 1978; R. Tyler & Wolf, 1974; U.S. Office of Personnel Management and ETS, 1980; Vernon, 1979; Willerman, 1979; Willerman & Turner, 1979). A new journal that started publication in 1977, *Applied Psychological Measurement*, proves to be largely devoted to issues about mental abilities, and yet another journal, *Intelligence*, has made its appearance. Psychologists are, or should be, challenged by such statements as one made by the editors of the journal *Cognition* that "there is no theory that unites the higher mental processes, so apparently mental tests are basically uninterpretable," although it is to be noted that these writers are puzzled about "why there is so much interest today in [research in individual differences] among otherwise serious scientists" (Mehler & Bever, 1973, p. 10). One can be assured, in any case, that competent personnel are in place to perform new research in mental ability testing.

What kind of research might such personnel conduct in order to advance knowledge and practice?

First of all, further research is needed on dimensions of individual differences in mental abilities, with particular attention to abilities, skills, and components that can be identified in performance on cognitive skills studied in cognitive psychology (Carroll, 1980b), in relation to more traditional measures of intelligence and scholastic aptitude. Some of these dimensions may be important enough to be included or recognized in new tests of mental abilities. But some of the traditionally established dimensions of intellectual ability need further clarification and, so to say, purification through a more thorough analysis of their makeup in terms of information-processing concepts.

Second, efforts should be devoted to the construction of more finely graded tests of intellectual skills, for example, the criterion-referenced types of tests that were mentioned in Section 2.2 as promising to be of real value in the educational process. To make this possible, some technical aspects of the mathematical and statistical theory of mental tests may need to be further developed, in particular, methods of assuring that item tasks are reasonably univocal in what they measure. Methods of determining test item homogeneity through factor analysis are still cumbersome (Bart, 1978; Muthén, 1978) and do not deal adequately (if at all) with the effects of chance success by guessing on item factor structure. The possibilities of integrating latent trait theory with componential analysis as developed by Sternberg (1977) need to be investigated.

Third, concentrated studies should be made of the development, growth, and enhancement through education and training of intellectual abilities as identified and measured by the more satisfactory tests that might be developed by the program of research suggested here. Much more information is needed on the conditions under which intellectual skills develop, or can be developed through appropriate intervention efforts, in the child, the adolescent, and the adult. This information must include knowledge on the extent to which different skills tend to have limits in their growth, and the extent to which any such limits can be predicted from measurements taken at earlier points.

Fourth, further information is needed on the role of identified intellectual abilities and skills in schooling and in the practical pursuits of life. Except for their purely scientific interest, there is little point in studying intellectual skills along the lines suggested here if they are not relevant to human activities and purposes.

There is every reason to believe that they are indeed relevant, however – at least some of them. Relevance needs to be determined not only through traditionally oriented studies of the predictive validity of tests against training and job criteria (with analysis of "validity generalization" as suggested by Hunter, 1980); it needs to arise also from detailed analyses of the intellectual components of activities in daily life, education, and jobs or professions (McCormick, 1976). For example, we know little about exactly what intellectual skills and operations come into play in, say, building a house, learning high-school algebra, or making a medical diagnosis.

Fifth, a theory of intelligence and cognitive skills needs to be set forth that will take account not only of the findings of studies such as those suggested here but also of more general psychological theories of the determinants of growth and learning. The picture of intellectual abilities that we have at present is chiefly static: we can factor-analyze or componentialize data from tests and experiments made on groups of persons at a given time and identify dimensions and components of individual differences, but such a picture fails to capture the dynamics of mental development and the varied influences that produce the observed differences. Test scores and other individual-difference parameters need to be conceived of as representing points on curves of individual growth (and decline?), rather than as points on a normal distribution in the population.

With these rather visionary ideas in mind, let us look at a number of topics from the standpoint of the way they have been approached in recent years.

THEORIES OF MENTAL ABILITIES

Even the more recent developments in factor analysis that have been reviewed herein – Guilford's structure-of-intellect model and Cattell's hierarchical model that specifies "fluid" and "crystallized" types of intelligence along with a traditional general factor – leave much to be desired in the way of a satisfactory theory of mental ability. Guilford's model is logically flawed, and vague in its definitions. Cattell has come much closer to offering a satisfactory psychological theory, with an elaborate array of special terminology and references to presumed psychological tendencies. Nevertheless, I believe that all this work suffers from several major deficiencies that are not commonly recognized.

First, the "factors" that are identified by the analytic techniques remain hypostatized end products of the research, rather than being considered as provisional intervening variables to be explained according to the dynamics of mental processes, and of antecedent conditions in the individual's constitution and life experiences. There is little *theoretical* interest in any factor, be it "general," "primary," or "group," unless one can offer an account of why the various performances loaded on the factor are correlated or otherwise linked. The finding of a correlation between two performances requires further analysis, because it could arise for any one of a number of reasons. The responses involved might have been learned together (for some quite arbitrary reason), *or* learning one of the performances might be prerequisite to the learning of the other performance, *or* the performances might indeed both depend upon some trait or capacity (like visual acuity or auditory sensitivity, or "thought power," if such exists).

Second, the data used in practically all the studies are mainly scores from tests and measurements that conform to very traditional formats. The tests usually consist of a collection of items that the researcher believed to have some homogeneity, but the actual degree of homogeneity is seldom investigated or even questioned. The scores are obtained by counting the number of items that the examinee has responded to "correctly" within some more or less arbitrary time limit. The responses are obtained at essentially one point of time, there being no effort to assess parameters of learning, memory, problem solving, concept formation, and so on over periods of time. Thus the kinds of materials that go to make up a factor analysis battery are usually limited in their diversity, even though superficially they may appear quite diverse in content. If a "general" factor is found to underlie the test intercorrelations, it is possibly rather narrow in its generality.

In the case of many studies where general factors are found, it would be hard to dismiss the hypothesis that the general factor simply reflects the fact that all its tests depend on the extent to which examinees have somewhere, sometime, mastered and retained the skills required to perform these tests – language skills, skills of attention and concentration, problem-solving algorithms, facts about the number system, and the like. The general factor could then be simply a measure of total learning; it could be attributed to an innate trait only if one could rule out *all* other possible variables that could account for differences: differential exposure to learning opportunities, different styles of child rearing and school instruction, and so on. Thus, when Eysenck (1973, p. 480) cites correlations among Thurstone's PMA tests as giving "the firmest support for the existence of a general factor of intellectual ability," he seems to ignore the possibility that the general factor could arise because people inevitably differ in the richness and variety of the intellectual experiences to which they have been exposed and from which they have profited.

The more general point is that researchers in mental abilities have rarely looked carefully at the measurements they take, tending to regard test scores as givens. This is true of factor analysts, with rare exceptions, and it is also true of test theorists, who seem mainly concerned to put together items, of whatever character and source, into a test that will have certain desirable properties – high reliability, normal score distribution, and so on. Take the matter of speededness in tests: Study after study in the factor-analytic literature, even to the present day, exhibits neglect of the fact, demonstrated by Davidson and Carroll (1945) and Lord (1956), that scores on tests with restricted time limits can be, and usually are, a function of both speed or rate of work and level of mastery. It is likely that the general factor that is often found in these studies is to some extent a function of individual differences in rate of work that enter into the performance of every test. It is encouraging, however, that papers by Furneaux and by White, reprinted in Eysenck's (1973) compilation, have redirected attention to this problem.

What is implied here is that we must make more detailed analysis of tests as complex tasks; I have suggested some ways of doing this (Carroll, 1976). More detailed analysis of tests will not be sufficient, however, unless more research is directed toward finding out how people learn to perform these tasks, and what conditions are favorable to that learning, whether in childhood or later on. Mental ability test scores are normally thought of as predictors of some kind of later learning success; too infrequently are they thought of as dependent variables exhibiting variance that demands explanation. For example, we have few studies in the genre of the one performed by McCullough (1939), who sought to find out how much improvement in certain group intelligence test scores could be produced by a 10-week course in reading. For most of the factors identified by Thurstone (1938a) we have little research evidence about the modifiability of test performances through education, training, or other types of interventions. Marjoribanks (1974) showed that home and school environmental variables predicted much of the variance in the PMA tests.

There are many other things that could be said, but cannot be said here, about ways in which psychometric specialists could reorient their research toward the formulation of a satisfactory theory of mental abilities. The needed technology is highly developed and readily available; what seems to be lacking is a general acceptance and understanding of the task.

THE HEREDITY VERSUS ENVIRONMENT ISSUE

The standard view within the testing profession, and among psychologists generally, has been for a long time that all measured mental abilities are a function of *both* genetic and environmental determinants, the contribution of neither of these being zero. Estimates of the heritability of intelligence range from about 40% to the figure accepted by Jensen (1972) and Eysenck (1973), 80%, unless we accept the figure suggested by Kamin (1974), namely, zero percent. The debates between Kamin and Jensen, and their respective supporters, have been so voluminous and technical that following and evaluating them could require the almost full-time attention of a specialist in genetic psychology. I do not claim to be such a specialist and therefore must rely on reviews and other writings that tend to make me believe that, although Jensen's views must be accepted with some caution, Kamin's claim that the heritability of intelligence cannot be shown to be greater than zero is unsupportable. Fulker (1975), for example, states that Kamin's account "lacks balanced judgment and presents a travesty of the empirical evidence in the field" (p. 519). Sandra Scarr-Salapatek (1976) calls Kamin's book "a disservice both to science and to the advancement of social equality" (p. 99). I am therefore not swayed from accepting the standard view mentioned above, although I find it difficult to accept a heritability estimate as high as 80%.

Before completely dismissing Kamin, however, I should remark that I have always thought that it would be difficult to assess the genetic influences on scores from tests that are so patently functions of specific learning experiences as typical IQ tests, with their burden of verbal and symbolic material. To this extent I would agree with Kamin that "there are no data sufficient for us to reject the hypothesis that differences in the way in which people answer the questions asked by testers are determined by their palpably different life experiences" (p. 176). But then, so would nearly all psychologists, unless Kamin meant that the differences were determined *only* by life experiences. Kamin continues, however:

That conclusion is silent with respect to another possible question. There may well be genetically determined differences among people in their cognitive and intellectual "capacities." To demonstrate this, psychologists would have to develop test instruments that provide adequate measures of such capacities. They have not as yet done this; they have only developed I.Q. tests. This book has been about – and only about – the heritability of I.Q. test scores. [P. 176]

Here Kamin must be corrected: Psychologists have developed more than IQ tests – they have developed tests and procedures for measuring a great variety of mental processes. But it just so happens that most of the relevant evidence on heritability, that is, in studies of twins and other kinds of kinship, is based on IQ scores, or on scores from scholastic aptitude and other tests that are closely similar to standard intelligence tests – for example, data of Loehlin and Nichols (1976) on National Merit Scholarship Qualifying Tests. There are few relevant data based on tests of primary and special abilities, as distinct from traditional intelligence tests (but see Cole, Johnson, Ahern, Kuse, McClearn, Vandenberg, & Wilson, 1979; Humphreys, 1970, 1974; Vandenberg, 1962; Vandenberg & Kuse, 1979). In future studies of heritability, it would be desirable to make more use of tests of differentiable mental abilities, or tests of capacity, learning rate, and the like. Vandenberg (1976) has already claimed to find genetic influences on learning tasks.

Given the difficulty of controlling environments, it will probably be very hard to provide convincing evidence for genetic influences even through twin or kinship studies. Longitudinal studies of twins reared apart are all but impossible. I would attach much more meaning and practical significance to studies designed to determine the actual degree of modifiability of the traits measured by mental tests, and the limits to which abilities could be increased. The technologies of factor analysis and test theory could make a significant contribution to such studies by providing tests and measures with desired characteristics of independence and homogeneity. If we find that tested abilities can be modified, we would know more about environmental effects and would acquire information of practical value in education. If they cannot, we would be inclined to favor a genetic hypothesis about them; we would at least acquire information useful in shaping educational and social policies.

Another promising line of attack on the heredity–environment issue, as it affects mental ability testing, is through studies of growth, using measures of differentiable mental abilities. Previous studies and analyses (Anderson, 1939; Bloom, 1964; Jensen, 1973a; R. Thorndike, 1966) have employed global IQ tests, for the most part. Just before his death, Thurstone (1955) completed a study of growth rates in Primary Mental Abilities, concluding that abilities increase at different rates; this kind of work needs to be followed up. It should be noted, however, that the so-called overlap hypothesis explored by Anderson (1939) and Bloom (1964), whereby ability appears to grow by random increments, is not as favorable to an environmentalist position as its advocates may think; it presents the problem of a "starting endowment," among other things. Also, the overlap hypothesis is only one of numerous models that could be advanced to account for the basic data, that is, correlations between ability measurements at different ages that decrease with increasing time between the age points correlated. Interesting alternative models are presented, for example, by Merz and Stelzl (1973), on the basis of the assumption that there is both accumulation and loss or forgetting of "processed experiences [verarbeitete Erfahrungen]."

THE PROBLEM OF RELEVANCE AND VALIDITY

Scores on mental ability tests tend to have at least moderate correlations with school and college academic grades, with the intellectual level of the occupation that the individual eventually follows, and, sometimes, with the level of success in that occupation. Why is this? The standard view in the profession is that performances on tests are predictive of later performances because they measure characteristics that are also relevant, in some way, to those later performances. In fact, in the development of any aptitude test it is standard procedure to identify, by a "job analysis" of the criterion performance, the kinds of abilities, knowledge, and skill required for successful performance, and then to develop tests to measure those characteristics. The validation of these tests, that is, the demonstration that they correlate significantly with criterion performance, is truly a form of hypothesis testing. There is nothing artifactual in the process, *pace* Putnam (quoted earlier).

There are, however, several weak links in the system. Tests are never perfect predictors, of course; there are both positive and negative errors of prediction, even though on the whole the predictions are correct. But the system depends crucially on the relative stability and unmodifiability of the aptitudes or other characteristics measured by the predictive instruments. One reason that scholastic aptitude tests are successful predictors is that the verbal and mathematical abilities they measure appear to be relatively stable and resistant to improvement, at least in the short term.

In the history of the mental testing movement, it has always been assumed that better predictive devices could be developed by using more exact and advanced knowledge of the nature of human abilities. This in fact has been, and continued to be, one of the practical motives behind the development of factor analysis, in both its methodological and its substantive aspects. It is also a motive for the improvement of test technology through the theory of tests.

Other than suggesting further work along these lines, I have no really new ideas about how the relevance of mental abilities in criterion performances can be better established. Some would even question the worthwhileness of that task. I may, however, point to several useful and in some ways novel ideas about aptitudes that have come to the fore in recent years. In 1963, I proposed to define aptitude by the relative amount of time that an individual would require to learn a task, subject matter, or skill under optimal instructional conditions; I regarded aptitude, defined in this way, as a function of basic traits and capacities as identified in factor analysis (Carroll, 1963). This idea has never been systematically tested, although I applied it (Carroll, 1974) to demonstrate that long-term school achievement data could be interpreted in terms of rates of progress as predicted by an aptitude measure. Bloom (1976) has modified this notion by characterizing aptitudes as "entry behaviors," and claims to have shown that these entry behaviors can be modified – in the sense that, under appropriate instructional conditions, students' rates of learning can be made to become more uniform, with the result that individual differences in terminal performance in a task are much reduced. Whether this idea could be applied in modifying aptitudes for school and college success is a question that should be studied extensively, using all the technology of factor analysis, test theory, and experimental design that is available.

OTHER PROBLEMS

Space does not permit an adequate review and discussion of the relevance of mental test technology to a number of other problems, such as that of possible cultural bias in tests used with minority groups, the decline of scholastic aptitude test scores, or the misuse of tests. To a large extent, such problems may be subsumed under the central problems already discussed. For example, it should be possible to resolve the problem of cultural bias by considering it within the general theory of mental abilities – looking into which traits and behaviors are most affected by cultural differences, investigating ways in which those traits and behaviors can be measured so as to minimize biasing effects, or studying ways of improving those traits or minimizing their effects in criterion performances.

THE THEORY–PRACTICE INTERFACE IN PERSPECTIVE:
A CONCLUDING STATEMENT

The notion that individuals differ in intelligence, mental capacity, or mental ability, and that such differences can be measured and studied scientifically, has been one of the important ideas of Western civilization for more than a century. For better or for worse, it has been particularly influential in the shaping of educational policy and in the actual management and conduct of schooling. The study of the development of this notion affords an interesting case in the history of science. Yet the complexity of the issues and the semantic overloads in the very term *intelligence* make it difficult to frame a discussion that is intended to be as judicious as possible on questions of what intelligence really is, what the relative influences of heredity and of environment on intellectual differences are, and how much mental abilities can be modified by human interventions. In this discussion, I use the term *intelligence* in the broadest and most neutral sense.

When the concept of intelligence as an object of scientific study was introduced by Galton in the late 19th century, it was intimately associated with the notion that intelligence was in large measure an inherited trait. It was natural that Galton's studies of the breeding of plants and animals, and of the inheritance of certain physical characteristics in human beings, led him to believe in the hereditary nature of intelligence. It was probably this belief that caused him to neglect the role of learning and experience in the formation of mental ability.

After the first hesitant and largely unsuccessful attempts of J. M. Cattell and others to measure intellectual traits through simple sensory and perceptual tasks, the concept of intelligence started to have an influence on school practice with Binet's development of procedures for diagnosing the mental conditions and prospects of slow learners. Although Binet did much to define intelligence as the manifestation of cognitive processes, he disavowed interest in the question of genetic origins of intelligence; in fact, he hoped that means could be found for improving the intelligence of mental defectives. Nevertheless, nearly all of those who used Binet's scale or its numerous adaptations were quick to assume that the mental growth rates it measured were greatly influenced by heredity. Increased scientific respectability was lent to the concept of intelligence as an inherited trait by the statistical studies of the Galton–Pearson–Spearman school, and it is significant that the study of intelligence and its measurement was the principal catalyst for the further development of statistical methods generally useful in the biological and behavioral sciences.

The gradual acceptance of a scientific concept of intelligence or mental capacity as a stable and probably inherited trait in individuals of all ages led to its use as a basis for mass testing, first in the selection of military personnel in World War I, and then in the schools. As an alternative to the individually administered Binet-type tests, group-administered paper-and-pencil tests were devised; in this process, subtle and largely unnoticed changes came about in the measurement properties and even the theoretical underpinnings of the tests. As methods for validating and standardizing tests became more refined, intelligence tests were eagerly seized upon by educators as a means of identifying promising students for selective schools and of assigning students to different levels of schoolwork difficulty. Intelligence testing was recognized as a scientific endeavor, and the notion of intelligence entered the public mind as a factor to be considered in the formulation of educational and social policies.

Examination and criticism of the concept of intelligence, either in- or outside professional circles in mental testing, were rarely deep. Outside the profession, debate was often based on misunderstandings of the facts and theories offered by test developers, and in any case a general science of human characteristics and behavior had not progressed sufficiently to serve as a basis for sound public discussion of the implications of mental ability testing. Within the profession, argumentation centered around the generality and relative immutability of intellectual differences, but techniques and models for studying these matters were simplistic, and alternatives or supplements to genetic explanations of data were not thoroughly explored. The claims of behaviorist psychologists, such as Watson, that human behavior is infinitely malleable were disbelieved, or patronizingly tolerated as "the *reductio ad absurdum* of a mindless environmentalism gone rampant" (Kamin, 1974, p. 178). Even in the public mind, environmental determinants of individual differences in intelligence were hard to believe in view of the obvious differences that could be observed among children in the same family, with presumably similar upbringing and advantages, and, at the same time, the obvious similarities in the mental capabilities of identical twins. Meanwhile, Brigham's recantation, in 1930, of his earlier hereditarian views and his development of a concept of "scholastic aptitude" distinct from intelligence were not well understood either by the mental testing profession or by educators in general. Tests perceived to be intelligence tests – regardless of the names given them by their creators – continued to be produced in standard molds, periodically revised, and utilized in great quantities. Perforce, nearly all studies of the relevance of mental ability tests for selecting and assigning students in schools, or of the effects of genetic and environmental factors on test performances, used scores on global tests of intelligence or scholastic aptitude as the variable of chief interest.

Since the middle 1930s, two lines of work have dominated the scientific study of individual differences: factor analysis and test theory. Factor analysis has been concerned with the decomposition of mental abilities into "factors," "primary mental abilities," or similar constructs. Test theory has been concerned with various statistical models and operations designed to produce certain desirable measurement properties in tests or test scores. In retrospect, these two types of scientific endeavor have had both productive and counterproductive features. Factor analysis has had at least the potentiality of facilitating the detailed understanding of what could be measured, and test theory has promoted the more accurate measurement of whatever could be measured. On the negative side, however, in factor analysis there has been too much interest in the identification of factors as end products of the research effort, and too little interest in explaining the factors identified in terms of their composition and antecedents. In test theory, there has been overemphasis on desirable measurement properties without corresponding consideration of what exactly was being measured – a pure trait or a mélange of correlated response tendencies. The two specialties drew apart, each failing to take adequate advantage of the achievements of the other. Both developed in such technically complex directions that their findings and theories became all but unintelligible to the practical test user, and even to many persons honestly seeking to construct better and more valid tests.

Until recently, the scene in intelligence testing was essentially one of stagnation. Buffeted by public criticisms of testing and the shocks of controversy about alleged elitist and even "racist" motives of the testing movement, the profession all but ceased working toward the development of better and more soundly based theories of intelligence and its uses. Some members of the profession believed that they could simply rest on their laurels. The overall decline in the utilization of intelligence tests in schools, the legal constraints on research with human subjects, the general public resistance to testing (for whatever reasons), and the inertia within the profession itself that resulted from complacency about the sufficiency of available methodologies and testing procedures and disquiet about misuses of these procedures made serious inroads on the ability of the testing profession to move forward. Large sectors of the profession were enmeshed in outmoded or at least debatable concepts of human behavior, particularly the assumption that mental abilities are relatively immutable even with extensive and prolonged experience or intervention and, furthermore, that they have almost overpowering genetic determinants.

The current upsurge of interest in the nature of intelligence and mental abilities, as exemplified in the putting together of this handbook, promises great things ahead. A new generation of researchers has appeared, with philosophies and backgrounds that are at least slightly different from those of earlier generations. The theories and tools now available are more favorable to progress.

These developments encourage me in my contention that intelligence, if seen in a proper light, is worthy of continued serious study, and that this study can have increasing relevance to problems of schooling and educational policy. The performances required on many types of mental ability tests – tests of language competence, of ability to manipulate abstract concepts and relationships, of ability to apply knowledge to the solution of problems, and even of the ability to make simple and rapid comparisons of stimuli (as in a test of perceptual speed) – have great and obvious resemblances to performances required in school learning, and indeed in many other fields of human activity. If these performances are seen as based on learned, developed abilities of a rather generalized character, it would frequently be useful to assess the extent to which a person had acquired such abilities. This testing could be for the purpose of determining the extent to which these abilities would need to be improved to prepare the person for further experiences or learning activities, or of determining what kinds and amounts of intervention might be required to effect such improvements. These determinations, however, would have to be based on more exact information than we now have concerning the effects of different types of learning experiences, including observation, practice, instruction, and so forth, on the improvement of these abilities. As matters stand now, we know very little about the parameters governing the growth of such individual attributes as language competence, reasoning ability, and speed of cognitive operations.

Both in the testing community and in the public mind, testing has tended to connote measurement designed chiefly to indicate the limits of an individual's potentiality at a given point, with the implication that those limits will persist. It is reasonable to believe that if researchers could adopt a different stance concerning the nature and role of intellectual abilities, namely, that intellectual skills and competences are a positive force in human activities – powers to be sought and measured – and that their development and application can be enhanced through education and training, many of the difficulties about ability tests that have come up in public discussion and litigation about test bias, the validity of tests for employment selection, and similar matters would be enormously reduced.

Even if performances on mental ability tests have at least some genetic determinants, as they probably do, they undoubtedly have very substantial "environmental" determinants – the environment being conceived of as comprising all the events and conditions outside the individual that can modify growth and change behavior. Environmental variance is for the most part the only kind of variance that we have a right to work with, but we need to know the limits to which, and the conditions under which, environmental manipulations can have positive effects. If the technological apparatus of factor analysis, test theory, and general experimental design can be directed toward the production of this kind of knowledge, and if this knowledge can be expressed and validated in a form that can be used by practitioners – a large order, perhaps, but feasible in principle – then the devoted efforts that have produced this apparatus will eventually have paid off.

NOTES

This chapter is a revised and updated version of a chapter that appeared originally under the title "On the Theory–Practice Interface in the Measurement of Intellectual Abilities," in P. Suppes (Ed.), *Impact of Research on Education: Some Case Studies*, pp. 1–105 (Washington, D.C.: National Academy of Education, 1978). That chapter was prepared as part of a project performed by the National Academy of Education pursuant to a contract (NIE-C-74-0116) from the National Institute of Education, U.S. Department of Health, Welfare, and Education. The present version is printed here by special permission of the National Academy of Education. The opinions expressed are solely those of the author; they do not necessarily reflect positions of either the National Institute of Education or the National Academy of Education.

1 Two years later, the psychologist E. G. Boring (1923), in an article in the *New Republic*, made the not entirely frivolous suggestion that "intelligence is what the tests test" – an admittedly "narrow definition, but a point of departure for a rigorous discussion... until further scientific discussion allows us to extend [it]" (p. 35).

2 The data, surprisingly enough to the modern reader, consisted of scores on tests of discriminative judgments of pitch, light, and weight, along with marks in several academic subjects. Spearman chose these tests after an extensive review of the work of Cattell and others who had attempted to use sensory judgments in measuring intelligence.

3 According to Hearnshaw's (1979) biography of Burt, however, "no evidence was taken [by the committee] from Burt or any other psychologist, and the findings of psychologists were subtly distorted" (pp. 116 ff.).

4 It is now generally agreed that Burt was in fact guilty of deliberate deceit or at least misrepresentation in some of his writings; see Dorfman (1978) and Hearnshaw (1979). Burt's misrepresentations do not, however, undermine the validity of the established knowledge in the fields with which he was concerned.

REFERENCES

Alexander, W. P. Intelligence, concrete and abstract. *British Journal of Psychology, Monograph Supplement*, 1935, 6(19).

American Psychological Association. Technical recommendations for psychological tests and diagnostic techniques. *Psychological Bulletin*, 1954, 51 (Supplement).

American Psychological Association. *Standards for educational and psychological tests and manuals*. Washington, D.C.: Author, 1966.

American Psychological Association. *Standards for educational and psychological tests.* Washington, D.C.: Author, 1974.

Anastasi, A. *Differential psychology: Individual and group differences in behavior* (3rd ed.). New York: Macmillan, 1958.

Anderson, J. E. The limitations of infant and preschool tests in the measurement of intelligence. *Journal of Psychology,* 1939, *8,* 351–379.

Angoff, W. H. (Ed.). *The College Board admissions testing program: A technical report on research and development activities relating to the Scholastic Aptitude Test and Achievement Tests.* New York: College Entrance Examination Board, 1971. (a)

Angoff, W. H. Scales, norms, and equivalent scores. In R. L. Thorndike (Ed.), *Educational measurement* (2nd ed.). Washington, D.C.: American Council on Education, 1971. (b)

Ash, P. The implications of the Civil Rights Act of 1964 for psychological assessment in industry. *American Psychologist,* 1966, *21,* 797–803.

Baker, K. H. Item validity by the analysis of variance: An outline of method. *Psychological Record,* 1939, *3,* 242–248.

Bart, W. M. An empirical inquiry into the relationship between test factor structure and test hierarchical structure. *Applied Psychological Measurement,* 1978, *2,* 331–335.

Baxter, B. (Ed.). American Psychological Association, Task Force on Employment Testing of Minority Groups: Job testing and the disadvantaged. *American Psychologist,* 1969, *24,* 637–650.

Bennett, G. K., Seashore, H. G., & Wesman, A. G. *Differential aptitude tests.* New York: Psychological Corporation, 1947–1975.

Bentler, P. M. Multivariate analysis with latent variables: Causal modeling. *Annual Review of Psychology,* 1980, *31,* 419–456.

Binet, A. Perceptions d'enfants. *Revue Philosophique,* 1890, *30,* 582–611.

Binet, A., & Simon, T. Méthodes nouvelles pour le diagnostic du niveau intellectuel des anormaux. *L'Année Psychologique,* 1905, *11,* 191–244.

Binet, A., & Simon, T. Le développement de l'intelligence chez les enfants. *L'Année Psychologique,* 1908, *14,* 1–94.

Binet, A., & Simon, T. L'intelligence des imbéciles. *L'Année Psychologique,* 1909, *15,* 1–147.

Birnbaum, A. Some latent trait models and their use in inferring an examinee's ability. In F. M. Lord & M. R. Novick, *Statistical theories of mental test scores* (Pt. 5). Reading, Mass.: Addison-Wesley, 1968.

Bloom, B. S. *Stability and change in human characteristics.* New York: Wiley, 1964.

Bloom, B. S. *Human characteristics and school learning.* New York: McGraw-Hill, 1976.

Bôcher, M. *Introduction to higher algebra.* New York: Macmillan, 1907.

Bock, R. D., & Wood, R. Test theory. *Annual Review of Psychology,* 1971, *22,* 193–224.

Boring, E. G. Intelligence as the tests test it. *New Republic,* 1923, *35,* 35–37.

Bridgman, P. W. *The logic of modern physics.* New York: Macmillan, 1927.

Brigham, C.C. Intelligence tests of immigrant groups. *Psychological Review,* 1930, *37,* 158–165.

Brim, O. G., Jr., Neulinger, J., & Glass, D. C. *Experiences and attitudes of American adults concerning standardized intelligence tests* (Tech. Rep. 1 on the Social Consequences of Testing). New York: Russell Sage Foundation, 1965.

Brody, E. B., & Brody, N. *Intelligence: Nature, determinants, and consequences.* New York: Academic Press, 1976.

Brown, W. Some experimental results in the correlation of mental abilities. *British Journal of Psychology,* 1910, *3,* 296–322.

Brown, W., & Thomson, G. *The essentials of mental measurement.* Cambridge: Cambridge University Press, 1921.

Buros, O. K. (Ed.). *The nineteen forty mental measurements yearbook* Highland Park, N.J.: Mental Measurements Yearbook, 1941.

Buros, O. K. (Ed.). *The third mental measurements yearbook.* New Brunswick, N.J.: Rutgers University Press, 1949.

Buros, O. K. (Ed.). *The fourth mental measurements yearbook.* Highland Park, N.J.: Gryphon Press, 1953.

Buros, O. K. (Ed.). *The fifth mental measurements yearbook.* Highland Park, N.J.: Gryphon Press, 1959.

Buros, O. K. (Ed.). *The sixth mental measurements yearbook.* Highland Park, N.J.: Gryphon Press, 1965.

Buros, O. K. (Ed.). *The seventh mental measurements yearbook*. (2 vols.) Highland Park, N.J.: Gryphon Press, 1972.

Buros, O. K. (Ed.). *Tests in print II: An index to tests, test reviews, and the literature on specific tests*. Highland Park, N.J.: Gryphon Press, 1974.

Buros, O. K. (Ed.). *The eighth mental measurements yearbook*. (2 vols.) Highland Park, N.J.: Gryphon Press, 1978.

Burt, C. Factor analysis by sub-matrices. *Journal of Psychology*, 1938, *6*, 339–375.

Burt, C. The education of the young adolescent: Psychological implications of the Norwood Report. *British Journal of Educational Psychology*, 1943, *13*, 126–140.

Buss, A. R., & Poley, W. *Individual differences: Traits and factors*. New York: Gardner Press, 1976.

Campbell, N. R. *An account of the principles of measurement and calculation*. London: Longmans, 1928.

Cancro, R. (Ed.). *Intelligence: Genetic and environmental influences*. New York: Grune & Stratton, 1971.

Carroll, J. B. A factor analysis of verbal abilities. *Psychometrika*, 1941, *6*, 279–307.

Carroll, J. B. The effect of difficulty and chance success on correlations between items or between tests. *Psychometrika*, 1945, *10*, 1–19.

Carroll, J. B. An analytical solution for approximating simple structure in factor analysis. *Psychometrika*, 1953, *18*, 23–38.

Carroll, J. B. The nature of the data, or how to choose a correlation coefficient. *Psychometrika*, 1961, *26*, 347–372.

Carroll, J. B. Factors in verbal achievement. In P. L. Dressel (Ed.), *Proceedings of the Invitational Conference on Testing Problems, 1961*, Princeton, N.J.: Educational Testing Service, 1962.

Carroll, J. B. A model of school learning. *Teachers College Record*, 1963, *64*, 723–733.

Carroll, J. B. Stalking the wayward factors: Review of J. P. Guilford & Ralph Hoepfner, *The analysis of intelligence*. *Contemporary Psychology*, 1972, *17*, 321–324.

Carroll, J. B. Fitting a model of school learning to aptitude and achievement data over grade levels. In D. R. Green (Ed.), *The aptitude–achievement distinction: Proceedings of the Second CTB/McGraw-Hill Conference on Issues in Educational Measurement*. Monterey, Calif.: CTB/McGraw-Hill, 1974.

Carroll, J. B. Psychometric tests as cognitive tasks: A new "Structure of Intellect." In L. B. Resnick (Ed.), *The nature of intelligence*. Hillsdale, N.J.: Erlbaum, 1976.

Carroll, J. B. Individual difference relations in psychometric and experimental cognitive tasks (Report No. 163. Chapel Hill: L. L. Thurstone Laboratory, University of North Carolina, April 1980. (NTIS No. ADA-086 057; ERIC Document Reproduction Service No. ED 191 891) (a)

Carroll, J. B. Measurement of abilities constructs. In United States Office of Personnel Management and Educational Testing Service, *Construct validity in psychological measurement: Proceedings of a Colloquium on Theory and Application in Education and Employment*. Princeton, N.J.: Educational Testing Service, 1980. (b)

Carroll, J. B., & Maxwell, S. E. Individual differences in cognitive abilities. *Annual Review of Psychology*, 1979, *30*, 603–640.

Cattell, J. M. Über die Zeit der Erkennung und Benennung von Schriftzeichen, Bildern und Farben. *Philosophische Studien*, 1885, *2*, 635–650. Translated in A. T. Poffenberger (Ed.), *James McKeen Cattell: Man of science*. Vol. 1: *Psychological research*. Lancaster, Pa.: Science Press, 1947.

Cattell, J. M. Psychometrische Untersuchungen. *Philosophische Studien*, 1886, *3*, 452–492. (a)

Cattell, J. M. The time taken up by cerebral operations. *Mind*, 1886, *11*, 222–242, 377–392, 524–538. (b)

Cattell, J. M. Mental tests and measurements. *Mind*, 1890, *15*, 373–381.

Cattell, J. M., & Farrand, L. Physical and mental measurement of the students of Columbia University. *Psychological Review*, 1896, *3*, 618–648.

Cattell, R. B. The measurement of adult intelligence. *Psychological Bulletin*, 1943, *40*, 153–193.

Cattell, R. B. Higher order factor structures and reticular vs. hierarchical formulae for their interpretation. In C. Banks & P. L. Broadhurst (Eds.), *Studies in psychology*. London: University of London Press, 1965.

Cattell, R. B. *Abilities: Their structure, growth, and action*. Boston: Houghton-Mifflin, 1971.

Chauncey, H., & Dobbin, J. E. *Testing: Its place in education today*. New York: Harper & Row, 1963.

Christie, T., & Griffin, A. The examination achievements of highly selective schools. *Educational Research*, 1970, *12*, 202–208.

Cole, R. E., Johnson, R. C., Ahern, F. M., Kuse, A. R., McClearn, G. E., Vandenberg, S. G., & Wilson, F. R. A family study of memory processes and their relations to cognitive test scores. *Intelligence*, 1979, *3*, 127–138.

College Entrance Examination Board. *Report of the Commission on Tests: I. Righting the balance*. New York: Author, 1970.

Conant, J. B. *The American high school today: A first report to interested citizens*. New York: McGraw-Hill, 1959.

Cooley, W. W., & Lohnes, P. R. *Multivariate procedures for the behavioral sciences*. New York: Wiley, 1962.

Coombs, C. H. A factorial study of number ability. *Psychometrika*, 1941, *6*, 161–189.

Cory, C. H., Rimland, B., & Bryson, R. A. Using computerized tests to measure new dimensions of abilities: An exploratory study. *Applied Psychological Measurement*, 1977, *1*, 101–110.

Crano, W. D., Kenny, D. A., & Campbell, D. T. Does intelligence cause achievement? A cross-lagged panel analysis. *Journal of Educational Psychology*, 1972, *63*, 258–275.

Crawford, A. B. *Incentives to study*. New Haven: Yale University Press, 1929.

Crawford, C. B. Determining the number of interpretable factors. *Psychological Bulletin*, 1975, *82*, 226–237.

Cremin, L. A. *The transformation of the school: Progressivism in American education, 1876–1957*. New York: Knopf, 1961.

Cronbach, L. J. Coefficient alpha and the internal structure of tests. *Psychometrika*, 1951, *16*, 297–334.

Cronbach, L. J. Five decades of public controversy over mental testing. *American Psychologist*, 1975, *30*, 1–14.

Cronbach, L. J., & Furby, L. How should we measure "change" – Or should we? *Psychological Bulletin*, 1970, *74*, 68–80.

Cronbach, L. J., Gleser, G. C., Nanda, H., & Rajaratnam, N. *The dependability of behavioral measurements: Theory of generalizability for scores and profiles*. New York: Wiley, 1972.

Cronbach, L. J., Rajaratnam, N., & Gleser, G. C. Theory of generalizability: A liberation of reliability theory. *British Journal of Mathematical and Statistical Psychology*, 1963, *16*, 137–163.

Davidson, W. M., & Carroll, J. B. Speed and level components in time limit scores: A factor analysis. *Educational and Psychological Measurement*, 1945, *5*, 411–427.

Doolittle, M. H. Method employed in the solution of normal equations and the adjustment of a triangulation. *U.S. Coast and Geodetic Survey Report*, 1878, pp. 115–120.

Dorfman, D. D. The Cyril Burt question: New findings. *Science*, 1978, *201*, 1177–1186.

Downey, M. T. *Carl Campbell Brigham: Scientist and educator*. Princeton, N.J.: Educational Testing Service, 1961.

DuBois, P. H. *A history of psychological testing*. Boston: Allyn & Bacon, 1970.

Dunlap, J. W. The Psychometric Society – Roots and powers. *Psychometrika*, 1942, *7*, 1–8.

Dvorak, B. J. The new USES General Aptitude Test Battery. *Journal of Applied Psychology*, 1947, *31*, 372–376.

Ebbinghaus, H. Über eine neue Methode zur Prüfung geistiger Fähigkeiten und ihre Anwendung bei Schulkindern. *Zeitschrift für angewandte Psychologie*, 1897, *13*, 401–459.

Egan, D. E. Testing based on understanding: Implications from studies of spatial ability. *Intelligence*, 1979, *3*, 1–15.

Ekstrom, R. B. *Cognitive factors: Some recent literature* (Project Rep. 73-30). Princeton, N.J.: Educational Testing Service, 1973.

Ekstrom, R. B., French, J. W., & Harman, H. H. Cognitive factors: Their identification and replication. *Multivariate Behavioral Research Monographs*, 1979, No. 79-2.

Ellison, M. L., & Edgerton, H. A. The Thurstone Primary Mental Abilities Tests and college marks. *Educational and Psychological Measurement*, 1941, *1*, 399–406.

Eysenck, H. J. (Ed.). *The measurement of intelligence*. Baltimore: Williams & Wilkins, 1973.

Eysenck, H. J. (with contributions by D. W. Fulker). *The structure and measurement of intelligence*. New York: Springer-Verlag, 1979.

Fechner, G. *Elemente der Psychophysik*, Leipzig: Breitkopf & Härtel, 1860.

Ferguson, G. A. Item selection by the constant process. *Psychometrika*, 1942, 7, 19–29.

Ferguson, G.A. On transfer and the abilities of man. *Canadian Journal of Psychology*, 1956, 10, 121–131.

Fincher, C. Is the SAT worth its salt? An evaluation of the use of the Scholastic Aptitude Test in the university system of Georgia over a thirteen-year period. *Review of Educational Research*, 1974, 44, 293–305.

Findley, W. G., & Bryan, M. M. *Ability grouping: 1970. Status, impact, and alternatives*. Athens: University of Georgia, Center for Educational Improvement, 1971.

Findley, W., & Bryan, M. *The pros and cons of ability grouping*. Bloomington, Ind.: Phi Delta Kappa Educational Foundation, 1975.

Finney, D. J. The application of probit analysis to the results of mental tests. *Psychometrika*, 1944, 9, 31–39.

Fisher, R. A. *Statistical methods for research workers*. Edinburgh & London: Oliver & Boyd, 1925.

Flanagan, J. C. (Ed.). *The aviation psychology program in the Army Air Forces* (Rep. 1, Army Air Forces Aviation Psychology Program Research Reports). Washington, D.C.: U.S. Government Printing Office, 1948.

Flanagan, J. C. *Flanagan aptitude classification tests*. Chicago: Science Research Associates, 1951–1960.

Flanagan, J. C. Truman Lee Kelley [obituary notice]. *Psychometrika*, 1961, 26, 343–345.

Flanagan, J. C., & Cooley, W. W. *Project talent: One year follow-up studies*. Pittsburgh: University of Pittsburgh, Project Talent, 1966.

Flanagan, J. C., Dailey, J. T., Shaycoft, M. F., Gorham, W. A., Orr, D. B., & Goldberg, I. *Design for a study of American youth, 1: The talents of American youth*. Boston: Houghton-Mifflin, 1962.

Flanagan, J. C., & Jung, S. M. *Progress in education: A sample survey, 1960–1970*. Palo Alto, Calif.: American Institutes for Research, 1971.

French, J. L. (Reviser). *Henmon-Nelson Tests of Mental Ability, 1973 revision*. Boston: Houghton-Mifflin, 1973.

French, J. W. The description of aptitude and achievement tests in terms of rotated factors. *Psychometric Monographs*, 1951, 5.

French, J. W. *Kit of selected tests for reference aptitude and achievement factors*. Princeton, N.J.: Educational Testing Service, 1954.

French, J. W., Ekstrom, R. B., & Price, L. A. *Kit of reference tests for cognitive factors*. Princeton, N.J.: Educational Testing Service, 1963.

Fulker, D. W. Review of Kamin's *The science and politics of I.Q. American Journal of Psychology*, 1975, 88, 505–519.

Gaito, J. Measurement scales and statistics: Resurgence of an old misconception. *Psychological Bulletin*, 1980, 87, 564–567.

Galton, F. *Hereditary genius: An inquiry into its laws and consequences*. New York: Appleton, 1869.

Galton, F. *Inquiries into human faculty and its development*. London: Macmillan, 1883.

Galton, F. Some results of the Anthropometric Laboratory. *Journal of the Anthropological Institute*, 1885, 14, 275–287.

Galton, F. Family likeness in stature. *Proceedings of the Royal Society of London*, 1886, 40, 42–63.

Galton, F. Co-relations and their measurement, chiefly from anthropometric data. *Proceedings of the Royal Society of London*, 1889, 45, 135–145.

Goddard, H. H. The Binet and Simon tests of intellectual capacity. *The Training School*, 1908, 5, 3–9.

Gordon, E. W., & Wilkerson, D. A. *Compensatory education for the disadvantaged*. New York: College Entrance Examination Board, 1966.

Goslin, D. A. *The search for ability: Standardized testing in social perspective*. New York: Russell Sage Foundation, 1963.

Green, B. F., Jr. The computer revolution in psychometrics. *Psychometrika*, 1966, 31, 437–445.

Green, D. R. (Ed.). *The aptitude–achievement distinction: Proceedings of the Second CTB/McGraw-Hill Conference on Issues in Educational Measurement*. Monterey, Calif.: CTB/McGraw-Hill, 1974.

Green, D. R., Ford, M. P., & Flamer, G. B. (Eds.). *Measurement and Piaget*. New York: McGraw-Hill, 1971.

Guilford, J. P. (Ed.). *Printed classification tests* (Res. Rep. 5, Army Air Forces, Aviation Psychology Program). Washington, D.C.: Government Printing Office, 1947.

Guilford, J. P. The structure of intellect. *Psychological Bulletin*, 1956, *53*, 267–293.

Guilford, J. P. *The nature of human intelligence*. New York: McGraw-Hill, 1967.

Guilford, J. P., & Hoepfner, R. *The analysis of intelligence*. New York: McGraw-Hill, 1971.

Guilford, J. P., & Zimmerman, W. S. *Guilford–Zimmerman Aptitude Survey*. Orange, Calif.: Sheridan Psychological Services, 1947–1956.

Gulliksen, H. *Theory of mental tests*. New York: Wiley, 1950.

Guttman, L. Multiple rectilinear prediction and the resolution into components. *Psychometrika*, 1940, *5*, 75–99.

Guttman, L. The quantification of a class of attributes: A theory and method for scale construction. In P. Horst (Ed.), *The prediction of personal adjustment*. New York: Social Science Research Council, 1941.

Guttman, L. Image theory for the structure of quantitative variates. *Psychometrika*, 1953, *18*, 277–296.

Guttman, L. Reliability formulas for non-completed or speeded tests. *Psychometrika*, 1955, *20*, 113–124.

Hakstian, A. R., & Cattell, R. B. *Comprehensive ability battery*. Champaign, Ill: Institute for Personality and Ability Testing, 1976.

Hakstian, A. R., & Cattell, R. B. Higher-stratum ability structures on a basis of twenty primary abilities. *Journal of Educational Psychology*, 1978, *70*, 657–669.

Harman, H. H., Ekstrom, R. B., & French, J. W. *Kit of factor reference cognitive tests*. Princeton, N.J.: Educational Testing Service, 1976.

Harnischfeger, A., & Wiley, D. E. *Achievement test score decline: Do we need to worry?* Saint Louis, Mo.: CEMREL, 1976.

Hearnshaw, L. S. *Cyril Burt: Psychologist*. Ithaca, N.Y.: Cornell University Press, 1979.

Helmholtz, H. von. Zählen und Messen, erkenntniss-theoretisch betrachtet. In H. von Helmholtz, *Wissenschaftliche Abhandlungen, III*. Leipzig: Barth, 1885.

Henmon, V. A. C., & Nelson, M. J. *Henmon–Nelson test of mental ability*. Boston: Houghton-Mifflin, 1932–1935.

Herrnstein, R. I. *I.Q. in the meritocracy*. Boston: Little, Brown, 1973.

Hills, J. R. Use of measurement in selection and placement. In R. L. Thorndike (Ed.), *Educational measurement* (2nd ed.). Washington, D.C.: American Council on Education, 1971.

Hofstadter, R. *Social Darwinism in American thought*. Philadelphia: University of Pennsylvania Press, 1944.

Hölder, L. O. Die Axiome der Quantität und die Lehre vom Mass. *Berichte, Sächsische Akademie der Wissenschaften, Math. nat. Klasse*, 1901, *53*, 1–64.

Holmen, M. G., & Docter, R. *Educational and psychological testing: A study of the industry and its practices*. New York: Russell Sage Foundation, 1972.

Holzinger, K. J., & Harman, H. H. Comparison of two factorial analyses. *Psychometrika*, 1938, *3*, 45–60.

Horn, J. L. On subjectivity in factor analysis. *Educational and Psychological Measurement*, 1967, *27*, 811–820.

Horn, J. L. Organization of abilities and the development of intelligence. *Psychological Review*, 1968, *75*, 242–259.

Horn, J. L. Human abilities: A review of research and theory in the early 1970's. *Annual Review of Psychology*, 1976, *27*, 437–485.

Horn, J. L. Human ability systems. In P. B. Baltes (Ed.), *Life-span development and behavior* (Vol. 1). New York: Academic Press, 1978.

Horn, W. O. *International Primary Factors Test Battery*. Stevens Point, Wis.: International Tests, 1973.

Horst, P. Relations among *m* sets of measures. *Psychometrika*, 1961, *26*, 129–149.

Hotelling, H. Analysis of a complex of statistical variables into principal components. *Journal of Educational Psychology*, 1933, *24*, 417–441, 498–520.

Hotelling, H. The most predictable criterion. *Journal of Educational Psychology*, 1935, *26*, 139–142.

Hoyt, C. Test reliability estimated by analysis of variance. *Psychometrika*, 1941, *6*, 153–160.

Humphreys, L. G. Analytical approach to the correlation between related pairs of subjects on psychological tests. *Psychological Bulletin,* 1970, *74,* 149–152.

Humphreys, L. G. The misleading distinction between aptitude and achievement tests. In D. R. Green (Ed.), *The aptitude–achievement distinction: Proceedings of the Second CTB/McGraw-Hill Conference on Issues in Educational Measurement.* Monterey, Calif.: CTB/McGraw-Hill, 1974.

Humphreys, L. G. The construct of general intelligence. *Intelligence,* 1979, *3,* 105–120.

Hunt, E. Varieties of cognitive power. In L. B. Resnick (Ed.), *The nature of intelligence.* Hillsdale, N.J.: Erlbaum, 1976.

Hunt, E., Frost, N., & Lunneborg, C. Individual differences in cognition: A new approach to intelligence. In G. Bower (Ed.), *Advances in learning and motivation* (Vol. 7). New York: Academic Press, 1973.

Hunt, J. M. *Intelligence and experience.* New York: Ronald Press, 1961.

Hunter, J. E. Construct validity and validity generalization. In United States Office of Personnel Management and Educational Testing Service, *Construct validity in psychological measurement: Proceedings of a Colloquium on Theory and Application in Education and Employment.* Princeton,N.J.: Educational Testing Service, 1980.

Husén, T. The concept of intelligence in applied psychology: Some introductory observations. *International Review of Applied Psychology,* 1975, *24,* 83–84.

Jäger, A. O. *Dimensionen der Intelligenz.* Göttingen: Verlag für Psychologie, Hogrefe, 1967.

Jencks, C., Smith, M., Acland, H., Bane, M. J., Cohen, D., Gintis, H., Heyns, B., & Michelson, S. *Inequality: A reassessment of the effect of family and schooling in America.* New York: Basic Books, 1972.

Jensen, A. R. How much can we boost IQ and scholastic achievement? *Harvard Educational Review,* 1969, *39,* 1–123.

Jensen, A. R. *Genetics and education.* New York: Harper & Row, 1972.

Jensen, A. R. *Educability and group differences.* London: Methuen, 1973. (a)

Jensen, A. R. *Educational differences.* London, Methuen, 1973. (b)

Jensen, A. R. *Bias in mental testing.* New York: Free Press, 1980.

Jones, L. V. The nature of measurement. In R. L. Thorndike (Ed.), *Educational measurement* (2nd ed.). Washington, D.C.: American Council on Education, 1971.

Jöreskog, K. G., & Lawley, D. N. New methods in maximum likelihood factor analysis. *British Journal of Mathematical and Statistical Psychology,* 1968, *21,* 85–96.

Kaiser, H. F. The varimax criterion of analytic rotation in factor analysis. *Psychometrika,* 1958, *2,* 187–200.

Kaiser, H. F. Varimax solution for Primary Mental Abilities. *Psychometrika,* 1960, *25,* 153–158.

Kaiser, H. F., & Caffrey, J. Alpha factor analysis. *Psychometrika,* 1965, *30,* 1–14.

Kamin, L. J. *The science and politics of I.Q.* Potomac, Md.: Erlbaum, 1974.

Keliher, A. V. *A critical study of homogeneous grouping* (No. 452, Contributions to Education). New York: Columbia University, Teachers College, 1931.

Kelley, T. L. *Statistical method.* New York: Macmillan, 1923.

Kelley, T. L. *The interpretation of educational measurements.* Yonkers-on-Hudson, N.Y.: World Book, 1927.

Kelley, T. L. *Crossroads in the mind of man: A study of differentiable mental abilities.* Stanford, Calif.: Stanford University Press, 1928.

Krantz, D. H., Luce, R. D., Suppes, P., & Tversky, A. *Foundations of measurement* (Vol. 1). New York: Academic Press, 1971.

Kuder, G. F., & Richardson, M. W. The theory of the estimation of test reliability. *Psychometrika,* 1937, *2,* 151–160.

Labov, W. The logic of nonstandard speech. *Georgetown University Monographs on Languages and Linguistics,* 1969, *22,* 1–43.

Lambert, C. M. Symposium on education of pupils for different types of secondary schools. VII: A survey of ability and interest at the stage of transfer. *British Journal of Educational Psychology,* 1949, *19,* 67–81.

Lamke, T. A., & Nelson, M. J. *The Henmon–Nelson Tests of Mental Ability* (Rev. ed.). Boston: Houghton-Mifflin, 1957–1958.

Levy, P. On the relation between test theory and psychology. In P. Kline (Ed.), *New approaches in psychological measurement.* London & New York: Wiley, 1973.

Linden, K. W., & Linden, J. D. *Modern mental measurement: A historical perspective.* Boston: Houghton-Mifflin, 1968.

Linn, R. L. A Monte Carlo approach to the number of factors problem. *Psychometrika*, 1968, *33*, 37–72.

Loehlin, J. C., & Nichols, R. C. *Heredity, environment, and personality: A study of 850 sets of twins*. Austin: University of Texas Press, 1976.

Loevinger, J. A systematic approach to the construction and evaluation of tests of ability. *Psychological Monographs*, 1947, *61*(4).

Loevinger, J. The attenuation paradox in test theory. *Psychological Bulletin*, 1954, *51*, 493–504.

Loevinger, J., Gleser, G. C., & DuBois, P. H. Maximizing the discriminating power of a multiple-score test. *Psychometrika*, 1953, *18*, 309–317.

Lohman, D. F. *Spatial ability: Individual differences in speed and level* (Technical Report No. 9). Stanford, Calif.: Stanford University, School of Education, Aptitude Research Project, October 1979.

Lord, F. M. A theory of test scores. *Psychometric Monographs*, 1952, 7.

Lord, F. M. Some perspectives on "the attenuation paradox" in test theory. *Psychological Bulletin*, 1955, *52*, 505–510.

Lord, F. M. A study of speed factors in tests and academic grades. *Psychometrika*, 1956, *21*, 31–50.

Lord, F. M. A theoretical study of two-stage testing. *Psychometrika*, 1971, *36*, 227–242.

Lord, F. M., & Novick, M. R. *Statistical theories of mental test scores*. Reading, Mass.: Addison-Wesley, 1968.

Loretan, J. O. The decline and fall of group intelligence testing. *Teachers College Record*, 1965, *67*, 10–17.

Lumsden, J. Test theory. *Annual Review of Psychology*, 1976, *27*, 251–280.

Marjoribanks, K. Environment as a threshold variable: An examination. *Journal of Educational Research*, 1974, *67*, 610–616.

Maruyama, G., & McGarvey, B. Evaluating causal models: An application of maximum-likelihood analysis of structural equations. *Psychological Bulletin*, 1980, *87*, 502–512.

McClure, W. E. The status of psychological testing in large city public school systems. *Journal of Applied Psychology*, 1930, *14*, 486–496.

McCormick, E. J. Job and task analysis. In M. D. Dunnette (Ed.), *Handbook of industrial and organizational psychology*. Chicago: Rand McNally, 1976.

McCullough, C. M. Relationship between intelligence and gains in reading ability. *Journal of Educational Psychology*, 1939, *30*, 688–692.

McDonald, R. P. A general approach to nonlinear factor analysis. *Psychometrika*, 1962, *27*, 397–415.

McNemar, Q. Lost: Our intelligence? Why? *American Psychologist*, 1964, *19*, 871–882.

Mehler, J., & Bever, T. G. Editorial. *Cognition*, 1973, *2*, 7–11.

Meili, R. Die faktorenanalytische Interpretation der Intelligenz. *Schweizerische Zeitschrift für Psychologie*, 1964, *23*, 135–155.

Merz, F., & Stelzl, I. Modellvorstellungen über die Entwicklung der Intelligenz in Kindheit und Jugend. *Zeitschrift für Entwicklungspsychologie und Pädagogische Psychologie*, 1973, *5*, 153–166.

Monroe, W. S. Educational measurement in 1920 and 1945. *Journal of Educational Research*, 1945, *38*, 334–340.

Mort, P. R., & Featherstone, W. B. The general uses of psychological tests. *Review of Educational Research*, 1932, *5*, 300–307.

Muthén, B. Contributions to factor analysis of dichotomous variables. *Psychometrika*, 1978, *43*, 551–559.

Norwood, C. *Curriculum and examinations in secondary schools: Report of the Committee of the Secondary School Examinations Council appointed by the President of the Board of Education in 1941*. London: H. M. Stationery Office, 1943.

Novick, M. R. The axioms and principal results of classical test theory. *Journal of Mathematical Psychology*, 1966, *3*, 1–18.

Otis, A. S. An absolute point scale for the group measure of intelligence. *Journal of Educational Psychology*, 1918, *9*, 238–261.

Otis, A. S. The Otis Correlation Chart. *Journal of Educational Research*, 1923, *8*, 440–448.

Pearson, K. *The grammar of science*. London: Walter Scott, 1892.

Pearson, K. Contributions to the mathematical theory of evolution. I: On the dissection of asymmetrical frequency curves. *Philosophical Transactions* (Ser. A), 1894, *185*, 71–110.

Pearson, K. Mathematical contributions to the theory of evolution. III. Regression, heredity and panmixia. *Philosophical Transactions* (Ser. A), 1896, *187*, 253–318.

Pellegrino, J. W., & Glaser, R. Cognitive correlates and components in the analysis of individual differences. *Intelligence*, 1979, *3*, 187–214.

Pellegrino, J. W., & Glaser, R. Components of inductive reasoning. In R. E. Snow, P-A. Federico, & W. E. Montague (Eds.), *Aptitude, learning, and instruction: Cognitive process analyses*. Hillsdale, N.J.: Erlbaum, 1980.

Peterson, J. *Early conceptions and tests of intelligence*. Yonkers-on-Hudson: World Book, 1925.

Pintner, R. *Intelligence testing: Methods and results* (2nd ed.). New York: Henry Holt, 1931.

Powers, D. E., & Alderman, D. L. The use, acceptance, and impact of *Taking the SAT–A test familiarization booklet* (Report RDR-78-79, No. 6, and RR-79-3). Princeton, N.J.: Educational Testing Service, February 1979.

Pruzek, R. M., & Coffman, W. E. *A factor analysis of the mathematical sections of the Scholastic Aptitude Test* (College Entrance Examination Board Research and Development Rep. 65-6, No. 10, and Research Bulletin 66-12). Princeton, N.J.: Educational Testing Service, 1966.

Putnam, H. Reductionism and the nature of psychology. *Cognition*, 1973, *2*, 131–146.

Rankin, P. T. Pupil classification and grouping. *Review of Educational Research*, 1931, *1*, 200–230.

Rasch, G. *Probabilistic models for some intelligence and attainment tests*. Copenhagen: Nielson & Lydiche, 1960.

Ravitch, D. The I.Q. Myth – Criticisms, complexities, contradictions. *New York Times*, April 20, 1975, Sec. D. p. 29.

Rayburn, W. G., & Hayes, E. J. Compensatory education: Effective or ineffective? *Journal of Counseling Psychology*, 1975, *22*, 523–528.

Resnick, L. B. (Ed.). *The nature of intelligence*. Hillsdale, N.J.: Erlbaum, 1976.

Richardson, S. C. Some evidence relating to the validity of selection for grammar schools. *British Journal of Educational Psychology*, 1956, *126*, 15–24.

Royce, J. R. (Ed.). *Multivariate analysis and psychological theory*. London & New York: Academic Press, 1973.

Rucci, A. J., & Tweney, R. D. Analysis of variance and the "second discipline" of scientific psychology: A historical account. *Psychological Bulletin*, 1980, *87*, 166–184.

Saunders, D. R. *An analytic method for rotation to orthogonal simple structure* (Research Bulletin 53-10). Princeton, N.J.: Educational Testing Service, 1953.

Scarr-Salapatek, S. Review of Kamin's *The science and politics of I.Q. Contemporary Psychology*, 1976, *21*, 98–99.

Schmid, J., & Leiman, J. M. The development of hierarchical factor solutions. *Psychometrika*, 1957, *22*, 53–61.

Sharp, S. E. Individual psychology: A study in psychological method. *American Journal of Psychology*, 1898–1899, *10*, 329–391.

Simon, B. *The politics of educational reform, 1920–1940*. London: Lawrence & Wishart, 1974.

Slack, W. V., & Porter, D. The Scholastic Aptitude Test: A critical appraisal. *Harvard Educational Review*, 1980, *50*, 154–175.

Smith, B. O. *Logical aspects of educational measurement*. New York: Columbia University Press, 1938.

Spearman, C. The proof and measurement of association between two things. *American Journal of Psychology*, 1904, *15*, 72–101. (a)

Spearman, C. "General intelligence," objectively determined and measured. *American Journal of Psychology*, 1904, *15*, 201–293. (b)

Spearman, C. Correlation calculated from faulty data. *British Journal of Psychology*, 1910, *3*, 71–295.

Spearman, C. *The nature of "intelligence" and the principles of cognition*. London: Macmillan, 1923.

Spearman, C. *The abilities of man*. London: Macmillan, 1927.

Spearman, C., & Jones, L. W. *Human ability: A continuation of "The abilities of man."* London: Macmillan, 1950.

Stanley, J. C. Analysis of unreplicated three-way classifications, with applications to rater bias and trait independence. *Psychometrika*, 1961, *26*, 205–219.

Stanley, J. C. Reliability. In R. L. Thorndike (Ed.), *Educational measurement* (2d ed.). Washington, D.C.: American Council on Education, 1971.

Stanley, J. C., & Wang, M. D. Weighting test items and test-item options: An overview of the analytical and empirical literature. *Educational and Psychological Measurement*, 1970, *30*, 21–35.

Stern, W. *Psychologische Methoden der Intelligenz-Prüfung*. Leipzig: Barth, 1912.

Sternberg, R. J. *Intelligence, information processing, and analogical reasoning: The componential analysis of human abilities*. Hillsdale, N.J.: Erlbaum, 1977.

Stevens, S. S. On the theory of scales of measurement. *Science*, 1946, *103*, 667–680.

Stevens, S. S. Mathematics, measurement, and psychophysics. In S. S. Stevens (Ed.), *Handbook of experimental psychology*. New York: Wiley, 1951.

Sullivan, E. T. Psychographic representation of results of the Stanford Revision of the Binet – Simon tests. *Journal of Delinquency*, 1926, *10*, 284–285.

Sullivan, E. T., Clark, W. W., & Tiegs, E. W. *California Test of Mental Maturity*. Los Angeles: California Test Bureau, 1936–1939.

Suppes, P., & Zinnes, J. L. Basic measurement theory. In R. D. Luce, R. R. Bush, & E. Galanter (Eds.), *Handbook of mathematical psychology* (Vol. 1). New York: Wiley, 1963.

Svensson, N. *Ability grouping and scholastic achievement: Report on a five-year follow-up study in Stockholm*. Uppsala: Almqvist & Wiksell, 1962.

Tatsuoka, M. M. Multivariate analysis in educational research. *Review of Research in Education*, 1973, *1*, 273–319.

Taylor, C. W. A factorial study of fluency in writing. *Psychometrika*, 1947, *12*, 239–262.

Taylor, W. L. "Cloze procedure": A new tool for measuring readability. *Journalism Quarterly*, 1953, *30*, 415–433.

Terman, L. M. *The measurement of intelligence*. Boston: Houghton-Mifflin, 1916.

Terman, L. M., & Merrill, M. A. *Measuring intelligence*. Boston: Houghton-Mifflin, 1937.

Terman, L. M., & Merrill, M. A. *Stanford–Binet intelligence scale*. Boston: Houghton-Mifflin, 1960.

Thomson, S., & DeLeonibus, N. *Guidelines for improving SAT scores*. Reston, Va.: National Association of Secondary School Principals, 1978.

Thorndike, E. L. *Introduction to the theory of mental and social measurements*. New York: Columbia University, Teachers College, 1904.

Thorndike, E. L., et al. Intelligence and its measurement: A symposium. *Journal of Educational Psychology*, 1921, *12*, 123–147, 195–216, 271–275.

Thorndike, E. L., Bregman, E. O., Cobb, M. V., Woodyard, E., & the staff of the Division of Psychology of the Institute of Educational Research of Teachers College, Columbia University. *The measurement of intelligence*. New York: Columbia University, Teachers College, Bureau of Publications, 1927.

Thorndike, R. L. *Personnel selection: Test and measurement techniques*. New York: Wiley, 1949.

Thorndike, R. L. Intellectual status and intellectual growth. *Journal of Educational Psychology*, 1966, *57*, 121–127.

Thorndike, R. L., & Hagen, E. *10,000 careers*. New York: Wiley, 1959.

Thurstone, L. L. *The nature of intelligence*. London & New York: Harcourt, Brace, 1924.

Thurstone, L. L. *Fundamentals of statistics*. New York: Macmillan, 1925. (a)

Thurstone, L. L. A method of scaling psychological and educational tests. *Journal of Educational Psychology*, 1925, *16*, 433–451. (a)

Thurstone, L. L. A law of comparative judgment. *Psychological Review*, 1927, *34*, 273–286.

Thurstone, L. L. The absolute zero in intelligence measurement. *Psychological Review*, 1928, *35*, 175–197.

Thurstone, L. L. *The reliability and validity of tests*. Ann Arbor, Mich.: Edwards Brothers, 1931. (a)

Thurstone, L. L. Multiple factor analysis. *Psychological Review*, 1931, *38*, 406–427. (b)

Thurstone, L. L. *The vectors of the mind*. Chicago: University of Chicago Press, 1935.

Thurstone, L. L. Primary mental abilities. *Psychometric Monographs*, 1938, *1*. (a)

Thurstone, L. L. *Tests for primary mental abilities: Experimental edition, 1938*. Washington, D.C.: American Council on Education, 1938. (b)

Thurstone, L. L. Current issues in factor analysis. *Psychological Bulletin*, 1940, *37*, 189–236.

Thurstone, L. L. *A factorial study of perception*. Chicago: University of Chicago Press, 1944.

Thurstone, L. L. *Multiple factor analysis*. Chicago: University of Chicago Press, 1947.

Thurstone, L. L. *The differential growth of mental abilities* (Psychometric Laboratory Rep. No. 14). Chapel Hill: University of North Carolina, 1955.

Thurstone, L. L., & Thurstone, T. G. The 1935 psychological examination. *Educational Record*, 1936, *17*, 296–317.

Thurstone, L. L., & Thurstone, T. G. *SRA Primary Mental Abilities, 1962 Edition*. Chicago: Science Research Associations, 1949–1965.

Thurstone, L. L., Thurstone, T. G., & Adkins, D. C. The 1938 psychological examination. *Educational Record*, 1939, *20*, 263–300.

Toops, H. A. Eliminating the pitfalls in solving correlation – A printed correlation form. *Journal of Experimental Psychology*, 1921, *4*, 434–446.

Toops, H. A. The status of university intelligence tests in 1923–24. *Journal of Educational Psychology*, 1926, *17*, 23–36; 110–124.

Tucker, L. R. Maximum validity of a test with equivalent items. *Psychometrika*, 1946, *11*, 1–13.

Tucker, L. R. Implications of factor analysis of three-way matrices for measurement of change. In C. W. Harris (Ed.), *Problems in measuring change*. Madison: University of Wisconsin Press, 1963.

Tuddenham, R. D. The nature and measurement of intelligence. In L. Postman (Ed.), *Psychology in the making*. New York: Knopf, 1962.

Tyler, L. E. *Individuality: Human possibilities and personal choice in the psychological development of men and women*. San Francisco: Jossey-Bass, 1978,

Tyler, R. W., & Wolf, R. M. (Eds.). *Crucial issues in testing*. Berkeley, Calif.: McCutchan, 1974.

United States Office of Personnel Management and Educational Testing Service. *Construct validity in psychological measurement: Proceedings of a Colloquium on Theory and Application in Education and Employment*. Princeton, N.J.: Educational Testing Service, 1980.

Vandenberg, S. G. The hereditary abilities study: Hereditary components in a psychological test battery. *American Journal of Human Genetics*, 1962, *14*, 220–237.

Vandenberg, S. G. Genetic factors in human learning. *Educational Psychologist*, 1976, *12*, 59–63.

Vandenberg, S. G., & Kuse, A. R. *Genetic determinants of spatial ability*. In M. A. Wittig & A. C. Petersen (Eds.), *Sex-related differences in cognitive functioning*. New York: Academic Press, 1979.

Vernon, P. E. *The structure of human abilities* (2nd ed.). London: Methuen, 1961.

Vernon, P. E. *Intelligence: Heredity and environment*. San Francisco: W. H. Freeman, 1979.

Wade, N. I.Q. and heredity: Suspicion of fraud beclouds classic experiment. *Science*, 1976, *194*, 916–919.

Walker, D. A. Answer pattern and score scatter in tests and examinations. *British Journal of Psychology*, 1931, *22*, 73–86.

Walker, D. A. Answer pattern and score scatter in tests and examinations. *British Journal of Psychology*, 1936, *26*, 301–308.

Walker, D. A. Answer pattern and score scatter in tests and examinations. *British Journal of Psychology*, 1940, *30*, 248–260.

Walker, H. M. *Studies in the history of statistical method*. Baltimore: Williams & Wilkins, 1929.

Warren, R., & Mendenhall, R. M. *The Mendenhall–Warren–Hollerith correlation method*. New York: Columbia University Statistics Bureau, 1929.

Werdelin, I. *Geometrical ability and the space factor in boys and girls*. Lund, Sweden: Gleerups, 1961.

Werts, C. E., & Linn, R. L. Path analysis: Psychological examples. *Psychological Bulletin*, 1970, *74*, 193–212.

Wherry, R. J. A modification of the Doolittle method: A logarithmic solution. *Journal of Educational Psychology*, 1932, *23*, 455–459.

Wherry, R. J., & Gaylord, R. H. The concept of test and item reliability in relation to factor pattern. *Psychometrika*, 1943, *8*, 247–264.

Wherry, R. J., & Winer, B. J. A method for factoring large numbers of items. *Psychometrika*, 1953, *18*, 161–179.

Whipple, G. M. *Manual of mental and physical tests*. Baltimore: Warwick & York, 1910.

Willerman, L. *The psychology of individual and group differences*. San Francisco: W. H. Freeman, 1979.

Willerman, L., & Turner, R. G. (Eds.). *Readings about individual and group differences*. San Francisco: W. H. Freeman, 1979.

Wissler, C. The correlation of mental and physical traits. *Psychological Monographs*, 1901, 3, 1–62.

Wolfle, D. Factor analysis to 1940. *Psychometric Monographs*, 1940, 3.

Wolfle, L. M. Strategies of path analysis. *American Educational Research Journal*, 1980, 17, 183–209.

Wood, B. D. *Measurement in higher education*. Yonkers: World Book, 1923.

Wright, S. Correlation and causation. *Journal of Agricultural Research*, 1921, 20, 557–585.

Wundt, W. *Beiträge zur Theorie der Sinneswahrnehmung*. Leipzig & Heidelberg: Winter, 1862.

Yerkes, R. M. (Ed.). Psychological examining in the United States Army. *Memoirs of the National Academy of Sciences*, 1921, 15.

Young, M. *The rise of the meritocracy, 1870–2033: An essay on education and equality*. London: Thames & Hudson, 1958.

Yule, G. U. On the theory of correlation. *Journal of the Royal Statistical Society*, 1897, 60, 812–854.

Yule, G. U. *An introduction to the theory of statistics*. London: Griffin, 1911.

PART II

Cognition, personality, and intelligence

3 *Attention, perception, and intelligence*

LYNN A. COOPER and DENNIS T. REGAN

Our goal in preparing this chapter has been to isolate basic attentional and perceptual contributions to intelligence. Relating the concepts "attention," "perception," and "intelligence" at either empirical or theoretical levels has not been an easy task. The notion that attentional and perceptual capabilities might determine in significant ways overall intellectual ability has been alive since the early days of systematic intelligence testing (see, e.g., Spearman, 1927; Thurstone, 1938). And this same view has been one of the essential premises underlying the recent and much-heralded unification of cognitive and differential approaches to the study of human intelligence (Carroll, 1976).

Nonetheless, providing a synthesis of these three psychological concepts has been difficult, at best. One problem that we have encountered is the lack of consensus in either the cognitive or the differential literature concerning their meaning. A discussion of alternative conceptualizations of the nature of attention, perception, and intelligence within cognitive psychology is beyond the scope of this chapter. Suffice it to say that some theorists have regarded attention as a filtering mechanism (e.g., Broadbent, 1958), whereas others make reference to a limited-capacity pool of information-processing resources (e.g., Norman & Bobrow, 1975). Still others view attention as skill, modifiable through practice (e.g., Neisser, 1976). The nature of perception is also a matter of some debate, with one approach emphasizing the direct pickup of environmental information (e.g., Gibson, 1966), and other approaches regarding perception as the outcome of a sequence of internal information-processing stages (e.g., Rumelhart, 1977a). The nature of intelligence is probably the most controversial of the three concepts, and Sternberg (Chapter 5) summarizes alternative attempts at a definition.

The view of the human organism that we adopt (and one that is currently popular within cognitive psychology) is of a system for processing and transforming environmental information, with component subprocesses being highly interactive and interdependent, rather than strictly sequential and independent. This interactive view of the information-processing system poses another problem for any analysis of attentional and perceptual contributions to intelligence. According to this account, it is difficult to isolate just where in the information-processing sequence attentional and perceptual factors most significantly influence intelligent behavior, and where "higher-level" cognitive and memorial factors begin to provide more powerful contributions to intelligence.

We have not attempted to solve these problems here. Rather, our strategy has consisted of carefully delimiting the areas of research and theory that we consider. For purposes of the present discussion, we have regarded as essentially synonymous

123

intelligence and measures of ability on which individuals differ. We have defined *attentional* and *perceptual* operations as those lowest-level processes that might contribute to such ability differences. Our discussion necessarily includes reference to certain cognitive operations that might not traditionally be regarded as attentional or perceptual in nature. However, we have tried to avoid consideration of issues that clearly involve higher-level operations such as learning and problem-solving.

The chapter contains two major sections. In the first, we summarize and evaluate research that has tried to uncover basic information-processing skills that account for individual differences in psychometric measures of ability. This work is the product of the recent effort to link cognitive and differential approaches to the study of individual differences in intelligence. We conclude that this attempt to isolate information-processing correlates of ability differences has met with mixed success. In particular, information-processing measures that do distinguish more from less able people often account for only a small portion of the variance in the ability differences. In Section 3.2, we consider the possibility that more flexible aspects of cognitive functioning may make more substantial contributions to individual differences in intelligence than do basic information-processing skills. The additional sources of individual differences that we consider in this section include strategies – or procedures for organizing cognitive processes – and attentional factors. We conclude with a general evaluation of the work that we review, and we outline what we see as promising and productive directions for future research.

3.1.   BASIC INFORMATION-PROCESSING SKILLS UNDERLYING PSYCHOMETRIC MEASURES OF ABILITY

It is a generally accepted view in cognitive psychology that ability or intelligence reflects both a person's knowledge of the world and some more basic, general set of skills for processing information that does not depend on the content of the information being processed. Much of the thrust of cognitive psychology's recent interest in intelligence has been directed toward isolating these basic processing skills and determining the extent of their relationship to traditional psychometric measures of ability. The nature of the question that the cognitive psychologist wishes to ask is put nicely in the title of a pioneering paper by Hunt, Lunneborg, and Lewis: "What Does It Mean to Be High Verbal?" (1975). That is, what might be the nature of the basic information-processing skills that distinguish lower scorers from higher scorers on tests of verbal ability?

In this section, we review and evaluate a selected set of recent experiments designed to uncover correlations between information-processing skills, seemingly related to attentional and perceptual mechanisms, and measures of ability. The plan of the section is as follows: First, we discuss several studies of the relationship between some information-processing tasks and measures of verbal ability, pointing out differences in the adequacy of the approaches of various types of investigation. Second, we provide a similar analysis of studies of the component processes underlying measures of reading ability. Third, we discuss in essentially the same way the nature of the information-processing skills that may be related to spatial ability. Finally, we attempt to synthesize the salient and replicable results of these investigations, and we provide an evaluation of the success of this general approach to studying human intelligence.

VERBAL ABILITY

One rather obvious strategy for exploring the relationships among information-processing skills and ability measurements might involve isolating a sample of subjects that differ in measured ability and then testing these subjects on a series of information-processing tasks. Measures of performance on the information-processing tasks could be derived, and then these performance measures could be correlated with the ability measurements. The hope, using this sort of approach, is that the pattern of correlations among the task performance measures and the ability measures might yield some coherent picture of just what aspects of which tasks are most strongly related to ability differences. Such an interpretable pattern of correlations might, in turn, help to uncover the basic processing skills that underlie ability.

As an example of this sort of research strategy, consider a series of studies by Lunneborg (1977). In these experiments, subjects were tested first on a variety of psychometric instruments, and then on a variety of information-processing tasks, many of which used response time as the dependent variable of interest. Correlations among the processing measures and the psychometric measures were then computed. Of chief concern to Lunneborg was the extent of the possible relationship between choice reaction time (presumably a reflection of processing speed) and the ability measures. Unfortunately, the results are difficult to interpret. In one study, the correlations of choice reaction time with ability measures were reasonably high (between $-.55$ and $-.28$, with faster times being related to higher measured ability), but these correlations virtually disappeared in two subsequent experiments. Had the pattern of correlations been consistent across experiments or within an experiment across sets of information-processing and ability measures, then undoubtedly more could have been learned from Lunneborg's study. What seems lacking in this approach is an attempt to specify just what information-processing skills the laboratory tasks are measuring and which such skills might be components common to a variety of the tasks. With a theory of the information-processing components of laboratory tasks as a guide, a selection of tasks with theoretically meaningful and, one hopes, shared components could be made, and predictions could be generated concerning relationships between the information-processing measures and the ability measures. What is clear from this study is that there is no guarantee that such a theory will fall out of the pattern of correlations among many tasks and many ability measures. In a subsequent experiment using much the same approach, Lunneborg (1978) did find more interpretable patterns of relationships among ability and information-processing measures. In this case, significant correlations between performance IQ and visual and nonlinguistic processing measures were found, whereas vocabulary and verbal IQ scores appeared to be more strongly related to measures of linguistic flexibility and reading time.

A somewhat more satisfying approach to investigating the relation between information-processing skills and measures of ability is illustrated by some of the experiments reported by Hunt and his associates (1975; see also Hunt, Frost, & Lunneborg, 1973). Their basic notion was that tests of verbal ability provide direct measures of verbal knowledge (e.g., meaning of words, size of vocabulary, rules of syntax) but only indirect measures of content-free information-processing efficiency. Nonetheless, high-scoring and lower-scoring groups of subjects might differ reliably in the speed and efficiency with which they carry out basic information-processing tasks. The subjects in the studies of Hunt and his colleagues were

University of Washington students who scored in the upper quartile ("high verbals") or lower quartile ("low verbals") on a composite verbal ability measure from a standardized test administered to high-school juniors. The laboratory tasks on which these subjects were tested involved a variety of more or less "standard" information-processing paradigms. The interesting point about the selection of tasks was that they represented an effort by the investigators to specify in advance what the information-processing demands of the tasks might be. Thus the investigators had a basis for predicting on which tasks the high verbal subjects should excel, and, further, for analyzing the nature of the information-processing skills that might lead to more efficient performance. One might quarrel both with the authors' analysis of the information-processing tasks and, particularly, with their claims concerning processing skills common to various tasks for they provide no external evidence for the relationships among the processing variables that they hypothesize are related. Nonetheless, this approach goes beyond the purely correlational method in attempting to specify in advance the information-processing skills underlying performance on the laboratory tasks.

For purposes of our analysis, only two of the tasks used by Hunt and his colleagues will be considered at length. We describe these experimental paradigms in some detail, as they have been used extensively in the work of others to be discussed in later sections. The first task was based on a procedure originally introduced by Posner and Mitchell (1967) and Posner, Boies, Eichelman, and Taylor (1969). The paradigm involves presentation of two letters that are identical in both name and typecase (A,A), identical in name but not in case (A,a), different in name but not in case (A,B) or different in both name and case (A,b). In one standard version of the procedure of Posner and his associates (1969), subjects are shown such letter pairs and are required to respond "same" as rapidly and accurately as possible if the two letters share a common name. Otherwise, the required response is "different." Of central interest is the difference between the time taken to respond "same" when the letters are identical in name only (A,a) and the time to respond "same" when they are physically identical (A,A) as well. The average difference in response time between name identical (NI) and physically identical (PI) instances, or the NI–PI difference, is on the order of 70 msec when groups of college students are tested as subjects (Posner et al., 1969).

One standard interpretation of this reaction-time difference is as follows: In the case of NI trials, the name associated with each visual pattern must be retrieved from memory in order for the subject to respond "same." Thus the NI–PI difference is a measure of the additional time needed to access the name of a letter code in memory. Variations on the standard Posner procedure – which themselves produce reliable NI–PI differences – include instructing the subject on separate blocks of trials to respond "same" on the basis of physical identity only or name identity only, and measuring the speed with which a deck of cards containing letter pairs can be sorted into "same" and "different" piles under physical identity or name identity instructions. In the 1975 study of Hunt and his associates, both the standard paradigm and the card-sorting modifications were used.

The results that Hunt and his co-workers (1975) obtained for the letter-matching task can be summarized as follows: For both the standard reaction-time version of the task and the card-sorting variant, high verbal subjects exhibited a smaller difference between NI and PI trials than did low verbal subjects. The magnitude of the NI–PI difference was about 64 msec for high verbals and 89 msec for low verbals.

(In subsequent work by Hunt and his colleagues, reviewed in Hunt, 1978, the magnitude of the NI–PI difference has been found to increase substantially when groups spanning a wider range of measured ability are tested; e.g., the NI–PI difference is as large as 310 msec for schoolchildren with mild mental retardation.) Hunt and his associates interpret this finding as indicating that high verbals have relatively faster access to overlearned material (letter names) in memory than do low verbals, and that this faster memory access to name codes is a basic information-processing skill that underlies verbal ability.

There are some potential problems with this interpretation, though, which plague not only the study by Hunt and his colleagues but also the work of other investigators to be reviewed later. First, although the interaction between level of verbal ability and type of letter-pair identity was indeed statistically significant, it is nonetheless true that high and low verbal subjects differed in mean response times on PI trials as well as on NI trials. (In the case of the standard reaction-time task, high verbals were about 18 msec faster than low verbals on PI trials, and the difference was about 44 msecs on NI trials.) The problem here is that the entire NI–PI difference between high and low verbal subjects cannot necessarily be attributed to differences in the efficiency of memory access. In addition, there may be general speed factors or differential speed-of-pattern-matching processes that contribute to the differences in both measured ability and reaction time.

A second problem with the interpretation of Hunt and his co-workers (1975) lies in the empirical basis for their claim that the NI–PI difference is an index of efficiency of memory retrieval of overlearned codes. In order to establish that speed of memory access, and not some other factor, really is an information-processing skill correlated with verbal ability, it would be desirable to show that individuals with small NI–PI differences (fast memory access) also show small reaction-time differences in some component of another information-processing task, where that component is also assumed to be an index of efficiency of retrieval of overlearned material. What this amounts to is establishing construct validity via an individual-differences analysis for processing components of tasks for which those components are assumed to be related. If such construct validity can be established, then the meaning of a relationship between processing time and measured ability is more readily interpretable. Hunt and his associates do not provide such an analysis of relationships among processing components in similar tasks.

The second task of interest used by Hunt and his colleagues (1975) was a modification of the "sentence–picture verification" paradigm introduced by Clark and Chase (1972). In this paradigm, the subject is first shown a sentence describing a spatial relation between two elements (e.g., *star* or *, and *plus* or +). The relational terms used in the initial description may contain either of the words *above* and *below*, and the description may or may not contain a negative. This pattern yields four basic sentence types in the initial descriptions: "star above plus," "star not above plus," "star below plus," and "star not below plus." Following presentation of the sentence, a test picture is presented that contains either of the configurations $_*^+$ and $^+_*$. The subject must indicate as rapidly and accurately as possible whether the initial sentence is true or false of the test picture. In the modification used by Hunt and his associates (1975), two measures of response time were obtained – the time the subject needed to encode or comprehend the initial sentence and the time needed to verify that the sentence was true or false of the picture, which was presented as soon as the subject indicated that encoding of the sentence was complete.

There are a number of theoretical analyses of the processes underlying perform-ance on this task, which we will consider in detail later (e.g., Carpenter & Just, 1975; Clark & Chase, 1972; Glushko & Cooper, 1978). For now, let us consider only the general analysis offered by Clark and Chase (1972) and by Hunt and his colleagues (1975). When the initial sentence is presented, the subject encodes it by forming an internal representation that will subsequently be compared with the picture. A num-ber of investigators have suggested that this internal representation is linguistic in nature and that the time it takes to form the representation is affected by the linguistic complexity of the sentence (see Clark & Chase, 1972; Trabasso, Rollins, & Shaughnessey, 1971). Furthermore, both the presence of a negative term and the presence of a "marked" form of a spatial comparative (in this case, *below* as opposed to *above*) are thought to increase linguistic complexity and hence to increase encod-ing time. Clark and Chase propose that the internal representation of the picture to be compared with the representation of the sentence is also linguistic in nature. Hence we might expect that the test picture would be converted into a representa-tion similar to that of the initial sentence and that processing time for verifying that the picture is true or false of the sentence would be affected by the linguistic variables that affect encoding of the sentence. If this analysis of the task is correct, then differences between the times to encode or to verify more or less complex sentence types measure the speed with which a subject can convert the sentence or picture stimulus material into a linguistic internal representation and then perform the comparison.

Hunt and his associates found no effect of linguistic markedness, but they did find both a significant effect of negation and a significant interaction between the size of the negation effect and verbal ability. High verbal subjects took about 55 msec longer to encode sentences containing a negative than sentences without a negative, and this difference rose to about 100 msec for low verbal subjects. The size of the negation effect differed across ability levels in the case of decision times also. High verbals required about 70 additional msec to compare a negative sentence with a picture, and low verbals required an additional 120 msec to make the same compari-son. The investigators interpret the differential size of the negation effect for differ-ent levels of measured ability as follows: The larger difference in time needed by low verbal subjects for encoding or comprehending negative than for encoding or com-prehending affirmative sentences could reflect a superior ability in the high verbals to convert a complex sentence into a corresponding internal representation. The difference between high and low verbals in the size of the negation effect for deci-sion latencies could reflect a superior efficiency in comparing a picture against a complex internal representation for the high verbal subjects.

We can question the interpretation of these results along much the same lines as we did the interpretation of the results of the letter-matching task. First, the differ-ential size of the negation effect could derive simply from a general tendency toward faster processing in the high verbal subjects. From the way in which Hunt and his co-workers present their data, it is not possible to determine whether the two ability groups are approximately equivalent in speed of encoding and/or comparing an affirmative sentence or whether the high verbal subjects excel in this base condition as well as in their relative sensitivity to negation. Second, the interpretation of the pattern of differences is tied to a particular theoretical analysis of the operations involved in the sentence–picture verification task. And Hunt and his associates provide no evidence for the validity of the assumed underlying processes, in that they do not show that subjects with relatively small negation effects also show small reaction-time effects in other tasks that are presumed to measure the efficiency with which more or less complex internal representations are encoded and compared against test stimuli. The general thrust of this second objection – that an interpretation of performance differences is critically dependent on the adequacy of one's theory of the processes underlying a given information-processing task – will become quite important when we come to consider further work that Hunt and his colleagues have done on an analysis of the relationship between patterns of ability and patterns of performance in the sentence–picture verification situation (Lansman, 1979; MacLeod, Hunt, & Mathews, 1978).

We conclude our discussion with an examination of what we consider two "model" sets of experiments on basic information-processing correlates of verbal ability, one by Chiang and Atkinson (1976) and one by Keating and Bobbitt (1978). The appealing feature of these studies is that the investigators attempt to demonstrate empirically the assumed theoretical relationships among component-processing parameters of various cognitive tasks. They do so by correlating individual subjects' values of parameters from models of the tasks across different tasks and within the same task. They inspect the pattern of correlations to determine whether there is adequate support for the theoretical analysis of the tasks (i.e., whether parameters that, theoretically, ought to be related are related empirically). Having established such construct validity for the processing parameters of the tasks, they then obtain correlations of these parameters with psychometric measures of ability to determine which basic information-processing skills relate to differences in ability.

In the Chiang and Atkinson study, the subjects were Stanford University undergraduates whose verbal and math scores on the Scholastic Aptitude Test (SAT) were available. The information-processing tasks on which the subjects were tested were a memory-search task (S. Sternberg, 1966) and a visual-search task. (A test of digit span was also included, but we will not consider the results here.) In the memory-search test, the subject is presented with a set of from one to five items (letters), and then with a test letter. The subject is required to report as rapidly and accurately as possible whether or not the test letter is contained in the set of letters in memory. Generally, the amount of time needed to make the response increases linearly with the number of items in the memory set (S. Sternberg, 1969). This linear reaction-time function (along with other aspects of the data usually obtained with this procedure) is taken as evidence that subjects perform the task by sequentially comparing the test item to each item in the memory set before making a positive or a negative response. The slope of this reaction-time function provides an estimate of the time required for each memory comparison, or the rate of scanning items in memory. The intercept of the reaction-time function reflects all other processes not involved in memory search – namely, encoding the test item, determining whether a match has been found, and executing the appropriate response.

The component-processing operations in the visual-search task are theoretically related to those in the memory-scanning task. In the visual-search paradigm, a single target item is presented first, and a display of from one to five items follows. The subject is required to search the display set and to determine as rapidly and accurately as possible whether the target is contained in the display set. As in the memory-search task, it is generally found that reaction time increases linearly with the size of the set of visual display items (Atkinson, Holmgren, & Juola, 1969; Estes & Taylor, 1964, 1966). The slope of this function is thought to reflect the time for each comparison of the target item with each display-set item and also the time needed to encode each item in the visual display. The intercept parameter in the visual-search task is taken as a measure of the time needed to make the yes–no decision and the time required to execute the response.

Chiang and Atkinson (1976) estimated the intercept and slope parameters for each of their individual subjects for both the memory-search and the visual-search tasks. When the individual subjects' parameter values were intercorrelated, a compelling pattern emerged. Correlations between the intercepts of the two tasks and the slopes of the two tasks were high (.968 and .832, respectively). However, there was virtually no correlation between the intercepts and the slopes within each task. That is, subjects who are characterized by rapid search rates manifest this skill in both memory- and visual-search conditions, and subjects who encode efficiently do so in both experimental situations. Furthermore, the lack of correlation between intercept and slope parameters in the same task shows that the correlation of parameters across tasks is a reflection of more than simple general processing speed. For a general speed factor should show up in a correlation of intercept and slope parameters, as well as in a correlation of each of these parameters in different tasks.

Despite the elegance of Chiang and Atkinson's analysis of the relationships among component-processing skills, the results of their attempt to relate these skills to psychometric measures of ability are quite disappointing. Unfortunately, they failed to obtain any significant correlations between the information-processing parameters and either the SAT verbal or the SAT math score. When the data were broken down by sex, some significant correlations emerged, but the pattern is extremely difficult to interpret. One possible reason for the failure to find relationships between processing components and ability could be that the range of measured ability of Stanford undergraduate students was rather narrow.

Some more positive evidence concerning the relationship between ability and information-processing skills has been found in a study by Keating and Bobbitt (1978). The ability measure used by these investigators was a composite score on the Standard and Advanced Raven Progressive Matrices (Raven, 1960, 1965). This test is generally regarded as a measure of problem-solving ability in that, unlike measures of verbal ability, it does not assess general or vocabulary knowledge. The subjects in the experiment were children from Grades 3, 7, and 11. The information-processing tasks used were the Posner letter-matching task (the card-sorting variation described earlier) and the memory-search task. In addition, tests of simple and choice reaction time were included. In the simple reaction-time task, the subject had to indicate as rapidly as possible whenever a light turned red. In the choice reaction-time task, the subject had to push one button when a green light appeared and another when a red light appeared, and to push the buttons as rapidly as possible.

The results of these experiments were subjected to a number of analyses. Analyses of variance generally showed significant main effects of age and ability levels, such that older and higher-ability subjects performed each of the tasks more efficiently than younger and lower-ability subjects. Of particular interest are some of the interactions between age and ability and certain task variables. For the letter-matching task, significant interactions emerged, such that the NI–PI difference was smaller for older than for younger subjects and also smaller for higher- than for lower-ability subjects. For the memory-scanning task, there was an interaction between memory-set size and ability, such that search rate was slower for lower-ability subjects.

Like Chiang and Atkinson (1976), Keating and Bobbitt (1978) attempted to provide construct validity for the component operations presumed to underlie the various information-processing tasks. To do this, they proposed a four-stage sequence of basic component processes consisting of (a) encoding, (b) operation, (c) binary decision (response selection), and (d) response execution. Various parameters of the information-processing tasks were assigned to one or more of the four sequential stages. Then individual subjects' values for these parameters were correlated across tasks. The hope was that variables assumed to involve common processing stages would correlate more highly than those that did not have any stages in common. Unlike Chiang and Atkinson, Keating and Bobbitt did not compute within-task correlations. The results of this analysis revealed that the intercorrelations among variables having common stages were higher than those among variables without stages in common (.66 and .30, respectively). The authors interpret the pattern of correlations as showing that there are basic information-processing operations that are tapped by the different tasks, but that, in addition, there exists a general speed factor that is reflected in the lower but often still significant correlations among variables without hypothesized common stages.

In their final analysis, Keating and Bobbitt assessed the relationship among three information-processing parameters and measured ability via multiple regression techniques. The information-processing parameters were measures of decision efficiency (choice reaction time minus simple reaction time), efficiency of memory retrieval of overlearned codes (NI–PI difference), and memory-search efficiency (slope of the memory-scanning function). With age partialed out, the information-processing measures accounted for only 15% of the variance in the ability scores, but this was a significant amount of added variance. More interestingly, when correlations were computed for each age group separately, the NI–PI difference was always the most effective variable, and it accounted for progressively more variance in measured ability as the age of the subjects increased (17%, 25%, and 32% of variance for the three groups in chronological order).

What, if any, systematic findings have emerged from a consideration of these various studies reflecting different approaches to assessing the relationship between basic information-processing skills and measures of verbal ability? Clearly, the most universal processing difference between the higher- and the lower-ability subjects in the work just reviewed is the difference between the time for matching letters identical in name only and letters that are, in addition, physically identical. Furthermore, this difference emerges despite procedural variations in the letter-matching task (the discrete trial reaction-time method and the card-sorting technique), and for both children (Keating & Bobbitt, 1978) and adults (Hunt et al., 1975). Thus far, we have interpreted this NI–PI difference as reflecting efficiency of memory access to overlearned material. In subsequent sections, as the difference appears in still other bodies of work, we shall consider whether this processing skill is specifically one of the letter-code access or whether it may reflect a more general process of memory access or even of flexibility in applying information-processing skills.

Another possible candidate for an operation underlying verbal ability is the speed with which items in memory can be compared with a test item. Keating and Bobbitt's (1978) finding of a decrease in the slope of the Sternberg memory-scanning function with increasing ability provides evidence for this notion, but the evidence is mixed at best. On the opposite side, we have Chiang and Atkinson's failure to find a relationship between slope and ability, and the report of Hunt and his associates

(1975) that the positive relationship reported earlier (Hunt et al., 1973) could not be replicated. And S. Sternberg (1975) has reported no relationship between scanning rate and measures of intelligence within normal university and high-school populations. The relationship of memory-comparison efficiency to ability may be a subtle one, however. Hunt (1978, 1980) has reviewed evidence suggesting a rather dramatic difference in memory-comparison processes when the groups considered come from populations more varied in their abilities than the normal college sample used by most investigators. For example, groups of subjects suffering from various forms of mental retardation show much steeper slopes in the memory-scanning experiment than do normal high-school and college students. Furthermore, Keating and Bobbitt (1978) report an almost significant interaction between age and ability in the slope of the memory-scanning function such that the effect of ability on scanning rate becomes less important as age increases. What this may mean is that general memory-comparison skills are well developed across ability levels within the normal range, but that these general skills are not available to the younger subject or to the subject more severely limited in ability.

A third possible skill that may be related to ability is simply overall processing speed. That is, more able people may just be faster at anything they do. We will consider seriously the general speed factor as a source of ability differences in later sections. At present, analyses such as those of Keating and Bobbitt (1978) suggest that although a general speed factor may exist, there are additional more specific processing skills that contribute to differences in verbal intelligence.

READING ABILITY

The ability to read rapidly and with high comprehension is a crucial aspect of "intelligent" behavior in any literate society. At a minimum, reading involves picking up visual information from a page of print and processing that information on a variety of levels so as to yield, eventually, understanding of the meaning of a passage. In this section we review and evaluate some of the literature that attempts to isolate the basic processes or components of reading that might differentiate highly skilled from less skilled readers. The recent literature on reading is voluminous, and our review will be highly selective.

We first discuss in detail a series of studies by Jackson and McClelland (1975, 1979; Jackson, 1978; see also McClelland & Jackson, 1978) that purport to demonstrate a very basic visual information-processing difference between average and very proficient readers. We highlight these studies because they combine elegance and care in experimental design and execution, clarity of exposition, and a consistent and intriguing pattern of results.

It has been known for over 70 years (Huey, 1908/1968) that reading takes place during pauses or fixations of the eye, and that faster readers make fewer fixations per page of text, although they spend about the same amount of time on each fixation. This suggests that faster readers may be able to process a larger amount of text per fixation, and a study by Gilbert (1959) supports the suggestion. Gilbert presented single lines of text for very brief periods, and found that faster readers could accurately report more of the text than slower readers. But precisely what is the nature of the advantage that enables fast readers to extract more information from a single fixation? The possibilities are numerous, and Jackson and McClelland (1975, 1979) designed their studies so as to narrow them down.

A word is in order about the measure of reading ability used in these studies. Groups of relatively fast and average readers are selected from a university population. These groups have nonoverlapping scores on a measure of Effective Reading Speed, which is the speed of reading the text material multiplied by the score on a very strict comprehension test. There is a persuasive rationale for using this measure of reading ability: The best readers should both read quickly and comprehend much. And, in fact, fast effective readers typically do score higher on both speed and comprehension. The groups are then put through a variety of tasks designed to tap particular processing abilities that might distinguish them.

In their first study, Jackson and McClelland (1975) replicated Gilbert's (1959) results and investigated the possibility that faster readers might pick up more from a single fixation because they have a visual sensory processing advantage. But faster readers actually showed no greater ability to pick up information presented at the periphery of the visual field, nor were their thresholds lower for detecting a single letter under conditions of pre- and postexposure patterned masking.

At the other extreme from basic sensory processes, fast readers might be better at filling in missing information on the basis of contextual cues. Or they might have superior understanding of the orthographic constraints of the English language, and thus be more effective at guessing "missing" letters in words. Finally, fast readers might simply be able to hold more material in short-term memory. But Jackson and McClelland (1975) found that fast readers maintained their superiority over slow readers even when forced to pick between two words differing in but a single letter, both of which fit the context of the previous sentence but only one of which had actually appeared. Contextual cues could not guide such a choice. Furthermore, fast readers could report accurately a larger percentage of a string of briefly presented random letters, so the superiority shows itself even when orthographic regularities are eliminated. This last result also suggests that the fast readers' visual processing advantage is independent of language comprehension processes responsible for our understanding the meaning of what is read. Finally and relatedly, greater short-term memory capacity does not seem responsible for the fast readers' superiority on the tasks just described, for they were not superior on an auditory version of the unrelated-letters task (Jackson & McClelland, 1979).

What, then, accounts for the superior performance of the more able readers in extracting information from a brief presentation of text or letters? The results thus far point to some relatively central processing capacity that seems visually specific; but attempting to identify what this capacity might be requires specifying a theory of reading. Jackson and McClelland (1979) do not attempt such a theory, but they share the central assumptions of many information-processing theories of reading (e.g., Estes, 1975; Frederiksen, 1978; Rumelhart, 1977b) that the processing of information in reading occurs simultaneously and interactively at many different levels of analysis, which are organized in a loose hierarchy. Constructing a conceptual representation of what is read (understanding the meaning of the text), it is argued, involves subprocesses corresponding to analysis of visual features, letter clusters, words, and semantic/conceptual meanings. The output of each level of encoding and analysis may serve as input to the level(s) above it, and may in turn be influenced by output from these higher levels. The problem becomes one of isolating level(s) of processing at which fast readers have an advantage.

To this end, Jackson and McClelland (1979) utilized a variety of matching tasks, in which the subject decided as quickly and as accurately as possible whether two presented stimuli were the same or different according to a specified criterion. The stimuli to be matched and the criterion for responding "same" were chosen to reflect different levels in the processing hierarchy leading to reading with comprehension. The matching tasks of primary interest were letters, where the subject is instructed to respond "same" if the letters have the same name (e.g., *A,a*) or are physically the same (e.g., *A,A;* after Posner et al., 1969); words, where the subject responds "same" if the words are synonyms; words, where the "same" response is given to homonyms; pseudowords, with a "same" response to homophones; and simple dot patterns, with a "same" response if the patterns are physically identical. The tasks thus were an attempt to reflect, respectively, the processes of forming letter codes, word meanings, verbal (articulatory) word codes, and visual codes. In addition to the matching tasks, the test battery included measures of listening comprehension and of verbal ability.

The results were that fast readers had shorter reaction times on all the matching tasks except dot patterns. This exception is important, for it indicates that the advantage of fast readers does not lie in more rapid encoding or comparison of any visual display. In the matching tasks that did show a fast–average reader difference, the magnitude of the difference was generally proportional to overall response time. But again, the dot-matching task, which had the longest response times, did not show a difference between readers of varying ability.

Given only these results, the fast-reader advantage could lie at any or all of the levels of processing presumably tapped by the various matching tasks. But Jackson and McClelland (1979) subjected their data to a variety of correlational, partial correlational, and regression analyses that clarify considerably the interpretation of the findings. The simple correlational analysis showed that the single strongest predictor of effective reading speed was a measure of listening comprehension, in which the subjects answered a set of questions about a passage read to them at normal speaking rate. The listening comprehension measure accounted for about half the variance in effective reading speed. This measure was also statistically independent of the reaction-time measures from the matching tasks. The strongest predictor of reading ability in this study, then, seems to be a modality-independent set of language comprehension skills for understanding and remembering meaningful discourse. A subsequent stepwise regression analysis, with variables entered in the order of the amount of unexplained variance in reading ability accounted for, confirmed that listening comprehension was the most powerful predictor of reading ability. We will discuss this listening comprehension variable in more detail later on.

The correlational analysis indicated that the reaction-time measure that most strongly predicted reading speed was on the letter name-match task, and the stepwise regression analysis confirmed that this reaction-time measure accounted for a significant proportion of the remaining variance when it was entered after listening comprehension. None of the other reaction-time measures accounted for significant residual variance. And the name-match reaction time continued to account for significant variance in reading speed even when listening comprehension and the other reaction-time measures were partialed out (Jackson & McClelland, 1979, tab. 7). Finally, a measure of verbal aptitude (School and College Aptitude Test, Series II, Form 1C) correlated approximately .45 with effective reading speed. However, once the name-match reaction-time variable was entered in the stepwise regression analysis, verbal aptitude failed to account for any of the residual variance.

These results strongly suggest that the letter name-match variable is the best measure of the component of reading ability that is picked up by the reaction-time matching tasks. In interpreting the difference on this task, Jackson and McClelland suggest that fast readers have swifter access to letter identity codes stored in long-term memory, a claim similar to the one that Hunt and his colleagues (1975) have made for high verbals. This explanation is consistent with the lack of any relationship between the reaction-time tasks and the listening comprehension task (letters were not involved in the latter), as well as with the obtained differences between fast and average readers on the synonym, homonym, and homophone tasks, if we make the reasonable assumption that letter identification is a component of fluent word identification (see e.g., Estes, 1975; McClelland, 1976).

In his doctoral thesis, Jackson (1978) attempted to clarify the nature of the name-match reaction-time advantage for fast readers by addressing two questions: Is the fast-reader advantage restricted to letter codes, or does it appear whenever any meaningful (nameable) visual stimulus is presented? Second, if the difference is found on other meaningful material besides letters (or words), is it attributable to differential practice with the nameable material, or does it occur even without differential amounts of practice? The second question has some implications for the possible beneficial effects of mere practice in identifying letters and words in improving the performance of poorer readers. If better readers come to the reading situation with an already existing superiority in ability to access memory codes for any meaningful pattern, regardless of familiarity with it, one would be less sanguine about the possibility that practice could close the gap between readers of differing ability.

Jackson (1978) replicated many of the results of the previous work by Jackson and McClelland (1979). In addition, he found that faster readers were quicker to indicate whether two line drawings were or were not members of the same general category (e.g., *toy, vegetable, musical instrument*). This category-match reaction-time variable correlated −.29 with the measure of effective reading speed (faster reaction times being associated with superior effective reading speed). Name-match reaction time correlated −.35 with reading speed. And category-match and name-match reaction times correlated .42 with each other. Each contributes significantly to effective reading speed when listening comprehension is partialed out. Most importantly, the two reaction-time tasks seem to be tapping the same component of reading ability, for when either is partialed out, the correlation of the other with reading speed drops essentially to zero. So the name-match reaction-time measure is an index of a very general processing ability to access rapidly a learned code in memory for any meaningful visual material.

That this ability is independent of practice with the particular visual material processed is strongly suggested by a second experiment (Jackson, 1978), in which the stimuli were an unfamiliar character set constructed by using features similar to those found in letters. None of the characters closely resembled existing letters, however. Fast readers showed no advantage in a physical identity-matching task. But when pairs (five pairs in total) of these characters were given one-syllable nonsense names, and the subjects were required to respond "same" if the two characters shown had the same name, fast readers showed roughly a 100-msec advantage over average readers on this task. This difference occurred despite the fact that the two groups did not differ in amount of practice with or prior exposure to the characters, in that both groups learned the names in the same small number of trials.

The upshot of this elegant body of research is that relatively proficient adult readers differ from less proficient ones in the rapidity with which they can execute a basic visual information-processing skill – that is, access from long-term memory to the name for any meaningful visual pattern. Letters appear to be the meaningful visual patterns involved in reading, but the information-processing skill at which proficient readers have an advantage is apparently much more general than the ability to access the names of letters. The results seem to suggest that better readers bring to reading a "talent" independent of practice with the particular material being viewed, and independent of the language comprehension skills that account for the bulk of the variance in reading ability in these studies. Though the results are impressively consistent from study to study, and make a coherent conceptual package, it is perhaps worth remembering that the correlation between reading ability and this processing skill as indicated by the various reaction-time tasks was generally in the .30 range, a figure that accounts for only about 10% of the variance in the data. And even this may be an inflated estimate, because the reading groups were selected to be nonoverlapping in ability.

The listening comprehension measure, on the other hand, did account for a very large proportion of the variance (typically about 50%) in effective reading scores in these studies. We might ask what particular skills are involved in listening comprehension that would contribute to reading ability, and the possibilities are clearly numerous. People who can comprehend discourse better may have better knowledge of word meanings, better short-term memory capacity (although this seems unlikely; see, e.g., Perfetti & Goldman, 1976), better ability to maintain continuous attention in the task of understanding (Jackson & McClelland, 1979), better ability to use structure and context of discourse so as to apply processing resources where they are most needed, or a variety of other advantages.

This last possibility was investigated in a series of studies by Perfetti and his colleagues (see especially Perfetti & Goldman, 1976; Perfetti & Lesgold, 1978). These authors utilized a variety of techniques to investigate the possibility that good and poor readers would be differentially sensitive to aspects of discourse structure that might be related to ease of comprehension of meaningful material. Specifically, they investigated the possibilities (a) that aspects of sentence and thematic structure of discourse would affect subjects' ability to comprehend and remember spoken or written material, and (b) that good readers would profit more from discourse organization than poor readers. They performed several experiments, and the findings converged in support of (a) but provided no evidence whatever for (b).

Consider memory for spoken or written material. Perfetti and Lesgold (1978) performed several "probe discourse experiments," in which the subject's task is to read (or listen to) material presented to him or her and to attempt to remember it. Every now and then, a probe word that has occurred recently in the text is presented to the subject, whose task is to report the word (called the target) that immediately followed the probe word in the text. It is possible to manipulate a variety of aspects of discourse structure between the target's position in the text and the occurrence of the probe test item, and thereby to see whether good and poor readers are differentially sensitive to them. Perfetti and colleagues did this in a variety of studies using as subjects, typically, third- to fifth-grade students of differing reading abilities but matched IQs.

As three examples of this manipulation (reported in Perfetti & Lesgold, 1978), they varied (a) the number of words intervening between target and probe test, and whether these words were within the same sentence or across sentence boundaries; (b) whether the context in which sentences were presented to subjects was normal or scrambled; and (c) whether the material intervening between target and probe test item referred to material already given earlier in the text, or introduced new material (see Haviland & Clark, 1974). In each of these cases, we would expect a main effect of discourse structure: Memory should be better for material within a sentence than across sentence lines, especially if a large number of words intervened between target and test. It should also be better for material presented in a meaningful context. And it should be better when given rather than new information intervened between target and test. All of these predictions were confirmed, presumably because in each case the material was easier to process when the discourse was more structured. We should also expect in each case a main effect of reading ability: Good readers should remember more from spoken or written passages than should poor readers. The results clearly supported this prediction as well. But are good readers more proficient because they are better able to take advantage of the structure of discourse? Perfetti and Lesgold's (1978) answer is an emphatic no. In no case was there a statistical interaction between reading ability and discourse structure. Poor readers' memory for the material was helped (or hindered) by discourse structure (or its absence) every bit as much as that of good readers. Determination of the precise nature of the listening comprehension differences between good and poor readers clearly awaits further investigation.

We turn, finally, to an information-processing approach to reading that retains the assumption that reading can be viewed as a set of interactive component processes, but adopts a different method from Jackson and McClelland's for identifying those processes and testing their relationship to reading ability. We highlight this work by Frederiksen (1978, 1979) because the theoretical approach and research methods clearly have promise, although the data base on which the conclusions rest needs expansion.

The component processes in reading hypothesized by Frederiksen are Perceptual Encoding, Decoding, and Lexical Access. Encoding is divided into two processes – Encoding of Graphemes and Encoding of Multiletter Units. Decoding is also divided into two separate processes – Phonemic Translation, which involves applying letter–sound correspondence rules to derive a phonological–phonemic representation, and Articulatory Programming, which refers to "automaticity in deriving a speech representation, in the assignment of stress and other prosidic features" (Frederiksen, 1978, p. 29). The component processes are assumed to be hierarchically organized, although Frederiksen (1978) explicitly states that the initiation of the "higher" processes need not necessarily await completion of earlier ones. With these assumptions about the nature of reading, Frederiksen's overall research goals were three: (a) to derive information-processing tasks that should be measures of these separate component processes, (b) to show, by factor analysis, that the hypothesized five processes do best represent the pattern of correlations among the tasks, and (c) to show that the factor structure actually is related to scores on standard tests of reading ability.

We do not here consider in detail the tasks selected (see Frederiksen, 1978). But the general idea was to choose tasks such that different conditions of a task (for example, responding "same" to name identical versus physically identical letters) should place different demands on one of the hypothesized processing components of reading (in the case, Grapheme Encoding). Then reaction-time differences were computed between conditions for several such tasks in the expectation that these differences should be highly correlated if the tasks tap the same component process. In certain cases, the reason why a particular reaction-time difference should tap a particular component process was unclear. Nevertheless, Frederiksen (1978) found that his hypothesized five-factor structure (one factor corresponding to each of the five hypothesized component processes) provided an impressive fit to the pattern of correlations among the 11 reaction-time differences computed. Further, he was able to show statistically that simpler, four-factor models did not provide an adequate fit.

Frederiksen (1978) tested the relationship between his component processes, as revealed in the factor structure for the chronometric tasks, and reading ability on a sample of 20 high-school sophomores, juniors, and seniors who represented a wide range of reading ability levels. Three measures of reading ability were assessed, and the multiple correlations of the five factors with the reading scores ranged from a low of .73 for the Gray Oral Reading Test to 1.00 for the Total Score on the Nelson–Denny Reading Test. These multiple correlations are particularly impressive when it is noted that none of the reaction-time tasks defining the factors involved reading anything more complex than a single word or pseudoword. The factors with the heaviest loading on reading scores in this sample were Encoding of Multiletter Units and Articulatory Programming, but we do not make much of these relative weights because the sample is so small and the findings clearly need to be replicated. For the same reason, we do not make an explicit comparison with the findings of Jackson and McClelland just discussed, save to mention that Frederiksen (1978) did find that the name identity versus physical identity letter-matching reaction-time difference significantly discriminated between good and poor readers. Also, if the Frederiksen results hold up, it should be possible to tap chronometrically what Jackson and McClelland have called listening comprehension with simple information-processing tasks. But the most attractive feature of Frederiksen's work is the explicit statement of a theory of reading as embodying particular component processes, along with the sophisticated methods for testing for the existence of those component processes and their relationship to reading ability.

On the basis of the work described, we can draw some general conclusions about the information-processing abilities that discriminate between relatively good and poor readers. The difference is clearly not to be found in low-level sensory capacities (Jackson & McClelland, 1975). Nor does it derive simply from more exposure to or greater familiarity with letters (Jackson, 1978). At the other extreme, good readers do not seem to differ from poor readers in high-level sensitivity to discourse structure (Perfetti & Lesgold, 1978), although this is not to say that good readers cannot more effectively utilize contextual cues in some circumstances (e.g., see Frederiksen, 1977). All of the extensive work by Jackson and McClelland converges on the point that good readers can more quickly access the name of any meaningful visual pattern, regardless of practice with it. And there is the very intriguing suggestion in Jackson and McClelland (1979) that this ability may totally account for the often-found association between measures of verbal ability and reading ability. Finally, there is the possibility (although we are skeptical) that measures of basic information-processing abilities, if carefully selected and tied to a component-processes theory of reading, may account for much more of the variance in reading ability than the approximately 10% or so generally found in the literature.

SPATIAL ABILITY

The term *spatial ability* is often thought to refer to competence in encoding, transforming, generating, and remembering internal representations of objects in space and their relationships to other objects and spatial positions. Psychometric tests providing measures of levels of spatial ability have been available since the time of Thurstone (1938). We will not undertake a review of the psychometric literature on tests of spatial ability here. Rather, we point to two recent reviews of psychometric and correlational studies of spatial ability (Lohman, 1979a; McGee, 1979) that indicate the existence of at least two separable but correlated major spatial factors and several minor ones.[1]

The first of these factors – Spatial Visualization – refers to the ability to manipulate representations of visual objects mentally. Tests measuring this ability load on Guilford's (1969) factor labeled Cognition of Figural Transformation. A typical item on one such test might require the testee to imagine a particular object having undergone a particular spatial transformation (e.g., a 90° rotation). The picture showing the result of that spatial transformation must then be selected from a number of alternative pictures. The second major spatial factor – Spatial Orientation – refers to the ability to determine spatial relationships with respect to an imagined orientation of one's own body. Tests measuring this ability load on Guilford's (1969) Cognition of Visual Figural Systems factor. A typical item on such a test might require the testee to determine which of a number of pictures of landscapes accurately shows what he or she would see from the cockpit of an airplane shown in another picture.

Tests of spatial ability have been shown to predict well certain aspects of job performance, technical-school success, and success in engineering, calculus, and other mathematics courses (see McGee, 1979; Smith, 1964, for reviews). From our point of view, tests of spatial ability provide an interesting place to look for attentional and perceptual correlates of intelligence for two reasons: First, the information-processing demands of these tests (e.g., imagining transformations on visual objects) seem, intuitively, to have much in common with ordinary perceptual processing. Second, unlike tests of verbal or reading ability, spatial ability tests do not seem particularly dependent on specific world knowledge. It might be in just this situation – when the contribution of knowledge is minimized – that the contribution of basic information-processing skills to ability measures could be most clearly revealed.

In the discussion that follows, we hope to accomplish several goals. First, we review some of the information-processing studies of tasks that seem to require skills similar to those tapped by items on tests of spatial ability. In particular, we provide evidence for sources of individual and group differences in performance on these tasks. Second, we examine studies that have specifically tried to relate measures of spatial ability to parameters of information-processing models for performance on tests of spatial ability. Finally, we attempt to make sense of the results of these studies, and we point to potential new directions in investigating the nature of spatial ability.

One information-processing task that has received considerable current attention and that bears similarity to visualization items on tests of spatial ability is the "mental rotation" task first studied by Shepard and Metzler (1971). In their initial experiment, Shepard and Metzler asked subjects to determine whether pairs of perspective drawings of three-dimensional objects were the same in shape or were mirror images. In addition to a possible difference in shape, the objects could differ in their portrayed orientations either in the picture plane or about an axis in depth. The most significant result of Shepard and Metzler's study was that the time required to make the same–different discrimination increased linearly with the difference in the portrayed orientations of the two objects in the pair. Shepard and Metzler interpreted these results as suggesting that subjects performed the task by imagining one object in the pair rotated into the orientation of the other object and then by comparing the transformed internal representation with the second object to determine whether there was a match or a mismatch in shape. Presumably, the slope of the reaction-time function provides an estimate of the rate at which this mental manipulation can be carried out, and the intercept provides an estimate of the time required to encode the two objects in the pair, to compare them following the mental rotation, and to select and execute the response of "same" or "different."

Subsequent studies of this process of mental rotation have shown that when familiar visual stimuli (e.g., letters of the alphabet) are shown individually in non-standard orientations, the time to determine whether they are normal or reflected versions increases monotonically with the extent of their departure from the canonical, upright position (Cooper & Shepard, 1973a, 1973b). In addition, linear reaction-time functions, indicating a process of mental rotation, have been demonstrated for stimuli such as random polygons (Cooper, 1975), and Cooper and Podgorny (1976) have shown that the rate of mental rotation of such polygons is unaffected by the complexity of the visual figures. Orderly relationships between decision time and extent and/or number of spatial transformations have not been limited to tasks in which the transformation is specifically one of rotation. For example, Shepard and Feng (1972) have reported that response time for "mental paper folding" items, similar to surface development items on tests of spatial ability, increases linearly with the number of transformations required to complete the items.

Models of the processes underlying these mental transformation tasks can be considered as characterizations of the operations involved when a given subject solves a given visualization item on a typical test of spatial ability. Is there any evidence from the information-processing literature for individual differences in mental transformation tasks that might ultimately be related to psychometrically measured spatial ability? In fact, in all of the studies just cited, substantial individual differences both in rate of mental transformation and in encoding, comparison, and response processes have consistently been found. For example, in the Cooper (1975) study, slopes of the linear function relating reaction time to angular disorientation (expressed in terms of rate of mental rotation) have ranged from 320° to 840° per sec for individual subjects, and intercepts have ranged from 300 to 1,000 msec. These differences are difficult to interpret from a psychometric viewpoint, however, because the number of subjects in each study has been small and the subjects have been selected from a population that undoubtedly would score high on tests of spatial ability (generally, university graduate students and faculty). Indeed, in the original Shepard and Metzler (1971) study, subjects were initially screened on the basis of a series of tests of spatial ability. In a subsequent study, Metzler and Shepard (1974) systematically investigated the effects of sex and handedness on mental rotation (again, with a small number of subjects), and no compelling or consistent patterns emerged in the data.

More recently, Kail and his associates (Kail, Carter, & Pellegrino, 1979; Kail, Pellegrino, & Carter, 1980) have used larger samples of subjects to investigate both developmental and sex differences in mental rotation studies. The developmental studies (Kail et al., 1980) – using subjects from Grades 3, 4, and 6 and from college – indicate that the rate of mental rotation increases with increasing chronological age, and also that the intercept of the reaction-time function decreases as age increases. In addition, these investigators found interactions between age and stimulus familiarity for encoding, comparison, and response processes (the intercept parameter). To the extent that one accepts the view that older subjects are generally more able, these results suggest that mental transformation processes are quicker and more efficient in those of higher ability.

Within a college population, Kail and his colleagues (1979) have examined sex differences in performance on a mental rotation task. To the extent that mental rotation tasks require the underlying processes that are measured in tests of spatial ability, such an investigation is quite reasonable. For there is a substantial body of literature documenting the superiority of males over females on psychometric tests of both the Visualization and the Orientation factor of spatial ability (see McGee, 1979, for a recent review of this literature). The results from the 1979 study by Kail and his co-workers can be summarized as follows: No differences were found between the sexes in the intercept of the reaction-time function, which presumably reflects the speed of encoding, comparison, and response processes. Somewhat curiously, given the psychometric literature, overall accuracy was also roughly equal for men and women. The extent to which the male and the female data were fit by linear functions was also equal, a finding which suggests that both sexes did indeed use a process of mental rotation in solving these spatial problems. The chief difference between the sexes was located in the slope of the reaction-time functions, with the men overall having a faster rate of rotation than the women. Closer examination of the data revealed that the variability of the slopes was considerably greater for women than for men, with about 30% of the distribution of slopes for women falling outside the distribution for men.

This study, then, is indirect support for the idea that speed of mental transformation is related to spatial ability. The support is only indirect, because no attempt was made to correlate psychometrically measured ability with parameters of performance on the mental rotation task for this set of subjects. The argument rests on the assumption that these subjects would show the sex differences in spatial ability that are characteristic of other populations. In any event, the studies of Kail and his associates and earlier studies of mental rotation provide compelling evidence for individual and group differences in the rate at which mental transformations on representations of visual objects can be carried out.

Several recent programs of research have taken the further step of attempting to relate measured spatial ability to parameters of information-processing tasks. We concentrate primarily on a series of studies by Egan (1976, 1978, 1979a, 1979b), although Lohman (1979b) has also reported an extensive if not readily interpretable study along these same lines. Egan's basic approach has been to recast items on tests of visualization and orientation abilities into an information-processing/latency framework. He then examines the relationship between overall accuracy on the psychometric tests and latency on the modified information-processing tasks. He goes on to develop process models of the operations underlying performance on the information-processing tasks, and he seeks to establish relationships between parameters of the process models and psychometric measures of spatial ability.

In all his studies, his subjects have been aviation officer candidates and naval flight officer candidates. An example of a psychometric test of orientation ability that Egan has used is the U.S. Navy's Spatial Apperception Test. In the standard version, the testee is shown a particular aerial view of a landscape, and must select from among five airplanes the one oriented so that a pilot in the cockpit would see that particular aerial view. In the information-processing/latency version of this task, one landscape paired with one airplane orientation is presented on each trial, and the subject must determine as rapidly as possible whether they are or are not correctly matched. An example of a psychometric test of visualization ability that Egan has used is the Guilford–Zimmerman Aptitude Survey's Spatial Visualization subtest. In the standard version, the testee must mentally rotate an alarm clock in a specified sequence, and then select which of five depicted clocks matches the final position in the sequence of transformations. In the latency version of this task, only one of the five alternative clocks is shown – paired with another clock and the specified sequence of transformations – and the subject must determine as rapidly as possible whether the test clock accurately depicts the result of the set of mental rotations.

In some initial studies, Egan (1976, 1978) found the following pattern of relationships among the accuracy and latency measures on the psychometric tests and the modified information-processing versions: Correlations among accuracy scores both across tests and between the psychometric and information-processing versions of a given test were generally high and positive. Also, latency scores correlated positively across information-processing tasks. However, the correlations between accuracy and latency measures were generally low and negative.[2] This failure to find a correlation between the accuracy and the reaction-time measures is not due to an unreliability in the reaction times, for reliability of the latency measures was generally as high as that of the accuracy measures. Further evidence for the independence of the accuracy and the reaction-time indexes derives from a factor analysis of the matrix of intercorrelations, in which the latency tasks and the accuracy measures clearly loaded on separate factors (Egan, 1978).

This pattern of results is puzzling, because the psychometric tests – on which overall accuracy is measured – are nonetheless taken under speeded or time-limited conditions. Thus the speed with which the mental operations underlying completion of individual items can be performed should presumably be reflected in the overall accuracy scores. There are several possible reasons for this lack of relationship between reaction time and accuracy. First, the two measures could be indexes of separate aspects of spatial ability. Second, the latency measure could have nothing to do with spatial ability, as measured on psychometric tests, but could rather reflect nothing more than some "general" speed factor. (We will consider this second possibility in some detail in a later section of the chapter.) The third and most interesting possibility is that, although accuracy and overall latency are not correlated, measured spatial ability still might correlate with one or more components of the reaction-time measure that reflect the time required for different mental operations.

To evaluate this third possibility, Egan (1978, 1979a, 1979b) developed process models of the mental operations in the reaction-time tasks and attempted to find relationships between spatial ability measures and different parameters of the models. We consider first his process model of the reaction-time version of the orientation task. Briefly, the model proposes that the subject first encodes the orientation shown in the aerial view and the orientation of the observer in the airplane cockpit in terms of a number of different spatial dimensions (in the case of items on this task, the dimensions would be extent of rotation about three different axes in space). The values of the two encoded representations on these spatial dimensions are then compared sequentially. As soon as a mismatch is found, the response "no" can be executed; the "yes" response can be executed only after all three dimensions have been compared and found to match. This model clearly predicts that the time taken to respond will increase as the number of dimensions on which the two pictures match increases. The slope of the reaction-time function should provide an estimate of the time for a single-dimensional comparison, and the intercept should reflect the time needed for encoding and response selection and execution.

Egan (1979a) found that the group data generally fit the model well, in that latency scores increased linearly with the number of matching spatial dimensions. But to what extent might accuracy scores or measures of spatial ability be related to either the rate of comparing spatial dimensions or the speed of encoding and response processes? Correlations of intercepts, slopes, and degree of linearity of the reaction-time functions with spatial ability measures revealed only two significant relationships. First, the degree to which the latency functions were linear was positively correlated with measured spatial ability. Second, for a subset of the subjects, the intercept parameter showed a significant negative correlation with ability measures. What these results suggest is that the basic information-processing skill contributing to high scores on spatial ability tests is efficiency or speed of encoding and response processes, rather than the efficiency with which spatial dimensions can be compared. The degree of linearity of the reaction-time functions may reflect the extent to which subjects were consistent in using the dimensional comparison strategy, and this, too, was positively related to measured spatial ability.

A similar and somewhat disappointing picture emerges from an analysis of the relationship between hypothesized information-processing parameters in the visualization task and psychometric measures of spatial ability. Egan's (1976, 1978, 1979b) information-processing/latency version of the visualization test is basically the mental rotation task already discussed. The intercept of the reaction-time function can be thought of as the time required to encode the two visual objects in the pair, to compare them following the mental rotation, and to select and execute the appropriate response. The slope provides an estimate of the speed of the actual process of mental transformation. (The model that Egan, 1976, 1978, 1979b, proposes for this task is slightly different from the account just given, of the component processes in mental rotation. It derives from Just and Carpenter's (1976) analysis of patterns of eye fixations while subjects perform a mental rotation task.)

As in his analysis of the orientation task, Egan (1979a) found support from the group data for his information-processing analysis of the visualization task, in that reaction time increased approximately linearly with the angular difference between the portrayed orientations of the two visual objects to be compared. However, correlations between the slopes of the functions for individual subjects and measures of spatial ability were generally quite low, whereas the correlation between intercept and accuracy (the ability measure) was a statistically significant $-.30$. Once again, it appears that efficiency of encoding and comparison processes – not rate of mental transformation – is a basic information-processing skill underlying spatial ability. One further aspect of Egan's data deserves mention. In addition to the latency versions of the psychometric tests, he included a two-choice reaction-time task. Latency scores on this task had generally low correlations with accuracy measures. This finding suggests that the significant correlation between intercept and ability in the mental rotation task really does reflect efficiency of visual coding and comparison operations, rather than response processes or a general speed factor, both of which are measured in the choice reaction-time task.

In summary, the Egan studies provide little support for the appealing notion that the speed with which mental transformations such as rotation or comparison of spatial dimensions can be carried out underlies measures of spatial ability. Rather, speed of encoding operations is related in a weak though statistically significant way to the ability measures. A similar conclusion can be drawn from the work of Pellegrino, Glaser, and their associates on the operations involved in the solution of geometric analogies (see Glaser & Pellegrino, 1978–1979; Mulholland, Pellegrino, & Glaser, 1980; Pellegrino & Glaser, 1980). In these studies, latencies for solving geometric analogies varying in difficulty – in terms of both the number of spatial transformations required and the number of visual elements that must be transformed – have been examined, and components of the latency measures have been correlated with psychometric measures of ability. A full consideration of this impressive body of work is beyond the scope of the present chapter. Two of the findings, however, are relevant to this discussion. First, measures of the rate of transformational processing were not significantly correlated with ability measures. Second, there was a significant negative relationship ($r = -.44$) between ability scores and intercepts of the reaction-time functions (see also R. Sternberg, 1977).

Our tentative conclusion that basic processes of visual coding, representation, and comparison may contribute more to spatial ability than seemingly more complex operations such as efficiency of mental transformation does not go unchallenged. One obvious problem with this analysis comes from the studies of developmental and sex differences in rate of mental rotation that were discussed earlier (Kail et al., 1979, 1980). Recall that in those studies both older subjects and, within an adult sample, male subjects were found to have shallower reaction-time functions (faster rates of mental rotation) than younger subjects or females. These findings suggest that spatial ability and transformation rate are related, in that adults are generally more able than children, and females tend to score lower on tests of spatial ability than do males. The argument is not conclusive, however, because no psychometric measures of spatial ability were available for the subjects in these studies; so a direct correlational analysis of mental rotation rate and ability score could not be performed.

A much more problematic finding comes from a recent study by Lansman (1979). In the portion of this study that is relevant to the present discussion, Lansman found a strong correlation between scores on a Visualization factor and slopes of reaction-time functions from a mental rotation task. (The correlation was $-.50$, with faster rotaters scoring higher on the ability measure than slower rotaters.) Furthermore, no significant correlations were obtained between this slope parameter and other ability factors, and efficiency of mental transformation was thus strongly implicated as a component of specifically spatial ability. Lansman also reported a significant correlation ($-.25$) between the spatial ability measure and the intercept parameter. Finally, in marked contrast to Egan's (1976, 1978) results, a high negative correlation emerged in Lansman's study between overall latency on the rotation task and accuracy on the spatial ability measure. It is difficult to interpret Lansman's results as reflecting an overall speed component in ability, because the reaction-time measures on the mental rotation task correlated almost exclusively with the Visualization factor, and not with other ability factors. We conclude, then, that there is reasonable evidence for a relationship between visual encoding processes and measured spatial ability, in that the correlation between ability and intercept is ubiquitous.[3] Any evidence for a relationship between mental manipulation speed and spatial ability needs to be established more firmly, however.

In concluding this section on spatial ability, we would like to point briefly to two potentially fruitful directions for research on basic information-processing skills underlying spatial ability measures. One research avenue might involve assessing the relationship between spatial ability and components of information-processing tasks not specifically derived from items on psychometric tests. In most of the studies reviewed herein, the information-processing tasks have been adaptations in a reaction-time framework of individual items on psychometric tests of spatial ability. Our understanding of the component processes underlying spatial ability might benefit from research examining other kinds of tasks that provide more general measures of visual encoding and comparison operations (e.g., same–different visual matching) in terms of the relationships of the processes in these tasks to measures of spatial ability. (See Lansman, 1979, however, for an unsuccessful attempt to relate parameters of a model of the sentence–picture verification task to spatial ability.)

A second research direction might involve exploring the relationship between the cognitive processes underlying more "ecologically valid" spatial information-processing tasks and psychometric measures of spatial ability. A topic of considerable current interest in cognitive psychology concerns the way in which information about the relationships among objects and locations in an environment is acquired, represented internally, and accessed for purposes of making judgments about that environment or for purposes of actual locomotion through the environment from one place to another (see, e.g., Baum & Jonides, 1979; Kosslyn, Pick, & Fariello, 1974; Loftus, 1976; Stevens & Coupe, 1978, to mention but a few recent studies).

This research effort to understand the nature of the mental operations and representations underlying "cognitive mapping" has proceeded by and large without a concern for determining possible relationships between the processes involved in generating and using cognitive maps and the processes contributing to measures of spatial ability. There are several exceptions to this general statement. For example, Kozlowski and Bryant (1977) have successfully correlated self-reports of "sense of direction" with performance on a task related to learning to locomote through an actual environment. Even more relevant for our purposes is a preliminary set of studies by Thorndyke and Stasz (1980). These investigators have been examining the factors that make particular persons more or less adept at learning to read maps of fictitious environments. On the basis of an initial study, they identified a variety of processing strategies that appeared to underlie effective map learning. In a subsequent experiment, Thorndyke and Stasz demonstrated (a) that certain of the learning strategies were trainable, and (b) that both map-learning performance and success in the use of learning strategies were positively related to a psychometric measure of spatial ability. These initial results are suggestive, and they underscore the potential utility of examining the relationship between the operations involved in learning and using representations of the environment and psychometric measures of spatial ability.

SUMMARY AND EVALUATION

Thus far we have considered in some detail a number of studies designed to uncover relationships between information-processing skills and measures of ability. The goal of this approach to studying individual differences is to provide a theoretical framework for the analysis of human intelligence. That is, rather than viewing ability as some "thing" or trait that is reflected in a global test score, we have tried to isolate basic perceptual and cognitive processes that distinguish higher- from lower-ability persons. To the extent that this effort is successful, we should be able to provide an account of the nature of the mental operations that make individuals intelligent. But how successful has this effort actually been? Here we briefly review the central findings from experiments on individual differences in verbal ability, reading ability, and spatial ability. We then point to problems in the interpretation of the results of these experiments, as well as to more general problems with the information-processing approach to an analysis of ability. Detailed and subtle methodological criticisms are beyond the scope of our discussion. However, several excellent methodological papers have recently appeared (see, e.g., Baron & Treiman, 1980; Carroll, 1978; Hunt & MacLeod, 1978; McClelland & Jackson, 1978).

Despite the relatively large amount of experimental work, few consistent findings have emerged from studies of the relationship between information-processing tasks and verbal ability. The one clear result, obtained by virtually all investigators, is that high verbal subjects show a smaller difference than do low verbal subjects between the time needed to determine that two letters of different cases share the same name and the time needed to determine that two physically identical letters are the same (the NI–PI difference). The general interpretation of this result is that high verbal subjects enjoy faster access to overlearned codes in memory (letter names) than do low verbal subjects. High verbal subjects may also have more rapid and efficient memory-scanning and comparison operations, particularly when the reference group is very low-ability subjects (Hunt, 1978) or children (Keating & Bobbitt, 1978).

Related to the NI–PI difference between high and low verbal subjects are findings on the Posner task: Studies of reading ability have consistently found that good readers can more quickly than poorer readers access the name of a letter code in memory. This ability, which accounts for about 10% of the variance in reading ability, is not restricted to letter codes. Better readers can more efficiently access the name of any meaningful visual pattern, even when practice with the pattern is held constant (Jackson, 1978). Though many investigations have indicated that modality-independent language comprehension skills account for the bulk of the variance in reading ability, Frederiksen (1978) has offered a component-process model of reading and has devised simple reaction-time tasks for isolating those processes which in one study accounted for nearly all the variance in reading ability in a sample of high-school students.

In the area of spatial ability, the picture is complicated by conflicting findings. However, one result that tends to emerge quite consistently is that the intercept of the function relating reaction time to extent of spatial transformation is significantly negatively correlated with spatial ability. An interpretation of this negative correlation is that high spatial subjects are faster at visual encoding and comparison operations than are low spatial subjects. It may also be that high spatial subjects are faster at performing mental transformations (measured by the slope of the reaction-time function), but the evidence is mixed (see, in particular, Egan, 1978; Lansman, 1979).

Even for the few information-processing differences that have been found to relate to individual differences in ability, there are problems of theoretical interpretation. We divide these problems into two general categories: problems relating to the possibility of a general speed factor and problems deriving from the adequacy of the theoretical analysis of the information-processing tasks. With regard to the possibility of a general speed factor, we should note that in virtually all of the information-processing tasks discussed, response time has been the chief dependent variable of interest; and correlations between reaction time and ability level or the magnitude of reaction-time differences that relate to ability have constituted the evidence for basic information-processing factors in intelligence. But could it not be the case that the efficiency of component-processing operations – presumably measured by the cognitive tasks – has little or nothing to do with measured ability? Rather, more able individuals could simply be faster at hitting response buttons than less able individuals, and hence the correlations between performance on reaction-time tasks and ability level could emerge.

It is very difficult to eliminate this possibility of a general speed difference between high- and low-ability subjects in the case of many of the experiments that we have discussed. However, in some of the studies, there is at least indirect evidence that overall speed is not the sole determinant of the relationship between performance on information-processing tasks and ability. For example, Jackson and McClelland (1979) failed to find a statistically significant reaction-time difference between fast and average readers in either a dot-pattern-matching task or a physical identity letter-matching task, but the times for the two groups did differ reliably on a name identity letter-matching task. Presumably, if the chief difference between the fast and average readers is one of general speed, then the time required for visual pattern matching (measured by the dot pattern and the physical identity letter-pattern tasks) – as well as the time needed for name identity letter matching – should have been less for the high- than for the lower-ability subjects. Another example of a finding that argues against a general speed factor comes from Egan (1978). Recall that he obtained very low correlations between choice reaction time and spatial ability while obtaining considerably higher correlations between ability and other reaction-time parameters from his information-processing tasks. Similarly, Keating and Bobbitt (1978) found higher correlations among reaction-time parameters that were theoretically related than among parameters that were not hypothesized to be related. Again, if overall response speed – rather than the efficiency of particular processing operations – underlies differences in ability, then all of these correlations between ability and reaction-time parameters and between the reaction-time parameters themselves should have been roughly equal.

There is evidence, though, that strongly suggests that a general speed factor may contribute substantially to the relationship between performance on information-processing tasks and ability. Jensen (1979) has amassed considerable evidence for correlations among various parameters from reaction-time tasks and general measures of ability. Indeed, by combining certain parameters in a multiple regression equation, Jensen shows that about 50% of the variance in measured ability can be accounted for. Perhaps more relevant to the issue of a general speed factor are Jensen's (1979; Jensen & Munro, 1979) own studies on the relationship of reaction time and movement time to intelligence. In this paradigm, the subject must lift a finger from a home key when one, two, four, or eight lights, arranged in a semicircle around the home key, go on. The subject must then turn off the light by touching a microswitch directly below it. The time taken to lift the finger off the home key, once the light has appeared, is defined as the subject's reaction time. The time taken actually to turn off the light, once the finger has been raised, is the subject's movement time. Jensen and Munro (1979) have reported a −.39 correlation between reaction time and scores on the Raven Standard Progressive Matrices (Raven, 1960) and a correlation of −.43 between movement time and Raven scores. Note that these correlations are as high as those obtained between ability measures and reaction-time parameters from information-processing tasks. Furthermore, it is difficult to argue that the operations that theoretically underlie performance on the informa-tion-processing tasks (encoding, memory access, etc.) are involved in the simple task that Jensen is studying. Jensen and Munro's data strongly suggest a relation-ship between overall speed and ability scores. However, the theoretical interpreta-tion of this relationship between speed and intelligence is not clear. From these data, Jensen (1979) concludes only that intelligence tests "tap fundamental processes involved in individual differences in intellectual ability and not merely differences in specific knowledge, acquired skills, or cultural background" (p. 1).

If one accepts the notion that relationships between processing parameters in cognitive tasks and ability measures reflect more than a general speed factor, then problems with the interpretation of these relationships still remain. This second set of problems concerns the theoretical adequacy of the analysis of the component processes required by the information-processing tasks. Stated simply, any in-terpretation of a reaction-time difference between groups in an information-process-ing task or a correlation of reaction time with ability will be only as good as the theory of the component operations underlying performance on the information-processing task. This is why, throughout, we have praised studies in which an attempt has been made to establish construct validity for processing operations in various cognitive tasks.

As an example of the relationship between theory in cognitive psychology and the interpretation of sources of individual differences, consider the sentence–picture verification task (Clark & Chase, 1972). Hunt and his associates (1975) found that high verbal subjects had a smaller effect of negation than did low verbal subjects on reaction times both for encoding an initially presented sentence and for comparing the sentence with a subsequently presented picture. Their interpretation of this difference was tied to then-current theory of the nature of the mental operations and representations involved in the sentence–picture verification situation. In subse-quent work, Lansman (1979) has explored further possible relationships between ability factors and performance on this task. She found that both the information-processing model proposed by Clark and Chase (1972) and a modification of this model introduced by Carpenter and Just (1975) accounted for about 97% of the variance in the group mean reaction-time data. She went on to perform an indi-vidual-difference analysis of the sort suggested by Underwood (1975) as a test of the adequacy of the information-processing models. This was accomplished by deriving parameters from the reaction-time data that, according to the two models, provided measures of essentially the same underlying mental processes, and then correlating these two parameters across individual subjects. The results of this analysis and the derivation of the model parameters are too complex to be considered in detail here. What Lansman found, essentially, was that two of the parameters that theoretically provided measures of the same mental process, according to both of the models, correlated only .03 across individuals. And, if the cognitive models of the sen-tence–picture verification task were indeed accurate, then these measures should have been highly correlated across individual subjects.

What Lansman's analysis suggests is that neither the Clark and Chase nor the Carpenter and Just model gives an adequate account of the processes underlying performance in the sentence–picture verification task. In the absence of an adequate theory of an information-processing task, any interpretation of individual differences in performance on the task becomes virtually impossible. (In Lansman's study, only weak relationships between ability factors and reaction-time parameters were found.) It should be noted that the sentence–picture verification paradigm is particularly vulnerable to this criticism. MacLeod and his colleagues (1978) have reported substantial individual differences in strategies used to compare sentences with pictures. Glushko and Cooper (1978) have also demonstrated that seemingly minor variations in temporal parameters of the task can lead to gross changes in strategies within individual subjects. The general point, however, which extends beyond the sentence–picture verification task, is that interpretation of information-processing differences and their relation to differences in ability is only as powerful and adequate as current theory in cognitive psychology.

There are several issues in the interpretation of processing differences that are related to the general point of the adequacy of models of cognitive tasks. One of these issues concerns the specificity of the processes that distinguish higher- from lower-ability persons. That is, when we find that a particular parameter of performance on a reaction-time task distinguishes high- from low-ability subjects, are we to attribute the underlying processing difference to some aspect of the task or to the efficiency of some more basic general mental operation? Often this is a difficult question to resolve. Consider, for example, Jackson and McClelland's (1979) finding that good and poor readers differed more, in reaction-time performance, on a homonym-matching task than on the standard Posner name identity letter-matching task. At first blush, this result suggests that phonological processes – presumably tapped by the homonym task – contribute more to differences in reading ability than does a general factor of access to overlearned codes in memory. However, when Jackson and McClelland partialed out the contribution of name identity matching to effective reading speed, the relationship between the homonyn task and ability became negligible. So the more general operation of memory access, rather than phonological processing per se, was responsible for the differences in reading ability. Another obvious example of this issue of general versus specific information-processing skills comes from the work of Jackson (1978), showing that retrieval of general conceptual categories, rather than specific access to letters names, mediates the difference between good and poor readers on performance in the Posner letter-matching task situation.

A second issue in interpreting the relationship between reaction-time and ability differences concerns the precise location of the source of individual variation in the information-processing sequence. To the extent that we adopt the view that component information processes are interactive and interdependent – rather than strictly serial or parallel and independent – then it will be difficult to determine just which processes contribute to individual differences in ability. For differences in lower-level processes, such as accessing learned information from memory, will influence the efficiency of operation of higher-level processes as well. McClelland and Jackson (1978) elaborate this point, with respect to the particular example of information-processing determinants of reading ability:

It is also worth noting that accessing information in memory may well influence other important components of the reading process as well. Within the context of models in which all components of the process are strongly interdependent (e.g., Rumelhart, 1977[b]) it is clear that accessing syntactic, semantic, and lexical information in memory must be an important determinant not only of comprehension itself, but of the actual process of picking up information from the printed page. Faster access to the semantic and syntactic properties of words picked up in one reading fixation will leave the faster reader in a better position to use contextual information to infer letters and words he has not fully processed from the page, and to guide the movements of the eye to an advantageous position for picking up information on the next fixation. Indeed, if we adopt an interactive model of reading, there is hardly any aspect of the reading process which will not be facilitated by more efficient access to information in memory. [Pp. 200–201]

The final issue that we mention concerning interpretation of information-processing skills underlying individual differences in ability is the temporal stability of the demonstrated or hypothesized processing differences. The studies reviewed here are essentially silent on this matter. Though certain reaction-time differences (e.g., the difference between the times for name identity and physical identity letter matching) have been shown to be stable correlates of verbal and reading ability across different variations of the matching task, different groups of adult subjects, and different developmental levels, there has been virtually no attempt to show that given groups of subjects that differ in ability continue to differ in the magnitude of an information-processing difference over time. The demonstration of such temporal stability of processing differences – alleged to constitute sources of individual differences in ability – would seem important to establish.

In concluding this section, we must note that, despite the initial promise of the attempt to combine psychometric and information-processing approaches to the study of individual differences, the magnitude of the relationships between ability measures and basic processing parameters appears to be small. Correlations between psychometric measures of ability and information-processing operations have hovered around .30. Why might it be that component information-processing skills fail to account for much of the variance in ability scores? There are several possibilities, all of which could be contributing to the weakness of these relationships.

One possibility is that the ability measures that have been correlated with performance differences on information-processing tasks are simply too global and that higher correlations could be obtained between processing parameters and more refined subscales of ability. Another possibility is that the information-processing tasks that have been studied are not sensitive enough to reveal sources of individual differences. A related idea (already discussed in some detail) is that models of these cognitive tasks are inadequate and lead to the selection of inappropriate processing parameters for correlational analyses with ability differences. Still a third possibility is that basic information-processing skills in fact are weak determinants of individual differences in ability. In the case of verbal ability, in particular, it is quite conceivable that general knowledge factors influence test scores more heavily than do component content-free perceptual and cognitive factors. At a more general level, it could be that, whereas differences in basic information-processing skills provide a reliable (if small) contribution to individual differences in ability, strategies for selecting component perceptual and cognitive operations and flexibility in attentional factors provide an even greater contribution. We consider this final possibility in more detail in the following section.

3.2.   THE ROLE OF STRATEGIES AND ATTENTION IN INDIVIDUAL DIFFERENCES
        IN ABILITY

The generally low correlations between basic information-processing parameters and individual differences in ability have led to the suspicion that other, more flexible aspects of cognitive functioning may make more substantial contributions to intelligence than do low-level processing skills. These additional aspects may include strategies – the methods that one selects for approaching a task or solving a problem – and general attentional factors. This point is certainly not a novel one. Hunt (1974), for example, has distinguished between two quite different strategies for completing items on the Raven Progressive Matrices test of general intelligence. One strategy is based on an algorithm that relies on Gestalt-like perceptual factors, and the other strategy is more analytic in nature. R. J. Sternberg (1977), too, has emphasized the importance of strategies, or the order in which component-processing operations are combined, in the solution of analogy items.

Recently, both Baron (1978) and Hunt (1978, 1980) have pointed to several sources of individual differences in intelligence. The basic distinction that Baron makes is between capacities, or unmodifiable information-processing limitations, and strategies, or modifiable procedures for organizing cognitive processes in acquiring knowledge and solving problems. Hunt's distinction is basically the same, but to the list of sources of individual differences in competence he adds general attentional resources, or "cognitive energy." Baron argues vigorously for the importance of strategies in ability differences, and he marshals considerable empirical evidence – primarily from developmental studies and work on human memory – in support of his argument.[4] He concludes this provocative paper by speculating about the nature of central strategies (those which transfer to both novel and familiar situations) that might make some people appear more intelligent than others. The central strategies that he considers most important include relatedness search, the strategy of searching memory for items related in some way to an item that is presented; stimulus analysis, the strategy of processing a stimulus in terms of its component parts or dimensions; and checking, the strategy of suppressing an initial response in order to evaluate other possibilities. Here we too emphasize the contribution of strategies to individual differences in performance. Our discussion has two parts: In the first, we provide evidence for a relationship between strategies and differences in measured ability; in the second, we selectively review evidence for qualitative individual differences in strategies whose relationship to intelligence is less clear. We conclude this section with a brief consideration of individual differences in attentional resources and mechanisms.

STRATEGIES

One reason why it is difficult to study strategies experimentally is that we rarely have a clear notion of what sorts of strategies are available for performing cognitive tasks until we observe compelling individual or group differences in patterns of data. Once we have isolated different strategies in this fashion, we can ask further questions concerning their trainability or manipulability by performing experiments in which different groups of subjects are instructed to use one strategy or another. A very nice set of studies following essentially this line of reasoning, and further, providing evidence about the relationship of strategies to ability, has recently been reported by MacLeod and his associates (1978) and by Hunt (1980). In the initial experiment, MacLeod and his colleagues had two aims. They were interested both in testing alternative models of the sentence–picture verification task and in relating performance on the task to psychometric measures of verbal, reading, and spatial abilities. Both of the models, one proposed by Clark and Chase (1972) and the other proposed by Carpenter and Just (1975), assume that subjects use a linguistic strategy in performing the task, in that they encode both the initially presented sentence and the subsequently presented picture into propositional representations for purposes of comparing the two. The models differ primarily in the nature of the matching operation, but both predict that the variables of negation and linguistic markedness should increase the time taken to perform the verification operation.

In the procedure followed in the study by MacLeod and his co-workers, the time taken to encode or comprehend the initial sentence and the time taken to perform the subsequent verification were measured separately. The fit of the Carpenter and Just model to the group mean verification-time data for different sentence types was impressive. The model accounted for 89.4% of the variance in reaction times. However, correlations for individual subjects between model predictions and verification times were quite variable, ranging from .998 to −.877. In order to investigate these individual differences in more detail, MacLeod and his colleagues divided their subjects into groups that were "well fit" and "poorly fit" by the model. The data from the well-fit group showed strong effects of the linguistic variables (captured in the different sentence types), whereas the data from the poorly fit group showed virtually no effect of the linguistic variables.

The failure to find linguistic effects in the poorly fit group suggests that they may use a fundamentally different strategy in comparing sentences and pictures. One such strategy – primarily spatial in nature – would involve generating a visual image of the relationship between the elements described in the sentence during the comprehension interval and then directly comparing this generated visual image against the picture during the verification interval. Contrast this with the "linguistic" strategy of converting the picture into a propositional representation for purposes of comparison with the linguistically encoded representation of the sentence. The use of these different strategies suggests several hypotheses concerning group differences in the pattern of reaction-time results. Specifically, the spatial strategy should require considerable processing time during comprehension – when a visual image of the elements related in the sentence is being generated – and little processing time during verification – when the generated image is being directly compared with the picture. The linguistic strategy should yield just the opposite pattern. During comprehension, the sentence is being linguistically encoded, and this encoding should be relatively rapid. During verification, however, the picture must be converted into a linguistic representation, and it must be compared with the internal representation of the sentence. The data provided by MacLeod and his associates confirm these predictions nicely. The poorly fit group had longer comprehension times than did the well-fit group, as they should were they using a spatial/imaginal strategy. And the poorly fit group also had shorter verification times than did the well-fit group, a finding that is again consistent with the proposed differences in their strategies.

Even more intriguing are the relationships that MacLeod and his colleagues found between strategy use and psychometric measures of ability. Partial correlations between verbal ability (with spatial ability held constant) and verification time were −.44 for the well-fit group and −.05 for the poorly fit group. Similar correlations with spatial ability were .07 for the well-fit and −.64 for the poorly fit group. There was a significant correlation (.55) between sex and verification time for the poorly fit group, but not for the well-fit group. This provides additional evidence that the poorly fit subjects were using a spatial strategy, in light of the relationship between sex and spatial ability. Finally, inspection of the actual test scores of the two groups of subjects revealed that they did not differ in verbal ability, but the poorly fit group had considerably higher spatial ability scores.

In conclusion, this study presents a variety of converging evidence concerning the use of alternative strategies in a "simple" information-processing situation. If strategy choice can alter performance so markedly on this sentence–picture verification task, then the potential impact of strategy selection on the solution of more complex problems, undoubtedly including items on tests of intelligence, may be great indeed. The relationships between strategy use and psychometric measures of ability are some of the most intriguing of the results from the study by MacLeod and his co-workers, particularly the finding that subjects with high spatial ability tended to rely on a visual strategy. Does this mean that strategy "selection" is in some sense automatic – dictated by one's relative ability and not under conscious control? The results of a recent study by Mathews, Hunt, and MacLeod (cited in Hunt, 1980) suggest quite the opposite. These investigators replicated the pattern of data from the original experiment by MacLeod and his colleagues, this time predicting (correctly) in advance, on the basis of psychometric scores, which subjects should adopt spatial and which should adopt linguistic strategies. In later phases of the experiment, the same subjects were instructed concerning use of the two strategies, and it was found that they could behave in accord with either of the strategies when instructed appropriately. Thus, although a person's choice of the type of strategy to apply – when this element is optional – may be related to relative ability, there nonetheless appears to be considerable flexibility and trainability in strategy selection.

This conjecture is supported by recent studies by R. J. Sternberg and Weil (1980). These investigators presented subjects with linear syllogisms of the form "X is taller than Y; Y is taller than Z; who is tallest?" They hypothesized that the strategies used by subjects to solve these problems would be related to their levels of verbal and spatial abilities. The hypothesis was confirmed, with response times of subjects who used a linguistic strategy being correlated with verbal ability, but not with spatial ability, scores. The reverse correlational pattern was obtained for subjects identified as using a spatial strategy for solving the syllogisms. Of additional interest in this study is the finding that instruction about which of several alternative strategies to adopt led to clear differences in the nature of the models that best fit the data.

There are other sources of evidence for qualitative individual differences in the perceptual and cognitive operations that are used to perform a given task. One of these sources comes from the literature on "cognitive styles." Detailed consideration of this large and complex literature is beyond the scope of our discussion (but see Messick, 1976, for a recent review). We mention this literature only because there are suggestions that certain cognitive styles may reflect strategy differences, and that these differences are related to intelligence. Witkin (1964) presents evidence that the "field-independence–field-dependence" dimension of cognitive style correlates with intelligence, with more intelligent subjects being more field-independent. Zelniker and Jeffrey (in press) suggest that the "impulsive–reflective" dimension of cognitive style in children derives from strategies for attending to global versus detailed aspects of visual stimuli. And there is some evidence, though conflicting, that reflective children (those who process stimulus details) score higher on nonverbal intelligence tests (Messer, 1976).

Another source of evidence for individual differences in perceptual and cognitive strategies comes from recent experiments in the information-processing tradition. In these experiments, strategy differences have typically not been related to psychometric measures of intelligence. We consider these experiments important, though, because they purport to demonstrate qualitative processing differences between subjects in relatively simple perceptual and cognitive tasks – tasks often similar to those used in the search for basic information-processing correlates of ability. To the extent that individual differences in strategies are apparent in even basic information-processing situations, we have reason to believe that they must operate as well in more complex forms of intellectual behavior. Here we review some of these experiments in more detail.

One set of studies on individual differences in modes of perceptual processing comes from the work of Cooper and her collaborators on visual same–different pattern matching (see, in particular, Cooper, 1976, 1980a, 1980b; Cooper & Podgorny, 1976). In the basic paradigm in which the processing differences were first discovered, subjects were required to determine as rapidly as possible whether two successively presented random polygons were the same or different in shape. The second (test) polygon presented either was identical to the first (standard) or differed by a random perturbation in shape. Further, the "different" probes varied in their rated similarity to the standards.

Inspection of the data on individual subjects revealed two distinctly different patterns. For the larger subset of subjects, "different" reaction time decreased monotonically as dissimilarity between the standard and the test shape increased. "Same" reaction time was intermediate in speed – faster than the slowest (most highly similar) "different" response, but slower than the fastest (most dissimilar) "different" response. For the smaller subset of subjects, "different" reaction time was unaffected by similarity of the test shape to the standard, and average "same" reaction time was faster than any average "different" time. This second group of subjects was also considerably faster overall than the first group. Furthermore, despite the marked differences in their reaction-time performance, the two groups of subjects did not differ in either the magnitude or the pattern of their errors. For both groups, error rate decreased monotonically with increasing dissimilarity between the standard and the test shape.

The constellation of differences in patterns of performance – involving overall response time, sensitivity of reaction time to similarity, relative speed of the "same" and the "different" responses, and the relationship between reaction time and error rate – led Cooper (1976, 1980a; Cooper & Podgorny, 1976) to argue that the two types of subjects used quite different mental operations in comparing a memory representation of a visual shape with another, externally presented visual test shape. The subjects who were affected by similarity could be using an analytic comparison strategy, comparing the memory representation of the standard and the visual test shape feature by feature. This would explain the decrease in reaction time with increasing dissimilarity, because the more features there are that distinguish the memory representation from the test stimulus, the earlier will the comparison process succeed in finding one or more of those differences. The subjects who were unaffected by similarity could be using a more holistic comparison strategy, performing a parallel, templatelike comparison, in an attempt to verify that the memory representation and the test shape are the same. This holistic "sameness" comparison would explain both why the "same" responses of these subjects are faster than their "different" responses and why the "different" responses are not affected by similarity. For the "different" response could be made by default if the "same" comparison fails, requiring no further stimulus analysis. (For more details concerning the nature of these hypothesized comparison strategies, see Cooper, 1976, 1980a.)

Having isolated these performance differences in a number of independent experiments, Cooper (1980a, 1980b) went on to consider the related questions (a) whether additional evidence for the nature of underlying comparison strategies could be obtained, and (b) whether a given person's comparison strategy could be changed by various stimulus and judgmental manipulations. Unlike the study by Mathews and her associates (cited in Hunt, 1980), Cooper's informal observation suggested that in the visual comparison task subjects could not modify their natural strategies by mere instruction about the nature of the alternative strategy.

On the other hand, Cooper was successful in a series of experiments in causing some subjects to change to an alternative strategy by creating information-processing demands that naturally drew upon one strategy type or the other. Some of the central findings can be summarized as follows: When the same–different task is modified to incorporate the explicit detection of differences between the standard and the test shapes (by requiring subjects to determine the approximate location of a differing feature), some "holistic" subjects will switch to an "analytic" strategy. Presumably this is because the detection of differing features is a natural part of the analytic strategy, but this information is not available to the holistic comparison operation. When the visual materials used in the comparison task are multidimensional stimuli (two alternative shapes of two alternative colors and sizes), then all subjects show results consistent with an analytic mode of processing. Presumably this is because stimuli composed of such separable dimensions (c.f. Garner, 1974) cannot be integrated into a holistic internal representation and used as a basis for visual comparison. On the other hand, when the visual materials used in the comparison task are photographs of human faces varying in their rated similarity, almost all subjects give results consistent with a holistic mode of processing. This finding is suggestive in light of the current belief that configural properties of faces make them difficult to analyze in terms of their component parts or features (see e.g., Carey & Diamond, 1977). So these and other findings (Cooper, 1980a, 1980b) indicate that individual subjects approach even this very simple visual information-processing task with preferred strategies that are, to some extent, manipulable with changes in judgmental requirements and variables of stimulus structure.

To what extent might there be a relationship between ability and choice or use of a holistic or analytic comparison strategy? It is very difficult to evaluate this question, because in Cooper's studies the sample sizes were quite small, and no psychometric measures of ability were available for these subjects. It is worth noting, however, that the subjects were drawn from a population that most likely is relatively homogeneous in ability scores. Many (in some studies, the majority) of the subjects were graduate students and faculty members at universities. It is also the case that the two types of processors did not differ in their overall magnitude or pattern of error rates; so neither strategy type produced more success at the task as indexed by the error rate measure. It could be argued that, as far as optimizing all aspects of performance is concerned, the holistic strategy is superior to the analytic strategy. For the holistic subjects have faster response times than the analytic subjects, they fail to show effects of similarity, and they function with no detectable cost in errors. The holistic subjects also seem more flexible in adopting alternative strategies than do the analytic subjects (Cooper, unpublished data). But this account is merely speculative, going beyond the data. Though any relationship between these processing strategies and ability remains elusive, the existence of marked individual differences in preferred modes of processing visual information seems relatively clear.[5]

Hock and his associates (Hock, 1973; Hock, Gordon, & Gold, 1975; Hock, Gordon,

& Marcus, 1974; Hock & Ross, 1975) have proposed an information-processing dichotomy in same–different visual pattern-matching tasks that, superficially, seems related to the holistic–analytic distinction proposed by Cooper (1976, 1980a, 1980b; Cooper & Podgorny, 1976). Basically, Hock's research strategy consists of manipulating some aspects of stimulus structure in a same–different comparison task. For example, Hock (1973) presented for same–different comparison pairs of dot patterns that could be either symmetrical or asymmetrical and familiar or unfamiliar (manipulated both by pretraining and by rotating pretrained patterns 180° from their familiar orientation). Mean "same" reaction-time differences attributable to the stimulus manipulations were then computed for each subject by determining, for individual subjects, the difference between reaction times to asymmetrical and to symmetrical patterns and the difference between reaction times to familiar and to unfamiliar (rotated) patterns. These reaction-time differences were then correlated, and when a statistically significant positive correlation was obtained, it was argued that there are individual differences in strategies for processing visual information. (Additional stimulus factors that Hock and his associates have investigated in essentially the same way include physically identical versus name identical letter pairs [Hock et al., 1975] and intactness versus embeddedness of familiar visual figures [Hock et al., 1974].)

Hock characterizes these putative individual differences as emphases on "structural" versus "analytic" modes of processing visual stimuli. The "structural" subjects are those who are affected by the stimulus manipulations, and they are thought to process visual material on the basis of configural information. The "analytic" subjects are relatively unaffected by the stimulus manipulations, and they are claimed to process visual material on the basis of component parts of features. There are two central questions that can be raised concerning Hock's classification of individuals as structural versus analytic processors of visual information. First, is there any reason to believe that this structural–analytic distinction corresponds to the holistic–analytic distinction proposed by Cooper? Second, and more important, just how compelling are Hock's evidence and arguments for individual differences in modes of perceptual processing?

With respect to the first issue, there are several reasons for questioning a possible relationship between the processing differences proposed by Hock and those proposed by Cooper. First, the differences that Hock reports are quantitative – inferred from correlational evidence – and are found for "same" response times only. The differences that Cooper reports are more qualitative – based on patterns of performance – and are obtained for both "same" and "different" response types. Second, the structural subjects in Hock's experiments (presumably corresponding to the holistic subjects in Cooper's experiments) are generally slower overall than the analytic subjects. Cooper finds just the opposite, with holistic subjects considerably faster than analytic ones. Third, and perhaps most conclusively, Cooper (unpublished data) performed an experiment using groups of holistic and analytic subjects in which the stimulus factors manipulated by Hock and his colleagues (1975) – orientation of letter pairs and physical versus name identity matches – were used. There was no systematic difference in the sensitivity of the reaction-time performance of the two groups of subjects to these stimulus factors.

With respect to the second issue, inspection of the data from Hock's experiments reveals that the evidence for group differences in performance is surprisingly weak. Arguments for the structural–analytic processing dichotomy derive from correlational evidence, and these correlations are generally based on a small number of subjects and frequently achieve only marginal levels of statistical significance (e.g., in Hock, 1973, $r = .60$, $p < .05$, $N = 24$; in Hock, Gordon, & Marcus, 1974, $r = .73$, $p < .001$, $N = 32$ for Experiment 1, but $r = .40$, $p < .05$, $N = 32$ for Experiment 2; in Hock & Ross, 1975, $r = .41$, $p < .05$, $N = 24$). Even more disturbing, in some cases these correlations appear to be the result of the presence of a small number of extreme observations (see, in particular, Carroll's 1978 reanalysis of the Hock, 1973, data after elimination of these extreme cases). There is another, quite different, reason for questioning Hock's division of subjects into structural and analytic groups: the lack of a theoretical basis for predicting which type of information processor should be relatively more affected by which sorts of stimulus manipulations. That is, the performance difference that Hock and his associates report is between subjects who are relatively more or less affected by stimulus manipulations. But they provide no independent reason for predicting that lack of sensitivity to stimulus variables should necessarily imply analytic as opposed to structural processing. We conclude, then, that the evidence and arguments for the structural–analytic processing difference are inconclusive, and that this difference, even if valid, bears little relation to the individual differences in modes of visual comparison reported by Cooper.

As a final candidate for a demonstration of possible qualitative individual differences in perceptual and cognitive processing – rather unlike the visual comparison differences already discussed – we consider the work of Day (1970, 1973a, 1973b). Day (1970) has reported that, when presented with components of words to the two ears at approximately the same time (e.g., *lanket* to one ear and *banket* to the other), people differ markedly in what they report hearing. Some report the two components as fused (i.e., they report hearing the word *blanket*), whereas others report the two components separately (i.e., they report hearing *lanket* and *banket* individually). When number of subjects is plotted against fusion rate, the distribution is strongly bimodal (Day, 1970), suggesting the possibility of qualitative individual difference in perceptual processing. Furthermore, people who tend to fuse items in this dichotic listening task are also poor at determining which of two items, presented separately to the two ears, arrived first (Day, 1970). They also have shorter digit spans than do nonfusers (Day, 1973a), and they are less successful at learning a secret language in which the *r* sounds in words must be pronounced as *l* sounds, and vice versa (Day, 1973b).

Day has attributed the source of individual differences to the way in which the two types of subjects encode information from the environment. The people who tend to fuse in the dichotic listening task, or the "language-bound" subjects, are thought to encode information through a linguistic filter. That is, they are unable to disregard rules of the language in processing external stimuli. Hence they tend to perceive separate inputs as forming English words, and they have difficulty with tasks such as the *r–l* reversal, in which the integrity of familiar linguistic material is destroyed. The individuals who report the two inputs separately are characterized as "stimulus-bound," or "language-optional." They are able to encode external stimuli quite accurately, and they are not affected by linguistic constraints except in situations in which using those constraints will actually improve their performance.

The language-bound–language-optional distinction has received considerable attention because the individual differences seem striking and they may be arising from very basic differences in strategies for perceiving external information. But how well has this dichotomy held up under systematic replication and various procedural modifications? Keele and Lyon (1975) undertook a study designed both to replicate Day's individual differences and to determine to what extent various tasks involving fusion were interrelated. The three tasks selected were (a) accuracy of judging which of two inputs to the individual ears, separated by 80 msec, occurred first (temporal order judgments), (b) accuracy of reporting inputs to one ear while ignoring inputs to the other ear, and (c) accuracy of discriminating whether the inputs to the two ears were the same word, or two word-component inputs, where the component inputs formed a word when fused. Presumably, the tendency to fuse inputs to the two ears should hurt performance on all three tasks.

Somewhat surprisingly, Keele and Lyon found that accuracies on the three tasks were only weakly related, with a maximum correlation of .38 between accuracy on temporal order judgments and accuracy on judging inputs from one ear only. In addition, they found that the three tasks gave very different estimates of the frequency of input fusion, with very little fusion (high accuracy) in the word-component discrimination task. Finally, distributions of number of subjects against error scores for each of the three tasks showed no evidence of the bimodality reported by Day (1970).

In an even more conclusive set of experiments, Poltrock and Hunt (1977) attempted a systematic replication of Day's findings using a large sample of subjects (in Experiment 1, $N = 60$; in Experiment 2, $N = 100$). Their results were clear: Neither dichotic fusion rates nor temporal order judgments showed evidence of bimodality. However, these two measures were significantly correlated, a finding which suggests that individuals may differ in their tendency to use linguistic rules in judging aspects of perceptual input. These findings lead us to conclude that the language-bound–language-optional distinction originally proposed by Day does not represent a qualitative difference between individuals in modes of processing perceptual information. Most likely, people do differ in the extent to which they rely on linguistic rules in interpreting sensory input; however, this individual-difference variable appears to be continuous and quantitative rather than discrete and qualitative in nature.

In summary, the general argument for a relationship between strategies and intelligence seems promising, though there are as yet few sources of relevant or conclusive data. Future demonstrations of qualitative individual differences in modes of perceptual and cognitive processing will be welcome, and it will be important to show whether and/or how these strategy differences distinguish more from less able people. We regard as particularly significant the questions of (a) the extent to which relative differences in ability determine both strategy choice and effectiveness in the use of a particular strategy, and (b) the extent to which strategies can be modified through instruction or by changing information-processing demands. This latter question has obvious implications for training people to perform more effectively, and studying this question will require research techniques rather different from those used to study basic information-processing contributions to ability differences.

ATTENTION

Yet another possible source of individual differences in ability might involve general attentional factors. The intuitively appealing notion that brighter people pay attention more effectively has been alive in psychology for a considerable period of time. Indeed, William James (1890/1950) speculated at length about the relationship between attention and intelligence, taking the position that "what is called sustained attention is the easier, the richer in acquisitions and the fresher and more original the mind" (p. 423).[6] Surprisingly, however, very little empirical work has been done on individual differences in attention and their possible relationship to ability. When we consider this relationship, two possibilities suggest themselves. One is that more able people can more effectively direct or sustain attention where required. Such people could be said to have greater "attentional flexibility." The other possibility is that more able people simply have more attentional resources, capacity for processing information, or cognitive energy (see Kahneman, 1973). Here we briefly consider some empirical work directed toward each of these possibilities.

Kahneman and his colleagues (Gopher & Kahneman, 1971; Kahneman, Ben-Ishai, & Lotan, 1973) have reported two provocative studies on individual differences in attentional flexibility and their relationship to various measures of ability. Their strategy was first to devise a test of subjects' ability to sustain or direct attention in response to a cue, and then to relate performance on the test to measures of complex psychomotor skills in the natural environment – piloting airplanes and driving buses. The test, which involved dichotic listening, consisted of two parts. In the first, messages were presented to both ears, and subjects had to report target items only when they occurred on the cued ear. Immediately following and during Part 1 of the test, subjects were cued about which ear was relevant for Part 2. Effectively, the cue instructed the subject whether to maintain attention on the same ear or switch to the other ear. The task again was to report target items occurring on the cued ear only. Correlations were computed between each of three test scores – omissions in Part 1 (failure to report a target on the attended ear), intrusions in Part 1 (reporting a target on the irrelevant ear), and total errors in Part 2 – and both the flying ability of pilots in the Israeli Air Force (Gopher & Kahneman, 1971) and the accident ratings of Israeli bus drivers (Kahneman et al., 1973). Total errors on Part 2 correlated most highly (approximately .36) with each of these criterion variables. The authors suggest that this relationship reflects individual differences in an ability common to both the requirements of the attention task in Part 2 and those of normal driving or airplane piloting. This is the ability to shift rapidly or maintain already directed attention in response to an external signal.

There are some problems with this interpretation of the data, however. We mention two. First, measures of both intelligence and errors on Part 1 were significantly (though more modestly) associated with the criterion variables and with errors on Part 2, and there was no attempt to establish (via partial correlation or other statistical techniques) the independent contribution of Part 2 errors to the behavioral criteria. Thus the relationship between Part 2 errors and the criterion variables could reflect some (perhaps motivational) factor much more general than attentional flexibility. Second, the argument that Part 2 errors provide a measure of attentional flexibility is based only on a logical analysis of the task, with no additional converging evidence. The idea of meaningful individual differences in attentional flexibility gains credence, however, from the results of a recent study by Keele, Neill, and de Lemos (1978). These investigators devised three tests of attentional flexibility (in addition to using a version of the Kahneman Part 2 test). The pattern of intercorrelations among performance on the various tests was somewhat complex, but there were suggestions of significant relationships among most of them. Thus, although further work is needed, it may be that there is a general trait of attentional flexibility on which people varying in ability differ.

Finally, we turn to the idea that people differ in the extent of their attentional capacity or resources. Both Baron and Treiman (1980) and Hunt (1980) have suggested that resource differences may be strongly related to intelligence. Indeed, Hunt has proposed that differences in attentional resources may make at least as large a contribution to differences in ability as does the efficiency of basic information-processing skills. He also suggests that a general factor of attentional capacity could account for the reasonably high correlations among various measures of intellectual ability. The concept of attentional resources is similar to Spearman's (1927) notion of "mental energy." According to Norman and Bobrow (1975), "Resources are such things as processing effort, the various forms of memory capacity, and communication channels. Resources are always limited" (p. 45). The basic idea is that more able people have more resources, and thus will perform more competently when multiple demands are placed on those resources.

What empirical evidence is there for individual differences in attentional resources? In investigating this question, the *dual-task* method is most frequently used (for details, see, e.g., Posner, 1978; Norman & Bobrow, 1975). In this method, multiple demands are placed on the information-processing system, and the extent and nature of performance breakdowns are observed. The multiple demands are in the form of two tasks that must be performed simultaneously or nearly so. The relationship between performance on the two tasks as one of them is made more difficult is frequently the dependent variable of interest. The application of the method to the question of individual differences in attentional resources is illustrated by two studies reported in Hunt (1980).

In the first, subjects did a hard or easy memory task while simultaneously performing a simple probe reaction-time task. There was a significant correlation across individual subjects of −.40 between probe reaction time while performing the easy memory task and proportion correct on the hard memory task. The logic for interpreting this correlation as the result of individual differences in attentional resources is as follows: The memory task and the probe reaction-time task compete for fixed resources. The more limited a subject's resources, the longer the probe reaction time will be even under the relatively undemanding conditions of the easy memory task. When the memory task becomes hard, more limited subjects (identified by the long reaction times in the easy memory condition) will have few resources left to do this difficult task, and their error rate will be high − hence the correlation. In a second study more directly related to ability differences, subjects simultaneously solved increasingly difficult problems on the Raven Progressive Matrices test and performed a simple psychomotor task. By the logic just applied, there should be a correlation between performance on the psychomotor test while doing relatively easy Raven items and the point at which the subject makes his or her first error as the items become more difficult. The correlation was −.30.

Both of the results from the Hunt (1980) paper are consistent with the position that people differ in general processing capacity, and that this difference is related to ability. But there are other interpretations of the data as well. It is possible that there are multiple, separate, minimally correlated pools of resources for performing different types of tasks. Demonstrating general capacity differences across individuals would seem to require showing within-subjects consistencies (and across-subjects differences) in the point of breakdown in performance if any two tasks that compete for attention are used. Recently, Sverko (1977) has attempted such a demonstration. He tested subjects on four quite dissimilar information-processing tasks, administered both singly and in all possible pair-wise combinations. The four tasks involved rotary pursuit, digit classification, mental arithmetic, and an auditory discrimination.

In order to assess whether the data provided evidence for the notion of a general capacity (in Sverko's terms, a "unitary time-sharing ability"), two analyses were done. First, the performance of subjects in each experimental condition (individual tasks and task pairings) was correlated with performance in all other conditions. This intercorrelation matrix was then subjected to a factor analysis. Sverko reasoned that if there was a general time-sharing or resource-related ability, then five factors should emerge in the analysis – four of them corresponding to the four specific tasks, and the fifth representing the more general ability. Instead, only four task-specific factors were found. In a second analysis, Sverko computed a total performance decrement score for each task pairing by adding the proportionate performance change when the tasks were paired, rather than undertaken individually. Correlations were computed between the decrement scores for the three task pairings that did not contain overlapping tasks (i.e., Tasks 1 and 2 versus Tasks 3 and 4, Tasks 1 and 3 versus Tasks 2 and 4, and Tasks 1 and 4 versus Tasks 2 and 3). If the various tasks were drawing on a common, limited resource pool, then the correlations should have been substantial. In fact, all correlations were extremely low, ranging from .060 to .068. These results provide rather compelling evidence against the notion of a truly general, unitary, transsituational time-sharing ability or resource pool.

How, then, are we to account for the findings reported in Hunt (1980), and those of other investigators who have argued for general attentional resources from experiments using the dual-task method? One possibility is that the notion of individual differences in attentional resources, processing capacity, or an ability like time-sharing still makes sense, but only if we view the idea of capacity in a less general way. That is, there could exist multiple, separate pools of resources each limited in capacity and only minimally intercorrelated. (See Hawkins, Church, & de Lemos, 1978, for a clear statement of this view as it relates to individual-differences research.) Capacity limitations, and hence performance decrements in the dual-task situation, will be observed only when two tasks compete for the same pool of resources. This is a difficult position to evaluate experimentally, for we have little in the way of a priori notions about which tasks should tap common, as opposed to separate, sources of capacity. At a minimum, this view is consistent with research on "structural interference" (see, e.g., Brooks, 1968) which suggests that limited resources may be specific to spatial and verbal processing.

Another possibility is that the attentional contribution to ability is a skill, dependent on practice, rather than a limited-capacity resource. According to this view, people could differ in their levels of performance on concurrent tasks primarily because of the extent of their relative practice at doing two things at once. Some provocative findings of Damos and Wickens (1977) suggest that at least some portion of differences in time-sharing performance – presumably reflecting capacity limitations – are indeed dependent on practice at combining any two activities. In this study, three groups of subjects were tested in a situation that involved combining two independent psychomotor tasks. Prior to the testing, one group had been trained on performing a short-term memory task and a digit-classification task simultaneously, a second group had been trained on performing the tasks sequentially, and a third group had received no training at all. Somewhat surprisingly, the group that had had previous training on the concurrent information-processing tasks showed superior performance on the concurrent psychomotor tasks. This result suggests that practice at combining any two tasks will transfer to other multiple-task situations. Note that this does not necessarily imply that there are no skill- or practice-independent individual differences in resources or processing capacity. Rather, these findings suggest that a person's level of practice at a given time may contribute to the effectiveness of that person's use of limited resources.

In conclusion, we find the idea of individual differences in attentional factors as possible determinants of ability differences to be an intriguing possibility. As we have noted, however, the relevant data base examining this relationship is meager indeed. Furthermore, interpretation of the sources of individual differences – particularly in the dual-task experiments – is problematic at best. But this should not be surprising. Quite apart from any concern for understanding attentional contributions to individual differences in intelligence, the question of the nature of capacity or resources is currently quite a controversial one in cognitive psychology more generally. Some theorists argue that a general, limited-capacity resource pool underlies attentional phenomena (see, e.g., Norman & Bobrow, 1975), whereas others argue for multiple, independent sources of capacity (see, e.g., Navon & Gopher, 1979). Still others (see Neisser, 1976; Spelke, Hirst, & Neisser, 1976) have argued that the entire notion of capacity limitations is misguided, and have emphasized instead the role of practice in developing skills at performing combinations of tasks. Perhaps the study of the relationship between ability and attentional factors – as promising as it might appear to be – should await further theoretical resolution within cognitive psychology concerning the nature of attention and processing resources.

3.3.   CONCLUDING REMARKS

Having reviewed a considerable body of literature on relationships between attentional and perceptual processes and intelligence or ability, what can we conclude? Our tentative answer is "surprisingly little," but there are some firmly established findings and some promising research directions. Our quest to relate these three concepts in cognitive and in differential psychology began with a consideration of the extent to which quantitative differences among people in basic information-processing skills correlated with differences in ability. Some of the research in this area is elegant indeed (see, e.g., the studies of Jackson, 1978, and Jackson & McClelland, 1979). And we distinguished among approaches that we viewed as more or less adequate. In particular, we found congenial those studies that, in addition to showing evidence for a relationship between information-processing parameters and ability, also provided construct validity for the information-processing components that were being correlated with the ability measures.

Nonetheless, the findings from this recent and substantial research effort have been often disappointing and sometimes conflicting. In verbal and reading ability, it seems clear that efficiency of memory access (for any conceptual category) differentiates more from less able people. In the area of spatial ability, encoding speed is related to proficiency, but speed of mental manipulation may or may not predict performance on psychometric measures. In addition, the few differences in information-processing skills that distinguish higher- from lower-ability subjects tend to account for only a small portion of the variance (typically about 10%) of performance on intelligence tests (though they discriminate more effectively between extreme groups on any intelligence dimension). Finally, interpretation of correlations between information-processing skills and ability is plagued with the problem of developing adequate theoretical accounts of the cognitive tasks that are being related to the intelligence measures.

We view as promising the idea that attentional and strategic factors may contribute substantially to ability differences, particularly in view of the low correlations between basic information-processing parameters and individual differences. With respect to individual differences in strategies – or procedures for selecting, combining, and executing information-processing operations – there are several important questions that beg for more empirical research. They include: At what levels can qualitative differences in processing modes or strategies be isolated? (Some of the work that we have reviewed suggests that strategy differences can be found in rather low-level information-processing operations, as well as in higher-level problem-solving situations.) To what extent do strategy differences relate to ability or derive from relative ability differences? To what extent are strategies trainable or manipulable by varying task demands? Again, with respect to the relationship between strategies and intelligence, to what extent is initial strategy selection – as opposed to the efficiency in using a strategy, once selected – correlated with ability?

Studying individual differences in strategies and their relationship to intelligence is difficult, and we mentioned earlier that it may require research approaches somewhat different from those standardly used in cognitive psychology. This is because we rarely know in advance what strategies will be more or less effective in what situations. Rather, we infer strategic differences from quantitative or qualitative differences between individual subjects in patterns of data. In two of the cases discussed earlier, evidence for strategies emerged initially from post hoc individual-differences analyses of performance on simple cognitive tasks. In the 1978 study by MacLeod and his associates, strategy differences were inferred from the wide range of individual subjects' correlations between reaction-time performance on the sentence–picture verification task and predictions of a particular model of the cognitive operations required by the task. In the Cooper (1976, 1980a) studies, differences in processing modes were inferred from qualitative differences in individual subjects' patterns of reaction-time and error performance in a visual comparison task.

But isolating strategy differences via such trial-and-error post hoc individual-differences analyses is hardly likely to be an effective research approach. We need, in addition, to provide an analysis of the nature of the alternative strategies and to determine in advance which subjects are likely to use which strategies in which situations. In the case of the studies by MacLeod and his associates and by Cooper such a second step was taken. Mathews and her co-workers (in a follow-up, reported in Hunt, 1980, on the 1978 MacLeod et al. experiment) were able to predict – on the basis of verbal and spatial ability scores – which subjects would use which strategies, and they were further able to manipulate strategy use through instruction. Cooper (1980a, 1980b) was able to gain independent evidence for qualitative strategy differences, first, by providing an analysis of the nature of the hypothesized strategies, and next, by constructing information-processing tasks whose demands naturally drew on one strategy type or another. To the extent that these new tasks forced certain subjects to change their patterns of performance (and, by inference, their visual comparison operations), evidence for differential strategy use was obtained. In the case of studies like Cooper's, it remains to relate strategy selection to intelligence, ability, or some criterion measure.

There are other ways in which strategies could be studied, and they depart somewhat from the standard information-processing tradition. One method might involve isolating groups of subjects that differ extensively on some criterion measure of interest (e.g., people who learn to get around in new environments easily versus people who habitually and continually get lost). We could then query these people concerning their strategies for learning spatial layouts. From the verbal reports, we could attempt to analyze the strategies in terms of more basic information-processing skills. We could then perform laboratory experiments in which subjects were instructed to use alternative strategies, and performance differences could be assessed. This approach is similar to that of Thorndyke and Stasz (1980), based on protocol analysis of a map-learning task. The method has distinct potential, but it suffers from two rather obvious problems. The first is that some strategies that we might wish to study — particularly those involving basic perceptual and cognitive processing — might not be available to conscious introspection and hence verbal report. The second is the possible difficulty of translating verbal reports of strategies into experimental manipulations. Still another method for studying strategies is essentially the one advocated by Baron (1978). This involves generating logical hypotheses concerning the nature of strategies that might lead to efficient, intelligent behavior. We could then design tasks that tap these strategies, or train subjects in the use of these strategies and observe relative changes in performance. The success of this approach depends, of course, on having the proper intuitions concerning the nature of the strategies that contribute to intelligence.

Finally, we wish to comment on the idea that attentional flexibility and/or amount of processing resources make important contributions to individual differences in ability. This is an intriguing possibility, and there already exists some relevant and suggestive research. We predict that the relationship between attentional factors and intelligence will be a very active research area for the next several years — particularly in light of the mixed success in establishing correlations between basic information-processing skills and ability. As promising as this direction might seem, we nonetheless have some misgivings. The approach to studying this question appears to involve translating a task currently fashionable within cognitive psychology — in the case of attentional resources, the dual-task method — into an individual-differences framework. This approach is reminiscent of the effort, reviewed herein, to establish correlations between basic information-processing tasks and psychometric measures of ability. As we have seen, interpretations of these relationships have sometimes suffered from an inadequate theoretical analysis of the cognitive operations underlying the information-processing tasks. In the case of tasks measuring demands on attentional resources, controversies over interpretation are even more apparent at this point (see, e.g., Kantowitz & Knight, 1976; Navon & Gopher, 1979).

What we fear is that research on attentional contributions to intelligence could experience a fate similar to that of some of the research on basic information-processing determinants of ability: namely, establishing that individual differences exist, but not knowing what those individual differences really mean. The general point that we make, in concluding, is that progress in research on individual differences in ability must parallel the adequacy of theory and of understanding of experimental paradigms in cognitive psychology. Any effective unity between cognitive and differential approaches must be grounded in a clear understanding of the nature of general mental operations, and the experimental tasks and situations suitable for isolating and investigating them. One thrust of this chapter has been that we do not expect such unity to emerge from investigations of the way in which people of varying ability perform on tasks that are themselves inadequately understood. What this implies is that meaningful work on the contributions of attention and perception to intelligence must await a clearer conceptualization within cognitive psychology itself of the nature of those mechanisms.

NOTES

Preparation of this chapter was supported in part by NSF grant BNS 76-22079 to the first author. We wish to thank Robert Vallone for his unstinting help in all phases of the preparation of the chapter.

1 Lohman (1979a) presents an impressive array of evidence for the existence of three major spatial factors – Space Relations, Visualization, and Orientation – as well as a host of minor factors.
2 This finding may puzzle cognitive psychologists who consistently find relationships between speed and accuracy in information-processing tasks. Indeed, even in Egan's (1976, 1978, 1979b) data, reaction time and error rate are positively correlated across experimental conditions. That is, for the group data from, e.g., the mental rotation task, both reaction time and error rate increase monotonically with angular difference in the orientations of the two visual objects being compared. It is only in the individual-differences analysis of overall accuracy on tests of spatial ability and latency on the information-processing versions of these tasks that virtually no correlation is found.
3 There is one exception to this generalization in the studies reviewed in this section. Kail et al. (1979) found slope differences between the male and female subjects, but they found no reliable intercept differences between the sexes.
4 Beyond the scope of our discussion is the considerable body of research on memory and retrieval strategies, some of which is reviewed by Baron (1978). We will also not consider some recent and intriguing work on developmental changes in strategies for attentional and perceptual processing (see, e.g., Kemler & Smith, 1978; Smith & Kemler, 1977, 1978).
5 Recently, Agari (1979) has attempted to replicate Cooper's (1976) individual differences in visual processing using a larger sample of subjects and a slightly shortened version of Cooper's task. Although Agari found that the processing parameters used to identify the different subject types were highly correlated, evidence for the sharp dichotomy reported by Cooper was not obtained. The reasons for this discrepancy remain obscure.
6 This quotation does not really do justice to James's (1890/1950) position on the relationship between attention and intelligence. To James, highly intelligent people were able to attend more effectively because of their superior mental abilities: "Geniuses are commonly believed to excel other men in their power of sustained attention – But it is their genius making them attentive, not their attention making geniuses of them" (p. 423). Contrast this position with the view that we are considering – viz., that individual differences in attentional factors may constitute determinants of ability differences.

REFERENCES

Agari, Tomiko. *Individual differences in visual processing of nonverbal shapes.* Unpublished master's thesis, University of Washington, Seattle, 1979.
Atkinson, R. C., Holmgren, J. E., & Juola, J. F. Processing time as influenced by the number of elements in a visual display. *Perception and Psychophysics,* 1969, 6, 321–326.
Baron, J. Intelligence and general strategies. In G. Underwood (Ed.), *Strategies in information processing.* London: Academic Press, 1978.
Baron, J., & Treiman, R. Some problems in the study of differences in cognitive processes. *Memory and Cognition,* 1980, 8, 313–321.
Baum, D. R., & Jonides, J. Cognitive maps: Analysis of comparative judgments of distance. *Memory and Cognition,* 1979, 6, 464–468.

Broadbent, D. E. *Perception and communication*. New York: Pergamon Press, 1958.

Brooks, L. R. Spatial and verbal components of the act of recall. *Canadian Journal of Psychology*, 1968, *22*, 349–368.

Carey, S., & Diamond, R. From piecemeal to configurational representation of faces. *Science*, 1977, *195*, 312–314.

Carpenter, P. A., & Just, M. A. Sentence comprehension: A psycholinguistic processing model of verification. *Psychological Review*, 1975, *82*, 45–73.

Carroll, J. B. Psychometric tests as cognitive tasks: A new "structure of the intellect"? In L. B. Resnick (Ed.), *The nature of intelligence*. Hillsdale, N.J.: Erlbaum, 1976.

Carroll, J. B. How shall we study individual differences in cognitive abilities? – Methodological and theoretical perspectives. *Intelligence*, 1978, *2*, 87–115.

Chiang, A., & Atkinson, R. C. Individual differences and inter-relationships among a select set of cognitive skills. *Memory and Cognition*, 1976, *4*, 661–672.

Clark, H. H., & Chase, W. G. On the process of comparing sentences against pictures. *Cognitive Psychology*, 1972, *3*, 472–517.

Cooper, L. A. Mental rotation of random two-dimensional shapes. *Cognitive Psychology*, 1975, *7*, 20–43.

Cooper, L. A. Individual differences in visual comparison processes. *Perception and Psychophysics*, 1976, *19*, 443–444.

Cooper, L. A. Spatial information processing: Strategies for research. In R. Snow, P. A. Federico, & W. E. Montague (Eds.), *Aptitude, learning and instruction: Cognitive process analyses*. Hillsdale, N.J.: Erlbaum, 1980. (a)

Cooper, L. A. Recent themes in visual information processing: A selected overview. In R. E. Nickerson (Ed.), *Attention and performance VIII*. Hillsdale, N.J.: Erlbaum, 1980. (b)

Cooper, L. A., & Podgorny, P. Mental transformations and visual comparison processes: Effects of complexity and similarity. *Journal of Experimental Psychology: Human Perception and Performance*, 1976, *2*, 503–514.

Cooper, L. A., & Shepard, R. N. Chronometric studies of the rotation of mental images. In W. C. Chase (Ed.), *Visual information processing*. New York: Academic Press, 1973. (a)

Cooper, L. A., & Shepard, R. N. The time required to prepare for a rotated stimulus. *Memory and Cognition*, 1973, *1*, 246–250. (b)

Damos, D., & Wickens, C. Development and transfer of timesharing skills. *Proceedings of Human Factors Society 21st Annual Meeting*, 1977.

Day, R. S. Temporal order judgments in speech: Are individuals language-bound or stimulus-bound? *Haskin's Laboratories Status Report*, 1970, *SR-21/22*, 71–87.

Day, R. S. Digit-span memory in language-bound and stimulus-bound subjects. *Haskin's Laboratories Status Report*, 1973, *SR-34*, 127–139. (a)

Day, R. S. On learning "secret languages." *Haskin's Laboratories Status Report*, 1973, *SR-34*, 141–150. (b)

Egan, D. E. *Accuracy and latency scores as measures of spatial information processing* (Research Report No. 1224). Pensacola, Fla: Naval Aerospace Medical Research Laboratories, February 1976.

Egan, D. E. *Characterizations of spatial ability: Different mental processes reflected in accuracy and latency scores* (Research Report No. 1250). Pensacola, Fla: Naval Aerospace Medical Research Laboratories, August 1978.

Egan, D. E. *An analysis of spatial orientation test performance*. Paper presented to the American Educational Research Association, San Francisco, April 1979. (a)

Egan, D. E. Testing based on understanding: Implications from studies of spatial ability. *Intelligence*, 1979, *3*, 1–15. (b)

Estes, W. The locus of inferential and perceptual processes in letter identification. *Journal of Experimental Psychology: General*, 1975, *1*, 122–145.

Estes, W. K., & Taylor, H. A. A detection method and probabilistic models for assessing information processing from brief visual displays. *Proceedings of the National Academy of Sciences*, 1964, *52*, 446–454.

Estes, W. K., & Taylor, H. A. Visual detection in relation to display size and redundancy of critical elements. *Perception and Psychophysics*, 1966, *1*, 369–373.

Frederiksen, J. R. *Knowledge derived from text: Applications in decoding and comprehension*. Paper presented at the annual meeting of the American Psychological Association, New York, September 1977.

Frederiksen, J. R. *A chronometric study of component skills in reading* (Report No. 3757 [2]). Prepared for the Office of Naval Research by Bolt Beranek and Newman Inc., January 1978.

Frederiksen, J. R. *Component skills in readers of varying ability*. Paper presented at the annual meeting of the American Educational Research Association, April 1979.

Garner, W. R. *The processing of information and structure*. New York: Wiley, 1974.

Gibson, J. J. *The senses considered as perceptual systems*. Boston: Houghton Mifflin, 1966.

Gilbert, L. Speed of processing visual stimuli and its relation to reading. *Journal of Educational Psychology*, 1959, *55*, 8–14.

Glaser, R., & Pellegrino, J. W. Cognitive process analysis of aptitude: The nature of inductive reasoning tasks. *Bulletin de Psychologie*, 1978–1978, *32*, 603–615.

Glushko, R. J., & Cooper, L. A. Spatial comprehension and comparison processes in verification tasks. *Cognitive Psychology*, 1978, *10*, 391–421.

Gopher, D., & Kahneman, D. Individual differences in attention and the prediction of flight criteria. *Perceptual and Motor Skills*, 1971, *33*, 1335–1342.

Guilford, J. P. *The nature of human intelligence*. New York: McGraw-Hill, 1969.

Haviland, S. E., & Clark, H. H. What's new? Acquiring new information as a process in comprehension. *Journal of Verbal Learning and Verbal Behavior*, 1974, *13*, 512–521.

Hawkins, H. L., Church, M., & de Lemos, S. *Time-sharing is not a unitary ability*. University of Oregon, Eugene: Center for Cognitive and Perceptual Research, June 1978.

Hock, H. S. The effects of stimulus structure and familiarity on same–different comparison. *Perception and Psychophysics*, 1973, *14*, 413–420.

Hock, H. S. Gordon, G. P., & Gold, L. Individual differences in the verbal coding of familiar visual stimuli. *Memory and Cognition*, 1975, *3*, 257–261.

Hock, H. S., Gordon, G. P., & Marcus, N. Individual differences in the detection of embedded figures. *Perception and psychophysics*, 1974, *15*, 47–52.

Hock, H. S., & Ross, K. The effect of familiarity on rotational transformation. *Perception and Psychophysics*, 1975, *18*, 15–20.

Huey, E. B. *The psychology and pedagogy of reading*. Cambridge, Mass.: MIT Press, 1968. (Originally published, New York: Macmillan, 1908.)

Hunt, E. B. Quote the Raven? Nevermore! In L. Gregg (Ed.), *Knowledge and cognition*. Hillsdale, N.J.: Erlbaum, 1974.

Hunt, E. Mechanics of verbal ability. *Psychological Review*, 1978, *85*, 109–130.

Hunt, E. Intelligence as an information processing concept. *Journal of British Psychology*, 1980, *71*, 449–474.

Hunt, E., Frost, N., & Lunneborg, C. Individual differences in cognition: A new approach to intelligence. In G. Bower (Ed.), *The psychology of learning and motivation* (Vol. 7). New York: Academic Press, 1973.

Hunt, E., Lunneborg, C., & Lewis, J. What does it mean to be high verbal? *Cognitive Psychology*, 1975, *7*, 194–227.

Hunt, E., & MacLeod, C. M. The sentence-verification paradigm: A case study of two conflicting approaches to individual differences. *Intelligence*, 1978, *2*, 129–144.

Jackson, M. D. *Memory access and reading ability*. Unpublished doctoral dissertation, University of California, San Diego, 1978.

Jackson, M., & McClelland, J. Sensory and cognitive determinants of reading speed. *Journal of Verbal Learning and Verbal Behavior*, 1975, *14*, 565–574.

Jackson, M. D., & McClelland, J. L. Processing determinants of reading speed. *Journal of Experimental Psychology: General*, 1979, *108*, 151–181.

James, W. *The principles of psychology* (Vol. 1). New York: Dover Publications, 1950. (Originally published, New York: Holt, 1890.)

Jensen, A. R. *Reaction time and intelligence*. Paper presented at the NATO Conference on Intelligence and Learning, York University, York, England, 1979.

Jensen, A. R., & Munro, E. Reaction time, movement time, and intelligence. *Intelligence*, 1979, *3*, 121–126.

Just, M. A., & Carpenter, P. A. Eye fixations and cognitive processes. *Cognitive Psychology*, 1976, *8*, 441–480.

Kahneman, D. *Attention and effort*. Englewood Cliffs, N.J.: Prentice-Hall, 1973.

Kahneman, D., Ben-Ishai, R., & Lotan, M. Relation of a test of attention to road accidents. *Journal of Applied Psychology*, 1973, *58*, 113–115.

Kail, R., Carter, P., & Pellegrino, J. The locus of sex differences in spatial ability. *Perception and Psychophysics*, 1979, *26*, 182–186.

Kail, R., Pellegrino, J., & Carter, P. Developmental changes in mental rotation. *Journal of Experimental Child Psychology*, 1980, *29*, 107–116.

Kantowitz, B., & Knight, J. L. On experimenter-limited processes. *Psychological Review*, 1976, *83*, 502–507.

Keating, D. P., & Bobbitt, B. L. Individual and developmental differences in cognitive-processing components of mental ability. *Child Development*, 1978, *49*, 155–167.

Keele, S. W. & Lyon, D. R. *Individual differences in word fusion: A methodological analysis.* Advanced Research Projects Agency, Order No. 2284, 1975.

Keele, S. W., Neill, W. T., & de Lemos, S. M. *Individual differences in attentional flexibility.* Arlington, Va.: Office of Naval Research, Personnel and Training Research Programs, May 1978.

Kemler, D. G., & Smith, L. B. Is there a developmental trend from integrality to separability in perception? *Journal of Experimental Child Psychology*, 1978, *26*, 498–507.

Kosslyn, S. M., Pick, H. L., Jr., & Fariello, G. R. Cognitive maps in children and men. *Child Development*, 1974, *45*, 707–716.

Kozlowski, L. T., & Bryant, R. J. Sense of direction, spatial orientation and cognitive maps. *Journal of Experimental Psychology: Human Perception and Performance*, 1977, *3*, 590–598.

Lansman, M. *Ability factors and the speed of information processing.* Paper presented at the NATO Conference on Intelligence and Learning, York University, York, England, 1979.

Loftus, G. R. Comprehending compass directions. *Memory and Cognition*, 1976, *6*, 416–422.

Lohman, D. F. *Spatial abilities: A review and reanalysis of the correlational literature* (Technical Report No. 8, Aptitude Research Project). Stanford, Calif.: Stanford University, School of Education, October 1979. (a)

Lohman, D. F. *Spatial ability: Individual differences in speed and level* (Technical Report No. 9, Aptitude Research Project). Stanford, Calif.: Stanford University, School of Education, October 1979. (b)

Lunneborg, C. E. Choice reaction time: What role in ability measurement? *Applied Psychological Measurement*, 1977, *1*, 309–330.

Lunneborg, C. E. Some information-processing correlates of measures of intelligence. *Multivariate Behavioral Research*, 1978, *13*, 153–161.

MacLeod, C. M., Hunt, E. B., & Mathews, N. N. Individual differences in the verification of sentence–picture relationships. *Journal of Verbal Learning and Verbal Behavior*, 1978, *17*, 493–508.

McClelland, J. Preliminary letter identification in the perception of words and non-words. *Journal of Experimental Psychology: Human Perception and Performance*, 1976, *1*, 80–91.

McClelland, J., & Jackson, M. Studying individual differences in reading. In A. Lesgold, J. Pellegrino, S. Fokkema, & R. Glaser (Eds.), *Cognitive psychology and instruction.* New York: Plenum, 1978.

McGee, M. G. Human spatial abilities: Psychometric studies and environmental, genetic, hormonal, and neurological influences. *Psychological Bulletin*, 1979, *86*, 889–918.

Messer, S. B. Reflection-impulsivity: A review. *Psychological Bulletin*, 1976, *83*, 1026–1053.

Messick, S. (Ed.). *Individuality in learning: Implications of cognitive styles and creativity for human development.* San Francisco: Jossey-Bass, 1976.

Metzler, J., & Shepard, R. N. Transformational studies of the internal representation of three-dimensional objects. In R. L. Solso (Ed.), *Theories in cognitive psychology: The Loyola Symposium.* New York: Wiley, 1974.

Mulholland, T. M., Pellegrino, J. W., & Glaser, R. Components of geometric analogy solution. *Cognitive Psychology*, 1980, *12*, 252–284.

Navon, D., & Gopher, D. On the economy of the human-processing system. *Psychological Review*, 1979, *86*, 214–255.

Neisser, U. *Cognition and reality.* San Francisco: W. H. Freeman, 1976.

Norman, D. A., & Bobrow, D. G. On data-limited and resource-limited processes. *Cognitive Psychology*, 1975, *7*, 44–64.

Pellegrino, J. W., & Glaser, R. Components of inductive reasoning. In R. E. Snow, P. A. Federico, & W. E. Montague (Eds.), *Aptitude, learning, and instruction: Cognitive process analysis.* Hillsdale, N.J.: Erlbaum, 1980.

Perfetti, C., & Goldman, S. Discourse memory and reading comprehension skill. *Journal of Verbal Learning and Verbal Behavior,* 1976, *15*, 33–42.

Perfetti, C. A., & Lesgold, A. M. Discourse comprehension and sources of individual differences. In M. Just & P. Carpenter (Eds.), *Cognitive processes in comprehension.* Hillsdale, N.J.: Erlbaum, 1978.

Poltrock, S. E., & Hunt, E. Individual differences in phonological fusion and separation errors. *Journal of Experimental Psychology: Human Perception and Performance,* 1977, *3*, 62–74.

Posner, M. I. *Chronometric explorations of mind.* Hillsdale, N.J.: Erlbaum, 1978.

Posner, M., Boies, S., Eichelman, W., & Taylor, R. Retention of visual and name codes of single letters. *Journal of Experimental Psychology Monograph,* 1969, 79(1, Pt. 2).

Posner, M., & Mitchell, R. Chronometric analysis of classification. *Psychological Review,* 1967, *74*, 392–409.

Raven, J. C. *Guide to the standard progressive matrices.* London: Lewis, 1960.

Raven, J. C. *Advanced progressive matrices, Sets I and II.* London: Lewis, 1965.

Rumelhart, D. E. *Introduction to human information processing.* New York: Wiley, 1977. (a)

Rumelhart, D. Toward an interactive model of reading. In S. Dornic (Ed.), *Attention and Performance, VI.* Hillsdale, N.J.: Erlbaum, 1977. (b)

Shepard, R. N., & Feng, C. A chronometric study of mental paper folding. *Cognitive Psychology,* 1972, *3*, 228–243.

Shepard, R. N., & Metzler, J. Mental rotation of three-dimensional objects. *Science,* 1971, *171*, 701–703.

Smith, I. M. *Spatial ability.* San Diego: Robert R. Knapp, 1964.

Smith, L. B., & Kemler, D. G. Developmental trends in free classification: Evidence for a new conceptualization of perceptual development. *Journal of Experimental Child Psychology,* 1977, *24*, 279–298.

Smith, L. B., & Kemler, D. G. Levels of experienced dimensionality in children and adults. *Cognitive Psychology,* 1978, *10*, 502–532.

Spearman, C. *The abilities of man.* New York: Macmillan, 1927.

Spelke, E., Hirst, W., & Neisser, U. Skills of divided attention. *Cognition,* 1976, *4*, 215–230.

Sternberg, R. J. *Intelligence, information processing and analogical reasoning: The componential analysis of human abilities.* Hillsdale, N.J.: Erlbaum, 1977.

Sternberg, R. J., & Weil, E. M. An aptitude × strategy interaction in linear syllogistic reasoning. *Journal of Educational Psychology,* 1980, *72*, 226–236.

Sternberg, S. High speed scanning in human memory. *Science,* 1966, *153*, 652–654.

Sternberg, S. The discovery of stages: Extension of Donders' method. *Acta Psychologica,* 1969, *30*, 276–315.

Sternberg, S. Memory scanning: New findings and current controversies. *Quarterly Journal of Experimental Psychology,* 1975, *27*, 1–32.

Stevens, A., & Coupe, P. Distortions in judged spatial relations. *Cognitive Psychology,* 1978, *10*, 422–437.

Sverko, B. *Individual differences in time sharing performance* (Tech. Rep. ARL-77-4). Champaign-Urbana: University of Illinois, Aviation Research Laboratory, January 1977.

Thorndyke, P. W., & Stasz, C. Individual differences in procedures for knowledge acquisition from maps. *Cognitive Psychology,* 1980, *12*, 137–175.

Thurstone, L. L. Primary mental abilities. *Psychometric Monographs,* 1938, *1*.

Trabasso, T., Rollins, H., & Shaughnessey, E. Storage and verification stages in processing concepts. *Cognitive Psychology,* 1971, *2*, 239–289.

Underwood, B. J. Individual differences as a crucible in theory construction. *American Psychologist,* 1975, *30*, 128–134.

Witkin, H. A. Origins of cognitive style. In C. Scheerer (Ed.), *Cognition: Theory, research, promise.* New York: Harper & Row, 1964.

Zelnicker, T., & Jeffrey, W. E. Attention and cognitive style in children. In G. Hale & M. Lewis (Eds.), *Attention and the development of attentional skills.* New York: Plenum, in press.

4   *Learning, memory, and intelligence*

WILLIAM K. ESTES

4.1.   INTRODUCTION

OVERVIEW

In this chapter I propose to treat intelligence, not as a static trait or ability, but as a set of related aspects of the structure and functioning of an individual viewed as an information-processing system. En route to understanding the role of various aspects of learning and memory in intellectual function, it would seem a sensible starting point to review the accumulation of systematic observations of human performance in various environmental situations that are taken to reflect differing degrees of intelligence. However, no such collection of materials proves to be available. The tradition has been, rather, to study correlations between intelligence-test scores and gross indexes of adaptive intellectual performance (success in school, occupational category, economic level) and rarely to go beyond correlational to causal analyses. Until the lack begins to be made up, we are left with the more indirect, though still possibly useful, strategy of examining in detail how success is attained on the psychometric tests, and relating the results to the concepts and theories of learning and information processing (Carroll, 1976; W. K. Estes, 1974; Pellegrino & Glaser, 1979; R. Sternberg, 1977).

In order to review this aspect of the study of intelligence as the field actually is, rather than as we might wish it to be, I will start by summarizing some general conclusions that can be drawn from some three-quarters of a century of research on the relations among learning ability, memory capacity, and intelligence and indicating principal contemporary trends in this research. Then I will turn to the question of the resources, in the form of concepts, theories, and methods, that the psychology of learning and memory has to contribute to research on intelligence. It will not be possible to be exhaustive, so the review will be selective, concentrating attention on models already shown to have relevance. In each case I ask first what the nature of the given process or mechanism is, then what is known regarding individual differences and their relationship to measured intelligence.

SOME DEFINITIONS

Before entering into the discussion of the way learning and memory enter into research on and interpretations of intelligence, we need some provisional definitions. *Learning* is generally taken to refer to the way organisms profit by experience so as, on the average at least, to increase adaptability to their environments (see, e.g., Hilgard, 1956). Within this rough characterization, specific usages differ among investigators with different backgrounds. Some psychologists prefer to stay close to an operational level and recognize no distinction between learning and the changes in behavior that enable one to tell when learning occurs. Thus, whereas many psychologists use the term *conditioning* to refer to a major category of basic forms of learning, others, for example, Gormezano and Kehoe (1975), prefer to identify *conditioning* strictly with the operations used in the original experimental demonstrations of Pavlov (1927).

Similarly, some of the most influential of the early learning theorists (e.g., Hull, 1937, 1943; Tolman, 1932) emphasize a distinction between the changes in performance that index learning and learning itself, an inferred process. Other investigators (notably Skinner, 1938, and his followers) identify learning with the systematic changes in behavior produced by its past consequences in the form of rewards and punishments (technically, *reinforcement*). At one time there was much controversy in the psychological literature concerning these definitional issues, but interest in them has waned and it seems fair to say that at the present time nearly all investigators of human learning and intellectual function, and many investigators of animal learning, take the term *learning* to refer to any process whereby organisms acquire information or knowledge, regardless of whether the information is immediately reflected in changes in behavior.

In contrast, there seems to have been less debate about the problem of defining *memory*, generally recognized to be an abstraction referring to an organism's capability of storing and retrieving information. In the contemporary literature, information stored in memory is conceived as entering into performance by way of such cognitive processes and operations as memory search, comparisons between memorial representations and products of perceptual processes, and decision making.

Thus, in brief, throughout this chapter I shall take *intelligence*, or intellectual performance, to refer to adaptive behavior of the individual, usually characterized by some element of problem solving and directed by cognitive processes and operations. *Learning* will be taken to refer to all systematic processes of acquiring information or knowledge, *memory* to the structures and processes involved in storing and retrieving information, and *cognitive operations* to the actions (usually inferred rather than observable) carried out on the contents of memory and the products of perception in the course of performing intellectual tasks.

CORRELATIONS BETWEEN LEARNING AND INTELLIGENCE

What kinds of relationships obtain between the study of learning and memory (henceforth termed *cognitive psychology*), on the one hand, and the study of intelligence, on the other? Several quite distinct traditions bear on the answer. Historically, the first significant interaction to appear was the inclusion of tests of memory, in particular the digit-span test, in some of the earliest intelligence scales (Binet & Simon, 1905, 1916). Binet thought that intelligence should be considered quite distinct from memory (which he tended to equate with *judgment*), but he somewhat inconsistently included the digit-span test in the original Binet–Simon scale – perhaps persuaded by empirical correlations he observed in his laboratory between digit span and other tasks included in the scale. Memory span was more extensively tapped in later revisions of the Binet–Simon scale, and in a great many of the other tests of intelligence that followed.

When the Binet scales were revised by Terman (1916) for what proved to be extremely widespread use in U.S. schools, the emphasis was almost entirely on diagnosing a child's inability to profit from instruction or ability to accelerate in the schools. In an analysis of a later revision (McNemar, 1942), the nature and interrelationships of the various subtests were examined in detail, and it proved, contrary to the intention of Binet and Simon, that the subtests that appeared in content to constitute measures of memory correlated as highly with other measures of mental age as the reliabilities would permit. The author concluded that "memory" as assessed by these subtests of the New Revision (Terman & Merrill, 1937) is not very different from the "general intelligence" being measured by the scale as a whole.

Perhaps because of these results, together with the fact that the earliest intelligence tests were developed for the purpose of assessing children's abilities to succeed in school, many investigators have tended to equate intelligence with learning ability. Thus it is not surprising that in the early 1900s there began to appear the first of a long succession of efforts to demonstrate significant correlations between measures of learning ability taken from simplified laboratory tasks and psychometric measures of intelligence. Scanning a half-century of this literature, from Spearman (1904) to Munn (1954), reveals little in the way of positive relationships. The most systematic studies of this period yielded only low and marginally significant correlations between measures of IQ and laboratory measures of learning (Woodrow, 1940). A critical and analytic review by Zeaman and House (1967) made the point that many of the low correlations may have been a consequence of restricted ranges of IQs entering into the correlations. With this methodological defect allowed for, they found some correlations in the range .40–.60 (measures of intelligence vs. rate of paired-associate learning) and concluded that there is at least a significant positive relationship, for subjects of equal mental age, between IQ and measures of verbal learning.

Although these correlational efforts bore little fruit, the ideas behind them persisted, and in fact Thorndike, Bregman, Cobb, and Woodyard (1926) made a Herculean effort to subsume both learning and intelligence under a single conception of associative capacity. This effort did not immediately prove very influential, but perhaps in part because of it, a few decades later the first learning theorists in the modern sense, followers of Skinner (1938) and Hull (1943), initiated two substantial lines of investigation (reviewed by W. K. Estes, 1970). One of these had to do with the application of reinforcement theories to the training of the mentally retarded; the other had to do with the search for differences between retarded and normal persons in basic properties of conditioning and elementary learning.

With the emergence of the information-processing approach to human cognition in the late 1960s, the prevailing orientation began to shift from correlational investigations toward theoretically directed experimental efforts to examine the ways in which cognitive processes and operations enter into performance in intellectual tasks. Long-term objectives of these efforts are focused less on assessing relative abilities than on understanding the many aspects and determinants of intellectual performance, on contributing actively to the remedying of intellectual deficits or disabilities, and on helping to augment intellectual power and efficiency for those who are not deficient but still short of achieving all they might wish. The principal focus of this chapter will be on reviewing the concepts and methods contemporary cognitive psychology has to contribute to this enterprise. After a review of the several relevant aspects of research on learning and memory, it will be possible to return to the problem of interactions between learning and intelligence at a m theoretical level.

4.2.   LEARNING AND LEARNING THEORY

LEVELS OF LEARNING

It has long been customary to classify forms of learning into lower versus higher processes, the lower levels mainly characterizing organisms that are younger in age or lower on the phylogenetic scale, the upper levels mainly characterizing organisms that are more mature or higher on the phylogenetic scale. Further, the lower levels of learning have tended to involve little or no distinction between learning and performance: Habituation has been regarded as simply a progressive reduction in response tendency to constant stimulation, classical conditioning as the substitution of a new stimulus for an original one in a reflex, and operant conditioning or law-of-effect learning as the increase in strength of a stimulus-response connection produced by reinforcement. In the course of research over many decades there has been a continual uncovering of previously unsuspected complexities in what were earlier regarded as the lowest and simplest forms of learning. Nonetheless, it will be useful to review briefly some of the principal traditional categories, roughly in increasing order of complexity, with special attention to the ways in which individual differences have been related to laboratory findings.

HABITUATION

Properties.   However levels of learning are defined, surely the lowest and in a sense most primitive variety of learning is the process termed *habituatory decrement*, which takes the form of a progressive loss of responsiveness to almost any regularly repeated stimulus. For example, if one produces a sudden sound, as a snap of the fingers, in the vicinity of even a very young infant, one observes a clear startle response. But just as surely, if the stimulus is repeated at regular intervals, the magnitude of the response will be seen to decrease rapidly to the point at which continuing repetition of the stimulus evokes no perceptible reaction at all. This phenomenon is observed with respect to all reflexes in all organisms that have been studied, from the lowest invertebrates to man (Harris, 1943; Humphrey, 1933). Habituation is not limited to unconditioned reflexes, however, but is observed also for conditioned and even for verbal stimuli (Syz, 1926).

At one time habituation received little attention in learning theory, being generally regarded as an isolated reflexological phenomenon of no great theoretical interest. That viewpoint was perhaps bound up with a tradition, persistent through much of the history of the psychology of learning down to the last couple of decades, of viewing the organism as though it began life as almost a tabula rasa so far as learning and memory are concerned. Everyone recognized that animals and even people begin life with a few built-in unconditioned reflexes, but beyond that, almost all of the behavior of the mature animal or person was conceived to be a result of learning processes that produce associations between arbitrary combinations of stimuli and responses. With the growing influence of ethology since mid-century (see, e.g., Hinde & Tinbergen, 1958; Lorenz, 1952; Shettleworth, 1972), it has come to be appreciated that organisms of all phylogenetic orders are genetically programmed with rather elaborate organizations of behavioral dispositions. These result in often striking commonalities in behavior among members of a species in spite of considerable variation in the environment (hence the term *species-specific behavior*).

Processes. Speaking a bit analogically, the species-specific behaviors or behavioral propensities may be taken to represent results of a process akin to learning that has gone on in the species in the course of evolution rather than in any individual in the course of ontogeny. However, these species-specific behaviors are adaptive only on the average over the range of environments in which a species is likely to find itself; in specific situations, behaviors called forth more or less automatically by stimuli as a consequence of these inherited predispositions may prove quite unadaptive. However well a response has served one's ancestors, one needs a way of giving it up if it does not work for oneself in a particular situation. The mechanism for accomplishing this end is evidently the almost ubiquitous process of habituatory decrement. Indeed, as soon as the adaptive significance of habituation beyond the reflex level began to be appreciated, investigators looked for habituatory processes in much more complex species-specific behaviors and found habituation occurring just as reliably and predictably at this level as at the level of reflexes (see, e.g., Hinde, 1970).

Because the functional properties of habituation are essentially the same at different stages of development and at different phylogenetic levels, it does not follow that the processes responsible are identical. Indeed, considering habituation as a process influencing selective attention in human beings as well as lower animals, Sokolov (1963) has proposed a theoretical interpretation of habituation in terms of what would be considered rather high-level cognitive operations. Sokolov's conception, in brief, is that upon each experience with a repeated stimulus, an individual forms an internal representation ("model"), which is then compared with the new inputs on successive trials. To the extent that the internal representation matches a new input, responsiveness declines (habituation occurs); to the extent that a new input deviates from the internal representation, the individual is alerted, and response tendencies are reinstated to their normal strength.

Individual differences. In view of the fact that a number of investigators have hypothesized that a deficit in inhibitory control of behavior is closely associated with mental retardation (Denny, 1964; Ross & Ross, 1976), it might be expected that individual differences in susceptibility to habituation should be related to individual differences in more complex intellectual functions, but to date there seem to be few studies addressed to this problem. McCall and Kagan (1970) have presented evidence that individual differences in rate of habituation show some stability over the first year of so of infancy and that they are correlated with other indexes of emerging cognitive activity, for example, responsiveness to novel stimuli. However, Clifton and Nelson (1976), in a review of relevant developmental studies, emphasize the numerous problems of experimental technique and control that remain to be solved before measures of habituation in young children can be satisfactorily interpreted in terms of learning as distinguished from performance or other processes.

CONDITIONING

Interpretation. At one time classical conditioning was considered to be almost as primitive a learning process as habituation; however, new findings resulting from interactions between the research traditions of conditioning and information processing begin to present a picture of conditioning as a considerably more complex process than it was once thought to be. For example, a number of investigators (Egger & Miller, 1962; Kamin, 1969; Rescorla & Wagner, 1972) have generated an impressive accumulation of evidence that conditioning is to an important extent a function of the information value of the conditioned stimulus.

In earlier theories, the necessary and sufficient condition for conditioning to occur was taken to be simply the occurrence of a conditioned stimulus, an unconditioned stimulus, and an unconditioned response in temporal contiguity. However, it turns out that little or no conditioning occurs unless, at the time when a potential conditioned stimulus is presented, the organism is in a state of uncertainty about whether an unconditioned stimulus will follow, and thus receives an increment of information when that unconditioned stimulus does indeed occur. Suppose, for example, that an originally neutral stimulus, say a tone, is presented to an animal and followed by a shock. The normal result is that after a very few such trials the tone will come to evoke conditioned reactions signifying that the animal has come to anticipate the shock upon occurrence of the tone. If, however, prior to these episodes a light had been paired with the shock to the point of becoming a reliable conditioned stimulus (i.e., a reliable predictor of the shock), and if then on a number of trials the tone and the light together were presented to the animal preceding the shock, a subsequent test would show that the tone had acquired no capacity to evoke conditioned reactions.

Because it is of obvious adaptive significance for all organisms to learn when otherwise neutral stimuli or events signify that biologically important stimuli or events are about to occur, it is understandable that conditioning has been widely considered to be a basic and almost ubiquitous form of learning. Further, in some of the lower organisms, classical conditioning appears to be the only way in which stimuli take on such signal value. However, in the case of higher organisms, and especially man, there is considerable room for disagreement about the role of conditioning. Some psychologists regard conditioning as a basic element or building block in more complex forms of learning (e.g., Hull, 1943); others consider it to be simply a special form of associative learning in which there happens to be an indicator response that is privileged in the sense that the response evoked by the signal stimulus normally is very similar to the response evoked by the unconditioned stimulus (Konorski, 1967). That somewhat extreme proposition is difficult to document rigorously, but nonetheless it is clear that elementary forms of associative learning at least closely akin to conditioning occur in man as well as in lower animals. However, in the case of man, it has been known since Pavlov (1927) that under ordinary circumstances conditioning is dominated by higher-order processes that are largely verbal in character.

Normal–retarded comparisons. Even though conditioning cannot be thought to play a great part in the intellectual activity of human beings, it has provided a convenient vehicle for research on early mental development and on differences in functioning between severely mentally retarded and normal persons. One reason, of course, is simply that conditioning experiments can be carried out regardless of the verbal capabilities of the subject. Another is that the course of conditioning is susceptible to the influence of higher cognitive processes, and thus the conditioning experiment provides a simplified situation in which these influences may be studied more clearly than they could be in more complex problem-solving situations (Ross & Ross, 1976). And, though the supposition remains to be confirmed, investigators continue to operate on the assumption that individual differences in parameters of conditioning may be more amenable to study in relation to underlying differences in neurophysiological structures or processes than would be the case for individual differences in more complex forms of learning.

To date, it must be said that a considerable body of research comparing properties of conditioning between mental retardates and normals has not proven extremely revealing. By and large, gross properties of conditioning, such as rate of acquisition of a conditioned response, have not proven to vary greatly over a wide range of intellect, from moderate retardation to normal adult levels (W. K. Estes, 1970; Ross & Ross, 1976). There have, however, been some hints of selective deficits in the retarded that may prove to be of theoretical significance. For example, in trace conditioning, that is, the paradigm in which there is a temporal gap between offset of a conditioned stimulus and occurrence of an unconditioned stimulus, retarded persons seem less able than normals to bridge the temporal gap. This and related findings led Ellis (1963) to propose that both younger normal and mentally retarded individuals are characterized by a "stimulus trace deficit," and that the course of decay of a stimulus trace, as indexed by such measures as rate of trace conditioning, provides a prime measure of some aspects of integrity of the central nervous system. Attempts to test the hypothesis did not lead to convincing confirmation, however, and later Ellis (1970) recast his idea in terms of individual differences in short-term memory function. By and large it appears that at present the study of conditioning does not have a great deal to contribute to our understanding of why and how some individuals learn so much more readily than others, but still it may continue to prove a useful, perhaps even increasingly useful, tool for efforts to relate elementary learning capabilities to variations in brain structure and biochemistry.

INSTRUMENTAL LEARNING

Behavioral and cognitive approaches. By *instrumental learning* I shall refer to simple forms of learning relative to rewards and punishments (henceforth subsumed together under the term *reinforcement*). Technically, a distinction is made in the research literature between operant conditioning, associated with free-responding situations, and instrumental conditioning, observed in situations closely akin to the classical conditioning experiment (see, e.g., Hilgard & Marquis, 1940). These terms refer to extremely impoverished situations in which the organism is confined in a small space with very few options for responding, and the organism's disposition to perform some one action (e.g., pressing a lever that operates a food magazine or removing a foot from an electrified grid) is selected to index the course of learning. Clearly these experimental arrangements are not typical of many that an organism, animal or man, would encounter in its normal environment, but they do provide rigorously controlled situations in which to study in detail the way actions come to depend on temporal and probabilistic aspects of reinforcement and the way levels of motivation and reinforcement magnitudes enter into the determination of performance.

There are sharp differences of opinion concerning the relationship between instrumental learning as studied in the laboratory and adaptive behavior outside the laboratory. For students of operant conditioning in the tradition of B. F. Skinner, reinforcement is the key to adaptive behavior; individual differences in adaptive behavior or intellectual function, even differences between mental retardates and normal adult human beings, are traceable to variations in individual histories of reinforcement (Bijou, 1966). Though this premise has been a matter of much debate, little research has been addressed directly to it. The general proposition may be indeed beyond test but, nonetheless, investigators of operant conditioning have shown that there is at least some substance to it by demonstrations that specific deficiencies in adaptive behavior, especially in the mentally retarded, can be overcome at least in part by carefully contrived instrumental learning regimes (Birnbrauer, 1976).

The contrasting theoretical position, characterizing investigators associated with cognitive psychology and information processing, is that most adaptive learning outside the laboratory is a matter of acquiring information concerning relationships between situations and actions and their outcomes, rather than of modifying response strengths, and that learning by observation, rather than by reinforcement, is the rule (Atkinson & Wickens, 1971; Bandura, 1971, 1977; W. K. Estes, 1969, 1971).

A common framework. For students of intelligence, it may be less advantageous to try to decide between these opposed positions than to seek a theoretical framework capable of embracing both. This framework will surely have to be based on recognition of levels of processes from the reflex to the verbal, with the higher generally dominating the lower (Grant, 1964; Pavlov, 1927; White, 1965). At all levels, adaptive behavior depends on the acquisition of information, in some sense, concerning relationships between actions and outcomes. At the lower levels, however, this information comes only from the actual performance of responses and the immediate experience of their rewarding or punishing consequences, whereas at the higher levels multiple sources of information are the rule and need not result from trial-and-error behavior. At the lower levels, it is difficult to make any operationally significant distinction among response tendencies, memories, and expectations. When a rat in a Skinner box is observed to press a lever that activates a food hopper, one is free to say that the animal remembers past experiences and expects its response to be followed by a reward; but on the other hand, nothing is obviously added by these embellishments to the simple description that the rewarded response tends to be repeated. With adult human beings, in contrast, memory for relationships between responses and reinforcements can be shown to be at least partially independent of dispositions to repeat the responses (see, e.g., Buchwald, 1969), and a person who remembers that an action has been followed by a reward may or may not judge repetition of that action to be the appropriate behavior upon recurrence of the situation (Nuttin & Greenwald, 1968).

As human behavior matures, memory comes to enter into instrumental learning at more abstract levels, transcending recall of the outcomes of particular episodes. One aspect of this generalized role of memory has to do with a person's expectation that his or her performance will meet the standards or criteria required for reinforcement. These expectations are in turn a function of the person's past history of successes and failures and the way they are represented in memory (Bandura, 1977; Bandura & Walters, 1963; Rotter, 1954).

The relevance of learning theory to research on intelligence flows in part from an almost universal characteristic of intellectual tasks, namely, that any given problem can be solved in alternative ways that reflect different levels of learning and performance. For example, such tasks as mastering discrimination problems or learning the correspondences between numbers in the decimal and binary number systems can be accomplished at the level of specific stimulus-response associations, which may suffice for some immediate purposes, or on the basis of conceptual relations, which will not only handle the immediate task but provide a superior basis for transfer to new problems (Kendler, 1979; Suppes & Ginsberg, 1962). On theoretical grounds, it seems clear that the extent to which a learner proceeds to the higher levels of intellectual functioning is determined by conditions of reinforcing feedback as related to the disparity between the degree of success he or she attains with a particular cognitive strategy and the degree of success he or she has learned or has been led to expect should be available. However, more research is needed to analyze the specific ways in which this interaction develops in relation to particular kinds of intellectual tasks.

The other principal aspect of the extended role of memory concerns the acquisition of information about constancies in the environment. For the mature human being, a major component of instrumental learning is the acquiring of information concerning how tasks and situations should be categorized so that one can anticipate when and how a successful action in a particular situation is likely again to be successful when the same or a similar situation is encountered.

In this connection, Nuttin (1953) has introduced an important distinction between what he terms *open* and *closed* tasks. A closed task is one in which the setting and the instructions give the learner no reason to expect that a relationship observed between an action and a reward on one occasion will carry over to other occasions, whereas an open task is one in which the learner is given reason to expect such carry-over.

Following up this idea, my associates and I have produced evidence that Nuttin's conception can be generalized from a dichotomy between types of tasks to an intrinsically important aspect of instrumental learning in general, having to do with the acquisition of information about environmental constancies. Developmentally, it appears that children of preschool age have very limited appreciation of these constancies, at least in the form they assume in typical experiments on children's learning. For example, the young child may give evidence of remembering that an action was followed by a reward on one occasion but may not realize that repetition of the action is likely to lead to repetition of the reward.

Even at the earlier ages studied, performance in a discriminative learning situation is improved if information concerning environmental constancies is supplied to the child in a sufficiently concrete form; with increasing age, this type of crutch becomes less and less necessary (K. W. Estes, 1976). Thus, with increasing age, children's learning becomes increasingly intelligent in the sense of taking more effective account of general information about constancies in the environment, but as yet almost nothing is known concerning the specific kinds of experiences responsible for this developmental trend.

The way judgments about environmental constancies can be expected to enter into adult learning is illustrated by the following study (W. K. Estes, 1972b). The experimental situation simulated an aircraft control station with the subject having the role of the controller and having the tasks of transmitting messages to the hypothetical pilot and of learning by experience whether a given message sent in a particular situation was effective and should be repeated when the situation recurred or was ineffective and should not. Overall data from the experiment showed apparently inconsistent behavior, in that subjects sometimes repeated a successful message (that is, one that appropriately modified the behavior of the hypothetical pilot so as to avoid a crash) when the situation recurred and sometimes did not. More detailed analysis showed, however, that when auxiliary information indicated that the message sent had been actually received by the pilot, successful messages were repeated, whereas when auxiliary information indicated that (as a consequence of noise in the communication channel) the intended message had been misperceived, the message tended not to be repeated.

Instrumental learning and intelligence. It might seem that instrumental learning differs from classical conditioning only in some technical aspects of the way reinforcers are related to responses; however, these two elementary learning paradigms have entered in very different ways into research on intelligence and mental development. For classical conditioning, the primary interest has been in comparing groups of different ages or intellectual levels, on the premise that "conditionability" might prove to be a basic learning capacity related to intelligence. But for instrumental learning, primary interest has been in demonstrating that similar functional relationships between performance and independent variables can be observed for organisms of very different phylogenetic or developmental levels and, for human beings, different levels of intelligence (Holz & Azrin, 1966; Krasner & Ullmann, 1965; Skinner, 1966). These latter efforts have met with some success, and, with regard to individual differences, it can be said with one qualification that speed and functional properties of instrumental learning appear almost unrelated to intelligence over the range from moderate mental retardation to normal levels in human beings. The qualification is that the learning must be observed in a situation where special measures have been taken to keep higher-order verbal processes from influencing the course of learning, so that the learner can be said to be unaware of the relationships between actions and outcomes (Spielberger, 1962). When such measures are not taken, the course of instrumental learning is importantly modified by verbal processes, and one must presume that significant relationships to conventional indexes of intelligence could be observed, though no relevant formal studies seem to have been reported.

SELECTIVE LEARNING

Learning and information processing.   A great many of the kinds of problem situations that provide criteria of intelligent behavior and means of testing intelligence involve both discrimination and choice. Relevant aspects of a problem situation must be discriminated from the irrelevant, and appropriate actions selected over those less appropriate. But though the successful exercise of discrimination and choice may be conditioned by genetic endowment, the manifestation of these capabilities certainly depends always on the background of learning.

In order to organize our thoughts about the bewildering variety of forms of selective learning in and out of the laboratory, it will be helpful to begin with some general categorizations, as outlined in Table 4.1. For traditional as much as logical reasons, all instances of selective learning must involve relationships between information input to the individual and actions having to do with retrieval and use of the information; but for research purposes it has seemed essential to concentrate for the most part on either the input or the output side separately – hence the column headings in Table 4.1, which reflect primary focus on stimulus aspects (e.g., discrimination), on response aspects (e.g., multiple-choice learning), or on the combination of the two (e.g., hypothesis selection).

The stimulus column deals with the way organisms learn to discriminate or identify objects and their attributes, the response column with learning to select responses on the basis of the values or probabilities of their consequences, and the interaction column with learning that results in hypotheses or rules, usually though perhaps not necessarily verbal in form, which prescribe the sequence of actions that should be initiated by each of a number of possible input patterns. Further, within each of these categories of learning, it is useful to distinguish structural aspects from operations performed on the structures.

Even though, to an observer, the input of information to an individual may appear continuous, progress toward understanding the human information-processing system proves to be tied up with growing appreciation of the ways in which active cognitive processes fractionate, categorize, and combine elements or aspects of stimulus inputs into structures that have unitary characteristics. Thus incoming stimulus information from visual displays or auditory messages appears to be apprehended in terms of attributes or critical features, from which are generated representations in memory of events, objects, or concepts. On the response side, structural aspects range from simple motor units (articulatory units) to organized action sequences. Operations performed on these structures take the form of selective attention or encoding in the case of stimulus units, decisions in the case of response units, and generation, sampling and testing of hypotheses in the case of structures that combine stimulus and response aspects, that is, rules or plans.

Perceptual and discrimination learning.   To develop in a little more detail the relations of these various aspects of learning to intelligence, it will be convenient to proceed serially across the columns of Table 4.1. Beginning on the input side, it may be noted first of all that there are two major subcategories, perceptual and discrimination learning, the former referring to the development of familiar recog-

Table 4.1. *Aspects of selective learning*

| Aspect | Input–output focus | | |
	Stimulus	Response	Interaction
Types of learning	Discrimination and perceptual learning	Multiple choice and probability learning	Hypothesis selection
Structures	Features, attributes, concepts	Action sequences, strategies	Rules, plans
Operations	Selective attention, encoding	Decision	Generation, sampling, testing of hypotheses

nizable perceptual units and the latter to the process of learning to distinguish relevant from irrelevant units or attributes in any given task.

Perceptual learning occurs to an important extent in early life, is a slow cumulative process depending on interaction between motor activities and observation of the environment, and may be regarded primarily as a prerequisite to, rather than a component of, intelligent behavior (Hebb, 1949). Little is known of a quantitative character about individual differences in perceptual learning as it occurs under normal conditions (that is, in the absence of severe sensory deprivation, brain damage, or the like), but data on some of the products of perceptual learning, for example, size constancy, suggest that over a wide range the process is almost unrelated to measures of intelligence (Gibson, 1969).

Discrimination, in contrast to perceptual, learning is an important component of cognitive activity of people at all ages, learning rate varying to a major extent with intelligence as well as with age. Whereas perceptual learning is a process of coming to identify familiar units, discrimination learning is a matter of learning relationships among these units.

A typical example of discrimination learning outside the laboratory would be learning the relationship between the red and green lights on a traffic signal and the movement of traffic. In earlier discrimination theories, for example, Spence (1937), the process was conceptualized simply as the strengthening and weakening of associations between stimuli and responses. Thus, as a consequence of rewards and nonrewards, a child's tendency to go in the presence of green would be strengthened and the tendency to go in the presence of red would be weakened, the drawing apart of these response tendencies being the index of discrimination learning.

In virtually all modern theories, however, discrimination learning is conceived as having at least two important aspects, one dealing with selective attention and the other connected with the learning of relationships between the products of attention and actions or consequences. These two aspects can be illustrated by a common research paradigm in which the learner might be trained, for example, on a discrimination based on some one property of a stimulus display – say, either color or form. The contingencies of such an experiment can conveniently be represented in the form of an attribute-by-value table. For example, suppose that on various trials of an experiment the learner was presented with either a circle or a triangle, the circle or triangle being colored either red or green, and the task defined by the experimenter being to learn always to make a positive response to red stimuli and to withhold the positive response to green stimuli. The table would be

	Circle	Triangle
Red	+	+
Green	−	−

Because reward (represented by a plus sign in the table) is related consistently only to color, responses on the basis of form of the stimulus would be rewarded only half the time. Thus, in this example, color would be considered a relevant and form an irrelevant dimension.

In current theories (e.g., Sutherland & Mackintosh, 1971; Trabasso & Bower, 1968; Zeaman & House, 1963), the learning would constitute first learning to attend to the appropriate dimension, color in this example, and then learning to associate a particular value on this dimension with reward or with the positive response. If the contingencies were changed so that form was relevant, the table might take the form

	Circle	Triangle
Red	+	−
Green	+	−

so that responses to circles would be rewarded and those to triangles non-rewarded, regardless of color. In this case, the first stage of learning would be a matter of coming to attend selectively to the form dimension, and the second process would be one of learning that, within this dimension, circle rather than triangle was associated with reward. By employment of an ingenious type of analysis of discrimination data termed *backward learning curves* in the framework of a theoretical model, Zeaman and House (1963) provided quite clear evidence that discovery of a relevant dimension typically occurs on an all-or-none basis. Further, they showed that the mentally retarded differ from normals more in their difficulty in giving up irrelevant in favor of relevant dimensions than in their speed of associating correct stimulus values with rewards.

Discrimination, selective attention, and mental development. Characteristically, discrimination learning is slow in the young child and in the mentally retarded and becomes very rapid in the normal adult. Important research questions have been why the learning is initially slow and what conditions must be present for it to become more rapid. One reason, at least at a descriptive level, for the initial slowness is that the immature or unintelligent learner tends to persist, sometimes over a very long sequence of trials, in responding on the basis of an initially preferred but actually irrelevant stimulus dimension. For young children, this dimension is most often spatial position, so that in the example the young child might begin by always choosing the stimulus placed on the left side of a left–right arrangement and thus would not discover the difference in relevance of the form and color dimensions. Progress toward solution of the discrimination problem will occur only if ultimately the subject spontaneously deviates from the positional responding, or is instigated to do so by the experimenter or instructor, and has an opportunity to observe and thus learn about the differential correlations of the other dimensions with reward.

Improvement in the efficiency of discrimination learning, as with problem solving, is thus evidently at least in part a matter of acquiring general knowledge of the environment to the effect that it is usually unnecessary to settle for chance levels of reward frequency (50% in the example), and that active search for relevant dimensions tends nearly always to be rewarded.

Methods of evaluating learner's tendencies to attend selectively to stimulus dimensions have come primarily from what are termed discrimination-shift studies. An important comparison can be illustrated by the example just given. Suppose that a group of subjects was given training on the first problem, that is, always being rewarded for a choice of the red stimulus rather than the green one, whether the form was triangular or circular. If, following training on this procedure, one subgroup of subjects was transferred to a new problem in which the same dimension was relevant – say, blue stimuli were rewarded and yellow nonrewarded – whereas the second group was transferred to a new problem in which a different dimension was relevant – say, large stimuli were rewarded and small unrewarded – the first group (having what is termed an *intradimensional shift*) would exhibit the faster learning on the second problem. The superiority of the intradimensional over the extradimensional shift is taken as evidence that, during training on the first problem, the learners came to attend selectively to the relevant dimension (color in the example), rather than to the irrelevant dimension (form in the example). Speed of learning to attend to relevant dimensions, as evidenced by the shift comparisons, increases as a function of age, and within a given age as a function of other indexes of intelligence (Zeaman & House, 1963, 1974).

Of course, problems involving only two distinguishable stimulus dimensions are common only in simplified laboratory situations. Normally, it is doubtless the rule for larger numbers of dimensions to undergo simultaneous variation in the course of most interesting forms of learning; and in the general case, an important constraint on speed of learning is imposed by capacity limitations on the individual's capability of dealing simultaneously with variation in multiple attributes. There seems to have been no research on the problem of measuring individual differences in such capacities, but there has been considerable work on the complementary problem of investigating strategies that people may employ in order to deal in a systematic way with variation in multiple-stimulus dimensions (see, e.g., Millward & Wickens, 1974; Trabasso & Bower, 1968). These strategies may take the form, for example, of partitioning the total set of dimensions varying in a given situation into subsets and then attending selectively to one subset after another in order to exclude the irrelevant and ultimately to focus on the relevant dimension or dimensions. It is clear that acquisition of or training in such strategies can play an extremely important role in contributing to efficiency in dealing with complex discriminations. Again, it would seem on theoretical grounds that there must be important reciprocal interactions between other aspects of intelligence and the learning of effective strategies; however, formal verification of this assumption and the working out of the details of the interaction remain open problems for research.

CONCEPT LEARNING

Discrimination and concept formation. A form of learning that might be expected to be of utmost importance for the understanding of intelligence is concept formation. Because events rarely repeat themselves exactly, and because, in any case, the number of events that a person experiences is too large for all events to be remembered and recalled individually, much of our knowledge of the world is organized by concepts.

In the early days of learning theory it was assumed, with what still seems good reason, that, at least in animals and children, concept formation could be regarded as a relatively direct extension of discrimination learning. A child learns, for example, to associate the word *red* with certain objects – an apple, a fire engine – and *green* with others – leaves, a green shirt or a dress – and then, after sufficient experience with various exemplars, comes to apply these color terms correctly to new objects; the procedure is much the same with the names of forms, numbers, and so on. Similar generalizations of discrimination learning are achieved by animals, the results in some instances yielding conceptual behavior rivaling that manifest in human beings. This last characterization applies most conspicuously to animals closest to man, for example, chimpanzees (Premack, 1976).

In his earliest major contribution to learning theory, Hull (1920) laid the experimental groundwork for extending analyses of conceptual learning in animals to the human level by training subjects, simply via differential reward and nonreward, to attach appropriate labels to sets of Chinese characters that included common features. But, for reasons that could not be explicated without a lengthy essay on the history of psychology, this fruitful and informative line of research treating concept learning as an outgrowth of discrimination lapsed into unpopularity in the 1950s. Thus, in his authoritative examination of research methods, Hilgard (1951) dismissed this line of research with a casual remark to the effect that research on animal learning has no relevance for the understanding of human concept formation. The principal basis for this view was the fact that animals are unable to introspect about their concepts and presumably are unable to learn the equivalent of the verbal rules that adult human beings not only learn but express. A consequence of this curt dismissal of a whole research tradition was that, when learning theory began to be applied to problems of mental development and mental retardation in the 1950s, concept learning was grossly underrepresented.

Concept identification. In research on concept formation from about 1950 to 1970, interest in the way new concepts are formed gave way almost completely to emphasis on the way familiar concepts are identified in new situations. This new wave of research was apparently sparked to an important extent by the work of Bruner, Goodnow, and Austin (1956), which treated concept identification, not as a learning process, but rather as a form of problem solving. It was assumed that people identify concepts by generating and testing hypotheses about which of a number of already familiar rules should be applied in a particular situation. This approach led to the development of a considerable body of theory concerning the way in which hypotheses are sampled and accepted or rejected on the basis of observations (Levine, 1975; Millward & Wickens, 1974; Trabasso & Bower, 1968).

In research carried out in this tradition, the experimental subject is typically presented, in a series of trials, with exemplars drawn from a collection of multidimensional stimuli, and he or she attempts to discover the principle the experimenter has in mind for categorizing the stimuli into groups (e.g., figures with rectilinear boundaries versus figures with curvilinear boundaries, objects that are large and red versus objects that are small and blue). The only source of information available to the subject comes from his or her attempts to formulate hypotheses about the relevant properties, sort the objects in accord with the hypotheses, and determine from the experimenter's responses (right versus wrong or the equivalent) whether a hypothesis should be accepted or rejected.

Categories and prototypes.   During the 1970s, the hypothesis-testing approach to concept formation in turn dropped from its position of preeminence. The reason was mainly the observation, which came to be made with increasing frequency, that the concepts with which people deal in ordinary environments are often not definable in hard and fast categories delineated by common properties. Children, for example, seem to have no difficulty in learning at early ages to distinguish cats from dogs, fruits from vegetables, toys from utensils, though in none of these cases is there any one property that sharply segregates all members of one class from all members of the other. The idea took form that in such cases concepts are learned, not by discovering properties common to classes of objects or events, but rather by forming mental representations, or prototypes, of the combination of attributes most characteristic of a class, and by judging whether newly encountered objects are exemplars of the class on the basis of their overall resemblance or similarity to the prototype.

Experimental evidence for this conception of prototype formation began to accumulate rapidly following the pioneering studies of Posner and Keele (1968, 1970), and converging support from anthropological sources was added in a very influential series of studies by Rosch (1975; Rosch & Lloyd, 1978). Finally, the long-attenuated relationship between studies of concept formation and learning theory has begun to be reestablished with the new approach of Medin and Schaffer (1978), which shows that a sophisticated theory of discrimination learning can provide the basis for an account of concept learning in situations involving "ill-defined categories."

Overall, it would seem that the ideas growing out of the various approaches to concept formation must be highly relevant to intellectual performance. However, the approaches associated with hypothesis testing, learning theory, and anthropological observations have so far focused primarily on theoretical and ideological issues, so that the potentialities of this research for the measurement and modification of intellectual abilities have received scant attention. On the brighter side, efforts toward relating concept formation to intelligence have begun to appear at the animal level (Premack, 1976), and a useful framework for pursuing these connections at the level of human mental performance may be available in the current work of Anderson (1976) and others on the application of production systems to the simulation of human problem solving (see Dehn & Schank, Chapter 7).

ACQUISITION OF KNOWLEDGE

Approaches. One must recognize a major conceptual gap between learning in the sense of improving choices among alternatives or developing discriminations and learning in the sense of the acquisition of knowledge as it occurs in advanced schooling, or in science or professional life. One cannot hope to describe what a physician, a mathematician, or a business administrator has learned about his or her field in terms of specific responses or even specific items of information. The result of long-term learning in these cases is an elaborate organized body of information *about* a topic or a field. Properties of these organized memory structures and analyses of the way information is retrieved from them constitute a currently active line of research in semantic memory (discussed subsequently) but there has been scarcely a start on the problem of describing or interpreting the course of acquisition.

In order to appreciate how complex organized memory structures enter into intellectual functioning, we will need to know how numerous biological, social, and experiential variables enter into the determination and modification of learning and how more elementary processes combine to generate more complex ones. But making a start toward the desired objective is difficult, because learning in the sense of the acquisition of knowledge occurs outside the laboratory under conditions so uncontrolled and variable as to defy analysis. Consequently there are few firm facts on which to base even the beginnings of theory construction. It may be that, in principle, the mechanisms and processes revealed by theoretically directed research on simple laboratory tasks can ultimately account for the acquisition of knowledge, but even if the possibility exists in principle it may be impossible to realize in practice. Just as we cannot account for the observed properties of water by any amount of study of its constituent molecules, hydrogen and oxygen, separately, we may be unable to account for important properties of the acquisition of knowledge by any amount of understanding of constituent learning processes studied in isolation. The issue cannot be decided by logical arguments, however, and it is important to push as far as it will go the attempt to account for complex cognitive performance in terms of simpler components.

This strategy is currently to be seen in two quite different approaches. One of these derives from learning and association theory. It includes the ambitious and still somewhat programmatic effort of Bindra (1976) to produce a whole new system of the scope of Tolman's or Hull's but capable of encompassing more complex forms of learning, and also various more limited efforts at remodeling some of the basic assumptions of association theory in a way that may permit elementary associative units to serve as more effective building blocks for complex structures (e.g., W. K. Estes, 1973a, 1976, 1979).

The second principal approach derives less from learning theory itself than from computer science and the analogies students of artificial intelligence have found between information processing in computers and cognitive function in human beings. This latter approach in its early stages is epitomized by the pi-

oneering work of Feigenbaum (1963) and Hunt (1962). Though addressed originally to somewhat different phenomena – paired-associate learning in the case of
Feigenbaum and concept learning in the case of Hunt – these approaches have
important aspects in common. In each case, accumulating knowledge is conceived to be represented in the memory system, not by a collection of stimulus-
response connections or pair-wise associations between ideas, but rather by a
treelike structure (termed a *discrimination net* by Feigenbaum, a *decision tree* by
Hunt) that organizes accumulating information in such a way that it can be
accessed by a series of simple interrogations, much as in the game of Twenty
Questions. Still more important, in each case learning is conceived as being not
simply a deposit of the information received on each trial of a learning series, but
rather the result of an interaction between each new input and the current state of
the system, so that what is learned from a new experience depends on what has
been learned from previous ones.

Interactive discrimination networks. To illustrate a little more concretely, consider the way Feigenbaum's EPAM (Elementary Perceiver and Memorizer) model
might handle the discrimination problem cited in an earlier example, in which the
learner was presented with stimuli either circular or triangular in form and either
red or green in color, with the contingency that red stimuli were always correct
and green incorrect regardless of form. Suppose that on the first stimulus presentation of a series a subject were shown a red circle in Position 1 and a green
triangle in Position 2,

$$P_1 \qquad P_2$$

$$RC \qquad GT$$

where R, G, C, and T denote *red, green, circle,* and *triangle,* respectively. The
learner might happen to attend to form on this initial presentation, in which case
the result of this trial would be the following simple tree structure representing
the learner's memory that, on presentation of a new display, the stimulus should
be tested for form (Is it circular?) and assigned a plus value if circular and a minus
value if triangular:

Test

C or T?

C / \ T

+ —

Actually, under the conditions of the experiment in the example, the structure
would not suffice to lead to correct judgments uniformly. After an additional trial
on which, say, a green circle was presented in Position 1 and a red triangle in
Position 2,

$$P_1 \qquad P_2$$
$$GC \qquad RT$$

the growing discrimination net would take the following somewhat more complex form:

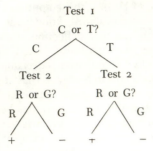

In this net, the first step upon presentation of a new display is to test for form (Is it circular or triangular?); then, regardless of the outcome, to test for color (Is it red or green?); and then to assign positive values to both red circles and red triangles as shown in the bottom row of the diagram. Here the learning process would stop, because this test sequence would generate correct judgments on all succeeding trials of the experiment, and there would be no need to incorporate information about position into the tree.

A difference in Hunt's model, oriented toward concept learning, is that the learner would focus on one or a subset of dimensions and record in the growing decision tree only the outcomes of tests on the dimensions that proved relevant. Thus, after the sequence of trials just given in the illustration, the decision tree would be very simple in form, including only a test for color and an assignment of a plus value if the outcome was red and a negative value otherwise:

Test

R or G?

R / \ G

+ −

Of course, the spirit of these models can hardly be captured by such simple examples. What is important is that the form of the memory structure resulting from a series of learning experiences and the way in which the accrual of information depends on continual testing of properties of new inputs against the current contents of memory apply to complex as well as to simple tasks. Thus, for example, if the model were being applied to a portion of an elementary biology course, a fragment of a discrimination net that might enable a student to answer such a question as "Is a whale a mammal?" might take the form

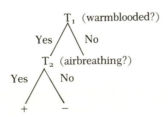

Hayes-Roth (1977) has formulated a model that accounts in some detail for the way the elements of such a structure become integrated into "knowledge assemblies" and the way they are accessed during performance of a task.

Learning-to-learn. Some problems that posed special difficulty for earlier learning theories are bypassed in these information-processing models. For example, it has long been a familiar fact that learners, whether animal or human, typically exhibit progressive increases in speed of learning upon repeated experiences with the same kind of material or task, this phenomenon being termed *learning-to-learn* or *learning set* (Harlow, 1949). There is no intrinsic reason within conditioning or associative learning theories why this phenomenon should occur, and consequently various special explanations were put forward (e.g., Medin, 1972; Restle, 1958). However, it is clear that in the information-processing models all learning involves learning-to-learn, because the information taken in on any given experience and the way it is organized depend on what has already been learned and the form of the existing memory structure. Learning is conceived as being an active process in which each new stimulus input gives rise to a series of tests to determine whether it can be appropriately categorized or diagnosed or whether its consequences can be predicted on the basis of information already in memory, with the information stored as a consequence of the given experience depending on the outcomes of these tests.

LEARNING AND INTELLIGENCE: RESEARCH DIRECTIONS AND NEEDED EMPHASES

From the appearance of the first reasonably well-articulated theories of learning in the 1940s, the assumption has been widely held that there must be close relationships between learning and intelligence, to the extent that some investigators, for example, Gagné (1968), have virtually identified intelligence with the cumulative products of learning. For the most part, however, research on learning and research on intelligence have proceeded on their own tracks with relatively meager interaction. The discreteness of these two major strands of research is certainly not optimal on either side, and there are reasons to think that even relatively modest changes in strategies or emphases might improve matters. I shall consider these possibilities from each standpoint in turn.

From learning to intelligence. First we may ask why research on learning has so rarely been oriented toward contributing to the understanding of intelligence. One reason is that research on learning is quite properly directed primarily toward the advancement of learning theory. For the most part, new research is generated by previous research, together with consideration of its relevance to theoretical issues. Even within that framework, however, there is a great deal of room for variation in strategies. It is all too easy to proceed on the comfortable but possibly unfounded assumption that all the significant properties of learning can be brought out by studying learning in an arbitrary selection of especially simplified situations. Just that tendency may have been responsible in part for the reluctance of investigators of intelligence – and, for that matter, education – to draw heavily on the fruits of learning research during its first half-century or so.

Findings arising from laboratory studies of learning were supposed to be extendable to more intrinsically interesting situations by virtue of transfer of training. Unfortunately, one of the best-established facts about transfer is that very often it stubbornly fails to occur, especially when one is dealing with problems of improving education, training the mentally retarded, or remedying learning disabilities. The historic distinction between learning and transfer, rather than lack of motivation among investigators of learning to contribute to practical applications, may be the real villain in the often-lamented isolation of learning theory from education.

Learning theorists have generally not responded well to scolding from outsiders about this isolation, but remedies may be emerging from within the discipline itself. Learning theories are concerned with the acquisition of skills and knowledge, which, however, must be brought into play in appropriate situations in order to be useful to the person who has done the learning.

One of the fruits of the flourishing sister discipline of cognitive psychology is increasing attention to and understanding of the way information accruing from learning experiences is organized in memory and the kinds of control processes that are involved in its retrieval. Such concepts as those of *retrieval cues* (Tulving, 1968, 1972) and *retrieval plans* (Raaijmakers & Shiffrin, 1981; Wood, 1972) help lead us to understand that the retrievability of learned information from memory depends to a major extent on the character of the information and the way it is organized. In other words, the problem of transfer cannot effectively be separated from the problem of what is learned. No simple formulas can be given for conducting research on learning that will take advantage of these principles, but illustrations of approaches that can serve to some extent as models are to be found, for example, in recent work of Anderson (1976) and Anzai and Simon (1979).

It is likely also that full utilization of learning research and theory for the study of intelligence cannot be expected to come from part-time efforts of investigators in the learning area, but rather may require the development of a new specialty cutting across learning, cognitive development, and the study of intelligence. The developmental approach is needed because there is no reason to think that the relevant learning processes can adequately be studied over the very short time spans of typical laboratory experiments, or independently of the stage of development of cognitive abilities. Direct contributions from emerging theories of intellect are needed because the relevant research on learning must be directed toward the conditions and rates of acquisition of the specific products of learning that enter into the tasks believed to index intelligence. Just as we now understand that research on the learning of language should not proceed independently of an understanding of linguistic competence (Chomsky, 1965), we have come to see that the learning of cognitive skills cannot proceed effectively in the absence of adequate characterizations of the skills themselves and the way they are organized and employed. The traditional psychometric approach to intelligence has not been fruitful in this respect, but more is to be anticipated from current investigations directed toward unraveling the components of intellectual performance (e.g., R. Sternberg, 1977).

From intelligence to learning.   The other side of the learning–intelligence interaction is that learning theory and investigations of learning may profit from, as well as contribute to, the study of intelligence. Learning in the sense of the formation of concepts or the acquisition of knowledge cannot be presumed ever to proceed independently of intelligence. The testing operations that are an integral part of learning must depend on processes of perception and judgment that permit the discrimination and identification of relevant attributes of a stimulus input and their categorization relative to motives or task demands. Similarly important are the continual comparisons of new inputs with information already in memory that guide the continuing growth of the memory structure during learning. Hence learning and intellectual function must be studied as continuously interacting components of the individual's whole cognitive system.

Implementing this general principle is not easy, but some useful methods are beginning to appear. One example is the insertion of memory probes into experiments on choice learning in order to monitor changes in the learner's state of information relevant to choices (Allen & Estes, 1972). A second is the use of probe questions during the course of associative learning to check on hypotheses about the specific cognitive processes implicated in the formation of associations (W. K. Estes, 1981). A third is the use of "think-aloud" protocols to track the moment-to-moment use of learning strategies in the course of problem solving (Ericsson & Simon, 1980).

The reciprocity between learning and intelligence has implications also for problems of measurement of ability. Quite possibly, the low correlations often observed between performance in laboratory learning tasks and criteria of intelligence may arise because the laboratory situations are so restricted as to preclude the operation of cognitive processes that, at least in the case of the mature human being, would enter into analogous kinds of learning outside the laboratory. One implication of this conclusion is that tests of learning ability that are to be applied to some practical purpose should be constructed so as to allow full play to all of the processes that might be involved in the criterion situation – quite a different orientation from the historical judgment that the tests should be sufficiently simplified to reveal the operation of some one basic capacity alone. Another implication is that learning ability and intelligence are not distinct capacities or aspects of the intellectual system. Rather, learning processes and the judgmental aspects of intelligence must be assumed to interact continually in the course of mental development, so that tests aimed at either aspect at a given time must be taken to reflect the past influences of both.

4.3.   MEMORY AND INFORMATION PROCESSING

VARIETIES OF MEMORY

A conspicuous shift in the literature on memory over the past few decades has been from the general use of the term *memory* to the use of *memories*. Thus, in current reports of work on research or theory, it rarely suffices to speak simply of memory; rather, one sees references to short-term memory, long-term memory, primary memory, secondary memory, and working memory, among a large number of varieties. There is by no means universal agreement on the various definitions and distinctions, but at the same time it seems clear that some categorizations are needed to enable one to organize and interpret the rapidly growing literature.

Some categorizations that I have found useful on the whole and will employ in this chapter are summarized in Figure 4.1. If the whole rectangle is taken to encompass all varieties of memory that we might recognize, the vertical line down the middle partitions these first of all approximately in accord with Tulving's

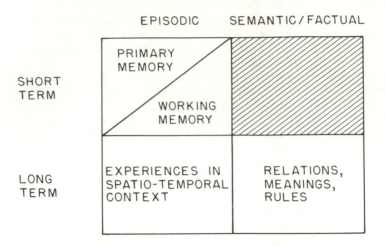

MEMORY   SYSTEMS

Figure 4.1.   Schema of some major categories of memory recognized in current theories. In some treatments the two long-term cells would be subsumed under the concept "secondary memory."

(1968) distinction between episodic and semantic memory. *Episodic memory* refers to memories of specific experiences, including information, not only about events that occurred, but about the time and the environmental context. Examples might range from one's recollection of the striking of a clock that is still echoing to memory of a childhood experience such as a christening or a birthday party and, in particular, would include memory of the events of an experimental trial in almost any laboratory experiment on memory. *Semantic memory,* in Tulving's classification, refers to information stored in memory concerning properties or relations that are independent of particular times or places – the definition of a word, the knowledge that the sky is generally blue and leaves in springtime are generally green, the distance from New York to Los Angeles, and so on. Much of this information is verbal in form, at least as recalled; hence the denotation *semantic*. The information need not be verbal, however, and thus the term *factual*, used by some investigators, is perhaps a better designation.

Considering now the horizontal lines through the middle of the rectangle in Figure 4.1, the intent is to partition memories orthogonally according to duration. One should not think of any hard-and-fast cutoff on the time dimension, but short-term memory refers to one's ability to maintain for a brief time a relatively rich representation of very recent events – a telephone number just obtained from directory service, a scene that has just been briefly portrayed on a TV screen, a fleeting expression on another person's face, a few words or a sentence just heard in the course of a conversation. Short-term memories are generally transient, being quickly degraded as a function of time unless maintained or refreshed by rehearsal or some other means. In contrast are long-term memories – for example, one's memory for salient experiences at a political meeting or a graduation ceremony, events described in newspapers or news broadcasts, material learned by

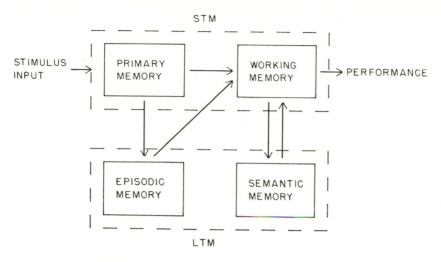

ACTIVATION PATHS

Figure 4.2. Assumed course of information flow through short- and long-term memory systems.

studying textbooks or attending lectures. These memories are referred to as long-term because normally they persist over extended periods of time unless interfered with in specific ways. Unlike short-term memories, which are necessarily episodic, long-term memories can be either for specific events in context (episodic) or for relations, rules, or principles (semantic or factual).

That picture is, however, a bit static. Some of the presumed interrelationships among the memory subsystems are illustrated in Figure 4.2. The flow of events is as follows. The stimulus input, for example, a passage of text read by the person in question or some words or a sentence heard, is processed and registered in the transient short-term memory system termed *primary memory*. Then several consequences may follow. Often, especially if this input is quickly followed by another equally complex one, the primary memory may simply be lost after a few seconds. On other occasions it may be "consolidated," that is, encoded in long-term episodic memory. At the same time, a comparison between attributes of the representation in primary memory and attribute information in long-term semantic/factual memory may reveal a match, in which case we would speak of the person's having recognized the stimulus input as belonging to a familiar category. In that event, and especially if the category is relevant to an ongoing task, some elements of the primary memory representation (usually numbers, letters, or words) may be maintained for a longer period in the short-term system by rehearsal.

SHORT-TERM MEMORY

Memory span. With that outline of the memory system in mind, we can proceed to the question of the relevance of specific memory subsystems to intelligence and intellectual behavior. Beginning with the short-term system, it can be said, first of all, that long before the various distinctions had been articulated in the psychological literature, immediate memory as represented in the familiar memory-span test was routinely included in scales of measurement of intelligence. It is curious, however, to note that this inclusion of memory-span tests in intelligence scales was initiated and continued in the absence of any substantial discussion of why immediate memory was thought relevant to intelligence. This omission is especially notable because the original tests of intelligence were intended to assess the ability of children to succeed in school, where virtually all instruction is presumably intended to deal with long-term memory for the materials learned. In fact, the originators of the intelligence-testing movement, Binet and Simon (1916), held that memory was an unimportant aspect or constituent of intelligence relative to "judgment," which they believed to be at the heart of intelligent behavior. Nonetheless, they included digit-span tests in their earliest scales, beginning with a mini-test for 3-year-old children that consisted simply of the examiner's asking the child to repeat two digits that had just been spoken by the examiner. In the Stanford revisions of the Binet scales (Terman, 1916; Terman & Merrill, 1937), tests of short-term memory were more extensively represented. Again, there was before the fact no substantial discussion of the reasons for this tactic, but the omission was rationalized in a sense by later demonstrations that the memory subscales correlated about as well with total score on the Stanford–Binet test and with the usual criteria as did other subtests (McNemar, 1942).

The memory-span test and related measures of short-term memory would surely not have been considered especially relevant to intellectual function by psychologists of any persuasion during the whole period from the first appearance of memory-span tests in intelligence scales to the paper by Miller (1956) that first related memory span to more complex aspects of cognitive performance. It is hardly an exaggeration to say that, throughout that half-century, human memory, as viewed by the public, by intelligence testers, and even by cognitive psychologists of the period, was regarded simply as a repository of information, with properties analogous to those of a storeroom in which items could be deposited and held until needed for some purpose. That statement might be qualified slightly with regard to long-term memory for complex material, as, for example, stories, in that a few investigators (in particular, Bartlett, 1932) noted that even though memory for experiences may begin as a passive receptacle of information, it does not generally remain so, but rather becomes complicated as a consequence of reconstructive and inferential processes. However, no such qualification seems needed in the case of the aspects of short-term memory captured by memory-span tests. The idea there was uniformly that memory span for just-apprehended items is a very limited-capacity receptacle and that the function of memory-span tests included in intelligence scales or other diagnostic testing is simply to determine what that capacity is for a given individual.

Within that frame of reference, assessments of memory span amounted simply to measurements of a static property of the subject; and it was difficult to understand why that property – the number of discrete items of information retainable for a short interval in immediate memory – should have any significant relation to intelligence or intellectual function. The continuing acceleration of research on short-term memory during the present decade, however, has led to some theoretical reorientation that puts the issue in quite different perspective. The possibility has emerged that tests of memory span may be significant, primarily for what they reveal concerning mental processes that enter into performance on the test. This reorientation was a consequence of growing concern with problems of encoding in memory (Melton & Martin, 1972) and with the depth or extent of processing of items of information entering the memory system.

Coding and levels of processing. Although reflecting also intellectual origins within the older traditions of conditioning and learning theory (see especially Lawrence, 1963), new interest in the way information becomes encoded in memory was a natural outgrowth of the information-processing movement and the computer metaphor. A typical course of events when information is being entered in a computer memory is for a message expressed in ordinary alphabetical characters to be typed in at the console of the computer, encoded by the receiving element (e.g., a teletype terminal) into a pattern of electrical signals transmittable over a cable, and then recoded in the central processor of the computer into a binary code that in turn determines the positive and negative orientations of tiny magnetic elements in the computer's core memory. The information can then be maintained indefinitely in the pattern of magnetic polarities. At some later time when the memory is "interrogated," this pattern determines the output of electrical signals that lead to the typing out of information, again in the form of letters of the alphabet, on a teletypewriter or the like.

Similarly, in the case of information entering human memory, it is conceived in information-processing theories that the letters or words seen or heard by an individual are converted by peripheral sensory systems into patterns of neural activity physically quite unlike the original stimulus patterns, and then in turn recoded in forms that can be maintained for relatively long periods in memory and, upon later interrogation, can lead to reconstruction of at least part of the originally received information. Almost nothing is known about the details of the neural encoding of stimulus information. However, it is the task of experimental psychology of memory to discover properties of the encoded information that are helpful in understanding such matters as the sources of capacity limitation on the rate of encoding or the characteristics of cognitive operations performed on the input material that lead to encodings of differing value for later retrieval of information.

In one theoretical paper that has been quite influential in shaping current research, Craik and Lockhart (1972) proposed that the amount or kind of intellectual effort put into the processing of stimulus information, and hence the form and depth of the processing, determines the type of memory code established and thereby the durability of the stored information and its availability for retrieval. Although reservations have been expressed about the concept of depth of processing as a satisfactory general framework for understanding short-term memory (Baddeley, 1978; Nelson, 1976), it has led to new and fruitful emphasis on the active role of the individual in determining how and in what form information becomes encoded in memory. Thus it is now realized that even so simple a task as the digit-span test may yield information, not only about the number of digits recallable, but about the depth and kind of information processing engaged in by the person being tested. To what extent individual differences in these respects reflect fixed capacities rather than strategies and habits produced by prior learning is unknown; however, the presumption that the answer is probably a mixture has led to new research efforts to analyze in detail the sources of individual differences in short-term memory performance (Belmont & Butterfield, 1971; Chi, 1976; Lyon, 1977).

One may well wonder how one can determine anything about the properties of encoding of information in memory in the absence of any way of getting directly at the patterns of neural firing, neuronal interconnections, or transmitter concentrations that are responsible. The answer is that the growth of theory significantly augments our ability to interpret such data as the patterns of errors people make when attempting to recall items, in ways that enable increasingly sharp tests of specific hypotheses about the nature of encoding of the items. In one of the earliest significant developments of this sort, Conrad (1964, 1965) reported that when people are presented visually with short sequences of letters to remember, the errors made in recall show that letters that sound alike are more likely to be confused with each other than letters that look alike, a finding which indicates that the information originally taken in by the eye has been converted to an encoded form having important auditory properties. It was tempting to leap to the conclusion that this recoding is done voluntarily by the person being tested because the auditorily encoded form is more resistant to forgetting than the visual. Further work has indicated, however, that the process is more automatic and more closely tied to sensory processing than might be suggested by that idea (W. K. Estes, 1973b; Peterson & Johnson, 1971). Nonetheless, the same studies show that, at least during the very early part of a retention interval, recall may be significantly augmented by the auditory coding. Continuing and progressively more analytic research along the same lines has shown that, even in very short-term memory, other properties and attributes, including temporal position (Lee & Estes, 1977), auditory stress patterns (Drewnowski & Murdock, 1980), and even some properties that would be termed categorical or semantic in nature (Craik & Levy, 1976; W. K. Estes, 1980), can be implicated to varying extents, depending on the conditions and nature of the individual's cognitive processing of the stimulus material.

Following even such a simple experience as seeing or hearing a single letter or single word, a person's short-term memory is evidently best described as including much information about the attributes or properties of the experience, rather than as being a repository for a single discrete item of information like the encoded representation of a letter in a computer's core memory (Drewnowski, 1980; W. K. Estes, 1980). Further, Drewnowski has shown another important way in which active intellectual processes can enter into even very simple tasks, with his conception of a priority ordering of attributes that is to an important extent under a person's voluntary control and that determines the order in which different attributes or properties of an experience are consulted by the person when he or she is attempting recognition or recall.

Working memory. Even more important with respect to the bearing of this work on intellectual function, the recognition that properties of encoding and the nature of cognitive processing may make some of the components of short-term memory much more readily available than others to enter into other cognitive activities such as problem solving has led to recognition of a dual function of short-term memory. It acts as a temporary retainer of just-perceived information that is being further processed into long-term memory, and at the same time as a mechanism for maintaining in an active state, perhaps by a rehearsal or recycling process, information drawn either from recent perception or from long-term memory that is actively involved in an ongoing task – hence the distinction shown in Figure 4.2 between the subsystems or aspects of short-term memory termed *primary memory* on the one hand and *working memory* on the other.

The conception of a working memory was a natural consequence of the reorientation of memory research in terms of information processing. Executive routines are basic to computer operating systems and thus to computer simulation models for intellectual function; and a working memory in some form is a basic constitutent of an executive routine, constituting the items of information and rules involved in a computation, solution of a problem, or the like.

In psychology, the term *working memory,* or *operational memory,* seems to have been first used in the modern sense by Posner and Rossman (1965), referring to a collection of items activated from long-term memory and kept in an active state during the solution of a problem. The concept seems to have appeared less as a consequence of new empirical evidence than as a logical requirement of an information-processing system. Posner (1967) remarks, "All human information processing requires keeping track of incoming stimuli and bringing such input into contact with already-stored material" (p. 267); however, he goes on to caution that "there is no reason to believe that the characteristics of the system involved in this process will be identical with those found in the usual short-term memory studies" (p. 268). Perhaps one difference is that short-term memory as implicated in a memory-span test may, but need not, involve rehearsal, whereas rehearsal appears to be an essential constituent of working memory (Baddeley, 1976).

The question whether primary memory and working memory are properly regarded as subsystems of a single limited-capacity short-term memory was explored systematically by Baddeley and Hitch (1974). These investigators looked for evidence on the question by having subjects engage in simple intellectual tasks during the retention interval of a short-term memory experiment and determining whether the characteristics of the task reduced the apparent capacity of short-term memory. Thus they looked for possible interference between the number of digits held in short-term memory (in preparation for a recall test) and performance on verbal reasoning, comprehension of text, or free recall. They found no interference when the number of digits being maintained was small enough, less than about four, but appreciable interference when the memory load was larger, with six or more digits being maintained simultaneously. Further, they found that phonological similarity of the items being held in short-term memory was a determiner of the amount of interference, as would be expected on the assumption of a common limited-capacity system. The observation that the maintenance of items in working memory apparently draws on information-processing capacity and is susceptible to phonetic similarity effects supported Baddeley's conception of working memory as a subsystem of short-term memory comprising an articulatory rehearsal loop.

Rehearsal and grouping strategies. The facts that older and more intelligent individuals both rehearse more and benefit more from rehearsal than younger and less intelligent ones may have to do in part with the way in which rehearsal is accomplished. There are good reasons to believe that rehearsal should not be equated simply with repetition. Thus the routinely observed increases in memory span with rehearsal must be primarily a consequence of the rehearsal of a number of members of a recently presented sequence together, leading to modification of the memory structure that, in turn, increases the subject's ability to recall the items together. It is not surprising, then, to find that one trend observed with age is a tendency for older children increasingly to rehearse items cumulatively (Chi, 1976).

One might expect also that the speed with which a person can encode recently heard or seen items in a rehearsable form would prove to be an important parameter in determining memory span. This expectation has been strongly confirmed. For example, Baddeley, Thomson, and Buchanan (1975) demonstrated a close relationship between memory span and reading rate for visually presented items; and the linear relation between number of items recalled and the time required to read them was eliminated when special measures were taken to suppress vocalization during the presentation of the items. Further, Nicolson (1980) has shown that in a situation where memory span was observed to increase substantially with age, the ratio of memory span to reading rate remained constant, a finding which suggests that the increases in span are attributable not to increases in memory capacity but to increases in the efficiency of encoding items into the rehearsal process.

Even given that a number of items are being rehearsed together, the process can differ in qualitative respects that may have important consequences. A number of recent investigators, for example, Craik and Watkins (1973) and Woodward, Bjork, and Jongeward (1973), have proposed a distinction between two major varieties of rehearsal. The first variety, primary, or maintenance, rehearsal, constitutes simple repetition of the recently presented items in sequence. Secondary, or elaborative, rehearsal involves not simply repetition but active grouping of the rehearsed items into relatively optimal clusters and attending to and encoding properties of the sequence such as repetitions of items, "trills," and the like (Restle & Brown, 1970).

The way in which rehearsal is assumed to contribute to retention is necessarily bound up with theories of what produces loss of information from memory. According to a decay theory, held by a number of the investigators who were prominent in initiating modern work on short-term memory, items recently registered in memory decay spontaneously as a function of time, the trace containing progressively less information until, after a few seconds, it can contribute nothing toward either recognition or recall (Broadbent, 1958; Brown, 1958). Associated with this conception of retention loss is the assumption that rehearsal simply refreshes the memory trace, in effect resetting the decay process so that it starts over again after each rehearsal of an item. To this conception, Atkinson and Shiffrin (1968) added the idea that, during rehearsal, items are more or less automatically transferred from transitory short-term to long-term memory.

The idea that rehearsal has the two consequences of refreshing memory traces and mediating the transition of items into long-term memory stores is an appealing one, but it has run into some complications. On the one hand, the idea of spontaneous decay as the mechanism of retention loss is based on a unitary strength model of the memory trace that has failed to find confirmation from studies of effects of repetition in short-term memory (Wells, 1974). But if the traces of recently perceived items do not decay, why should they need refreshing? Perhaps a better view is that the generation of the name of an item in the course of rehearsal produces a new memory trace having other properties than the original and being less likely to suffer interference from inputs of new items.

With regard to the matter of automatic transition from short- to long-term memory as a consequence of rehearsal, rather ingenious techniques employed by Craik and Watkins (1973) and Woodward and associates (1973) indicate that primary rehearsal has virtually no effect on long-term recallability of items, though it may produce measurable increases in later recognition. Elaborative rehearsal, on the other hand, certainly does further the transition from short- to long-term memory. One of the most elementary aspects of elaborative rehearsal is the breaking up of a continuously presented input sequence into groups for rehearsal. It has frequently been found that groups of about three items are relatively optimal for rehearsal (W. K. Estes, 1972a; Wickelgren, 1964). Thus, if seven digits were presented in a digit-span test with a sequence such as 6, 1, 7, 4, 9, 5, 3, a person might attempt to rehearse the sequence of seven all together, or might group the items as 6, 1, 7; 4, 9; 5, 3, and the latter would almost certainly prove the more effective procedure.

Differences in memory span among normal adults are evidently not largely attributable to differences in grouping strategies (Lyon, 1977), but variations in memory span with age and differences between retarded individuals and normals certainly are related to variations in the use of grouping. Spitz (1966), for example, has shown that memory-span performance of retarded individuals can be substantially increased by experimentally inducing grouping. And Ericsson, Chase, and Faloon (1980) have shown that an evidently normal person was able to increase his memory span far beyond ordinary bounds by systematic application of grouping and other elaborative strategies.

Just why grouping proves so advantageous has not yet been fully explained. One suggestion, not easily tested in a rigorous way, is that there are irreducible capacity limitations on the number of articulatory units that can be maintained in a single rehearsal loop (Baddeley, 1976). Another idea is that the constituent members of a rehearsal group become associated with common retrieval cues (perhaps representations of aspects of the context in which rehearsal occurs), with the consequence that, at the time of later recall, reinstatement of even a single member of such a group may lead to recall of the entire group as a unit (W. K. Estes, 1974; Jones, 1976). This assumption that members of a rehearsal group enter into a hierarchical associative structure with certain unitary properties is rather closely related to the conception of coding of clusters of items that has been elaborated by Johnson (1972), and to the well-known concept of "chunking" originated by Miller (1956). The present situation, then, is that grouping strategies are undeniably effective, that a number of suggestions about the mechanisms involved have some support, but that no wholly satisfactory theory is yet available.

MEMORY IN INFORMATION PROCESSING

The notion of an active working memory as an integral component of an information-processing system has been taken up in the most recently developed models for a number of aspects of intellectual function; and application of the models has in turn yielded new empirical findings documenting this newer conception of short-term memory as a constellation of structures and processes, rather than a

passive repository. For example, Gilmartin, Newell, and Simon (1976) implemented the conception of a short-term memory under strategy control in their
computer simulation model for performance in a variety of short-term recall tasks.
Their model combines, in a way, older and newer conceptions of short-term memory. They conceived the system as comprising a linear array of eight cells, each
capable of holding a symbol, such as a letter, or a chunk (that is, a small group of
symbols encoded as a single character). The rest of short-term memory capacity
was conceived as being taken up with control information, that is, indicators or
pointers to strategies employed, such as searching long-term memory for items
resembling or related to those currently in short-term memory, rehearsing items
or groups of items in working memory, and outputting items or groups of items
when called for.

   Gilmartin and his associates applied their model only to a simple forward-recall
task, but the kind of short-term memory system conceived in the model has been
brought into closer relation with theoretical treatments of more complex tasks in a
series of studies by Simon and his collaborators. In one of these, Simon (1976)
undertook the task of identifying the basic abilities underlying intellectual performance in a task such as extrapolating sequential patterns (e.g., inducing the
rule for extending arithmetic or geometric series). Such a task, in Simon's analysis, requires the ability to perceive relations ("same," "next," "complement") and
a working short-term memory capable of storing ordered sequences of up to four
or five characters and of being scanned for relationships among the items. With
regard to other forms of problem solving that have been treated in terms of Newell
and Simon's general problem solver (Newell & Simon, 1972), Simon (1978) emphasizes the serial character of problem solving as conceived in the model and the
degree to which performance of such a problem solver, human as well as computer simulation, is limited by the capacity of short-term memory. (The time required
to transfer items in and out of short-term working memory is estimated to be
about 200 msec per item, and the time required to transfer and store a chunk of
information in long-term memory is estimated to be on the order of 5–10 sec.)
Simon proposes that these capacity limitations on a short-term system account for
the fact that human problem solvers typically do not backtrack from the current
node (knowledge state) in the sequence of cognitive operations involved in attempting to solve a problem.

   Other than formal problem solving, perhaps the comprehension of language
would be the form of cognitive activity most widely taken to tax information-
processing capabilities fully. During the past few years, research literature on
experimental studies and related models of comprehension of text has begun to
accumulate (see, e.g., Kintsch, 1978). Here again, as formal models begin to
appear, an active short-term working memory appears as an essential ingredient.
For example, in a model under development by Kintsch and his associates
(Kintsch & Van Dijk, 1978; Kintsch & Vipond, 1979), the "meaning elements" of
a text that an individual is reading are conceived as being organized into a coherent "semantic text base" characterized by propositions and their arguments.
In the first stage of comprehension during reading of a text, the incoming information is conceived as being converted into a list (or sequence) of propositions
representing the meaning of the text, coherence being achieved by overlap of the
arguments of successive propositions, that is, commonality in the subjects or
objects of the sentences expressing the propositions, or the like. The rate of

processing is, then, limited by the capacity of the reader's short-term working memory to retain in an active state the representations of several propositions at a time, so that the necessary comparisons can be made. When, in the course of reading, a number of propositions have been entered into the memory system, a small sample are assumed to be selected and entered in a short-term working memory where they are maintained in an active state, and only these are available to be connected with those appearing in the next input.

These treatments indicate the functional properties the short-term working memory system must have in order to account for the empirically observed properties of human problem solving and comprehension within the models currently being developed to interpret these major types of intellectual performance. And now a word is in order concerning the relationship between the short-term memory system as it appears in models for complex intellectual performance and this system as it appears in the models and experimental approaches involved in specific lines of laboratory investigation. One must expect, first of all, that the system as manifested in simplified laboratory tasks will appear much less rich in structure and process than the system as represented in models of comprehension and problem solving. Indeed, one of the reasons for heavy reliance on simplified laboratory tasks is that the whole system, in interaction with the other information-processing structures and operations involved in problem solving or comprehension, is too complex to be comprehended adequately by any one manageably simple model or to be investigated by any one experimental approach.

It is to be expected that, in any one line of laboratory investigation, many properties of the system will be held constant or relegated to the background so far as possible while some one aspect is intensively investigated. Thus the model of Atkinson and Shiffrin (1968), which provided the basis for the representations of short-term memory in the work of Kintsch and Simon just discussed, first implemented a clear theoretical distinction between long- and short-term memory stores, with a subset of the latter being maintained in an active state by rehearsal and with reciprocal transfer of items between the two stores. Research carried out within the framework of their model was directed primarily toward the accumulation of evidence for these basic properties and toward working out the distinction between the structural aspects of the system responsible for its capacity limitations and the "control processes," that is, the aspects under the active control of the individual. These studies achieved their purposes to an impressive degree, but necessarily left open details of how the rehearsal mechanism operates and how an individual searches short-term memory for items needed in a particular task. The former of these aspects was the subject of detailed investigation by Atkinson and Shiffrin (1971) and Craik and Watkins (1973), among others, and the search process was the focus of a major and chronologically parallel line of investigation instigated originally by S. Sternberg (1966), and carried forward by S. Sternberg (1975), Theios (1973), and Wescourt and Atkinson (1976), among others.

The early studies in this series exploited a simple recognition experiment in which a person is presented first with a "memory set" of a few visually or auditorily presented letters and then with a probe letter, the task being to judge whether the probe letter was in the memory set. This work yielded evidence for a very simple form of memory search in which the representation of the probe is compared serially with the representations of each of the items of the memory set at a constant rate, the search either continuing until all items have been examined (exhaustive search) or terminating when a match is found between the probe and an element of the memory set (self-terminating search). A flurry of attempts to determine experimentally once and for all whether the search, or scanning, process is exhaustive or self-terminating proved almost fruitless, and later work (e.g., Schneider & Shiffrin, 1977) has indicated quite clearly that many details of the way scanning is done fall in the category of control processes that can be modified to an important extent by instructions or by the subject's previous learning.

Implications for measurement. Some of the implications of this rapidly growing body of research and theory on short-term memory for the problems of measuring memory capacity and relating it to criteria of intelligence should be almost obvious. It can hardly be too strongly emphasized that, just as the short-term memory system is proving much too complex to be comprehended in any single type of experiment, its functional properties are too numerous and enter into different tasks in too many different combinations to make it reasonable to hope to obtain any meaningful measure of the capacity of the system from a single score such as that resulting from a digit-span test. The fact that these scores correlate significantly with total intelligence-test scores or with criteria of intelligence must evidently be taken to signify that performance even in the apparently simplest test situations reflects a number of interacting processes.

Recognition of this likelihood has several important implications. On the one hand, it may ultimately increase the diagnostic value of these tests by permitting the interpretation of test performance in more theoretically meaningful terms (W. K. Estes, 1974). At the same time, one is forced to recognize that the whole idea of concentrating on the improvement of aspects of measurement by "purifying" subtests of elementary capacities may be on the wrong track. The more promising approach may be to attempt to devise tests of specific functions, such as the operation of short-term working memory, by assessing the performance of the relevant subsystem in the context of more complex tasks (W. K. Estes, 1981).

INDIVIDUAL DIFFERENCES AND DEVELOPMENTAL TRENDS IN
SHORT-TERM MEMORY

Because performance on short-term memory tasks is commonly used as a constituent of various diagnostic tests, one may anticipate that people do differ substantially in such performance, that the differences tend to be consistent over time and to generalize to some extent across tasks, and that performance will be found to vary systematically with age and to differ on the average between groups of people judged to be grossly different in intellectual capabilities (i.e., between mental defectives and normals). Early research addressed to the testing of these expectations yielded a number of results that are instructive even if not always as precise as desirable.

An early study that stands out by virtue of the quantity of data collected and the extensiveness of the analyses performed is an investigation of growth of memory in schoolchildren by Bolton (1891–1892). Digit-span tests were given to samples of children ranging from third grade to high school. A systematic increase in digit span with age was observed, but with the function becoming apparently asymptotic, beyond the sixth grade, at a memory span of approximately six digits. A three-by-three table relating level of digit-span performance to teachers' ratings of general standing in school showed a positive but apparently rather low correlation. Considering the confounding of school grade with other measures of intelligence and the lack of sensitivity of the crude correlational analysis, these findings provide scant basis for the rather strong conclusion that memory span increases with age rather than intelligence, a conclusion echoed in later reviews of this literature, for example, Spearman (1904). However, Spearman went on to comment that the issue was not definitely closed, in view of the inadequacy of the experimental and statistical methods used up to that time, and noted that Binet obtained a more positive relationship between digit span and other indicators of intelligence (a finding that perhaps accounts for the inclusion of digit span in the Binet–Simon scale).

A much later review, by Batchelder and Denny (1977), found the digit-span test still under investigation for the same problems, though with more sophisticated statistical methods. Correlations between span and total score on the remaining subscales of the Wechsler Adult Intelligence Test were found to run in the neighborhood of .75 and were coupled with significant group differences for college students versus unselected adults and for retardates versus normals. Batchelder and Denny proposed "span ability" as an index of the structural, or innate, basis of intelligence.

Much of the work currently being reported on relations between short-term memory and intelligence falls very directly in the traditions set by the earliest studies, though with some increasing variation in the tasks examined, and in some respects with more refined analyses of the data. Whereas research on the relation of short-term memory to intelligence was almost wholly empirically based for the first 60 years or so, in recent years new lines of investigation have been motivated increasingly by theoretical developments. A notable example was the Atkinson and Shiffrin (1968) model, which both provided a conceptual framework within which structures and processes presumed to be implicated in digit span and related tasks could be represented and also suggested new experimental paradigms for their analyses.

In one of these associated experimental developments, Atkinson and his associates (Phillips, Shiffrin, & Atkinson, 1967) introduced a modification of the memory-span task that provided for evaluating memory by means of recognition rather than recall. Presumably recognition should provide a more sensitive measure of the state of memory, because recall is subject to various kinds of production deficiencies and other complications at the level of performance. In the recognition paradigm, as modified by Ellis (1970) for use with children and mental retardates, the subject viewed the front of a console on which was arranged a row of nine circular windows. A set of projectors behind the console could display numerals in any of the windows individually in any desired order and for any prescribed exposure duration. In the basic experiments, a random sequence of digits was selected for a trial, and the digits were exposed one after another in the row of windows from left to right, with a constant exposure time for each digit and a constant interval between exposures of successive digits. A retention interval followed the termination of the display in the last window, and then a test digit appeared in a single window that was centered at the top of the panel, the subject's task being to indicate in which window of the row of nine the test digit had appeared.

Studies by Phillips and his associates (1967) and by Ellis and Hope (1968) provided support for the idea that a person's ability to indicate the position in which the test or probe digit had appeared may be taken to reflect short-term memory independently of the production processes involved in recall, and opened new possibilities for empirically distinguishing the contributions of structural and control processes. In work pursuing this idea, Ellis (1970) compared the performances of normal and retarded individuals at different rates of stimulus presentation. Large average differences between normal and retarded subjects were observed, but the pattern proved of more interest than the overall difference. When the data were plotted in the form of serial-position curves, that is, functions indicating the proportion of correct responses at each of the nine positions in the display, large differences were observed between normals and retardates at the early positions, but no difference appeared at the last position. This result has been taken to indicate that very short-term sensory memory is essentially independent of other aspects of intelligence. The differences observed at the earlier positions, together with the fact that the performance of the normal subjects was more strongly influenced by presentation rate than was that of the defective subjects, were taken by Ellis to support the idea that memory capacity, at least for very short-term retention, may differ little between normal and retarded individuals. The retardates are characterized by a deficiency in the rehearsal strategies that are required to permit transformation of information from very short-term sensory memory to forms capable of maintaining longer-term recall or recognition. The relevance of the temporal spacing of the items during presentation of the to-be-remembered set is that wider temporal spacing allows greater opportunity for rehearsal during the presentation of the sequence.

Considerable evidence indicates that the tendency to utilize this opportunity for rehearsal increases with age and is much greater for normal than for retarded persons of a given age. The advantageous effects of rehearsal are exhibited mainly at the earlier positions in the serial-position curve for two reasons; one is that items presented at the last positions are still represented in short-term sensory memory and can usually be recalled without having been rehearsed, and the other is that the earliest items in the sequence have the greatest number of opportunities to be rehearsed during the course of the input. Studies by Rundus and Atkinson (1970) and by Hogan (1975) show clearly that efficiency of recall of items is directly related to the amount of rehearsal they have had.

Though several lines of converging evidence (reviewed by Chi, 1976) indicate that the effective use of rehearsal is strongly and directly related to both age and intelligence, a fully satisfactory explanation of these trends is not yet available. Presumably individuals learn to rehearse because the advantageous results of rehearsing in various tasks prove rewarding. Thus the failure to use rehearsal, which is termed *production deficiency* in the classification of Flavell (1970), and is characteristic of children before the age of about 5 years, may be closely tied up with the children's not having developed necessary skills in performing rehearsal.

The learning process needed to overcome the production deficiency and lead to normal adult performance must include at least two principal components – learning when to rehearse and learning how to rehearse. To the extent that a deficiency is localized in the former component, one might expect that inducing rehearsal would lead to immediate increases in efficiency of recall. This implication has been borne out in a number of studies. For example, Keeney, Cannizzo, and Flavell (1967) showed that with 6- and 7-year-old children, inducing rehears-al among those whose recall was deficient because they did not rehearse raised performance to a level similar to that of children of the same age who initially did rehearse. However, from a practical standpoint, efforts of this sort have often proven disappointing, because when young children or mentally deficient indi-viduals have been induced to rehearse, they do not automatically continue doing so even in the same task unless prompted further by the experimenter (Hagen, Hargrave, & Ross, 1973); and they do not automatically transfer an acquired rehearsal tendency from one task situation to another.

The hypothesis suggests itself that rehearsal is generally initiated by a self-instruction, this instruction being an item of information, probably verbal in form, that is stored in memory and becomes effective only if retrieved at the point in performance of a task when rehearsal is needed. When rehearsal is initiated by a suggestion from an experimenter or instructor, this suggestion or instruction may become associated with the context in which it occurs in the memory system of the person being instructed. However, with any change in the situation, or even the passage of time in the given situation, the context must be expected to change and no longer to provide an effective retrieval cue for the instruction to rehearse. Thus it must be expected that effective training to overcome a production defi-ciency must include measures calculated to associate the instruction to rehearse with elements or attributes of the various tasks or situations in which rehearsal is likely to be called for.

Research on individual differences in memory abilities has been importantly influenced during the past decade, and will undoubtedly be even more strongly influenced in the future, by the important distinction introduced by Atkinson and Shiffrin (1968) between structural and control processes in memory. The former category refers to aspects of memory that are independent of experience and that impose limits on the capacity and efficiency of operation of the system. Presum-ably individual differences in the structural aspects would be set by individual anatomical and physiological characteristics, innately determined to some major extent. Control processes refer to aspects of the system that do result from train-ing and individual experience and are presumably under voluntary control – for example, the use of mnemonics, strategies of memory search and recall, and rehearsal.

Because both structural and control processes must be implicated in every test used to assess memory or memory abilities, it follows that all of the results on individual differences, at least up to about 1970, must have utilized measures of abilities in which structural and control processes were confounded. Conse-quently, no conclusions can reasonably be drawn from that body of work regard-ing individual differences in aspects of memory that should be relatively per-sistent over time and independent of particular experiences – presumably the objective of nearly all work on measurement of cognitive abilities that might underlie intelligence.

A major task for continuing research, then, is to find effective ways of separat-ing the roles of structural and control processes and to devise ways of determining their separate contributions to cognitive performance. A first step is simply to seek to identify ways in which control processes might be expected to enter into al-ready familiar tests or tasks. This tactic was followed, for example, by Belmont and Butterfield (1971) in the case of short-term memory tasks that had been used to analyze differences between normal and retarded individuals. Showing that control processes contribute importantly to performance on such tasks is a necessary step, and progress in that direction has been quite rapid. It does not follow from such demonstrations, however, that individual differences in performance on the tasks are due wholly to differences in control processes.

Several approaches are available for the attempt to move further toward separating the contributions of the two kinds of processes. One is simply to try to eliminate one component, and in the present context this necessarily means attempting to eliminate the role of control processes and then ascertain whether the individual differences of interest are eliminated. Following this tactic, Lyon (1977), for example, showed that individual differences among normal adults in short-term memory span were not eliminated in spite of efforts to induce all of the subjects to utilize the same rehearsal and grouping strategies. Essentially the same approach was used and the same result obtained by Huttenlocher and Burke (1976) with respect to variation in memory span as a function of age of children. This approach has the weakness, of course, that one cannot know whether all of the control processes relevant to a task have been identified and eliminated.

An alternative strategy with some advantages is to consider, instead, patterns of correlations of different tasks with the same criterion. Then it may be possible to relate the patterns to the presumed contributions of known types of structural and control processes to the tasks. Here Hunt (1978) has reported some quite striking results. His criterion was score on a verbal intelligence scale for college-age subjects. When groups with high and low verbal ability scores (dubbed "high and low verbals") were compared for short-term retention as determined by the Brown–Peterson task, significant differences were found in measures of retention of both item and order information. However, in each case the retention curves were parallel for the high and low groups, a finding which suggests that they reflected differences in efficiency of encoding the items in memory rather than differences in maintenance of the information during the retention interval (which might be presumed to be the aspect more subject to differences in control processes).

In a related set of comparisons, Hunt analyzed differences between high and low verbals on a task bearing more directly on encoding or decoding efficiency. The measure was obtained from the letter-matching task utilized by Posner and his colleagues in the accumulation of evidence for distinct levels of encoding of visually perceived letters (see, e.g., Posner, 1978). When two letters presented simultaneously are identical in form (e.g., *A,A* or *a,a*) and the subject's task is to indicate quickly whether they are the same or different letters, the judgment is presumably based on the comparison of the two visual patterns and is referred to as *physical match*. If, however, the two letters differ in case (e.g., *A,a* or *B,b*), the judgment that the members of a pair denote the same letter must depend on encoding of the visual information to a higher level, presumably in the form of the names of the letters – hence the designation *name match*. Hunt assumed that the speed of physical matches may be taken to reflect only structural processes having to do with the encoding and comparison of visual patterns, whereas the speed of name matches reflects the efficiency of encoding the information to a level that makes contact with representations of letters in long-term memory. Consequently, the difference in speed between name and physical matches for an individual could be taken to be a useful measure of speed of verbal encoding and access to long-term memory.

Bringing together a number of relevant studies in the literature, Hunt showed a very strong relationship between this name–physical measure and presumed level of verbal ability in different subject groups, as, for example, in high or low verbal university students, 10-year-old children, elderly adults, and mentally retarded persons. In still another set of comparisons, Hunt considered efficiency of retrieval from short-term memory as indexed by the slope of the set-size function in the Sternberg memory-scanning task and again found a strong relationship between this measure and groups known or presumed to differ widely in verbal ability (though he found no significant correlation within the normal range). These results would seem to provide considerable support for the view that measures of short-term memory are related to criteria of intelligence, not because the number of items retainable in a short-term store is an important aspect of intelligence, but rather because the tasks used are sensitive to individual differences in speed and efficiency of elementary cognitive processes and operations that enter into the accomplishment of complex as well as simple intellectual tasks.

The remaining important method that has been put forward for separating control from structural processes is investigation of the effects of extensive training that might be expected to produce major changes in control processes while leaving structural processes unaffected. Many of the early studies following this approach have yielded negative results, but these should be accepted with caution, because the assumption that control processes depend on experience does not imply that they are necessarily extremely labile and sensitive to the small variations in amount of training that are usually involved in single experiments. Recent work of LaBerge (1975) and Shiffrin and Schneider (1977) utilizing considerably more extensive amounts of training has shown that significant shifts can be produced in patterns of data that would be taken to reflect different contributions of structural and control processes. Thus it seems likely that, for significant results bearing on individual differences to be obtained via this strategy, substantially larger amounts of training will need to be used than have been characteristic of most published studies.

Overall, several tentative conclusions seem justified by the presently available body of research on individual differences in short-term memory. One is that individual differences in control processes are undeniably important in simple as well as complex tasks and that efforts to modify these by training procedures often yield significant results. The satisfaction with these successes must be restrained, however, until more progress has been made on the critical problem of making the results of such training persist over appreciable periods of time, and generalize from one task to another. Finally, there is substantial evidence that individual differences on measures of memory and correlations of these with criteria of intelligence are significantly related to individual differences in measures of rather elementary cognitive processes that are not known to be susceptible to training or sensitive to individual differences in specific learning histories.

It follows that scores on the tests of memory that are included in intelligence scales or used in connection with neurological testing, inextricably confounding the contributions of control and structural processes, can be of little diagnostic value, and that refinement of the tests by purely psychometric methods is unlikely to improve matters greatly. Progress apparently can be achieved, however, by research carried out within the framework of information-processing models that relate both structural and control processes to intellectual function.

Relation to cognitive competence. "The amount of knowledge one possesses is a good guide to general cognitive competence" (Hunt, 1978, p. 110). This view is borne out by the wide use of tests of general information in intelligence scales, but it is not yet reflected in any substantial amount of research bearing on the role of long-term memory in intellectual function or its relation to psychometric intelligence. The reason is perhaps simply matter of temporal lag. The major burst of research and theoretical activity concerned with short-term memory that followed the appearance of Broadbent's (1958) book and continued through the 1960s has already led to an appreciable literature on the relationship of short-term memory to various aspects of intelligence (reviewed in an earlier section of this chapter). Important new models and methods for exploring the organization of human long-term memory and the nature of retrieval of information from it began to appear less than 10 years ago (an important date being the appearance of Collins and Quillian's 1972 network model). This research area is currently highly active, but attempts to relate the work to intelligence have as yet scarcely begun to appear. It seems highly likely, however, that the lack will be made up during the coming decade.

It was noted in an earlier section that the process of learning to acquire knowledge has just begun to be subject to analysis. Further, the relevant abilities, like those implicated in other forms of slow learning, are not effectively measured by any existing methods. Tests of general information can provide useful assessments of a person's current state of knowledge and thus provide useful predictions concerning intellectual performance. However, the relative ability of different people to acquire knowledge is not tapped by such tests unless the people can be assumed to have had equal opportunities to learn prior to the administration of the tests, a criterion that can rarely if ever be realized (W. K. Estes, 1970).

The aspect of knowledge receiving most attention in contemporary cognitive psychology is neither the process of acquisition nor the relevant capacities, but rather the way information is organized in and retrieved from long-term memory (for major reviews, see Anderson, 1976; Collins & Loftus, 1975; Smith, 1978).

From association to clustering. From its inception in the work of Ebbinghaus (1885/1913) until about 1950, a great part of research on human verbal learning and memory was carried out either with paired associates or with serial lists. The first paradigm is essentially a simulation of learning to associate people's names and faces; the second is an analog of learning the successive landmarks on a route.

It once seemed that learning in these situations could adequately be conceptualized in terms of simple associations or connections between items (Ebbinghaus, 1885/1913; Thorndike, 1913). During an experience with a paired-associate item, for example, the stimulus member of a pair would become associated with a response member, the result being that on later occasions presentation of the stimulus member alone would evoke memory of the response member.

Similarly, each of the successive items in a serial list was conceived as being associated with or connected to the next. For serial learning, at least, this simple scheme proved less than adequate upon further analysis (e.g., McGeoch & Irion, 1952).

The deficiencies were magnified when free recall began to take over as the favored paradigm in about 1950. The free-recall experiment simulates a very common aspect of intellectual tasks, that of remembering lists of items without regard for order – for example, the moves allowed for a chess piece or the names of the instructions available for the writing of a computer program. In the simplest form of the free-recall experiment, the experimenter presents a subject with an unordered list of words, for example, *dog, car, red, blue, cat, house, barn, deer,* and so on, and then tests the subject for his or her ability to recall the items (regardless of order).

In the most direct extension of the earlier association theories to the situation, one might suppose that, during the presentation of the list, the representation of each word in memory would become associated with the one that followed it, and that on a subsequent test recall of the first word would lead in succession to recall of the remainder of the items of the list in order. However, some of the most conspicuous results of free-recall experiments show this conception to be entirely inadequate. One of these results is that presenting the words of the list in a different random order on each trial of such an experiment does not render cumulative learning of the list inordinately difficult, as it ought to do according to the interitem conception. Further, it is characteristic for subjects, following the first presentation of a list, to recall the items in an order closely related to the input order, but on successive further presentations to move to a mode of recall that does not reflect the input order of any trial at all, but rather tends to group together items having semantic or categorical relationships (as *dog, cat, deer* in the example just given).

Hierarchical organization. It appears that the items of a list do not simply become associated with each other, if indeed they do so at all, but rather must become associated with one or more common elements or focuses, each of which has the capability of evoking recall of a cluster of items or even all of the items of the list. These common focuses have been termed *nodes* (Anderson & Bower, 1973) or *control elements* (W. K. Estes, 1972a, 1976) of an associative network in neo-association models; they correspond on the psychological side to the concept of retrieval cue that has become influential as a consequence of the work of Tulving (1968).

A very special case of the concept of retrieval cue would be the stimulus member of a paired-associate item. More generally, the idea is that in any learning situation, and in particular, those studied with respect to free recall, some cue in the situation, which might be one of the words of a free-recall list, a category label for a cluster of words in such a list, or some element or aspect of the context in which the list was presented, serves the function in a test situation of evoking recall of all of the words associated with it. According to the revised association model, if a learner simply listened passively to a list of words, we might expect the resulting associative structure to take a form like that shown in Figure 4.3*A*. Representations of the various words and the context in which they occurred would be associated with a common node or control element, and on a later test,

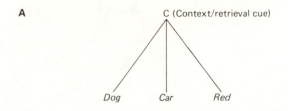

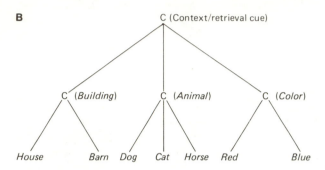

Figure 4.3.   Associative structures: *A*, multiple associations of words of a free-recall list to a common control element; *B*, expansion of the multiple-association structure into a hierarchical organization.

reinstatement of some portion of the context might activate the control element and lead to recall of the words.

There are several reasons why this simple associative structure would not lead to efficient recall. Firstly, there are sharp limits on the number of items that can simultaneously be maintained in a high state of availability. Evidence reviewed by Mandler (1967) suggests that the limit is about five unconnected words (that is, words that do not form a meaningful unit). Secondly, as each of the words is recalled, it may tend to arouse its own associates, which are not, in general, members of the list; for example, recalling the word *dog* might activate memory of the name of the learner's own household pet, and this in turn perhaps the names of members of the family, and thus lead the learner outside the set of items to be recalled. The substantial body of research on free recall shows that educated adults in our society achieve high levels of performance by organizing retrieval cues and list items into more efficiently associative structures than that shown in Figure 4.3*A* (Mandler, 1967; Tulving, 1968).

For example, when hearing the illustrative list given as an example here, the learner might note that several of the items belonged to the category *animal* and several to the category *color,* and might proceed to rehearse these category names along with the items themselves. The resulting associative structure might take the form shown in Figure 4.3*B,* in which the context and the category names are associated with a common node or control element, but with each of the category names serving as a lower-level control element for the appropriate individual items. At the time of a test for recall, reinstatement of the context would first activate representations of the category names in memory, and these in turn would activate memory of the constituent items. Now the limitation on capacity is circumvented, in that any individual control element need have only a small number of associates maintained in a high state of availability. Models of this type characterize the current approaches of Anderson and Bower (1973) and Collins and Loftus (1975).

The idea that this type of schema might also characterize the organization of an individual's long-term semantic memory may seem somewhat speculative, but it has been brought down to earth by an experimental approach originating with Quillian (1968), which utilizes reaction times to explore relationships within collections of words or concepts that are related in semantic memory by subordinate and superordinate category labels.

An important type of intellectual performance that should be expected to depend heavily on the organization of long-term memory is comprehension of verbal material. During the past decade there has been substantial progress toward the experimental analysis of simpler forms of comprehension, in particular, sentence comprehension. In what has come to be a standard experimental task, either pictorial or verbal material is presented for study and then the subject is tested for comprehension by means of the presentation of sentences concerning the material, to which a response such as "true" or "false" is to be made as quickly as possible. Reaction times for these responses are the principal data used to test hypotheses about memory organization.

In a simple but useful procedure used by Freedman and Loftus (1971), the subject is presented on each trial with a noun followed by a letter, and his or her task is to give as quickly as possible a word beginning with the given letter that belongs to the category indicated by the noun. An example would be *animal, h,* to which a frequent response would be "horse." According to the basic associative model presented in Figure 4.3, presentation of the category name, *animal* in the example, reinstates a portion of the context in which the associated word has occurred in the past. The effect is to bring the representations of items in memory associated with the same control element into a state of increased availability, so that subsequent presentations of one of the associated cues, in this case the letter *h,* could lead to retrieval of an associated word in the cluster with short latency.

Detailed understanding of the relationships involved has been advanced appreciably by a painstaking study performed by Loftus and Suppes (1972), who examined the effects of a number of variables such as frequencies of occurrence of the category name in English, length of the category name, size of the category, and frequency in English of words within a category.

Individual differences in semantic memory. Just as with short-term memory, it seems that the understanding of the nature and organization of long-term memory, especially in relation to individual differences, may be furthered by a separate consideration of structural and control processes. This distinction has not yet been implemented substantially in relation to long-term memory, but there are indications that attempts in this direction may prove fruitful.

Research on semantic memory has led to several formal models of considerable descriptive power (Carpenter & Just, 1975; Chase & Clark, 1972; Smith, Shoben, & Rips, 1974); and Hunt and his associates have undertaken the task of attempting to relate these models and the parameters represented in them to individual differences in verbal ability (Hunt, 1978). One important result of Hunt's work is the finding that, within a group of college-student subjects, the performance of some proved to be well described by one and the performance of others by another of the alternative models, and these subgroups yielded quite different patterns of correlations between their average sentence verification times and scores on verbal ability tests. It appears that these models may primarily represent organizations of control processes characteristic of particular individuals or groups, and that the possibility of effective measurement of structural aspects of human long-term memory awaits new approaches.

Measuring abilities and their interrelationships is a useful enterprise in itself, but it is desirable to go beyond measurement and attempt to diagnose, perhaps even remedy, the source of poor performance by persons with learning disabilities or disadvantaged cultural backgrounds. A good example of the potentialities in this latter approach has been reported by Cole, Gay, Glick, and Sharp (1971). These authors were studying cognitive functioning in the members of the Kpelle tribal group in Liberia. Upon testing people from this culture, either nonliterate or schooled subjects, with 20-item lists of either rather easily classifiable or not easily classifiable words, they found small differences among groups differing in age or education, with generally very poor performance – less than 50% recall, little improvement over successive trials, and no evidence of the use of category names as retrieval cues. It would have been easy simply to write off this performance, which is far below that observed for persons of comparable age in the United States, as evidence of inferior memory capacity among the Kpelle. However, Cole and his associates proceeded instead to look for causes of the inferior performance in the background of the subjects, and arrived at the hypothesis that the Kpelle in the course of their daily activities have occasion to organize recall more often in terms of the locations of groups of objects than in terms of category names. In a simplified experimental situation set up to check on this possibility, the investigators found that under conditions arranged to be conducive to the use of locational retrieval cues, recall increased very substantially over trials and reached a level of about 80%.

Thus it will be seen that the progress of theory in this area has taken us a substantial step past the idea of memory as being simply the expression of a capacity. In order to understand performance in tasks involving memory, one needs always first of all to analyze the task to discover the kinds of retrieval cues that will be available to bridge the changes in context between the time of learning and the time of test for recall, and secondly, to look at the past history of the person being studied for evidence about the types of retrieval cues he or she habitually uses and the conditions of their use. Further, a test of memory, whether intended to assess achievement or to measure ability, provides an opportunity for the person tested to exhibit retrieval strategies that he or she has learned to use with a given type of material. People may differ in memory capacity, but we have reason to assume that test scores reflect differences in capacity only if we know that the people compared are using the same retrieval strategies.

This newer view of intellectual tests helps us also to understand why some of the almost absurdly simple tasks used in intelligence tests may predict differences in intellectual performance in school and everyday life. Take, for example, the word-naming task, which is a subtest at year 10 of the Stanford–Binet Intelligence Scale. The person tested is simply required to name as many different words as possible in 1 min, without using sentences or counting. How could performance in this task possibly reflect important aspects of intellectual ability? We know that vocabulary is an important aspect of intelligence, but surely this task cannot provide a meaningful estimate of vocabulary size in view of the extremely tiny sample obtained and the major extent to which the words given must be influenced by accidental circumstances. Yet it is a well-documented fact that correlations of scores on this subtest with total test score and with criteria of validity such as school performance are of the same order of magnitude as those involving subtests with more obvious intellectual content.

The first step toward a solution of this paradox is to note that, even in the simplest task, it is possible for individuals to perform at quite different levels of behavioral organization, and that the mode of response to a test problem will tend to reflect the way in which an individual has learned to approach tasks outside the testing situation or laboratory. To illustrate, let us consider portions of the protocols that might be generated by two hypothetical children in the word-naming task. Child A begins with the sequence of words *chair, table, dinner, time, clock,* whereas Child B begins *chair, table, bed, desk, shoe, glove, shirt, dress.* Even the briefest inspection suggests that the two children are approaching the task in quite different ways. In any associative theory of memory, it is assumed that words become associated with objects and also with other words during a person's experience. And in the case of the protocol of Child A, it appears that the responses given simply reflect these elementary associations. We might surmise that the chair in which the child was sitting gave rise to the first word, the word *chair* led to *table* by a strongly established association, and so on through the remainder of the sequence. But the protocol for Child B shows much more evidence of organization. It is as though the bringing to mind of the word *chair* led the child to think of a category designation, perhaps *furniture,* and that he then proceeded to three other members of the category, then shifted to another category, which was again suggested by an object in the immediate surroundings, but continued to enumerate members of the category rather than following out the incidental chains of associations set off by each individual word. We can be sure that a subject following the strategy of Child B will in general produce many more words in a given time, in part because he or she can much more readily keep track of the words already given and avoid repetitions.

Word naming is doubtless not a common task in everyday life, but there must be numerous occasions on which the organized retrieval strategy exhibited by Child B in the example proves useful. Almost anyone studying the use of language must have wondered how it is possible for a person to call up promptly virtually any member of a vocabulary that may run to thousands of words. Surely we cannot assume that all of these thousands of potential verbal responses are kept simultaneously in a high state of availability, and, in fact, there is much evidence to the contrary. However, we may note also that, in the use of language, words generally are not called for in a random sequence. Rather, features of the situation or context call for a word of a given type, and then specific cues require selection from the subclass. Suppose, for example, that someone asks the question, "What is the color of Jane's eyes?" Hearing the word *color* brings a subset of words, the color names, into a state of high availability for the listener; then, when the question is complete, a choice among these can be made promptly.

These considerations lead us to assume that the associative structure reflected in the type of performance exhibited by Child B in the illustration reflects a hierarchical organization of the type illustrated in Figure 4.3B. Individual words are associated with each other, not by direct linkages, but rather by common associates such as class or category names. Further, these category names, which serve as retrieval cues or control elements, may appear on different levels. I shall not pursue the details here, but perhaps I have gone far enough to convey the idea that the significance of the word-naming test as an indicator of intellectual ability arises not because it directly measures any simple capacity, or even provides a measure of vocabulary size, but rather because performance in the task yields evidence about the level of organization at which the subject operates in situations calling for the use of language.

Aspects of long-term memory in problem solving. Because the problems most commonly studied in experimental or computer simulation studies of problem solving (the Towers of Hanoi, the missionaries and cannibals, water jug problems, etc.) are barren of content, discussions of problem solving often carry the impression that the only relevant aspect of long-term memory is the collection of representations of rules and operations that must be utilized in the course of solving the problems. In current models based on the general approach of Newell and Simon's (1972) general problem solver, the rules and the representations of the conditions under which they are to be applied are stored in memory in the form of production systems (Chase, 1978; Simon, 1978), and efficiency in problem solving is conceived as depending on appropriate sequencing of these productions – sequencing that in turn reflects the ordering of pointers to the productions in a "stack," essentially a working-memory buffer.

In most problem solving of importance outside the laboratory, however – mathematical reasoning, scientific problems, decision problems arising in business or government – factual knowledge is essential to the formulation and solution of the problems. In all such cases, both of the principal aspects of long-term memory are relevant: episodic memory as the source of analogies between a current problem and others that the person has solved in the past, and semantic memory as the store of information concerning concepts and relationships relevant to a current problem.

In most of the influential contemporary theories of long-term memory, both episodic and semantic information is represented in associative networks in which nodes, or control elements, corresponding to episodes or concepts, are interconnected by associative pathways (e.g., Anderson, 1976; Anderson & Bower, 1973; Collins & Loftus, 1975; W. K. Estes, 1976; Norman & Rumelhart, 1975). In the case of episodic memory, the elements in the network are representations of events in spatio-temporal contexts, and the tendency for activation to spread from one element to another along associative pathways is conceived as depending on the similarity or commonality of the spatio-temporal contexts of the episodes. In the case of semantic memory, the elements of a network may be conceived as being multidimensional memory traces having much the properties of lists of features or attributes. Activation is conceived as spreading from one element to another along associative pathways as a function of the frequency and recency of previous activations and of the similarity or overlap of the feature lists.

With regard to efficiency in problem solving, the demands on episodic and semantic memory are somewhat different. Undoubtedly, the expert problem solver in any area – medical diagnosis, the solution of physics or computer programming problems, or whatever – exploits an ability to identify and remember problems previously encountered whose solutions or methods of solution are germane to the case currently under consideration.

The function of experience is to build up the stock of potentially useful episodic memories, and the function of training or education is to improve the ability to utilize relevant or deep, rather than irrelevant or superficial, properties of a problem situation when bringing to mind potentially relevant analogies (Chi, Feltovich & Glaser, 1981).

In studies of the solutions of physics problems by experienced physicists, as compared to solutions by students who presumably have the same relevant knowledge but much less experience, it is found that the physicists characteristically tend to categorize a new problem and look for analogies on the basis of physical principles, whereas the less-experienced students look for analogies on the basis of more superficial aspects of the problems, often perceptual properties of the situation.

With regard to semantic memory, within wide limits it seems clear that the sheer quantity of information stored in memory is not a matter of great importance, because an individual can draw on recorded information in books or computer files. However, the problem solver in any practical area does need to have a sufficient stock of semantic information to be able to call on other sources effectively and to have representations of concepts and "pointers" to other sources of information so organized as to be readily accessible.

One of the principal limitations of the human memory system, compared to the computer, is the very much slower speed of access to human memory, characteristically on the order of hundreds of milliseconds per item for human memory, compared to very small fractions of milliseconds for the computer. The matter of access speed is critical because the retrieval of items of information from human long-term memory evidently has to proceed to a great extent by means of serial searches of segments of associative networks (Shiffrin, 1970; Simon, 1978). Because the number of concepts represented in semantic memory must be very large, even for a school child (let alone a normal adult), problem solving would be extremely slow and uncertain if relevant items of information had to be retrieved from semantic memory by serial searches of large networks.

Studies of the mechanisms of free recall (Shiffrin, 1970; Tulving, 1968) and of reaction times for retrieval operations (thoroughly reviewed by Chase, 1978) have suggested two principal ways in which the slowness of memory search is circumvented. One is a tendency to organize groups of related concepts or other elements often accessed together into clusters or categories in such a way that the elements of a cluster can be accessed simultaneously by way of a common associate, for example, a category label. The second device is the formation of hierarchical retrieval structures, presumably by means of elaborative rehearsal. It appears that hierarchical organization becomes the norm in the normal adult, and especially so in persons expert at some type of problem solving, at two levels – the long-term organization of vocabulary and concepts and the short-term organization of material relevant to a particular task.

With regard to long-term organization, the work of Rosch (1975) on natural categories provides considerable support for the idea that a person's information about his or her normal environment tends to be organized in a hierarchical structure, with relatively higher-order categories (e.g., *living thing, animal, inanimate object*) near the top of the hierarchy, basic object categories (*tree, table, pencil*) at an intermediate level, and finer subordinate categories at the lowest levels.

Although the categories having to do with objects and properties of the normal environment appear to be organized in a similar hierarchical fashion for all people in a culture, the same cannot be assumed to be true for the specialized knowledge required for solution of problems. Rather, a critically important function of education and experience in specific kinds of problem solving may be the organization and reorganization of relevant aspects of semantic memory into efficient retrieval structures. In the studies of expert and novice solvers of physics problems by Chi and her associates (1981), for example, evidence from "think-aloud" protocols confirmed the expected differences in organization of relevant semantic memory for these two types of solvers.

COGNITION AND INTELLIGENCE

With the results of the preceding reviews of specific topics in hand, it is possible to go further than in the introduction to this chapter toward outlining the interrelationships among various aspects of cognition – learning, information processing, intellectual motivation – and intelligence. The simplest schema that might suffice in the present state of research and theory is portrayed in Figure 4.4, a modification of one presented elsewhere in a discussion of these interactions (W. K. Estes, 1981).

It will be noted, first of all, that the rubric *intelligence* appears nowhere in the schema. This venerable, but never fully defined, term is taken to refer to the entire constellation of properties, constituents, and determiners of intelligent behavior, considered in turn to denote adaptive behavior regulated by cognitive functions (cf. Charlesworth, 1976). By *cognitive functions* I refer to such activities as perceiving relationships, comparing and judging similarities and differences, coding information into progressively more abstract forms, classification and categorization, and memory search and retrieval.

However, having available in one's repertoire various cognitive rules and operations is necessary, but not sufficient, for intelligent behavior. It is necessary for these rules to be activated in problem situations, situations that must in turn require both retrieval and motivation. Thus, although the fact has often slipped from attention, it has been recognized from the time of Binet (and was perhaps first strongly emphasized by Lewin, 1940) that motives must be considered on a par with the more intellectual determiners of intelligent behavior. The relevant motives cannot in general be identified with simple biological drives and the like. Rather, they must be viewed as organized components of the cognitive system, incorporating products of earlier learning together with affective dispositions, and entering into cognitive function in ways that are not yet well understood (Bower, 1975).

The principal point that Figure 4.4 is meant to emphasize is the highly interactive character of the system we are dealing with when we study either cognition or intelligence. Intelligent behavior, whether in problem solving, comprehension, or creativity, is implemented by cognitive operations, which draw in turn on the products of past learning. However, the course of learning, especially learning in

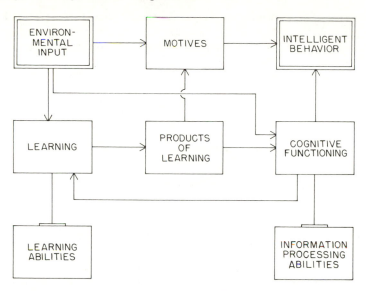

Figure 4.4.   Assumed interrelationships of principal abilities, processes, and cognitive structures entering into the determination of intelligent behavior.

the sense of acquisition of knowledge or development of intellectual skills, is modified by cognitive control processes. Both learning and cognitive performance appear to be constrained by capacity limitations. These may to some extent reflect individual differences in structural rather than control processes, and thus may be conditioned by innate differences in structures, but there is little reason to believe that existing psychometric methods can assess these sources of variation in performance independently.

Appraisals of intelligence, or of either learning or information-processing abilities taken separately, always involve indirect inference. The behavior we tap when we give tests or scales of intelligence falls in the dependent variable box at the upper right of the diagram and must *always* be assumed to depend on all of the other factors portrayed. Thus to measure any one component it is necessary either to hold all of the others constant, which may often be impossible of realization, or to understand the interactions well enough to partial out the effects of components other than the one that is being measured [W. K. Estes, 1981, p. 12]

With regard to the two main types of abilities, the problems are somewhat asymmetric, with the information-processing abilities generally being somewhat less difficult to appraise separately. One reason is that intelligence tests tap performance during a short interval of time, within which the amount of learning that goes on may be assumed to be negligible. The products of previous learning are always important, but these may sometimes be handled by allowing different amounts of previous time and training for different persons in order to produce a common background of knowledge relevant to the test. On the other hand, when the objective is to test learning ability, behavior must necessarily be followed over a longer period of time. Thus one must contend with the important feedback loop from cognitive functioning to learning, which means that cognitive functions that themselves depend on information-processing abilities influence the speed and perhaps also the quality of learning. It would seem, then, that progress toward untangling the multiple determinants of individual differences in intelligent behavior can come only within the framework of more comprehensive theories of the whole interactive cognitive system.

REFERENCES

Allen, G. A., & Estes, W. K. Acquisition of correct choices and value judgments in binary choice learning with differential rewards. *Psychonomic Science*, 1972, 27, 68–72.
Anderson, J. R. *Language, memory, and thought*. Hillsdale, N.J.: Erlbaum, 1976.
Anderson, J. R., & Bower, G. H. *Human associative memory*. Washington, D.C.: V. H. Winston, 1973.
Anzai, Y., & Simon, H. A. The theory of learning by doing. *Psychological Review*, 1979, 86, 124–140.
Atkinson, R. C., & Shiffrin, R. M. Human memory: A proposed system and its control processes. In K. W. Spence & J. T. Spence (Eds.), *The psychology of learning and motivation: Advances in research and theory* (Vol. 2). New York: Academic Press, 1968.
Atkinson, R. C., & Shiffrin, R. M. The control of short-term memory. *Scientific American*, 1971, 225(2), 82–90.
Atkinson, R. C., & Wickens, T. D. Human memory and the concept of reinforcement. In R. Glaser (Ed.), *The nature of reinforcement*. New York: Academic Press, 1971.
Baddeley, A. D. *The psychology of memory*. New York: Basic Books, 1976.
Baddeley, A. D. The trouble with levels: A reexamination of Craik and Lockhart's framework for memory research. *Psychological Review*, 1978, 85, 139–152.
Baddeley, A. D., & Hitch, G. Working memory. In G. H. Bower (Ed.), *The psychology of learning and motivation: Advances in research and theory* (Vol. 8). New York: Academic Press, 1974.
Baddeley, A. D., Thomson, N., & Buchanan, M. Word length and the structure of short-term memory. *Journal of Verbal Learning and Verbal Behavior*, 1975, 14, 575–589.
Bandura, A. Vicarious and self-reinforcement processes. In R. Glaser (Ed.), *The nature of reinforcement*. New York: Academic Press, 1971.
Bandura, A. *Social learning theory*. Englewood Cliffs, N.J.: Prentice-Hall, 1977.
Bandura, A., & Walters, R. H. *Social learning and personality development*. New York: Holt, Rinehart, & Winston, 1963.
Bartlett, F. C. *Remembering: A study in experimental and social psychology*. Cambridge: Cambridge University Press, 1932.
Batchelder, B. L., & Denny, M. R. A theory of intelligence: I. Span and the complexity of stimulus control. *Intelligence*, 1977, 1, 127–150.
Belmont, J. M., & Butterfield, E. C. What the development of short-term memory is. *Human Development*, 1971, 14, 236–248.
Bijou, S. W. A functional analysis of retarded development. In N. R. Ellis (Ed.), *International review of research in mental retardation* (Vol. 1). New York: Academic Press, 1966.
Bindra, D. *A theory of intelligent behavior*. New York: Wiley, 1976.
Binet, A., & Simon, T. Sur la nécessité d'établir un diagnostic scientifique des états inférieurs de l'intelligence. *L'Année Psychologique*, 1905, 11, 163–190.
Binet, A., & Simon, T. *The development of intelligence in children*. Baltimore: Williams & Wilkins, 1916.
Birnbrauer, J. S. Mental retardation. In H. Leitenberg (Ed.), *Handbook of behavior modification and behavior therapy*. Englewood Cliffs, N.J.: Prentice-Hall, 1976.
Bolton, T. L. The growth of memory in school children. *American Journal of Psychology*, 1891–1892, 4, 362–380.
Bower, G. H. Cognitive psychology: An introduction. In W. K. Estes (Ed.), *Handbook of learning and cognitive processes* (Vol. 1). Hillsdale, N.J.: Erlbaum, 1975.
Broadbent, D. E. *Perception and communication*. New York: Pergamon Press, 1958.
Brown, J. Some tests of the decay theory of immediate memory. *Quarterly Journal of Experimental Psychology*, 1958, 10, 12–21.
Bruner, J. S., Goodnow, J. J., & Austin, G. A. *A study of thinking*. New York: Wiley, 1956.

Buchwald, A. M. Effects of "right" and "wrong" on subsequent behavior: A new interpretation. *Psychological Review*, 1969, 76, 132–143.

Carpenter, P. A., & Just, M. A. Sentence comprehension: A psycholinguistic processing model of verification. *Psychological Review*, 1975, 82, 45–73.

Carroll, J. B. Psychometric tests as cognitive tasks: A new "structure of intellect". In L. B. Resnick (Ed.), *The nature of intelligence*. Hillsdale, N.J.: Erlbaum, 1976.

Charlesworth, W. R. Human intelligence as adaptation: An ethological approach. In L. B. Resnick (Ed.), *The nature of intelligence*. Hillsdale, N.J.: Erlbaum, 1976.

Chase, W. G. Elementary information processing. In W. K. Estes (Ed.), *Handbook of learning and cognitive processes* (Vol. 5). Hillsdale, N.J.: Erlbaum, 1978.

Chase, W. G., & Clark, H. H. Mental operations in the comparison of sentences and pictures. In L. W. Gregg (Ed.), *Cognition in learning and memory*. New York: Wiley, 1972.

Chi, M. T. H. Short-term memory limitations in children: Capacity or processing deficits. *Memory and Cognition*, 1976, 4, 559–572.

Chi, M. T. H., Feltovich, P. J., & Glaser, R. Categorization and representation of physics problems by experts and novices. *Cognitive Science*, 1981, 5, 121–152.

Chomsky, N. *Aspects of the theory of syntax*. Cambridge, Mass.: MIT Press, 1965.

Clifton, R. K., & Nelson, M. N. Developmental study of habituation in infants: The importance of paradigm, response system, and state. In T. J. Tighe & R. N. Leaton (Eds.), *Habituation: Perspectives from child development, animal behavior, and neurophysiology*. Hillsdale, N.J.: Erlbaum, 1976.

Cole, M., Gay, J., Glick, J., & Sharp, D. W. *The cultural context of learning and thinking*. New York: Basic, 1971.

Collins, A. M., & Loftus, E. F. A spreading-activation theory of semantic processing. *Psychological Review*, 1975, 82, 407–428.

Collins, A. M., & Quillian, M. R. How to make a language user. In E. Tulving & W. Donaldson (Eds.), *Organization of memory*. New York: Academic Press, 1972.

Conrad, R. Acoustic confusions in immediate memory. *British Journal of Psychology*, 1964, 55, 75–84.

Conrad, R. Order error in immediate recall of sequences. *Journal of Verbal Learning and Verbal Behavior*, 1965, 4, 161–169.

Craik, F. I. M., & Levy, B. A. The concept of primary memory. In W. K. Estes (Ed.), *Handbook of learning and cognitive processes* (Vol. 4). Hillsdale, N.J.: Erlbaum, 1976.

Craik, F. I. M., & Lockhart, R. S. Levels of processing: A framework for memory research. *Journal of Verbal Learning and Verbal Behavior*, 1972, 11, 671–684.

Craik, F. I. M., & Watkins, M. J. The role of rehearsal in short-term memory. *Journal of Verbal Learning and Verbal Behavior*, 1973, 12, 599–607.

Denny, M. R. Research in learning performance. In H. A. Stevens & R. Heber (Eds.), *Mental retardation: A review of research*. Chicago: University of Chicago Press, 1964.

Drewnowski, A. Attributes and priorities in short-term recall: A new model of memory span. *Journal of Experimental Psychology: General*, 1980, 109, 208–250.

Drewnowski, A., & Murdock, B. B., Jr. The role of auditory features in memory span for words. *Journal of Experimental Psychology: Human Learning and Memory*, 1980, 6, 319–332.

Ebbinghaus, H. *Memory* (H. A. Ruger & C. E. Bussenius, Trans.). New York: Teachers College, Columbia University, 1913. (Originally published, 1885.)

Egger, M. D., & Miller, N. E. Secondary reinforcement in rats as a function of information value and reliability of the stimulus. *Journal of Experimental Psychology* 1962, 64, 97–104.

Ellis, N. R. The stimulus trace and behavioral inadequacy. In N. R. Ellis (Ed.), *Handbook of mental deficiency*. New York: McGraw-Hill, 1963.

Ellis, N. R. Memory processes in retardates and normals: Theoretical and empirical considerations. In N. R. Ellis (Ed.), *International review of research in mental retardation* (Vol. 4). New York: Academic Press, 1970.

Ellis, N. R., & Hope, R. Memory processes and the serial position curve. *Journal of Experimental Psychology* 1968, 77, 613–619.

Ericsson, K. A., Chase, W. G., & Faloon, S. Acquisition of a memory skill. *Science*, 1980, 208, 1181–1182.

Ericsson, K. A., & Simon, H. A. Verbal reports as data. *Psychological Review*, 1980, 87, 215–251.

Estes, K. W. An information-processing analysis of reinforcement in children's discrimination learning. *Child Development*, 1976, 47, 639–647.

Estes, W. K. Reinforcement in human learning. In J. T. Tapp (Ed.), *Reinforcement and behavior*. New York: Academic Press, 1969.

Estes, W. K. *Learning theory and mental development*. New York: Academic Press, 1970.

Estes, W. K. Reward in human learning: Theoretical issues and strategic choice points. In R. Glaser (Ed.), *The nature of reinforcement*. New York: Academic Press, 1971.

Estes, W. K. An associative basis for coding and organization in memory. In A. W. Melton and E. Martin (Eds.), *Coding processes in human memory*. Washington, D.C.: V. H. Winston, 1972. (a)

Estes, W. K. Reinforcement in human behavior. *American Scientist*, 1972, 60, 723–729. (b)

Estes, W. K. Memory and conditioning. In F. J. McGuigan & D. B. Lumsden (Eds.), *Contemporary approaches to conditioning and learning*. Washington, D.C.: V. W. Winston, 1973. (a)

Estes, W. K. Phonemic coding and rehearsal in short-term memory for letter strings. *Journal of Verbal Learning and Verbal Behavior*, 1973, 12, 360–372. (b)

Estes, W. K. Learning theory and intelligence. *American Psychologist*, 1974, 29, 740–749.

Estes, W. K. Structural aspects of associative models for memory. In C. N. Cofer (Ed.), *The structure of human memory*. San Francisco: W. H. Freeman, 1976.

Estes, W. K. Cognitive processes in conditioning. In A. Dickinson & R. A. Boakes (Eds.), *Mechanisms of learning and motivation: A memorial volume to Jerzy Konorski*. Hillsdale, N.J.: Erlbaum, 1979.

Estes, W. K. Is human memory obsolete? *American Scientist*, 1980, 68, 62–69.

Estes, W. K. Intelligence and learning. In M. P. Friedman, J. P. Das, & N. O'Connor (Eds.), *Intelligence and learning*. New York: Plenum, 1981.

Feigenbaum, E. A. The simulation of verbal learning behavior. In E. A. Feigenbaum & J. Feldman (Eds.), *Computers and thought*. New York: McGraw-Hill, 1963.

Flavell, J. H. Developmental studies of mediated memory. In H. W. Reese & L. P. Lipsitt (Eds.), *Advances in child development and behavior* (Vol. 5). New York: Academic Press, 1970.

Freedman, J. L., & Loftus, E. F. Retrieval of words from long-term memory. *Journal of Verbal Learning and Verbal Behavior*, 1971, 10, 107–115.

Gagné, R. M. Contributions of learning to human development. *Psychological Review*, 1968, 75, 177–191.

Gibson, E. J. *Principles of perceptual learning and development*. New York: Appleton-Century-Crofts, 1969.

Gilmartin, K. J., Newell, A., & Simon, H. A. A program modeling short-term memory under strategy control. In C. Cofer (Ed.), *The structure of human memory*. San Francisco: W. H. Freeman, 1976.

Gormezano, I., & Kehoe, E. J. Classical conditioning: Some methodological-conceptual issues. In W. K. Estes (Ed.), *Handbook of learning and cognitive processes* (Vol. 2). Hillsdale, N.J.: Erlbaum, 1975.

Grant, D. A. Classical and operant conditioning. In A. W. Melton (Ed.), *Categories of human learning*. New York: Academic Press, 1964.

Hagen, J. W., Hargrave, S., & Ross, W. Prompting and rehearsal in short-term memory. *Child Development*, 1973, 44, 201–204.

Harlow, H. F. The formation of learning sets. *Psychological Review*, 1949, 56, 51–65.

Harris, J. D. Habituatory response decrement in the intact organism. *Psychological Bulletin*, 1943, 40, 385–422.

Hayes-Roth, B. Evolution of cognitive structures and processes. *Psychological Review*, 1977, 84, 260–278.

Hebb, D. O. *The organization of behavior: A neuropsychological theory*. New York: Wiley, 1949.

Hilgard, E. R. Methods and procedures in the study of learning. In S. S. Stevens (Ed.), *Handbook of experimental psychology*. New York: Wiley, 1951.

Hilgard, E. R. *Theories of learning* (2nd ed.). New York: Appleton-Century-Crofts, 1956

Hilgard, E. R., & Marquis, D. G. *Conditioning and learning*. New York: Appleton-Century, 1940.

Hinde, R. A. Behavioural habituation. In G. Horn & R. A. Hinde (Eds.), *Short-term changes in neural activity and behaviour*. Cambridge: Cambridge University Press, 1970.

Hinde, R. A., & Tinbergen, N. The comparative study of species-specific behavior. In A. Roe & G. G. Simpson (Eds.), *Behavior and evolution*. New Haven: Yale University Press, 1958.

Hogan, R. M. Interitem encoding and directed search in free recall. *Memory and Cognition*, 1975, *3*, 197–209.

Holz, W. C., & Azrin, N. H. Conditioning human verbal behavior. In W. K. Honig (Ed.), *Operant behavior*. New York: Appleton-Century-Crofts, 1966.

Hull, C. L. Quantitative aspects of the evolution of concepts. *Psychological Monographs*, 1920, 28(123).

Hull, C. L. Mind, mechanism, and adaptive behavior. *Psychological Review*, 1937, *44*, 1–32.

Hull, C. L. *Principles of behavior*. New York: Appleton-Century-Crofts, 1943.

Humphrey, G. *The nature of learning*. New York: Harcourt, 1933.

Hunt, E. *Concept learning: An information processing problem*. New York: Wiley, 1962.

Hunt, E. Mechanics of verbal ability. *Psychological Review*, 1978, *85*, 109–130.

Huttenlocher, J., & Burke, D. Why does memory span increase with age? *Cognitive Psychology*, 1976, *8*, 1–31.

Johnson, N. F. Organization and the concept of a memory code. In A. W. Melton & E. Martin (Eds.), *Coding processes in human memory*. Washington, D.C.: V. H. Winston, 1972.

Jones, G. V. A fragmentation hypothesis of memory: Cued recall of pictures and of sequential positions. *Journal of Experimental Psychology: General*, 1976, *105*, 277–293.

Kamin, L. J. Selective association and conditioning. In N. J. MacKintosh & W. K. Honig (Eds.), *Fundamental issues in associative learning*. Halifax, N.S.: Dalhousie University Press, 1969.

Keeney, T. J., Cannizzo, S. R., & Flavell, J. H. Spontaneous and induced verbal rehearsal in a recall task. *Child Development*, 1967, *38*, 953–966.

Kendler, T. S. The development of discrimination learning: A levels-of-functioning explanation. In H. W. Reese & L. P. Lipsitt (Eds.), *Advances in child development and behavior* (Vol. 13). New York: Academic Press, 1979.

Kintsch, W. Comprehension and memory of text. In W. K. Estes (Ed.), *Handbook of learning and cognitive processes* (Vol. 6). Hillsdale, N.J.: Erlbaum, 1978.

Kintsch, W., & Van Dijk, T. A. Toward a model of text comprehension and production. *Psychological Review*, 1978, *85*, 363–394.

Kintsch, W., & Vipond, D. Reading comprehension and readability in education practice and psychological theory. In L.-G. Nilsson (Ed.), *Perspectives on memory research*. Hillsdale, N.J.: Erlbaum, 1979.

Konorski, J. *Integrative activity of the brain*. Chicago: University of Chicago Press, 1967.

Krasner, L., & Ullmann, L. P. *Research in behavior modification: New developments and implications*. New York: Holt, Rinehart, & Winston, 1965.

LaBerge, D. Acquisition of automatic processing in perceptual and associative learning. In P. M. A. Rabbitt & S. Dornic (Eds.), *Attention and performance* (Vol. 5). New York: Academic Press, 1975.

Lawrence, D. H. The nature of a stimulus: Some relationships between learning and perception. In S. Koch (Ed.), *Psychology: A study of a science* (Vol. 5). New York: McGraw-Hill, 1963.

Lee, C. L., & Estes, W. K. Order and position in primary memory for letter strings. *Journal of Verbal Learning and Verbal Behavior*, 1977, *16*, 395–418.

Levine, M. *A cognitive theory of learning: Research in hypothesis testing*. Hillsdale, N.J.: Erlbaum, 1975.

Lewin, K. Intelligence and motivation. In the National Society for the Study of Education's 39th Yearbook, *Intelligence: Its nature and nurture. Part I: Comparative and critical exposition*. Bloomington, Ill.: Public School Publishing Co., 1940.

Loftus, E. L., & Suppes, P. Structural variables that determine the speed of retrieving words from long-term memory. *Journal of Verbal Learning and Verbal Behavior*, 1972, *11*, 770–777.

Lorenz, K. Z. *King Solomon's ring*. New York: Crowell, 1952.

Lyon, D. R. Individual differences in immediate serial recall: A matter of mnemonics? *Cognitive Psychology*, 1977, *9*, 403–411.

Mandler, G. Organization and memory. In K. W. Spence & J. T. Spence (Eds.), *The psychology of learning and motivation: Advances in research and theory* (Vol. 1). New York: Academic Press, 1967.

McCall, R. B., & Kagan, J. Individual differences in the infant's distribution of attention to stimulus discrepancy. *Developmental Psychology*, 1970, 2, 90–98.

McGeoch, J. A., & Irion, A. L. *The psychology of human learning*. New York: Longmans, Green, 1952.

McNemar, Q. *The revision of the Stanford–Binet scale*. Boston: Houghton Mifflin, 1942.

Medin, D. L. The role of reinforcement in discrimination learning set in monkeys. *Psychological Bulletin*, 1972, 77, 305–318.

Medin, D. L., & Schaffer, M. M. Context theory of classification learning. *Psychological Review*, 1978, 85, 207–238.

Melton, A. W., & Martin, E. *Coding processes in human memory*. Washington, D.C.: V. H. Winston, 1972.

Miller, G. A. The magical number seven, plus or minus two: Some limits on our capacity for processing information. *Psychological Review*, 1956, 63, 81–97.

Millward, R. B., & Wickens, T. D. Concept-identification models. In D. H. Krantz, R. C. Atkinson, R. D. Luce, & P. Suppes (Eds.), *Contemporary developments in mathematical psychology: Learning, memory, and thinking* (Vol. 1). San Francisco: W. H. Freeman, 1974.

Munn, N. L. Learning in children. In L. Carmichael (Ed.), *Manual of child psychology* (2nd ed.). New York: Wiley, 1954.

Nelson, T. O. Reinforcement and human memory. In W. K. Estes (Ed.), *Handbook of learning and cognitive processes* (Vol. 3). Hillsdale, N.J.: Erlbaum, 1976.

Newell, A., & Simon, H. A. *Human problem solving*. Englewood Cliffs, N.J.: Prentice-Hall, 1972.

Nicolson, R. The relationship between memory span and processing speed. In M. P. Friedman, J. P. Das, & N. O'Connor (Eds.), *Intelligence and learning*. New York: Plenum, 1981.

Norman, D. A., & Rumelhart, D. E. *Explorations in cognition*. San Francisco: W. H. Freeman, 1975.

Nuttin, J. *Tâche, réussite, et échec*. Louvain, Belgium: Publications Universitaires, 1953.

Nuttin, J., & Greenwald, A. G. *Reward and punishment in human learning*. New York: Academic Press, 1968.

Pavlov, I. *Conditioned reflexes*. London: Oxford University Press, 1927.

Pellegrino, J. W., & Glaser, R. Cognitive correlates and components in the analysis of individual differences. *Intelligence*, 1979, 3, 187–214.

Peterson, L. R., & Johnson, S. T. Some effects of minimizing articulation of short-term retention. *Journal of Verbal Learning and Verbal Behavior*, 1971, 10, 346–354.

Phillips, J. L., Shiffrin, R. M., & Atkinson, R. C. Effects of list length on short-term memory. *Journal of Verbal Learning and Verbal Behavior*, 1967, 6, 303–311.

Posner, M. I. Short-term memory systems in human information processing. *Acta Psychologica*, 1967, 27, 267–284.

Posner, M. I. *Chronometric explorations of mind*. Hillsdale, N.J.: Erlbaum, 1978.

Posner, M. I., & Keele, S. W. On the genesis of abstract ideas. *Journal of Experimental Psychology*, 1968, 77, 353–363.

Posner, M. I., & Keele, S. W. Retention of abstract ideas. *Journal of Experimental Psychology*, 1970, 83, 304–308.

Posner, M. I., & Rossman, E. Effect of size and location of informational transforms on short-term retention. *Journal of Experimental Psychology*, 1965, 70, 496–505.

Premack, D. *Intelligence in ape and man*. Hillsdale, N.J.: Erlbaum, 1976.

Quillian, M. R. Semantic memory. In M. Minsky (Ed.), *Semantic information processing*. Cambridge, Mass.: MIT Press, 1968.

Raaijmakers, J. G. W., & Shiffrin, R. M. Search of associative memory. *Psychological Review*, 1981, 88, 93–134.

Rescorla, R. A., & Wagner, A. R. A theory of Pavlovian conditioning: Variations in the effectiveness of reinforcement and nonreinforcement. In A. H. Black & W. F. Prokasy (Eds.), *Classical conditioning II: Current research and theory*. New York: Appleton-Century-Crofts, 1972.

Restle, F. Toward a quantitative description of learning set data. *Psychological Review,* 1958, *65,* 77–91.

Restle, F., & Brown, E. R. Serial pattern learning. *Journal of Experimental Psychology,* 1970, *83,* 120–125.

Rosch, E. Cognitive representations of semantic categories. *Journal of Experimental Psychology: General,* 1975, *104,* 192–233.

Rosch, E., & Lloyd, B. B. *Cognition and categorization.* Hillsdale, N.J.: Erlbaum, 1978.

Ross, L. E., & Ross, S. M. Cognitive factors in classical conditioning. In W. K. Estes (Ed.), *Handbook of learning and cognitive processes* (Vol. 3). Hillsdale, N.J.: Erlbaum, 1976.

Rotter, J. B. *Social learning and clinical psychology.* Englewood Cliffs, N.J.: Prentice-Hall, 1954.

Rundus, D., & Atkinson, R. C. Rehearsal processes in free recall: A procedure for direct observation. *Journal of Verbal Learning and Verbal Behavior,* 1970, *9,* 99–105.

Schneider, W., & Shiffrin, R. M. Controlled and automatic human information processing: I. Detection, search, and attention. *Psychological Review,* 1977, *84,* 1–66.

Shettleworth, S. J. Constraints on learning. *Advances in the Study of Behavior,* 1972, *4,* 1–68.

Shiffrin, R. M. Memory search. In D. A. Norman (Ed.), *Models for memory.* New York: Academic Press, 1970.

Shiffrin, R. M., & Schneider, W. Controlled and automatic human information processing: II. Perceptual learning, automatic attending, and a general theory. *Psychological Review,* 1977, *84,* 127–190.

Simon, H. A. Identifying basic abilities underlying intelligent performance of complex tasks. In L. B. Resnick (Ed.), *The nature of intelligence.* Hillsdale, N.J.: Erlbaum, 1976.

Simon, H. A. Information-processing theory of human problem solving. In W. K. Estes (Ed.), *Handbook of learning and cognitive processes* (Vol. 5). Hillsdale, N.J.: Erlbaum, 1978.

Skinner, B. F. *The behavior of organisms: An experimental analysis.* New York: Appleton-Century, 1938.

Skinner, B. F. Operant behavior. In W. K. Honig (Ed.), *Operant behavior.* New York: Appleton-Century-Crofts, 1966.

Smith, E. E. Theories of semantic memory. In W. K. Estes (Ed.), *Handbook of learning and cognitive processes* (Vol. 6). Hillsdale, N.J.: Erlbaum, 1978.

Smith, E. E., Shoben, E. J., & Rips, L. J. Structure and process in semantic memory: A featural model for semantic decisions. *Psychological Review,* 1974, *81,* 214–241.

Sokolov, Ye. N. *Perception and the conditioned reflex.* Oxford: Pergamon Press, 1963.

Spearman, C. "General intelligence," objectively determined and measured. *American Journal of Psychology,* 1904, *15,* 201–293.

Spence, K. W. The differential response in animals to stimuli varying within a single dimension. *Psychological Review,* 1937, *44,* 430–444.

Spielberger, C. D. The role of awareness in verbal conditioning. In C. W. Eriksen (Ed.), *Behavior and awareness.* Durham, N.C.: Duke University Press, 1962.

Spitz, H. H. The role of input organization in the learning and memory of mental retardates. In N. R. Ellis (Ed.), *International review of research on mental retardation* (Vol. 2), New York: Academic Press, 1966.

Sternberg, R. J. *Intelligence, information processing, and analogical reasoning: The componential analysis of human abilities.* Hillsdale, N.J.: Erlbaum, 1977.

Sternberg, S. High-speed scanning in human memory. *Science,* 1966, *153,* 652–654.

Sternberg, S. Memory scanning: New findings and current controversies. *Quarterly Journal of Experimental Psychology,* 1975, *27,* 1–32.

Suppes, P., & Ginsberg, R. Application of a stimulus sampling model to children's concept formation with and without overt correction responses. *Journal of Experimental Psychology,* 1962, *63,* 330–336.

Sutherland, N. S., & Mackintosh, N. J. *Mechanisms of animal discrimination learning.* New York: Academic Press, 1971.

Syz, H. C. Psycho-galvanic studies on sixty-four medical students. *British Journal of Psychology,* 1926, *17,* 54–69.

Terman, L. M. *The measurement of intelligence.* Boston: Houghton Mifflin, 1916.

Terman, L. M., & Merrill, M. A. *Measuring intelligence.* Boston: Houghton Mifflin, 1937.

Theios, J. Reaction time measurements in the study of memory processes: Theory and data. In

G. H. Bower (Ed.), *The psychology of learning and motivation: Advances in research and theory* (Vol. 7). New York: Academic Press, 1973.

Thorndike, E. L. *Educational psychology* (Vol. 2). New York: Teachers College, Columbia University, 1913.

Thorndike, E. L., Bregman, E. O., Cobb, M. V., & Woodyard, E. *The measurement of intelligence.* New York: Teachers College, Columbia University, 1926.

Tolman, E. C. *Purposive behavior in animals and men.* New York: Appleton-Century, 1932.

Trabasso, T., & Bower, G. H. *Attention in learning: Theory and research.* New York: Wiley, 1968.

Tulving, E. Theoretical issues in free recall. In T. R. Dixon & D. L. Horton (Eds.), *Verbal behavior and general behavior theory.* Englewood Cliffs, N.J.: Prentice-Hall, 1968.

Tulving, E. Episodic and semantic memory. In E. Tulving & W. Donaldson (Eds.), *Organization of memory.* New York: Academic Press, 1972.

Wells, J. E. Strength theory and judgments of recency and frequency. *Journal of Verbal Learning and Verbal Behavior,* 1974, *13,* 378–392.

Wescourt, K. T., & Atkinson, R. C. Fact retrieval processes in human memory. In W. K. Estes (Ed.), *Handbook of learning and cognitive processes* (Vol. 4). Hillsdale, N.J.: Erlbaum, 1976.

White, S. H. Evidence for a hierarchical arrangement of learning processes. In L. P. Lipsitt & C. C. Spiker (Eds.), *Advances in child development and behavior* (Vol. 2) New York: Academic Press, 1965.

Wickelgren, W. A. Size of rehearsal group and short-term memory. *Journal of Experimental Psychology,* 1964, *68,* 413–419.

Wood, G. Organizational processes and free recall. In E. Tulving & W. Donaldson (Eds.), *Organization of memory.* New York: Academic Press, 1972.

Woodrow, H. Interrelations of measures of learning. *Journal of Psychology,* 1940, *10,* 49–73.

Woodward, A. E., Jr., Bjork, R. A., & Jongeward, R. H., Jr. Recall and recognition as a function of primary rehearsal. *Journal of Verbal Learning and Verbal Behavior,* 1973, *12,* 608–617.

Zeaman, D., & House, B. J. The role of attention in retardate discrimination learning. In N. R. Ellis (Ed.), *Handbook of mental deficiency.* New York: McGraw-Hill, 1963.

Zeaman, D., & House, B. J. The relation of IQ and learning. In R. M. Gagné (Ed.), *Learning and individual differences.* Columbus, Ohio: Merrill, 1967.

Zeaman, D., & House, B. J. Interpretation of developmental trends in discriminative transfer effects. In A. D. Pick (Ed.), *Minnesota Symposia in Child Psychology* (Vol. 8) Minneapolis: University of Minnesota Press, 1974.

5 Reasoning, problem solving, and intelligence

ROBERT J. STERNBERG

Reasoning, problem solving, and intelligence are so closely interrelated that it is often difficult to tell them apart. Consider, for example, the following arithmetic word problem:

I planted a tree that was 8 in. tall. At the end of the first year it was 12 in. tall; at the end of the second year it was 18 in. tall; and at the end of the third year it was 27 in. tall. How tall was it at the end of the fourth year?

This arithmetic word problem obviously requires "problem solving" for its solution. The problem is labeled as one of "reasoning" on the test in which it appears. And the test in which it appears is one of "intelligence": the Stanford–Binet Intelligence Test (Terman & Merrill, 1937). The same fluidity of boundaries among the three constructs is equally in evidence for any of a number of problems on the Stanford–Binet. For example, "reconciliation of opposites" requires a person to indicate in what way two opposites, such as *heavy* and *light*, are alike. In the conventional senses of the terms, reconciliation of opposites requires reasoning, problem solving, and intelligence.

Whatever *intelligence* may be, *reasoning* and *problem solving* have traditionally been viewed as important subsets of it. Almost without regard to how *intelligence* has been defined, *reasoning* and *problem solving* have been part of the definition. Consider some methods for defining *intelligence,* and the roles *reasoning* and *problem solving* have played in each.

One time-honored approach to discovering the meaning of a construct is to seek expert opinion regarding its definition. The editors of the *Journal of Educational Psychology* did just this in their 1921 symposium on experts' conceptions of intelligence. Almost all of the definitions provided by the 14 experts mentioned *reasoning* and *problem solving* at least implicitly. For example, Terman's (1921) definition of *intelligence* as the ability "to carry on abstract thinking" (p. 128) might be viewed as a definition of intelligence in terms of abstract reasoning, and Pintner's (1921) definition of intelligence as the ability "to adapt [one]self adequately to relatively new situations in life" (p. 139) might be viewed as a definition of intelligence in terms of practical problem solving.

A second approach to the definitional problem might be viewed as a quantitatively more sophisticated version of the first. Sternberg, Conway, Ketron, and Bernstein (1981) applied factor analysis to definitional data collected from people-in-the-street, and followed up these analyses with a comparable factor analysis of definitional data collected from experts in the field of intelligence. The motivating idea was to discover related sets of behaviors, or "factors," in people's conceptions of intelligence. Problem-solving behavior was an important factor in the conceptions of both groups.

A third approach to the problem differs from the first two in that it analyzes *intelligent behavior* rather than *people's conceptions of intelligent behavior*. The distinction between the two must be kept clear, because people's conceptions of what they do and of the organization of what they do may differ from what the people actually do, and from the organization of what they actually do. This third approach, which has been widely used in the human-abilities field, is factor analysis of ability tests. Traditionally, psychometricians (specialists in psychological measurement) have sought to discover the nature of intelligence by searching for common sources of individual-differences variation in performance on large collections of tests consensually believed to measure intelligence. Reasoning and problem solving have played important parts in virtually every theory of intelligence that has been factor-analytically derived. The earliest factor-analytic theory of intelligence, for example – Spearman's (1904, 1923, 1927) – posited a general source of individual-differences variation, *g*, common to the whole range of ability tests. Two "principles of cognition" heavily implicated in *g*, eduction of relations (e.g., "What is the relation between *lawyer* and *client*?") and eduction of correlates (e.g., "What word completion would result in an analogous relation from *doctor*?"), are almost certainly important components of reasoning. Likewise, in Thurstone's (1938) theory of intelligence, reasoning was one of seven primary mental abilities (and in some versions of Thurstone's theory, two of eight, because inductive reasoning and deductive reasoning could be split into separate factors). Guilford's (1967) theory of the structure of intellect also drew heavily upon reasoning operations. Guilford's "cognition of relations," for example, appears to be essentially identical to Spearman's "eduction of relations." The importance of reasoning and problem solving to psychometric theories of intelligence is not surprising when one considers that some of the best-known tests of intelligence comprise reasoning or problem-solving items exclusively or almost exclusively, for example, the Miller Analogies Test, Raven's Progressive Matrices, and Cattell's Culture Fair Test of *g*.

A fourth approach, information-processing analysis, is like the psychometric approach in its application to quantitative indexes of intelligent behavior (rather than to quantitative indexes of conceptions of intelligent behavior), but differs from the psychometric approach in its use of stimulus variation rather than individual-differences variation as the means of isolating elementary units of intelligence. The motivating idea in information-processing analysis is to decompose performance on tasks into elementary information-processing components, and then to show the interrelations among the components used to solve various tasks requiring intelligent performance. In this approach, too, reasoning and problem solving have been found to be critical ingredients of intelligence (Simon, 1976; Sternberg, 1977b, 1979b).

There seems to be little doubt that reasoning and problem solving play important roles in conceptions of intelligence, almost without regard to the derivation of these conceptions: These roles are important as subsets of intelligent behavior. But what is the relationship between reasoning and problem solving, and even more important, what are they, in and of themselves? Unless we seek to stipulate the meanings of these terms from scratch, we need to look at the relationship between them to understand the ways in which the terms have been used, and we find that the distinction between them has always been fuzzy at best. Certain kinds of problems have been studied under the rubric of "reasoning," others under the rubric of "problem solving," and it seems to be primarily a historical accident whether a given kind of problem has been classified as one, the other, or both. Problem solving seems to require reasoning, and reasoning seems to require problem solving. For example, it is a matter of "analogical reasoning" to complete the item *Happy* is to *ecstatic* as *sad* is to ? but a matter of "analogical problem solving" to indicate in what ways current civilization resembles civilization during the declining days of the Roman Empire.

The remainder of this chapter will be divided into four major sections. The first will present a metatheoretical framework in terms of which theory and research on reasoning and problem solving can be understood. The next two sections will present critical reviews of the literatures on reasoning and problem solving, respectively. Although the division of literature is largely arbitrary, it is nevertheless convenient. Because it would require a book-length volume to do justice to the breadth of literature in each area, the emphasis in these reviews will be upon depth in the coverage of a selective subset of each literature. No attempt will be made to cover either literature in its full breadth and scope. The final section will discuss how reasoning and problem solving relate to intelligence.

5.1.   A METATHEORETICAL FRAMEWORK FOR THEORY AND RESEARCH ON
        REASONING AND PROBLEM SOLVING

This section proposes a metatheoretical framework for theory and research on reasoning and problem solving: It is divided into two parts, the first discussing the basic psychological constructs that constitute the framework and the second listing and discussing questions that a theory within this framework ought to be able to answer.

BASIC PSYCHOLOGICAL CONSTRUCTS

The proposed metatheoretical framework is based upon the notion of the *component*. In the framework, reasoning and problem solving are understood and interrelated in terms of the components they comprise. A component is an elementary information process that operates upon internal representations of objects or symbols (Sternberg, 1977b, 1979b; see also Newell & Simon, 1972). The component may translate a sensory input into a conceptual representation, transform one conceptual representation into another, or translate a conceptual representation into a motor output. Each component has three important properties associated with it that may be measured by mathematically (or simulatively) estimated parameters: *duration, difficulty*, and *probability of execution*. In other words, a given component consumes a certain amount of real time in its execution, has a certain probability of being executed correctly, and has a certain probability of being executed at all.

Components perform at least five kinds of functions (Sternberg, 1979a, 1980e): *Metacomponents* are higher-order control processes that are used for planning a course of action, for making decisions regarding alternative courses of action during reasoning or problem solving, and for monitoring the success of the chosen course of action. *Performance components* are processes that are used in the execution of a reasoning or problem-solving strategy. *Acquisition components* are processes used in learning how to reason or to solve problems. *Retention components* are processes used in retrieving previously stored knowledge, whether it be knowledge needed during reasoning or problem solving or knowledge regarding the reasoning or problem-solving algorithm itself. *Transfer components* are processes used in generalization, that is, in carrying over knowledge from one reasoning or problem-solving task to another. This chapter will concern itself primarily with components of the first two kinds (metacomponents and performance components).

Components performing each of the five kinds of functions just named can be classified according to three levels of generality (Sternberg, 1979a): *General components* are required for performance of all tasks within a given task universe; *class components* are required for performance of a proper subset of tasks that includes at least two tasks within the task universe; and *specific components* are required for the performance of single tasks within the task universe. A component's level of generality will depend upon the task universe under consideration: A component that is "general" in a very narrow range of tasks may be "class" in a broader range of tasks. The components considered in this chapter are all either general or class components in the domain of reasoning and problem-solving tasks.[1]

QUESTIONS RAISED BY THIS FRAMEWORK

This metatheoretical framework suggests a number of questions that a theory of reasoning or problem-solving performance ought to be able to answer:

1. *What kind or kinds of problems does the theory deal with*? The answer to this question would seem to be evident from the name of a theory, but my reading of the literatures on reasoning and problem solving suggests that it is almost never obvious. Theorists specify only rarely either the full universe or the subsets of the universe that are and are not covered by their theories.

How might one go about selecting tasks that are worthy of theoretical and empirical analysis? Two ways seem to have been common in the past. I will summarize them here, show ways in which they are inadequate, and propose a third way.

First, consider the task-selection procedures used by differential psychologists employing factor-analytic and other correlational techniques. Differential psychologists seem traditionally to have used either or both of two means for deciding what tasks to include in psychometric assessment batteries (Sternberg, 1979b). The first means is to sample broadly from the universe of available tasks purported to measure the construct or constructs of interest. The problem with this task-selection procedure is that it merely places the burden of task selection upon one's predecessors, who may have placed the burden on their predecessors, and so on. The second means of task selection used by differential psychologists is to choose tasks on the basis of their correlations with other tasks that are somehow related to the task of interest. If one selects only tasks that are perfectly intercorrelated with each other (across subjects), then the resulting tasks will probably differ from each other only trivially. At the other extreme, choosing tasks that are uncorrelated will result in tasks having nothing in common. A more common practice in the differential literature, especially when the investigator is evaluating correlations of tests with factors, has been to set an arbitrary lower limit, such as .30. In addition to being arbitrary, however, such a limit seems to invite consideration of a plethora of tasks, some of which may be trivial variants of other tasks and of no theoretical or practical interest in their own right. More important, this means of selecting tasks, and the one preceding it, lack any kind of theoretical motivation. We started off seeking a way in which theory would dictate or at least guide the selection of tasks. We have ended up with a statistical but atheoretical means of task selection that will dictate the scope of the theory. I do not wish to rule out correlational procedures entirely as an aid to task selection. But their function should be one of aiding rather than controlling.

Second, consider the task-selection procedures followed by information-processing psychologists using computer simulation, response time, and related procedures to understand reasoning or other psychological constructs. Newell (1973) has pointed out the dismal state of task-selection procedures among information-processing psychologists: Information-processing psychology has seemed, at times, to be a psychology more of cute tasks that have tantalized researchers than of mental phenomena in which tasks serve as a means toward understanding. We develop a psychology of "tasks" rather than of the mind. I do not wish to rule out tantalizing tasks from the domain of psychological research, nor do I wish to rule out correlational procedures. Tasks usually maintain the interests of psychologists at least in part because they can lead to theoretically fruitful lines of research. A task of no theoretical interest will probably last only a short time in the psychologists' toy chest. But the functional autonomy of tasks from psychological theory seems to serve no constructive purpose, and when tantalization dictates rather than aids task selection, it is serving an improper function.

Third, consider the means of task selection advocated here. In this approach, tasks are selected on the basis of four criteria originally proposed by Sternberg and Tulving (1977) in a different context: quantifiability, reliability, construct validity, and empirical validity (Sternberg, 1979a).

The first criterion, quantifiability, assures the possibility of the "assignment of numerals to objects or events according to rules" (Stevens, 1951, p. 1). Quantification is rarely a problem in research on reasoning. Occasionally, psychologists are content to use subjects' introspective reports or protocols as their final dependent variable. The protocols, used in and of themselves, fail the test of quantification. If, however, aspects of the protocols are quantified (see, e.g., Newell & Simon, 1972) and thus rendered subject to further analysis, these quantifications can be acceptable dependent variables so long as they meet the other three criteria.

The second criterion, reliability, measures true-score variation relative to total-score variation. In other words, it measures the extent to which a given set of data is systematic. Reliability needs to be computed in two different ways, across item types and across subjects. Because the two indexes are independent, a high value of one provides no guarantee or even indication of a high value of the other. Each of these two types of reliability can be measured in two ways, at a given time or over time.

The third criterion, construct validity, assures that the task has been chosen on the basis of some psychological theory. The theory thus dictates the choice of tasks, rather than the other way around. A task that is construct-valid is useful for gaining psychological insights through the lens provided by some theory of cognition.

The fourth criterion, empirical validity, assures that the task serves the purpose in the theory that it is supposed to serve. Thus, whereas construct validity guarantees that the selection of a task is motivated by theory, empirical validity tests the extent to which the theory is empirically supportable. Empirical validation is usually performed by correlating task performance with an external criterion.

2. *What performance components are posited by the theory?* A theory of reasoning or problem solving should state the performance components required for or optionally used in the solution of items of the kinds accounted for by the theory. Investigators differ, of course, in the source of their ideas regarding the components used. They may do an implicit task analysis by going through a task themselves; they may use verbal reports supplied by subjects after testing; they may use thinking-aloud protocols supplied by subjects during testing; they may use their intuitions to expand or modify previous theories.

One of the first things an investigator will want to test is whether the performance components posited by the theory as being involved in task performance are indeed used by subjects performing the reasoning or problem-solving task. A mathematical parameter can be assigned to each information-processing component in a given theory. Parameters may be of three kinds: Latency parameters represent the duration of each component; error parameters represent the difficulty of each component; probability parameters represent the probability that the component will be executed in a given task situation. A given model assumes that parameters of a given kind combine in a specific fashion. The combination rule is usually testable (see Sternberg, 1977b).

Response time is hypothesized to equal the sum of the amounts of time spent on each of the various components. Hence a simple linear model predicts response time to be the sum across the various components of the number of times each component is performed (as an independent variable) multiplied by the duration of that component (as an estimated parameter) (Sternberg, 1977a).

Proportion of response errors is hypothesized to equal the (appropriately scaled) sum of the difficulties encountered in executing each component. A simple linear model predicts proportion of errors to equal the sum across the different components of the number of times each component is performed (as an independent variable) multiplied by the difficulty of that component (as an estimated parameter). This additive combination rule is based upon the assumption that each subject has a limit on processing capacity (or space; see Osherson, 1974). Each execution of a component uses up capacity. Until the limit is exceeded, performance is flawless except for constant sources of error (such as motor confusion, carelessness, momentary distraction, etc.). Once the limit is exceeded, however, performance is at a chance level (Sternberg, 1977a).

An alternative model of item difficulty is linear with respect to logarithms of item-easiness values rather than with respect to the raw easiness (or difficulty) values. In this model, the probability of answering an item correctly is equal to the product of the probabilities of performing each of the components correctly. For example, if there are two components that are theorized to be involved in performance of a task, and the probabilities of executing the two components correctly are .90 and .60, respectively, the probability of answering the problem correctly is .90 × .60, or .54. Stated in another way, the log of the probability of answering the problem correctly is equal to the sum of the logs of the probabilities of performing each of the components correctly. Although this model of item difficulty is probably the more widely used in information-processing research, I think it is often inappropriate in the domain of reasoning, and probably in many other domains as well. The model assumes that probabilities of erroneous (or correct) executions of components are independent across components.

The probability of choosing a particular one of the various possible responses to a problem is assumed to be equal to the sum of the probabilities of using or combining components in each of the possible ways that can lead to that response. Obviously, the probabilities for the various responses to the problem must sum to unity.

Information-processing components can be isolated through a number of techniques, some of which are described in Sternberg (1978b). Means for evaluating the success of these and other techniques are described in Sternberg (1978c).

3. *Upon what representation or representations do these components act?* I doubt that there is any known test that is reasonably conclusive in distinguishing one representation for information from another. Empirical tests of alternative represen-

tations always make assumptions about information processing, because observable behavior is always the result of some set of processes acting upon some representation or representations. An information-processing model can be shown to be wrong, but can never be shown to be right, because some other information-processing model may make the same empirical predictions as a model that is not falsified. If the information-processing assumptions underlying a test of representation are wrong, then the test of the representation is of dubious validity. But if the information-processing assumptions underlying a test are not falsified, it is still possible for the representation to be wrong, because the processing assumptions may not be correct, or an alternative representation may exist that performs as well or better under the nonfalsified processing assumptions. At best, then, one can argue for the plausibility of a representation, but not for its ultimate correctness.

4. *By what combination rule or rules are the components combined?* By combination rule, I refer to the order in which components are combined, and to the use of serial versus parallel processing, exhaustive versus self-terminating processing, and independent versus nonindependent processes. The items in these latter three distinctions can be referred to as the "mode" of information processing. Order and mode apply to execution of different components, and to multiple executions of the same component.

Consider first the combination of different component processes. Suppose that two component processes, x and y, are used in the solution of a reasoning or problem-solving item. These components may be executed in either of two (2!) different orders. Moreover, the components may be executed in various modes: First, the processes may be executed serially (x, then y) or in parallel (x and y simultaneous). If, for example, x is inference from A to B in an analogy of the form A is to B as C is to D, and y is mapping from A to C, then either mapping may be executed immediately after inference is executed, or the two operations may be done simultaneously. When more than two processes are involved, some combination of serial and parallel processing may be used. Second, the processes may be executed exhaustively (both x and y always performed) or with self-termination (y executed only if execution of x fails to yield a solution). For example, in the analogy *He* is to *she* as *him* is to (a. *hers*, b. *theirs*), application of the rule that connects *he* to *she* from *him* to each answer option will probably fail to yield a solution, because neither option is quite ideal. But justification of one option as preferable to the other but nonideal will yield *hers* as the preferred solution. In this case, justification is needed only if application fails to solve the analogy. Third, execution of each process may be independent of execution of each other process (the use or amount of use of x is uncorrelated across item types with the use or amount of use of y) or nonindependent of execution of each other process (the use or amount of use of x is correlated across item types with the use or amount of use of y). For example, if the number of attributes to be inferred from A to B of an analogy is correlated with the number of attributes to be mapped from A to C, the amounts of use of inference and mapping will be nonindependent: Larger numbers of inferences will be associated with larger numbers of mappings. Processes that are maximally nonindependent (perfectly correlated) in occurrence will be completely confounded, and hence incapable of being disentangled experimentally. Optimal distinguishability between processes occurs when their use is uncorrelated across item types. The same distinctions that apply for executions of different component processes apply as well for multiple executions of the same component process.

5. *What are the durations, difficulties, and probabilities of component execution?* A complete theory of human reasoning or problem solving should be able to specify not only the component processes used in reasoning or problem solving, but also the durations, difficulties, and probabilities of execution of these components. Component properties depend upon many facets of the task and its context. Thus the absolute durations of various component processes are of some interest in themselves, but are of less interest than the durations of certain processes relative to certain other processes or the duration of a given process under a variety of experimental conditions. Durations, difficulties, and probabilities of component executions can all be estimated as parameter values via mathematical modeling or computer simulation.

6. *What metacomponents are used in this form of reasoning?* I have identified six metacomponents used in reasoning and problem solving (Sternberg, 1980e): selection of performance components for task solution, selection of one or more representations upon which these components are to act, selection of a strategy for combining the components, decision about whether to maintain a given strategy, selection of a speed–accuracy trade-off, and solution monitoring (i.e., keeping track of progress being made toward a solution). Metacomponents activate and receive feedback from the other kinds of components. Brown (1978) and Brown and DeLoache (1978) have suggested an overlapping list. Are metacomponents really needed in a theory of reasoning or problem solving? Various kinds of "meta" have become fashionable in today's research, and one might well wonder whether they are anything more than a passing fashion. Several lines of evidence suggest that metacomponents really are needed, however (see Sternberg, 1980e). Methods for isolating them are described in Sternberg (1979c).

7. *What are the effects of (a) problem format, (b) problem content, and (c) practice upon reasoning and problem solving?* Effects of problem format, content, and practice upon reasoning and problem solving can be inferred from separate internal and external validation of data for different levels of each of these variables.

Internal validation consists of the attempt to explain between-items stimulus variation in terms of an underlying model of task performance. The internal validation procedure should be applied separately to each problem format, content, and level of practice of interest. Use of these procedures for each level of each variable of interest enables one to determine specific effects of each level, for example, whether the strategy used later in practice is the same as the one used earlier in practice. *External validation* consists of the attempt to explain between-subjects variation in terms of performance on previously validated measures that are outside the immediate paradigm of interest. The external validation procedure should be applied so that separate correlations of various scores from the experimental task and the reference tests are computed for each format, content, and level of practice. If the results of internal and external validation converge, one has a strong case for the particular argument being made. If the results diverge, alternative explanations of the obtained data must be considered.

8. *What are salient sources of individual differences in reasoning or problem solving at a given age level, and how do these sources of individual differences manifest themselves?* Again, there are two ways to answer this question – from the standpoint of internal validation and from the standpoint of external validation. Investigation of individual differences via internal validation is facilitated if it is possible to model individual data just as one models group data. Such modeling is

usually possible for latency data if each individual contributes observations to each item data point; it is usually not possible for error and response-choice data, simply because the number of observations needed to obtain reliable probability data is prohibitive for individual subjects. If individual data are available and sufficiently reliable, one treats each individual subject as a level of a subjects variable, just as one might treat each individual item content as a level of a content variable. It is thus possible to observe what aspects of the modeling are salient sources of variation across subjects, such as the components used; the representations upon which the components act; the strategy or strategies by which components are combined; the durations, difficulties or probabilities of execution; the consistency with which strategies are used; and so on. Investigation of individual differences via external validation involves the demonstration that identified sources of individual differences are related to patterns of individual differences in external criteria. Thus, whereas internal validation localizes the sources of variation, external validation helps interpret them and test their generalizability beyond the experimental task or tasks being investigated.

9. *What are significant sources of cognitive development in reasoning or problem solving across age levels, and how do these sources manifest themselves?* The sources of cognitive development, or differences across age levels, are the same as those within age levels, although the importance of various sources of individual-differences variation may be different across age levels and within age levels. In the present case, one treats the data of subjects at each age as a level of an age variable. Instructions, and sometimes the task, must be made suitable for the various age levels. For example, an analogies test that measures reasoning at a higher age level might well measure vocabulary at a lower age level.

An understanding of the development of reasoning and problem solving requires an understanding of how acquisition, retention, and transfer components operate in reasoning and problem-solving tasks, and of how these kinds of components and the various other kinds of components interrelate.

In general, acquisition (retention, or transfer) of a reasoning or problem-solving skill will be facilitated by factors such as increased need for the skill, variability of reasoning or problem-solving contexts in which the skill is required, importance of the skill to solving the reasoning or problem-solving item, recency of need for the skill, helpfulness for the performance of the skill of the reasoning or problem-solving context in which the skill is required, and helpfulness of previously stored information to the implementation of the skill in the reasoning or problem-solving situation (see Sternberg, 1979a). The importance of one or another factor will vary with the particular skill and the particular context in which the skill is required.

10. *What is the relationship between a given form of reasoning and other forms of reasoning?* The question posed here is one of how an investigator demonstrates commonalities between tasks in the various kinds of components and in the representations and strategies used in reasoning and problem solving. At least four tests of identity between pairs of constructs can be employed. Outcomes of these tests can suggest, but not prove, identity. First, one can demonstrate that the same information-processing model applies across tasks. Second, one can test whether values of a given parameter differ significantly across tasks; if the values do not differ, the plausibility of the argument that the parameter is the same in each task is increased. Third, one can show that any manipulation that has a certain effect upon a given component in one task has a comparable effect upon a given component in another

task. Fourth, one can show that the correlation across subjects between two parameters in two tasks is close to perfect (or, in theory, to the reliability of measurement of subjects' scores).

11. *What is the relationship between a given form of reasoning or problem solving and general intelligence?* In order to investigate this relationship, one uses the external validation strategy described earlier for relating one form of reasoning to another. One correlates performance on the task, or the components of the task, with general intelligence as measured by some test or tests that satisfy the investigator's criteria for an acceptable index of intelligence. (See Sternberg, 1977b, 1979a, 1979b, 1980a, for my own proposed conceptualization of intelligence.)

12. *What are the practical implications of what we know about a particular kind of reasoning or problem solving?* Some investigators would argue that practical implications are of no interest to them. I believe that a theory or task is of no interest if, ultimately, it bears no relation at all to practical concerns. The relation may be only tenuous at a given time, or the practical implications of a theory may be of the sort that will become clear only after a long period of time. But I do not think the issue of practical applications should be ignored altogether, lest we find ourselves studying arcane and obscure tasks that have no interest to anyone except ourselves. Unfortunately, we presently know almost nothing about the relations of components of laboratory tasks to real-world performance.

Consider how the metatheoretical framework described in this section might be applied to diagnostic and prescriptive problems in educational theory and practice.

Suppose we know that a certain child is a poor reasoner. We might know this because of the child's low scores on psychometric tests of reasoning ability or because of the child's poor performance in school on problems requiring various kinds of reasoning. The kinds of analyses suggested here yield a number of indexes for each child (or adult) that can help localize the source of difficulty. These sources correspond to the basic sources of individual differences already described. One can discover whether certain components needed to solve one or more kinds of reasoning problems are unavailable, or available but not accessed when needed; whether the child is using a suboptimal strategy – that is, one that is time-consuming, inaccurate, or unable to yield any solution at all; whether the child finds execution of certain components especially difficult or time-consuming; whether the child is inconsistent in his or her use of strategy; or whether the child fails in metacomponential decision making about problem solution.

In the prescriptive domain, the first question to be addressed is whether a given information-processing strategy can be taught. One can find this out by teaching the strategy to a group of subjects, modeling the subjects' data, and determining whether the pattern of response time or error rate data conforms to the predictions of the model. The data for each individual subject, as well as for the group, can be modeled on this basis. This kind of quantitative modeling procedure makes it possible to perform a very direct test of whether subjects have learned a particular model of information processing, in that one actually assesses exact fit between predictions and data. The fit of the trained strategy model to the data can be assessed through external as well as internal validation techniques. If, for example, subjects are taught to use a model of reasoning that is essentially spatial in nature, certain component scores should be theorized to correlate with scores on standard psychometric tests of spatial ability. The second question to be addressed is whether a particular model of information processing is more efficacious, on the average, than alternative models. The question can be answered simply by comparing response times and error rates under various training conditions that have been demonstrated to be successful in imparting the proposed strategy model to the subjects. A third question is whether certain strategies are more efficacious for people with certain patterns of abilities, whereas other strategies are more efficacious for people with different patterns of abilities. This question can be answered through either correlational or analysis-of-variance methodology. In the former methodology, task or component scores are correlated with scores on standard ability tests. If scores obtained using one strategy show high correlations with one kind of ability, and scores obtained using another strategy show high correlations with a different kind of ability, then one has evidence that the efficacy of a given strategy depends upon the ability pattern of the subjects using that strategy. In the latter methodology, one compares latency or error scores for subjects high and low in targeted abilities under various strategy training conditions, searching for an interaction between the strategy and aptitude patterns of the subjects. Interactions can be particularly strong when there are reasonably large proportions of subjects who are high in an ability called for by one strategy and low in an ability called for by another strategy, and vice versa.

The twelve questions just posed are obviously not the only ones that might be asked, nor are they necessarily the "right" ones to ask. They do seem to provide, however, a reasonable basis for testing the completeness of a theory of reasoning or problem solving falling under the general metatheoretical framework outlined in the first part of this section.

5.2.   REASONING AND INTELLIGENCE

Reasoning may be characterized as an attempt to combine elements of old information to form new information. The old information may be external (from books, magazines, newspapers, television, etc.), internal (stored in memory), or a combination of the two. The new information may be implicit but not obvious in the old information, as is the case when deductive reasoning is performed, or it may be nowhere contained in the old information, as is the case when inductive reasoning is performed. Although it can be shown that the distinction between deduction (reasoning from given premises to a logically certain conclusion) and induction (reasoning from given premises to a reasonable but logically uncertain conclusion) is actually a fuzzy one (Skyrms, 1975), I shall maintain the distinction here as a matter of convenience, much as a distinction is maintained between reasoning and problem solving.

INDUCTIVE REASONING

The scope of inductive reasoning

In inductive reasoning, the information contained in the premises of a problem is insufficient to reach a conclusion. As a result, one can reach inductively probable conclusions, but not deductively certain ones. A number of different kinds of inductive-reasoning problems have been studied, among them:

1. *Analogies,* for example, *lawyer* is to *client* as *doctor* is to ? Analogies can be composed from any of a number of different kinds of content (e.g., verbal, geometric,

schematic-picture) and any of a number of different kinds of formats (e.g., fill-in-the-blank, true–false, multiple-choice). Although it is usually the last term that the subject has to induce, analogies can be presented in formats where one of the other terms is missing, or even where several of the other terms are missing (e.g., Lunzer, 1965). Reviews of the literature on analogical reasoning can be found in Dawis and Siojo (1972) and in Sternberg (1977b), as well as later on in this chapter. Among the original reports of theory and research on analogical reasoning are those of Ace and Dawis (1973); Achenbach (1970a, 1970b, 1971); Evans (1968); Feuerstein (1979); Gallagher and Wright (1977, 1979); Gentile, Kessler, and Gentile (1969); Gentile, Tedesco-Stratton, Davis, Lund, and Agunanne (1977); Grudin (1980); Johnson (1962); Kling (1971); Levinson and Carpenter (1974); Lunzer (1965); Meer, Stein, and Geertsma (1955); Mulholland, Pellegrino, and Glaser (1980); Reitman (1965); Rips, Shoben, and Smith (1973); Rumelhart and Abrahamson (1973); Shalom and Schlesinger (1972); Spearman (1923); Sternberg (1977a, 1977b); Sternberg and Gardner (1982); Sternberg and Nigro (1980); Sternberg and Rifkin (1979); Tinsley and Dawis (1972); Whitely (1973, 1977, 1979a, 1979b); Whitely and Barnes (1979); Whitely and Dawis (1973, 1974); Williams (1972); Willner (1964); and Winston (1970). This set of references does not include those from the voluminous literature on matrix problems, which are similar, but not identical, to analogies.

2. *Series completions,* for example, 2, 5, 8, 11, ? Series completions, like analogies, can be composed for a variety of contents (e.g., verbal, geometric, numerical, schematic-picture) and can be stated in any of a number of different forms (e.g., fill-in-the-blank, true–false, multiple-choice). Usually the subject's task is to fill in the term following the last given one (extrapolation task), although one or more terms may be missing from the middle rather than from the end of the series (interpolation task). A review of the literature can be found in Jones (1971). Some of the original theoretical and empirical reports on series completions include those of Egan and Greeno (1974); Ernst and Newell (1969); Gregg (1967); Holzman, Glaser, and Pellegrino (1976); Jones (1971); Klahr and Wallace (1970); Kotovsky and Simon (1973); Lashley (1951); Leeuwenberg (1969); Pellegrino and Glaser (1980); Psotka (1975, 1977); Restle (1967, 1970, 1972); Restle and Brown (1970a, 1970b); Simon (1972); Simon and Kotovsky (1963); Simon and Lea (1974); Simon and Newell (1974); Simon and Sumner (1968); Sternberg (1979b); Sternberg and Gardner (1982); Thurstone (1938); Vitz and Todd (1969); and Williams (1972).

3. *Classifications,* for example, "Which of the following words does not belong with the others? *cat, elephant, unicorn, wolf.*" Classifications can be presented in verbal form, or in any of the forms applicable to the other kinds of induction problems already considered (numbers, geometric forms, schematic pictures). Although the problems are usually presented in the "odd-man-out" format used in the example, they are sometimes presented so that subjects are required to find more than one item that does not belong with the others (e.g., Cattell & Cattell, 1963), or so that subjects are required to indicate which of several answer options fits best with a set of given items (e.g., Sternberg & Gardner, 1982).

For whatever reason, the psychometric classification task has not been subjected to a great deal of experimental analysis. This is surprising, because its role in the psychometric tradition has been as prominent as that of series completions, and because the processes involved in this kind of problem would seem to be of equal interest. Although the problem in its psychometric form has not been widely studied, there has been enormous interest in the psychological literature on classificatory and categorization behavior. Some perceptual approaches to this area are reviewed in Reed (1972), and some conceptual approaches are reviewed in Rosch (1977). Some original reports that deal with the psychometric classification problem are those of Pellegrino and Glaser (1980), Sternberg (1979b), Sternberg and Gardner (1982), and Whitely (1979a, 1979b).

These three kinds of induction problems are not the only ones that have been studied, of course. A large literature exists on matrix problems (e.g., H. Burke, 1958; Esher, Raven, & Earl, 1942; Gabriel, 1954; Hunt, 1974; Jacobs & Vandeventer, 1971a, 1971b, 1972; Linn, 1973), as well as on causal inference (e.g., Ajzen, 1977; Carroll & Siegler, 1977; Chapman, 1967; Chapman & Chapman, 1967, 1969; Fischhoff, 1976; Gollob, Rossman, & Abelson, 1973; Kelley, 1967, 1972; Lyon & Slovic, 1976; Mill, 1843; Nisbett & Borgida, 1975; Nisbett, Borgida, Crandall, & Reed, 1976; Nisbett & Ross, 1979; Scriven, 1976; Smedslund, 1963; Taylor & Fiske, 1978; Tversky & Kahneman, 1974, 1977; Wason, 1968; Wason & Johnson-Laird, 1972). Other kinds of induction problems have been and might be studied as well, some of which at first glance do not even appear to be induction problems. Metaphorical comprehension, for example, can be seen as a special case of inductive reasoning (Miller, 1979; Sternberg, Tourangeau, & Nigro, 1979; Tourangeau & Sternberg, 1981). For the purposes of the present review it will be sufficient to present a case study of just one kind of inductive reasoning that psychologists of all persuasions seem to agree is a critical element of intelligence, reasoning by analogy.

A case study of inductive reasoning: the analogy

NATURE OF THE PROBLEM.   An analogy is a problem of the form *A* is to *B* as *C* is to *D* (*A:B: :C:D*), where, in most instances, the last term is omitted and must be filled in, selected from among answer options, or confirmed in a true–false situation. An analogy can be made arbitrarily difficult by making the terms difficult to encode. For example, the analogy *Philology: languages: :mycology:*(a. *flowering plants*, b. *ferns*, c. *weeds*, d. *fungi*) requires only minimal reasoning ability, but is difficult because very few people know that *mycology* is the study of fungi. Analogies that derive their difficulty from the complexity of the terms rather than from the relations between terms or between relations do not necessarily measure inductive-reasoning ability (see Sternberg, 1977b). Our concern here will be with analogies that derive their difficulty from their reasoning aspects rather than from their vocabulary aspects.

Performance on analogies satisfies the four criteria described in the preceding section of the chapter. First, performance can be quantified in terms of response latency, error rate, or distribution of responses given among the possible responses that might be given. Second, performance on analogical reasoning tasks can be measured reliably. Sternberg (1977a) reported reliabilities across items of .97 and .89 for people-piece and geometric analogies respectively, and standard psychometric tests including sections measuring analogical reasoning typically report reliabilities across subjects in the .80s and .90s (e.g., Miller Analogies Test Manual, 1970). The construct validity of performance on tests of analogical reasoning is unimpeachable. One of the first theorists of general intelligence, Spearman (1923), used analogies as the prototypes for intelligent performance. Spearman exemplified his three basic principles of cognition through the use of the analogy. The ability to perceive second-order relations, or relations between relations, has served as the touchstone marking the transition between concrete and formal operations in Piaget's (1970) theory of intelligence; and analogies, because they require the ability to perceive relations between relations for their solution, can serve as a useful measure for distinguishing concrete-operational from formal-operational children (Sternberg & Rifkin, 1979). Finally, analogies have played a major role in information-processing theories of intelligence. Reitman (1965) and Sternberg (1977b) have used analogies as cornerstones for information-processing theories of intelligence, and other investigators have also seen analogies as fundamental to information-processing notions of intelligence (e.g., Pellegrino & Glaser, 1980; Whitely, 1979a, 1979b). Thus analogies have played a central part in the theorizing of differential, Piagetian, and information-processing theories of intelligence. Indeed, at least two books have been written that deal almost exclusively with analogies and their relationship to intelligence (Piaget with Montangero & Billeter, 1977; Sternberg, 1977b).

PERFORMANCE COMPONENTS.   All theorists seem to agree that analogical reasoners must *encode* analogy terms, that is, translate them into internal representations upon which further mental operations can be performed, and that these reasoners must complete analogy solution by *responding* with an answer to a given problem. Theorists have expressed their major disagreement over the roles of three intermediate comparison operations, called *inference, mapping,* and *application,* and over whether any additional operations need to be added to this list. Consider first the disagreements revolving around these three critical operations. I will use as an example analogy *lawyer:client: :doctor:*(a. *patient,* b. *medicine*).

A first theory claims that inference, mapping, and application, as well as encoding and response, are all used in analogy solution. The reasoner (a) encodes the terms of the analogy, (b) infers the relation between *lawyer* and *client* (a lawyer renders professional services to a client), (c) maps the higher-order relation between the first half of the analogy and the second (both deal with individuals who render professional services), (d) applies a relation analogous to the inferred one from *doctor* to each answer option, choosing the correct option (a *doctor* renders professional services to a *patient,* not to a *medicine*), and (e) responds (Sternberg, 1977a, 1977b). A second theory claims that only inference and application, in addition to encoding and response, are used in analogy solution; mapping is not used (Johnson, 1962; Shalom & Schlesinger, 1972; Spearman, 1923). The various theorists use different labels for what are here called inference and application. Johnson refers to the inductive operation and the deductive operation, Shalom and Schlesinger to the formation of the connection formula and the application of the connection formula, and Spearman to the eduction of relations and the eduction of correlates. A third theory claims that inference and mapping, but not application, are used in analogy solution. In this theory mapping of the higher-order relation between the two halves of the analogy, rather than application, is used as the final comparison operation that determines which answer correctly solves the analogy (Evans, 1968; Winston, 1970).

Whitely and Barnes (1979) have argued that application in fact needs to be split into two subcomponents. In the first, which retains the name *application,* the subject uses the relation inferred in the domain (first half) of the analogy as mapped to the range (second half) of the analogy to form a conception of the ideal solution. In the second subcomponent, which Whitely and Barnes call *confirmation,* the subject compares each of the answer options (in analogy formats where answer options are indeed presented) to the ideal solution. This modification was originally proposed by

Sternberg (1977b, pp. 192–193) and rejected. Sternberg and Gardner (1982) have agreed with Whitely and Barnes, however, that application should be subdivided. Like Whitely and Barnes, they have referred to the construction of the ideal solution as *application;* they have referred to the comparison of each given option to the other options as *comparison,* following Sternberg (1977b).

Sternberg (1977b) has argued that an additional, optional operation needs to be added in order to complete the theories described. This operation is one of *justification.* It is used when none of a set of presented answer options is perceived as strictly "correct." In this event, the subject justifies one answer as closest to the ideal of the available options.

REPRESENTATION OF INFORMATION. A wide variety of specific representations of information in analogical reasoning have been proposed by various theorists. One reason for this variety is that analogy-solving computer programs have been a favorite among those with interests in computer simulation and artificial intelligence (e.g., Evans, 1968; Reitman, 1965; Williams, 1972; Winston, 1970), and computer theories require a detailed specification of representation. Each computer program, of course, uses a representation that differs at least somewhat from that of other computer programs. However, if we consider only general classes of representations, rather than specific examples of these classes, we find that two major classes of representations have been proposed: an attribute-value representation and a spatial representation. My current belief is that in solving analogies, subjects probably draw to some extent upon both kinds of representations, and possibly upon other kinds of representations as well: The subjects perceive their task as one of solving analogies, and will represent information in whatever way or ways will elucidate relationships between terms or between pairs of terms. If theorists of analogical reasoning can conceive of alternative ways of representing information for the solution of a given analogy, there is no reason to believe that subjects cannot do likewise. Ultimately, it is quite possible that different "surface" representations are intermappable into a single "deep" representation.

An *attribute-value representation* of one kind or another has been used by all of the computer theorists and by Sternberg (1977a, 1977b). Consider, for example, how an attribute-value representation could account for the representation of information during the solution of the analogy *Washington:1: :Lincoln:*(a. 10, b. 5) (Sternberg, 1977a):

Washington might be encoded as [(president (first)), (portrait on currency (dollar)), (war hero (Revolutionary))]

1 might be encoded as [(counting number (1)), (ordinal position (1st)), (amount (1 unit))]

Lincoln might be encoded as [(president (16th)), (portrait on currency ($5)), (war hero (Civil))]

10 might be encoded as [(counting number (10)), (ordinal position (10th)), (amount (10 units))]

5 might be encoded as [(counting number (5)), (ordinal position (5th)), (amount (5 units))]

The attribute-value representation can be extended to pictorial as well as verbal kinds of items. A black square inside a white circle, for example, might be represented as [(shape (square)), (position (surrounded)), (color (black))], [(shape (circle)), (position (surrounding)), (color (white))]. The attribute-value representation can also be extended to continuous values. Terms of animal-name analogies, for example, such as *tiger* in the analogy *tiger:cat: :wolf:*(a. *zebra*, b. *dog*), can be represented in the form [(size (x)), (ferocity (y)), (humanness (z))], where x, y, and z represent amounts of size, ferocity, and humanness, respectively.

A *spatial representation* of information has been used by Rumelhart and Abrahamson (1973); Rips, Shoben, and Smith (1973); and Sternberg and Gardner (1982). In each case the domain of stimuli has consisted of animal names, although Rumelhart and Abrahamson reported that they had formulated analogies based upon terms of a color space, with equal success. The spatial representation assumes that for each term of an analogy problem, one can locate a point in a multidimensional conceptual space, and that for any analogy problem of the form $A:B: :C:?$ there exists an ideal solution point in the multidimensional space that serves as the optimal completion of the analogy. It has been found that a three-dimensional space, with dimensions of size, ferocity, and humanness, well represents a large set of mammal names (Henley, 1969).

No one has directly tested the validities of these alternative representations for information, nor is it clear how their validity could be tested directly: Representations have been assumed rather than tested.

COMBINATION RULES.   Investigators have sought to test models predicting response latencies, response errors, and response choices. Because different combination rules have been used in each case, each will be considered separately.

Consider first the prediction of *response latencies* via models of real-time information processing. Sternberg (1977a) tested the three basic theories of analogical reasoning described earlier, using justification where appropriate. Application had been split into the two subcomponents in model tests for one of three experiments (see Sternberg, 1977b), but because model performance with the additional parameter clearly did not warrant addition of the extra parameter, use of comparison was discontinued. All models were assumed to be strictly linear and additive. Sternberg's (1977a) data supported the theory with all three of the operations, inference, mapping, and application.

Sternberg (1977a, 1977b) compared four variants of the proposed model that differed in the order and mode of component execution. In each case information processing was assumed to be strictly serial (mostly as a matter of convenience and simplicity), and parallel models were not tested; executions of the various processes demanded by the problems were manipulated in order to remove significant dependencies. All variants of the basic model assumed that encoding of all attribute-values of a given term occurred in immediate succession. Models differed in which of the operations – inference, mapping, and application – were exhaustive and which were self-terminating. The data were interpreted as giving strongest support to a variant in which inference was exhaustive and mapping and application were self-terminating. Values of R^2 were .92, .86, and .80 for people-piece, verbal, and geometric analogies, respectively. Slightly less support went to a model in which inference, mapping, and application were all self-terminating. Much less support went to two other models. A subsequent experiment with people-piece stimuli confirmed this order of model fits (Sternberg & Rifkin, 1979).

Mulholland and his associates (1980) also tested fits of models to latency data, in their case for geometric analogies. Their model differed in form from those discussed previously in that it separated out only encoding, transformation operations (e.g., inference), and response. A simple additive model accounted for 95% of the variance in the latency data. When an interaction term was added that multiplied the number of attribute values to be encoded by the number of attribute values to be compared, model fit increased slightly but significantly. The investigators argued that the interaction should be taken into account, at least for large numbers of subjects. The interaction term suggests that encoding and comparison do not proceed independently.

Sternberg and Nigro (1980) fitted alternative models to latency data for verbal analogies that were constructed from a wide variety of possible conceptual relations. These investigators were particularly interested in what role, if any, word association plays in the solution of verbal analogies. With just three parameters – encoding, justification, and response (which were used for consistency in numbers of parameters across the age levels that were studied) – Sternberg and Nigro were able to account for 85% of the variance in their adults' latency data. Word association was found to play no significant role in the solution processes of the adult subjects.

Sternberg and Gardner (1982) fitted a mathematical model to latency data obtained from subjects solving animal-name analogies. These authors were the first to use independent variables in prediction of latency data that were based upon a spatial representation (in contrast to the preceding studies, which all assumed attribute-value representations). Their model, which included only encoding, comparison, justification, and response (for comparability to other induction tasks that were studied) accounted for 77% of the variance in the latency data.

Consider next the prediction of *error rates* in analogy solution. Several investigators have sought to predict the bases for differential error rates across their various item types.

Sternberg (1977a, 1977b) used the same basic additive model to predict error rates that he had used to predict solution latencies. The only difference was in the dependent variable. Proportion of response errors was hypothesized to equal the (appropriately scaled) sum of the difficulties encountered in executing each component operation. A simple linear model predicted proportion of errors to be the sum across the different component operations of the number of times each component operation is executed (as an independent variable) multiplied by the difficulty of that component operation (as an estimated parameter). The model was successful in accounting for error rates in people-piece and geometric analogy experiments, but not in a verbal analogies experiment. Values of R^2 were .59, .50, and .12 in the three respective experiments.

Mulholland and his colleagues (1980) used a different model to account for their error data. These investigators claimed that their data showed independence and additivity of error probabilities associated with separately transformed elements. Error rates can thus be understood as the simple accumulation of independent, incorrect executions of information processes, any one of which leads to an error in response. The authors' logarithmic model accounted for an impressive 93% of the variance in their error data. The one thing to keep in mind in using or evaluating a model such as this one is that probabilities of errors owing to different kinds of accumulated operations must be independent. Such a model would not be tenable if certain operations depended for their validity upon other, earlier-executed operations, for example, if application depends upon inference, and both inference and application depend upon encoding.

Consider finally the prediction of probabilities of various *response choices* in analogy solution. The first ones to predict response choices were Rumelhart and Abrahamson (1973). These authors used animal-name analogies and had subjects rank order options. They assumed that information could be represented in a multidimensional space. In order to predict response choices, Rumelhart and Abrahamson adapted Luce's (1959) choice rule to the choice situation in the analogy; the details of this choice rule need not concern us here. They further specified that the monotone decrease in the likelihood of choosing as best a particular answer option x_i follows an exponential decay function with increasing distance from the ideal point (best possible solution in a multidimensional space) of the analogy. Finally, they specified that once subjects have ranked a given alternative as first, they reapply the choice rule to the remaining alternatives to choose an option as second ranked, and continue to reapply the rules until all options have been rank ordered. Rumelhart and Abrahamson conducted three ingenious experiments designed to test the validity of their model of response choice in analogical reasoning. In the first experiment, they set out to demonstrate that subjects rank order options in accordance with the assumptions just described. In a second experiment, they tested the prediction of their model that the probability of choosing any particular response alternative x_i as the best alternative depends upon the ideal solution point and upon the alternative set, but not upon the particular terms in the analogy itself. Thus all possible analogies with a given ideal point and alternative set should yield the same distribution of responses over the alternatives, regardless of the terms of the analogy. The data from the second experiment were somewhat consistent with the prediction. The third experiment used a concept-formation design in which subjects were required to acquire concepts for three new mammals, "bof," "dax," and "zuk." Subjects were taught these new concepts by an anticipation method. Rumelhart and Abrahamson found that after about five learning trials, subjects were able to use the imaginary mammal names just as they were able to use regular mammal names in solving analogies.

Sternberg and Gardner (1982) replicated Rumelhart and Abrahamson's Experiment 1 in the context of an experiment designed to show interrelationships between various forms of inductive reasoning. Their model fits were highly comparable to those of Rumelhart and Abrahamson, providing further support for the validity of the response-choice model under the assumption of a multidimensional representation of information.

DURATIONS, DIFFICULTIES, AND PROBABILITIES OF COMPONENT EXECUTION.   Consider first *durations* of component execution. For maximum interpretability, I shall consider durations as the amounts of time spent per component per problem, rather than the amount spent per attribute or some other unit that depends upon the form of representation used. Consider, for example, the data of Sternberg (1977a, 1977b). Sternberg estimated latency parameters in each of his people-piece, verbal, and geometric analogy experiments. Estimates were for the model found to provide the best fit to the data – the one with inference, mapping, and application – and for the model variant found to provide the best fit – the one with inference exhaustive, and mapping and application self-terminating. Several aspects of the parameter estimates are worth mentioning. First, as would be expected, performance components are of longer durations for analogies with successively greater overall latencies, except for response, which is and should be approximately constant, regardless of the difficulty of the analogies. Second, encoding of analogy terms takes the greatest proportion of time in every case, even though its absolute time changes considerably with item content. Third, the amount of time spent in analyzing relations between attributes was relatively short in the people-piece experiment (30%) and in the verbal analogy experiment (29%), where simple, obvious attributes were used, but relatively long in the geometric analogies experiment (57%), where the attributes were much less obvious. Finally, although the amount of time spent on response was about the same in each case, the proportion of time decreased considerably as analogy difficulty increased.

Next consider *difficulties* of component execution. Sternberg (1977b) found that only self-terminating components contributed significantly to the prediction of error rates for the people-piece analogies. In other words, errors were due for the most part to incomplete processing in self-terminating components.

Consider finally parameter estimates obtained in the prediction of the probability distribution for *response choices* in analogical reasoning. Rumelhart and Abrahamson (1973), on the one hand, and Sternberg and Gardner (1982), on the other, obtained similar values of α, the slope of an exponential function, for the same analogies administered to different subjects.

METACOMPONENTS. Consider again the six metacomponents of reasoning and problem solving identified earlier, and what we know about each of them in the domain of analogical reasoning.

Selection of performance components. All of the adults I have studied in a number of experiments on analogical reasoning have been willing and able to select components of analogical reasoning from the full set described earlier. Although some subjects may select only a subset of the components in the full model for use during analogical reasoning, this seems primarily to be a matter of choice rather than of component availability: The components required for analogical reasoning seem to be accessible to most adults of normal mental capacity.

Selection of representation(s). People seem to be able to use alternative or even multiple representations for information in analogical reasoning. Sternberg (1977b), for example, reported that an additive (overlapping) clustering representation actually provided a better fit to the group error-rate data for mammal-name analogies than did a spatial representation. In an additive clustering representation, mammals are grouped in clusters such as "rodent pests" (rat, mouse), "cat family" (cat, lion, tiger, leopard), "doglike animals" (dog, wolf, fox), "wild predators" (cat, lion, tiger, leopard, wolf, fox), and so on (Shepard & Arabie, 1979). In the Sternberg (1977b) data, the additive clustering model proposed accounted for 56% of the variance in the error data, whereas the spatial model proposed accounted for only 28%. Michael Gardner and I have replicated this finding for the same analogies but for different subjects in unpublished data we have collected. Nevertheless, the spatial representation fits response-choice data extremely well, and it is not even clear how the additive clustering representation could be applied to data of this sort. I am inclined to regard the two kinds of modeling as elucidating different aspects of subjects' reasoning about the mammal names. If the results of fitting both kinds of representations are sensible, then it is quite possible that both are "correct": They elucidate different aspects of the ways in which subjects conceive of relations between elements in a given data set.

Selection of strategy for combining components.   Many of the most important theoretical questions about analogical reasoning concern strategy selection, although very few of them have yet been answered. Let us take the question whether subjects can use inherent properties of analogies to simplify their processing of information when the need arises. Consider, for example, the analogy, *snow:blood: :white:red.* The models described earlier would all call for inference of the relation between *snow* and *blood;* some of these models would then call for mapping of the relation between *snow* and *blood,* on the one hand, and between *white* and *red,* on the other. But one important property of analogies is that, as proportions, they can be viewed as relating (A,C) to (B,D) as well as (A,B) to (C,D). In this analogy, certainly it would be to the subject's advantage to infer the relation between *snow* and *white,* and then to map the relation between *snow* and *white,* on the one hand, and that between *blood* and *red,* on the other. Sternberg (1977b, pp. 232–233) tested this model variant for verbal analogies, and found a slight improvement in fit over that obtained for the standard strategy, suggesting that subjects might flexibly alter their strategy so that if the semantic relation between the first and third terms is closer than that between the first and second, then they infer the relation between A and C – the first and third terms – and map the relation between (A,C) and (B,D). Grudin (1980) has presented even stronger data arguing for this flexibility in strategy.

Decision whether to maintain a strategy.   We currently have no evidence that subjects change their strategy for analogy solution with practice. Hence, as far as we know, subjects generally do decide to maintain whatever strategy they have started with.

Selection of a speed–accuracy trade-off.   At the present time, we know that a micro-trade-off between speed and accuracy is found in analogical reasoning: Greater speed is attained at some cost in accuracy (Sternberg, 1977b). Data currently being collected by Miriam Schustack and me also indicate that it is possible to induce a macro-trade-off between speed and accuracy, at least when the analogies are presented tachistoscopically. In other words, different instructions regarding the relative importance of speed and accuracy can result in differential speed–accuracy trade-offs. More interesting than the question whether a trade-off can be induced, however, is the question where the loci of the trade-off reside. Schustack and I seek to discover these loci in our experiment.

Solution monitoring.   We do not yet know just how subjects monitor their solution of analogy problems, but we know that they do monitor their performance. This monitoring manifests itself through the justification component, which is executed when none of the response options fit the subject's ideal conception of what the answer to an analogy should be. Justification seems to take the form of checking and possibly reexecuting previously executed operations. Subjects seek to find either errors of commission (an operation was executed incorrectly) or errors of omission (an operation was executed incompletely, so that failure to encode an important attribute or to conceive of an important relation resulted).

PROBLEM FORMAT, PROBLEM CONTENT, AND PRACTICE.   Problem format, problem content, and practice all have been found to affect analogical reasoning performance. Consider first the effects of *problem format.*

Some investigations have been based upon true–false analogies (Ingram, Pellegrino, & Glaser, 1976; Mulholland et al., 1980; Sternberg, 1977a, 1977b). The format is of questionable merit when the analogy attributes are nonobvious and ill-defined, as in the verbal analogies of Ingram and his associates and of Sternberg. I now believe the format may be inappropriate for such analogies, because it is not clear that for analogies with ill-defined attributes, any one completion is strictly correct (at least for the terms available in the English language). For example, is the analogy *white:black: :big:short* true or false? In some senses of the words *big* and *short,* it is true; in others, it is false. Ingram and his co-workers found that analogies with completions that were "near misses" had longer latencies than analogies that were either clearly true or obviously false, and they proposed a model that could handle this finding. Other investigators have used two-option forced-choice analogies (Sternberg, 1977a, 1977b, for geometric analogies; Sternberg & Rifkin, 1979). Sternberg (1977b) has described two extreme strategies that might be used in scanning options in the forced-choice format. Still other investigators have used four-option multiple-choice analogies (Rumelhart & Abrahamson, 1973; Sternberg & Gardner, 1982; Whitely & Barnes, 1979). The strategies subjects use in solving problems of this nature seem to be very complex.

Lunzer (1965) presented analogies that had either just one term missing (which could be *A, B, C,* or *D*) or two terms missing (*C* and *D, A* and *B, B* and *C,* or *A* and *D*). As would be expected, analogies with a single term missing were easier to solve than analogies with two terms missing. Those with *C* and *D* missing or with *A* and *B* missing were found to be less difficult than those with *B* and *C* missing or with *A* and *D* missing. Presumably, this was because, for the latter two kinds of problems, there was no single relation linking the missing pair: Each of the two missing terms was involved in a different relation within the analogy.

Levinson and Carpenter (1974) presented verbal problems in two forms – as analogies and as quasi-analogies. An analogy took the form exemplified by *Bird* is to *air* as *fish* is to ? A quasi-analogy took the form exemplified by "A bird uses air; a fish uses ?" The quasi-analogies thus supplied the relationship, whereas the analogies did not. There were no significant differences in performance on the two types of problems for the oldest subjects tested, who were 15 years old (but see the section on between-ages differences that follows).

Sternberg and Nigro (1980) presented analogies to subjects in each of the following three forms:

1. *Narrow:wide: :question:(trial, statement, answer, ask).*
2. *Win:lose: :(dislike:hate), (ear:hear), (enjoy:like), (above:below).*
3. *Weak:(sick: :circle:shape), (strong: :poor:rich), (small: :garden:grow), (health: :solid:firm).*

Numbers of answer options ranged from two to four. Adult subjects were fastest on the first form and slowest on the last form (but see the section on between-ages differences that follows). However, error rates were highest for the second form. Adult subjects solved the problems exhaustively, in the sense that they passed through all of the answer options sequentially before selecting a response.

Johnson (1962) used what he called a method of "serial analysis" in his presentation of verbal analogies. Analogies were presented tachistoscopically, with trials divided into two parts. In the first part, subjects received the first half of the analogy. They had as long as they wanted to view this half of the problem, and when they were done studying it, they initiated the second part of the trial. In this part of the trial, subjects received the second half of the analogy. They terminated this part of the trial by responding to the analogy as quickly as possible. Response latency was longer for the second half of the trial (mean latency = 6.68 sec) than for the first half (mean latency = 3.33 sec).

Sternberg (1977b) extended Johnson's method of serial analysis in a method of "precueing." Analogies were presented in two parts. The first part could consist of no terms, one term, two terms, or three terms. The second part of the trial always consisted of the full analogy. Sternberg found that cue times – latencies for the first part of the trial – increased with greater amounts of precueing in the first part of the trial, and that solution times – latencies for the second part of the trial – decreased.

Consider now effects of *problem content*. Sternberg (1977a, 1977b) found verbal analogies to be more difficult than people-piece analogies, and geometric analogies to be more difficult than verbal analogies. This ordering probably said more about the particular instantiations of content Sternberg used than about intrinsic properties of the content, because no attempt was made to equate concepts in any way. As mentioned earlier, for example, verbal analogies can be made arbitrarily difficult by using terms that pose vocabulary or general information demands beyond the capacities of many subjects solving the problems. Tests such as the Miller Analogies Test are difficult largely because the vocabulary and general information demands are so high (Sternberg, 1977b, 1978).

Tinsley and Dawis (1972) did an experiment that specifically set out to equate conceptual difficulty of items with two different kinds of content. In their items, the same objects were presented verbally and figurally, so that the only difference between the two sets of analogies they studied was in the content vehicle through which the objects were expressed. These authors found no significant difference in difficulty between the two contents, and they also found a correlation of .86 between the 30 items constituting each form of the test. Unfortunately, all subjects received both types of analogies in immediate succession, with the verbal analogies always coming first. As a result, it is difficult to know to what extent the results were affected by the fact that each subject received each item twice in rapid succession and by the fact that order of presentation and item content were confounded.

Johnson (1962) presented items that were intended to be difficult because of vocabulary demand in either the first half or the second half of the analogy. For example, *feline* is to *canine* as *cat* is to ? was presumed to be difficult because of the vocabulary demand in the first half of the item, whereas *lose* is to *win* as *liability* is to ? was presumed to be difficult because of the vocabulary demand in the second half. In all three item formats – response production, multiple-choice, and multiple-choice with options containing only the first letter of the option – items were more difficult (higher response latency and higher error rate) if the greater vocabulary demand was in the first half of the trial. (Recall that Johnson divided his trials into two parts, a part in which the first half was presented and a part in which the second half was presented.) Johnson found that more time was spent on the first part of the trial for items where the vocabulary load was in the first part than for items where the vocabulary load was in the second part; he found that more time was spent on the second part of the trial for items where the vocabulary load was in the second part than for items where the vocabulary load was in the first part.

Consider finally the effects of *practice* upon analogy solution. Sternberg (1977b) compared performance during a first session of people-piece analogy solution to performance during a fourth (and final) session. As would be expected, latencies and error rates decreased from the first session to the fourth. All components showed shorter latencies during the fourth session than during the first except for inference. There was no evidence of strategy change across sessions: Fits of the various models and variants of models were almost identical in the two sessions. The most interesting difference in results showed up during external validation of scores: In the first session, no correlations of latencies for the second (solution) part of the trial with reasoning tests were significant; in the fourth session, more than half of the correlations were significant, and many of them were of high magnitude, reaching into the .60s and .70s. Thus subjects changed in their rank order of the effectiveness with which they could solve the analogies. Sternberg (1977b) noted that this pattern of difference in the correlations is related to previous findings. Nobel, Nobel, and Alcock (1958) used tests from the Thurstone Primary Mental Abilities battery to predict individual differences in trial-and-error learning. They found that prediction was higher for total correct scores than for initial correct scores. These data suggested that the higher correlations resulted from performance during later trials. Fleishman and Hempel (1955) and Fleishman (1965) found that the percentage of variance accounted for in motor tasks by traditional psychometric tests increased with practice on the motor tasks. These results led Glaser (1967) to conclude that psychometric test scores are more highly correlated with performance after asymptote is reached than with performance during initial trials of practice.

Vygotsky (1962) noted that mental testing is usually based upon performance on tasks for which no explicit training has been given. He suggested that it might be more appropriate to measure performance after training and practice rather than before, at the upper rather than at the lower threshold of performance, because "instruction must be oriented toward the future, not the past" (p. 104). The present data are consistent with Vygotsky's notions, and with Ferguson's (1954) notion of intelligence as "performance at some crude limit of learning" (p. 110).

INDIVIDUAL DIFFERENCES WITHIN AGE LEVEL (ADULTS). Sternberg (1977b) found substantial individual differences in the speeds at which the various performance components of analogical reasoning are executed, and in the degree to which subjects used any systematic strategy at all. No substantial individual differences were found in components or forms of representation used, and no one else has found such individual differences either. Sternberg also failed to find clear-cut individual differences in strategies for combining components, other than that some people appeared to use the third variant of the model described earlier (inference exhaustive, mapping and application self-terminating) and that other people appeared to use the fourth variant (inference, mapping, and application self-terminating).

Whitely and Barnes (1979), on the other hand, have interpreted data they have collected as evidencing important differences in strategy among adults. These authors used a "simulation task" to study verbal analogical reasoning. In this task, analogies were composed of pronounceable nonwords, for example, *lyomon: firmani: :dulciver:(bansher, ponto, nax, squish)*. (*Squish* is actually a word, although it was one of their stimuli.) The terms were supposed to refer to animals that could evolve on other planets. In the simulation task, subjects could require information about any of the analogy terms in any order. Information consisted of a picture of the animal and a list of five properties of the animal. Whitely and Barnes's results suggest that substantial strategy differences may occur in analogical reasoning.

Some unpublished data monitoring subjects' eye movements during analogical reasoning have been collected by Richard Snow at Stanford, and these data also suggest strategy differences. The Whitely–Barnes data, however, are still inconclusive. First, it is not yet clear whether what subjects do during the simulation task actually "simulates" what they do during normal solution of verbal analogies. Both Reitman (1965) and Sternberg (1977b) found that subjects had only the foggiest idea of how they went about solving verbal analogies, and the fact that scores on Whitely and Barnes's simulation task correlated only .20 ($p < .05$) with scores on a psychometric verbal analogies test might lead one to question whether the two tasks do indeed draw upon the same strategies and other elements of reasoning. In drastically reducing their rate of work, subjects may also be changing their style of work. Second, the artificiality of the stimuli may lead to specialized strategies not applicable to ordinary analogy problems. The way information is encoded about a "squish" may or may not correspond to the way in which it is encoded about a real animal. Whether or not the simulation task measures the same kind of reasoning as the standard analogical reasoning task, the form of reasoning it does measure seems to be potentially interesting in its own right, combining as it does the needs for learning of concepts and for reasoning with those concepts.

DIFFERENCES ACROSS AGE LEVELS.   A great deal of developmental work has been done in the domain of analogical reasoning, and it is possible to touch upon only a fraction of that work here.

Piaget, with Montangero and Billeter (1977), has suggested three stages in the development of reasoning by analogy. Understanding of these stages requires some knowledge of the paradigm these investigators used to study the development of analogical reasoning. They presented 29 children between the ages of 5 and 13 with sets of pictures and asked the children to arrange the pictures into pairs. The children were then asked to put together those pairs that went well together, placing groups of four pictures into two-by-two matrices that represented relations of analogy among the four pictures. Children who had difficulty at any step of the procedure were given prompts along the way. Children who finally succeeded were presented with a counter-suggestion to their proposed solution, by which the investigators hoped to test the strength of the children's commitment to their proposed response. At all steps along the way, children were asked to explain their reasons for grouping things as they did. In the first proposed stage of Piaget's model, characterizing the performance of children of ages 5–6, children can arrange pictures into pairs, but the children ignore higher-order relations between pairs. Thus, although these children can link A to B or C to D, they cannot link (A,B) to (C,D). In the second stage, characterizing the performance of children from about 8 to 11 years of age, children can form analogies, but when challenged with counter-suggestions, they readily rescind their proposed analogies. Piaget interprets this finding as evidence of only a weak or tentative level of analogical reasoning ability. In the third stage, characterizing the performance of children of ages 11 and above, children form analogies, are able to state explicitly the conceptual bases of these analogies, and resist counter-suggestions from the experimenter.

Lunzer (1965) presented children aged 9–17+ with verbal analogies taking the various forms described earlier (e.g., just the A term missing, just the C term missing, the A and B terms missing, and A and D terms missing). Lunzer found that children had great difficulty with even the simplest analogies until about 9 years of age, and did not show highly successful performance until the age of 11. Lunzer concluded that even the simplest analogies require recognition of higher-order relations that are not discernible to children who are not yet formal-operational. The suggestion of three stages in Lunzer's work (before age 9, between ages 9 and 11, after age 11) seems correspondent to Piaget's suggestion regarding three stages of reasoning by analogy.

Gallagher and Wright (1977, 1979) have done research comparing the relative abilities of children in Grades 4 to 6 to provide what these investigators called "symmetrical" or "asymmetrical" explanations of analogy solutions. Symmetrical explanations showed awareness of the higher-order relation linking (*A,B*) to (*C,D*). Asymmetrical explanations ignored this relation, dealing either with only the (*C,D*) relation or with both the (*A,B*) and the (*C,D*) relations, but in isolation from each other. Percentages of symmetrical responses increased with age and were associated with higher levels of performance on the analogies.

Levinson and Carpenter (1974) presented verbal analogies (e.g., *Bird:air: :fish:?*) and quasi-analogies (e.g., "A bird uses air; a fish uses ?") to children of 9, 12, and 15 years of age. The standard analogies required recognition of the higher-order analogical relationship; the quasi-analogies essentially supplied this relationship. The investigators found that whereas 9-year-olds could answer significantly more quasi-analogies than analogies correctly, 12- and 15-year-olds answered approximately equal numbers of each kind of item. Moreover, whereas performance on the standard analogies increased monotonically across age levels, performance on the quasi-analogies did not increase. These results provide further evidence for the ability of formal-operational children, but not concrete-operational children, to use second-order relations in the solution of verbal analogies.

Sternberg and Rifkin (1979) investigated the development of analogical reasoning processes with two kinds of schematic-picture analogies. One kind was the people-piece analogy used by Sternberg (1977a, 1977b); the other kind was also a schematic figure of a person. But whereas the people-piece analogies were composed of perceptually integral attributes, the schematic-figure analogies were composed of perceptually separable attributes (see Garner, 1974). In the perceptually integral attributes, the levels of one attribute depend upon levels of other attributes for their existence. For example, in the people pieces, it is impossible to represent a level of height without representing some level of weight (two of the attributes), and vice versa. In the perceptually separable attributes, levels of attributes are not dependent in this way. For example, in the schematic figures, it is possible to represent the color of a hat without representing the type of footwear a figure has on. For analogies with perceptually integral attributes, subjects became more nearly exhaustive in their information processing with increasing age. This tendency appears to be a general higher-order strategy in cognitive development (Brown & DeLoache, 1978), and appears to be associated with dramatic decreases in error rate over age (Sternberg, 1977b; Sternberg & Rifkin, 1979). Moreover, it was found that although fourth-graders, sixth-graders, and adults solved the analogies by mapping the higher-order relation between the two halves of the analogies, second-graders did not. Once again, then, we have support for a late-developing ability to recognize and utilize higher-order relations. For the analogies with perceptually separable attributes, subjects at all ages used the same fully self-terminating strategy, the one that second-graders used for the perceptually integral attributes. Mapping was not used, or was used for a constant amount of time across item types. (The two outcomes are experimentally indistinguishable.) Thus it appears that for analogies with integral attributes, strategy changes with age, whereas for analogies with separable attributes, it does not change.

Some investigators have been particularly interested in the role word association plays in children's solutions of analogies. The pioneering studies in the role of association in analogy solution were done by Achenbach (1970a, 1970b, 1971), who found that children in the intermediate and early secondary-school grades differ widely in the extent to which they use word association as a means of choosing one from among several response options. Moreover, the extent to which children use word association serves as a moderator variable in predicting classroom performance: Correlations between performance on IQ tests and school achievement were substantially lower for children who relied heavily on free association to solve analogies than for children who relied primarily on reasoning processes. Gentile and his associates (1977) further investigated children's associative responding, using Achenbach's CART (Children's Associative Responding Test). They found that associative priming can have a marked effect on test scores, leading children either toward or away from correct solutions. Sternberg and Nigro (1980) found that third- and sixth-graders used word association to a significant extent in the solution of verbal analogies, but that ninth-graders and adults did not.

Sternberg and Nigro (1980) were interested not only in whether children use word association, but also in how they use it in analogy solution. They found that in analogies with the three formats they used (described earlier), word association is used to guide search among options, with higher-association responses being examined before lower-association ones. The ninth-graders and adults, however, did not use word association in this way, or in any other way that was discernible from their data.

RELATIONSHIPS BETWEEN ANALOGICAL REASONING AND OTHER KINDS OF REASONING. Several investigators have asserted that the processes used in solving analogies are used as well in solving other kinds of induction problems, such as series completions and classifications (Greeno, 1978; Pellegrino & Glaser, 1980; Sternberg, 1977b, 1979c, 1979d). Sternberg and Gardner (1982) conducted two experiments designed to test this assertion. These experiments used animal-name analogies (including those of Rumelhart & Abrahamson, 1973, e.g., *tiger:chimpanzee: :wolf:*[a. *raccoon*, b. *camel*, c. *monkey*, d. *leopard*]); series completions (e.g., *squirrel:chipmunk:*[a. *raccoon*, b. *horse*, c. *dog*, d. *camel*]), where the subject's task was to indicate which of four completions would follow next in a series; and classifications (e.g., *zebra, giraffe, goat,* [a. *dog*, b. *cow*, c. *mouse*, d. *deer*]), where the subject's task was to indicate which of the options fit best with three terms in the item stem.

In the first experiment, subjects were asked to rank order each of four answer options for goodness of fit. Correlations were .99 between the data sets for analogies and series completions, .97 between the data sets for analogies and classifications, and .98 between the data sets for series completions and classifications. The fits of the exponential model to each of the data sets were also very good: $r = .97$ for analogies, $r = .98$ for series completions, and $r = .99$ for classifications. Moreover, parameter estimates were quite similar across the three tasks. The results suggest commonalities in decision rules for response choice across the three inductive-reasoning tasks. The second experiment of Sternberg and Gardner used the same items, except that the number of answer options was reduced from four to two. Subjects were nonoverlapping with those in the first experiment. The main dependent variable in this experiment was solution latency rather than response choice. The authors fitted a four-parameter model to data sets from each of the three tasks. The model fitted the data for each task reasonably well: $r = .88$ for analogies, $r = .82$ for series completions, and $r = .78$ for classifications. Only the estimated value of the justification parameter differed significantly across tasks. Individual parameter estimates were too unreliable for individual-differences analysis. These data were interpreted as providing further support for a unified model of performance in the three inductive reasoning tasks.

In an innovative approach to modeling cognitive abilities, Whitely (1979b) fitted a three-component latent trait model to data for a verbal analogy and a verbal classification test (see also Whitely, 1979a). Whitely (1979c) then used this latent trait model as a basis for covariance modeling (Jöreskog, 1969, 1970; Jöreskog & Sörbom, 1978) intended to account for individual differences in analogy and classification performance, as well as differences in item difficulties. The same basic model provided a good fit to data for both the verbal analogies and the verbal classifications tasks, although parameter estimates differed.

Further support for the possible unity of performance components in at least some induction tasks is provided by the success of computer programs such as Williams's (1972) Aptitude-Test Taker and Simon and Lea's (1974) General Rule Inducer (GRI) program, both of which can solve induction problems of a variety of types. The success of these programs shows that a single set of processes can be sufficient for solving various kinds of induction problems, although of course it does not show that people actually use a single set of processes.

RELATIONSHIP BETWEEN ANALOGICAL REASONING AND INTELLIGENCE. Theorists such as Spearman (1923), Piaget (1970; Piaget, with Montangero & Billeter, 1977), and Reitman (1965) have argued for many years that intelligence and analogical reasoning are intimately connected. Spearman's three principles of cognition were based upon three processes he believed to be involved in reasoning by analogy; Piaget's concrete- and formal-operational stages are differentiated in children by the children's ability to solve analogies; and Reitman's theory of intellectual functioning is based upon solution of analogies. Moreover, empirical data collected by these investigators and others have been consistent with the strong claims made regarding the centrality of analogical reasoning in intelligent functioning. Factor-analytic investigations such as those conducted by Spearman (1904, 1927), for example, have consistently shown analogy items to be among the highest in their loadings on g, or general intelligence. Some recently collected data have provided further insights into the information-processing relationships between analogical reasoning and intelligence.

Sternberg (1977b) found that each of the major "reasoning operations" in analogical reasoning – inference, mapping, application, justification – can correlate with performance on tests of general intelligence when the attributes of the analogies being solved are nonobvious. As would be expected, faster component execution was associated with higher scores on the psychometric tests. Sternberg also found an association between encoding speed and measured intelligence, except that the association went the opposite way: Slower encoding was associated with higher measured intelligence. Sternberg interpreted this finding in metacomponential terms: Brighter subjects spend relatively longer in encoding the stimuli in order to facilitate their execution of subsequent performance components that will draw upon the results of the encoding. Evidence from his studies supported this interpretation. Even the response constant shows a strong correlation with measured intelligence: Faster speed of response was associated with higher measured intelligence. This basic finding has since been replicated in the analogies task (Mulholland et al., 1980) and in other tasks as well (Egan, 1976). This finding may have a metacomponential interpretation also: The response constant includes confounded within it all sources of response variation that are constant across items. Strategy planning, solution monitoring, and other metacomponents are likely to be constant in duration across item types, and hence to be confounded with the response constant. These sources of variation may be responsible for the correlation of the response constant with IQ. Sternberg (1979c) has gone so far as to suggest that the metacomponents underlying the variation are the most important elements to be reckoned with in a theory of intelligence. Finally, Sternberg (1977b) found that for verbal analogies, at least, greater systematicity (as measured by higher internal consistency of individual-subject data) in use of a strategy in solving analogies was associated with higher intelligence. All of these findings have received developmental confirmation to support the data obtained with adults. All component latencies show a general decrease with age, except for encoding, which after an initial decrease (owing, presumably, to cognitive development in encoding skills) shows a subsequent increase in latency (Sternberg & Rifkin, 1979); and systematicity in strategy utilization also increases with age, at least for some types of analogies (Sternberg & Nigro, 1980; Sternberg & Rifkin, 1979).

Whitely (1976, 1977) has also shown significant relationships between measured intelligence and performance in analogical reasoning. In her 1976 study, she found significant multiple correlations (in the .30s, .40s, and .50s) between scores on verbal analogies expressing different semantic relations and scores on standard measures of mental ability. In her 1977 study, she found correlations ranging up to the .60s between numbers correct on an analogies test and scores on the Differential Aptitude Test and the Lorge–Thorndike Intelligence Test. Correlations for latencies of analogy solution were somewhat lower, but still statistically significant for items that were answered correctly.

To summarize, the history of theory and research on relationships between analogical reasoning and intelligence shows the two to be strongly related. Indeed, according to some theorists, an understanding of intelligence requires an understanding of analogical reasoning: Spearman (1923), Reitman (1965), and Sternberg (1977b) all based parts of their theories of intelligence on their theories of reasoning by analogy.

PRACTICAL RELEVANCE.   Sternberg (1977b) has argued that reasoning by analogy is pervasive in everyday experience. "We reason analogically whenever we make a decision about something new in our experience by drawing a parallel to something old in our experience. When we buy a new pet hamster because we liked our old one or when we listen to a friend's advice because it was correct once before, we are reasoning analogically" (p. 99).

Oppenheimer (1956) has pointed out the signal importance of analogy in scientific reasoning of the kind done by scientists and even nonscientists on an everyday basis:

Whether or not we talk of discovery or of invention, analogy is inevitable in human thought, because we come to new things in science with what equipment we have, which is how we have learned to think, and above all how we have learned to think about the relatedness of things. We cannot, coming into something new, deal with it except on the basis of the familiar and old-fashioned. The conservatism of scientific enquiry is not an arbitrary thing; it is the freight with which we operate; it is the only equipment we have. [Pp. 129–130]

Analogical reasoning also plays an important role in legal thinking, where it may be called "reasoning by example" (Levi, 1949):

The basic pattern of legal reasoning is reasoning by example. It is reasoning from case to case. It is a three-step process described by the doctrine of precedent in which a proposition descriptive of the first case is made into a rule of law and then applied to a next similar situation. The steps are these: similarity is seen between cases; next the rule of law inherent in the first case is announced; then the rule of law is made applicable to the second case. This is a method of reasoning necessary for the law, but it has characteristics which under other circumstances might be considered imperfections. [Pp. 1–2]

Analogical reasoning can be successfully trained. Feuerstein, Schlesinger, Shalom, and Narrol (1972) and Feuerstein (1979) have presented the results of an extensive training program for verbal and figural analogies that constitute part of Feuerstein's Learning Potential Assessment Device (LPAD). Feuerstein and his colleagues have used two basic kinds of training, which might be termed "performance-componential" and "metacomponential." In an experiment involving 551 children (including urban, upper-middle-class schoolchildren; urban, lower-class schoolchildren; and educable mentally retarded children), Feuerstein (1979) found significant effects of verbal and figural training of both kinds. The largest gains were made, however, by children receiving both kinds of training together.

Whitely and Dawis (1973) described a cognitive intervention for improving the estimate of latent ability measured from analogy items, and Whitely and Dawis (1974) tested this and other interventions on high-school students. There were six conditions varying amount of practice, instruction, and feedback. The "practice" groups did not perform better than the controls, but the "instruction" groups did perform better. Experimental groups receiving feedback did not perform better than groups not receiving it, but the group receiving semantic category instruction in addition to feedback performed significantly better than the comparable group not receiving category instruction. These and other results suggested that the category instruction was critical to improved performance.

Sternberg and Ketron (1982) have found that it is possible to train many subjects to use the variants of the models described earlier. Subjects are shown how to use the strategies to solve analogies composed of schematic pictures; and left to their own devices, the subjects can continue to use these strategies. Instruction was successful for analogies with integral attributes, but not for analogies with separable attributes.

Are certain strategies better for some people and other strategies better for others? There is some evidence that is at least suggestive that this is the case. Sternberg and Rifkin (1979) and Sternberg and Nigro (1980) have found that older subjects tend to be more nearly exhaustive in their information processing. More nearly exhaustive strategies tend to increase accuracy, but at the expense of requiring a greater memory load during analogy solution. The data suggest that subjects should be encouraged to use a strategy that is maximally exhaustive but that does not exceed the capacity of their working memory in its demands. With developments in technology for measuring working-memory capacity (see Case, 1978a, 1978b), it may be possible eventually to individualize instruction in analogy solution in a way that maximizes individual analogy performance.

To recapitulate, the proposed metatheoretical framework can be and has been applied to the understanding of one form of inductive reasoning, reasoning by analogy. We now turn to a consideration of how the framework can be applied to the study and understanding of deductive reasoning.

DEDUCTIVE REASONING

The scope of deductive reasoning

In deductive reasoning, the information contained in the premises of a problem is logically (although not necessarily psychologically) sufficient to reach a valid conclusion. A number of different kinds of deductive-reasoning problems have been studied, among them:

1. *Linear syllogisms,* for example, "John is taller than Pete; Pete is taller than Bill; who is tallest?" In these problems, a logically valid conclusion is implied by the premises only if it is assumed that the relations linking the terms are transitive. For example, the relation "taller than" would satisfy transitivity, whereas the relation "plays better tennis than" might not. The problems may be presented in either verbal or nonverbal form and, in either case, may be embellished by the addition of negatives (e.g., "John is not as tall as Pete") or even additional premises. When premises are added, the problems are usually referred to as linear ordering or transitive inference problems, and indeed, linear syllogisms may be viewed, strictly speaking, as one of many possible kinds of linear ordering problem. Reviews of the literature on linear syllogistic reasoning can be found in Johnson-Laird (1972) and in Sternberg (1980b), as well as later in this chapter. Some of the original sources include Clark (1969a, 1969b, 1971, 1972b); DeSoto, London, and Handel (1965); Donaldson (1963); Handel, DeSoto, and London (1968); Hunter (1957); Huttenlocher (1968); Huttenlocher and Higgins (1971); Huttenlocher, Higgins, Milligan, and Kauffman (1970); Huttenlocher and Strauss (1968); Keating and Caramazza (1975); Lutkus and Trabasso (1974); Mayer (1978, 1979); Piaget (1921, 1928, 1955, 1970); Potts (1972, 1974); Potts and Scholz (1975); Riley and Trabasso (1974); Shaver, Pierson, and Lang (1974); Sternberg (1980a, 1980b, 1980c); Trabasso (1975); Trabasso and Riley (1975); Trabasso, Riley, and Wilson (1975); and Wood, Shotter, and Godden (1974).

2. *Categorical syllogisms,* for example, "All dorfles are dingbats. Some dunkits are dorfles. Can one conclude that some dunkits are dingbats?" Premises of categorical syllogisms, like those of linear syllogisms, can be presented in either affirmative or negative form (e.g., "No dorfles are dingbats" or "Some dunkits are not dorfles"). Premises of categorical syllogisms, unlike those of linear syllogisms, however, are almost never presented in pictorial form, and as a result, the syllogisms have not been presented to very young (preoperational) children. The syllogisms may be presented with more than two premises, in which case they are called *sorites,* or *set inclusion problems.* Reviews of the literature on cateogrical syllogistic reasoning can be found in Guyote and Sternberg (1981) and in Wason and Johnson-Laird (1972). Some of the original sources include Begg and Denny (1969); Ceraso and Provitera (1971); Chapman and Chapman (1959); Dickstein (1975, 1976, 1978); Erickson (1974, 1978); Frase (1966a, 1966b, 1968); Gilson and Abelson (1965); Griggs

(1976, 1978); Henle (1962); Henle and Michael (1956); Janis and Frick (1943); Johnson-Laird (1975); Johnson-Laird and Steedman (1978); Kaufman and Goldstein (1967); Lefford (1946); Lippman (1972); McGuire (1960); Morgan and Morton (1944); Revlin and Leirer (1978); Revlis (1975a, 1975b); Richter (1957); Roberge and Paulus (1971); Sells (1936); Simpson and Johnson (1966); Sternberg and Turner (1981); Wason and Johnson-Laird (1972); Wilkins (1928); Wilson (1965); and Woodworth and Sells (1935).

3. *Conditional syllogisms,* for example, "If Conrad the Clown performs, people laugh; Conrad the Clown performs; can one conclude that people laugh?" As is the case with categorical syllogisms, premises may be negated (e.g., "If Conrad the Clown performs, people do not laugh," or "Conrad the Clown does not perform"). The premises may also be strung together to form an arbitrary number of items. Problems are almost always presented verbally. Reviews of the literature can be found in Guyote and Sternberg (1981) and in Wason and Johnson-Laird (1972). Some of the original sources include Guyote and Sternberg (1978); Kodroff and Roberge (1975); Marcus and Rips (1979); Osherson (1974, 1975); Paris (1973); Rips and Marcus (1977); Roberge and Paulus (1971); Staudenmayer (1975); Staudenmayer and Bourne (1977); Taplin (1971); Taplin and Staudenmayer (1973); Taplin, Staudenmayer, and Taddonio (1974); Wason and Johnson-Laird (1972).

These three kinds of syllogistic reasoning are not, of course, the only kinds of deductive reasoning that have been or might be studied, but they account for a fairly large proportion of the literature on deduction. Other kinds of deduction problems are considered by Wason and Johnson-Laird (1972), and a good logic text such as Copi (1978) reviews a wide range of types of deduction problems. Rather than attempting to survey this entire literature here within the framework proposed in the preceding section, I shall review just one literature – that on linear syllogistic reasoning – as an example of the form such a review takes. Space considerations and the scope of this chapter simply do not permit a review of the entire range of literature on deductive reasoning.

A case study of deductive reasoning: the linear syllogism

NATURE OF THE PROBLEM. In a linear syllogism, a person is presented with two premises, each describing a relation between two items, one of which overlaps between premises. The person's task is to use the overlap to determine the relation between the two items not occurring in the same premise, and then to answer a question requiring knowledge of this relation. In the item "Sue is older than Lil; Lil is older than Ann; who is oldest?" the person must deduce that Sue is older than Ann, and hence that Sue is oldest of the three girls.

An often-used domain of linear syllogisms consists of 2^5, or 32 item types, obtained by allowing each of the three adjectives in the problem (one in each premise and one in the conclusion) to be at either one pole (e.g., *old*) or the other (e.g., *young*); by allowing the premises to be either affirmative (as in this case) or negative equative (e.g., "Lil is not as old as Sue"); and by allowing the correct answer to the item to be in either the first premise (as in this case) or in the second (as would be obtained by reversing the order of the premises). The premise adjectives are usually not psychologically symmetrical. One form (in this case, *old*) is simpler in certain senses to describe than the other form (in this case, *young*). The simpler form is the one that constitutes the name of the scale (in this case, *oldness* rather than *youngness*, or in a similar case, *tallness* rather than *shortness*). The simpler form is referred to as *unmarked*, whereas the more complex form is called *marked*.

Although the 32 items formed in this way constitute the standard domain of linear syllogisms, they are not the only possible linear syllogisms. Additional items may be formed by allowing just one or the other premise to be negated, or by allowing problems to be indeterminate, that is, specifying only a partial rather than a full ordering, such as "Sue is older than Lil; Sue is older than Ann; who is oldest?" The theories to be described here need augmentation in order to deal with the additional complexities created by items of these kinds.

Performance on linear syllogisms satisfies the four criteria for a "worthwhile" measure described in the preceding section. First, performance can be quantified by measurement of either response latency or error rate. Second, it can be measured reliably: Reliabilities of latencies (across item types) are generally in the high .80s or low .90s (Sternberg, 1980c, 1980d). Third, construct validity has been demonstrated numerous times in various ways: The linear syllogism plays an important part in Piaget's (1921, 1928, 1955) developmental theory of intelligence, because the ability to perform transitive inferences is alleged to differentiate preoperational from concrete-operational children; the problem plays an important role in DeSoto's theory of people's predilections for linear orderings (DeSoto, 1961; Desoto et al., 1965), in that the problem permits formation of a single, linear ordering; the problem plays an equally important role in Clark's (1969b, 1973) theory of linguistic processes in verbal comprehension, in that the processes alleged to be used in solving linear syllogisms are alleged also to be used in a large variety of verbal comprehension tasks; and the problem plays a central role in my own unified componential theory of human reasoning (Sternberg, 1978a, 1979b), in that the processes used are alleged to be used in a variety of deduction tasks, and the task itself falls into the task hierarchy that constitutes the organization of the theory. Finally, the empirical validity of performance on the problem has been demonstrated repeatedly. Burt (1919) used the problem in measuring the intelligence of schoolchildren, and performance on the problem has been found to be highly correlated with performance on verbal, spatial, and abstract reasoning ability tests (Shaver et al., 1974; Sternberg, 1980c; Sternberg & Weil, 1980): Correlations with such tests generally fall in the .30–.60 range.

PERFORMANCE COMPONENTS. Theorists differ in their views regarding the performance components used in solving linear syllogisms. Three views will be discussed here, based upon three different models of linear syllogistic reasoning. The three models are a spatial model based upon the models of DeSoto and his associates (1965) and Huttenlocher (Huttenlocher, 1968; Huttenlocher & Higgins, 1971), a linguistic model based upon the Clark (1969b) model, and a linguistic–spatial mixed model described by Sternberg (1980d). Although the first two information-processing models are based upon previous models, they are not isomorphic to these previous models, in that the first two models were not presented by their original formulators in "componential" terms. The present models do seem to capture the major intuitions of the models as originally proposed.

The models all agree that there are certain encoding, negation, marking, and response operations that contribute to the latency with which a subject solves a linear syllogism. All full linear syllogisms contain certain terms and relations to be encoded, and require a response. Only some linear syllogisms contain premises with negations and marked adjectives. Although the models agree on the presence of these performance components, they disagree about which of these components are spatial and which are linguistic. The three models of linear syllogistic reasoning will be presented with reference to an example of a relatively difficult linear syllogism: "*C* is not as tall as *B; A* is not as short as *B;* who is shortest?" The correct answer is *C*, and by convention, *A* will always refer to the extreme item at the unmarked end of the continuum, and *C* to the extreme item at the marked end of the continuum. Each of these models can be represented in flow-chart form, and detailed descriptions of the various models are presented elsewhere (Sternberg, 1980d). Johnson-Laird (1972) has proposed slightly different flow charts for two of the models, the spatial and the linguistic ones. I describe here in detail only the mixed model, which is best supported by the available data (Sternberg, 1980c, 1980d). (Those not interested in these details may wish to skip the remainder of this section.)

In the linguistic–spatial *mixed model,* linguistic decoding of the problem is followed by its spatial recoding. The subject begins the solution by reading the first premise. In order for the premise to be understood, it must be formulated in terms of the kind of deep-structural propositions proposed by the linguistic model. Encoding a marked adjective into this deep-structural format takes longer than encoding an unmarked one. Also, the presence of a negation requires a reformulation of the deep-structural proposition. Thus "*C* is not as tall as *B*" is originally formulated as (*C* is tall+; *B* is tall) and is then reformulated as (*B* is tall+; *C* is tall), as in the linguistic model. Once the deep-structural propositions for the premise are in final linguistic form, the terms of the propositions are seriated spatially. If there is a marked adjective, the subject takes additional time in seriating the relation spatially in the non-preferred (usually bottom-up) direction. If the adjective is not marked, then the premise is seriated in the preferred (usually top-down) direction. Note that whereas a negation is processed linguistically, a marked adjective is processed first linguistically (in comprehension) and later spatially (in seriation). After seriating the first premise, the subject repeats the steps just described for the second premise.

In order for the subject to combine the terms of the premises into a single spatial array, the subject needs the pivot available. Either the pivot is immediately available from the linguistic encoding of the premises or it must be found spatially. According to the mixed model, there are two ways in which the pivot can become available immediately: (a) It is the single repeated term from all previous linguistic encodings; or (b) it is the last term to have been linguistically encoded. These rules have different implications for affirmative and negative premises.

In problems with two affirmative premises, the pivot is always immediately available, because each premise has been linguistically encoded just once. One term, the pivot, is distinctive from the others in that more than one relational tag has been associated with it, one from its encoding in the first premise and one from its encoding in the second premise. The second principle therefore need not even be applied. Indeed, it is applied only if the first principle fails.

The use of distinctiveness as a cue to the identity of the pivot fails in problems with at least one negative premise. In these problems, each premise containing a negation is encoded in two ways – in its original encoding and in its reformulated encoding in which the roles of the terms have been reversed. The pivot is therefore no longer the only term with more than one relational tag associated with it, and it thus loses its distinctiveness. The subject must therefore search for the term with the largest number of relational tags, unless he or she can apply the second principle.

When the distinctiveness principle fails, the subject attempts to link the first premise to the last term to have been encoded in working memory. If this term of the second premise happens to be the pivot, the link is successful, and the subject can proceed with problem solution. Pivot search can thus be avoided if the last term to have been encoded is the pivot. But if this term is not the pivot, the link cannot be made, and the subject must search for the pivot – the term with the largest number of relational tags. This search for the pivot takes additional time.

Once the pivot has been located, the subject seriates the terms from the two spatial arrays into a single spatial array. In forming the array, the subject starts with the terms of the first premise and ends with those of the second premise. The subject's mental location after seriation, therefore, is in that half of the array described by the second premise. The subject next reads the question. If there is a marked adjective in the question, the subject will take longer to encode the adjective and to seek the response at the nonpreferred (usually bottom) end of the array. The response may or may not be immediately available. If the correct answer is in the half of the array where the subject just completed seriation (his or her active location in the array), then the response will be available immediately. If the question requires an answer from the other half of the array, however, the subject will have to search for the response, mentally traversing the array from one half to the other and thereby consuming additional time.

One final search operation is used optionally under special circumstances. If the subject has constructed a sharp spatial encoding, then he or she is now ready to respond with the correct answer. If the subject's encoding is fuzzy, however, the subject may find that he or she is unable to respond with a reasonable degree of certainty. The subject therefore checks his or her tentative response as determined by the spatial representation with the encoding of that response term in the linguistic representation. If the question and response are congruent, the check is successful, and the subject reformulates the question to ascertain whether it can be made congruent with the response. Only then does he or she respond.

To summarize, the performance components needed for solution of linear syllogisms according to the linguistic–spatial mixed model are premise reading, encoding of terms in the preferred relation, encoding of terms in the nonpreferred relation (which may be viewed as an augmentation of the preceding component), reversal of terms in the encoded relation for negated premises, seriation of terms in the preferred direction, seriation of terms in the nonpreferred direction (which may be viewed as augmentation of the preceding component), pivot search, seriation of terms for the combined premises, question reading, response search, establishment of congruence between question and response (optional), and response.

All of the models are rather detailed, and it is easy to lose the forest among the trees. Thus some overall comparison among the three models may help put them into perspective. The models all agree that marked adjectives and negations should increase solution latency. They disagree, however, about why solution latency is increased. According to the spatial model, solution latency is increased because processing of negations and marked adjectives requires a more complex encoding of information into a visualized spatial array. According to the linguistic model, the additional time results from increased difficulty in a linguistic encoding process.

According to the mixed model, negations require a more complex linguistic encoding process, whereas marked adjectives require first more complex linguistic encoding and then more complex spatial encoding.

The models also agree that some form of pivot search (for the middle term in the array) is needed under special circumstances. The models disagree, however, about what these circumstances are. In the spatial model, pivot search is required for premises that are not end-anchored, that is, for premises in which the first term is the middle rather than an end of a spatial array. Absence of end-anchoring necessitates a search through the visualized spatial array. In the linguistic model, pivot search results from compression of the first premise in the deep-structural encoding (i.e., the first term of the first premise, but not the second, is stored in working memory). If the term that was dropped from working memory in compression happens to be the pivot term, then the subject has to retrieve that term back from long-term memory. In the mixed model, pivot search is required if the reformulated deep-structural version of a negative second premise does not have the pivot in its latter (and hence most recently available) proposition.

The spatial and mixed models agree that the terms of the two premises are combined into a single, unified representation. This combination is accomplished through a seriation operation in which each of two partial spatial arrays is unified into a single array. The linguistic model disagrees, positing that functional relations from the two premises are stored separately.

The linguistic and mixed models agree in the need for an operation to establish congruence between question and answer, but in the mixed model, the establishment of congruence is optional. It is used only when the spatial encoding of terms is of insufficient quality to permit the subject to respond to the problem with a reasonable degree of certainty. No operation for the establishment of congruence exists in the spatial model.

In the spatial model, subjects are hypothesized to prefer working in a certain direction (usually top-down) between as well as within premises. Generally, this preference means that extra time will be spent in seriation if the term at the preferred end of the array does not occur in the first premise. No corresponding "additional latency" exists in either the linguistic or the mixed model.

In the linguistic model, subjects search the deep-structural propositions for the term that answers the question. In a spatial array, it is obvious which term corresponds to which question adjective. For example, the tallest term might be at the top, the shortest term at the bottom. In linguistic propositions, there is no such obvious correspondence, so that the subject must check both extreme terms relative to the pivot, seeking the correct answer.

In the mixed model, subjects have to search for the response to the problem if their active location in their final spatial array is not in the half of the array containing the response. Subjects mentally traverse the array to the other half, looking for the response. No corresponding operation exists in either the spatial or the linguistic model.

Finally, the models agree that the final operation is a response process, whereby the subject selects his or her answer.

These are not the only models of linear syllogistic reasoning that have been or might be proposed. Hunter (1957) and Quinton and Fellows (1975), for example, have presented alternative models that can also be cast in "componential" terms.

The three models presented seem to be the major models of current interest, however, and are probably the ones worthy of the closest attention, at least at the present time.

In order to compare the relative abilities of the models to account for performance of human subjects on linear syllogisms, it is necessary first to postulate a combination rule. Discussion of the relative merits of the models will therefore be postponed until combination rules have been discussed.

REPRESENTATION OF INFORMATION.   Theorists disagree about the form of representation subjects use for information stored, manipulated, and retrieved in the course of linear syllogistic reasoning. The basic controversy has been over whether information is represented spatially, linguistically, or both spatially and linguistically. Spatial theorists argue that information is represented in the form of a spatial array that functions as an internal analogue to a physically realized or realizable array. Linguistic theorists argue that information is represented in the form of linguistic, deep-structure propositions of the type originally proposed by Chomsky (1965). Mixed model theorists argue that both forms of representation are used, with the linguistic form of representation serving its primary function during initial decoding of the problem, and with the spatial form of representation serving its primary function during later recoding of the problem. A resolution of this controversy not only would enlighten us with regard to transitive inference, but might further shed light on the kinds of arguments that are valuable in distinguishing between subjects' use of spatial or imaginal representations, on the one hand, and linguistic or propositional representations, on the other (see Anderson, 1976; Kosslyn & Pomerantz, 1977; Pylyshyn, 1973).

Let us first consider evidence in favor of a *spatial representation*. Eight principal kinds of evidence have been adduced in favor of a spatial representation for information.

Introspective reports.   Many subjects in various experiments have reported using spatial imagery to solve transitive inference problems such as linear syllogisms (Clark, 1969a; DeSoto et al., 1965; Huttenlocher & Higgins, 1971).

Need for spatial array to combine premise information.   At some point during the course of problem solution, subjects must comprehend the higher-order relation between the two lower-order relations expressed in the individual premises. Such comprehension is tantamount to making the transitive inference needed to solve the problem. Spatial imagery theorists have specified at a reasonable level of detail how such comprehension can take place (see Huttenlocher, 1968; Huttenlocher & Higgins, 1971). Linguistic theorists, however, have not specified in reasonable detail how the transitive inference is actually made. Clark (1971) has admitted that the "linguistic theory is not complete. For one thing, it does not fully specify how information from the two premises are [*sic*] combined" (p. 513).

Comparability of data patterns for purported imaginal arrays to those for physical arrays.   One of Huttenlocher's main arguments in favor of spatial imagery has been that "the difficulty of solving different forms of [linear] syllogisms parallels the difficulty of arranging real objects according to comparable instructions" (Huttenlocher, Higgins, Milligan, & Kauffman, 1970). A series of experiments has shown that the two types of items do indeed show parallel patterns of data (Huttenlocher, Eisenberg, & Strauss, 1970; Huttenlocher, Higgins, Milligan, & Kauffman, 1970; Huttenlocher & Strauss, 1968).

Symbolic distance effects. Data reported by Potts (1972, 1974), Mayer (1978, 1979), and Trabasso and his colleagues (Trabasso & Riley, 1975; Trabasso et al., 1975) seem strongly to implicate some kind of spatial process in linear ordering problems. In a typical experiment, subjects are taught a linear ordering of items that takes the form (A, B, C, D, E, F). Subjects are trained only on adjacent pairs of items; yet they are able to judge the untrained relation between B and E more rapidly than they are able to judge the trained relation between C and D: The further apart the two items are, the easier the judgment turns out to be. This symbolic distance effect is compatible with the kind of "internal psychophysics" proposed by Moyer (1973) and by Moyer and Bayer (1976), whereby a spatial analogue representation is constructed for the array, and elements of this analogue representation are compared to one another.

Serial position effects. In the linear ordering experiments just described, subjects are trained on all adjacent pairs of items in the linear ordering. Trabasso and his colleagues (Lutkus & Trabasso, 1974; Riley & Trabasso, 1974; Trabasso et al., 1975) have found that errors made during training and retraining exhibit a serial-position effect with respect to position of the pairs in the linear ordering: Maximum errors occur on middle pairs, and fewer errors occur on pairs nearer the ends of the ordering. This serial-position effect is interpreted as prima facie evidence for an underlying spatial array (see Bower, 1971).

Directional preferences within linear orderings. In many of the adjective pairs used in linear syllogism problems, one adjective of a bipolar pair results in more rapid or more accurate solutions than the other. For example, use of the adjectives *taller* and *better* results in facilitated performance relative to the adjectives *shorter* and *worse* (Handel et al., 1968). These authors have proposed that faster solution for the adjectives *taller* and *better* can be accounted for by the facts that (a) *taller–shorter* is represented along a continuum proceeding from top to bottom and *better–worse* is represented along a continuum proceeding from right to left, and (b) people proceed more readily in a downward direction than in an upward direction, and more readily in a rightward than in a leftward direction (p. 513).

End-anchoring effects. Investigators of transitive inference have repeatedly found end-anchoring effects in their data (see DeSoto et al., 1965; Huttenlocher, 1968). End-anchoring effects are observed when it is easier to solve a transitive inference problem presented from the ends of an array inward than it is to solve the problem presented from the middle of the array outward. Such effects are consistent with a spatial representation of information.

Correlations with spatial visualization tests. Shaver and his colleagues (1974) have reported correlations across subjects between errors in the solution of linear syllogisms and scores on tests of spatial visualization. These correlations varied in magnitude, but an impressive number of them reached statistical significance. These correlations were interpreted as evidence that spatial imagery is used in the solution of linear syllogisms.

With eight kinds of evidence converging on the same conclusion, one is tempted to accept the conclusion without further ado. Yet none of the eight kinds of evidence proves to be conclusive considered either by itself or in conjunction with the remaining kinds of evidence.

Consider first *introspective reports*. Introspective reports of the use of imagery are common, and are acknowledged even by the most prominent linguistic theorist (Clark, 1969b). A long-standing question in psychology, however, has been whether such reports can be accepted at face value (see, e.g., Ericsson & Simon, 1980; Nisbett & Wilson, 1977). Although such reports are definitely suggestive, they are certainly not conclusive. Consider next *combination of premise information, symbolic distance effects, serial-position effects*, and *end-anchoring effects*. Can a linguistic representation account for any or all of these effects? The answer appears to be affirmative: A small modification and extension of a linguistic representation suggested by Holyoak (1976) will predict all of these effects. Consider next *comparability of data patterns for imaginal and physical arrays*. Huttenlocher's argument that data patterns for reasoning with purported imaginal arrays are very similar to those for placement with actual physical arrays presents a reasonable case for the analogy between the two kinds of arrays. The correspondence does not always hold, however (Clark, 1969b, 1972a). Consider now *directional preferences*. In general, adjectives that encourage top–bottom or right–left processing are also those that are linguistically unmarked. Thus linguistic theory also predicts facilitated processing for these adjectives. Consider finally *correlations with spatial tests*. Available correlational evidence from the study by Shaver and his associates (1974) provides convergent validation for the spatial hypothesis, but does not provide discriminant validation with respect to one or more alternative hypotheses. In other words, errors on the linear syllogisms task might well have correlated with tests of spatial visualization ability because of a general factor that pervades performance on both spatial and linguistic ability tests. In order to provide a stronger test of the spatial hypothesis, one would have to show high correlations between linear syllogism and spatial test performance coupled with low correlations between linear syllogism performance and linguistic test performance.

Consider now evidence favoring a *linguistic representation* of information in linear syllogistic reasoning. Three principal kinds of evidence have been adduced in its favor.

The first, the *principle of primacy of functional relations*, states that "functional relations, like those of subject, verb, and direct object, are stored, immediately after comprehension, in a more readily available form than other kinds of information, like that of theme" (Clark, 1969b, p. 388). This principle forms the basis for the linguistic representation of information in terms of base strings and underlying deep-structural transformations on these base strings. Clark has not offered any direct experimental evidence to support the principle, although he does claim indirect support from several sources (Donaldson, 1963; Piaget, 1928).

The second kind of evidence is the *principle of lexical marking*. According to Clark's (1969b) lexical marking principle, "the senses of certain 'positive' adjectives, like *good* and *long*, are stored in memory in a less complex form than the senses of their opposites" (p. 389). The "positive" adjectives are the unmarked ones, and their opposites are the marked ones. If, as Clark claims, marked adjectives are stored in memory in a more linguistically complex form than is needed for unmarked adjectives, then one might well expect the encoding of marked adjectives to be more time-consuming than the encoding of unmarked adjectives, and indeed, all studies of linear syllogistic reasoning that have investigated both marked and unmarked adjectives have found longer latencies or more errors associated with items containing marked adjectives than with items containing unmarked adjectives. This evidence therefore seems on its face to support the principle of lexical marking.

The third kind of evidence is the *principle of congruence*. According to Clark (1969b), "Information cannot be retrieved from a sentence unless it is congruent in its functional relations with the information that is being sought" (p. 392). If information from the premises is not congruent with the information being sought, then additional time will be needed to establish congruence between the question and response. Suppose, for example, the question is "Who is best?" and the answer is *A*. If *A* were encoded from a premise such as "*A* is better than *B*," then solution should be relatively rapid, because *A* was encoded in terms of the comparative *better* and the question asks who is *best*. Suppose that, instead, the relevant premise were "*B* is worse than A," which, according to Clark, can be expanded to "*B* is worse than *A* is bad." This premise does not contain information congruent with the question. The question can be answered only if it is reformulated to read, "Who is least bad?"

Evidence in favor of a linguistic representation of information is at least as flimsy as that in favor of a spatial representation. First, the observational evidence to support the *principle of primacy of functional relations* is suggestive at best, and certainly no stronger than subjects' direct introspective reports of spatial imagery. At present, the principle seems to stand more as a presupposition for the remaining two principles than as a principle that is testable in its own right. Second, the mere existence of a marking effect as predicted by the *principle of lexical marking* does not in itself argue for a linguistic representation for information. As noted earlier, a number of investigators have noticed that the unmarked form of a bipolar adjective pair is generally the form that would be expected to appear at the top of a spatial array (DeSoto et al., 1965; Huttenlocher & Higgins, 1971). If an adjective pair could be found in which the marked form suggested the top of a spatial array and the unmarked form suggested the bottom of a spatial array, then, according to Clark (1969b), it would be possible to disentangle the spatial and linguistic accounts of the marking effect. Such an adjective pair is found in *deep–shallow*, where *deep*, the unmarked adjective in the pair, suggests the lower end of a spatial array. Clark (1969b) has reported that when subjects are presented with linear syllogisms containing the adjective pair *deep–shallow*, the standard marking effect is obtained. However, another critical adjective pair, *early–late*, is reported by Clark (1969b) to show results opposite to those predicted by lexical marking. Finally, consider again the *principle of congruence*. Spatial theorists are skeptical that the available data provide adequate support for this principle. In a series of recent experiments, Potts and Scholz (1975) obtained a congruence effect under some circumstances but not under others. Clark's (1969b) data provide only weak support for the principle of congruence. My own data (Sternberg, 1980c) suggest that the "principle of congruence" holds when items are presented in standard form, but not when they are presented premise by premise, with subjects pacing the rate of premise presentation. I believe the reason for the difference can be found in the relative quality of encodings in the two kinds of experimental situations (see the description of processes in the mixed model presented earlier).

Finally, let us consider evidence in favor of a *dual linguistic–spatial representation*. In a series of studies (Sternberg, 1980c, 1980d; Sternberg & Weil, 1980), subjects have received linear syllogisms plus psychometric tests of verbal and spatial abilities. The psychometric tests were factor-analyzed in order to yield two orthogonal factors of measured verbal and spatial abilities. Overall response latencies and latencies for individual components of information processing (determined according to the linguistic–spatial mixed model) were then correlated with the factor scores. In every one of six experiments, overall latencies were significantly correlated with both verbal and spatial factors. The absolute and relative magnitudes of the correlations with the two factors differed across experiments, but were all in the .30–.60 range. Moreover, latency parameters hypothesized to represent the durations of processes operating upon a linguistic data base generally correlated with verbal but not spatial ability; latency parameters hypothesized to represent the durations of processes operating upon a spatial data base generally correlated with spatial but not verbal ability; and confounded latency parameters that represented components operating upon both kinds of data bases generally correlated with both abilities. These results seem consistent with the notion that subjects use both linguistic and spatial representations in their solutions of linear syllogisms.

To conclude, there is some evidence that subjects use a spatial representation, and some evidence that subjects use a linguistic representation. In each case, the evidence argues in favor of the use of one kind of representation, but not in opposition to the use of the other kind. The entire body of evidence in favor of one or the other kind of representation is thus fully consistent with the use of both kinds, and the results from the Sternberg studies seem to argue that subjects do indeed use both linguistic and spatial representations in their solution of linear syllogisms. The Sternberg results provide further evidence regarding which performance components of the mixed model operate upon which kind of representation. In general, "linguistic" parameters show correlations with linguistic but not spatial ability tests, "spatial" parameters show the reverse pattern, and confounded parameters show correlations with both.

COMBINATION RULE.   In a series of six experiments comparing the three alternative models for untrained adult subjects (Sternberg, 1980c, 1980d; Sternberg & Weil, 1980), all components were assumed to be executed in the order specified in the earlier description of models; all of the models were tested with an additive combination rule, that is, a rule assuming strictly serial information processing; and the mixed model was best in each case. Values of R^2 between predicted and observed latency data ranged from .74 to .88 for the mixed model, with a median of .83. The range for the spatial model was .57–.66, with a median of .58. The range for the linguistic model was from .59 to .69, with a median of .62. Averaged across the four experiments of Sternberg (1980d), the root-mean-square deviations (RMSD) of observed from predicted values were 28 csec for the mixed model, 55 csec for the spatial model, and 52 csec for the linguistic model. All parameters of the mixed model were statistically significant in each of the six experiments (except for negation in one experiment), although many parameters of the other models were nonsignificant across the various experiments. Although under some circumstances the mixed model had one more parameter than the alternative models, the superiority of the mixed model remained even when the extra parameter was deleted. Overall, then, these data can be interpreted as providing rather strong support for the mixed model. Unfortunately, mine are the only data comparing the three models, because the mixed model has only very recently been proposed.

DURATIONS, DIFFICULTIES, AND PROBABILITIES OF COMPONENT EXECUTION. Parameter estimates for the mixed model were relatively stable across experiments (providing further support for the tenability of the mixed model), although most of the estimates of latency could be reduced by giving subjects instructions that encouraged speedy solution (Sternberg, 1980c).

There turned out to be unexpected complexities in the modeling of error rates, the explanation of which would be beyond the scope of this chapter. Estimates of parameters for predicting error rates are presented in Sternberg (1980c). Response probabilities were not modeled, because under standard instructions telling subjects to respond as quickly as possible without making errors, error rates ran only about 1%.

METACOMPONENTS. Consider the six metacomponents of reasoning and problem solving identified in the previous section, and what we know about each one.

Selection of performance components for task solution. Analyses of individual model fits indicate that about 70–75% of subjects spontaneously choose the components of the mixed model, about 10–15% spontaneously choose those of the linguistic model, and about 10–20% spontaneously choose those of the spatial model. Some subjects, of course, use none of these models. Individual differences in the strategy components subjects spontaneously choose to use in solving linear syllogisms do not correspond in a systematic way to ability patterns (Sternberg & Weil, 1980).

Selection of representation(s). When correlations of latency scores with ability factor scores are analyzed for subjects using each of the various models, it is found that scores for subjects using the linguistic model components correlate with verbal ability scores but not with spatial ability scores; scores for subjects using the spatial model components correlate with spatial ability scores but not with verbal ability scores; and scores for subjects using mixed model components correlate with both verbal and spatial ability scores (Sternberg & Weil, 1980).

Selection of strategy for combining components. The linear models that have been tested all assume serial processing for combining components. These models provide a good, although imperfect, fit to the data. Because nonlinear (and hence nonserial) models have not been tested, we really do not know how many subjects are strictly serial and how many use at least some parallel processing in their solution of the problems.

Decision about whether to maintain a strategy. Data to be described shortly suggest that subjects generally stick with the strategy they start with. It is interesting to note that when a change in strategy is induced through experimental instructions, subjects react in different ways as a function of their initial success with the strategy they are using. The probability of their adopting a trained strategy that differs from the mixed strategy most of them use appears to be inversely related to the subjects' prior success with the mixed strategy. In other words, subjects who find themselves performing effectively ("winning") with the mixed strategy are less likely to switch to the trained alternative strategy, despite instructions to do so. They seem to know that they have a winning strategy, and to decide on this basis to stick with it (Sternberg & Weil, 1980).

Selection of a speed–accuracy trade-off.   Subjects can be instructed to alter their speed–accuracy trade-off function in order to increase rate of information processing at the expense of accuracy of information processing. In one experiment, speed-emphasis instructions reduced mean latency of response from the typical 7–7½ sec to a faster 6 sec, at the cost of an increase in error rate from 1% to 7%. The distribution of model use was unaltered by the speed instructions, even though no explicit mention was made of the use of any one model or another. When subjects speed up, most of the increase in rate of response is isolated in encoding operations. Pivot search, response search, and response also show some decrease in latency. Negation, marking, and noncongruence are only minimally affected (Sternberg, 1980c).

Solution monitoring.   The extent to which subjects monitor their performance during linear syllogistic reasoning is unknown. In general, subjects are able to give only a very vague account of how they went about solving the problems. Most can report whether or not they used imagery, but not much more. Their inability to describe their solution processes does not mean they do not monitor their performance, however, because solution monitoring can be conducted below the level of consciousness.

EFFECTS OF PROBLEM FORMAT, PROBLEM CONTENT, AND PRACTICE.   Each of the variables of problem format, problem content, and practice has received at least some study, so that we are in a position to assert at least tentatively some effects of these variables on performance in a linear syllogistic reasoning task.

Consider first *problem format*. Two basic procedures have been used in timing of performance. The most common procedure is to present the problems for as long as subjects take to solve them. The subject's response to a problem terminates its presentation (Clark, 1969b; Hunter, 1957; Huttenlocher, 1968; Sternberg, 1980a, 1980b, 1980c). An alternative and less common procedure is to present the linear syllogism for a period of 10 sec. If a subject is able to solve the problem correctly in this amount of time, his or her response is counted as correct; otherwise it is counted as an error (Clark, 1969a; DeSoto et al., 1965; Keating & Caramazza, 1975). The difference in procedure has a major effect upon inferences about subjects' processing strategies (Sternberg, 1980b). The former procedure tends to favor interpretation of the results in terms of the mixed model, whereas the latter procedure tends to favor interpretation in terms of the linguistic model. If, however, the time limit at the deadline is changed, the results may favor the mixed model. Thus the deadline determines what the results look like, for reasons discussed elsewhere (Sternberg, 1980c).

Two basic procedures have also been used with regard to presentation of the premises and question. Some investigators have presented both premises plus the question simultaneously (e.g., Clark, 1969a, 1969b; Hunter, 1957). Others have presented the premises separately, or else have presented the premises together but the question separately (e.g., Huttenlocher, 1968; Potts & Scholz, 1975). Still others have used both procedures (Sternberg, 1980d), and have even presented the question before the premises. The mixed model was always best. It seems that establishment of congruence is required only when the premises and question are presented simultaneously. In this case premise encoding tends to be less thorough and thus more in need of later verification (Sternberg, 1980d).

Consider next *problem content*. The effects of relational terms (usually adjectives) have been most thoroughly investigated by DeSoto and his associates (1965) and Handel and his co-workers (1968). Two characteristics of the relational terms have received the most attention: differences in directional preference between and within bipolar pairs, and differences in difficulty between and within bipolar pairs.

With regard to directional preferences, the research of DeSoto and his colleagues and of Handel and his associates has suggested that subjects tend to order certain relational pairs, such as *better–worse, father–son*, and *more–less*, vertically in spatial arrays. *Better, father*, and *more* are generally represented at the upper end of each array. Other relational pairs, such as *earlier–later* and *faster–slower*, tended to evoke horizontal spatial arrays, with *earlier* and *slower* at the left end of each array. In still other relational pairs, such as *cause–effect, farther–nearer*, and *lighter–darker*, most subjects are inconsistent in their directional preferences.

With regard to directional difficulties, Handel and his colleagues tested subjects with problems containing a number of different relational pairs. Although these investigators did not explicitly test differences in item difficulty as a function of spatial direction, it is clear from their data that relational terms for which subjects were inconsistent in their spatial directions were more difficult to process than were relational terms for which subjects were consistent. Within relational pairs, DeSoto and his co-workers and other investigators have found that items are easier when presented with the adjective of a pair that encourages top–bottom rather than bottom–top processing, or left–right rather than right–left processing.

Consider finally effect of *practice*. Most theorists seem to assume that subjects are constant in their strategy. Not all theorists make this assumption, however. Citing the theory and data of Wood (1969), Wason and Johnson-Laird (1972) have proposed that

the inexperienced subject represents the premises in a unified form (with or without imagery) because this is likely to be the normal practical mode of dealing with the relational information. But by dint of sheer repetition this approach is likely to give way to a purer and more formal strategy geared to the specific constraints of the problem.... In short, subjects seem likely to pass from an approach analogous to the IMAGE theory to one analogous to the LINGUISTIC theory. [P. 122]

According to this hypothesis, one would expect subjects to follow a spatial model early during their experience with linear syllogisms, and to switch later to a linguistic model.

Shaver and his associates (1974) have proposed a strategy-change hypothesis that reverses the sequence just described. They noted that Johnson-Laird (1972) "hypothesized that imagery is abandoned in favor of a linguistic strategy after practice with three-term series problems. The opposite temporal sequence is indicated by our results, suggesting that in this case at least, imagery provided the 'more economical and specialized' strategy" (p. 373). According to this hypothesis, then, subjects are assumed to follow a linguistic strategy early during their experience with linear syllogisms, and to switch later to a spatial strategy.

Sternberg (1980d) tested these strategy-change hypotheses in two ways. The first was to compare fits of the various models for earlier sessions of practice with those for later sessions of practice. It was found that the mixed model was superior to the alternative models, without regard to session of practice, and that it was superior by roughly the same amount in each case. The second way of testing the hypothesis was to compare correlations of latency scores with verbal and spatial scores for early and late sessions of practice. If a strategy change were occurring, one might expect the magnitudes of the correlations with spatial (or verbal) ability to decrease over sessions, and those of the correlations with verbal (or spatial) ability to increase over sessions. In fact, the relative magnitudes of the correlations remained about the same over sessions, again providing no evidence consistent with a strategy shift.

INDIVIDUAL DIFFERENCES WITHIN AGE LEVEL (ADULTS).   The general componential framework we have been using reveals a number of sources of individual differences. First, subjects differ in the components they use for solving linear syllogisms. The large majority of subjects appear to use the components of the mixed model, but nontrivial numbers use the components of either the spatial or the linguistic model. These models, it must be remembered, are only approximations to subjects' actual strategies. The data of virtually all the subjects have reliable variance not accounted for by any of the models (Sternberg, 1980d). Second, subjects differ in their representations of information: Some appear to use only a linguistic representation, others only a spatial representation; most appear to use both kinds (Sternberg & Weil, 1980). Third, subjects appear to differ in the consistency with which they employ any strategy at all: The internal consistency reliability of individual data sets varies widely across subjects. Thus subjects differ not only in the model which best fits their individual data sets, but in the extent to which any model can and does fit their data set at all. Fourth, subjects differ widely in the rates at which they execute the various performance components, with the largest individual differences occurring in the encoding and response operations (Sternberg, 1980d). Finally, subjects differ in their accuracy of component execution (Shaver et al., 1974).

DIFFERENCES ACROSS AGE LEVELS.   Investigators have differed in their claims regarding what model is used by children of various ages in solving linear syllogisms or other kinds of transitive inference problems, but with the exception of Piaget (1921, 1928, 1955), they have been remarkably consistent in their claims that there is no evidence of strategy change across ages (Bryant & Trabasso, 1971; Hunter, 1957; Keating & Caramazza, 1975; Riley, 1976; Riley & Trabasso, 1974; Sternberg, 1980b; Trabasso, 1975). And even Piaget makes no claims of changes in strategies for children at or above the level of concrete operations. Sternberg's (1980b) data are the only ones that compare the spatial, linguistic, and mixed models, as well as the algorithmic model of Quinton and Fellows (1975), across age levels. The mixed model outperforms the others at the Grade 3, 5, 7, and 11 levels. At Grade 9, there is an inversion, with the linguistic model outperforming the mixed model. This inversion, however, can be localized to the first session of practice; in the second session, the mixed model performs better. Whether this represents a true phenomenon or a quirk in the data cannot be known, although this one inversion seems to fit into no particular pattern.

As one might expect, both solution latencies and error rates decrease with increasing age: Mean latencies (in seconds) for the 32 standard linear syllogisms are 14.51, 11.98, 10.02, 9.88, and 7.54 in Grades 3, 5, 7, 9, and 11, respectively; mean error rates are .40, .25, .23, .18, and .16 for the respective grades. The largest decrease in latency across grade levels is in the response component. The other components also show generally decreasing trends, although the rates of decrease are much slower than that of the response component (Sternberg, 1980b).

RELATIONSHIP BETWEEN LINEAR SYLLOGISTIC REASONING AND OTHER KINDS OF REASONING. As would be expected, performance on linear syllogisms is significantly correlated with performance on other kinds of reasoning tasks. Sternberg (1980d) reported a correlation of −.52 between latencies for linear syllogisms and scores on tests of abstract reasoning ability. (Negative correlations result from correlating latencies, where lower scores indicate superior performance, with test or factor scores, where higher scores indicate superior performance.) Although my colleagues and I have not correlated performance on linear and categorical syllogisms directly, the fact that both show high correlations with spatial ability tests would suggest that they would show high correlations with each other as well (Guyote & Sternberg, 1981; Sternberg, 1980d).

These high correlations can be explained at least in part within the present componential metatheoretical framework. First, linear syllogisms require at least some of the same performance components as do related kinds of problems, such as categorical syllogisms: Both require encoding of premise information, decoding of negations, combination of information from pairs of premises, and response. Second, linear syllogisms are like categorical syllogisms and certain other kinds of reasoning problems in their requirement of a spatial representation of information for solution (at least for most people). Third, the problems share many metacomponents with other kinds of reasoning problems. Whether or not the performance components are the same, in each case, the decision must be made about what performance components to use, and similarly, decisions must be made regarding combination rule, representation, speed–accuracy trade-off, and so on. Thus, even if the content of the decisions differs, the acts of deciding are required in each case. Finally, the acquisition, retention, and transfer components used to learn, remember, and generalize performance on various kinds of reasoning tasks are probably highly overlapping, and thus lead to increased correlations between tasks owing to the similar psychological histories of the tasks.

RELATIONSHIP BETWEEN LINEAR SYLLOGISTIC REASONING AND INTELLIGENCE. Because all of the various kinds of reasoning tests mentioned have been used in standard batteries for the assessment of intelligence, and because performance on linear syllogisms is rather highly correlated with performance on these other reasoning tasks, there is empirical evidence of the usefulness of linear syllogisms as psychometric measures of intelligence. Linear syllogisms have also played major roles in the two other major traditions of theory and research on intelligence, the Piagetian tradition and the information-processing tradition. In the Piagetian tradition, as mentioned earlier, linear syllogisms have served as a basis for distinguishing preoperational children from concrete-operational ones. In the information-processing tradition, theorists have argued that the processes used in linear syllogistic reasoning are central to intelligent language comprehension (Clark, 1973), to imaginal representation of linear orderings (DeSoto et al., 1965), and to deductive reasoning in general (Sternberg, 1980d), which is an important aspect of intelligence.

PRACTICAL RELEVANCE.   Virtually all of the theorists who have studied linear syllogisms have done so at least in part because of the practical importance of the processes underlying linear syllogistic reasoning, whether for everyday language comprehension or for any other purpose. Sternberg (1980d) has given an example of how transitive inference is used in many of the situations of everyday life. Consider the plight of a customer eating at a restaurant. He or she is faced with what may be a bewildering choice of meals. Because the customer has neither the time nor the patience to compare every possible meal in order to determine which he or she prefers, the customer relies upon a strategy of transitive inference, deciding that if, for example, pizza is preferred to an omelette, and an omelette is preferred to a garden salad, then pizza is preferred to the garden salad. Without transitive inference, every possible paired comparison would have to be done in order to be sure that one's preferred meal was being ordered. Consider another example, the task college admissions officers face in filling a small number of slots in the entering class from a large number of applications for those slots. Were the admissions officers not to make transitive inferences, the number of paired comparisons that would be required to weigh each candidate against every other candidate would be far beyond all reasonable bounds.

Sternberg and Weil (1980) were interested in whether particular strategies for solving linear syllogisms can be trained, and in whether an aptitude–strategy interaction exists in linear syllogistic reasoning whereby the efficacy of a particular strategy depends upon a person's pattern of verbal and spatial abilities. If the answers to both of these questions were affirmative, then it might be possible to train people to use a strategy that would be optimal for their pattern of abilities. In fact, the answers to both questions were affirmative.

To recapitulate, the proposed metatheoretical framework can be and has been applied to the understanding of one form of deductive reasoning, linear syllogistic reasoning. Similar analyses have been performed for other forms of deductive reasoning (e.g., categorical and conditional syllogistic reasoning), but the purpose of this chapter is to show how the framework can be applied to a variety of problems, and so we will now turn to a consideration of rather different kinds of problems.

5.3.   PROBLEM SOLVING AND INTELLIGENCE

Problem situations – the bases for problem-solving behavior – have been characterized in a number of different ways. Johnson (1955) has suggested that a problem situation exists when an individual's first goal-directed response is unrewarding. Köhler (1925) has suggested that a problem situation exists when an individual must take an *Umweg*, or detour, to reach a goal. Vinacke (1952) has taken a similar position, claiming that a problem situation exists when there is an "obstacle" to overcome. Woodworth and Schlosberg (1954) have argued that a problem situation exists when an individual has a goal, but no clear or well-learned route to the goal. Still other definitions have been proposed by Humphrey (1951), Maltzman (1955), Ray (1955), Russell (1956), Underwood (1952), and van de Geer (1957). According to Duncan (1959), who reviewed what was once "recent research on human problem solving," "the defining characteristics most frequently mentioned are the integration and organization of past experience when the definition refers to all of thinking, and the dimension of discovery of correct response when reference is made to problem solving specifically" (p. 397).

The definition I prefer is one offered by Raaheim (1974), which finds its historical roots in an earlier definition by Morgan (1941). Morgan suggested that a problem situation exists when there are some elements or conditions that are known and some other elements or conditions that are unknown, and the solution depends upon a discovery of how to deal with the unknown factors of the situation. In Raaheim's words, a problem situation is a "deviant member of a series of earlier situations of the same sort" (p. 22). Thus one always has some basis for dealing with the problem on the basis of past experience, but not enough of a basis to provide an immediate solution.

Problems may be subdivided in any of a number of ways (see, e.g., Greeno, 1978). A convenient way of subdividing them, and the one that I will use for the present purpose, is in terms of "well-defined" and "ill-defined" problem spaces (see Newell & Simon, 1972). A problem with a well-defined problem space is one for which the steps to solution can be clearly specified by the experiment and, ultimately, by the problem solver. Problems of this kind often require a series of small transformations on the problem input to yield the problem output. The particular difficulty is usually not in achieving any one step, but in achieving a coordinated set of steps that will yield the desired outcome. A problem with an ill-defined problem space is one for which the steps to solution cannot be clearly specified by either the experimenter or the problem solver. Problems of this kind usually require one or two major insights about the problem input to yield the problem output. The particular difficulty is usually in achieving these insights. Once they are achieved, solution of the problem becomes more or less automatic. As is true for so many distinctions, well-defined and ill-defined problem spaces are better conceived of as representing directions on a continuum than as representing a crisply conceived dichotomy. Solution of the former kind of problem will almost always be facilitated by one or more insights about the problem or about certain steps of the problem; solution of the latter kind of problem usually requires some small steps as well as the large ones.

PROBLEMS WITH WELL-DEFINED PROBLEM SPACES

The scope of problems with well-defined problem spaces

In problems with well-defined problem spaces, it is possible to specify in some detail a problem space the traversal of which will result in a correct solution. A number of different kinds of problems with well-defined problem spaces have been studied, among them:

1. *Missionaries and cannibals problem.* The missionaries and cannibals problem is one of a number of "river-crossing problems" in which a group of travelers must be transported across a river from one bank to another. What makes the task problematical is that the boat can hold only a limited number of travelers, and that certain combinations of travelers are not permitted: In the missionaries and cannibals version, for example, the number of cannibals cannot be allowed to exceed the number of missionaries, because when the cannibals outnumber the missionaries, the cannibals eat the missionaries. An essentially identical problem has been studied using

"hobbits" and "orcs," and very similar problems have been studied using men and elves, and silver and gold talismans. A closely related problem uses jealous husbands and wives. Problems of this general kind have been studied by Ernst and Newell (1969); Greeno (1974); Jeffries, Polson, Razran, and Atwood (1977); Reed and Abramson (1976); Reed, Ernst, and Banerji (1974); Simon and Reed (1976); and Thomas (1974). A selective review of the literature appears later in this section.

2. *Water jugs problem.* The water jugs problem can take various forms, but in all forms, the goal of problem solving is to transfer water between or among a set of jugs so as to accomplish some desired goal state. For example, one might be given a 5-gal. jug and an 8-gal. jug, and be asked how it is possible to put precisely 2 gal. in the 5-gal. jug. Either jug can be filled from a nearby sink, and water can be poured from one jug to another, but the jugs do not have gradations of measurement marked on them, and no measuring devices are available except the jugs themselves (Ernst & Newell, 1969). In a slightly different version, a mother sends her boy to the river to bring back exactly 3 pt. of water. She gives the boy a 7-pt. can and a 4-pt. can. The subject's task is to show how the boy can measure exactly 3 pt. of water (Terman & Merrill, 1937). In a more difficult version of the same kind of problem, a subject is told to consider three jugs of varying capacity, for example, Jugs A, B, and C, and is told that A will hold 8 units, B will hold 5 units, and C will hold 3 units. Initially, A is full and B and C are empty. The subject's task is to determine how it is possible to divide the contents of the largest jug equally between the largest and the middle-sized jugs (see Atwood & Polson, 1976; Luchins, 1942). Problems of this general kind have been studied by Atwood and Polson (1976), Ernst and Newell (1969), Luchins (1942), and Mortensen (1973).

3. *Tower of Hanoi problem.* In the Tower of Hanoi problem, the subject is presented with three pegs arranged in a linear order and *n* disks (with *n* usually about 4 or 5). The *n* disks are graded in size, and are initially stacked on the left peg, with successively larger disks closer to the bottom of the peg. The subject's task is to transfer the disks from the left-hand peg to the right-hand one. The basic constraints are that disks can be transferred one at a time from any peg (left, middle, right) to any other, that one can remove a disk only from the top position on a given peg, and that one can never place a larger disk on top of a smaller one. Various isomorphs of the basic problem have also been studied, using such vehicles as a tea ceremony and three five-handed monsters holding three crystal globes. In every case, the goal is to transfer objects in a minimum number of moves. The Tower of Hanoi problem and its isomorphs have been studied by Egan and Greeno (1974), Ernst and Newell (1969), Hayes and Simon (1974, 1976a, 1976b), and Simon (1975).

This list of problems is obviously far from complete; it deals with only a limited class of problems with well-defined problem state spaces. Nevertheless, it constitutes a reasonable sampling of the kinds of problems with well-defined state spaces that have been studied.

A case study of problem solving in a well-defined problem space: the missionaries and cannibals problem

NATURE OF THE PROBLEM.   In a typical version of the missionaries and cannibals problem, the subject must figure out how to transport three missionaries and three cannibals across a river. A boat is available for transportation, but it will hold only two people at a time. It is also possible to use the boat to transport just a single person at a time. The number of cannibals on either side of the river can never be allowed to exceed the number of missionaries, because, in this event, the cannibals will eat the missionaries. A somewhat more difficult version of the problem uses five missionaries and five cannibals and a boat that will hold up to three persons at a time. Several variants of the problem have been used, all of which pose essentially the same problem to the subjects: hobbits and orcs, elves and men, and silver and gold talismans.

Performance on the missionaries and cannibals problem has not yet been shown to satisfy all of the criteria proposed earlier, although the means for making this demonstration are readily available. Let us consider each criterion for task selection in turn.

Performance on the task is certainly quantifiable, and in a number of different ways. One overall measure of performance is simply the total number of moves needed to solve the problem; another is the total amount of time spent in solving the problem. Each of these overall measures can be broken down further. The total number of moves can be broken down into numbers of legal and illegal moves; and the number of legal moves can be further broken down into the number of correct moves (those that move the subject closer to the solution) and the number of incorrect moves (those that do not lead toward the solution). For each of these numbers of moves, one can also measure the total amount of time spent on moves of that kind. Another way of quantifying performance is by the number of times a given state is entered, where a state is defined by the number of missionaries and cannibals on each of the two sides of the river and by the position of the boat with respect to the two sides. Similarly, one can measure the total amount of time spent in each state. These states can be subdivided, of course, according to whether they are legal or illegal (e.g., more cannibals than missionaries on one side of the river), and measurements can be done separately for legal and illegal states. More refined measures are also possible for particular kinds of analyses, but it should be clear at this point that quantification of performance on these problems can be done in several different ways.

No one has explicitly tested the reliability of performance in the missionaries and cannibals problem. Indirect tests, however, have indicated high alternate-forms reliabilities across isomorphs (Jeffries et al., 1977) and instructional conditions (Simon & Reed, 1976).

Construct validity of performance on the missionaries and cannibals problem can be inferred from a number of different sources. The conclusion from all these sources is that performance on this task can and should be accounted for by a general theory of problem solving. Ernst and Newell (1969) showed that their General Problem Solver (GPS) program, which they took to be a theory of problem solving, was capable of solving the missionaries and cannibals problem using the same basic strategies as were used in the solution of other kinds of well-structured problems.

The construct validity of performance on the missionaries and cannibals problem is also supported by the analyses of Jeffries and her associates (1977), who have argued that the strategy subjects use in solving this problem is a special case of a more general strategy that can be used in solving other problems of this general kind (sometimes called MOVE problems), such as the water jugs problem.

The one criterion for task selection on which evidence is conspicuously missing is that of empirical validity. We do not know, at this time, whether any of the indexes of performance on the missionaries and cannibals problem are correlated with indexes of performance on the other tasks of interest that are not trivially different. For example, it would be of interest to know whether missionaries and cannibals performance is related to IQ or to planning ability of some sort (e.g., construction of flow charts in computer programming). As has been shown earlier, empirical validity cannot be taken for granted: Tasks that one would expect to be empirically valid (e.g., animal-name analogies) sometimes show disappointing correlations with external measures.

PERFORMANCE COMPONENTS.   Three complete models of performance on the missionaries and cannibals problem have been proposed: the GPS model of Ernst and Newell (1969), a modification of the GPS model that seems better able to account for strategies used by human subjects (Simon & Reed, 1976), and the model of Jeffries and her colleagues (1977), which also shares certain features with GPS, but is less closely derived from GPS than is the model of Simon and Reed. I shall describe in detail here only the Simon–Reed model.

According to Simon and Reed's model, subjects may use either or both of two basic strategies in the solution of the missionaries and cannibals problem. If they use both strategies, then they do so sequentially, with strategy change occurring either suddenly (strategy shift) or gradually (strategy learning). A given strategy may incorporate both systematic and random elements. In other words, a subject may choose among alternative courses of action on the basis of a preference ordering determined by the strategy, or the subject may select one of the alternatives at random (with equal probabilities assigned to all alternatives considered). So-called random behavior may be interpreted as its name implies – as genuinely random behavior – or as behavior based on a mixture of other strategies not incorporated into the proposed model. The authors opt for the second interpretation, although the preferred interpretation does not affect the outcome of applying the model to the data. Subjects are also assumed to seek to avoid, to a specifiable extent, reversing a move they have just made, that is, going backward so that the problem state is what it was prior to the move that led to the current state.

The first strategy is a *balance* strategy. In this strategy, subjects select that legal move which balances the number of missionaries with the number of cannibals on each side of the river. The authors suggest that use of such a strategy is motivated by subjects' awareness that the number of cannibals cannot be permitted to exceed the number of missionaries on a given side. Subjects soon also realize as an implication of this rule that the number of missionaries cannot exceed the number of cannibals on either side, unless the opposing side has no missionaries at all (to be eaten by the cannibals).

The second strategy is a *means–ends* strategy. Use of this strategy entails a subject's preferring that move which takes the maximum number of persons across the river on odd-numbered moves, or the minimum number of persons back across the river on even-numbered moves. This strategy seeks to reduce as much as possible the difference between the goal state (all persons across the river) and the current state of problem solving.

REPRESENTATION OF INFORMATION.   Investigators studying the missionaries and cannibals problem have all represented information needed and used during problem solving in terms of a problem state space. This particular state space is for a problem with three missionaries, three cannibals, and a boat that can hold a maximum of two persons. Slightly more complicated state spaces are needed for more difficult versions of the problem (e.g., five missionaries, five cannibals, and a boat holding a maximum of three persons). In Thomas's (1974) notation, each state is specified by a three-digit code, where the first digit represents the number of missionaries on the starting side, the second digit represents the number of cannibals on the starting side, and the third digit represents the location of the boat (1 if it is on the starting side, 0 if it is on the opposite side). One interesting and surprising feature of the space is its near "linearity": At all but two states, only two legal moves exist, the correct move and a move that will result in the subject's retreating to the previous state. A branching exists at the other two states, but either branch can lead to the correct next state. The state space becomes somewhat more complicated if illegal states are added (see, e.g., Jeffries et al., 1977, p. 414), but such states are cul de sacs from which subjects have no choice but to retreat immediately (lest they fail to solve the problem). The state space becomes more complicated in versions of the problem using more missionaries and cannibals (see, e.g., Simon & Reed, p. 88).

All investigators studying the missionaries and cannibals problem have made it clear that representations of the sort they have used are "formal" representations that may or may not correspond to what subjects have in their heads. Certainly subjects are not aware of this form of representation, because they are almost never aware of the linearity of the space, and because it would not be possible for them to hold the entire space in their working memories.

Thomas (1974) was interested in testing whether subjects' actual representations corresponded to the formal representation just given. He noted that GPS, Ernst and Newell's (1969) theory of problem-solving, did in fact use the formal state space as the basis for problem-solving performance. Two separate tests of the hypothesis were made. The results indicated that the formal state space is insufficiently rich as a representation of subjects' knowledge. The information available to a subject in a given state exceeds the three items of information characterizing that state (i.e., number of missionaries and cannibals on the original side plus position of boat). Whatever the states of the problem space may represent, they are not representative of separate stages of information processing. Subjects have some kind of higher-order representation that integrates or crosscuts stages.

Greeno (1974) reached the same conclusion as Thomas, although for a different reason. Two of Greeno's experimential conditions were a "correction condition," in which subjects were given corrective feedback if they made an error, and a "noncorrection prevent backward" condition, in which subjects were not given corrective feedback when they made errors, but in which they were immediately informed if they made a move that took them backward in the state space. Greeno found that although performance in these two conditions was identical in the two hardest states (321 and 110), performance was worse in the correction condition than in the noncorrection in the two relatively easy states that follow the two hardest states. Greeno interpreted this result as indicating that subjects in the noncorrection condition do some looking ahead from the difficult states, but that subjects in the correction condition are not able to do this because of disruption from the corrective feedback. Thus subjects in the noncorrection condition, at least, seemed to be organizing their responses at a level beyond that of individual states of the space.

COMBINATION RULES.   Consider first how the basic components of problem solving in the Simon–Reed model are combined. In this model, it is hypothesized that all subjects begin solution using the balance strategy and a "random element," and at some point switch to the means–ends strategy and a random element. There is a certain probability of switching strategy at each move through the state space. At each move there is also a probability that a given subject will guard against returning to a previous state (which Simon & Reed refer to as an antiloop strategy), and this probability increases over time. The probability that a subject will select his or her move according to the selected strategy rather than according to the random element also increases over time. Differences in problem-solving behavior as a function of experimental condition (e.g., prior practice with the missionaries and cannibals problem or receipt of a hint about how the problem should be solved) are produced by effects of the parameters of the model, namely, change in strategy-switching probability, initial probabilities of moving according to strategy rather than at random, probability of testing for a loop back to a previous state, and the rates at which these latter two probabilities change. There are thus five parameters to be combined in the model.

Simon and Reed tested this model in two experiments. In one experiment, subjects either were or were not given a subgoal (information regarding the placement of the boat and the numbers of missionaries and cannibals across the river); in a second experiment, performance was measured on a first trial of performance and on a second trial (replication) of performance. Predictions of the model were determined through a computer simulation. The proposed model accounted for 90%, 88%, 74%, and 79% of the variance in the legal-move data in the four respective experimental conditions. The authors interpreted these data as providing a reasonable level of support for the model.

In the final paragraphs of their article, Jeffries and her associates compare their model to that of Simon and Reed, and this comparison is obviously of interest here. The two models have in common their claims that people do not plan multistep sequences, that people use means–ends analysis and memory for states previously entered, and that when all else fails, people choose a move at random. The most striking difference between the models is that the Simon–Reed model assumes that subjects change strategies at some point during their experience with the problem, whereas the model of Jeffries and her colleagues assumes that a single, more complex strategy can account for problem solving throughout the course of a subject's experience with the problem. The latter model seems to say more about and place greater demands on memory for the problem-solving process, and it also assumes that subjects engage in later steps (i.e., stages of problem solving) only if earlier steps fail to yield a next move. Jeffries and her co-workers note that both models account quite well for obtained data, but that neither their data set nor that of Simon and Reed provides sufficient data to distinguish between models. Because both models seem to be accounting for the same kinds of data, it is not clear to me why this is the case. In terms of values of R^2, or percentage of variance accounted for in the data, the model constructed by Jeffries and her colleagues does better on these authors' data set than Simon and Reed's model does on *their* data set. Comparison of R^2 across experiments, however, and often even within experiments, is fraught with difficulties, and the greater predictive efficacy of the model of Jeffries and her co-workers might be due in part to its seemingly greater complication. At present, therefore, there seems to be no basis for distinguishing between the two models.

DURATIONS, DIFFICULTIES, AND PROBABILITIES OF COMPONENT EXECUTION. No one has attempted to account for latencies of components of problem solving during solution of the missionaries and cannibals problem, and hence no latency parameters have been estimated or even proposed. The parameters that have been estimated address aspects of problem solving that make various moves more or less difficult and that affect probabilities of entering various states.

In the Simon–Reed model fitting, there were "no known systematic procedures for finding best estimates of the model's parameters in order to fit it to a set of data" (p. 90). Hence Simon and Reed "tuned" the parameter estimates with the aid of data from the control condition of their first experiment, in which subjects were asked simply to solve the missionaries and cannibals problem without any hints or prior experience with the problem. Tuning consisted of adjusting parameters until the data from human subjects and from the simulation were almost perfectly congruent. Parameter estimates were psychologically plausible.

METACOMPONENTS. Our understanding of the metacomponents of problem solving in the solution of the missionaries and cannibals problem is rather minimal, and there are some metacomponents about which we know nothing.

Selection of performance components. Subjects' selection of performance components is motivated by several considerations. The first is the subjects' desire to attain balance between the number of missionaries and the number of cannibals on a given side. If the numbers are not monitored, one runs the risk of creating a situation in which the cannibals can eat the missionaries. In the Simon–Reed model, it is this consideration that leads to the use of a "balance" strategy early during problem solving. A second consideration is the subjects' desire to attain the final state as quickly as possible. Subjects presumably have the (correct) intuition that the missionaries and cannibals problem is one that can lead to infinite looping whereby a solution is never attained, and that one way of counteracting this possibility is to keep pursuing moves that lead to closer approximations to the end state. In the Simon–Reed model, this consideration leads to the use of a means–ends strategy later during problem solving.

Selection of representation(s). We know that subjects do not represent information about the missionaries and cannibals problem solely in terms of the formal state space (Greeno, 1974; Thomas, 1974). But we do not know how subjects do represent information, or even into what kinds of units the representation is parsed. There are some pragmatic considerations that, from the subject's point of view, would seem to place constraints upon the kind of representation that might be used. First, subjects could never hold the entire formal state space or any analogue of it in working memory. The representation that subjects use must somehow chunk information in a way that permits them to retain a local context and some sense of where they are in the global scheme of things, but that does not require retention of large numbers of states in working memory. Second, the representation must be one that is easily retrievable and modifiable. The missionaries and cannibals problem requires frequent access of processes to the representation(s) upon which these processes act, and because subjects almost certainly do not have the full psychological state space represented when they start problem solving, they must be able to add to and delete from their representation on a fairly regular basis as they glean new information about the problem. Third, the representation must be one that somehow permits unitization of several pieces of information, some of which are different in kind. Obviously, the subject must be able somehow to unitize information about the number of missionaries and cannibals on a given side, and about the position of the boat. But the subject will also need some integration of this information with his or her memory of the previous state, lest the previous state be reentered; also, the subject must be able to hold in working memory the present and at least partial information about the previous state while performing tests on the legality of the state he or she proposes to enter; finally, the subject must be able to remember which of the next possible states have already been tested for legality, lest the same state be tested again and again.

Selection of a strategy for combining components. The balance strategy and the means–ends strategy can at best be viewed as substrategies or components embedded in the context of an overall strategy for the solution of the missionaries and cannibals problem. This overall strategy includes different elements, depending upon the model to which the subject adheres (Simon & Reed's, Jeffries et al.'s, or some other). One question that inevitably arises is that of how a subject is able to put together such a complex package of information in the absence of prior experience (for most subjects) with problems of this kind. The data of Greeno and of Thomas suggest perhaps three or four stages of information processing in solving the missionaries and cannibals problem, and the models we have considered actually postulate numbers of stages at this level. It seems plausible that subjects consciously plan only three or four aspects of their information processing. The other aspects of processing that are necessary for solution of the problem may be immediate concomitants or consequents of these three or four basic aspects, combined with the structure of the problem. In other words, the basic decisions needed to solve the problem and the inherent nature of the problem guide the subject into making a fairly large number of decisions that he or she may not even be aware of, or of the need for. Were this not the case, the complexity of the models – particularly that of Jeffries and her associates – would be difficult to accept in a "performance model" of information processing. What might be the basic decisions that, once made, could lead almost automatically to the need for the remaining decisions?

First, the subject needs to decide upon an implicit "evaluation function," which in turn leads to selection of a strategy and a way of implementing that strategy. Second, the subject must decide what information is needed to start moving forward and to keep moving forward, namely, knowledge of numbers and positions of missionaries and cannibals, and of the position of the boat, for the present and the immediately preceding move. Third, the subject must decide to check for illegality, and he or she must work out a system for doing so; this decision leads in turn to a means for selecting a next move from among the available alternatives. These basic decisions seem to force the need for all of the other decisions that will have to be made during the course of problem solving.

Decisions about whether to maintain a strategy. It is obviously a matter of theoretical debate (between Simon & Reed on the one hand and Jeffries et al. on the other) whether subjects decide to change strategy midway through their solving of the missionaries and cannibals problem. What is a clear-cut decision in the model of

Simon and Reed, however, is a fuzzy one in the model of Jeffries and her colleagues, because of the continuous nature of the evaluation function in the latter model.

Selection of a speed–accuracy trade-off. There is no evidence at all regarding speed–accuracy trade-off. Reed (Reed & Abramson, 1976; Reed et al., 1974) has collected latency data, but not speed–accuracy trade-off data.

Solution monitoring. It is difficult for subjects to monitor their solution processes in the missionaries and cannibals problem, because they do not have the total state space available to them, and because later states do not always resemble the final state more closely than do earlier states. At best, subjects can infer whether the drift of the states they are entering is toward the goal state, even if individual states do not always appear to be in this direction. The two most difficult states – 110 and 321 – appear to be ones in which extensive solution monitoring occur (Greeno, 1974; Thomas, 1974). These are the states with the maximum number of possible alternative responses (five). In the case of state 321, it is the single state in the problem (for three missionaries and three cannibals) where it is possible to make a backward move that does not return one to the state just left. Hence subjects seem more likely to assess at these points whether they are indeed progressing toward their goal. Thomas found that when he informed subjects at state 110 that they were "on the right track," and that the problem was "solvable from here," it improved their performance considerably. In effect, the experimenter performed the solution monitoring for the subject.

PROBLEM FORMAT, PROBLEM CONTENT, AND PRACTICE. Consider first the effects of *problem format*. The standard format for presentation of the missionaries and cannibals problem has been to present subjects with the basic information required for solving the problem, and then to ask them to trace through the steps that are needed to go from the initial state to the goal state. There have been several basic variations on this format.

Thomas (1974) provided one group of subjects with feedback at state 110 that told the subjects that they were on the right track. This feedback increased the proportion of correct moves out of this state from .49 in a control group without feedback to .64 in the experimental (feedback) group, and decreased the number of backward and restarting moves from .26 to .15. Although these effects were in the predicted directions, they were not statistically significant.

Greeno (1974) had three different feedback conditions. In a first group, subjects were informed after errors that allowed orcs (the analogues to cannibals) to eat hobbits (the analogues to missionaries). In a second group, subjects were informed after errors that allowed orcs to eat hobbits, and also after moves that would produce backtracking through the state space. A third group consisted of subjects who were also informed after both kinds of errors, but who were further informed which response was correct. These subjects differed from the other subjects, then, in not having to experiment with other moves. Greeno found that the mean number of errors allowing orcs to eat hobbits was 9.6 in the first group, 9.9 in the second group, and 6.6 in the third group. The difference among groups was not significant, and the reduction in "eating" errors in the third group was attributed by Greeno to the subjects' being told the correct move and thereby being prevented from making more than one error in a given trial. The total number of backward moves was 12.7 in the first group, 6.7 in the second group, and 4.7 in the third group. The value for the first group differed significantly from the values for the other two groups, but the values for the other two groups did not differ significantly from each other.

Reed and Abramson (1976) performed two experiments that varied information about problem states across groups of subjects. In their first experiment, they used three missionaries and three cannibals for the test problem. Subjects received either no subgoal information, subgoal information about a subgoal that would be reached early during problem solution, or subgoal information about a subgoal that would be reached late during problem solution. The numbers of legal and illegal moves did not vary across groups, nor did solution time. Subjects given the earlier subgoal did reach that subgoal in significantly fewer moves and with significantly shorter latency than did subjects given the later subgoal; but overall performance on the problem was unaffected. Thus the differential effect of subgoal location was limited to performance before that early subgoal was reached, and the difference was washed out when indexes of performance for the total problem were considered. In their second experiment, using five missionaries and five cannibals, subjects were given an early subgoal or no subgoal at all. The subgoal significantly reduced the mean number of legal moves from 27.6 to 20.3, significantly reduced the number of illegal moves from 5.5 to 3.7, and significantly reduced mean solution time from 883 sec to just 437 sec. The mean number of legal moves to the subgoal state and the time to reach that state were also significantly reduced. The authors suggested that the subgoal facilitated overall performance in the second experiment but not in the first experiment because it caused a greater reduction in the size of the state space for the second problem. Although the minimum number of moves needed to achieve a solution is the same in both versions, the number of "false" moves is far greater in the larger version of the problem, and so it is a more difficult problem. Thus providing subgoal information in the larger version of the problem provides more information about moves the subject should not make. The authors conclude that a subgoal is probably not very effective in a problem space consisting of many states in which only one legal forward move can be made.

As mentioned earlier, several types of *problem content* have been used in studies of the missionaries and cannibals problem. There have been two basic kinds of manipulations. The first concerns the kinds of individuals to be transported – missionaries and cannibals, hobbits and orcs, elves and men, or silver and gold talismans. Jealous husbands and wives have been used in a problem that is similar (homomorphic) but not identical (isomorphic) to the missionaries and cannibals problem, and so this variant of the problem will not be considered here. The second kind of manipulation concerns the numbers of individuals to be transported, which has been either three of each kind or five of each kind.

The data of Jeffries and her co-workers (1977) directly address the relative difficulties of the various content isomorphs. These authors used hobbits and orcs, two variants of elves and men, and silver and gold talismans. They found no significant differences in numbers of legal moves across isomorphs. They did find significant differences in numbers of illegal moves and in numbers of errors, however. In particular, the numbers of illegal moves and errors were lowest in the hobbits–orcs condition, and highest in the silver–gold talisman condition. The two variants of the elves–men problem showed almost identical patterns of data for illegal moves and errors. The authors were able to localize the differences to the two problem states with the highest numbers of illegal moves. Thus problem content appears to have local rather than global effects.

The data of Reed and Abramson (1976) permit a direct comparison between the difficulty of the missionaries and cannibals problem for three and the difficulty for five individuals of each kind. For their control groups (standard problem presentation format), the mean number of legal moves was 20.0 in the 3MC (three missionaries and three cannibals) group and 27.6 in the 5MC group; the comparable means for illegal moves were 4.1 and 5.5; the comparable means for solution time were 361 sec and 883 sec. Clearly, the 5MC condition was considerably more difficult than the 3MC.

Quite a bit of research has been done on the effects of *practice* upon efficacy of problem solving in the missionaries and cannibals problem. Thomas (1974) was interested in part–whole transfer in problem solving. In one group, subjects simply solved the problem as presented in standard format. In a second group, subjects first solved the problem from the halfway point until the end; they then re-solved the problem, starting this time at the beginning. Thomas found two unexpected things. First, initial practice on the latter half of the problem did not facilitate later performance on that part of the problem (when the second group re-solved the problem), but this initial practice did facilitate later performance on the first part of the problem, that part on which the subject had not received prior practice. Second, the control group (the one that received the problem in the standard format) showed negative transfer with respect to the part–whole group from the first part of the problem to the second; that is, they required more moves to solve the second part of the problem (15.5) than did the subjects who solved the second part of the problem without yet having solved the first part (12.0). Thomas explained these findings in terms of "context effects," state-specific effects, and a psychological state space that did not correspond to the formal state space. But the explanations proposed by Thomas did not go very far toward removing the mystery surrounding these two surprising findings.

Greeno (1974) had subjects solve the hobbits–orcs problem repeatedly until they made no errors on two successive trials. Groups differed in feedback they received for their performance (as described earlier). Greeno found that subjects learned from positive information indicating which response was correct, rather than from elimination of errors in performance or from sampling of new strategies after commission of errors. Analysis of acquisition data was consistent with an hypothesis of all-or-none learning at individual states in the problem space, except for one state. Greeno used an elves and men version of the problem, as well as the hobbits and orcs version, and obtained essentially parallel results.

Reed and his colleagues (1974) investigated effects of practice, although their particular focus was upon transfer between the missionaries and cannibals problem and the jealous husbands and wives problem. The formal state space for the latter problem is the same as that for the former, if husbands are substituted for missionaries, and wives for cannibals. There is a critical difference between problems, however (which incidentally points out how the formal state space cannot capture all aspects of a problem needed in actual problem solving). In the jealous husbands and wives problem, husbands and wives are paired, such that wives must always be with their own husbands, if they are with any men at all. In the missionaries and cannibals problem, there is no such pairing. Reed and his associates refer to the two problems as "homomorphic," meaning that there is a many-to-one mapping from the missionaries and cannibals problem (where any pairing is possible) to the jealous husbands and wives problem (where only one pairing is possible). The authors sought to discover whether there would be significant transfer between problems, that is, whether practice with one would facilitate performance with the other.

The authors conducted three experiments. In the first, subjects were required to solve both problems, with half of the subjects starting with the missionaries and cannibals problem and the other half starting with the jealous husbands and wives problem. In the second experiment, subjects solved the same problem twice; this experiment thus investigated transfer within rather than across problems. In the third experiment, the procedure was identical to that followed in the first, except that the authors inserted an additional paragraph into the instructions informing subjects just how the two problems were related. In the first experiment, there was virtually no transfer from solution of the first problem to solution of the second. The second experiment was an attempt to find out why the results of the first experiment were so disappointing. Reed and his associates judged that for transfer to occur across problem types, it would at least have to occur within problem type. They therefore set out to find out if such transfer within problem type occurred. Averaged across problems, the authors found that there was a significant decrease in solution latency and in number of illegal moves, but not in total number of moves. Follow-up tests revealed that the effect was highly significant for practice on the jealous husbands and wives problem, but was only marginally significant for the missionaries and cannibals problem. The second experiment showed that at least some within-problem transfer took place, and so did not isolate the reason for the failure of transfer to occur in the first experiment. The third experiment provided a way of testing whether the reason for the failure was subjects' inability to see how the two problems are related. In this experiment, the authors found that with solution latency and number of illegal moves as the dependent variables, there was significant and substantial transfer from the jealous husbands and wives problem to the missionaries and cannibals problem, but not vice versa. With total number of moves as the dependent variable, there was no evidence of transfer. This experiment thus suggested that for transfer to occur, it was necessary for the more difficult problem to be presented first, and for subjects to be informed of the relationship between this problem and the less difficult one.

In an attempt to find out how transfer occurred, Reed and his co-workers asked subjects to indicate which of four strategies best described the relationship between their strategies in solving the first and their strategies for the second problem. Most subjects indicated that they "occasionally" used their memory for the first problem as a basis for solving the second problem, but that they usually attempted to solve the second problem independently of the first. Some subjects indicated that they did not use their memory for the first problem at all, but rather solved the second problem independently. Only a handful of subjects remembered "most" of their earlier moves, and none remembered all.

Simon and Reed (1976), of course, were very interested in practice effects on performance, and had one set of conditions in which subjects solved the missionaries and cannibals problem twice in succession. They found a substantial decrease in number of legal moves from the first trial of solution to the second.

INDIVIDUAL DIFFERENCES WITHIN AGE LEVEL (ADULTS). None of the investigators who have studied the missionaries and cannibals problem have been particularly concerned with individual differences. Nevertheless, the data of Reed and his associates (1974) are strongly suggestive of the existence of individual differences, at least when more than one trial is given: Subjects indicated several different levels of use of the first problem in solving the second problem. As always, individual differences may be responsible for differences in findings across the various studies that have been done.

DIFFERENCES ACROSS AGE LEVELS. The missionaries and cannibals problem has not been studied developmentally; so there is no information available on developmental differences. The problem does seem susceptible to developmental investigation, however, perhaps from the secondary-school age level upward.

RELATIONSHIPS BETWEEN SOLUTION OF THE MISSIONARIES AND CANNIBALS PROBLEM AND SOLUTION OF OTHER KINDS OF PROBLEMS. The apparent lack of interest in individual differences among investigators who have studied the missionaries and cannibals problem has led to a virtual absence of data across subjects regarding relationships between subjects' ability to solve the missionaries and cannibals problem and their ability to solve other kinds of problems. Such individual-differences analyses would be motivated by at least two theories – that of Ernst and Newell (1969) and that of Jeffries and her associates (1977) – which claim that the processes used in solving the missionaries and cannibals problem are highly overlapping with the processes used to solve other kinds of problems.

Jeffries and her co-workers, for example, claim that people working on transformation (MOVE) problems such as the missionaries and cannibals problem or the water jugs problem

consider only single-step move sequences, using two criteria for selecting successors: (i) select moves that lead to "better" states, where better is defined in terms of a means–ends evaluation, and (ii) avoid moves that lead to states recognized as previously visited. The details of how states are evaluated and the order in which moves are considered are specific to a particular task. [P. 436]

In this model, the memory processes are identical to those proposed by Atwood and Polson (1976) in their model of performance in the water jugs problem, and the move-selection process (stage model) is also very similar to that of Atwood and Polson. To the extent that there are differences between models, they are in the specifics (as opposed to the form) of the evaluation function. Such specifics would necessarily vary, because different items of information necessarily require different specific means of evaluation. Jeffries and her colleagues compared parameters estimated from performance in their missionaries and cannibals isomorphs to performance obtained on the water jugs problem (Atwood & Polson, 1976). Values of parameters were quite close. There is thus at least tentative evidence of generality of processes across two members of the class of MOVE problems, namely, the missionaries and cannibals problem and the water jugs problem. The work of Ernst and Newell (1969) suggests that the generality in methods of problem solving might extend even further. At least some correlational investigation ought to be done to determine whether patterns of individual differences, as well as parameter values, are similar across the various kinds of MOVE problems. An obvious next step in a program of research investigating the missionaries and cannibals problem would be to study individual differences, and to relate them across this task, the water jugs task, and perhaps the Tower of Hanoi task.

RELATIONSHIP BETWEEN PERFORMANCE ON THE MISSIONARIES AND CANNIBALS PROBLEM AND INTELLIGENCE.   Perhaps because of the lack of interest in individual differences among investigators studying the missionaries and cannibals problem, no one has attempted to correlate scores for various aspects of performance on the problem with scores on any kind of general intelligence test. I believe this to be unfortunate, because there seems to be an implicit assumption in the work that performance on the missionaries and cannibals problem taps at least some fundamental aspects of problem solving; and presumably, such fundamental aspects of problem solving would be important in any well-conceived notion of intelligence. An investigation of the relationship between missionaries and cannibals performance and measured intelligence could be an obvious part of the kind of individual-differences research mentioned previously.

PRACTICAL RELEVANCE.   The question of practical relevance has also received short shrift in the literature on the missionaries and cannibals problem. I am unable to find any discussion at all in the literature regarding what practical relevance performance on the problem might have. On the one hand, certain aspects of performance on the problem would seem to be called for in everyday problem solving: the setting of subgoals, the need to represent information in a way that moves one forward and not backward in problem solving, the use of some kind of evaluation function to choose among alternative next moves in problem solving, and so on. On the other hand, the problem seems artificial in at least some important ways: in the contrived nature of the task (regardless of which isomorph is used); in the seemingly arbitrary constraints that are placed upon accomplishment of the task (cannibals eating missionaries if they outnumber the missionaries; a boat that only holds two individuals); in the simple nature of the problem state space, in which for most moves (in the 3MC problem) there is only one legal move in the forward direction and one legal move in the backward direction; and in the clarity with which "legal" and "illegal" moves are defined. These limitations may or may not reduce or even undermine the ecological validity of the task as a representative case of real-world problem solving. Investigation of the task's ecological validity, or at least external validity of some kind, is sorely needed.

   To recapitulate, the proposed metatheoretical framework can be and has been applied to the understanding of one kind of problem solving, a kind in which the problem state space is well defined. We now turn to a consideration of how the framework can be applied to the study and understanding of problem solving in an ill-defined state space.

PROBLEMS WITH ILL-DEFINED PROBLEM SPACES

The scope of problems with ill-defined problem spaces

In problems of this kind, it is difficult (at least in our present state of knowledge about problem solving) to specify in any detail a problem space the traversal of which will result in an adequate solution. Several kinds of problems with ill-defined problem spaces have been studied, among them:

1. *Hatrack problem.* In the original form of this problem (Maier, 1933), subjects are asked to construct a hatrack in an experimental room. The room (as described by Hoffman, Burke, & Maier, 1963) is 8 ft. high in most places, and contains various items such as electrical conduits, lighting fixtures, fuse boxes, beams, and minor irregularities in floor and ceiling. The only equipment explicitly made available to subjects consists of two 1-in. by 2-in. poles, one 6 ft. in length and the other 7 ft. in length, and a 3-in. C-clamp. Subjects are told that the hatrack they construct must be sturdy enough to support a heavy coat and a hat. In the more difficult version of the problem, subjects are told that they must construct the hatrack in a specified part (near the center) of the room. The solution is achieved by using the C-clamp to wedge the two poles firmly against the floor and ceiling. The two poles are allowed to overlap just enough so that they will stay firmly in place when clamped together. The clamp not only holds the poles together, but also serves as the hook on which the hat and coat can be hung. In the easier version of the problem, subjects are allowed to construct the hatrack anywhere in the room. In this case, various elements of the room can be used in fashioning a solution. Hoffman and associates (1963) classified solutions as being of five types:

> Base: a solution in which one board is used as a support to hold the second one vertically, with the clamp joining them at the floor level;
> Balance: a solution in which the boards are leaned on each other in an X or T shape with the clamp joining them;
> Support: any solution using a part of the room (walls, pipes, ceiling beams, etc.) to hold up the construction (limited to the use of the ceiling pipes and beams during the test problem);
> Ceiling suspension: a solution in which the boards are wedged between the ceiling and ceiling pipes or beams, with the clamp joining them or appended to the joined ends;
> Floor–ceiling: the correct solution, in which the boards are wedged between floor and ceiling and joined tightly by the clamp.

This problem (in its two versions as well as minor variants of them) has been studied by R. Burke and Maier (1965); R. Burke, Maier, and Hoffman (1966); Hoffman and associates (1963); Judson, Cofer, and Gelfand (1956); Maier (1933, 1945, 1970); Maier and Burke (1966); Raaheim (1974); and Saugstad (1955).

2. *Two-string problem.* In the original form of this problem (Maier, 1931), subjects are brought into a large room containing many objects, such as poles, ring stands, clamps, pliers, extension cords, tables, and chairs. The experimenter hangs two cords from the ceiling. One hangs near the center of the room, the other near a wall. The cords are of sufficient length to reach the floor. Subjects are told that their task is to tie the ends of the two strings together. It soon becomes apparent to subjects that the cords are far enough apart so that it is not possible to hold both in one's hands simultaneously. Subjects must therefore use the materials in the room to attain a solution to the problem. This problem and its variants have been studied by Duncker (1945), Maier (1930, 1931, 1933, 1945, 1970), Maier and Burke (1966), Maier and Janzen (1968), Raaheim (1974), and Saugstad (1955, 1957, 1958).

3. *Radiation problem.* This problem, originally proposed by Duncker (1926), is usually posed in the following form: "Given a human being with an inoperable stomach tumor, and rays which destroy organic tissue at sufficient intensity, by what procedure can one free him of the tumor by these rays and at the same time

avoid destroying the healthy tissue which surrounds it" (Duncker, 1945, p. 1)? Proposals for solving the problem are usually of three basic kinds (Duncker, 1945). One kind attempts to avoid contact between the rays and the healthy tissue. For example, subjects might suggest that the rays be sent down a free path to the stomach, such as the esophagus; that healthy tissue be removed from the path of the rays, as by inserting a cannula; that a protective wall be inserted between the rays and the healthy tissue; or that the tumor somehow be displaced toward the surface, as by pressure. A second kind of solution attempts to desensitize the healthy tissue. For example, subjects might suggest that a desensitizing chemical be injected into the tumor victim, or that the victim be immunized by adaptation to weak rays. The third kind of solution attempts to lower the intensity of the rays on their way through healthy tissue. The preferred answer is of this kind, namely, that weakened rays originating from several different sources be sent through the body so that the rays all converge upon the tumor. At this point, and only at this point, will the rays be of sufficient intensity to destroy tissue, which in this case will be tumor tissue. The radiation problem has been studied by Duncker (1926, 1945) and by Gick and Holyoak (1980).

These three examples of problems with ill-defined problem spaces provide only a minimal sampling of the problems of this kind that have been studied. They are sufficient, however, to permit a contrast to the kind of problem considered earlier, that with a well-defined problem space. There are several salient differences between the two kinds. First, problems with ill-defined problem spaces seem to depend for their solution upon the attainment of a single major insight. Indeed, problems of this sort are often referred to as "insight problems." Problems with well-defined problem spaces seem to depend for their solution upon the attainment of a sequence of relatively more minor insights. No one striking realization marks the difference between success and failure in problem solving, as it can in insight problems. Second, in problems with well-defined problem spaces, it is possible to represent the problem space as a sequence of discrete and well-articulated states. It is this property that leads to the description "well-defined problem spaces." In problems with ill-defined problem spaces, it is not possible to represent the problem space as a sequence of discrete and well-articulated states. Third, in problems with well-defined problem spaces, the end state is similar or identical in kind to the starting state. For example, in the missionaries and cannibals problem, both the starting the end states specify numbers of missionaries and cannibals on each side of a river bank. The two states differ only in the number of each kind of individual on each side. In problems with ill-defined problem spaces, the end-state is different in kind from the starting state. For example, in the hatrack problem, the end state posits the existence of a hatrack. The hatrack does not yet exist in the starting state, nor is it clear how the input in the starting state can be transformed to create a hatrack.

Insight problems were a popular subject of study for Gestalt psychologists, whose major concerns (such as the specification of the circumstances under which insight occurs) differed in many respects from those of modern-day information-processing psychologists. As a result, much of the research that was done on insight problems was addressed to questions that no longer seem terribly interesting today; and many of the questions that do seem interesting were simply never considered. Because the reviews presented in this work are guided by theoretical questions purported to be of interest to modern-day psychologists, much of the discussion presented here will propose what needs to be studied, rather than reviewing what has already been studied that is not of contemporary interest.

A case study of problem solving in an ill-defined problem space: the hatrack problem

NATURE OF THE PROBLEM.   The hatrack problem requires experimental subjects to construct a hatrack out of two poles of unequal length and a C-clamp. In the easier version of the problem, subjects are allowed to use various structural features in the experimental room (ceiling beams, lighting fixtures, fuse boxes, etc.) to aid in construction of the hatrack. In the harder version of the problem, nothing can be used except the given elements. In this case, the solution is attained by connecting the poles with the C-clamp and wedging them against the floor and ceiling. The C-clamp is used as the hook on which to hang a hat and coat.

Consider how performance on the hatrack problem meets the various criteria proposed earlier. First, performance on the problem can be quantified in a number of different ways. These include the time to solution, the proportion of solutions that meet the constraints originally set out by the problem, the probability distribution of various solutions, and the proportion of subjects proposing any solution at all.

Second, it is unfortunately difficult or impossible to measure the reliability of most, but not all, indexes of performance on the hatrack problem. Test–retest reliability cannot be feasibly measured, because once a person has solved the hatrack problem, it is spoiled as a future measure of problem-solving skill. In this problem, once the solution is obtained, it is trivially easy to obtain the solution in subsequent trials. It is also unclear how, if at all, internal consistency reliability could be measured, because, in general, measures of performance are available only for performance in the final state. It would be possible to measure reliability for performance on insight problems in general, as opposed to one specific insight problem, by constructing a test that consisted of multiple problems of this kind, and by computing internal consistency of performance on such a test.

Third, there are data supporting a favorable assessment of the construct validity of performance on the hatrack problem. Investigations of the problem have served several theoretical purposes:

1. The problem has been used in investigations of whether problem solving of the kind required by the hatrack problem can be understood solely in terms of *reproductive thinking,* or whether it must be understood in terms of *productive thinking* as well. A major advocate of the former position, Saugstad (1955), would argue that individual differences in problem solving can be understood solely in terms of past learning of the elements or functions needed for solving a given problem. Availability of these functions is sufficient for problem solving in the new situation. In effect, the problem is solved by a "mechanism of equivalent stimuli." A major advocate of the latter position, Maier (Hoffman et al., 1963; Maier, 1933, 1945; Maier & Burke, 1966), would argue that individual differences in problem solving must be understood in terms of reasoning with past learning as well as in terms of the learning itself. The ability to combine previously learned elements is critical to solution of a given problem. Raaheim (1974) has taken a position intermediate between these two, although closer to Maier's. According to Raaheim, problem solving is an activity

in which an individual attempts to dispense with deviating elements in a problem situation in order to make the new problem situation equivalent to situations encountered in the past.

2. Hoffman and associates (1963) used the hatrack problem to investigate whether an experimenter's (positive or negative) evaluations of subjects' performance on an earlier and easier problem affects their performance on a later and more difficult problem. The easier problem was the easier version of the hatrack problem, and the more difficult problem was the harder version of the same problem.

3. R. J. Burke and colleagues (1966) used the hatrack problem to study the question of what makes for a good hint in problem solving. Hints varied in whether they were given before or after problem solving began. A major purpose of the investigation was to discover and classify the various functions hints can serve in facilitating and impeding problem solving.

4. Maier (1933) used the hatrack problem to test whether instructions on overcoming ingrained sets and habits could facilitate problem solving. Experimental subjects were given such instructions as "Keep your mind open for new combinations and do not waste time on unsuccessful attempts," and "Do not be a creature of habit and stay in a rut. Keep your mind open for new meanings" (p. 147). Control subjects were not given instructions of this kind. Instructions did facilitate performance.

Fourth, we need to consider the empirical validity of performance on the hatrack problem. Evidence (to be presented later) is scanty and only modestly encouraging. But the tests of empirical validity that have been performed (Burke & Maier, 1965) have been so weak that one must be hesitant to draw any conclusions solely on the basis of the previously established results.

To conclude this section, there is at least some justification for the study of the hatrack problem as an index of problem-solving ability or skill. The evidence supporting the usefulness of the problem as an object of study is weaker than that for other kinds of problems (or reasoning items) I have considered. The weaker evidence must be viewed in the context of the fact that most investigations of the problem were done a number of years ago, when the theoretical questions of primary interest were different from those that are of primary interest today. I would view the evidence as incomplete rather than as unfavorable. The major questions one might today like to have answered remain unanswered and for the most part unasked.

PERFORMANCE COMPONENTS.   There is no research identifying components of information processing in the hatrack problem. I am prepared to speculate, however, that the performance components involved in solution of this problem are highly overlapping with, if not identical to, those involved in certain forms of inductive reasoning, such as reasoning by analogy. Indeed, Maier's view of problem solving in insight problems might be viewed as one of problem solving by analogy. The major difference between insight problems and standard analogy problems would seem to be that the components are much more difficult to apply to insight problems than to standard analogy problems. In the analogies, the structure of the problems is clearly defined, whereas in the insight problems it is not.

The subject must first *encode* the problem as it is posed and the materials that are presented to the subject as means to solve the problem. In the hatrack problem, these materials include the two poles and the C-clamp. Many, if not most, subjects will not initially encode as relevant two critical elements of the problem solution, namely, the floor and the ceiling of the experimental room. Next, the subject must *infer* how elements of hatracks with which he or she has been familiar have functioned in these previously known hatracks. These elements must then be *mapped* onto the elements of the present situation. If no mapping is immediately available, as will most likely be the case, then it will be necessary for the subject to map elements of hatracklike structures onto the current situation in an attempt to find elements from analogous structures (flag poles, pole lamps, etc.) that can be mapped onto the elements of the current situation. Once the mapping is completed (and this is almost certainly the most difficult operation to complete), the subject must figure out how to *apply* the current elements in a way that is analogous to that inferred for past elements so that the present elements can also be combined into a hatrack. In the event that the subject generates multiple possible solutions, the subject must *compare* them and decide which is most viable. The subject must then attempt to *justify* the best (or only) solution as close enough to an ideal to be minimally acceptable. If the solution is acceptable, the subject *responds* with it. Otherwise, the subject must try to find another solution, repeating earlier problem-solving operations.

This view of problem solving during solution of the hatrack problem contains within it both a theoretical implication and a practical implication. The theoretical implication is that problem solving in insight problems (i.e., problems with ill-defined problem spaces) is primarily analogical. The problems are particularly difficult to solve because the subject must perceive some very nonobvious relationships. The basic terms of the analogy are *Elements of hatracks and hatracklike structures I have known:hatracks and hatrack-like structures I have known::elements of the present situation:a new hatrack* (the nature of which has to be figured out). The practical implication is that problem solving in insight problems can be studied in ways comparable to those used for studying reasoning by analogy. The method of precueing, in particular, would seem to be relevant. Subjects could be precued with information sufficient for performing various operations (encoding, inference, mapping, application, comparison, justification) and combinations of operations, and the effects of these precues on ease or difficulty of problem solving could then be assessed. The method could be used with precueing information providing needed knowledge for performing each of the successive operations (as has been done in reasoning by analogy), or it could be used with precueing information providing needed knowledge for performing combinations of operations that are not necessarily successive in information processing.

REPRESENTATION OF INFORMATION. None of the research that has been done on the hatrack problem has explicitly addressed the question of how information is represented in memory. Some form of representation is needed that can account for people's ability to draw analogies to past experiences in order to figure out how the elements of the experimental situation can be combined into a hatrack. In particular, the representation must be able to account for the fact that the elements of the present situation have never been combined in this particular way before, and no previous hatrack has even been encountered that was constructed of just these elements.

Schank (1979) has proposed a kind of memory structure that expands upon earlier ideas from organization theory (Bower, 1971; Tulving, 1966) and that seems suitable for the present purpose. In this structure, information is stored in the form of "memory organization packets," or MOPs.

The purpose of a MOP is to provide expectations that enable the prediction of future events on the basis of previously encountered structurally similar events.... The ability of MOPs to make useful predictions in somewhat novel situations for which there are no specific expectations but for which there are relevant experiences from which generalized information is available, is crucial to our ability to understand. [Schank, 1979, p. 46].

A MOP might be expected to exist for the hanging of a hat on a hatrack. According to Schank, a given MOP will usually have "strands" corresponding to (a) reasons for the MOP's existing if it is a state, or reasons for doing the MOP if it is an action; (b) enabling conditions for the state or action; (c) results of doing the MOP if it is an action; (d) normative methods of achieving or satisfying a given state; (e) the specific goals the state or action relates to and those which it affects; (f) associated states; and (g) associated actions. Accessing the MOP for "hanging a hat on a hatrack" will probably not enable one to solve the hatrack problem. The subject presumably must enter a MOP for some associated state or action in order to access the elements necessary for creating a hatrack. For example, a likely associated state is a flag pole or pole lamp, the latter of which is supported by its tight fit to both floor and ceiling. The analogy to the present situation might provide the clue for solution of the problem.

COMBINATION RULES.   Specific alternative strategies for solving the hatrack problem have not been explicitly investigated in previous research. An analysis of the task situation, however, suggests at least several plausible approaches to the problem, any one or combination of which might be used in solving the hatrack problem.

Focusing upon elements of present situation.   In this strategy, the subject focuses upon the elements of the present situation and tries to conceive of how these elements might somehow be combined to create a hatrack. The subject would thus think about what uses a C-clamp and a pair of poles might have in creating a hatrack.

Focusing upon elements of previously encountered hatracks.   This strategy entails the subject's focusing upon elements of previously encountered hatracks. The strategy is in some respects the opposite of the first one. In the first strategy, the subject tries to relate the new elements to elements of old hatracks. In this second strategy, the subject tries to relate old elements of previously known hatracks to elements of the new hatrack. The subject may reflect upon hatracks he or she has known, trying to find one that is of a construction that might be roughly suitable in the present instance.

Focusing upon elements of prototypical hatracks and their variants.   In this strategy, one frees oneself from specific past instantiations of hatracks, and tries to construct one or more hatracks that are prototypical, but that do not correspond to any specific hatracks one has previously seen.

Focusing upon a receptive state of mind.   A fourth strategy is to try to clear one's mind of any particulars at all, and to attain a receptive state of mind. In this strategy, the subject essentially waits for a flash of insight to strike. Information processing, to the extent that it exists at all during this strategy, is below consciousness and not subject to introspective report.

Strategy usage and effectiveness might be inferred in at least two different ways. One way would be to have subjects think aloud as they solve the hatrack problem, and attempt to classify their strategy usage on the basis of the protocols thereby obtained. Effectiveness of the strategies could be inferred by noting how often each strategy leads to an acceptable solution. A second way would be to train subjects to use particular strategies or combinations of strategies, and to compare rates of success in problem solving with those for subjects who are untrained. Presumably, training subjects to use the strategy they are already using should have no differential effect upon success rate, whereas training subjects to use alternative strategies would be likely to have some differential effect. This paradigm also permits a direct comparison of the effectiveness of the various strategies that have been trained.

DURATIONS, DIFFICULTIES, AND PROBABILITIES OF COMPONENT EXECUTION. No one has tested any information-processing models of performance on the hatrack problem, and, to my knowledge, the sketchy model proposed earlier (in Items 2–4) is the only model that has been proposed. Maier (1945; Hoffman et al., 1963) has analyzed problem difficulty in more global respects however. Maier (1945) found that 12 of 25 subjects with no prior experience on the hatrack problem or similar problems were able to solve the hatrack problem in 30 min. Hoffman and associates (1963) also studied subjects with no prior experience, and broke down performance by time to solution. They found that of 30 subjects given 30 min to solve the hatrack problem, 8 solved the problem within 5 min, 13 solved it within 10 min, 14 solved it within 15 min, 15 solved it within 20 min, 15 solved it within 25 min, and 15 solved it within 30 min. Thus, almost all subjects who reached a satisfactory solution did so within 10 min.

METACOMPONENTS. Hoffman and co-workers (1963) examined numbers of subjects who proposed each of five different solutions (presumably reflecting different strategies) during the first 10 min of experience with the problem. The first four strategies for making a hatrack were deemed to be incorrect; the last was deemed to be correct. Because subjects could attempt more than one solution, the sum of the number of attempts exceeds 30 (the number of subjects). Of these 30 subjects, 16 proposed a "base" solution, in which one board was used as a support to hold the second one vertically, with the clamp joining the boards at the floor level; 16 proposed a "balance" solution, in which the boards were leaned on each other in an X or T shape with the clamp joining them; 7 proposed a "support" solution, in which a part of the room (e.g., walls, pipes, ceiling beams, etc.) was used to hold up the construction; 8 proposed a "ceiling-suspension" solution, in which boards were wedged between ceiling and ceiling pipes or ceiling beam, with the clamp joining them or appended to the joined ends; and 13 proposed a "floor–ceiling" solution – the correct solution – in which the boards were wedged between floor and ceiling and joined tightly by the clamp.

Raaheim (1974) examined numbers of subjects who repeated unsuccessful attempts at solution various numbers of times. He found that of 37 subjects who never reached a solution (out of a total of 60 subjects), 9 subjects repeated unsuccessful attempts from 1 to 4 times, 19 subjects repeated unsuccessful attempts from 5 to 8 times, and 9 subjects repeated unsuccessful attempts from 9 to 14 times. Raaheim queried why presumably intelligent university students would repeat time and again solutions that had been designated by the experimenter "unsuccessful." He concluded that

> the most likely answer is that they are trying to solve a task *other* than the one intended by the experimenter. While the instructions aim at *some construction,* a nameless, unusual, but sturdy and quite ingenious sort of thing, the subjects nearly all very intensively try to find a way of *replacing the type of hatrack they know of* from their past experience. [P. 49]

Thus these subjects fail in their initial definition or conceptualization of the problem task.

PROBLEM FORMAT, PROBLEM CONTENT, AND PRACTICE.   Two major variations have been attempted in problem format. One variation is where in the room the hatrack must be constructed. In the easier variant, the hatrack can be constructed anywhere in the room, so that the subject can make use of various features of the room to facilitate construction. In the harder variant, the hatrack must be constructed in the center of the room, so that only the clamp and the two poles are available. A second variation is in whether the problem is presented with the actual materials or in written form. Raaheim (1974) found that the proportion of subjects writing down the correct solution (4/64) was about the same as the proportion of subjects choosing the correct solution first when using the actual materials (4/60).

Because the hatrack problem is content-bound (i.e., it is about a hatrack), no alternative contents have been explored.

Practice effects of various types have been widely studied in the literature on the hatrack problem. Research on practice effects has taken several different forms. Most of this research has dealt not with practice effects per se, but with whether "availability of functions" necessary for solution of a problem such as the hatrack problem is sufficient to guarantee solution of that problem. On the one hand, Saugstad (1955) has suggested that if a subject has available all of the functions (items of knowledge) necessary to solve a problem, then solution will be more or less automatic. On the other hand, Maier (Hoffman et al., 1963) has argued that availability of the necessary functions for solving a problem is not sufficient to guarantee solution of the problem: The subject may or may not be able to put together these functions into a workable strategy for solution.

One way of exploring this issue has been through a transfer paradigm. Hoffman and co-workers assigned 90 subjects at random to one of three conditions. In a no-experience condition, subjects were given the difficult version of the hatrack problem (construct it in the center of the room) immediately upon entering the experimental room. In two prior experience conditions (varying in type of reinforcement), subjects were given the easy version of the problem first (construct it anywhere in the room), and were encouraged to construct as many different types of hatracks as they could. Subjects with prior experience on the easier version of the problem performed significantly worse than subjects with no prior experience: Whereas only 25% of the subjects in the former groups solved the problem, 50% of the subjects in the latter group did. Hoffman and associates interpreted these results as showing that providing subjects with a great variety of functions can inhibit problem-solving performance by establishing misleading problem-solving sets. Thus, whereas the prior-experience groups must have had at least as many functions as the group with no prior experience, they performed more poorly because the correct functions were not automatically utilized.

Maier (1945) used a somewhat different transfer paradigm. In his experiment, 75 subjects were equally divided into three groups, and all were asked to solve the hatrack problem. In one group (a control group), subjects tried to solve the hatrack problem as soon as they entered the experimental room. In a second group, subjects were asked to help build two structures that could be used in the two-string problem and that could each be used as a hatrack. Subjects were told that the purpose of building this structure was to get them adjusted to the real problem situation. Subjects were taken to another end of the experimental room, and were asked to construct a hatrack in a certain spot. The two-string structures were left standing. In the third group, procedures were the same as in the second group, except that the two-string structures were disassembled before the subject was asked to build the hatrack. Performance was best in the group in which subjects were shown the two-string structure and in which the structure was left standing (18/25 reached solution). Performance was intermediate in the group in which subjects were shown the two-string structure and the structure was disassembled (12/25 reached solution). Performance was worst in the group in which subjects were not shown the two-string structure (6/25 reached solution). Thus, in this experiment, prior experience helped, but was clearly not sufficient for solution of the hatrack problem. There were still substantial numbers of subjects who did not reach a solution, despite prior experience that made available to them all of the functions needed for solution of the hatrack problem.

Another paradigm for studying effects of availability of functions is one that employs hints toward problem solution. Maier and Burke (1966) used one such paradigm. Subjects (135 male college students) were initially given 15 min to solve the hatrack problem. Those failing to solve the problem were given one of two hints. One hint informed the subjects that the ceiling of the room was part of the solution; the other hint informed the subjects that the clamp must serve as the hat (or coat) hook. Subjects were then given an additional 20 min to solve the problem. After this portion of the experiment ended, subjects were given an "availability-of-functions" test. They were taken into another experimental room in which the correct floor –ceiling solution to the hatrack problem had been constructed. Each subject was given a piece of paper on which to list as many functions or uses of this structure as he or she could possibly think of. Subjects were given five min to complete this task. Fifty subjects who had previously failed to solve the hatrack problem were then returned to the first experimental room, and again asked to construct a hatrack. Of the 135 subjects, 51 solved the problem without a hint; 34 solved the problem after a hint was given; and 50 never solved the problem. Thus the hint did seem to facilitate performance. Subjects in the three groups were strikingly similar in their available functions. All but one of the 135 subjects recognized the structure as a potential hatrack, coatrack, hanger, and so on. But of the 50 subjects who failed to solve the hatrack problem initially and were then asked to solve it after the availability-of-functions test, 7 were still unable to solve the problem, despite the fact that all 7 had listed the necessary function for the structure they had seen in the availability-of-functions test. Thus, for these subjects at least, availability of functions was insufficient to guarantee solution of the hatrack problem.

INDIVIDUAL DIFFERENCES WITHIN AGE LEVEL (ADULTS).   Evidence has already been
cited to the effect that individuals differ in their success in solving the hatrack
problem, and in the solutions they propose. Maier (1933) found a significant sex
difference in success in problem solution: Men performed significantly better than
women. Maier (1945) replicated this difference, and found that the difference held
up whether or not subjects had experience with the two-string type of structure
before solving the hatrack problem.

DIFFERENCES ACROSS AGE LEVELS.   I have been unable to locate any developmental
investigations of performance on the hatrack problem.

RELATIONSHIPS BETWEEN PERFORMANCE ON THE HATRACK PROBLEM AND ON OTHER
PROBLEMS.   No direct correlational studies appear to have been carried out relating
performance on the hatrack problem to performance on other insight problems, such
as the two-string problem and the water jugs problem. I would argue that the
processes, representations, and combination rules described earlier (Items 2–4)
would be applicable to these and other types of insight problems. Hence I would
expect performances on the various problems to be about as highly intercorrelated as
the probably not very high reliabilities of the performances would allow. R. J. Burke
and Maier (1965) correlated success on the hatrack problem (evaluated simply as
pass–fail) with success on various kinds of pencil-and-paper tests measuring skills
that would loosely fall into the problem-solving domain: ideational fluency, spontaneous flexibility, adaptive flexibility, redefinition. Only one of seven correlations
was significant, and this maximal correlation of .19 was scarcely impressive in magnitude. Raaheim (1974) found that level of activity in the hatrack problem correlated
significantly with success in solving the problem, but nevertheless claimed that the
hatrack "problem" is not a problem at all. Recall that, according to Raaheim, a
problem situation is "the deviant member of a series of earlier situations of the same
sort" (p. 22):

> It may be argued that the Hatrack situation must *not* be looked upon by the subjects as a
> problem of how to build a more or less ordinary looking hatrack by some extraordinary means.
> Rather it must be looked upon as a task of constructing something quite different from what is
> usually used for hanging up coats. But then, if it is not the problem of making a hatrack, is the
> situation facing the individual any problem situation at all? Is there any series of situations
> from the past to which the present one may be said to belong, i.e., a series of situations that fits
> in with the solution wanted by the experimenter? If not, the Hatrack task does not fall within
> the category of tasks encompassed by our definition of problem situations. [P. 49]

Raaheim claims that the hatrack situation can be turned into a problem situation by
giving subjects one or more hints that relate the situation to previous situations with
which they are familiar.

RELATIONSHIP BETWEEN PROBLEM SOLVING ON THE HATRACK PROBLEM AND INTEL-
LIGENCE.   R. J. Burke and Maier (1965) correlated performance on the hatrack
problem (success vs. failure in solution) with scores on the verbal and mathematical
sections of the Scholastic Aptitude Test. The correlations were trivial (each was
−.04). These are the only correlational data that I have been able to find. On the one
hand, they fail to support the notion that there is any relationship between hatrack
problem solving and measured intelligence. On the other hand, the measure of

performance is so crude (pass–fail) and the range of student ability probably so restricted (subjects were University of Michigan undergraduates) that Burke and Maier's test of the relationship between problem solving and intelligence seems wholly inadequate.

PRACTICAL RELEVANCE.   Maier (1933) investigated whether it is possible to improve performance on insight problems, including the hatrack problem, by giving subjects a prior lecture on problem-solving skills. The lecture covered 13 points, 3 of which were specific hints on how to solve the problems:

(1)   Locate a difficulty and try to overcome it. If you fail, get it completely out of your mind and seek an entirely different difficulty.
(2)   Do not be a creature of habit and stay in a rut. Keep your mind open for new meanings.
(3)   The solution-pattern appears suddenly. You cannot force it. Keep your mind open for new combinations and do not waste time on unsuccessful attempts. [P. 147]

The training was successful in significantly improving problem-solving performance. It was approximately equally beneficial for good and poor reasoners, but was more beneficial for women than for men.

The hatrack problem has been studied almost exclusively by psychologists whose theoretical concerns differ considerably from the ones proposed here as of major importance, and from the ones that concern most contemporary information-processing psychologists. The practical relevance of previous research on the hatrack problem does not appear to be particularly great, but one cannot thereby infer that research could not be done on the problem that would have greater practical relevance. Research into the nature of insight; into the generalizability of the components, representations, and strategies used in solving the hatrack problem; and into metacomponential decision making in problems with ill-defined problem spaces would all seem to have potential practical relevance. Because most problems encountered in the real world do have ill-defined problem spaces, it seems that research into such problems may eventually have greater practical payoff than research into the more tractable problems with well-defined problem spaces.

5.4.   REASONING, PROBLEM SOLVING, AND INTELLIGENCE

I have reviewed in this chapter only a small segment of the literature that could sensibly be viewed as dealing with reasoning, problem solving, and intelligence. But I believe the literature I have reviewed is fairly representative of work in the field. If there are biases in coverage, and almost certainly there are, they are probably toward greater coverage of work that I consider to be rather theoretically motivated and that is concerned with how reasoning and problem solving relate to general aspects of cognition and intelligence. A major purpose of the chapter has been to support the view that the interface between reasoning, problem solving, and intelligence can be profitably studied by considering the answers to 12 questions; these answers seem to constitute a reasonably coherent and complete account of the psychological phenomena of interest in a given domain of research. Obviously, these are not the only questions that might be posed, and some of these might be combined or deleted. But the set seems to work reasonably well in generating coverage of a task domain.

Intelligence is an amorphous concept, but if one accepts a global definition of it as adaptability to the varied situations in which one may find oneself then the study of reasoning and problem solving appears to provide a good entrée into the study of intelligence, because nontrivial adaptation inevitably will require reasoning and problem solving in various forms and guises. I argue that at least some of these forms and guises draw upon the components, strategies, and representations considered in this chapter.

Not all reasoning and problem-solving tasks seem to be equally good measures of intelligence. Raaheim (1974) has proposed that problems of intermediate difficulty appear to be the best measures. My own emphasis would be somewhat different. I would claim that the best tasks to study are those that are "nonentrenched," but that rely on processes, representations, and strategies shared with real-world tasks. By nonentrenched tasks, I mean ones that require strategy planning and execution of a kind that requires nonroutine thinking and behaving. My view, for which I claim no originality, is that intelligence is in large part the ability to acquire and think with new conceptual systems and to solve novel kinds of tasks.

This view seems consistent with many of our everyday notions about intelligence, if not with all of our research about it. A student is likely to be considered more intelligent if he or she can master a new kind of course (say, calculus or a foreign language) than if he or she can master another course that differs in substance but not in kind from courses taken previously. The student is likely to be considered more intelligent if he or she can solve new kinds of problems, rather than merely solving problems very similar to those that have been encountered numerous times in the past.

According to this view, a problem such as the hatrack problem should seem to provide an excellent way of measuring intelligence, and yet there is no evidence that it does so. In fact, I doubt that the hatrack problem does provide a very good measure of intelligence in the usual sense of the term. On the one hand, I believe that the attainment of insights into novel kinds of problems is an essential ingredient of intelligence. On the other hand, I doubt that there is any general ability that could be labeled "insight." Different people seem to have their best insights into different kinds of problems. And the class of problems represented by the construction of a hatrack from two poles and a C-clamp is probably not a particularly interesting one in terms of which to study people's insights. In this view, then, ecological validity of content is potentially of great relevance. If one wishes to study a scientist's or a business executive's insights, one would do best studying these insights in the domain to which they are normally applied in that person's day-to-day environment. Probably some tasks (such as analogies) measure intellectual functioning of such a basic kind that ecological validity is less important. But if one's goal is to study the ability to handle new kinds of situations successfully, then one probably should make sure that the situations are both new and of the kind that a given person will be likely to encounter. Performance in such situations seems to be exactly the kind that should be studied by those interested in the interface of reasoning, problem solving, and intelligence.

NOTES

Preparation of this chapter was supported by Contract N0001478C0025 from the Office of Naval Research to Robert J. Sternberg.
1 The various kinds of components, their interrelations, and their roles in a subtheory of intelligence are discussed in much greater detail in Sternberg (1980e).

REFERENCES

Ace, M. C., & Dawis, R. V. Item structure as a determinant of item difficulty in verbal analogies. *Educational and Psychological Measurement*, 1973, *33*, 143–149.

Achenbach, T. M. Standardization of a research instrument for identifying associative responding in children. *Developmental Psychology*, 1970, *2*, 283–391. (a)

Achenbach, T. M. The children's associative responding test: A possible alternative to group IQ tests. *Journal of Educational Psychology*, 1970, *61*, 340–348. (b)

Achenbach, T. M. The children's associative responding test: A two-year followup. *Developmental Psychology*, 1971, *5*, 477–483.

Ajzen, I. Intuitive theories of events and the effects of base-rate information on prediction. *Journal of Personality and Social Psychology*, 1977, *35*, 303–314.

Anderson, J. R. *Language, memory, and thought.* Hillsdale, N.J.: Erlbaum, 1976.

Atwood, M. E., & Polson, P. G. A process model for water jug problems. *Cognitive Psychology*, 1976, *8*, 191–216.

Begg, I., & Denny, J. Empirical reconciliation of atmosphere and conversion interpretations of syllogistic reasoning. *Journal of Experimental Psychology*, 1969, *81*, 351–354.

Bower, G. H. Adaptation-level coding of stimuli and serial position effects. In M. H. Appley (Ed.), *Adaptation-level theory.* New York: Academic Press, 1971.

Brown, A. L. Knowing when, where, and how to remember: A problem of metacognition. In R. Glaser (Ed.), *Advances in instructional psychology* (Vol. 1). Hillsdale, N.J.: Erlbaum, 1978.

Brown, A. L., & DeLoache, J. S. Skills, plans and self-regulation. In R. Siegler (Ed.), *Children's thinking: What develops?* Hillsdale, N.J.: Erlbaum, 1978.

Bryant, P. E., & Trabasso, T. Transitive inferences and memory in young children. *Nature*, 1971, *232*, 456–458.

Burke, H. R. Raven's Progressive Matrices: A review and critical evaluation. *Journal of Genetic Psychology*, 1958, *93*, 199–228.

Burke, R. J., & Maier, N. R. F. Attempts to predict success on an insight problem. *Psychological Reports*, 1965, *17*, 303–310.

Burke, R. J., Maier, N. R. F., & Hoffman, L. R. Functions of hints in individual problem-solving. *American Journal of Psychology*, 1966, *79*, 389–399.

Burt, C. The development of reasoning in school children. *Journal of Experimental Pedagogy*, 1919, *5*, 68–77.

Carroll, J. S., & Siegler, R. S. Strategies for the use of base-rate information. *Organizational Behavior and Human Performance*, 1977, *19*, 392–402.

Case, R. Intellectual development from birth to adolescence: A neo-Piagetian interpretation. In R. Siegler (Ed.), *Children's thinking: What develops?* Hillsdale, N. J.: Erlbaum, 1978. (a)

Case, R. Piaget and beyond: Toward a developmentally based theory and technology of instruction. In R. Glaser (Ed.), *Advances in instructional psychology* (Vol. 1). Hillsdale, N.J.: Erlbaum, 1978. (b)

Cattell, R. B. & Cattell, A. K. S. *Test of g: Culture Fair, Scale 3.* Champaign, Ill.: Institute for Personality and Ability Testing, 1963.

Ceraso, J., & Provitera, A. Sources of error in syllogistic reasoning. *Cognitive Psychology*, 1971, *2*, 400–410.

Chapman, L. J. Illusory correlation in observational report. *Journal of Verbal Learning and Verbal Behavior*, 1967, *6*, 151–155.

Chapman, L. J., & Chapman, J. P. Atmosphere effect re-examined. *Journal of Experimental Psychology*, 1959, *58*, 220–226.

Chapman, L. J., & Chapman, J. P. Genesis of popular but erroneous psychodiagnostic observation. *Journal of Abnormal Psychology*, 1967, *72*, 193–204.

Chapman, L. J., & Chapman, J. P. Illusory correlation as an obstacle to the use of valid psychodiagnostic signs. *Journal of Abnormal Psychology*, 1969, *74*, 271–280.

Chomsky, N. *Aspects of the theory of syntax.* Cambridge, Mass.: MIT Press, 1965.

Clark, H. H. The influence of language in solving three-term series problems. *Journal of Experimental Psychology*, 1969, *82*, 205–215. (a)

Clark, H. H. Linguistic processes in deductive reasoning. *Psychological Review*, 1969, *76*, 387–404. (b)

Clark, H. H. More about "Adjectives, comparatives, and syllogisms": A reply to Huttenlocher and Higgins. *Psychological Review*, 1971, *78*, 505–514.

Clark, H. H. Difficulties people have answering the question "Where is it?" *Journal of Verbal Learning and Verbal Behavior*, 1972, *11*, 265–277. (a)

Clark, H. H. On the evidence concerning J. Huttenlocher and E. T. Higgins' theory of reasoning: A second reply. *Psychological Review*, 1972, *79*, 428–432. (b)

Clark, H. H. Semantics and comprehension. In T. A. Sebeok (Ed.), *Current trends in linguistics*. (Vol. 12): *Linguistics and adjacent arts and sciences*. The Hague: Mouton, 1973.

Copi, I. M. *Introduction to logic* (5th ed.). New York: Macmillan, 1978.

Dawis, R. V., & Siojo, L. T. *Analogical reasoning: A review of the literature. Effects of social class differences on analogical reasoning* (Tech. Rep. 1). Minneapolis: University of Minnesota, Department of Psychology, 1972.

DeSoto, C. B. The predilection for single orderings. *Journal of Abnormal and Social Psychology*, 1961, *62*, 16–23.

DeSoto, C. B., London, M., & Handel, S. Social reasoning and spatial paralogic. *Journal of Personality and Social Psychology*, 1965, *2*, 513–521.

Dickstein, L. S. Effects of instructions and premise order on errors in syllogistic reasoning. *Journal of Experimental Psychology: Human Learning and Memory*, 1975, *1*, 376–384.

Dickstein, L. S. Differential difficulty of categorical syllogisms. *Bulletin of the Psychonomic Society*, 1976, *8*, 330–332.

Dickstein, L. S. Error processes in syllogistic reasoning. *Memory and Cognition*, 1978, *6*, 537–543.

Donaldson, M. *A study of children's thinking*. London: Tavistock, 1963.

Duncan, C. P. Recent research on human problem solving. *Psychological Bulletin*, 1959, *56*, 397–429.

Duncker, K. A qualitative (experimental and theoretical) study of productive thinking (solving of comprehensible problems). *Journal of Genetic Psychology*, 1926, *33*, 642–708.

Duncker, K. On problem-solving. *Psychological Monographs*, 1945, *58*(5, Whole No. 270).

Egan, D. E. *Accuracy and latency scores as measures of spatial information processing* (Research Rep. No. 1224). Pensacola, Fla.: Naval Aerospace Medical Research Laboratories, 1976.

Egan, D. E., & Greeno, J. G. Theory of rule induction: Knowledge acquired in concept learning, serial pattern learning, and problem solving. In L. W. Gregg (Ed.), *Knowledge and cognition*. Hillsdale, N.J.: Erlbaum, 1974.

Erickson, J. R. A set analysis theory of behavior in formal syllogistic reasoning tasks. In R. L. Solso (Ed.), *Theories of cognitive psychology: The Loyola Symposium*. Hillsdale, N.J.: Erlbaum, 1974.

Erickson, J. R. Research on syllogistic reasoning. In R. Revlin & R. E. Mayer (Eds.), *Human reasoning*. New York: Wiley, 1978.

Ericsson, K. A., & Simon, H. A. Verbal reports as data. *Psychological Review*, 1980, *87*, 215–251.

Ernst, G. W., & Newell, A. *GPS: A case study in generality and problem-solving*. New York: Academic Press, 1969.

Esher, F. J. S., Raven, J. C., & Earl. C. J. C. Discussion on testing intellectual capacity in adults. *Proceedings of the Royal Society of Medicine*, 1942, *35*, 779–785.

Evans, T. G. A program for the solution of geometric-analogy intelligence test questions. In M. Minsky (Ed.), *Semantic information processing*. Cambridge, Mass.: MIT Press, 1968.

Ferguson, G. A. On learning and human ability. *Canadian Journal of Psychology*, 1954, *8*, 95–112.

Feuerstein, R. *The dynamic assessment of retarded performers: The learning potential assessment device, theory, instruments, and techniques*. Baltimore: University Park Press, 1979.

Feuerstein, R., Schlesinger, I. M., Shalom, H., & Narrol, H. *The dynamic assessment of retarded performers: The learning potential assessment device, theory, instruments and techniques*. Vol. 2: *LPAD analogies group test experiment* (Studies in cognitive modifiability, Report No. 1). Jerusalem: Hadassah Wizo Canada Research Institute, 1972.

Fischhoff, B. Attribution theory and judgment under uncertainty. In J. H. Harvey, W. J. Ickes, & R. F. Kidd (Eds.), *New directions in attribution research*. Hillsdale, N.J.: Erlbaum, 1976.

Fleishman, E. A. The prediction of total task performance from prior practice on task components. *Human Factors*, 1965, *7*, 18–27.

Fleishman, E. A., & Hempel, W. E., Jr. The relation between abilities and improvement with practice in a visual discrimination reaction task. *Journal of Experimental Psychology,* 1955, *49,* 301–312.

Frase, L. T. Belief, incongruity, and syllogistic reasoning. *Psychological Reports,* 1966, *18,* 982. (a)

Frase, L. T. Validity judgments of syllogisms in relation to two sets of terms. *Journal of Educational Psychology,* 1966, *57,* 239–245. (b)

Frase, L. T. Associative factors in syllogistic reasoning. *Journal of Experimental Psychology,* 1968, *76,* 407–412.

Gabriel, K. R. The simplex structure of the Progressive Matrices Test. *British Journal of Statistical Psychology,* 1954, *7,* 9–14.

Gallagher, J. M., & Wright, R. J. *Children's solution of verbal analogies: Extension of Piaget's concept of reflexive abstraction.* Paper presented at the annual meeting of the Society for Research in Child Development, New Orleans, 1977.

Gallagher, J. M., & Wright, R. J. Piaget and the study of analogy: Structural analysis of items. In J. Magary (Ed.), *Piaget and the helping professions* (Vol. 8). Los Angeles: University of Southern California, 1979.

Garner, W. R. *The processing of information and structure.* Hillsdale, N.J.: Erlbaum, 1974.

Gentile, J. R., Kessler, D. K., & Gentile, P. K. Process of solving analogy items. *Journal of Educational Psychology,* 1969, *60,* 494–502.

Gentile, J. R., Tedesco-Stratton, L., Davis, E., Lund, N. J., & Agunanne, B. A. Associative responding versus analogical reasoning by children. *Intelligence,* 1977, *1,* 369–380.

Gick, M. L., & Holyoak, K. J. Analogical problem solving. *Cognitive Psychology,* 1980, *12,* 306–355.

Gilson, C., & Abelson, R. P. The subjective use of inductive evidence. *Journal of Personality and Social Psychology,* 1965, *2,* 301–310.

Glaser, R. Some implications of previous work on learning and individual differences. In R. M. Gagné (Ed.), *Learning and individual differences.* Columbus, Ohio: Merrill, 1967.

Gollub, H. F., Rossman, B. B., & Abelson, R. P. Social inference as a function of the number of instances and consistency of information presented. *Journal of Personality and Social Psychology,* 1973, *27,* 19–33.

Greeno, J. G. Hobbits and orcs: Acquisition of a sequential concept. *Cognitive Psychology,* 1974, *6,* 270–292.

Greeno, J. G. Natures of problem-solving abilities. In W. K. Estes (Ed.), *Handbook of learning and cognitive processes* (Vol. 5). Hillsdale, N.J.: Erlbaum, 1978.

Gregg, L. W. Internal representations of sequential concepts. In B. Kleinmuntz (Ed.), *Concepts and the structure of memory.* New York: Wiley, 1967.

Griggs, R. A. Logical processing of set inclusion relations in meaningful text. *Memory and Cognition,* 1976, *4,* 730–740.

Griggs, R. A. Drawing inferences from set inclusion information given in text. In R. Revlin & R. E. Mayer (Eds.), *Human reasoning.* New York: V. H. Winston, 1978.

Grudin, J. Processes in verbal analogy solution. *Journal of Experimental Psychology: Human Perception and Performance,* 1980, *6,* 67–74.

Guilford, J. P. *The nature of human intelligence.* New York: McGraw-Hill, 1967.

Guyote, M. J., & Sternberg, R. J. A transitive-chain theory of syllogistic reasoning. *Cognitive Psychology,* 1981, *13,* 461–525.

Handel, S., DeSoto, C. B., & London, M. Reasoning and spatial respresentations. *Journal of Verbal Learning and Verbal Behavior,* 1968, *7,* 351–357.

Hayes, J. R., & Simon, H. A. Understanding written problem instructions. In L. W. Gregg (Ed.), *Knowledge and cognition.* Hillsdale, N.J.: Erlbaum, 1974.

Hayes, J. R., & Simon, H. A. Understanding complex task instructions. In D. Klahr (Ed.), *Cognition and instruction.* Hillsdale, N.J.: Erlbaum, 1976. (a)

Hayes, J. R., & Simon, H. A. The understanding process: Problem isomorphs. *Cognitive Psychology,* 1976, *8,* 165–190. (b)

Henle, M. On the relationship between logic and thinking. *Psychological Review,* 1962, *69,* 366–378.

Henle, M. & Michael, M. The influence of attitudes on syllogistic reasoning. *Journal of Social Psychology,* 1956, *44,* 115–127.

Henley, N. M. A psychological study of the semantics of animal terms. *Journal of Verbal Learning and Verbal Behavior,* 1969, *8,* 176–184.

Hoffman, L. R., Burke, R. J., & Maier, N. R. F. Does training with differential reinforcement on similar problems help in solving a new problem? *Psychological Reports*, 1963, *13*, 147–154.

Holyoak, K. J. *Symbolic processes in mental comparisons.* Unpublished doctoral dissertation, Stanford University, 1976.

Holzman, T. G., Glaser, R., & Pellegrino, J. W. Process training derived from a computer simulation theory. *Memory and Cognition*, 1976, *4*, 349–356.

Humphrey, G. *Thinking: An introduction to its experimental psychology.* New York: Wiley, 1951.

Hunt, E. Quote the raven? Nevermore! In L. W. Gregg (Ed.), *Knowledge and cognition.* Hillsdale, N.J.: Erlbaum, 1974.

Hunter, I. M. L. The solving of three term series problems. *British Journal of Psychology*, 1957, *48*, 286–298.

Huttenlocher, J. Constructing spatial images: A strategy in reasoning. *Psychological Review*, 1968, *75*, 550–560.

Huttenlocher, J., Eisenberg, K., & Strauss, S. Comprehension: Relation between perceived actor and logical subject. *Journal of Verbal Learning and Verbal Behavior*, 1970, *9*, 334–341.

Huttenlocher, J., & Higgins, E. T. Adjectives, comparatives, and syllogisms. *Psychological Review*, 1971, *78*, 487–504.

Huttenlocher, J., Higgins, E. T., Milligan, C., & Kauffman, B. The mystery of the "negative equative" construction. *Journal of Verbal Learning and Verbal Behavior*, 1970, *9*, 334–341.

Huttenlocher, J., & Strauss, S. Comprehension and a statement's relation to the situation it describes. *Journal of Verbal Learning and Verbal Behavior*, 1968, *7*, 300–304.

Ingram, A. L., Pellegrino, J. W., & Glaser, R. *Semantic processing in verbal analogies.* Paper presented at the annual meeting of the Psychonomic Society, St. Louis, November 1976.

Jacobs, P. I., & Vandeventer, M. The learning and transfer of double-classification skills by first graders. *Child Development*, 1971, *42*, 149–159. (a)

Jacobs, P. I., & Vandeventer, M. The learning and transfer of double-classification skills: A replication and extension. *Journal of Experimental Child Psychology*, 1971, *12*, 140–157. (b)

Jacobs, P. I., & Vandeventer, M. Evaluating the teaching of intelligence. *Educational and Psychological Measurement*, 1972, *32*, 235–248.

Janis, I., & Frick, F. The relationship between attitudes toward conclusions and errors in judging logical validity of syllogisms. *Journal of Experimental Psychology*, 1943, *33*, 73–77.

Jeffries, R., Polson, P. G., Razran, L., & Atwood, M. E. A process model for missionaries–cannibals and other river-crossing problems. *Cognitive Psychology*, 1977, *9*, 412–440.

Johnson, D. M. *The psychology of thought and judgment.* New York: Harper & Row, 1955.

Johnson, D. M. Serial analysis of verbal analogy problems. *Journal of Educational Psychology*, 1962, *53*, 86–88.

Johnson-Laird, P. N. The three-term series problem. *Cognition*, 1972, *1*, 57–82.

Johnson-Laird, P. N. Models of deduction. In R. Falmagne (Ed.), *Reasoning: Representation and process.* Hillsdale, N.J.: Erlbaum, 1975.

Johnson-Laird, P. N., & Steedman, M. The psychology of syllogisms. *Cognitive Psychology*, 1978, *10*, 64–99.

Jones, M. R. From probability learning to sequential processing: A critical review. *Psychological Bulletin*, 1971, *76*, 153–185.

Jöreskog, K. G. A general approach to confirmatory maximum likelihood factor analysis. *Psychometrika*, 1969, *34*, 183–202.

Jöreskog, K. G. A general method for analysis of covariance structure. *Biometrika*, 1970, *57*, 239–251.

Jöreskog, K. G., & Sörbom, D. *LISREL IV: Estimation of linear structural equation systems by maximum likelihood methods.* Chicago: National Educational Resources, 1978.

Judson, A. J., Cofer, C. N., & Gelfand, S. Reasoning as an associative process: II. "Direction" in problem solving as a function of prior reinforcement of relevant responses. *Psychological Reports*, 1956, *2*, 501–507.

Kaufman, H., & Goldstein, S. The effects of emotional value of conclusions upon distortions in syllogistic reasoning. *Psychonomic Science*, 1967, *7*, 367–368.

Keating, D. P., & Caramazza, A. Effects of age and ability on syllogistic reasoning in early adolescence. *Developmental Psychology*, 1975, *11*, 837–842.

Kelley, H. H. Attribution theory in social psychology. In D. Levine (Ed.), *Nebraska Symposium on Motivation* (Vol. 15). Lincoln: University of Nebraska Press, 1967.

Kelley, H. H. *Attribution in social interaction*. Morristown, N.J.: General Learning Press, 1972.

Klahr, D., & Wallace, J. G. The development of serial completion strategies: An information processing analysis. *British Journal of Psychology*, 1970, *61*, 243–257.

Kling, R. E. A paradigm for reasoning by analogy. *Artificial Intelligence*, 1971, *2*, 147–178.

Kodroff, J. K., & Roberge, J. J. Developmental analysis of the conditional reasoning abilities of primary-grade children. *Developmental Psychology*, 1975, *11*, 21–28.

Köhler, W. *The mentality of apes*. London: Routledge & Kegan Paul, 1925.

Kosslyn, S. M., & Pomerantz, J. R. Imagery, propositions, and the form of internal representations. *Cognitive Psychology*, 1977, *9*, 52–76.

Kotovsky, K., & Simon, H. A. Empirical tests of a theory of human acquisition of concepts for sequential events. *Cognitive Psychology*, 1973, *4*, 399–424.

Lashley, K. S. The problem of serial order in behavior. In L. A. Jeffreys (Ed.), *Cerebral mechanisms in behavior: The Hixon Symposium*. New York: Wiley, 1951.

Leeuwenberg, E. L. L. Quantitative specification of information in sequential patterns. *Psychological Review*, 1969, *76*, 216–220.

Lefford, A. The influence of emotional subject matter on logical reasoning. *Journal of General Psychology*, 1946, *34*, 127–151.

Levi, E. H. *An introduction to legal reasoning*. Chicago: University of Chicago Press, 1949.

Levinson, P. J., & Carpenter, R. L. An analysis of analogical reasoning in children. *Child Development*, 1974, *45*, 857–861.

Linn, M. C. The role of intelligence in children's responses to instruction. *Psychology in the Schools*, 1973, *10*, 67–75.

Lippman, M. Z. The influence of grammatical transform in a syllogistic reasoning task. *Journal of Verbal Learning and Verbal Behavior*, 1972, *11*, 424–430.

Luce, R. D. *Individual choice behavior*. New York: Wiley, 1959.

Luchins, A. S. Mechanization in problem solving. *Psychological Monographs*, 1942, *54* (6, Whole No. 248).

Lunzer, E. A. Problems of formal reasoning in test situations. *Monographs of the Society for Research in Child Development*, 1965, *30*(2, Serial No. 100), 19–46.

Lutkus, A. D., & Trabasso, T. Transitive inferences in preoperational retarded adolescents. *American Journal of Mental Deficiency*, 1974, *78*, 599–606.

Lyon, D., & Slovic, P. Dominance of accuracy information and neglect of base rates in probability estimation. *Acta Psychologica*, 1976, *40*, 287–298.

Maier, N. R. F. Reasoning in humans: I. On direction. *Journal of Comparative Psychology*, 1930, *10*, 115–143.

Maier, N. R. F. Reasoning in humans: II. The solution of a problem and its appearance in consciousness. *Journal of Comparative Psychology*, 1931, *12*, 181–194.

Maier, N. R. F. An aspect of human reasoning. *British Journal of Psychology*, 1933, *24*, 144–155.

Maier, N. R. F. Reasoning in humans: III. The mechanisms of equivalent stimuli and of reasoning. *Journal of Experimental Psychology*, 1945, *35*, 349–360.

Maier, N. R. F. What makes a problem difficult? In N. R. F. Maier (Ed.), *Problem solving and creativity in individuals and groups*. Belmont, Calif.: Brooks/Cole, 1970.

Maier, N. R. F., & Burke, R. J. Test of the concept of "availability of functions" in problem solving. *Psychological Reports*, 1966, *19*, 119–125.

Maier, N. R. F., & Janzen, J. C. Functional values as aids and distractors in problem solving. *Psychological Reports*, 1968, *22*, 1021–1034.

Maltzman, I. Thinking: From a behavioristic point of view. *Psychological Review*, 1955, *62*, 275–286.

Marcus, S., & Rips, L. J. Conditional reasoning. *Journal of Verbal Learning and Verbal Behavior*, 1979, *18*, 199–224.

Mayer, R. E. Qualitatively different storage and processing strategies used for linear reasoning tasks due to meaningfulness of premises. *Journal of Experimental Psychology: Human Learning and Memory*, 1978, *4*, 5–18.

Mayer, R. E. Qualitatively different encoding strategies for linear reasoning premises: Evidence for single association and distance theories. *Journal of Experimental Psychology: Human Learning and Memory*, 1979, 5, 1–10.

McGuire, W. J. A syllogistic analysis of cognitive relationships. In M. J. Rosenberg & C. I. Hovland (Eds.), *Attitude organization and change*. New Haven: Yale University Press, 1960.

Meer, B., Stein, M., & Geertsma, R. An analysis of the Miller Analogies Test for a scientific population. *American Psychologist*, 1955, 10, 33–34.

Mill, J. S. *A system of logic, ratiocinative and inductive*. London: J. W. Parker, 1843.

Miller, G. A. Images and models, similes and metaphors. In A. Ortony (Ed.), *Metaphor and thought*. Cambridge: Cambridge University Press, 1979.

Miller Analogies Test manual. New York: Psychological Corporation, 1970.

Morgan, J. J. B. *Psychology*. New York: Farrar & Rinehart, 1941.

Morgan, J. J., & Morton, J. T. The distortion of syllogistic reasoning produced by personal convictions. *Journal of Social Psychology*, 1944, 20, 39–59.

Mortensen, U. Models for some elementary problem solving processes. In A. Elithorn & D. Jones (Eds.), *Artificial and human thinking*. San Francisco: Jossey-Bass, 1973.

Moyer, R. S. Comparing objects in memory: Evidence suggesting an internal psychophysics. *Perception and Psychophysics*, 1973, 13, 180–184.

Moyer, R. S., & Bayer, R. H. Mental comparison and the symbolic distance effect. *Cognitive Psychology*, 1976, 8, 228–246.

Mulholland, T. M., Pellegrino, J. W., & Glaser, R. Components of geometric analogy solution. *Cognitive Psychology*, 1980, 12, 252–284.

Newell, A. You can't play 20 questions with nature and win. In W. Chase (Ed.), *Visual information processing*. New York: Academic Press, 1973.

Newell, A., & Simon, H. A. *Human problem solving*. Englewood Cliffs, N.J.: Prentice-Hall, 1972.

Nisbett, R. E., & Borgida, E. Attribution and the psychology of prediction. *Journal of Personality and Social Psychology*, 1975, 32, 932–943.

Nisbett, R. E., Borgida, E., Crandall, R., & Reed, H. Popular induction: Information is not necessarily informative. In J. S. Carroll & J. W. Payne (Eds.), *Cognition and social behavior*. Hillsdale, N.J.: Erlbaum, 1976.

Nisbett, R. E., & Ross, L. *Human inferences: Strategies and shortcomings in social judgment*. Englewood Cliffs, N.J.: Prentice-Hall, 1979.

Nisbett, R. E., & Wilson, T. D. Telling more than we can know: Verbal reports on mental processes. *Psychological Review*, 1977, 84, 231–259.

Nobel, C. E., Nobel, J. L., & Alcock, W. T. Prediction of individual differences in human trial-and-error learning. *Perceptual and Motor Skills*, 1958, 8, 151–172.

Oppenheimer, J. R. Analogy in science. *American Psychologist*, 1956, 11, 127–135.

Osherson, D. N. *Logical abilities in children*. Vol. 2: *Logical inference: Underlying operations*. Hillsdale, N.J.: Erlbaum, 1974.

Osherson, D. N. *Logical abilities in children*. Vol. 3: *Reasoning in adolescence: Deductive inference*. Hillsdale, N.J.: Erlbaum, 1975.

Paris, S. G. Comprehension of language connectives and propositional logical relationships. *Journal of Experimental Child Psychology*, 1973, 16, 278–291.

Pellegrino, J. W., & Glaser, R. Components of inductive reasoning. In R. E. Snow, P. A. Federico, & W. Montague (Eds.), *Aptitude, learning, and instruction: Cognitive process analysis* (Vol. 1). Hillsdale, N.J.: Erlbaum, 1980.

Piaget, J. Une forme verbal de la comparison chez l'enfant. *Archives de Psychologie*, 1921, pp. 141–172.

Piaget, J. *Judgment and reasoning in the child*. London: Routledge & Kegan Paul, 1928.

Piaget, J. *The language and thought of the child*. New York: Meridian Books, 1955.

Piaget, J. *Genetic epistemology* (E. Duckworth, Trans). New York: Columbia University Press, 1970.

Piaget, J. (with J. Montangero & J. Billeter). Les correlats. In *L'Abstraction réfléchissante*. Paris: Presses Universitaires de France, 1977.

Pintner, R. Contribution to "Intelligence and its measurement: A symposium." *Journal of Educational Psychology*, 1921, 12, 139–143.

Potts, G. R. Information processing strategies used in the encoding of linear orderings. *Journal of Verbal Learning and Verbal Behavior*, 1972, 11, 727–740.

Potts, G. R. Storing and retrieving information about ordered relationships. *Journal of Experimental Psychology*, 1974, *103*, 431–439.

Potts, G. R., & Scholz, K. W. The internal representation of a three-term series problem. *Journal of Verbal Learning and Verbal Behavior*, 1975, *14*, 439–452.

Psotka, J. Simplicity, symmetry, and syntely: Stimulus measures of binary pattern structure. *Memory and Cognition*, 1975, *3*, 434–444.

Psotka, J. Syntely: Paradigm for an inductive psychology of memory, perception, and thinking. *Memory and Cognition*, 1977, *5*, 553–560.

Pylyshyn, Z. W. What the mind's eye tells the mind's brain: A critique of mental imagery. *Psychological Bulletin*, 1973, *80*, 1–24.

Quinton, G., & Fellows, B. "Perceptual" strategies in the solving of three-term series problems. *British Journal of Psychology*, 1975, *66*, 69–78.

Raaheim, K. *Problem solving and intelligence*. Oslo: Universitetsforlaget, 1974.

Raven, J. C. *Progressive Matrices: A perceptual test of intelligence, 1938, individual form*. London: Lewis, 1938.

Raven, J. C. *Guide to the standard progressive matrices*. London: Lewis, 1960.

Ray, W. S. Complex tasks for use in human problem-solving research. *Psychological Bulletin*, 1955, *52*, 134–149.

Reed, S. K. Pattern recognition and categorization. *Cognitive Psychology*, 1972, *3*, 383–407.

Reed, S. K., & Abramson, A. Effect of the problem space on subgoal facilitation. *Journal of Educational Psychology*, 1976, *68*, 243–246.

Reed, S. K., Ernst, G. W., & Banerji, R. The role of analogy in transfer between similar problem states. *Cognitive Psychology*, 1974, *6*, 436–450.

Reitman, W. *Cognition and thought*. New York: Wiley, 1965.

Restle, F. Grammatical analysis of the prediction of binary events. *Journal of Verbal Learning and Verbal Behavior*, 1967, *6*, 17–25.

Restle, F. Theory of serial pattern learning: Structural trees. *Psychological Review*, 1970, *77*, 481–495.

Restle, F. Serial patterns: The role of phrasing. *Journal of Experimental Psychology*, 1972, *92*, 385–390.

Restle, F., & Brown, E. R. Serial pattern learning. *Journal of Experimental Psychology*, 1970, *83*, 120–125. (a)

Restle, F., & Brown, E. R. Organization of serial pattern learning. In G. H. Bower (Ed.), *The psychology of learning and motivation* (Vol. 4). New York: Academic Press, 1970. (b)

Revlin, R., & Leirer, V. O. The effects of personal biases on syllogistic reasoning: Rational decision from personalized representations. In R. Revlin & R. E. Mayer (Eds.), *Human reasoning*. Washington: V. H. Winston, 1978.

Revlis, R. Syllogistic reasoning: Logical decisions from a complex data base. In R. Falmagne (Ed.), *Reasoning: Representation and process*. Hillsdale, N.J.: Erlbaum, 1975. (a)

Revlis, R. Two models of syllogistic reasoning: Feature selection and conversion. *Journal of Verbal Learning and Verbal Behavior*, 1975, *14*, 180–195. (b)

Richter, M. The theoretical interpretation of errors in syllogistic reasoning. *Journal of Psychology*, 1957, *43*, 341–344.

Riley, C. A. The representation of comparative relations and the transitive inference task. *Journal of Experimental Child Psychology*, 1976, *22*, 1–22.

Riley, C. A., & Trabasso, T. Comparatives, logical structures, and encoding in a transitive inference task. *Journal of Experimental Child Psychology*, 1974, *17*, 187–203.

Rips, L. J., & Marcus, S. Suppositions and the analysis of conditional sentences. In M. A. Just & P. A. Carpenter (Eds.), *Cognitive processes in comprehension*. Hillsdale, N.J.: Erlbaum, 1977.

Rips, L., Shoben, E., & Smith, E. Semantic distance and the verification of semantic relations. *Journal of Verbal Learning and Verbal Behavior*, 1973, *12*, 1–20.

Roberge, J. J., & Paulus, D. H. Developmental patterns for children's class and conditional reasoning abilities. *Developmental Psychology*, 1971, *4*, 191–200.

Rosch, E. Human categorization. In N. Warren (Ed.), *Advances in cross-cultural psychology* (Vol. 1). London: Academic Press, 1977.

Rumelhart, D. E., & Abrahamson, A. A. A model for analogical reasoning. *Cognitive Psychology*, 1973, *5*, 1–28.

Russell, D. H. *Children's thinking*. Boston: Ginn, 1956.

Saugstad, P. Problem-solving as dependent on availability of functions. *British Journal of Psychology*, 1955, *46*, 191–198.

Saugstad, P. An analysis of Maier's pendulum problem. *Journal of Experimental Psychology*, 1957, *54*, 168–179.

Saugstad, P. Availability of functions: A discussion of some theoretical aspects. *Acta Psychologica*, 1958, *14*, 384–400.

Schank, R. C. *Reminding and memory organization: An introduction to MOPs* (ARPA Tech. Rep. No. 170). New Haven: Yale University, Department of Computer Science, 1979.

Scriven, M. Maximizing the power of causal investigations: The modus operandi method. In G. V. Glass (Ed.), *Evaluation studies: Review annual* (Vol. 1). Beverly Hills, Calif.: Sage Publications, 1976.

Sells, S. B. The atmosphere effect: An experimental study of reasoning. *Archives of Psychology*, 1936, *29*, 3–72.

Shalom, H., & Schlesinger, I. M. Analogical thinking: A conceptual analysis of analogy tests. In R. Feuerstein, I. M. Schlesinger, H. Shalom, & H. Narrol (Eds.), *Studies in cognitive modifiability* (Report 1, Vol. 2). Jerusalem: Hadassah Wizo Canada Research Institute, 1972.

Shaver, P., Pierson, L., & Lang, S. Converging evidence for the functional significance of imagery in problem solving. *Cognition*, 1974, *3*, 359–375.

Shepard, R. N., & Arabie, P. Additive clustering: Representation of similarities as combinations of discrete overlapping properties. *Psychological Review*, 1979, *86*, 87–123.

Simon, H. A. Complexity and the representation of patterned sequences of symbols. *Psychological Review*, 1972, *79*, 369–382.

Simon, H. A. The functional equivalence of problem solving skills. *Cognitive Psychology*, 1975, *7*, 268–288.

Simon, H. A. Identifying basic abilities underlying intelligent performance of complex tasks. In L. Resnick (Ed.), *The nature of intelligence*. Hillsdale, N.J.: Erlbaum, 1976.

Simon, H. A., & Kotovsky, K. Human acquisition of concepts for sequential patterns. *Psychological Review*, 1963, *70*, 534–546.

Simon, H. A., & Lea, G. Problem solving and rule induction: A unified view. In L. W. Gregg (Ed.), *Knowledge and cognition*. Hillsdale, N.J.: Erlbaum, 1974.

Simon, H. A., & Newell, A. Thinking processes. In D. H. Krantz, R. D. Luce, R. C. Atkinson, & P. Suppes (Eds.), *Contemporary developments in mathematical psychology* (Vol. 1). San Francisco: W. H. Freeman, 1974.

Simon, H. A., & Reed, S. K. Modeling strategy shifts in a problem-solving task. *Cognitive Psychology*, 1976, *8*, 86–97.

Simon, H. A., & Sumner, R. K. Pattern in music. In B. Kleinmuntz (Ed.), *Formal representation of human judgment*. New York: Wiley, 1968.

Simpson, M. E., & Johnson, D. M. Atmosphere and conversion errors in syllogistic reasoning. *Journal of Experimental Psychology*, 1966, *72*, 197–200.

Skyrms, B. *Choice and chance* (2nd ed.). Encino, Calif.: Dickenson, 1975.

Smedslund, J. The concept of correlation in adults. *Scandinavian Journal of Psychology*, 1963, *4*, 165–173.

Smith, E. E., Shoben, E. J., & Rips, L. J. Structure and process in semantic memory: A feature model for semantic decisions. *Psychological Review*, 1974, *81*, 214–241.

Spearman, C. "General intelligence," objectively determined and measured. *American Journal of Psychology*, 1904, *15*, 201–293.

Spearman, C. *The nature of "intelligence" and the principles of cognition*. London: Macmillan, 1923.

Spearman, C. *The abilities of man*. New York: Macmillan, 1927.

Staudenmayer, H. Understanding conditional reasoning with meaningful propositions. In R. Falmagne (Ed.), *Reasoning: Representation and process*. Hillsdale, N.J.: Erlbaum, 1975.

Staudenmayer, H., & Bourne, L. E., Jr. Learning to interpret conditional sentences: A developmental study. *Developmental Psychology*, 1977, *13*, 616–623.

Sternberg, R. J. Component processes in analogical reasoning. *Psychological Review*, 1977, *84*, 353–378. (a)

Sternberg, R. J. *Intelligence, information processing, and analogical reasoning: The componential analysis of human abilities*. Hillsdale, N.J.: Erlbaum, 1977. (b)

Sternberg, R. J. Componential investigations of human intelligence. In A. Lesgold, J. Pellegrino, S. Fokkema, & R. Glaser (Eds.), *Cognitive psychology and instruction*. New York: Plenum, 1978. (a)

Sternberg, R. J. Isolating the components of intelligence. *Intelligence*, 1978, 2, 117–128. (b)

Sternberg, R. J. Intelligence research at the interface between differential and cognitive psychology. *Intelligence*, 1978, 2, 195–222. (c)

Sternberg, R. J. Developmental patterns in the encoding and combination of logical connectives. *Journal of Experimental Child Psychology*, 1979, 28, 469–498. (a)

Sternberg, R. J. The nature of mental abilities. *American Psychologist*, 1979, 34, 214–230. (b)

Sternberg, R. J. Six authors in search of a character: A play about intelligence tests in the year 2000. *Intelligence*, 1979, 3, 281–291. (c)

Sternberg, R. J. Stalking the I.Q. quark. *Psychology Today*, 1979, 13, 42–54. (d)

Sternberg, R. J. Componentman as vice-president: A reply to Pellegrino and Lyon's analysis of "The components of a componential analysis." *Intelligence*, 1980, 4, 83–95. (a)

Sternberg, R. J. The development of linear syllogistic reasoning. *Journal of Experimental Child Psychology*, 1980, 29, 340–356. (b)

Sternberg, R. J. A proposed resolution of curious conflicts in the literature on linear syllogistic reasoning. In R. Nickerson (Ed.), *Attention and performance VIII*. Hillsdale, N.J.: Erlbaum, 1980. (c)

Sternberg, R. J. Representation and process in linear syllogistic reasoning. *Journal of Experimental Psychology: General*, 1980, 109, 119–159. (d)

Sternberg, R. J. Sketch of a componential subtheory of human intelligence. *Behavioral and Brain Sciences*, 1980, 3, 573–584. (e)

Sternberg, R. J., Conway, B. E., Ketron, J. L., & Bernstein, M. Peoples' conceptions of intelligence. *Journal of Personality and Social Psychology: Attitudes and Social Cognition*, 1981, 41, 37–55.

Sternberg, R. J., & Davis, J. C. Student perceptions of Yale and its competitors. *College and University*, 1978, 53, 262–278.

Sternberg, R. J., & Gardner, M. K. A componential interpretation of the general factor in human intelligence. In H. J. Eysenck (Ed.), *A model for intelligence*. Berlin: Springer-Verlag, 1982.

Sternberg, R. J., & Ketron, J. L. Selection and implementation of strategies in reasoning by analogy. *Journal of Educational Psychology*, 1982, 74, 399–413.

Sternberg, R. J., Ketron, J. L., & Powell, J. S. Componential approaches to the training of intelligence. In D. K. Detterman & R. J. Sternberg (Eds.), *How and how much can intelligence be increased?* Norwood, N.J.: Ablex, 1982.

Sternberg, R. J., & Nigro, G. Developmental patterns in the solution of verbal analogies. *Child Development*, 1980, 51, 27–38.

Sternberg, R. J., & Rifkin, B. The development of analogical reasoning processes. *Journal of Experimental Child Psychology*, 1979, 27, 195–232.

Sternberg, R. J., Tourangeau, R., & Nigro, G. Metaphor, induction, and social policy: The convergence of macroscopic and microscopic views. In A. Ortony (Ed.), *Metaphor and thought*. Cambridge: Cambridge University Press, 1979.

Sternberg, R. J., & Tulving, E. The measurement of subjective organization in free recall. *Psychological Bulletin*, 1977, 84, 539–556.

Sternberg, R. J., & Turner, M. E. Components of syllogistic reasoning. *Acta Psychologica*, 1981, 47, 245–265.

Sternberg, R. J., & Weil, E. M. An aptitude–strategy interaction in linear syllogistic reasoning. *Journal of Educational Psychology*, 1980, 72, 226–234.

Stevens, S. S. Mathematics, measurement and psychophysics. In S. S. Stevens (Ed.), *Handbook of experimental psychology*. New York: Wiley, 1951.

Taplin, J. E. Reasoning with conditional sentences. *Journal of Verbal Learning and Verbal Behavior*, 1971, 10, 219–225.

Taplin, J. E., & Staudenmayer, H. Interpretation of abstract conditional sentences in deductive reasoning. *Journal of Verbal Learning and Verbal Behavior*, 1973, 12, 530–542.

Taplin, J. E., Staudenmayer, H., & Taddonio, J. L. Developmental changes in conditional reasoning: Linguistic or logical? *Journal of Experimental Child Psychology*, 1974, 17, 360–373.

Taylor, S. E., & Fiske, S. T. Salience, attention, and attribution: Top of the head phenomena. In
    L. Berkowitz (Ed.), *Advances in experimental social psychology* (Vol. 11). New York:
    Academic Press, 1978.
Terman, L. M. Contribution to "Intelligence and its measurement: A symposium." *Journal of
    Educational Psychology*, 1921, *12*, 127–133.
Terman, L. M., & Merrill, M. A. *Measuring intelligence.* Boston: Houghton Mifflin, 1937.
Thomas, J. C., Jr. An analysis of behavior in the hobbits–orcs problem. *Cognitive Psychology*,
    1974, *6*, 257–269.
Thurstone, L. L. *Primary mental abilities.* Chicago: University of Chicago Press, 1938.
Thurstone, L. L., & Thurstone, T. G. *SRA Primary Mental Abilities.* Chicago: Science Re-
    search Associates, 1962.
Tinsley, H. E. A., & Dawis, R. J. *The equivalence of semantic and figural test presentation of
    the same items* (Tech. Rep. No. 3004). Minneapolis: University of Minnesota, Center for
    the Study of Organizational Performance and Human Effectiveness, 1972.
Tourangeau, R., & Sternberg, R. J. Aptness in metaphor. *Cognitive Psychology*, 1981, *13*,
    27–55.
Trabasso, T., Representation, memory, and reasoning: How do we make transitive inferences?
    In A. D. Pick (Ed.), *Minnesota Symposium on Child Psychology* (Vol. 9). Minneapolis:
    University of Minnesota Press, 1975.
Trabasso, T., & Riley, C. A. On the construction and use of representations involving linear
    order. In R. L. Solso (Ed.), *Information processing and cognition: The Loyola Symposium.*
    Hillsdale, N.J.: Erlbaum, 1975.
Trabasso, T., Riley, C. A., & Wilson, E. G. The representation of linear order and spatial
    strategies in reasoning: A developmental study. In R. Falmagne (Ed.), *Reasoning: Repre-
    sentation and process.* Hillsdale, N.J.: Erlbaum, 1975.
Tulving, E. Subjective organization and effects of repetition in multi-trial free-recall learning.
    Journal of Verbal Learning and Verbal Behavior, 1966, *5*, 193–197.
Tversky, A., & Kahneman, D. Judgment under uncertainty: Heuristics and biases. *Science*,
    1974, *185*, 1124–1131.
Tversky, A., & Kahneman, D. Causal schemata in judgments under uncertainty. In M. Fish-
    bein (Ed.), *Progress in social psychology.* Hillsdale, N.J.: Erlbaum, 1977.
Underwood, B. J. An orientation for research on thinking. *Psychological Review*, 1952, *59*,
    209–220.
van de Geer, J. P. *A psychological study of problem solving.* Haarlem: Uitgeverij De Toorts,
    1957.
Vinacke, W. E. *The psychology of thinking.* New York: McGraw-Hill, 1952.
Vitz, P. C., & Todd, T. C. A model of learning for simple repeating binary patterns. *Journal of
    Experimental Psychology*, 1969, *75*, 108–117.
Vygotsky, L. S. *Thought and language* (E. Hanfmann & G. Vakar, Eds. and trans.). Cambridge,
    Mass.: MIT Press, 1962.
Wason, P. C. "On the failure to eliminate hypotheses... " – A second look. In P. C. Wason & P.
    N. Johnson-Laird (Eds.), *Thinking and reasoning.* Harmondsworth, England: Penguin,
    1968.
Wason, P. C.. & Johnson-Laird, P. N. *Psychology of reasoning: Structure and content.* London:
    B. T. Batsford, 1972.
Whitely, S. E. *Types of relationships in reasoning by analogy.* Unpublished doctoral disserta-
    tion, University of Minnesota, 1973.
Whitely, S. E. Solving verbal analogies: Some cognitive components of intelligence test items.
    Journal of Educational Psychology, 1976, *68*, 234–242.
Whitely, S. E. Information-processing on intelligence test items: Some response components.
    Applied Psychological Measurement, 1977, *1*, 465–476.
Whitely, S. E. Latent trait models in the study of intelligence. *Intelligence*, 1979, *4*, 97–132. (a)
Whitely, S. E. *Modeling aptitude test validity from cognitive components* (NIE 79-2 Tech.
    Rep.). Lawrence, Kans.: University of Kansas, Department of Psychology, 1979. (b)
Whitely, S. E. *Multicomponent latent trait models for information-processes on ability tests.*
    (NIE 79-1 Tech. Rep.). Lawrence, Kans.: University of Kansas, Department of Psychol-
    ogy, 1979. (c)
Whitely, S. E., & Barnes, G. M. The implications of processing event sequences for theories of
    analogical reasoning. *Memory and Cognition*, 1979, *1*, 323–331.

Whitely, S. E., & Dawis, R. A cognitive intervention for improving the estimate of latent ability measured from analogy items (Tech. Rep. No. 3010). Minneapolis: University of Minnesota, Center for the Study of Organizational Performance and Human Effectiveness, 1973.

Whitely, S. E., & Dawis, R. V. The effects of cognitive intervention on latent ability measured from analogy items. *Journal of Educational Psychology,* 1974, *66,* 710–717.

Wilkins, M. C. The effect of changed material on ability to do formal syllogistic reasoning. *Archives of Psychology,* 1928, *16*(102).

Williams, D. S. Computer program organization induced from problem examples. In H. A. Simon & L. Siklossy (Eds.), *Representation and meaning: Experiments with information processing systems.* Englewood Cliffs, N.J.: Prentice-Hall, 1972.

Willner, A. An experimental analysis of analogical reasoning. *Psychological Reports,* 1964, *15,* 479–494.

Wilson, W. R. The effect of competition on the speed and accuracy of syllogistic reasoning. *Journal of Social Psychology,* 1965, *65,* 27–32.

Winston, P. H. *Learning structural descriptions from examples* (AI TR-231). Cambridge, Mass.: MIT, Artificial Intelligence Laboratory, 1970.

Wood, D. J. *The nature and development of problem-solving strategies.* Unpublished doctoral dissertation, University of Nottingham, 1969.

Wood, D., Shotter, J., & Godden, D. An investigation of the relationships between problem solving strategies, representation and memory. *Quarterly Journal of Experimental Psychology,* 1974, *26,* 252–257.

Woodworth, R. S., & Schlosberg, H. *Experimental psychology.* New York: Holt, Rinehart, & Winston, 1954.

Woodworth, R. S., & Sells, S. B. An atmosphere effect in formal syllogistic reasoning. *Journal of Experimental Psychology,* 1935, *18,* 451–460.

6 *Personality and intelligence*

JONATHAN BARON

The field of personality research, including the study of *cognitive style*, the part of personality most directly related to intellectual functioning, is perceived by outsiders to be in a state of crisis. It appears to many scholars that the standards of rigor and scholarship in the rest of psychology have improved, leaving personality theory behind. Most workers in this field are perceived by outsiders as simply insensitive to this concern, and most of those few who seem sensitive (e.g., Mischel, 1977) have little to say about intelligence. It is my view, however, that reports of the death of personality theory are premature, that it is too important an area to be left entirely to personality theorists, and most importantly that intelligence itself consists partly of what must be called intellectual personality traits (Baron, 1981). I have been led to this view not from any commitment to personality theory itself but rather by reflection on the nature of intelligence and its manifestations.

In the course of this chapter I first discuss my point of view, which is based on that of Dewey (1933), who describes the nature of good thinking. This section draws extensively on Baron (in press). Next I apply this point of view to several issues in the study of personality and intelligence, including cognitive styles, stage theories of development, and the relation of styles to psychopathology. I then consider the implications of some issues in the study of personality for the study of intelligence, including correlations between personality and IQ, intelligence as a perceived trait, the social context of intelligence, the generality of intellectual personality traits, and personality change and its relation to the training of intelligence. I conclude with recommendations for research.

6.1. REFLECTIVE THINKING AND INTELLIGENCE

The theory of good thinking would seem to be a reasonable part of any complete theory of intelligence. A general theory of intelligence ought to say what it means to do something intelligently: to speak intelligently, to carry out a calculation intelligently, and so on. The ability to *think* intelligently is a more crucial ability than the others, however. By thinking well, a person may learn to manage his own capacity limits as if they were external problems to be overcome. We sometimes say even of a person who has largely lost the ability to learn (e.g., through brain damage) that "he is still intelligent despite his loss," but we would be reluctant to say the same of a person who had largely lost the ability to think. Thinking is, in a sense, the most essential expression of intelligence.

The next few sections of this chapter explore the possible form of a theory of reflective thinking in the tradition of Dewey. After reviewing Dewey's theory itself, I shall discuss how the theory can be brought up to date, and I shall sketch a new version. I shall argue that thinking in all its manifestations has a single description, which is not so abstract as to be useless. Following Dewey, I propose a general normative (prescriptive) model of the phases of reflective thinking. Associated with each phase are at least one parameter governing the operation of that phase and at least one rule for setting the optimum value of that parameter. People in general may tend to deviate from the optimum in a particular direction, and some people may be more prone to such biases than others. Because the parameters of thinking can vary on either side of an optimum, we should be more concerned with their normal level than with their possible outer limits. I note that the present approach leads to a concern with propensities rather than with capacities. Propensities, unlike capacities, are to some extent under voluntary control and are thus more subject to influence through education. Propensities may be taken as cognitive styles; thus the theory I sketch may provide a framework for the study of cognitive styles. There is also some reason to think that propensities may be general. Propensities are affected by values, expectations, and habits, which in turn are affected by emotions, and all of these factors must be considered when we try to change propensities or to understand their origins.

DEWEY'S "HOW WE THINK" AS A NORMATIVE THEORY OF THINKING

Dewey (1933) tried to characterize a type of thinking, which he called *reflective thinking*. The term refers to only one of the word's many senses, namely, thinking that tries to reach a goal, to resolve a state of doubt, or to decide on a course of action, in contrast to thinking as the content of the stream of consciousness, or *to think* as a synonym for *to believe*. To say that thinking is reflective is also to say that it is the kind of thinking one ought to do whenever easily applied or habitual rules of behavior do not suffice. Reflective thought involves an initial state of doubt or perplexity (a problem) and an active search of previous experiences and knowledge for material that will resolve the doubt.

There may, however, be a state of perplexity and also previous experiences out of which suggestions emerge, and yet thinking may not be reflective. For the person may not be sufficiently *critical* about the ideas that occur to him.... To many persons both suspense of judgment and intellectual search are disagreeable; they want to get them ended as soon as possible. They cultivate an over-positive and dogmatic habit of mind, or feel perhaps that a condition of doubt will be regarded as evidence of mental inferiority.... To be genuinely thoughtful, we must be willing to sustain and protract the state of doubt which is the stimulus to thorough inquiry, so as not to accept an idea or make positive assertion of a belief until justifying reasons have been found. [Dewey, 1933, p. 16]

One advantage of reflective thought over "merely impulsive and merely routine activity" is that it "enables us to act in a deliberate and intentional fashion to attain future objects or to come into command of what is now distant and lacking." Reflective thinking allows us to choose courses of action that succeed in attaining otherwise unattainable goals, and it makes us more likely to adopt true beliefs rather than false ones.

A theory of good thinking must not confine itself to the form of the thinking itself: "ability to train thought is not achieved merely by knowledge of the best forms of thought.... Moreover, there are no set exercises in correct thinking whose repeated performance will cause one to be a good thinker. The information and the exercises are both of value. But no individual realizes their value except as he is personally animated by certain dominant attitudes in his own character" (1933, p. 29). Dewey includes such "attitudes" as open-mindedness, wholeheartedness, and "responsibility" as necessary. ("To be intellectually responsible is to consider the consequences of a projected step; it means to be willing to adopt these consequences when they follow reasonably from any position already taken. Intellectual responsibility secures integrity; that is to say, consistency and harmony in belief") (p. 32).

As for the form of reflective thought itself, Dewey suggests five phases: (a) suggestion of an initial solution or action, which is not carried out because of a feeling of doubt; (b) intellectualization of the difficulty into a problem to be solved (what we would now call formation of a problem representation); (c) the use of one suggestion after another as hypotheses, which guide further reasoning; (d) reasoning in the narrow sense, that is, "the mental elaboration of the idea or supposition as an idea or supposition"; and (e) the testing of the hypotheses in action and in thought. These phases are intended as descriptions of actual steps taken, not as formal constraints.

What conclusions should we reach about this theory today? It might appear to some that the theory lacks content, because it seems hard to imagine any alternative to it. However, one notable alternative is provided by Newell (e.g., 1980), who has also tried to describe thinking in general terms. Newell's theory, based on computer models, has treated thinking as a matter of finding one's way through a "problem space" with allowable moves and a well-defined goal. Newell's theory calls attention to different aspects of thinking and to different ways of drawing analogies between thinking tasks. Whatever else may be said for Dewey's theory in contrast to Newell's, I believe that it will provide a better basis for a theory of cognitive style.

One element missing from Dewey's theory is a set of rules for the proper use of each phase of thinking. The rules might concern the proper setting of certain parameters, such as the number of hypotheses to consider or the amount of time to spend thinking. With these rules, the theory could provide us with a standard rather than just a framework. We might also seek deviations in one direction or the other from the optimum value of the parameter for each phase. People may differ in their propensity to deviate in one direction or the other or in the magnitude of their deviation. These differences in propensities may constitute cognitive styles.

THE PHASES OF REFLECTIVE THOUGHT

I now provide a sketch of a theory of reflective thinking modeled after Dewey's theory. I list five phases of thinking, modeled after Dewey's: problem recognition, enumeration of possibilities, reasoning (search for, or recognition of, evidence bearing on the possibilities), revision (use of the evidence), and evaluation of the possibilities to decide whether more thinking is required. For each phase I discuss one or two relevant parameters that govern operation of that phase and one or two rules for optimal setting of these parameters. The rules are standards by which to judge the correctness of thinking, not necessarily rules for a person to try to follow. Heuristics, or rules of thumb suitable for the latter purpose, however, may often be derived from the more formal rules (as suggested by Nisbett & Ross, 1980).

Phase 1. Problem recognition. A state of perplexity or doubt is recognized. This recognition acts simply as a stimulus to begin thinking. The cause of the doubt may be the automatic occurrence of one of the later phases, for example, the appearance in mind of evidence against a possibility. Problem recognition may also occur when the situation is novel, so that no previously acquired rule of behavior applies. (Note that the occasions for thinking are only a subset of those for intentional acts in Irwin's, 1971, sense. In most such cases, there is so little doubt as to which of a set of possible acts will lead to a preferred outcome that there is no need to think.)

Performance in some situations is limited by the tendency to find problems. Once the problem is found, the solution may be time consuming or even difficult, but the uniqueness of the achievement may depend mainly on finding the problem. This is often true in science and in the arts. It may also hold in the moral realm, where failure to recognize a moral problem may be the crucial determinant of immoral behavior (Arendt, 1965). Possibly one of the greatest sources of individual variation lies in the sheer amount of thinking that takes place, an amount that depends partly on the tendency to recognize problems. In general, people are probably too "thought-less" (Langer, 1978), but there may be pathological individuals who think too much (Shapiro, 1965).

The rule for this phase (like many other rules) is that the main parameter, the tendency to recognize problems, should be set so as to maximize ultimate expected value. (I leave until later the question of how value is to be determined; for now, it suffices to say that both the values of society and the subjective values of the individual are relevant.) People who live in highly predictable environments, where optimal behavior may be determined without thinking, will do best with a low setting of this parameter; others require a higher setting.

Phase 2. Enumeration of possibilities. Some number (usually one, sometimes zero, sometimes several) of possibilities are listed. Possibilities may concern beliefs that might be adopted or actions that might be taken. I shall collapse these cases, because there is no reason to distinguish them. (A choice of actions may reduce to a choice of beliefs as to which action will lead to the best outcome.) One possibility is often that about which doubt was originally raised. In some cases, it is advantageous to enumerate several possibilities before seeking evidence about any of them. In particular, evidence could be selected with a view to deciding among the possibilities. This is the essential wisdom behind the "method of multiple working hypotheses" in science (Chamberlain, 1897/1965).

Given a problem such as deciding on a chess move or on a purchase, one person may begin by listing all the possibilities before evaluating any, whereas another may evaluate one at a time until a possibility proves satisfactory. This parameter, the number of possibilities generated before any evidence is considered, should again be chosen to maximize expected value. For each number of possibilities enumerated, there is an expected loss of effort, an expected amount of subsequent effort required to meet a certain standard of quality or certainty of the possibility finally chosen, and possibly also a change in the expected probability of meeting the standard, with attendant value consequences. (Note that the difficulty of generating possibilities is a given, about which I have nothing to say except that it determines the "effort" term in the rule.) The value of this parameter may depend on the standard of evaluation. If the standard is strict, failure to enumerate possibilities may result in failure to choose the best one. This rule, of course, is so complex that no one can attempt to follow directly (unless it is someone who is planning the "thinking" to be done by a large organization). If people understand the underlying principle, however, they will be sensitive to the effects of possibility enumeration in repeated tasks (e.g., chess games), and they will have a better chance of learning how to set the parameter in each case.

When adding possibilities to the set under consideration, a person may tend to choose those that have been tried before or, at the other end of the scale, those that are new. Stereotypy in this sense – unwillingness to try new actions or beliefs – is the equivalent of rigidity in the sense of Luchins and Luchins (1959). Schwartz (1982) has studied some determinants of stereotypy in a task in which several different sequences of behavior, all determined by a simple rule, lead to reward. Subjects tend to discover one of these sequences and keep to it, preferring the reward to the chance to learn about the other sequences through variation.

The rule for the selection of novel versus familiar possibilities would be based on the expected cost (effort) and value of each. The cost of novel possibilities may depend on the difficulty of thinking of them, which may depend on individual capacities. (On the other hand, some people, like the author, may find recalling old possibilities so difficult that starting over each time is actually easier!) Related heuristics are, on the one hand, "think of a related problem" (Polya, 1945), or, on the other, "try something new."

Phase 3. Reasoning.   Possibilities are evaluated by search for, or recognition of, evidence for or against them. One type of evidence against a possibility is the emergence of another possibility to be added to the list of those under consideration. People seek evidence by consulting their memories, asking questions, or doing experiments.

Other things equal, it is better to select evidence that provides more "information" in some sense. Several demonstrations (e.g. Wason, 1968) have been interpreted as showing a "confirmation bias" in such situations, in which the thinker seeks uninformative evidence that allows him to maintain his preferred possibility. The error may be at other phases, however, such as the enumeration of possibilities. To discover whether there really are errors in this phase of this type of task, we need a normative rule that takes the results of earlier phases into account. Savage (1954) suggests such a rule, namely, that evidence should be selected (once again) to maximize expected value. The value of a piece of information is the expected value of the decision made with that information minus the expected value of the decision made without it. This rule tells us not only which of several pieces of information to select (when there is some cost in selecting more than one) but also whether or not to select a given piece. It thus determines the optimal setting of the parameter that sets the probability of choosing evidence. A heuristic corresponding to Savage's rule is to ask oneself, "What difference would it make if I knew this?"

When one possibility is initially favored over others, we can ask whether a person seeks evidence likely to strengthen that possibility or to weaken it. This question arises only when it is possible to seek evidence of one sort or another, which is the case when one is seeking examples or counterexamples in memory (Baron, 1981) but usually not when one seeks external evidence, as in performing a scientific experiment. Again, this parameter should be set so as to maximize expected value. A heuristic rule consistent with the general rule is that one should set the parameter according to the kind of possibility one is evaluating: If the possibility is a proposition about general truth, one should be biased toward counterevidence; if it is a proposition about possibility or plausibility, one should be biased toward confirming evidence; and otherwise one should be neutral. It seems likely that people are generally more biased toward confirming evidence than they ought to be.

Phase 4. Revision.   The list of possibilities is revised on the basis of evidence. Revision may mean addition or deletion of possibilities or modification of members of the list or of strengths assigned to them. When it is appropriate to assign strengths to possibilities, indicating one's prior commitment to each, and to evidence, indicating the effect of each piece of evidence on each possibility, a normative rule for revision has been stated by Shafer (1976) under very general assumptions. Under certain conditions, this rule reduces to Bayes's theorem, in which strengths are interpreted as probabilities of the usual sort. An implication of these rules is that the order in which evidence is presented (for a possibility relevant to a particular point in time) should not matter. In particular, the strength assigned to a belief already held should reflect the evidence on which that belief is based, so that new evidence will be weighed appropriately. A related heuristic is that one should keep track of the evidence for one's most important beliefs. (Scholars cite references in part for precisely this purpose.) Another rule of thumb might be, "Regard the strength of a possibility as if it were itself a strength of evidence, so that you combine new evidence with old on equal terms."

Much research has explored the extent to which people revise beliefs appropriately. In general, the finding has been that people are insensitive to evidence (Nisbett & Ross, 1980, ch. 8). We might call this a kind of rigidity (a different kind from that studied by Luchins & Luchins, 1959) in the setting of the parameter that determines sensitivity to evidence. There are cases in which people seem to be insensitive to relevant prior beliefs, for example, beliefs about characteristics of populations (Tversky & Kahneman, 1974). In these cases, however, typically the relevant belief is *not* represented as a possibility at the time when the thinking is done.

In other cases, the phase of revision may consist of modification of possibilities rather than their addition, deletion, or change in strength. The prototypical case is artistic creation, where the single possibility is a product, such as a musical theme, a line in a poem, or a painting. The idea of revision of a product does not occur automatically to every artist, especially not to one who believes that spontaneous creation confers special status on a work. Other examples (Baron, 1981) include formation of representations of problems, discovery of generalizations in such fields as philosophy and linguistics, and ordinary writing. In the case of generalizations, the evidence often consists of counterexamples to a tentatively stated principle or rule (Baron, 1981).

Phase 5. Evaluation.   The current set of possibilities is evaluated to decide whether the process should continue. If so, the thinker goes back to Phase 2 or 3; if not, the best possibility is chosen. This choice requires a method for evaluation of the goodness of the possibilities, and the same method will normally be used as part of the process of deciding whether to continue thinking as well.

In ordinary problem solving, such as trying to locate a reference or find the bug in a computer program, one is usually faced with a choice of continuing to work on the problem or giving up, where giving up involves some default option, such as going to the library or rewriting part of the program. In other cases, when evaluation is the critical phase, such as in deciding what kind of product to buy, the question is whether to continue to collect evidence or to make the choice on the basis of the evidence at hand. The same choice arises in many laboratory tasks designed to measure impulsiveness (Kagan, 1966). The rule for this phase is that one should stop working on a problem when the expected value would be reduced by continuing to work. This decision, of course, involves one's belief about the probability of success or improvement that will result from further work. A heuristic simply enables one to ask oneself whether further work is likely to pay; this question alone might eliminate many cases of impulsiveness or obsessive decision making.

An important parameter of thinking determines how soon one stops thinking, relative to the optimum dictated by the rule. There is some evidence (Baron, 1981; Messer, 1976) that most people are too impulsive, that is, that they tend to set to stop thinking too soon. However, to my knowledge, no previous research on impulsiveness (including my own) has attempted to measure or control the relevant values. (For some purposes we may want to distinguish between impulsiveness and nonpersistence. In essence, the time a person spends thinking may depend – in addition to other factors – on whether or not at least a single possibility is available. When no possibility is available, we might call a person nonpersistent who gives up too early, so that we reserve the term *impulsive* for cases in which a possibility is actually chosen.)

Let me now make a few general points about the phases and rules that I have described. First, they are called phases rather than stages because their timing is highly flexible. They can be spread over years (in the case of hypothetic–deductive reasoning) or collapsed into a few seconds. They can overlap in time, and one event might be part of two different phases. Parts of one reflective thought process may involve another whole sequence, for example, the working out of an experiment.

Second, the general normative model plays different roles in different cases. In some cases, it provides a formal and precisely testable model for the specific case. In other cases, it serves as a more general guide. In these cases, use of the model as an instructional tool would help a student avoid drastic errors in approach to the task.

Third, the parameters may be used to measure individual differences, that is, as measures of cognitive styles (in a sense). When they are used in this way, the main question is whether people differ in a parameter consistently across situations. Of course, the answer to this question could change if education changes (and, e.g., if it is effective in teaching performance to some people more than to others). We may also ask how the parameters correlate with each other and with potential determinants. There is no reason, however, to expect these parameters to function as factors and no reason to expect correlations among them in any particular pattern.

Fourth, in some cases, the rules I have stated may be used to teach good thinking as well as to judge it. The basic rules would be used only in the most formal kind of thinking (e.g., evaluation of public policy alternatives), and the everyday thinker would have to settle for rules of thumb and corrective heuristics. Invention of good heuristics may depend on knowledge of the rules and perhaps also of common blocks to following them. There is a special value for education in our being able to state rules of good thinking, whether these are formal rules or heuristics. The teaching of thinking, like the teaching of other skills, ultimately involves prompting people to do the right thing and giving them practice doing it. Other functions of education, such as the inculcation of values, beliefs, and aesthetic responses, are relevant to the teaching of skills only indirectly, to the extent that these things affect what a person does. Rules are statements of what the student is to do, and they are thus the most direct kind of statement of the goal of teaching thinking.

I have so far suggested some parameters of thinking and some general rules for setting these parameters appropriately. The rules usually concern the weighing of values, and the parameters are usually interpretable as biases that indicate the degree and direction of the discrepancy from the rule-determined optimum. The values, for example, the negative or positive value of thinking itself, play an important role. The question of *whose values* is thus important, as there may be conflict between the values of the individual at the moment and the values of others or between the values of the same person at a different time. For example, for political purposes, it might help if everyone did more thinking about the issues that confront humanity, but the individuals involved may find such thinking unpleasant, preferring instead to base their political actions on emotion or on the authority of respected others. On a more mundane level, some children may dislike schoolwork and may refuse to think because of their immediate values, although their values would dictate otherwise if they could see the whole course of their lives. For present purposes, it is of interest to use different sets of values in judging thinking. In particular, it is of interest to know whether a person is performing consistently with his own values at the time; if so, any inconsistency with the behavior dictated by other values can be explained in terms of the discrepancy in the values themselves. Of course, there is more to be said about this matter, but this is not the place to say it.

THE RELATION OF REFLECTIVE THINKING TO CAPACITIES

The study of individual differences in processes relating to intelligence has been concerned mostly with capacities, such as working-memory capacity or memory-access speed, rather than propensities. The setting of the kinds of parameters that I have listed is a matter of choice, however, a matter subject to some voluntary control, hence involving propensity rather than capacity. For example, instructions that tell a person to enumerate more possibilities before evaluating any, to weigh evidence more heavily relative to his prior beliefs, or to set a higher standard for quality of his decisions ought to affect what he does somewhat. This difference has four implications: Propensities are teachable in ways that capacities are not; a propensity need not take an extreme value in order to be set optimally; propensities are best measured in normal circumstances rather than in optimal circumstances; and special problems arise in determining whether people in general have biases on one side of optimality. In this section, I discuss each of these implications in turn.

When I say that the rules of good thinking ought to be teachable, I do not mean that they are unaffected by biological limits on information processing or by individual differences in such limits. I mean only that there is some choice involved in a person's value of a parameter and that the way in which this choice is made might be teachable. My reason for thinking that the parameters listed are corrigible is that it is easy to imagine changing any one of them in response to instruction. They are all stylistic in the sense that they are to some extent under control. For example, a person can be instructed not to act on the first idea that comes to mind, to ask whether a piece of evidence makes any difference before taking the trouble to collect it, to experiment with novel solutions to problems, or to ask whether further thinking might be helpful before giving up on a problem. If a person does not follow such instructions, it would probably be because he does not believe that they will help, not because he is unable. For this reason we tend to be somewhat suspicious of people who act impulsively and then excuse themselves by saying, "I couldn't help myself; I didn't want to do what I did, but I just found myself doing it."

Another characteristic shared by these propensities (the kinds of parameters I listed) is that their optimum point – like the ideal amount of salt in a stew – need not be at one end of the continuum of possible values. Thus an instruction to change the setting of a parameter may be helpful. This is not the case for parameters that represent capacities. For example, it would ordinarily not help people to tell them that the parameter governing their working-memory capacities is too low. In any test of this capacity, the object is obviously to have as large a working memory as possible (given reasonable effort). Of course, practice might still help improve the capacity, at least in specific situations (see Baron, in press), but the same is true for stylistic parameters. Propensities may be affected by practice as well as by simple instruction, so that they provide larger targets for the educator to hit.

Because propensities are potentially under voluntary control, they must be measured without the subject's awareness that they are being measured. After all, we would not want our measures to be contaminated by the degree to which the subject tried to impress us. We assume that greater generality is to be found if we measure a propensity without such contamination. Tests of propensities resemble measures of speed of walking rather than measures of speed of running; we measure the former under normal conditions, the latter under optimal conditions. Many tests now in use have this character, including the Rorschach inkblot test and tests of cognitive style that involve choosing which two of three stimuli go together best (Kogan, 1976; Smith & Kemler, 1977). In at least one sense of the term, these measures may be considered to be measures of style rather than of ability.

Current intelligence tests are not supposed to have this character. For example, the scoring of such tests usually considers both time and errors, so that subjects cannot affect their scores significantly by making more impulsive responses. When it is found that the score on a test can be influenced by such changes, the test is usually considered to be flawed.

Finally, it is difficult to specify with regard to propensities what it might mean to say that people are generally too impulsive, too rigid, or too stereotyped. Surely there are situations in which people are not impulsive enough, not rigid enough, and so forth. There are several answers to this problem. Most simply, the real question concerns the match between intellectual adjustment – the setting of the parameters – and environmental demands (including demands that result from culture and from the physical environment). Thus any claim about people would be specific to a particular place and time, and the solution to the mismatch could as well be a change in environment (e.g., building machines that understand our idiosyncrasies) as a change in people themselves. Any test of people's lack of adjustment would have to be based on some sort of sample of environmental demands, or on measures of a person's general adjustment, however crude these measures must be. For example, some evidence that people are too impulsive consists in findings that less impulsive people are better adapted according to such criteria as school grades and absence of objectionable behavior (Messer, 1976).

Another kind of answer requires the discovery of correctable inconsistencies between people's desires and their behavior. Nonoptimality in thinking may result from certain fallacies or biases that are clearly seen to be irrational once they are understood (assuming that people are willing to make judgments at all about methods of thought). Instruction that teaches people to guard against these fallacies may be effective in improving thinking. For example, McCauley and Stitt (1978) found that people's stereotypes of black Americans were not exaggerated, as many theories of stereotypes would suggest they ought to be. Perhaps the subjects were aware enough of the dangers of stereotyping to guard against its excessive use. There is some evidence that people can be taught to avoid other sorts of fallacies, the knowledge of which is less widespread, such as overconfidence (Koriat, Lichtenstein, & Fischhoff, 1980). Some of these fallacies – like children's tendency to confuse number and length – may be the result of universal developmental processes; if so they should be acknowledged to be a property of people in general. In sum, when people are taught a rule or a rule of thumb, they may find that they gain, in the long run, by following it. The existence of such gains is the most important test of any effort to teach rules for thinking.

GENERALITY

Rules of the sort I have listed are supposed to be useful in all situations in which habit or easily followed rules will not suffice. Thus any propensity to deviate from the rule in a particular direction could also be a highly general personality trait or style. What reason is there to think that propensities may be general?

First, the propensity may be influenced by a general capacity of the sort just discussed. Little can be said about this possibility because so little is known about the generality of individual differences in capacities. (Baron & Treiman, 1980, discuss the methodological difficulties in acquiring such knowledge.)

Second, a propensity may become general through transfer between situations. Because transfer is often hard to demonstrate, researchers have often been skeptical about the possibility of general transfer (e.g., Hayes, in press).

Still, transfer is not the only way in which a propensity may become general through learning. In particular, people might be given – or might give themselves – general instructions. Suppose, for example, that we tell a person, "When trying to decide whether to continue thinking, weigh the expected gain from further thought against the cost of the effort involved in thinking." This is a highly general instruction, and we might test a person's ability to follow it in any situation involving thought. If people given this instruction can follow this rule in any such situation, we might say that they have learned it. The only question now is whether they would remember to follow the rule when removed from our presence in space or time.

Most experiments on transfer of learning (e.g., of strategies for learning arbitrary material) do not provide general instructions. Rather, the subject is given instructions for the specific case in which the original learning is observed. To show transfer, subjects must figure out for themselves the general instruction as it applies to a new case, *and* they must think of the original case when confronted with the new case, even though they are given no reason to do so. (In some transfer experiments, subjects are at least told that they are learning something that will be useful elsewhere, but still no effort is made to tell them exactly what that something is.) Thus there is reason to be more hopeful about the possibility of general rules than we would be from looking at the transfer literature alone. That literature is simply inconclusive about this possibility.

Although the question of generality is much discussed in the personality literature and will recur later in this chapter, it is appropriate to ask why the issue merits consideration. One question of interest is whether a propensity can be modified in general. If the propensity in question functions as a general trait – as a measure of individual differences that are consistent across situations – then we have one argument for the possibility of general modifiability. It is not conclusive evidence, however, for the generality of the trait may be due to general biological influences. Further, if the propensity does not function as a general trait, we cannot conclude that it is not modifiable in general. Knowledge of the relevant rule may be so rare that the variations in such knowledge are insignificant. What is or is not a general trait may change as education changes, both in what it teaches and in how well it succeeds in teaching everyone equally.

DETERMINANTS OF FOLLOWING THE RULES

I must distinguish between two parts of the kind of theory I am proposing. One part concerns the rules that good thinkers follow. The other part concerns the factors that cause them to follow or not to follow those rules. Here I shall briefly discuss the second part. We have little relevant knowledge, but it may help to analyze the possibilities in general and in a couple of cases.

First, it must be acknowledged that propensities of the sort I have described may be affected by biological factors. For example, a child may be impulsive to some extent because of impatience or inability to attend to one thing for a sufficient amount of time. These problems may be innate or the result of brain damage. (Educational interventions may still be helpful, however; Meichenbaum, 1977.) I say no more about these factors, because I (and others, I suspect) know little about them.

In general, propensities may be affected by values, expectations, and habits. Values (preferences) and expectations work together (Irwin, 1971). If a person desires some goal and expects that a certain behavior will achieve that goal, he will tend to produce the behavior. As I have noted, values may lead to poor thinking if the values of the individual are not, in some sense, as they ought to be. For example, a person may place too low a value on his own thinking, compared with its value to others. Like values, expectations may fail to correspond with reality in correctable ways. Habits are elicited by situations rather than goals and are not under the control of expectations (in Skinner's terms, are not affected by availability of reinforcement). Habits are thus automatic in this sense (although not necessarily in the sense that they require little effort or in the sense that they cannot be controlled). Practice may be involved in the formation of habits in a way in which it is not involved in the control of other behavior.

Although all factors that affect propensities must exert their effects through effects on values, expectations, and habits, it is worth considering some other, less direct, influences as well. Some insight may come from consideration of factors thought to affect two manifestations of decreased propensity to think effectively: learned helplessness in humans (Alloy & Seligman, 1979) and impulsiveness (Messer, 1976). Learned helplessness results from learning that one cannot control the outcome in some situation. Helplessness experiences (and depression, which is thought to operate in similar ways) impair subsequent learning to control an outcome. Impairment may occur in several ways. The subject may be hindered in learning about the new contingency, a deficit that could itself have several causes. He may be less prone to take any intentional action; the impairment may be a motor one, or more generally, it may be a deficit in initiation of intentional action. (The latter deficit would account for helplessness effects on learning *not* to do something; inhibition of what one would otherwise do is itself a kind of voluntary act.) This decreased propensity may itself result from an induced emotional state. Even if the subject learns the response–outcome contingency normally, he may be less likely to infer that it will continue to hold. This deficient inference may be the result of a general belief that situations in which one can control outcomes are not stable. Finally, helplessness may reduce one's motivation to seek pleasure or avoid pain, in turn perhaps a direct result of an induced emotional state. Each of these different causes of reduced manifestation of learning has different consequences for remediation of the deficit (and indeed it may be partly through these consequences that the deficits may be distinguished; see Dweck, 1975).

Impulsiveness as treated in the literature is the tendency to respond quickly, and to make many errors as a result, in situations that require thinking. It is typically measured in a complex perceptual–matching task (Kagan, 1966; see Messer, 1976, for a review). (The opposite of impulsiveness is *reflectiveness,* but this is clearly a poor term, since Dewey's use of *reflective* corresponds more closely to the original meaning.) Impulsiveness or its opposite may be a matter of habit. For example, children who are taught to answer quickly when asked a question may continue to do so long after childhood, and they may even transfer this style to new situations such as school examinations. Impulsiveness may also be a matter of values, either too low a value on accuracy or a negative value on thought, relative to the value of one's thought to others. Such values, in turn, may result from beliefs or more general values. Impulsive people may believe that the appearance of self-confidence is more important than accuracy itself in obtaining other ends such as the respect of other people. They may be unafraid in general and unafraid of making mistakes in particular. They may be motivated to maintain their self-esteem, which would be hurt by a failure occurring after some effort but not by a failure resulting from impulsiveness. ("I could have done it if I had tried.") Impulsiveness may also result from expectations of the same sort that might account for learned helplessness. For example, impulsive people may expect further thought not to increase the probability of success. Such an expectation might result (correctly or incorrectly) from prior failure experiences. More generally, any cause of learned helplessness could also cause impulsiveness when the task used to measure impulsiveness involves repeated trials with feedback. Repeated trials imply an opportunity to learn the contingency between the subject's thought and performance in the task.

Four comments warrant attention here. First, all of these possible causes of impulsiveness (or helplessness, for that matter) are practically relevant only when one is interested in remediating the impulsiveness. The damage done by impulsiveness, in the context of a normative theory of thinking, is the same regardless of its cause. Second, the cause of impulsiveness in an individual cannot be inferred from correlational studies involving groups. For example, it seems that anxiety about performance is negatively correlated with impulsiveness; yet it is still possible that anxiety causes impulsiveness in some people. Third, the causes of impulsiveness may be situation-specific. For example, people may be anxious only in certain situations. Still, the same *kinds* of factors may affect general propensities, if these exist. Fourth, the analogy between learned helplessness and impulsiveness may be useful, because the determinants of the former, at least, have received considerable attention. Adherence to the rules of good thinking in general, however, is not always analogous to the manifestation of learning to control an outcome. In particular, failure to control an outcome generally implies a failure to take intentional action. Failure to follow the rules of good thinking, on the other hand, may be compatible with all sorts of intentional actions. Such actions may be less effortful than good thinking, but in other cases, such as that of the student memorizing a proof instead of trying to understand it, the effort to avoid thinking may be greater than the effort involved in the thinking itself.

INTERIM SUMMARY AND PROSPECTUS

A list of the main points I have made so far may be helpful. First, Dewey's theory provides a useful analysis of the phases of reflective thinking. This analysis is sufficiently general to include most if not all kinds of intelligent thought. Second, it is possible to specify general normative rules for the use of each phase and definitions of parameters. The rules are analogous to, and include, some of the rules of decision making under uncertainty, such as Bayes's theorem (when it applies). Third, the following of these rules reflects choice as well as capacity. Thus propensities to follow a rule or to deviate from it in a certain way are subject to education in a way that capacities are not. One important empirical question is whether people can follow and can remember to follow a general instruction. Fourth, because of the voluntary nature of propensities, measurement of good thinking should concern itself with normal behavior as well as with optimal behavior. Finally, propensities may be affected by values, expectations, and habits, which in turn may be affected by emotions, all of which need to be considered in any full account of why people have any particular propensities.

I have thus far constructed a framework for an inquiry about the relation between intelligence and personality. I will now consider the status in the literature of two categories of questions: those concerning implications of the study of intelligence, as I conceive of it, for the study of personality and those concerning the implications of the study of personality for the study of intelligence. In the former category, I discuss cognitive styles and suggest interpretations for stage theories of personality development (Kohlberg, 1969; Loevinger, Wessler, & Redmore, 1970; Perry, 1971). I also consider the question of "neurotic styles" (Shapiro, 1965). The second category includes correlations between measures of intelligence and of personality, the nature of intelligence as a trait perceived by people in general, the social context of intelligence, the generality of personality traits, and the modifiability of traits and motives. I shall conclude by suggesting directions for future research and theorizing.

6.2.   IMPLICATIONS FOR PERSONALITY THEORY

COGNITIVE STYLES

The concept of cognitive style emerged largely from ego psychology (e.g., Gardner et. al., 1959) and showed the influence of Gestalt psychology. Ego psychology, in turn, was an outgrowth of psychoanalytic psychology; most of its adherents were psychoanalysts, and its primary concern was pathology rather than normal personality. Historically, cognitive styles and cognitive controls had about the same theoretical status within ego psychology as did defense mechanisms. Whereas the latter were functions of the ego that defended it against unacceptable impulses external to it, the former were functions of the ego in its own right. It was a tenet of ego psychology that these functions played a greater role in personality development than Freud had given them. In particular, cognitive styles and controls, that is, characteristic modes of perceiving and thinking, could affect the choice of defense mechanisms and consequently the choice of pathological symptoms.

The concern of clinical psychology with ego mechanisms is evident quite early in the extensive use of the Rorschach (1942) inkblot test, which was seen from the outset as a test of perceptual and associative processes. The late 1940s (e.g., Klein & Schlesinger, 1949) witnessed an increase in the attention given to individual differences in performance on tasks used to study perception. For example, Klein and Schlesinger (1951) reported individual differences in the range of interstimulus intervals over which apparent motion is perceived, and they related these differences to Rorschach responses. (Such results might be ignored today partly because the differences in apparent-motion perception can be ascribed to response bias rather than to true perceptual differences. Still, as Erdelyi, 1974, notes, response bias itself may be of interest, if, for example, effects on it are consistent across laboratory and nonlaboratory situations.) Another concern of the same period was the effects of motives on perception (e.g., Bruner & Goodman, 1947), a concern that characterized the "new look" school of perceptual research.

One early measure of cognitive style was Gardner's (1953) object-sorting test, in which the subject was asked to sort an array of heterogeneous objects into groups. Subjects differed in the number of groups they formed, and these individual differences were consistent across types of material classified. This style dimension led to several others, such as Pettigrew's (1958) measure of category width, in which the subject indicates the maximum and minimum values of, for example, the speed at which birds can fly. This scale was subsequently reinterpreted as having to do with risk taking (extreme width corresponding to caution – in case the direction is not obvious – Kogan & Wallach, 1964).

Another early style dimension was based on Holzman's (1954; Holzman & Klein, 1954) leveling–sharpening distinction. The basic task involved a demonstration of individual differences in a type of assimilation error. Subjects were asked to estimate the absolute sizes of squares presented in a series. As the series progressed, larger squares replaced the smaller ones, so that the average size of the squares increased. "Levelers" were insensitive to the progressive change and thus gave drastic underestimates of the sizes of the later squares. This tendency was ascribed to imprecise memory traces; it was consistent across other perceptual tasks, including the Rorschach (Holzman & Gardner, 1959).

Block and Petersen (1955) took a more empirical approach to the study of personality effects on perception. They gave subjects a line-length discrimination task, and they measured decision time and confidence for both easy and difficult discriminations. Subjects were divided into those who were overconfident, those who were underconfident, and those whose confidence appropriately varied with the difficulty of the discrimination. Subjects were rated with the California Q-Sort (Block, 1961), a general personality test based on the precepts of ego psychology. Different items distinguished different groups of subjects. For example, subjects who were overconfident were characterized by "Is rigid; inflexible in thought and action." Many of the characteristic items, however, were not so sensible; for example, those who decided quickly were characterized by "Has a slow personal tempo; responds, speaks, and moves slowly." In a related study, Johnson (1957) found that subjects were consistent across several tasks in speed and in confidence and that those who decided quickly had higher confidence. These studies are of interest because they are related to subsequent work on reflection–impulsivity. The latter study suggests that impulsivity may result from overconfidence, that is, a bias toward positive evaluation of the result of the thinking done so far.

The tradition of style research based on ego psychology has continued along two lines, the first being correlational studies of task performance and personality measures, and the second clinical studies of individual cases. Useful reviews of the correlational studies especially as they bear on development of style, may be found in Kagan and Kogan (1970) and Kogan (1973, 1976). This tradition has led to extensive research on a few style measures, such as field dependence versus independence, and reflection–impulsivity (to be discussed later), and a proliferation of other style measures, the most recent of which is a measure of understanding visual metaphor (Kogan et al., 1980).

An interesting monograph in the clinical tradition is Shapiro's (1965) *Neurotic Styles*. Shapiro argues that neurotic symptoms are partly determined by broad styles of thought and behavior, which are often as pathological in their own right as the symptoms they produce. These styles concern not only attention – in the earlier tradition – but also the degree of intentional control over action. The obsessive and paranoid styles are characterized by strong self-control and lack of spontaneity, whereas the hysterical and impulsive styles are characterized by yielding to impulses. The paranoid is sharp in attention to detail; for example, one patient who feared being hypnotized "just happened to notice" a book on hypnotism on a shelf many feet away in his therapist's office. The hysteric is broad in attention, registering overall impressions rather than details and manifesting poor memory for detail as a result. I shall return to Shapiro's account.

Despite the compelling quality of Shapiro's examples, his account suffers from the same problem that is associated with much of the experimental research on cognitive style, namely, the theoretical concepts are expressed in metaphorical language, without any attempt at precision. The most extreme example of this imprecision is perhaps from Witkin's description of *differentiation* (a descendant of leveling–sharpening). The original form of this concept, *field dependence*, was fairly clear and promised to become even clearer. For example, Linton (1955) showed consistent individual differences in "the effect of the perceptual field on response to selected elements within the field" across the rod-and-frame test (in which the subject must adjust a rod to the vertical despite the tilt of a surrounding frame and of his own chair), the embedded-figures test (in which the subject must find a camouflaged figure), and a few measures of "conformity." When the concept was extended, however, it became less clear: "Differentiation refers to the complexity of structure of a psychological system. One of the main characterizations of greater differentiation is specialization of function; another is clear separation of self from nonself" (Witkin, 1965). This statement tempts me to ask just what a structure is, how complexity is defined, let alone measured, what a system is, how self could *not* be separate from nonself, and so forth. (Further reading of this literature provides only answers couched in the same terms.) By this point, differentiation was still measured by the rod-and-frame task, the embedded-figures test, and a figure-drawing test that registered the degree of detail.

That these or any cognitive measures can predict the form of a patient's neurosis is of some interest, but their ability to specify "complexity of structure of a system," let alone "separation of self from nonself," is not clear. Despite such imprecision, the theoretical constructs tend to assume a life of their own; instead of seeking to understand the logical dimensions of cognitive style, researchers have tended to concentrate on improving the measurement of differentiation.

Often the justification for these vague terms is that they are labels of factors that result from factor analysis of a pattern of intercorrelations of tests. There are at least two problems here: First, most of the measures of cognitive style used in experiments yield scores that are at best only correlates of the dimension at issue, even in the restricted situation examined. The embedded-figures test, for example, is supposed to measure the ability to ignore irrelevant background, but it is clearly also influenced by the ability to search quickly and flexibly through a perceptual display in which many elements might constitute the figure to be found. Correlations among measures may be due to these spurious influences as well as to real ones. When perceptual measures involving accuracy are used, as in both the embedded-figures test and the rod-and-frame test, we must remember that Spearman (1904) showed that measures of perceptual accuracy are generally intercorrelated. In fact, Widiger, Knudson, and Rorer (1980) found that the standard measures of differentiation or analytic style correlate highly (e.g., .62) with nonverbal tests of general ability such as Raven's Progressive Matrices.

The second problem with factor analysis is that – if we suppose each measure to be affected by only a single variable – the absence of extremely high loadings of measures of the same factor would suggest that the factor itself was measuring something other than that which is measured by any of the individual tests. Thus the nature of the factor itself cannot be precisely defined, in the absence of extremely high loadings, even if the measures themselves are so defined. The relevance of factors to theoretical issues must thus remain unclear.

Although the entire literature on cognitive style has become distasteful to those who now call themselves cognitive psychologists, some work on cognitive style is harder to criticize. For example, Kagan, Lapidus, and Moore (1978), define reflection–impulsivity in the following terms:

Some children are careful in examining the differential validity of several response alternatives and hence make fewer errors; others are less careful and, as a result, make more errors.

The . . . dimension is only applicable to those problem situations where (a) the child believes an aspect of intellectual competence is being evaluated, (b) the child has a standard for the quality of his performance . . . , (c) the child understands the problem and believes he or she knows how to achieve its solution, (d) several equally attractive response alternatives are available, and (e) the correct answer is not immediately obvious and therefore the child must evaluate the differential validity of each potential solution hypothesis. [P. 1006]

Although it is not clear to me what *available* means, and therefore whether the dimension applies only to multiple-choice problems (which I think would be unnecessarily limiting), we have here almost a clear definition. In fact, children are consistent in choosing to be accurate or fast across different tasks that meet these criteria (Messer, 1976).

The work on reflection–impulsivity also fits into the framework I outlined earlier. Although the definition refers to behavioral indexes – time and errors relative to other subjects in the same task – it is hard to see how people can vary on this trade-off consistently across tasks unless we assume that they differ in the evalua-tion phase I described. In addition, the evidence (see Baron, 1981; Messer, 1976) suggests that individual differences are indeed consistent across tasks. If im-pulsivity is as great a problem as it seems to be in educational settings, explicit efforts to reduce it (e.g., Meichenbaum, 1977) seem warranted. It would be of interest to know whether the difficulty is primarily in the assignment of values (e.g., to thinking, to being correct), in the expectation of success from further thinking, in habit, or in emotions that affect these things.

Three criticisms of the work on reflection–impulsivity seem noteworthy. First, and least important, because the research has not always been characterized by an effort for clarity, it has tended to invite the same suspicion that has greeted other style research. Second, the dimension is a single one, and it would be better if it were embedded in a set of dimensions that could be viewed together as some kind of coherent whole. Third, the evaluative quality of the dimension (Kogan, 1976), with reflection considered better, has not been adequately supported. Al-though reflective subjects appear to be better adapted in a variety of ways (Mes-ser, 1976), it has not been shown that reflectiveness affects adaptation causally nor that people are generally too impulsive according to any normative standard. (This problem is complicated by difficulties in the measurement of reflection–im-pulsivity as practiced. Traditionally, subjects have been classified by a median split for time and errors, and the main comparisons have involved the fast–inaccu-rate and slow–accurate groups. Block, Block, & Harrington, 1974, have argued that the split by errors alone can account for most results when this method is used. New methods, based on multiple regression, examination of separate cor-relations, or subtraction of z scores – see Kagan and associates (1978) – seem to have solved this problem (see Kagan et al., 1978; Mitchell & Ault, 1979; Smith, Baron, & Smith, 1981). Nevertheless, reliability of the two component scores is still sometimes a problem (see Baron & Treiman, 1980.)

The framework I outlined earlier may solve the last two of these problems. The parameters of thinking may be seen as dimensions of cognitive style, and the outline of the phases of thinking allows us to list a number of such dimensions that together might constitute a complete set. The third problem must be solved through measurement or manipulation of values; in practice this may be difficult, but in principle the problem is clear. To show that people are too impulsive, we must establish that their impulsiveness hinders them in reaching their own goals (collectively or as individuals). One way to demonstrate such impairment is to turn people into "money pumps," as was done by Fischhoff, Slovic, and Lichten-stein (1977) in their study of overconfidence. Subjects gave odds that their an-swers to general information questions were correct and then made bets based on the odds they gave; their overconfidence led to actual loss of money (which was given back). This kind of method, that is, demonstration of general biases toward irrationality in most people, provides an alternative to demonstrations based on correlations between measures of style and measures of adaptation, which are often explainable in terms of extraneous influences. In the present case, one could provide explicit payoffs that would determine an optimum point (deter-mined for each subject on the basis of the expectations for success that subjects ought to have) on the trade-off between speed and accuracy. (The payoff should not be so great, however, that it moves the subject away from normal behavior.)

Some studies of individual differences in thinking would be counted as studies of cognitive style except that they fall outside the mainstream tradition. Two of these studies are of particular interest here because they illustrate certain aspects of the approach I have recommended in the first part of this paper. I shall describe them in a little more detail than usual, because they are, I think, unfairly neglected in other discussions of style research.

Brim, Glass, Lavin, and Goodman (1962) adopted a view of the phases of thinking similar to the one I have proposed, with Dewey as their model. Their phases were: "(1) identification of the problem; (2) obtaining necessary information; (3) production of possible solutions; (4) evaluation of such solutions; (5) selection of a strategy for performance; and (6) actual performance of an action or actions, and subsequent learning and revision" (1962, p. 9). (I would switch the order of Phases 2 and 3, to permit the possibilities to affect the selection of evidence. Phases 5 and 6 seem to me to be another episode. Also, the phases described by Brim and his colleagues are designed to account only for choice of actions, whereas mine are supposed to apply as well to adoption of beliefs.) The researchers gave subjects problems with the intention of examining individual differences in their Phases 4 and 5. For example, subjects, all of whom were parents, were asked how they would deal with a hypothetical 10-year-old son if they discovered that he had been engaging in petty theft (without getting caught). Subjects were given six reasonable alternatives (e.g., ignore the theft, explain the end results of crime, deprive the boy of television) and were asked to write out the results of each action, to estimate the probability (and the timing) and the subjective value (to the parent) of each outcome, and to rank the alternative actions (and provide contingency plans, if they wished). Subjects were scored for number of outcomes listed and other variables, including, most interestingly, the degree of conformity to the principle of maximum expected utility in their ranking of the alternative actions. In general, there was mixed evidence (i.e., sometimes significant, sometimes not, depending on the subgroup) that tested intelligence (and other personality measures) was correlated with a tendency to consider unfavorable outcomes as well as favorable ones, conformity to the expected utility principle, and number of outcomes considered. There were many other results concerning social class, sex, ethnic group, and other personality measures. Although this study contained so many measures that its results must be considered suggestive at best (except for the overall result that decision processes *are* predictable from personality measures), it is noteworthy in its use of a normative standard and a prior framework that specified the styles of interest. (Unfortunately the extensive use of factor analysis in this study only obscures the value of this framework, which is suitable for development of a priori hypotheses.)

A second interesting study is that of Ramanaiah and Goldberg (1977), who asked each subject to predict college grades, intelligence, leadership, or sociability of 160 students from a number of variables such as high-school grades, test scores, number of hours that the student was employed, and sex. Each subject's predictions were then fitted by a multiple regression equation for that subject, which specified the best linear combinations of the input variables that would produce that subject's judgments. Ramanaiah and Goldberg found individual differences, which were consistent across different judgments, on such measures as linear predictability (the goodness of fit of the regression equation), differentiation (the variance of the predictions), and confidence in the predictions made. These measures could be predicted by personality measures; for example, those subjects who were low in confidence showed "indecisiveness" (omission of items) in the Minnesota Multiphasic Personality Inventory. Interestingly, accuracy of prediction was not consistent across the two cases where it could be judged. Thus, the stylistic aspects of this task were more general than those aspects involving ability to do the task. Like the study made by Brim and associates that I just described, the study by Ramanaiah and Goldberg is based on a framework, to some extent a normative one, that allows a priori specification of a set of cognitive styles. The task used here is more limited, however. Many of the measures have no counterpart in most other studies of thinking.

To summarize, I think that the study of cognitive style is still a worthwhile enterprise. We need clear definition, preferably within a framework that specifies a set of related styles, consideration of the subject's own values and expectations, and use of normative standards as points of comparison. The potential uses of style measures will become clearer in the sections to follow, I hope. For example, such measures might serve as ways of evaluating education and as ways of understanding the effects of development and culture on intellectual performance. Style measures might also predict the success of different educational techniques, but I believe this use is made considerably more complicated if the possibility of changing styles is considered as part of some of the techniques.

STAGE THEORIES OF DEVELOPMENT

Another area in which the view I have sketched bears on personality theory is in the area of ego development, broadly defined. A number of different theories share the assumption that there are stages of development of thinking about ethics, social relationships, knowledge, and personal commitment. Major influences on this tradition are Piaget (1932), Erikson (1950, 1959), and Maslow (1954, 1962). Although Piaget and Erikson proposed stages that everyone, by and large, is supposed to go through, the theories I shall discuss assume, following Maslow, that most people do not go through the full sequence. These theories therefore become theories of individual differences among adults as well as of developmental differences. Like the cognitive-style literature just discussed, these theories also posit broad dispositions of thinking that cut across all the domains of the life of a person, including the formation of life plans. I shall suggest that many of the facts that support these theories can be accounted for equally well by a theory based on the application of thinking, as I have defined it, to these domains. If I am correct, these facts at least somewhat support the idea that the training of thinking is important (see Baron, 1975, for the same argument stated in different terms).

Loevinger, Wessler, and Redmore (1970; see also Holt, 1980) discuss the general concept of ego development and show how its stages may be measured in a sentence completion test. The test is taken as a projective measure of impulse control, interpersonal style, conscious preoccupations, and cognitive style. There are six levels, and the highest two are rarely reached. Here are some examples for each stage, with the subject's completion to the right of each dash:

> Stage 2: impulsive – "tends to dichotomize the world…"
> A good mother – is nice.
> Usually she felt that sex – is good for me because I get hot.
> Being with other people – gives me the creeps.

Stage 3: conformist – "Formulas... tend to be stated in absolute terms, without contingencies or exceptions."

A good mother – always understands her children.

Being with other people – makes you feel like you belong.

When people are helpless – I feel sorry for them.

Stage 4: conscientious – "will often combine alternatives that are polar opposites"

A good mother – conceals the fact.

A woman should always – be a lady in the parlor and a whore in the bedroom.

Being with other people – is one way of finding you're not the only one with problems.

Stage 5: autonomous – "construes conflicting alternatives as aspects of many-faceted life situations."

Usually she felt that sex – was delightful, intriguing, and very, very boring.

I feel sorry – for those who do not appreciate the beauty of nature.

Sometimes she wished that – she had things she would not be happy with if she had them.

Stage 6: integrated – "responses combine separate thoughts that would otherwise be rated [stage] 5."

A good mother – is kind, consistent, tender, sensitive, and always aware a child is master of its own soul.

The worst thing about being a woman – cannot be generalized, as one woman makes an asset of the same situation decried by another.

My main problem is – I am afraid, I lack courage to be what I want to because it is different from what my parents feel I should be.

There is a general movement from simplistic, one-sided statements to statements that recognize apparent contradictions to statements that recognize other kinds of complexity. There is also a widening of concerns, from immediate feelings to life plans and identity.

Although some of this scale concerns content, for example, the widening concerns, some of it (naturally, the part I have emphasized) concerns thought as well. It is likely that the more mature responses to the test items result from more thinking or better thinking according to the norms described earlier. For example, statements about complexity may result from the discovery of counterevidence against an initial possibility (for an answer to the item). Because the quality of a person's answers have little consequence for him, this quality probably reflects automatic use of the phases of thinking, rather than use that is measured relative to the expected gain.

Kohlberg (1969, 1970) proposes a sequence of stages for moral development in particular, based on Piaget's and Loevinger's theories, and he argues that these stages are actually manifestations of more general developmental patterns. Kohlberg is concerned only with moral "reasoning," although he argues (on the basis of some empirical evidence) that the stage of thinking can influence behavior when the situation is unambiguous and when different kinds of reasoning naturally lead to different substantive conclusions. Kohlberg measures the stage of moral reasoning by giving people dilemmas that can be argued either way at almost any stage. For example, one dilemma concerns a man who has a chance to steal a drug that he cannot afford to buy and that might save his wife's life. The subject is interviewed, and his statements on various issues are scored, such as the value of life, the authority of government, and the motives for engaging in moral action. The scores are based on the *type* of underlying principle to which the subject appeals. In the lowest, "preconventional," stages, morality is confused with self-interest or avoidance of punishment; for example, the reason for not stealing the drug would be to avoid jail. (Note that the self-interest is not that of the subject but that of the character in the dilemma; thus this sort of response reflects a principle of reasoning rather than the distortion of reasoning by the subject's self-interest.) In the "conventional" stages, morality is confused with conventions, with emotions or feelings, or with societal norms or laws. The person might refrain from stealing to avoid disapproval or to support the system of society. In the "postconventional" stages, morality is based on principles that transcend conventions, principles such as utilitarianism or justice based on an implicit social contract. At one of these stages, a reason not to steal would be that doing so would be to violate a social contract that in the long run saves more than a single life.

Kohlberg's dilemmas, despite the stated emphasis on reasoning, may actually elicit less reasoning than the sentence-completion items do. People are frequently faced with moral questions, and most people have developed a stock of principles that are simply retrieved and applied. Most people, when faced initially with Kohlberg's dilemmas, feel little doubt or perplexity, because they do not question the first principle that comes to mind as an answer to the question. (Of course, it may be that they *should* question that first principle, but my point is that we are rarely able to see what would happen if they did.) Although different principles statistically result from thinking of different kinds, possibly this need not be the case. People who apply a "high-stage" principle may have learned that principle from someone else, and people who apply a low-stage principle may have figured it out for themselves after considerable thought of a high quality (but limited, perhaps, by lack of relevant experiences or by inability to recall them).

Miriam Glassman and I (in unpublished work) have found it possible to score moral reasoning according to a scheme based roughly on the phases listed above. It turns out that individuals who use high-stage principles, in Kohlberg's sense, *are* also more likely to report counterevidence spontaneously and to change, in response to evidence they think of, the first statement they offer. Still, this is not necessarily the case. It seems to me that anyone who wants to teach moral reasoning – as Kohlberg does – would do well to teach the application of thinking, as I have described it, to moral questions. Indeed, Rawls (1971, ch. I, 9) describes the method of the moral philosopher as being essentially the revision of tentative principles on the basis of counterexamples, where the import of the examples is determined by our intuition about clear cases.

In a third relevant project, Perry (1971) interviewed Harvard students each year for several years about general issues in their studies and their lives. He found he could classify their responses according to a developmental scheme based on a student's attitude toward truth in his studies and the development of their life goals and commitments concerning religion, morality, politics, personal relationships, and work. The thinking of each student was generally consistent across these different domains. Students moved through the stages as they stayed in college, although some began at a fairly high stage, and many never completed the progression. At the earliest stages, truth was defined by authority, and professors who argued both sides of an issue were seen as obstructive. Commitments, as well, were defined by the person's own past history, family, and so on. In the middle stages, students became aware of relativism and the possibility of making a good argument against almost any possibility, whether it concerned an issue in a course or a decision about life. This realization often began when students understood how some of their professors were arguing (thinking out loud?) and discovered that they as students could earn better grades by doing the same in their papers. The students then realized that "complex thinking" could be extended to matters beyond the classroom – to problems not previously thought to be problems – hence the "freshman identity crisis," which, of course, often occurs in the junior year. Finally, students became aware of the need to make a commitment in spite of the possibility of counterevidence. These final commitments were often identical in content to those with which the student had entered (commitments to medical school, Judaism, etc.), but the new commitments were consistent with better understanding of the paths not chosen. Perry's work is simply the best evidence I have seen for the value of thinking. Unfortunately, Perry has no evidence concerning changes in thinking itself, so it is possible that the changes were all the result of application of thinking to new areas. If so, this difference would occur in the "problem recognition" phase only. Still, that may not be a trivial change at all.

In sum, much of the evidence that supports developmental-stage theories of personality may be accounted for by changes in the phases of thinking, particularly the phases involving problem recognition, search for evidence, and evaluation. These theories make a highly suggestive claim that thinking may influence the aspects of a person's life that are most important for that individual and for others, such as personal commitments and morality.

STYLES AND PATHOLOGY

In this section I will reexamine Shapiro's (1965) suggestion that different pathologies may be characterized by pathological styles, which may sometimes be so extreme as to constitute pathology in their own right. I shall suggest that there may be extreme forms of bias in some of the phases, and these may correspond to part of Shapiro's suggested styles. In contrast to a general deficiency of thinking, in which all biases characteristic of normal people are exaggerated (e.g., extreme impulsiveness, rigidity, and failure to discover problems), the deficiencies I shall discuss may result from imbalances, that is, extreme values on some parameters but not on others. Although this account does not do justice to Shapiro's full characterization of each style, it might, by limiting itself to the domain of reflective thinking, be more amenable to empirical investigation while continuing to capture at least some part of the phenomenon. I shall discuss a few pathologies classified according to traditional diagnostic criteria; however, I should note that pathological styles, in their own right, might ultimately require new diagnostic categories. It is noteworthy that Beck (1976) has also called attention to distorted forms of thinking characteristic of different types of neurotic pathology.

The clearest example may be paranoia, in particular, the tendency of paranoid patients to form delusions. It is actually quite difficult to define a delusion, the difficulty being that we would not want to include just any manifestly false belief. The definition of *delusion* as a strong belief that is objectively false might even be too broad. Such a definition would include false beliefs formed in a supportive social context or in a physical environment that provided limited evidence (e.g., belief in the world's flatness or in Newton's laws). A definition of delusions in terms of the way beliefs are formed would not have these problems. I think we would want to call a belief delusional when its strength is out of proportion to the evidence for it, as the evidence would be perceived by the subject without the distorting effect of the belief itself (if any). Once an initial possibility is considered, a delusion may result from rigidity as I have defined it, that is, from insensitivity to subsequent evidence (or from biased search for evidence). If there is a general style characteristic of delusional people, it ought to appear in laboratory measures of this sort of rigidity (or biased search). This idea is, of course, no surprise. The only novelty lies in my suggestion that we may interpret delusions in a more general framework of possible distortions of thought. Note that delusional people need not be found just in mental hospitals. The extent to which delusions impair functioning may depend on their content. Thus delusions of persecution and grandeur might make a person particularly bothersome to others, whereas delusions about politics, medicine, the supernatural, and so forth might be tolerated and in some circles even encouraged.

The obsessive style characterized by Shapiro (1965) may also be interpreted in my framework. One interesting characteristic of obsessives is their recurrent doubting, which shows itself both in inability to make a decision and in recurrent regrets once a decision has been made. Such doubting may contribute to the maintenance of pathological behavior, such as checking rituals (going back to the house repeatedly to make sure the gas was turned off). Still, this form of thinking may persist in some patients even when the behavior itself is modified through therapy. When pathological behavior recurs after therapy, its cause may be the underlying style of thinking rather than (or in addition to) unconscious conflicts. We may most simply interpret this style as the opposite of the paranoid style, namely, *over*sensitivity to evidence, particularly counterevidence. It is also possible that this style represents a deficit at the evaluation phase, so that the criterion for stopping thinking is too stringent. Then, too, the style may result from stereotypy, with hypotheses recurring so frequently that they eventually occur automatically. Alternatively, it may result from a bias toward recall of evidence that conflicts with the possibility in mind (when there is only one). The precise characterization of this style requires examining its "phenomenology" in the light of my framework and, ultimately, doing experiments to test the generality of the style.

Hyperactivity is characterized by both impulsiveness in mental tasks and inability to sustain attention in vigilance tasks as well as by overactive behavior. Conceivably the impulse to leap up and run around may cause all of the other symptoms. It is also possible, however, that the distortions of thinking are separate and that they survive the effect of maturation on the motor behavior itself (Weiss & Hechtman, 1979). The simplest hypothesis about these distortions is that there is a bias toward cessation of thinking at the evaluation phase. This bias shows itself both as impulsivity in Kagan's sense and as nonpersistence in continuous tasks. In hyperactivity, clearly, biological factors are likely to contribute to stylistic distortion, although this contribution would not imply that the style was unmalleable through training (as Meichenbaum, 1977, argues that it is).

Although thinking is an important part of personality, it is not the only part that can go wrong. Pathologies of other aspects of functioning may affect thinking and the use of thinking, aside from other effects they have. One interesting set of pathologies is involved in the formation and execution of plans, whether they relate to taking a snack from the refrigerator or to the way to conduct one's life. Semmer and Frese (1979) have shown how pathologies may be characterized as deficits of plans or of planning, and Frese (1981) has suggested that people may be characterized by "action styles," by analogy with cognitive styles. For example (mine, not Frese's), the hysterical style (Shapiro, 1965) is characterized by frequent statement (formation) of plans that are not carried out. As a result, perhaps, hysterical personalities never accomplish very much, although one would never suspect this inertia from a brief discussion with one. Action styles may thus characterize aspects of pathology that are not captured by the framework I have outlined. They are also, of course, related to cognitive styles in a variety of ways, which it would take me too far afield to describe.

A second area that may affect thinking and its use concerns defense mechanisms. There may be styles of defense that parallel cognitive and action styles. Vaillant (1977) has shown how differences in defensive style may contribute to success or failure in work and in close personal relationships. He interviewed a sample of 95 Harvard graduates as part of a longitudinal study begun 30 years earlier, in 1942. The adjustment at the time of the interview could be predicted from the defensive styles as determined from data collected over the course of the study. Poorly adjusted subjects tended to use "immature" defenses, such as projection, hypochondriasis, and fantasy, whereas well-adjusted subjects tended to use "mature" defenses, such as suppression ("postponing but not avoiding" a difficult issue that must be dealt with) and anticipation ("realistic anticipation of or planning for future inner discomfort"). These findings and the case histories that illustrate them suggest a large role for defense mechanisms in the ultimate application of intelligence to the conduct of one's life and work. The same defenses may play a role in thinking itself. The very decisions and behaviors that make for success or failure in life may result from good or bad thinking.

In sum, various pathological symptoms may in part stem from disorders of thinking. We might characterize these disorders in terms of extreme values of the parameters of thinking I have listed. The thinking disorders might be pathological in their own right. It ought to be possible to apply the framework I have outlined to the study of the nature, diagnosis, and possibly even the treatment of such distortions. Failure to treat them might account for some of the failures in treatment of the more specific pathologies they produce.

6.3.   IMPLICATIONS FOR THE STUDY OF INTELLIGENCE

I now turn to the ways in which personality theory and methods are relevant to the study of intelligence. I discuss five such connections: correlations between measures of intelligence and personality, intelligence as a perceived trait, the social context of intelligence, the generality of traits, and the malleability of traits. In general these connections are important if I am correct in saying that the parameters of thinking can have the status of personality traits. If so, we can bring to these parameters all the questions that have been asked about other traits, and there is some value in doing so.

CORRELATIONS BETWEEN MEASURES OF PERSONALITY AND OF INTELLIGENCE

The first question that might occur to a reader of the title of this chapter is, "OK, what's the relation?" This is a good question. It would be nice to know whether personality affects the development of intelligence, whether certain personality traits are affected by the same genetic or environmental factors that affect aspects of intelligence, and whether intelligence affects personality, either by making a person better adapted in some way and thus making him happier or by affecting a person's perception of the world and the beliefs and motives that result from that perception. There is in fact an enormous literature on this matter, but I shall have very little to say about it. Most of this literature involves looking for correlations between measures of intelligence, usually IQ tests, and measures of personality, often personality tests, but sometimes more objective indicators of adjustment or success. The problem is that it is difficult to learn anything from such research. Neither intelligence nor most aspects of personality can be measured with high validity, so such correlations may be, in every case I know of, ascribed to artifactual influences (even plausible ones) of other variables on the measures. The problem of measurement of intelligence may even be worse than that of measurement of personality traits, because at least some of these traits (e.g., delay of gratification) are clearly defined, but intelligence is not.

One longitudinal study of the effects of intelligence on adaptation was begun by Terman in 1922 (Sears, 1977; Terman & Oden, 1959). One thousand children with IQs over 150 have now been followed up to the age of retirement. In general, the differences between the subjects and the population as a whole on objective measures of adaptation are rather small, although there are indeed some; for example, the subjects were less likely than most people to become alcoholics or criminals. (They were no less likely to enter mental hospitals.) The subjects did tend to do more intellectually demanding work than most people, and even those who did not tended to have challenging hobbies or to be active socially or politically. The problem with this study is that IQ scores are correlated with social class and with social class of parents. Social class – and concomitant aspects of life, such as who one's friends and neighbors are and where one goes to school – may account for all of the effects found.

More recently, Jencks and associates (1972) attempted to analyze effects of family background, social class, education, and "cognitive skills" on income and occupational status by using the statistical technique of path analysis. According to this method, when all other factors are held constant, cognitive skills (scores on intelligence or aptitude tests) do affect educational attainment (perhaps only because the tests are used to determine admission), and even when education is held constant, along with the other variables, cognitive skills have some effect on income. Still, path analysis makes no allowance for unreliability or for invalidity of the measures (Baron & Treiman, 1980; Lord, 1969). For example, the aspect of social class that is effective may be poorly measured by sociological indexes. Thus social class may still account for all the results.

Many studies have examined correlations between IQ tests and personality measures given at the same time in life. For example, Samuel (1980) found, as had several of the studies he cites, that intelligence correlates negatively with "trait" anxiety (i.e., anxiety that is stable over time, as opposed to "state" anxiety, that aroused by the situation), negatively with sadness, positively with ability to concentrate, and positively with internality, a person's belief that he can control his fate (as measured by a questionnaire). Other studies have found that IQ correlates with creativity (when the range of IQ considered is sufficient to permit it to correlate with anything; Barron, 1957), with children's ability to delay gratification (Mischel & Metzner, 1962), and with *n Ach* (need for achievement; Robinson, 1961).

In every case, the interpretation of these correlations is unclear. Correlations with anxiety and sadness may be due to effects of these emotions on intelligence, to the effects of education on adaptation (with the uneducated being sad and anxious because of their lack of worldly success), or to effects of these emotions on the ability to deal with testing situations. Correlations with creativity and ability to concentrate may have to do with direct effects of these traits on the ability to take intelligence tests or perhaps with some real overlap in these traits and the abilities that ought to be called intelligence. Correlations with achievement motivation and internality may stem from effects of these motives and beliefs on real intelligence, from their effects on the learning of material included on IQ tests (but not on real intelligence), or from the adaptation of one's beliefs and motives to one's capacities. (A person who is innately athletic is likely to develop a motive to achieve athletically, because most people like to do what they are good at, and to develop a belief that, with enough effort, anyone else could learn to hit a topspin backhand or kick a 50-yd. field goal.) Finally, correlations with delay of gratification may be due to effects of strict child rearing on both intelligence and personality, to effects of rate of development (inasmuch as this study involved children) – which is not necessarily predictive of adult intelligence – to effects of intelligence on ability to calculate one's own interest, or to effects of ability to delay gratification on intelligence or on the acquisition of the knowledge measured by IQ tests.

There are ways to avoid some of these problems of interpretation. For example, some studies (e.g., Kagan et al., 1958) have looked at the correlates of changes in IQ over time, thus holding constant some of the troublesome factors such as family background. Honzik and MacFarlane (1973) looked at the correlates of change in IQ between 18 and 40 years of age. Personality ratings were based on extensive case files collected before the age of 18. Subsequent increases in IQ correlated negatively with the "tendency to arouse liking and acceptance in people," negatively with "gregarious, emphasizes being with others," and negatively with "behaves in a sex-appropriate manner." Although these correlations at first appear interesting and surprising, artifactual explanations again exist. For the first two variables, possibly people who choose extroverted, social pursuits as adults continue to develop their intelligence in this domain, which is given only cursory treatment in most IQ tests, whereas those who choose bookish, introverted pursuits receive much exposure to just the sort of verbal and mathematical material that the tests include. Thus the effects may arise from the tests rather than from intelligence itself. The sex-typing result must be considered in the light of historical change. During the period of the study (and, indeed, at this writing), there was a social division, roughly along class lines, with respect to sex roles. Those who believe less strongly in traditional sex roles may be likely to pursue formal and informal educational opportunities of the sort that would affect their IQ test scores (and perhaps their intelligence itself). In other words, this result might change in the course of history.

In mentioning such questions of interpretation, I do not mean to suggest that the tests I have described are useless or that the questions are unanswerable. Even IQ tests and aptitude tests, for all our doubts about what they measure, are likely better than the alternatives as ways of diagnosing mental retardation or determining which people will probably succeed in college. Some of the questions may be answerable when we have clear measures of components of intelligence – such as those based on the framework I have outlined – as well as clear measures of personality. In conjunction with training studies, such measures may prove quite informative about cause and effect.

INTELLIGENCE AS A PERCEIVED TRAIT

When the study of intelligence measurement began, subjective ratings of the intelligence of others were used as a criterion against which tests were validated. The surprising finding in Spearman (1904) was that measures of sensory capacities were correlated with teachers' ratings of children's intelligence. Both Binet and Simon (1916) and Terman (1916) used teacher ratings to validate their tests. Sternberg, Conway, Ketron, and Bernstein (1981) also note that we often trust subjective judgments of intelligence more than we trust supposedly more valid objective tests (e.g., when we make admissions decisions) and that people use their concepts of intelligence as guides to train their children. They suggest further that a major purpose of the theory of intelligence is to influence everyday conceptions of intelligence; indeed, this may be one of the main functions of all psychological theory, as most practitioners of psychology are lay people.

There are only a few studies of people's concepts of intelligence (see Sternberg et al., 1981, for a more complete review). Wober (1974) asked members of different tribes in Uganda to fill out semantic differential forms that indicated the connotations that the native word for intelligence had for members of each tribe. Tribes differed. For example, to some groups the word meant "fast," for others, "slow." Wiggins, Hoffman, and Taber (1969) asked nonstudent subjects to judge intelligence on the basis of descriptions of the sort that might be available to a college admissions committee. Each subject's judgments were predicted by a multiple regression equation, the coefficients of which indicated how heavily that subject weighed each kind of available information. Subjects differed in the factors they considered important, and these differences were related to characteristics of the subjects. One group of subjects (selected by a procedure involving factor analysis) tended to downplay a measure of English effectiveness (relative to other groups); this group did particularly well on a test of numerical ability. Another group relied particularly heavily on measures of responsibility and study habits (which were actually not very valid in real life); this group was characterized by high scores on measures of authoritarianism, ethnocentrism, and religious conventionalism and by low scores on an intelligence test. (The author is reminded of his own membership on an admissions committee, the members of which show different attitudes toward grades, tests, and research that relate to their own respective undergraduate records.) If people's conceptions of intelligence were affected by such attitudes, and if these conceptions were used as standards for child rearing, they could be involved in the perpetuation of cognitive styles and belief systems across generations.

Sternberg and associates (1981) asked lay people to list characteristics of *intelligence, everyday intelligence,* and *academic intelligence.* Subjects obtained in a college library listed similar characteristics for *academic intelligence* and *intelligence,* but this similarity was less apparent on the lists of subjects obtained in a supermarket or railroad station. In a second experiment, subjects were asked to judge behaviors listed in Experiment 1 for importance in defining their concept of an "ideally" intelligent person, characteristicness of such a person, characteristicness of their concept of intelligence, or characteristicness of themselves. Subjects were "experts" (i.e., researchers) as well as lay people. Answers of lay people and experts were much the same, as were answers to the different questions. (Sternberg et al. did not try to predict individual differences in ratings from personality measures, as had Wiggins et al., although they did look at – but did not report in detail – the predictive value of tested intelligence.) Although there were slight differences from group to group or for different kinds of intelligence, the common core seemed to have to do with (a) problem solving, (b) verbal ability, and (c) practical or social intelligence. Items typical of these three factors were: (a) able to apply knowledge to problems at hand, displays common sense, approaches problems thoughtfully; (b) reads with high comprehension, is verbally fluent, learns rapidly; (c) sizes up situations well, displays interest in the world at large, accepts others for what they are. Lay people were given an intelligence test, and the scores on this test were correlated ($r > .5$) with the closeness of the self-characteristicness ratings to the (expert) prototype (list of weights of behaviors) of the ideally intelligent person. Finally, descriptions of individuals were compiled by selecting items from the same list. Ratings made of the intelligence of the people so described were correlated ($r > .96$) with predictions made from the various prototypes.

Neisser (1979) has argued that the concept of intelligence is, and can be, no more than just such ratings of characteristic features. He argues that intelligence is thus a "Roschian" (i.e., Wittgensteinian, family-resemblance) concept, with many characteristic features but with no defining ones. In fact, in the study by Sternberg and associates, although the attributes could be ranked in order of characteristicness (from "able to apply knowledge to problems at hand" to "likes to read," etc.), apparently no core attributes separated themselves from the others by a quantum leap, even among the experts. This finding would seem to support Neisser's claim, but I must make two points about the study's relevance to this claim.

First, subjects were never asked to give defining (i.e., necessary) features. Some training in philosophy might be needed before a subject could answer such a question, even if it were asked. For example, a person would have to use the philosopher's strategy of looking for counterexamples in order to know that literacy, let alone good reading, cannot be a defining feature. If there are defining features, they are probably not immediately accessible. Further, if Putnam (1975) is correct, even defining features have little to do with people's concepts about categories in nature, and the problem of eliciting information about such concepts might be quite severe. In essence, people regard concepts such as *water* as properly defined only within the context of a theory of nature, which the person himself understands only weakly unless he is an expert. Putnam's view accounts for our intuition that a chemist could convince us that a red metallic substance was in fact water in a new form or that a colorless, tasteless, transparent (etc.) liquid was not really water. In the case of intelligence, "experts," when they reflect, may have the same attitude as lay people, believing that the real experts do not yet exist.

Second, the present state of the concept of intelligence has no implications about its future state. A good theory of intelligence might clarify the concept not only for experts but also for lay people. As matters stand, it seems plausible (although I know of no evidence) that the concept of intelligence has changed historically as a result of the development of intelligence tests.

It would be interesting to examine people's conceptions of the defining attributes, or the essence, however expressed, of intelligence, if it is possible to elicit such information. Many people are capable of providing a detailed account of their own intellectual strengths and weaknesses, complete with accounts of which basic causes or enduring traits produce which superficial manifestations. We might call this an account of the *structure* of an individual's intellectual personality (although I hate to suggest yet another use for this word). Perhaps people can also make such judgments of other people's personalities and of ideal types (e.g., an ideally intelligent person, etc.). This sort of a "model" (Stevens & Collins, 1980) of another person might be used for such purposes as judging someone's suitability for a position or educating someone (e.g., one's child). It is also of interest to know how accurate such structural models are. This question may be hard to answer directly, but one could at least assess the agreement of the models held by mother, father, and adolescent, for example.

I have mentioned the importance of judgments of intelligence, and of the concepts behind these judgments, for child rearing and for decisions about people's potential. (Note that the same concepts may be used to judge one's own potential, for better or for worse.) Before I leave this topic, I should make two comments about the validity, first, of judgments of personality traits in general, and second, of the implicit theories behind such judgments.

First, these judgments are not useless; in particular, it is possible to use them to predict the behavior of the people judged, often quite well, in a variety of situations (Hogan, DeSoto, & Solano, 1977). The basis for prediction, however, is best determined empirically, by actual evidence of predictive power in the situation in question for similar people. One cannot tell from the name of a variable whether or not it will be useful for predicting a given behavior.

Second, such judgments do not prove especially valid as measures of what they are supposed to measure (rather than of something else that is as useful predictively). In particular, there are several well-documented biases that affect the judgment process itself. Many of these, such as the tendency of raters to give "socially desirable" answers, and to say yes when asked whether a trait applies to a person, are avoidable at least sometimes. One that is not so easily avoided is the halo effect, or in its more general form, the tendency of raters to make judgments largely on the basis of an implicit theory, which holds that the trait in question should be related to a known trait. For example, when asked whether we think someone is clever, we might base our judgment on the fact that the person always carries a book, because we believe that cleverness is correlated with large amounts of reading. Alternatively, when asked to judge intelligence, we might base our judgment on style of speech (e.g., dialect). When raters are asked to complete large personality inventories, the situation is even worse. Given that personality judgments are usually made from memory, that memory is limited, and that raters are encouraged to answer every item on a scale, regardless of whether they recall any specific instances of relevant behavior or not, many judgments are, not surprisingly, intelligent guesses rather than actual generalizations from experience. Schweder and D'Andrade (1979) provide not only an excellent statement of this problem but also some empirical evidence: Trait judgments made from memory tend to correlate as predicted by implicit theories to a greater extent than do judgments of behavior made on the spot.

These criticisms do not imply that rating data should never be used. They do suggest that such data should be supplemented with more objective data, at least when the precise nature of what is being measured is at issue. Implicit theories of personality may also affect the extraction of evidence on which the implicit theories are based. The same biases that affect judgments could thus impair the accuracy of the implicit theories (Nisbett & Ross, 1980). Good psychological research could help to bring these theories into line with reality.

THE SOCIAL CONTEXT OF INTELLIGENCE

The ability to think is developed in a social context, and thinking functions in a social context. We might productively ask about the match between development and function. For example, societies, or institutions, may differ in their reliance on thinking itself. In most armies, the soldier is trained to do a certain set of tasks; by contrast, the scientist is expected to solve new problems, and thinking is expected to be part of the job. Specialization of labor, and credentials, are the social methods for avoiding thought, and these methods compete with the encouragement of thinking as ways of organizing society. Different aspects of intelligence are relevant to different social organizations. The ability to learn, to become expert, is relevant to specialization; the ability to think is relevant to what might be called the *liberal* view, in the sense of placing more trust in individuals to adapt to new circumstances and to conduct their own affairs.

It would seem natural to study such phenomena through comparison of thinking and learning in different cultures. Cross-cultural cognitive psychology at present, however, seems to be caught up in an ideological war against the apparent implications of some of its own findings. For example, Wagner (1978) and Sharp, Cole, and Lave (1979) have shown that schooling (in Morocco and in rural Mexico) seems to affect performance of novel tasks such as learning a list of items in order or classifying a set of objects according to a consistent rule. The latter study found that the classification effect was not dependent on familiarity of the material; the effects were just as great when types of corn were used instead of abstract forms. The question about these results (Cole's reply in Sharp et al., 1979) is whether they tell us about effects of schooling on intelligence in general or whether their implications are restricted to one type of intelligence among many, namely that used in schools. Such a question might be answered by more careful experimentation, perhaps with tasks that are based on some sort of theory (e.g., tasks chosen to measure the kinds of propensities I have discussed). Still, the idea that cultural effects on abilities are of limited generality has become a working assumption of most cross-cultural cognitive psychology, so that the search for cultural effects on highly general abilities or styles has largely been called off. This state of affairs, I think, is unfortunate, because the existence of cultural differences in very general propensities can teach us about the effects of possible changes, for better or worse, in our own culture.

Outside the field of cross-cultural cognitive psychology, there is some relevant literature. Calhoun (1973) examined the history of intelligence in the region around New York from colonial times to the end of the 19th century. He argued that the "cognitive style" of whole populations is affected by beliefs and practices

in education and child rearing and that the style manifests itself in the achievements of the culture. He argued that the decline of a certain verbal culture over
the period, and an increase in the ability to think visually, accounted for some
American achievements in building ships and bridges. These shifts were also
apparent from stylistic changes in sermons, which reflected the style not only of
the preachers but also of the audiences. The general changes were ascribed partly
to trends in education – toward more regimentation – and in child rearing (where
developments were too complex to describe briefly). I doubt that the details of
Calhoun's account will survive scrutiny. The enterprise strikes me as a useful
one, however, and Calhoun's general assumptions about historical changes in
thinking are consistent with the point of view I present here.

The study of cultural and historical differences in achievement motivation has
seen exactly the sort of enterprise that Calhoun's account might inspire, in the
domain of motivation rather than that of cognitive style. The study of achievement
motivation itself began with Murray's (1938) attempt to list the major human
motives or needs. Need achievement, or *n Ach,* was one of a list of 28, which also
included need dominance, need sex, and need affiliation. Murray defined *n Ach* as
"the desire or tendency to do things as rapidly and/or as well as possible" (1938, p.
164). Achievement motivation is thus closely related to many of the motives that
operate in the framework I have outlined; however, it is a broader concept, involving motives that are socially defined (e.g., achievements respected by others) as
well as those defined in terms of thought itself. One measure of *n Ach,* which
came to be the primary one, was based on stories made up in response to a set of
ambiguous pictures, the Thematic Apperception Test. The scoring system developed for this test was flexible enough to be applied to other material. McClelland
(1961) attempted to measure the achievement motivation characteristic of various cultures at various times in their history by applying the system to readers
used by children learning to read. Stories from 23 countries collected between
1920 and 1929 were able to predict economic growth in those countries between
1929 and 1950 (in terms of deviation from growth otherwise expected). Achievement themes in 1950 readers again predicted subsequent (but not prior) economic growth. Similarly, de Charms and Moeller (1962) found that achievement
themes in U.S. readers increased until 1890 and then declined. There was a
parallel, but slightly delayed, rise and fall in the number of patents per capita
issued by the patent office!

There is other cross-cultural research on cognitive style. For example, Salkind,
Kojima, and Zelnicker (1978) compared children in Israel, Japan, and the United
States in reflection–impulsivity as measured by a matching test (the Matching
Familiar Figures Test). Among 5-year-olds, the Japanese were the most reflective
and the Israelis the most impulsive. By age 10, the groups completely reversed;
the interpretation of these trends is not clear. It would be of interest to seek style
measures from a greater variety of cultures, perhaps using Rorschach test data
(available from many cultures) as an index of reflection–impulsivity. The same
kinds of analyses done by McClelland could then be performed.

The child-rearing antecedents of intelligence have received some study (e.g.,
Carew, 1980). Typically, however, "intelligence" is indexed by IQ test scores,
which are heavily affected by vocabulary, especially in children. Thus, it is not
surprising that such intelligence scores are affected by provision of opportunity to

learn meanings of new words (Carew, 1980). I know of no studies of the antecedents of thinking in the sense in which I have defined it.

Blank (1973), whose view of "the abstract attitude" is very similar to my own view of good thinking, has developed a preschool program designed to teach such thinking. The main technique is a tutorial dialogue between teacher and pupil, in which the teacher asks questions corresponding to each of the phases of thinking: Can you think of . . . ? Why do you think that? Can you think of anything else? Are you sure? Pupils are supposed to internalize these questions and thus to learn how to think for themselves. The program is successful in increasing IQ scores and later school performance, but Blank herself recognizes that these measures should not be as sensitive to the program's effects as direct measures of what was taught. Unfortunately, no such measures were available.

My own informal – and of course heavily biased – observations and interviews suggest that college students who can think well have usually been exposed to a tutorial sort of dialogue in their homes. Typically, parent–child disagreements about even the most trivial matters are resolved by arguments, in which the child must give reasons, answer counterarguments, and so on. On the other hand, parents sometimes report that efforts to engage in such discussions result in friction and bad feelings. These two observations suggest a research question: What social factors govern the acceptability of intellectual challenges, both inside and outside the home? Who is allowed to make such challenges? How must they be phrased to avoid insult? Why? What is the insult to be avoided? The issue has to do with the nature of good manners in intellectual discussions, but of course manners exist for a reason. The worst outcome of such research could be a finding that good thinking in a culture cannot arise without its members suffering the shame of occasional failure, particularly when they are children.

THE GENERALITY OF TRAITS

I have suggested that the parameters of thinking I listed can be viewed as personality traits, as dimensions of individual differences. In recent years, there has been considerable discussion about the status of personality traits in general. Although the most persistent critics of traits have often explicitly exempted cognitive styles from their criticisms (Mischel, 1973), it is still worthwhile to examine the issues for what they can teach us. (The exemption may be unfair; style measures may show greater consistency only because they are more reliable [Epstein, 1979], and Mischel's arguments do not logically depend on absolute levels of consistency.) The following is my own reconstruction of these issues, based largely on the following sources: Allport (1966); Bem and Allen (1974); Bem and Funder (1978); Block, Weiss, and Thorne (1979); Epstein (1979); Hogan, DeSoto, and Solano (1977); Jackson and Paunonen (1980); Kenrick and Stringfield (1980); Mischel (1973, 1977); Shweder (1977); and Shweder and D'Andrade (1979). These articles are only entry points into a vast literature, however.

I shall take a trait to be an inferred stable disposition to behave a certain way in a certain class of situations, relative to the way others would behave. For our purposes, examples of traits may be impulsivity, rigidity, interest in mathematics, interest in word puzzles, and desire to please others. For practical purposes, a personality psychologist might give a test of interest in mathematics, say, to help a person decide whether to pursue a career in computer programming. For theoretical purposes, we might use a test of this sort to ask questions about the antecedents or consequences of certain traits.

The argument in its simplest form concerns the validity of traits, that is, the correlation between exhibiting the behavior in different situations where it might be manifest. The evidence suggests that traits are stable over time, as long as they are measured in the same situations. A person who is outgoing in school at age 6 is likely to be outgoing in school at age 16. The problem is that the same person may be an introvert at home. Prediction of the "same" behavior across "different" situations tends to be poor. In practice, when someone wants to predict the behavior of people, such as the adjustment of mental patients after leaving the hospital (Mischel, 1977), in many cases it is more useful to examine the situation than the traits of the person. Further, there is reason to think that people, including psychologists, are unreasonably biased in favor of using traits rather than situations to explain or predict the behavior of *other* people (although there is dispute about the evidence for this claim; see Hogan et al., 1977). The extreme form of this view, which nobody holds, is called *situationism,* the view that behavior is totally determined by the situation a person is in and that apparent differences in traits are artifacts of phenomena like perception of the test situation.

One problem concerns our definition of behaving "the same." Suppose we measure intellectual performance in four situations: two kinds of math problems and two kinds of verbal puzzles. One problem in each content area requires sustained thought, and the other requires speed, so that an impulsive person would not be impaired in the latter. Now, suppose that within a sample of people, some are consistently interested in math problems, others are interested in verbal puzzles, others are impulsive, and others are reflective. If we try to predict performance within problems of the same content, for example, from one kind of math problem to the other, we will do poorly for those subjects who are consistently impulsive or reflective. Conversely, if we try to predict performance across problem types (speed vs. thought), we will do poorly for people consistent only in interest. In sum, it is simply impossible for everyone to be consistent on every dimension in every situation. Given this general problem, we might be more successful if we tried to find out *which* dimensions are consistent for a given individual before we tried to make predictions for that person. We might ask the individual, or a close friend, to provide us with information. When this procedure is followed, consistency across situations improves considerably (Bem & Allen, 1974; Kenrick & Stringfield, 1980).

It might still be argued, however, that the main determinant of behavior is neither traits nor situations but rather their interaction. This view takes two forms (Mischel, 1973). One, exemplified by psychoanalytic theory, holds that there are deeper consistencies behind apparent inconsistencies, so that, in principle, we ought to be able to find traits that will yield considerable consistency, if we do not simply assume that these traits correspond to observable behavior in a direct way. The deeper consistencies themselves may be of several types, but they all imply that the possible interactions between persons and situations are at least statistically limited. I have followed this path in my proposal for parameters as traits. For example, I would measure impulsiveness not simply in terms of time and errors but rather in terms of this trade-off relative to the subject's values in the situation. Thus, apparent cross-situational inconsistency in impulsiveness could be consistent with a deeper consistency in one's bias *relative* to one's values. If the values themselves are somewhat general, then behavior in a given situation can be predicted from two general traits.

The other interactionist view holds that there is no such deeper consistency. Although people are consistent on the same dimension in the same situation, they are simply idiosyncratic in the way they behave elsewhere. Proponents of this view do not deny that people have elaborate rules for their own behavior and that they follow these rules. Rather, they contend that there are as many such rules as there are people and that little order characterizes them (Mischel, 1977).

It is hard to see any other way of interpreting these questions except as ways of asking, "What accounts for most of the variance?" At the simplest level, the alternatives are situations and traits. At the next level, the answers are idiosyncratic or systematic interactions based on deeper traits, that is, interactions that are predictable from knowledge of how people with a given set of deep traits perform in a given situation. Mischel (1973) notes that the simpler question is silly (despite the large empirical effort invested in answering it) because it cannot be answered in general. Undoubtedly we can find some cases in which situations are the best predictors and other cases in which traits are. If we want to know which possibility prevails in general, we must have an unbiased sample of cases, and there is no way to create such a sample. (We can, of course, ask about the predictive value of trait terms within a certain general class. If we take much of personality research to concern itself with trait terms in ordinary language, we are likely to find that such terms perform approximately as well, predictively, as any other yet devised, especially when subjects have a chance to identify their consistent traits. This finding may be of some interest to those who believe there is something to learn from the psychology of the commonsense actor, e.g., Sabini & Silver, 1981.)

I believe that the same criticism applies to the two versions of the interactionist position. It seems likely that in some cases deep regularities *can* be found, especially when the superficial descriptions originally used are inadequate. We could, if necessary, construct such cases artificially by inventing unnatural personality descriptions, such as *glorf*, which means "hits other children on the playground or eats worms." We might find that glorf predicts eating of bottle caps only by children who do not carry weapons. We might postulate "deeper" traits, such as aggressiveness and fondness for eating strange objects. This example is merely intended to suggest that the contrast between deep and superficial consistency relates more to the adequacy of our terms than to people themselves. If we choose inadequate terms at the outset, terms that do not "carve personality at the joints," we will be forced to find deeper traits if we seek consistency. The fact that we do not think of things this way is a sign of our confidence in the personality terms of our common language.

Suppose that we want to invent intellectual traits (styles), at any level of depth, that do show consistency; must we rely on common language? To begin with, we could ask how traits might become general in the first place. Consistencies in style across situations may depend in part on the effect of consistencies in capacities, because capacities affect styles. We know very little about this effect; even the few studies that might be relevant in understanding such consistencies (e.g., Sternberg, 1977) may be contaminated by consistencies in experience and prior practice in different domains (Baron & Treiman, 1980). Otherwise, consistencies may result from consistencies in any of the factors that affect styles, such as preferences, expectations, and habits. Any of these influences may transfer to novel situations and may thus become general to the extent that they do (Baron & Treiman, 1980). Because transfer is likely to be imperfect, consistency is likely to be imperfect. Still, the dimensions that show the greatest consistency are likely to be those along which transfer is most likely to occur. Traits may also become general as a result of training. A parent who wants to teach a child honesty, for example, may teach the child to be honest in a variety of situations. The child may learn honesty only situation by situation, but the trait will still appear to be quite general.

Finally, people may create their own general traits by constructing rules for themselves and teaching themselves to follow these rules, just as parents do for children. There is great room for idiosyncrasy here. If we want to discover the most useful traits, we might begin by asking people, or even ourselves, about the rules we follow. The nature of traits may change with culture or history. Educational programs themselves may create traits. For example, efforts to teach mathematics to the general public seem to have achieved variable success, so that in cultures where such instruction is attempted, there is considerable variation in, interest in, and knowledge of mathematics. The same may occur as a result of efforts to teach thinking. In sum, it may be said that the existence or nonexistence of general traits has no logical bearing on the question of whether general propensities are teachable. If a general trait exists, it may do so for reasons unrelated to learning. If it does not exist, it may come to exist when circumstances change. Nonetheless, the study of general traits may have other uses, for example, in the selection of people for special programs designed to modify those traits.

PERSONALITY CHANGE

If the teachable part of intelligence includes intellectual personality traits, and if personality traits can be changed, then intelligence can be changed. A great deal of evidence indicates that personality can in fact be changed even as late as adolescence or adulthood. Some evidence comes from programs designed to reach fairly large numbers of people with resources similar to those of schools. The techniques used by these programs might be useful, suitably modified, for teaching intelligence.

The most dramatic case of personality change is brainwashing, or "coercive persuasion" (Lifton, 1961; Orne, 1978). Typical brainwashing techniques involve removal of all signs of the victim's identity, such as clothing characteristic of a group, forms of address and, of course, possessions. After a period of severe deprivation, the victim is asked to write a confession in exchange for the opportunity to satisfy elementary needs. The confession is written at first only to achieve this end. After a brief respite, the victim is told that the confession is inadequate, that it does not fit the captors' "knowledge" of the person's transgressions and the cycle begins again. For the purpose of writing a "satisfactory" confession the victim must work harder and harder to assume the role that the captors have prescribed. The line between pretense and reality is never discretely crossed, but eventually the victim takes on a new identity and ideology that in some cases survive for months after "rescue." Of course, this is an extreme case, but it does suggest a few general points about personality change. First, "Where the hand leads, the heart follows." Role playing and pretending may be one way to adopt a new role or identity. Second, personalities or identities have a kind of stability that resists change, so that efforts to weaken present identity may be helpful in allowing change to occur. Third, substantial changes in personality may require the agent of change to exert substantial power over the subject. Such power is not usually available in schools but is normally available to parents, particularly when children are young. The advantages of early rather than later intervention may lie largely in the fact that power is more easily exercised when the subject is young. On the other hand, as individuals develop, the power of others over them may be replaced by their power over themselves, so that individuals' capacity to change their own personalities, once they decide to do so, is increased.

Several courses have been designed to increase the achievement motivation of those planning a career in business (Aronoff & Litwin, 1966; Kolb, 1965; McClelland, 1961; reviewed by de Charms, 1968). One of the techniques used requires the participants to make up stories and score the stories for achievement themes. Such themes include "success in completion with some standard of excellence," and "attainment of a long-term achievement goal." This exercise is performed repeatedly, so that the participants learn to produce such stories. The general principle "Where the hand leads, the heart follows" seems to be at work here as well. Another technique involves the use of games that are models of achievement situations, for example, ordering goods for a factory. In this game, the players actually assemble the goods into toys, and they must try to order just the right amount of goods to keep pace with their rate of assembly, which must also remain high, in order to turn a profit. Other techniques involved mutual support of the participants in the style of t-groups, and efforts to create the impression that the intended change was part of a "step up" to a higher social class. In general, these courses have been successful not only in changing the scores on tests of achievement motivation – which is not surprising at all, given that these tests were used in training – but also in promoting actual achievement in business. De Charms (1976) has run a similar program that has successfully changed academic motivation in students. Although these courses purport to change motivation only, they are still relevant to the training of cognitive styles. As I argued, one of the determinants of such styles may in fact be motivations or preferences.

In fact, there is evidence that programs for disadvantaged preschool children affect subsequent academic achievement at least in part through their effects on expectations and motives. A follow-up evaluation of eight experimental programs (Consortium for Longitudinal Studies, 1979) showed that these programs affected the children's attitudes toward themselves. When asked to tell "something you've done that makes you feel proud of yourself," children in the programs were more likely than controls to give achievement-related responses. This effect, in turn, may have been the result of changes in parents' expectations for their children, which were also found to have occurred.

Personality change also occurs in psychotherapy. The techniques used here are so varied and so well studied that it would be foolish even to attempt a review in a few pages. Still, one useful technique common to many forms of therapy is the monitoring of activities outside the therapy session. The patient is given some sort of instruction, perhaps implicit, and reports at the next session on his success in following it. This tactic may have the effect of encouraging the patient to remember to follow the instruction when it is appropriate to do so.

Finally, Dweck (1975) has been able to remove the debilitating effect of failure on subsequent performance in children's problem solving. Children who were subject to such a learned helplessness effect were taught to attribute their failure to lack of effort rather than to other factors such as lack of ability. Such attribution retraining is a promising technique whenever a pattern of undesirable behavior is caused by a certain set of beliefs concerning causes and effects.

The techniques that I have mentioned throughout this chapter are: role playing, identification of the change with a social goal, modeling, tutorial dialogue, games, assignment with review, and attribution retraining. Other techniques are discussed in more detail in Segal, Chipman, and Glaser (in press). These techniques may be worthy of study in their own right.

6.4.   CONCLUSION

In this chapter I have sketched a theory of thinking, which may serve as a framework for discussion of individual differences in thinking. The theory specifies a number of phases, each with at least one associated parameter, such as the tendency to recognize a problem, the number of hypotheses enumerated before any evidence is considered, the tendency to consider habitual hypotheses as opposed to new ones, the tendency to search for confirming versus disconfirming evidence, responsiveness to evidence as opposed to prior beliefs, and stringency of the criterion for stopping the whole process. Each of these parameters has an optimal setting that is determined by a rule, usually one that takes into account values and expectations. For example, the rule for the last parameter is that one should stop thinking when the expected payoff from further thinking becomes less than the cost. The expected payoff is a function of one's opinion that further thought will improve the value of one's decision and also indicates the value of that improvement. The expected cost is the cost of the effort of thinking (or the fun of thinking, on the other side of zero) and of the time involved. We may determine the optimum with respect to either the subject's values of the moment or the values of others. In a given situation a person may have a characteristic setting of this parameter, on one side of the optimum or the other. The person's propensity to set the parameter at one place or another, relative to the optimum, may be general across (at least some class of) situations; if so, it would be appropriate to call the propensity a cognitive style. The parameter governing the stringency of evaluation is roughly equivalent to the style of reflection–impulsivity (where values are never considered).

The theory provides a framework for systematic enumeration and measurement of cognitive styles, thus remedying a flaw in the current study of styles. It also provides an account of evidence that purportedly shows stages of ego development. It suggests ways of considering the pathology of thinking and the styles of thinking that may shape the "choice" of neurosis.

My consideration of various topics in personality theory in their relation to intelligence prompts me to make some suggestions for research. First, we might appropriately ask which thinking parameters are set optimally – according to both individual and group values – and, for those that are not generally optimal, on which side they tend to deviate. The simplest technique to use for this purpose is the laboratory experiment with explicit (but not necessarily monetary) payoffs. Once this work has been done, individual differences in the various parameters should be sought. The best way to demonstrate such differences is to show consistency across tasks of different kinds. Thereafter we might attempt to identify the determinants of propensities to deviate from the optimum, partly by measurement of the various components of each rule. For example, the subject's expectation for the value of further thinking, values, and so forth could be determined. This technique will inform us only about the most proximal determinants, however; for example, it cannot tell us much about emotional factors (which exert their effects indirectly). Manipulation of various factors is also possible, to find out whether the subject is undersensitive or oversensitive to any of them. Correlational studies may be of some use as well, but we must avoid the trap of taking a correlation as evidence of a single cause. For example, if impulsive people are less anxious than reflective ones, we cannot conclude that nobody is impulsive because of anxiety about failure. Experiments in which anxiety is manipulated in individual subjects can tell us whether the latter mechanism exists.

Another set of questions concerns the use of thinking in specific domains, such as moral reasoning, belief formation, work, and interpersonal relationships. Research on these questions would help establish the importance of thinking in each area (see, for example, Perkins, 1980; Steinlauf, 1979).

We might also investigate the relation between the parameters of thinking and other aspects of intelligence, such as biological capacities. For example, the enumeration of hypotheses, and the search for evidence, are undoubtedly limited by ability to retrieve information from memory as well as by other factors. The study of people's conceptions of intelligence seems particularly fruitful. It would be of great interest to know how much these conceptions err in consequential ways. People may have beliefs about how to think, for example, that are positively harmful when applied to their own thinking or to the thinking of their children. Alternatively, people may know more about good thinking than they put into practice.

The framework that I have provided may also be used to analyze cultural changes, cultural differences, and effects of child-rearing practices on intellectual development. Such studies must be correlational rather than experimental (for ethical reasons), but they can still provide ways of understanding these various domains. Thus the study of change through history may be of interest to the historian, if not to the psychologist.

Finally, we might formulate questions of the following sort: How do traits become general? How does personality change? How is good thinking learned? These questions appear to be scientific, but I think they are better viewed as matters of engineering. The answers may change with the invention of new educational technologies, new child-rearing methods, and new cultural institutions. Work on the other questions I have listed suggests the nature of such change, but the psychological researcher who wants to be truly helpful in answering such questions must be willing to take on the role of the inventor. Of course, any new invention must be evaluated, and here the researcher can be useful as well.

I conclude with a word of caution. One implication of the view I have outlined is that the development of intelligence is intimately connected with other aspects of personality development, because thinking is affected by values, emotions, and so forth. Thus a full understanding of intellectual development may require substantial understanding of personality development itself. As Meehl (1978) noted, however, there are severe limits on the extent to which we can ever understand personality development in full. For example, personality is often subject to "divergent causality," in which small, essentially random, events have large impacts: "... an object in unstable equilibrium can move slightly to the right instead of the left, as a result of which a deadly avalanche occurs. ..." A similar problem is that of the "random walk": "At several points that are individually minor but collectively critical determinative, it is an almost 'chance' affair whether the patient does *A* or not *A*, whether his girl friend says she will or will not go out with him on a certain evening, or whether he happens to hit it off with the opthalmologist that he consults about some peculiar vision disturbances that are making him anxious about becoming blind, and the like. If one twin becomes psychotic after such a random walk, it is possible that he was suffering from what was only, so to speak, 'bad luck'..." (1978, pp. 809–811). It might be that a great deal of personality, our interests, our beliefs, may be so determined, including the part that affects our intelligence.

NOTES

Part of this chapter is based on an editorial in *Intelligence* (1981) on which I received many helpful comments. Judy Baron and Robert Sternberg made useful suggestions about the present chapter.

REFERENCES

Alloy, L. B., & Seligman, M. E. P. On the cognitive component of learned helplessness and depression. In G. Bower (Ed.), *The psychology of learning and motivation.* (Vol. 13). New York: Academic Press, 1979.

Allport, G. W. Traits revisited. *American Psychologist,* 1966, *21,* 1–10.

Arendt, H. *Eichmann in Jerusalem.* New York: Viking, 1965.

Aronoff, J., & Litwin, G. Achievement motivation training and executive advancement. Unpublished manuscript, 1966.

Baron, J. Some theories of college instruction. *Higher Education,* 1975, *4,* 149–172.

Baron, J. Reflective thinking as a goal of education. *Intelligence,* 1981, *5,* 291–309.

Baron, J. What kinds of intelligence components are fundamental? In J. Segal, S. Chipman, & R. Glaser (Eds.), *Thinking and learning skills.* (Vol. 2). Hillsdale, N.J.: Erlbaum, in press.

Baron, J., & Treiman, R. Some problems in the study of differences in cognitive processes. *Memory and Cognition,* 1980, *8,* 313–321.

Barron, F. Originality in relation to personality and intellect. *Journal of Personality,* 1957, *25,* 730–742.

Beck, A. T. *Cognitive therapy and the emotional disorders.* New York: International Universities Press, 1976.

Bem, D. J., & Allen, A. On predicting some of the people some of the time: The search for cross-situational consistencies in behavior. *Psychological Review,* 1974, *81,* 506–520.

Bem, D. J., & Funder, D. C. Predicting more of the people more of the time: Assessing the personality of situations. *Psychological Review,* 1978, *85,* 485–501.

Binet, A., & Simon, T. Méthodes nouvelles pour le diagnostic du niveau intellectuel des anormaux. *Année Psychologique,* 1905, *11,* 191–244.

Binet, A., & Simon, T. [*The development of intelligence in children*] (E. S. Kite, Trans.). Baltimore: Williams and Wilkins, 1916.

Blank, M. *Teaching learning in the preschool.* Columbus, Ohio: Merrill, 1973.

Block, J. *The Q-sort method in personality assessment and psychiatric research.* Springfield, Ill.: Charles C Thomas, 1961.

Block, J., Block, J. H., & Harrington, D. M. Some misgivings about the Matching Familiar Figures Test as a measure of reflection–impulsivity. *Developmental Psychology*, 1974, 5, 611–632.

Block, J., & Petersen, P. Some personality correlates of confidence, caution, and speed in a decision situation. *Journal of Abnormal and Social Psychology*, 1955, 51, 34–41.

Block, J., Weiss, D. S., & Thorne, A. How relevant is a semantic similarity interpretation of personality ratings? *Journal of Personality and Social Psychology*, 1979, 37, 1055–1074.

Brim, O. G., Glass, D. C., Lavin, D. E., & Goodman, N. *Personality and decision processes.* Stanford, Calif.: Stanford University Press, 1962.

Bruner, J. S., & Goodman, C. Value and need as organizing factors in perception. *Journal of Abnormal and Social Psychology*, 1947, 42, 33–44.

Calhoun, D. *The intelligence of a people.* Princeton, N.J.: Princeton University Press, 1973.

Carew, J. V. Experience and the development of intelligence in young children at home and in day care. *Monographs of the Society for Research in Child Development*, 1980, 45 (6–7, Social No. 187).

Chamberlain, T. C. The method of multiple working hypotheses. *Science*, 1965, 148, 754–759. (Originally published, 1897.)

Consortium for Longitudinal Studies. *Lasting effects after preschool.* (Publication OHDS 79-30178). Washington, D.C.: Department of Health, Education and Welfare, 1979.

Darlington, R. B., Royce, J. M., Snipper, A. S., Murray, H. W., & Lazar, I. Preschool programs and later school competence of children from low-income families. *Science,* 1979, 208, 202–204.

de Charms, R., & Moeller, G. H. Values expressed in American children's readers: 1800–1950. *Journal of Abnormal and Social Psychology*, 1962, 64, 135–142.

de Charms, R. *Personal causation.* New York: Academic Press, 1968.

de Charms, R. *Enhancing motivation in the classroom.* New York: Irvington, 1976.

Dewey, J. *How we think: A restatement of the relation of reflective thinking to the educative process.* Boston: Heath, 1933.

Dweck, C. S. The role of expectations and attributions in the alleviation of learned helplessness. *Journal of Personality and Social Psychology*, 1975, 31, 674–685.

Epstein, S. The stability of behavior: I. On predicting most of the people much of the time. *Journal of Personality and Social Psychology*, 1979, 37, 1097–1126.

Erdelyi, M. H. A new look at the New Look: Perceptual defense and vigilance. *Psychological Review*, 1974, 81, 1–25.

Erikson, E. H. *Childhood and society.* New York: Norton, 1950.

Erikson, E. H. Identity and the life cycle. *Psychological Issues*, 1959, 1 (1). (Monograph)

Feuerstein, R., Rand, Y., Hoffman, M. B., & Miller, R. *Instrumental enrichment.* Baltimore: University Park Press, 1980.

Fischhoff, B., Slovic, P., & Lichtenstein, S. Knowing with certainty: The appropriateness of extreme confidence. *Journal of Experimental Psychology: Human Perception and Performance,* 1977, 3, 552–564.

Frese, M. Personal communication, 1981.

Gardner, R. W. Cognitive styles in categorizing behavior. *Journal of Personality*, 1953, 22, 214–233.

Gardner, R. W., Holzman, P. S., Klein, G. S., Linton, H. B., & Spence, D. P. Cognitive control. *Psychological Issues*, 1959, 1 (4). (Monograph)

Hayes, J. R. Three problems in teaching general skills. In J. Segal, S. Chipman, & R. Glaser (Eds.), *Thinking and learning skills.* (Vol. 2). Hillsdale, N.J.: Erlbaum, in press.

Hogan, R., DeSoto, C. B., & Solano, C. Tests, traits, and personality research. *American Psychologist*, 1977, 32, 255–264.

Holt, R. R. Loevinger's measure of ego development: Reliability and national norms for male and female short forms. *Journal of Personality and Social Psychology*, 1980, 39, 909–920.

Holzman, P. S. The relation of assimilation tendencies in visual, auditory, and kinesthetic time-error to cognitive attitudes of leveling and sharpening. *Journal of Personality*, 1954, 22, 375–394.

Holzman, P. S., & Gardner, R. W. Leveling and repression. *Journal of Abnormal and Social Psychology*, 1959, 59, 151–155.

Holzman, P. S., & Klein, G. S. Cognitive system-principles of leveling and sharpening: Individual differences in assimilation effects in visual time-error. *Journal of Psychology*, 1954, 37, 105–122.

Honzik, M. P., & MacFarlane, J. W. Personality development and intellectual functioning from 21 months to 40 years. In L. F. Jarvik & C. Eisdorfer (Eds.), *Intellectual functioning in adults*. New York: Springer, 1973.

Hunt, E. Mechanics of verbal ability. *Psychological Review*, 1978, *85*, 271–283.

Irwin, F. W. *Intentional behavior and motivation: A cognitive theory*. Philadelphia: Lippincott, 1971.

Jackson, D. N., & Paunonen, S. V. Personality structure and assessment. *Annual Review of Psychology*, 1980, *31*, 503–551.

Jencks, C., Smith, J., Ackland, H., Bane, M. J., Cohen, D., Gintis, H., Heyns, P., & Michelson, S. *Inequality: A reassessment of the effect of family and schooling in America*. New York: Basic Books, 1972.

Johnson, L. C. Generality of speed and confidence in judgment. *Journal of Abnormal and Social Psychology*, 1957, *54*, 264–266.

Kagan, J. Reflection–impulsivity: The generality and dynamics of conceptual tempo. *Journal of Abnormal Psychology*, 1966, *71*, 17–24.

Kagan, J., & Kogan, N. Individual variation in cognitive processes. In P. Mussen (Ed.), *Carmichael's manual of child psychology* (Vol. I). New York: Wiley, 1970.

Kagan, J., Lapidus, D. R., & Moore, M. Infant antecedents of cognitive functioning: A longitudinal study. *Child Development*, 1978, *49*, 1005–1023.

Kagan, J., Sontag, L. W., Baker, C. T., & Nelson, V. L. Personality and I.Q. change. *Journal of Abnormal and Social Psychology*, 1958, *56*, 261–266.

Kahneman, D., Slovic, P., & Tversky, A. *Judgment under uncertainty: Heuristics and biases*. Cambridge: Cambridge University Press, 1980.

Kenrick, D. T., & Stringfield, D. O. Personality traits and the eye of the beholder: Crossing some traditional philosophical boundaries in the search for consistency in all of the people. *Psychological Review*, 1980, *87*, 88–104.

Klein, G. S., & Schlesinger, H. J. Where is the perceiver in perceptual theory? *Journal of Personality*, 1949, *18*, 32–47.

Klein, G. S., & Schlesinger, H. J. Perceptual attitudes toward instability: Prediction of apparent movement responses from Rorschach responses. *Journal of Personality*, 1951, *19*, 289–302.

Kogan, N. Creativity and cognitive style: A life-span perspective. In P. B. Baltes & K. W. Schaie (Eds.), *Life-span developmental psychology: Personality and socialization*. New York: Academic Press, 1973.

Kogan, N. *Cognitive styles in infancy and early childhood*. Hillsdale, N.J.: Erlbaum, 1976.

Kogan, N., Connor, K., Gross, A., & Fava, D. Understanding visual metaphor: Developmental and individual differences. *Monographs of the Society for Research in Child Development*, 1980, *45* (1, Serial No. 183).

Kogan, N., & Wallach, M. A. *Risk taking: A study in cognition and personality*. New York: Holt, Rinehart & Winston, 1964.

Kohlberg, L. Stage and sequence: The cognitive-developmental approach to socialization. In D. Goslin (Ed.), *Handbook of socialization theory and research*. New York: Rand McNally, 1969.

Kohlberg, L. Stages of moral development as a basis of moral education. In C. M. Beck, P. S. Crittenden, & E. V. Sullivan (Eds.), *Moral Education: Interdisciplinary Approaches*. Toronto: University of Toronto Press, 1970.

Kolb, D. A. Achievement motivation training for underachieving high-school boys. *Journal of Personality and Social Psychology*, 1965, *2*, 783–792.

Koriat, A., Lichtenstein, S., & Fischhoff, B. Reasons for confidence. *Journal of Experimental Psychology: Human Learning and Memory*, 1980, *6*, 107–118.

Langer, E. Rethinking the role of thought in social interaction. In J. Harvey, W. Ickes, and R. Kidd (Eds.), *New directions in attribution research*. Hillsdale, N.J.: Erlbaum, 1978.

Lifton, R. J. *Thought reform and the psychology of totalism: A study of brainwashing in China*. New York: Norton, 1961.

Linton, H. B. Dependence on external influence: correlates in perception, attitudes, and judgement. *Journal of Abnormal and Social Psychology*, 1955, *51*, 502–507.

Loevinger, J. The meaning and measurement of ego development. *American Psychologist*, 1966, *21*, 195–217.

Loevinger, J., Wessler, R., & Redmore, C. *Measuring ego development* (2 vols.). San Francisco: Jossey-Bass, 1970.

Lord, F. W. Statistical adjustments when comparing preexisting groups. *Psychological Bulletin,* 1969, *72,* 336–337.

Luchins, A. S., & Luchins, E. H. *Rigidity of behavior.* Eugene, Oreg.: University of Oregon Press, 1959.

Maslow, A. H. *Motivation and personality.* New York: Harper, 1954.

Maslow, A. H. *Toward a psychology of being.* Princeton, N.J.: Van Nostrand, 1962.

McCauley, C., & Stitt, C. L. An individual and quantitative measure of stereotypes. *Journal of Personality and Social Psychology,* 1978, *36,* 929–940.

McClelland, D. C. *The achieving society.* Princeton, N.J.: Van Nostrand, 1961.

McClelland, D. C., & Winter, D. G. *Motivating economic achievement.* New York: Free Press, 1971.

Meehl, P. E. Theoretical risks and tabular asterisks: Sir Karl, Sir Ronald, and the slow progress of soft psychology. *Journal of Clinical and Consulting Psychology,* 1978, *46,* 806–834.

Meichenbaum, D. *Cognitive behavior modification: An integrative approach.* New York: Plenum, 1977.

Messer, S. B. Reflection–impulsivity: A review. *Psychological Bulletin,* 1976, *83,* 1026–1052.

Mischel, W. Toward a cognitive social learning reconceptualization of personality. *Psychological Review,* 1973, *80,* 252–283.

Mischel, W. On the future of personality measurement. *American Psychologist,* 1977, *32,* 246–254.

Mischel, W., & Metzner, R. Preference for delayed reward as a function of age, intelligence, and length of delay interval. *Journal of Abnormal and Social Psychology,* 1962, *64,* 425–431.

Mitchell, C., & Ault, R. L. Reflection–impulsivity and the evaluation process. *Child Development,* 1979, *50,* 1043–1049.

Murray, H. A. *Explorations in personality.* New York: Oxford University Press, 1938.

Neisser, U. The concept of intelligence. *Intelligence,* 1979, *3,* 217–227.

Newell, A. Reasoning, problem solving, and decision processes: The problem space as a fundamental category. In R. Nickerson (Ed.), *Attention and performance VIII.* Hillsdale, N.J.: Erlbaum, 1980.

Nisbett, R., & Ross, L. *Human inference: Strategies and shortcomings of social judgment.* Englewood Cliffs, N.J.: Prentice-Hall, 1980.

Orne, M. Coercive persuasion. Unpublished manuscript, University of Pennsylvania, 1978.

Perkins, D. Difficulties in everyday reasoning and their change with education. Unpublished manuscript, Harvard University, 1980.

Perkins, D. General cognitive skills: Why not? In J. Segal, S. Chipman, & R. Glaser (Eds.), *Thinking and learning skills.* (Vol. 2). Hillsdale, N.J.: Erlbaum, in press.

Perry, W. G., Jr. *Forms of intellectual and ethical development in the college years: A scheme.* New York: Holt, Rinehart and Winston, 1971.

Pettigrew, T. F. The measurement and correlates of category width as a cognitive variable. *Journal of Personality,* 1958, *26,* 532–544.

Piaget, J. *The moral judgment of the child.* Glencoe, Ill.: Free Press, 1932.

Polya, G. *How to solve it.* Princeton, N.J.: Princeton University Press, 1945.

Putnam, H. *Mind, language, and reality.* London: Cambridge University Press, 1975. (Collected papers.)

Ramanaiah, N. V., & Goldberg, L. R. Stylistic components of human judgment: The generality of individual differences. *Applied Psychological Measurement,* 1977, *1,* 23–29.

Rawls, J. *A theory of justice.* Cambridge, Mass.: Harvard University Press, 1971.

Robinson, P. The measurement of achievement motivation. Unpublished doctoral dissertation, Oxford University, 1961.

Rorschach, H. [*Psychodiagnostics*] (P. Lemkau & B. Kronenberg, trans.). Bern, Switzerland: Huber, 1942.

Sabini, J., & Silver, M. *Moralities of everyday life.* London: Oxford University Press, 1981.

Salkind, N. J., Kojima, H., & Zelnicker, I. Cognitive tempo in American, Japanese, and Israeli children. *Child Development,* 1978, *49,* 1024–1027.

Samuel, W. Mood and personality correlates of IQ by race and sex of subject. *Journal of Personality and Social Psychology*, 1980, *38*, 993–1004.

Savage, L. J. *Foundations of Statistics*. New York: Wiley, 1954.

Schwartz, B. Reinforcement induced behavioral stereotypy: How not to teach people to discover rules. *Journal of Experimental Psychology: General*, 1982, *111*, 23–59.

Schweder, R. A., & D'Andrade, R. G. Accurate reflection or systematic distortion? A reply to Block, Weiss, and Thorne. *Journal of Personality and Social Psychology*, 1979, *57*, 1075–1084.

Sears, R. S. Sources of life satisfaction of the Terman gifted men. *American Psychologist*, 1977, *32*, 119–128.

Segal, J., Chipman, S., & Glaser, R. (Eds.), *Thinking and learning skills*. Hillsdale, N.J.: Erlbaum, in press.

Semmer, N., & Frese, M. Handlungstheoretische Implikationen für kognitive Therapie. In N. Hoffman (Ed.), *Grundlagen kognitiver Therapie*. Bern: Huber, 1979.

Shafer, G. *A mathematical theory of evidence*. Princeton, N.J.: Princeton University Press, 1976.

Shapiro, D. *Neurotic styles*. New York: Basic Books, 1965.

Sharp, D., Cole, M., & Lave, C. Education and cognitive development: The evidence from experimental research. *Monographs of the Society for Research in Child Development*, 1979, *44*(1–2, Serial No. 178).

Shweder, R. A. Likeness and likelihood in everyday thought: Magical thinking and everyday judgments about personality. In P. N. Johnson-Laird & P. C. Wason (Eds.), *Thinking: Readings in cognitive science*. Cambridge: Cambridge University Press, 1977.

Smith, J. D., Baron, J., & Smith, C. A. Reflection–impulsivity in young adults. Unpublished manuscript, University of Pennsylvania, 1981.

Smith, L. B., & Kemler, D. G. Developmental trends in free classification: Evidence for a new conceptualization of perceptual development. *Journal of Experimental Child Psychology*, 1977, *24*, 279–298.

Spearman, C. "General intelligence" objectively determined and measured. *American Journal of Psychology*, 1904, *15*, 201–293.

Steinlauf, B. Problem-solving skills, locus of control, and the contraceptive effectiveness of young women. *Child Development*, 1979, *50*, 268–271.

Sternberg, R. J. *Intelligence, information processing, and analogical reasoning*. Hillsdale, N.J.: Erlbaum, 1977.

Sternberg, R. J. The nature of mental abilities. *American Psychologist*, 1979, *34*, 214–230.

Sternberg, R. J. Sketch of a componential subtheory of human intelligence. *Brain and Behavioral Sciences*, 1980, *3*, 573–614.

Sternberg, R. J., Conway, B. E., Ketron, J. L., & Bernstein, M. People's conceptions of intelligence. *Journal of Personality and Social Psychology*, 1981, *41*, 37–55.

Stevens, A. L., & Collins, A. Multiple conceptual models of a complex system. In R. E. Snow, P.-A. Federico, & W. E. Montague (Eds.), *Aptitude, learning, and instruction* (Vol. 2). Hillsdale, N.J.: Erlbaum, 1980.

Terman, L. M. *The measurement of intelligence*. Boston: Houghton Mifflin, 1916.

Terman, L. M., & Oden, M. H. *The gifted group at mid-life: Thirty-five years follow-up of the superior child*. Stanford: Stanford University Press, 1959.

Tversky, A., & Kahneman, D. Judgment under uncertainty: Heuristics and biases. *Science*, 1974, *185*, 1124–1131.

Vaillant, G. E. *Adaptation to life*. Boston: Little, Brown, 1977.

Wagner, D. A. Memories of Morocco: The influence of age, schooling, and environment on memory. *Cognitive Psychology*, 1978, *10*, 1–28.

Wason, P. C. "On the failure to eliminate hypotheses..." – A second look. In P. C. Wason & P. N. Johnson-Laird (Eds.), *Thinking and reasoning*. Harmondsworth: Penguin, 1968.

Weiss, G., & Hechtman, L. The hyperactive child syndrome. *Science*, 1979, *205*, 1348–1354.

Wickelgren, W. A. *How to solve problems*. San Francisco: Freeman, 1974.

Widiger, T. A., Knudson, R. M., & Rorer, L. G. Convergent and discriminant validity of measures of cognitive style and abilities. *Journal of Personality and Social Psychology*, 1980, *39*, 116–129.

Wiggins, N., Hoffman, P. J., & Taber, T. Types of judges and cue utilization in judgments of intelligence. *Journal of Personality and Social Psychology*, 1969, *12*, 52–59.

Witkin, H. A. Psychological differentiation and forms of pathology. *Journal of Abnormal Psychology*, 1965, 70, 317–336.

Wober, M. Towards an understanding of the Kiganda concept of intelligence. In J. W. Berry & P. R. Dasen (Eds.), *Culture and cognition: Readings in cross-cultural psychology*. London: Methuen, 1974.

7 *Artificial and human intelligence*

NATALIE DEHN AND ROGER SCHANK

7.1. INTRODUCTION

The field of *artificial intelligence* (henceforth AI) started as the study of machine intelligence – the design and construction of intelligent machines. AI has since, we believe, matured into an effective methodology for studying *human* intelligence. That by studying machines we should learn about people may seem at first to be incongruous, if not outright wrongheaded. However, we will see that – and why – this has turned out to be far from the case.

The present chapter, then, discusses how AI research can lead to progress in the understanding of human intelligence and ways in which it has already done so. It should be noted from the start, however, that AI's primary concern with human intelligence is a different concern from what is studied in *psychology* under that name. AI is concerned with the operation of human intelligence – with how intelligence *works*.

Section 7.2 traces the evolution of early AI, or machine intelligence, into a field of human intelligence research. Not all of AI, of course, took this path – some very active research efforts that evolved from the same origins and are therefore also called artificial intelligence grew in different directions and now have rather different focuses. This survey, however, will touch only lightly on areas of AI that have little to say about human intelligence. The promising work now under way in several of these areas is best evaluated within the framework of the goals of those fields, which fall beyond the scope of this chapter.[1] Our survey, then, is not a general survey of AI but rather, as the title suggests, a survey of that AI most relevant to human intelligence.

Having seen how early AI developed into the subfield of modern AI that is the focus of this survey, we will consider, in section 7.3, the role that the computer plays in human-intelligence-oriented AI and, perhaps more important, the role that it does not play. Section 7.4 will then return to a consideration of early AI and of the issues originally regarded as significant, in preparation for section 7.5, which discusses the issues of current concern and their sources. Section 7.6 considers the implications of AI for more traditional research concerns (matters of general intelligence and individual differences), and section 7.7 provides a brief summary.

7.2. FROM MACHINE INTELLIGENCE TO HUMAN INTELLIGENCE RESEARCH

AI has its roots in the early days of computers, when excitement about the machines' seemingly human capabilities was so intense that little distinction was made between intelligent and unintelligent computers. The most basic capabilities of com-

352

puters, those of performing arithmetic and of making logical decisions, were viewed then as signs of intelligence.

Programming a computer to perform a new task was basically a matter of specifying a *procedure* in terms of steps, or subtasks, that the computer could already perform. As more and more programs were written, both the computer's repertory of subtasks and human expertise in specifying such procedures increased. Thus the number and complexity of tasks that computers were capable of accomplishing grew quickly.[2]

The kinds of tasks people attempted to write programs to accomplish varied widely – and whereas some of these attempts succeeded, others did not. Some failures were due simply to insufficient technical skill on the part of the programmer, but other failures had far more serious implications. A pattern was slowly emerging: It was easiest to program computers to do types of work that most people found very hard, such as long, detailed mathematical calculations, whereas it was most difficult to program machines to perform operations of which even a small child or mentally defective adult was capable, such as understanding language or recognizing objects or situations. The significance of this pattern, however, was not fully appreciated for some time.

Views as to what constitutes an intelligent program have changed considerably during the last two or three decades. Many programs that were once considered intelligent or almost intelligent are no longer so regarded. At least part of this shift is due to a changing definition of intelligence – a change driven, in large part, by experience with these programs. The construction of a program satisfying existing formal criteria for intelligence has typically resulted in a refinement of those criteria in order to exclude it.

Machine intelligence, thus, was originally regarded primarily as an *alternative* to human intelligence; each of these two forms of intelligence would have, it was expected, its own idiosyncratic strengths and weaknesses. There were hopes, fed by the superior speed and accuracy with which computers performed certain tasks that humans judged difficult, that machine intelligence might even eventually generally surpass its human counterpart.

Though most early AI research focused on the capabilities of machine-specific intelligence, there was also some interest in intelligence more broadly construed. The difficulty in clarifying the true meaning of intelligence, it was thought, was due to there being but one example of an intelligent being, namely the human. The development of alternate forms of intelligence, it was hoped, would help us overcome our "provincialism" and would thus enable us to understand intelligence in the most general sense.

In subsequent years, AI developed in several directions. Much of the interest in extending the capabilities of computers was channeled into computer science proper. From the standpoint of computer science, AI has largely been the territory on the other side of an advancing frontier; research in AI extends the field of computer research, yielding to it domains once, but no longer, associated with AI. Another path that AI took, however, led to human intelligence research.

Although there was some interest in human cognition in early AI (see, for instance, Newell & Simon, 1961), it took the failure of many early machine intelligence efforts to cause a general shift in orientation. Some efforts, true, led to successful spinoffs in the form of useful "application programs," such as MACSYMA, a symbolic integration program (Moses, 1967; Slagle, 1961), but the attainment of machine *intelligence* remained elusive. These primarily negative results, however, also proved useful in bringing a growing, helpful *understanding* of what would not work. Arrogance about the potential superiority of machine-specific intelligence slowly gave way to a growing respect for human intelligence and its operation. Characteristics of human intelligence and memory that had at first seemed to be weaknesses began to be recognized as strengths, fundamental to the robustness and generality of human intelligence.

One such characteristic is the human tendency not to consider carefully all aspects of a problem or to work out all alternatives before deciding on an answer but rather to isolate a few aspects of the problem that seem most important or interesting, to concentrate on those, and largely to ignore the rest. Such an approach sounds, at first, rather sloppy and unreliable, especially compared with that which is generally programmed into computers, of giving careful consideration to *all* factors before making any determination. The traditional-computer approach can guarantee that the *best* answer be found (if there is one) and is error free; the human approach will lead to but an *acceptable* answer (if that!) and is error prone.

This difference explains the initial success of computers in doing many of their first tasks – they *were* more accurate and more reliable than people – yet the same difference also indicates why humans performed other work so much more effectively than computers. People excelled, as computers did not, at solving problems involving situations too complex ever to be considered fully. The complexity could arise either from the amount of input data associated with the problem (perhaps a visual scene, the sound of someone's voice, or a social situation) or from the number of possibilities that could be cognitively generated in reasoning from the problem to the solution. Humans, given their sloppy modes of thought, never even *try* full consideration and hence never even notice the difficulty of problems that are complex in this sense. Computers that were programmed to consider the entire problem thoroughly, however, would drown in deliberation as a result. Although computers can make simple logical decisions very fast, when there are far too many such decisions to be made, no reasonable amount of speed can possibly help.

Thus for problems that are sufficiently small in this special sense, traditional *algorithmic* computer techniques are superior to human *heuristic* methods. Examples of such problems include financial record keeping, mathematical calculations and, more generally, any of the other well-known and now traditional uses of computers. The problems that are too large, however, interestingly enough, encompass virtually all of those confronted by humans in daily life – from understanding language to deciding what to do next to deciding how to handle a social situation.

For the first class of problems, using a faster computer results in faster (and/or more) answers; for the second class, no conceivable improvements in technology can help. Therefore artificial intelligence is now turning more and more toward attempted simulation of human methods.

There are mixed motives in this shift. For those researchers who are primarily task-oriented it is that human methods currently appear to be the best or only available tool and therefore must do until some more clever means is thought of. For hard-line machine-specific-intelligence researchers, a model of human intelligence can serve as a useful base from which, it is hoped, machine intelligence can eventually transcend human intelligence. Those who have been avoiding human methods only because there seemed to be easier computer methods available are beginning to shift as that proves not to be the case.

As attempts at human simulation reveal more and more about human cognitive mechanisms, there has been, within AI, a rapidly growing appreciation of and fascination with the operation of human intelligence. AI is now, in this sense, beginning to converge with the research of cognitive psychologists. A still greater convergence is taking place under the aegis of cognitive science, which has further attracted philosophers, anthropologists, social psychologists, linguists, and developmental psychologists.

Much of the AI research on human intelligence is taking place in the subfield of *natural language processing*. Natural language has played an especially important role in AI because attempts at building systems with natural language processing capabilities have confronted researchers with the issues central to an understanding of intelligence. As we will see, most of the progress in natural language processing, although necessary for building programs with natural language capabilities, has been not especially linguistic-specific but, rather, concerned with more basic and general issues of intelligence.

Machine-oriented research continues, however, in the AI subfields of *pattern recognition* (Duda & Hart, 1973), *game playing* (Berliner, 1977; Levy, 1976; Newell, Shaw, & Simon, 1958; Nilsson, 1969; Samuel, 1959, 1967), *vision* (Duda & Hart, 1973; Horn, 1975; Marr, 1978, 1979; Ullman, 1979; Waltz, 1975; Winston, 1975), *speech recognition* (Hayes-Roth, Mostow, & Fox, 1978; Lea, 1980; Reddy, 1975), *theorem proving* (Fikes & Nilsson, 1971; Green, 1969), and *robotics* (Finkel, 1976; Miller, 1977). Substantial and impressive progress has been made within such fields, but the current thrust of such work is primarily in directions not directly relevant to human intelligence.

It is not, however, completely appropriate to discriminate among AI research orientations purely on the basis of *task*, because cognitive issues can be found in virtually *any* task. Still, different tasks do tend to force different theoretical issues to the fore. Thus, for instance, although some work relevant to intelligence is being done in chess-playing research (Berliner, 1974), most of the progress in this area deals with rather different issues. Similarly, though many of the fundamental issues of memory and knowledge organization *were* encountered in computer *vision* work (as we will see), most work in vision is now concerned with low-level issues.

A major part of AI, but one of only minor relevance to human intelligence, is *expert systems*, or *knowledge engineering* (Bernstein, 1977; Feigenbaum, 1977). This field has led to a number of impressive and useful programs, including:

> MYCIN (Shortliffe, 1976), which helps physicians diagnose and treat infections;
> INTERNIST (Pople, 1977), which solves diagnostic problems in internal medicine;
> MOLGEN (Martin et al., 1977), which plans experiments in molecular genetics;
> DENDRAL (Buchanan, Sutherland, & Feigenbaum, 1969), which helps organic chemists analyze mass spectrograms;
> CRYSALIS (Englemore & Nii, 1977), which infers protein structures from electron density maps.

These programs and others have performed impressively in comparison with human experts. They draw upon the techniques of traditional AI in their highly symbolic representation of knowledge and in their heuristic processing. The significance of such programs in their own right, and their role in a *general* history of AI, should not be underestimated

Still, from the standpoint of human intelligence research, expert systems are little more than spinoffs of AI. Although these systems rely heavily on domain knowledge culled from the rules that human experts have introspectively discovered, expert systems are still basically in the tradition of old machine intelligence work, showing (a) an interest in making the program *better* than human experts and (b) a consequent willingness to use techniques that violate psychological plausibility.

From the standpoint of intelligence research, direct concern with hard tasks, such as spectral analysis, is premature. All human experts have rich and varied knowledge bases before they even begin to acquire their special expertise. Experts certainly make use of some very domain-specific techniques. Still, as humans, they are general purpose in their cognitive capabilities; it is unlikely that they do not, in drawing upon and applying their expertise, make heavy use of their more basic cognitive mechanisms.

7.3.   THE ROLE OF THE COMPUTER PROGRAM IN HUMAN-INTELLIGENCE-
        ORIENTED ARTIFICIAL INTELLIGENCE

The computer was clearly central to AI when its primary concern was machine intelligence, but to understand the relevance of modern AI research to *human* intelligence, we must understand both the roles that the computer program does now play and those that it does not *now* play in AI. Let us begin by considering the former.

The building of programs is of methodological importance, as a scientific tool for the refinement and debugging of theories of intelligence. First, the very writing of the program reveals hidden assumptions and lack of clarity in the underlying theory and indicates where further thought is needed. Thus, the writing of AI programs can both help detect and help correct inadequacies in theories of intelligence. Second, the program, once written, can serve as experimental apparatus. One can thus "try the theory out," exploring its explanatory value. The lessons gained from such testing can help the researcher greatly in understanding the phenomena under study. Programs serving as experimental apparatus are, of course, based on existing theories of the phenomena under study and hence are almost invariably "wrong." Frequently a researcher, aware that a theory is wrong before the program is even written, will write it anyway, though, because the computer program will clarify *where* the theory is wrong, *how* it is inadequate, *what* is irrelevant, and *what else* is needed. Third, the program, once written and tested, can serve as a demonstration of the theory it embodies, as an aid to the communication and explanation of that theory.

The power of program writing and testing in promoting theory development is far greater than might at first be apparent. As each cycle of writing and testing a program increasingly illuminates significant aspects of a phenomenon, the initial theory wanes in significance. Many AI research efforts have used extremely naive theories as starting points. An initially simple theory, however, can evolve into a theory that is more complete. This evolution results from the application of knowledge gained from each successive cycle of program development (see, e.g., Schank, 1978a).

In order to illustrate more clearly the role that computer programs play in theory development, let us consider more explicitly the nature of programs and the aspects most relevant to AI and to intelligence research.

Computer programs *specify processes*. They are written in such a way that a computer can take the specification and actually perform the task specified. They can also be written in such a way as to allow people thus to observe how (i.e., by what process) the programs produce their results. In running a program, one can observe both *what* the program does and *how* it does it.

Computer programs are thus *process models,* modeling the process by which a task is accomplished. When a human reads a story, for instance, and understands its significance, he or she is doing so via some process. A program reading that story would need to do so via some process also. To the degree that the program's process seems to be the same as that of a human, the program is serving as a process *model.*

The fact that a computer program is unlike a human on some levels of abstraction is irrelevant to the program's usefulness as a *process* model, just as it is irrelevant that a mannequin (modeling human appearance) does not have internal organs. If the processes used by the human and by the program differ substantially, then the program is a bad model; however, even bad models, if examined carefully, can lead to successively better models.

As a process model, a program has predictive as well as explanatory power. Differences in process are usually reflected in behavioral differences. Conversely, similarities in process should be reflected in further similarities in behavior, including side effects. Unintentional replication of side effects can provide independent support for a process. One of the most important classes of side effects that can be unintentionally replicated consists of mistakes in hard or tricky cases. When a computer program makes a humanlike mistake in understanding a story or in falling for an optical illusion, that mistake is confirming evidence for the underlying process. Of course, when the program makes a "computerlike" mistake, one that no person would ever make, that error is disconfirming evidence for the model.

A program doing something intelligent is thus like a person doing something intelligent. This is not to deny the profound differences that exist between computers and humans but merely to deny that they are relevant at the level of abstraction of theoretical interest – in humans *or* computers – namely the level of *cognition.* (This matter is discussed, with some rigor, in Pylyshyn, 1980.) Of course, these differences *do* affect some levels that are of instrumental importance and hence affect the ease (technical and moral) with which cognitive scientists can probe, examine, and modify such systems.

If we return, then, to the question of what role computers do and do not play in artificial intelligence, we can now see that in an important sense AI is no longer concerned with computers at all. Intelligence must be embodied before it can be applied or detected, and a computer program serving as a good process model of aspects of human intelligence is merely embodying the human mind in a different form.

Artificial intelligence in this sense is therefore not about anything artificial but is simply about intelligence. Computers play a strong supporting role, with programs being an efficacious part of the AI methodology, but they do not play the central role that they did in AI research concerned with *machine* intelligence.

7.4.   ISSUES AND APPROACHES OF EARLY ARTIFICIAL INTELLIGENCE

Let us now reexamine early AI from the standpoint of issues and approaches, paying special attention to those from which later issues and approaches developed.

HEURISTICS

The step from algorithms to heuristics is commonly regarded as the point at which AI began to be a field distinct from the rest of computer science. Heuristics are basic to any intelligent program – indeed, to any intelligent process – but mundane, unintelligent programs (such as payroll and accounting packages) are still by and large algorithmic. The role of *heuristics* (as contrasted with *algorithms*) in intelligent processing is important enough that it is worth considering in some detail exactly what an algorithm is, what a heuristic is, and what their relative merits are.

Knuth (1973) defines *algorithm* as "a finite set of rules which gives a sequence of operations for solving a specific type of problem," with the following five important features.

1.   *Finiteness*. The algorithm always terminates after a finite number of steps.
2.   *Definiteness*. "Each step of an algorithm must be precisely defined; the actions to be carried out must be rigorously and unambiguously specified for each case."
3.   *Input*
4.   *Output*
5.   *Effectiveness*. "All the operations to be performed in the algorithm must be sufficiently basic that they can *in principle* be done exactly and in a finite length of time" (Knuth, 1973 pp. 4–6; italics added).

One of the most exciting features of computers when they first came out was their ability to execute algorithms. Mathematicians had developed many algorithms for solving various problems, but executing them by hand was very time consuming and error prone; although the algorithm *itself* was guaranteed to give the right solution, errors in *executing* one of thousands or millions of steps could invalidate the entire execution. Computers performed the task quickly and accurately.

Heuristics are also finite sets of rules that give sequences of operations for solving specific types of problems, but they differ from algorithms in that they do not specify exactly how to solve an entire problem and they do not guarantee that it will always lead to a correct answer. Heuristics are suggestions, helpful but not infallible.

Heuristics can usefully be thought of as *test–action pairs* (Davis & King, 1975; Newell, 1973), *test* being a description of the conditions under which the rule is appropriate and *action* signifying the step to be taken when the test is satisfied. For instance, consider the rule: If you are hungry, get something to eat. This rule would remain inactive until one became hungry and would then suggest a solution to one's problem (hunger).

Note that this heuristic (a) does not specify a complete solution (it neither tells one *how* to get food nor what to do once one has it); (b) does not guarantee a solution (one can eat something and still be hungry); and (c) is not infallible (it is not always appropriate to eat when one is hungry). Nonetheless, it is a good and useful rule. Together with many other heuristics (such as: To get something to eat, go to a restaurant; or: To get something to eat, go food shopping and prepare food in kitchen), it is a good way of solving a common problem.

Although mathematicians, scientists, and engineers use algorithms for solving some very well defined problems, most people use heuristics for solving most everyday problems. The vast majority of the decisions we make each hour are made heuristically, and even when a problem allowing algorithmic solution arises, it is usually surrounded by a great many more problems requiring heuristic solution. Thus we may decide the unit price of an item at the grocery store by applying arithmetic algorithms, but the decision of whether the item is then worthwhile (or the prior decision of whether the item is interesting enough to warrant such computation) is generally made by less formal and reliable methods. The lack of absolute reliability usually does not matter; in most cases, the cost of recovering from errors, if and when they occur, is much less than the cost of avoiding them with absolute certainty in the first place.

Designing algorithms is very hard and requires considerable intelligence. *Execution* of algorithms is not hard – arithmetic is easy, once you know how – but *learning* algorithms is hard. Learning algorithms is difficult for most people because of the organization of human memory, as we will see in section 7.5. We will also see why some people learn them much more easily than other people do.

Although one might validly evaluate those people who *learn* algorithms easily as more intelligent than those who do not, most computers that execute algorithms never had to undergo this learning stage. They bypass that process altogether, though at a very great expense of extensibility, as we shall see. The sophisticated human memory organization that makes us so slow to absorb new algorithms proves well worth the expense for a *general* problem solver.

Given that algorithms *guarantee* the *right* answer, one might be led to believe that algorithms were somehow more closely associated with intelligence than heuristics are. Heuristics may seem a sloppy, second-rate way of solving a problem, far inferior to algorithmic methods, but we will now see why this is not the case. Algorithms have far more limited application than at first it might (and did) appear.

One major shortcoming of algorithms (and the first one noticed historically) is computational. Although algorithms are guaranteed to take no more than a finite number of steps, *finite* does not mean *reasonable* – $10^{1,000,000,000,000,000,000}$ is certainly a finite number, but an algorithm requiring that many steps would be completely impractical. The number of steps that can practically be done depends, of course, on both the time available for finding the solution and the time required per step. Before computers, algorithms were of limited usefulness because they took so long to execute, and only a relatively small number of types of problems were simple enough to be solved algorithmically (by hand). With computers executing thousands, and later millions, of arithmetic and logical operations per second, algorithms promised to become more useful again. The number of problems with feasible algorithms became much greater with the first computers and continues to grow as computers grow in speed; the maximum possible speed of computers is bounded, however, by physical limits. That computers were so much faster at executing algorithms than prior methods merely temporarily masked what remained a rather severe problem: No matter how many *times* faster a computer is, mere speed will not help in executing the amounts of computation that can be generated by combinatorial or exponential explosion. The danger of such explosions lurks wherever there are sequences of decisions to be made, as we will see in the following section.

Heuristics were recognized early in AI as the most feasible way of handling tasks requiring intelligence. The fuller significance of heuristic processing would only become clear once the significance and implications of intelligent memory organization became recognized, but five of the most significant limitations of algorithms recognized early in AI – reasons why heuristics were seen as being needed in their stead – are the following.

1. Most problems are not well enough defined to allow the formulation of an algorithm to solve them. Professional programmers (who write algorithmic programs

to solve other people's business or scientific problems) encounter this difficulty constantly and must spend much time with the expert posing the original form of the problem, in order to reformulate and clarify the problem into one that can be dealt with. Frequently the effort fails, with the realization that the original ill-formulated problem was too confused and self-contradictory to be cleaned up. (Many messy problems are, nonetheless, quite amenable to heuristic approaches.) Of the thousands of decisions a person makes each day, the vast majority pertain to such ill-formulated problems, and except when such a decision is critically important, it is simply not worth the effort even to try to clarify the problem.

2. Once a problem is cleanly specified, it is still usually extremely difficult to find an algorithm to solve it. The process of designing an algorithm is not itself algorithmic, and most people do not have very good heuristics for algorithm design. One of the major things people learn when they begin to program is heuristics for algorithm design; it is not a skill most people acquire from other sources (so it is clearly not a skill most people normally apply).

3. Learning an algorithm someone else has designed may be easier than designing it oneself but is still generally quite difficult. Therefore, even when an algorithm is known to be known, people frequently still rely on heuristics rather than learning and applying the algorithm. (Both learning and inventing are easier for heuristics than for algorithms, for reasons that will become clearer in section 7.5.)

4. Even when an algorithm is known in principle, it frequently cannot be applied because it is too expensive of some resource. For instance, there is an algorithm for playing games with well-defined moves that is guaranteed always to select the best possible move against a good opponent (it does not take into account the possibility that a stupid move by the opponent may open up an even stronger position but rather plays with the conservative assumption that the opponent always makes his or her best move). This technique actually works for very simple games, like tic-tac-toe or nim, but a game as complex as chess would require so large a number of steps that one would encounter theoretical limits such as the amount of time left before the expected collapse of the universe and the total number of particles in the universe. The number of steps *is* still finite, but it is very, very large.

5. Even when it is physically possible to apply algorithmic methods, it is frequently still too expensive to be desirable, given the worth of accomplishing the task, especially when far cheaper heuristics are available.

Realizing that virtually all *intelligent* problem solving (formal and informal) is done heuristically is essential to any realistic approach to intelligence.

REPRESENTATION

Much of the effort in early AI research was expended on *problems of computer representation* – both those relating to the use of a computer at all and those on the more abstract level of intelligent problem solving.

Low-level computer representation issues. Before a computer could begin to perform a task, it had to understand the nature of that task. Typically, there was a program embodying knowledge about how to solve any of a class of problems (such as a kind of puzzle). The program "expected" to be told of a particular instance of that class.

At a minimum, a *representation* was needed that would adequately discriminate among possible variants of input problems (such as the different possible chess moves). The program would then have knowledge of how to manipulate the input specifications in a series of "reasoning steps" in such a way as to end up with a representation of the answer. In addition to the input representation of the problem and the output representation of the solution, there was generally also a need for *internal representation,* a means of capturing how the program was thinking about the problem. For instance, in chess, there were problems of specifying the opponent's move to the computer (input representation), of communicating the program's decided move to the opponent (output representation), and also of representing the chess game itself in progress. How the game (or other problem or task) was *represented* was tightly coupled with how the program could make its *decisions.*

Artificial intelligence representation issues. The representation of a problem greatly affects the approach one takes to thinking about it. Alternate adequate representations for problems include some that are much better than others (as judged by the complexity of the set of decisions it requires to be made). For instance, two ways of representing a chess position are (a) the Cartesian view of the chess board itself, specifying by row and column the coordinates of each piece, and (b) the relativistic perspectives of the individual pieces, that is, a set of views of the board, as seen from each piece, of the squares and pieces that may be reached by an offensive maneuver or that pose a defensive threat.

Humans as well as computers are affected by the form of representation. For instance, many paradoxes are based on the obfuscation of something very simple by a bad representation. Also, solving a given problem can be a very different experience, depending on whether it is posed in English, by a graph, by a diagram, by an equation, or by a physical model. People, however, are capable of reformulating badly represented problems into alternative representations more amenable to solution.

How people reformulate problems is a challenging question for research. Early AI found it hard enough to build programs that could solve problems when given a good representation. Before such programs could be developed, however, good representations had to be found or developed. Thus representation was a major area of research in early AI.

REASONING

Another very hard problem in early AI was that of developing programs that could reason. "Innate" to computers (i.e., built into the hardware itself) was the capacity to make simple logical decisions, but most problems require a series of such minuscule decisions before they can be solved. Very impressive progress was made in devising techniques amenable to computer capabilities, but reasoning processes that seemed easy, even obvious, for humans remained very hard to accomplish using any of these early techniques.

A large part of the explanation for this difficulty proved to be that early AI researchers were actually making problem solving harder for computers than it was for people. In an attempt to simplify the problem of reasoning, knowledge was discarded as a complication, and reasoning tasks that minimized the need for prior knowledge were chosen. The mechanisms developed made no use of knowledge; some even carefully distilled all knowledge out.

Researchers avoided giving programs knowledge beyond general know-how for the task, partly because encoding knowledge in a form that the computer could use posed many representational difficulties and AI was already addressing several very difficult issues. A second reason was that knowledge was not believed to be important to the general *mechanisms* of intelligence.

Yet another reason involved a suspicion that prior knowledge was cheating; if someone *knew* enough that was relevant, then little intelligence was needed to solve the problem, the most extreme case being when the person explicitly knew the answer. *Canning* (i.e., having answers directly preassociated with expected inquiries) was used in some early computer programs and can actually cope with some constrained problems, but this technique most quickly encounters problems of computational explosion and is also unable to take context into account; it is thus unsuited for any problem requiring intelligence.

Heuristically guided trial-and-error search.   If we analyze the complexity of problems that people, but not early computers, could do, we find that such problems typically entail a series of choices. The alternatives one has at any given point in the decision-making process depend on what choices one has made so far; any decisions, in turn, affect future options.

A nice way of representing a conclusion and the path of decisions that has led to it is a data structure known as a *tree*. In the case of a simple game like tic-tac-toe, for instance, if one goes first, there are nine possible squares in which to put one's mark. Because each such move can lead to a different situation, we may consider each such possibility a different branch.

For each of the nine branches, or first moves, the opponent has eight alternatives, eight squares left in which to put his mark. We can represent this situation as eight branches stemming from each of the nine branches. We thus have 8×9, or 72, possible two-move sequences so far. For each of the eight of each of the nine branches or two-move sequences, seven possible squares now remain to be marked. We thus have a tree of depth 3, with nine branches coming from the root, eight stemming from each of the nine, and seven branches from each of the eight, which we may mathematically describe as $7 \times 8 \times 9$ branches at level 3.

If we fill out the remainder of the tree down to a total of nine levels, however, the branching does not remain quite so symmetrical. Any branch representing a situation in which one of the players has placed three marks in a row terminates, with no further subbranching, because the game is over and there are no more decisions to be made.

Given such a tree, we can consider the leaves (a *leaf* being a termination point with no branches emerging out from it). Each leaf represents a final game configuration (not unique) and also defines (via the path from the root to the leaf) a complete game history (unique). The tree thus represents a *game space* of all possible games of tic-tac-toe. Making decisions can thus be viewed as moving along the tree from the root to a leaf, and each decision as selecting a subbranch of the current branch for further traversal, with the aim of arriving at the particular leaf (or any of a set of leaves) representing won games (or other types of solutions).

If one could see the full tree laid out before one, it could act as a street map, unambiguously indicating which branches lead to any particular place. More typically, however, one cannot see the full tree – it is far too big! The problem therefore becomes a matter of how to navigate, and this is the essence of *heuristically guided search*. The heuristics are rules that suggest ways to turn or when to go back and try something different. The discovery of such heuristics was, together with the development of representations, a central aspect of early AI.

Trees graphically illustrate the number of possibilities inherent in a process entailing successive decisions. Our tic-tac-toe tree suffers from combinatorial explosion: The width of the tree starts off at 1 at the root (level 0), becomes 9 at level 1, $9 \times 8 = 72$ at level 2, $9 \times 8 \times 7 = 504$ at level 3, and so forth. There are thus 9! or 352,880 ways to fill all nine squares (many games present fewer possibilities because the game terminates when one player places three marks in a row). Tic-tac-toe illustrates a relatively slow form of growth in being merely combinatorial (because the number of options was steadily going down). More typically, such decision trees grow exponentially.

The interesting danger of computational explosion is that it causes problems rather suddenly to become uncontrollable. One can have a method that performs quite well until the problem becomes just a little larger, when the method suddenly and dramatically ceases to be of practical use.

One of the advantages of AI computer models is that though computers can run simulations many *times* faster than humans can by hand, computers are as vulnerable to the limitations imposed by exponential growth as we are – we simply boggle somewhat sooner than they. It just takes them a little longer before they boggle. Computer simulations can thus help discriminate between reasonable and unreasonable difficulty. Any technique involving exponential growth is simply *not* the method used by humans unless the technique is always used only in a restricted way, so that the problem never grows large (i.e., the tree remains shallow).

The term *pruning* refers to the simplification of a search space by writing off an entire branch as unpromising, thereby eliminating it from further consideration. Because of the exponential growth of trees (in number of branches per level), a single pruning decision can be very significant. The closer to the root a pruning decision is made, of course, the greater the effect.

The conceptual process just described takes us to the heart of the difference between early machine intelligence and human intelligence. On a computer most real problems blow up unless the length of the decision sequence is kept very short, because the number of possibilities grows uncontrollably.

The problem of how to prune does not go away if we ignore it. It is simply not possible to visit the entire tree, so without good heuristics guiding trial-and-error searching, the problem solver has, by default, implicitly pruned by the ordering of the branches on the tree. (Branches late in the list will never be reached.) Heuristically guided trial-and-error search tries to do better than chance.

This very hard problem of how to prune all the more frustrated early AI research because of the ease with which people seemed to zero in on solutions. Much later in AI, pruning reemerged as the problem of *interest* (knowing what to pay attention to). When we discuss more recent research in human-intelligence-oriented AI, we will see the role that the organization of human memory plays in this process.

Theorem proving. Another technique used in computer reasoning was formal logic, which had certain advantages of abstraction but shared the computational problems of tree methods and had as a further disadvantage too strong a conception of "truth."

Formal definitions and truth conditions have played an important role in mathematics, but such concepts were badly overextended. This overextension may have been partially due to a confusion of level in the early AI interest in logic. A physical computer itself is based on principles of logic, but as we saw in section 7.2, the details of instantiation are irrelevant to the processes being embodied.

Still, whatever the reason for interest in truth conditions, they are completely inadequate for dealing with the kinds of real world problems that people normally solve. Logic is very sensitive to inconsistency; for instance, a single contradiction within a system makes it possible to "prove" anything. The ability to handle inconsistency, and a kind of sloppiness that simply cannot be tolerated by traditional formal logical systems, proved to be *central* to intelligence. Thus, formal logic was a dead end as a means of representing any problems requiring intelligence (other than logic-based mathematics itself). Efforts in theorem proving were to prove useful in the history of AI, though, in clarifying the irrationality and sloppiness inherent in any truly intelligent system.

Problem reduction.   Another attempt to direct computer reasoning processes used a technique known as *problem reduction*. Behind this approach was the very elegant idea of *recursion*, a method in which one solves a problem by solving subproblems that can include (smaller) versions of the original problem.

General Problem Solver (GPS) is an early AI program and theory developed by Newell, Simon, and Shaw (Newell & Simon, 1961). It was based on the assumption that there are task-independent, general problem-solving mechanisms that can be cleanly separated from knowledge of the task environment.

Newell and Simon describe the essence of GPS as follows:

The main methods of GPS jointly embody the heuristic of means–end analysis . . . typified by the following kinds of common sense argument:

> I want to take my son to nursery school. What's the difference between what I have and what I want? One of distance. What changes distance? My automobile. My automobile won't work. What is needed to make it work? A new battery. What has new batteries? An auto repair shop. I want the repair shop to put in a new battery; but the shop does not know I need one. What is the difficulty? One of communication. What allows communication? A telephone . . . , and so on.

[1972, p. 416]

Although the informal example given above is fairly naturalistic and typical of the problems intelligent people actually solve in day-to-day life, GPS was actually used and tested in such formal domains as crypto-arithmetic (i.e., solving such problems as *PLEASE + SEND = MONEY* for the digits encoded as *P, L, E, A, S, N, D, M, O*, and *Y* such that the numeric equation holds true) and symbolic logic.

Note further that although the nursery-school *problem* is naturalistic, the solution suggested begins to sound strained. An intelligent person truly concerned with taking a son to school in time is likely to know enough not to bog down with auto mechanics until the son has safely reached his destination. Although the example of the nursery school may have been intended as a slight exaggeration to illustrate means–ends analysis most effectively, it does suggest some genuine problems that the GPS approach encounters.

Problem reduction improved upon left-to-right theorem provers in that it gave the reasoning process direction. Means–ends analysis is a very useful and generally valid heuristic; however, without auxiliary sources of guidance, this technique is likely to lead to the loss of perspective, as in the nursery-school case.

7.5.   ISSUES OF HUMAN INTELLIGENCE AS SEEN FROM CURRENT ARTIFICIAL
INTELLIGENCE

Most of the issues of concern to current AI human intelligence research arose through the reformulation of issues motivating early AI programs – reformulations driven by the diagnostic failures of these programs. This, and the unique perspective provided by AI's methodological use of computers, has led AI to focus on a set of issues different from that on which the intelligence subfield of psychology focuses. (There is, however, significant overlap of interest between AI and other subareas of cognitive, social, and developmental psychology.)

We will now discuss these central areas of intelligence research in current AI, showing the roots of each issue in earlier AI. We will, in the process, discuss both *what* AI has to say about human intelligence and *why* AI has uncovered as much as it has about human intelligence.

UNDERSTANDING

Understanding is basic to intelligence. This statement may seem a truism until we remember that, well after the decline of Skinner's theories, intelligence is still *measured* by responses to stimuli. We give students, or subjects, problems to solve, and if they respond with mostly correct answers, we judge them intelligent; if their answers are mostly wrong, then we consider them unintelligent. For all our pretheoretic intuitions of what we mean by *intelligence, understanding* can still sound frighteningly unempirical and elusive, because it is hard to reach a human subject except through input–output (I/O) behavior. AI has given us a way of probing understanding itself – of watching the process involved, watching further processes resulting from that primary process, and examining the knowledge and memory representations that mediate between them.

The roots of the AI research topic of *understanding* can, like those of most current issues of AI, be found in early AI. These roots are found, though, in the *absence* of understanding in early programs and in the *problems* that this absence created. Through these early programs, we have developed a much better sense of what understanding is *not* – and hence of what it is. We will see, for instance, that understanding entails making inferences and results in the ability to make further inferences.

There are, of course, a great many possible levels of understanding; we will shortly see how different kinds of inference lead to different depths of understanding. We will also see how one's understanding is affected by prior knowledge and by the organization of this knowledge in memory. Existing AI programs are still very limited in their understanding capabilities, compared with humans, but progress is being made. More significant than how well current programs understand relative to humans, however, are discoveries about the nature of understanding that have been made in the process of building such programs.

Early AI programs were, basically, limited to performing clever manipulations on their input until they arrived at the correct output. Designing these clever manipulations was frequently a feat of extreme intelligence and deep understanding on the part of the AI researchers involved, and the resulting programs frequently gave a strong *illusion* of intelligence; still, there was little genuine understanding or intelligence *in the programs themselves*. Of course the very fact that they were able to create so effective an illusion was importantly diagnostic in the development of a theory of understanding. There were also some important glimmerings of genuine understanding. For instance, implicit already in the understanding shown by early programs was the use of *expectations* to guide processing of input; this technique would not, however, be an explicitly recognized aspect of understanding for some time.

A convenient and sensible way of handling or avoiding the problem of understanding in the absence of anything better was to rely on task criteria. It was assumed that making a program perform a task previously performed only by intelligent humans (such as symbolic integration, theorem proving, or chess) would necessarily and automatically involve intelligence on the part of the program. Some such tasks, such as geometric analogy (Evans, 1963), had actually been used to test intelligence in humans, to discriminate between more and less intelligent individuals. (Further examples can be found in Minsky, 1963, and Feigenbaum & Feldman, 1963.) The task criterion was made further appealing by the apparent ease with which the proposed intelligence of a program could be empirically verified. Verification of the intelligence of programs was viewed as important, particularly because of the (then justified) skepticism with which many people greeted machine intelligence.

The tendency to ignore the problem of genuine understanding was further encouraged by the orientation of most early AI researchers toward *machine* intelligence, which then dominated the field. Until AI researchers developed a better understanding of the limits of raw computing power, there would be a great temptation to believe that cognitive shortcuts were possible, that they could circumvent understanding, and that sheer power could substitute for selectivity. That was, of course, true for many problems, but those, almost by definition, are not *AI* problems.

One of the most notorious failures of the early days of computers was machine translation (Automatic Language Processing Advisory Committee, 1966; Bar Hillel, 1960; Locke & Booth, 1955; Oettinger, 1960). In the late 1950s, attempts were made to build programs that could translate a natural language text in one language into another, using dictionaries to find corresponding words of one language in the other and grammars to rearrange the word order and to perform other syntactic transformations. What the machine translation programs lacked, however, was any sense of the *meaning* of the texts they were translating. In retrospect, this was clearly an unpromising approach, given that a major problem with *human* translators is their inability to produce an intelligent translation of material they do not understand, such as technical material outside their specialty. At this time, however, brute force was still considered a promising technique for machine intelligence. The machine translation project was finally abandoned as a failure because it did not produce acceptable translations.

Apart from the actual task failure of the early AI attempt at machine translation, the method was theoretically futile – the program was simply manipulating symbols, without any idea of what they stood for. That was the fundamental problem with the approach, as we will see when we consider later and more successful forays into natural language processing and machine translation. More recent work has shown that once a program *understands* a text, retelling it in a language different from the original (i.e., translating it) is not appreciably harder than paraphrasing it in the original language (given that the program can generate in general in the target language).

To demonstrate this, we can consider the following paraphrases composed by a program called SAM (Cullingford, 1978; Schank & Abelson, 1977). The program read the original story *for understanding* and then retold it (in the language specified) from its memory of the conceptual story, without referring back to the original text. The English and the Spanish summaries that follow are unedited versions of the computer program's output, both made up from the same understanding of the original text. The input story was taken from a local newspaper and was selected because the program knew about vehicle accidents.

Input text:

Friday evening a car swerved off Route 69. The vehicle struck a tree. The passenger, a New Jersey man, was killed. David Hall, 27, was pronounced dead at the scene by Dr. Dana Blauchard, medical examiner. Frank Miller, 32, of 593 Foxon Rd, the driver, was taken to Milford Hospital by Flanagan Ambulance. He was treated and released. No charges were made. Patrolman Robert Onofrio investigated the accident.

English summary:

AN AUTOMOBILE HIT A TREE NEAR HIGHWAY 69 FOUR DAYS AGO. DAVID HALL, AGE 27, RESIDENCE IN NEW JERSEY, THE PASSENGER, DIED. FRANK MILLER, AGE 32, RESIDENCE AT 593 FOXON ROAD IN NEW HAVEN, CONNECTICUT, THE DRIVER, WAS SLIGHTLY INJURED. THE POLICE DEPARTMENT DID NOT FILE CHARGES.

Spanish summary:

UN AUTO CHOCO CONTRA UN ARBOL CERCA DE LA CARRETERA 69 EL VIERNES AL ANOCHECER. DAVID HALL, DE 27 ANOS, QUE VIVIA EN NEW JERSEY, EL PASAGERO, SE MURIO. FRANK MILLER, DE 32 ANOS, QUE VIVIA EN 593 CALLE FOXON EN NEW HAVEN, CONNECTICUT, EL CHOFER, QUEDO UN POCO HERIDO. EL DEPARTAMENTO DE POLICIA NO ACUSO A NADIE.

[Carbonell, Cullingford, & Gershman, 1978, p. 19]

Some cross-cultural differences can potentially create problems in translation, but the deeper the understanding of the translator, the better able the translator is to handle them intelligently. Such a problem in fact arises in the example above, from the text "No charges were made." In Spanish-speaking countries, the legal procedure for dealing with a serious accident is somewhat different from that in Connecticut: Whereas in the United States filing charges is one of the first steps that would be taken after an accident in which a crime is suspected, in Hispanic countries the police generally first make an accusation and only file charges after several days of investigation. The program was intelligent in translating this sentence as "EL DEPARTAMENTO DE POLICIA NO ACUSO A NADIE," because it reflects an understanding of "the police did not file charges" as "no criminal prosecution was initiated." Given this understanding, it expressed the idea in *Spanish* by mentioning the corresponding first (non-)action.

The importance of understanding this sentence is even greater if the translator is to paraphrase it intelligently in Russian. In Russia, fault for a collision must always be assigned, and it is the responsibility of the authorities to find someone to blame. Therefore, naive translation of "the police did not file charges" would be understood by most Russians as meaning that there was a cover-up (Carbonell, Cullingford, & Gershman, 1978).

Understanding is thus crucial to intelligent translation. It is, in fact, essential to a wide range of intelligent cognitive activity, the scope of which is suggested by the following examples.

Natural language. We have already seen that the attempt to do translation without understanding was futile and misguided. Understanding is also necessary, however, for a wide range of other natural language activities, including *question answering* (Kolodner, 1980; Lehnert, 1978), *conversation* (Reichman, 1978; Schank & Lehnert, 1979), *story understanding* (Dyer & Lehnert, 1980), and *story generation* (Dehn, 1981a; Meehan, 1976).

Vision. Minsky argued in his classic "frames paper" (Minsky, 1975) that understanding is essential to the process of vision. A major motivation for his development of *frame theory* was the results of his computations of the resources that the brain would need if vision were simply a matter of recording an uninterpreted mass of tiny dots of color, as in a television or magazine picture. His results indicated that the resources needed for vision *without* understanding lay well beyond the outer limits of neurophysiological plausibility; his theory of vision based on understanding required far less, resources well within reasonable limits. His theory also made two important predictions: (a) that we hallucinate stereotypical details that do not exist and (b) that we do not always notice everything that *is* there. There is accumulating experimental evidence for both predictions (Allport & Postman, 1958; Bartlett, 1932; Bower, Karlin, & Dueck, 1975; Bransford & Johnson, 1972; Brewer & Treyens, 1981; Reicher, 1969). Thus, understanding appears to be essential to visual processing.

Game playing. One of the cognitive domains that has been most explored without benefit of understanding is game playing, but even here, understanding is an important part of *intelligent* behavior. A chess master understands the significance of a board position or of a move; it has rich symbolic significance for this person. Strategy, or even tactics, require understanding of the game situation.

Situations. Understanding is also central to processing real world situations. A robot detecting a person prone on the floor needs to *understand* the situation in order to behave intelligently – needs to determine, for instance, whether the person is asleep, relaxing, or dead; without such understanding, the robot is likely to take highly inappropriate and unintelligent action. Similarly, if one perceives that the person sitting next to oneself is drawing a knife, one needs to understand whether that person is preparing to use it as a weapon or in some more innocuous way, before one can react intelligently.

The problem of understanding situations has emerged in AI not only in robotic problem solvers (Fahlman, 1974; Fikes & Nilsson, 1971; Sacerdoti, 1974, 1977, 1979; Sussman, 1975) but also in story processing (Schank & Riesbeck, 1981).

Music and other art forms. Music needs to be understood in order to be processed intelligently, whether the processing consists of performance, analysis, pleasure listening, or creative composition. Without understanding, attempts at composition, for example (Hiller & Isaacson, 1959), are futile. (Some AI theories of musical understanding are discussed in Bamberger, 1976a, 1976b; Laske, 1977; Meehan, 1978; Minsky, 1981; Smoliar, 1971).

The importance of understanding to intelligent behavior may be clearest when it is absent. Many programs have successfully *mimicked* intelligent behavior without actually being intelligent. One of the best-known examples is ELIZA (Weizenbaum, 1966), a program mimicking Rogerian psychotherapists. Consider, for instance, the following fragment from a conversation (via computer terminal) of a person with ELIZA.

ELIZA: What seems to be your problem?
Patient: My mother drinks too much.
ELIZA: Who else in your family drinks too much?

ELIZA's follow-up question sounds very intelligent – as it would be if it were based on the background knowledge and inference that we are so tempted to read into it. Implicit in normal human understanding of this dialogue is that the mother consumes too much alcohol (rather than simply too much fluid); it is also implicit that her ability to fulfill her family roles is probably greatly impaired by this problem, that her problem may be partially caused by other family tensions, and that it may, in turn, lead to further family stress. Were the program actually making such inferences, we would be justified in claiming that it understood (at least to some extent) the patient's complaint and that its response was intelligent.

The ELIZA program did *not* understand what was told it, however, even to the extent that a layman might, and certainly not as a psychiatrist would. The program generated its responses by using a set of rules that simply manipulated the input *text*, bypassing understanding altogether. For instance, the response "Who else in your family" was basically a canned response triggered by *key-word recognition* of the word *mother*. The same rejoinder would have been triggered by *father* or *brother* or any other words on a list of names of family relations associated with that rule, but the program itself was not making any generalization. It did not have the concept of a mother, family, alcoholism, or of how alcoholism could affect family relations. It was simply manipulating symbols, using patterns of text cleverly predicted by its designer.

INFERENCE

Reading a story with any intelligence at all involves being able to infer events and states that were implied by the story, even if they were not explicitly spelled out. For instance, one simply has not understood "John went to three drug stores yesterday" if one does not infer that John was attempting to buy something normally sold in drugstores and that his first two attempts failed to procure it (Cullingford, 1978).

Inference is by no means limited to intelligent processing of language – it is an essential part of any understanding, such as that of the robot confronted with the prone person, the visual inference of hidden lines, or the like. Our examples, however, will primarily draw on natural language both because this area has been rather thoroughly explored and because such examples are easier to present.

Rieger (1975) proposed 16 general classes of inferences that could be made from a conceptualization (the meaning of a sentence).

1. Specification inferences
        John picked up a rock.
        He hit Bill.
        JOHN HIT BILL WITH THE ROCK.
        John and Bill were alone on a desert island.
        Bill was tapped on the shoulder.
        JOHN TAPPED BILL.
2. Causative inferences
        John hit Mary with a rock.
        JOHN WAS PROBABLY MAD AT MARY.

3.   Resultative inferences
       Mary gave John a car.
       JOHN HAS THE CAR.

4.   Motivational inferences
       John hit Mary.
       JOHN PROBABLY WANTED MARY TO BE HURT.

5.   Enablement inferences
       Pete went to Europe.
       WHERE DID HE GET THE MONEY?

6.   Function inferences
       John wants the book.
       JOHN PROBABLY WANTS TO READ IT.

7.   Enablement-prediction inferences
       Dick looked in his cook book to find out how to make a roux.
       DICK WILL NOW BEGIN TO MAKE A ROUX.

8.   Missing enablement inferences
       Mary could not see the horses finish.
       She cursed the man in front of her.
       THE MAN BLOCKED HER VISION.

9.   Intervention inferences
       The baby ran into the street.
       Mary ran after him.
       MARY WANTS TO PREVENT THE BABY FROM GETTING HURT.

10.   Action prediction inferences
       John wanted some nails.
       HE WENT TO THE HARDWARE STORE.

11.   Knowledge-propagation inferences
       Pete told Bill that Mary hit John with a bat.
       BILL KNEW THAT JOHN HAD BEEN HURT.

12.   Normative inferences
       Does Pete have a gall bladder?
       IT'S HIGHLY LIKELY.
       John saw Mary at the beach Tuesday morning.
       WHY WASN'T SHE AT WORK?

13.   State duration inferences
       John handed a book to Mary yesterday.
       Is Mary still holding it?
       PROBABLY NOT.

14.   Feature inferences
       Andy's diaper is wet.
       ANDY IS PROBABLY A BABY.

15.   Situation inferences
       Mary is going to a masquerade.
       SHE WILL PROBABLY WEAR A COSTUME.

16.   Utterance-intent Inferences
       Mary could not jump the fence.
       WHY DID SHE WANT TO?

[Rieger, 1975, 193–195]

Most of the inferences in the examples above are easily *recognized* as plausible inferences, but they are substantially harder to notice when they have not been pointed out. AI's methodology has helped us to be more aware of the pervasiveness of inferencing and also to determine particular inferences needed.

A clear case in point is some mistakes made by TALE-SPIN (Meehan, 1976), a program that makes up Aesop-like stories. The TALE-SPIN program was designed with the inference rules it was expected to need, but several important rules were initially omitted because they were so obvious as to be virtually invisible. The program, however, indicated what was missing in the "mis-spun tales" it produced. The following (from Meehan, 1976) presents four examples of stories resulting from undebugged inference rules; the stories and story fragments were authored by TALE-SPIN (and quoted by Meehan), and the explanations are Meehan's.

1

> One day Joe Bear was hungry. He asked his friend Irving Bird where some honey was. Irving told him there was a beehive in the oak tree. Joe threatened to hit Irving if he did not tell him where some honey was.

Joe has not understood that Irving really has answered his question, albeit indirectly. Lesson: answers to questions can take more than one form. You've got to know about beehives in order to understand that the answer is acceptable. Also, it's polite to give some details when you answer a question. ("Do you know what time it is?""Yes.") So now Irving says that there's honey in the hive and that so-and-so (a bee) owns the honey.

2

> One day Joe Bear was hungry. He asked his friend Irving Bird where some honey was. Irving told him there was a beehive in the oak tree. Joe walked to the oak tree. He ate the beehive.

A further refinement is to unscramble an acceptable answer in the proper fashion, remembering a little better what the original question was.

3

In the early days of TALE-SPIN, all the action focused on a single character. Other characters could respond to him only in very limited ways, when they were asked direct questions, for example. There was no concept of "noticing": If people walk into our room, they need not always announce their presence. You see them. The following story was an attempt to produce "The Ant and the Dove," one of the Aesop fables.

> Henry Ant was thirsty. He walked over to the river bank where his good friend Bill Bird was sitting. Henry slipped and fell in the river. He was unable to call for help. He drowned.

That *was not* supposed to happen. Falling into the river was deliberately introduced to cause the central "problem" of the story. Had Henry been able to call Bill for help, Bill would have saved him, but I had just modified DO-MTRANS so that being in water prevents speech, which seemed reasonable. Since Bill was not asked a direct question, he did not notice his friend drowning in the river. "Noticing" is now an inference from change of location . . . and Bill sees Henry in the river, deduces that Henry's in danger, and rescues him.

4

Here are some rules that were in TALE-SPIN when the next horror occurred. If A moves B to location C, we can infer not only that B is in location C, but that A is also. If you're in a river, you want to get out, because you'll drown if you do not. If you have legs, you might be able to swim out. With wings, you might be able to fly away. With friends, you can ask for help. These sound reasonable. However, when I represented "X fell" as "gravity moved X," I got this story:

> Henry Ant was thirsty. He walked over to the river bank where his good friend Bill Bird was sitting. Henry slipped and fell in the river. Gravity [having neither legs, wings, nor friends] drowned.

[1976, pp. 127–129]

In our discussion of the need to understand a text in order to translate it intelligently, we saw how same-language paraphrase similarly reflected one's understanding. A paraphrase can also serve to show the inferences that were made. Below is another example of a story understood by SAM, with the paraphrase it produced when instructed to spell out all the details it inferred.

Original story: John went to New York by bus. On the bus he talked to an old lady. When he left the bus, he thanked the driver. He took the subway to Leone's. On the subway his pocket was picked. He got off the train and entered Leone's. He had some lasagna. When the check came, he discovered he could not pay. The management told him he would have to wash dishes. When he left, he caught a bus to New Haven.

Computer paraphrase: JOHN WENT TO A BUS STOP. HE WAITED AT IT A FEW MINUTES. HE ENTERED A BUS. THE DRIVER GOT THE TICKET FROM JOHN. HE WENT TO A SEAT. HE SAT DOWN IN IT. WHILE JOHN WAS ON THE BUS AN OLD LADY AND JOHN TALKED. THE DRIVER TOOK JOHN TO NEW YORK. HE WENT TO THE DRIVER. WHEN GETTING OFF THE BUS JOHN THANKED THE DRIVER. JOHN GOT OFF IT.

HE ENTERED A STATION. HE PUT A TOKEN INTO THE TURNSTILE. HE WENT TO THE PLATFORM. HE WAITED AT IT A FEW MINUTES. HE ENTERED A SUBWAY CAR. A THIEF WENT TO JOHN. THE THIEF PICKED JOHN'S POCKET. HE WENT. JOHN WENT TO THE SEAT. HE SAT DOWN IN IT. THE DRIVER TOOK JOHN TO LEONE'S.

HE ENTERED LEONE'S. HE LOOKED AROUND INSIDE IT. HE SAW HE COULD GO TO A TABLE. HE WENT TO IT. HE SAT DOWN IN THE SEAT. HE ORDERED SOME LASAGNA. THE WAITER INDICATED TO THE CHEF JOHN WOULD LIKE HIM TO PREPARE SOMETHING. THE CHEF PREPARED THE LASAGNA. THE WAITER GOT IT FROM THE CHEF. THE WAITER WENT TO THE TABLE. HE SERVED THE LASAGNA TO JOHN. HE BECAME FULL.

HE ASKED THE WAITER FOR THE CHECK. JOHN GOT IT FROM THE WAITER. JOHN DISCOVERED HE WAS UNABLE TO PAY THE CHECK. THE MANAGEMENT TOLD JOHN HE WOULD HAVE TO WASH THE DISHES. HE ENTERED THE KITCHEN. HE WASHED THE DISHES. HE LEFT LEONE'S.

HE WENT TO THE BUS STOP. HE WAITED AT IT A FEW MINUTES. HE ENTERED THE BUS. THE DRIVER GOT THE TICKET FROM JOHN. HE WENT TO THE SEAT. HE SAT DOWN IN IT. THE DRIVER TOOK JOHN TO NEW HAVEN. HE GOT OFF THE BUS.

[Schank & Abelson, 1977, pp. 178–179]

Normally people do not retell stories in such long, boring detail, but they do privately make such inferences as part of their normal understanding of the story.

A deeper level of understanding (displaying greater intelligence) is recognizing the point of a story and is thus demonstrated by the ability to give a short but apt paraphrase. This is yet a different kind of inference – inferring the significance. Such understanding is demonstrated by a program called FRUMP (Dejong, 1979), which skimmed a United Press International news story and produced a summary.

Original story: The United States welcomed Soviet Foreign Minister Andrei Gromyko Thursday with a statement it will continue to abide by the expiring Strategic Arms Accord so long as Russia also observes its provisions.

The Administration told Congress in a letter it will issue a "unilateral statement" pledging the United States to observe the 1972 SALT I agreement even after its Oct. 3 expiration date.

The decision was conveyed to Sen. John Sparkman, D-Ala., Chairman of the Senate Foreign Relations Committee, diplomatic sources said. It sparked immediate concern among some senators, including Sen. Henry Jackson, D-Wash.

At the State Department, Secretary of State Cyrus Vance began a first round of talks with Gromyko in an effort to break the current stalemate in U.S. Soviet Strategic Arms Limitation Talks and open the way to a new accord.

Gromyko was scheduled to meet President Carter Friday. The Soviet official said on arrival Wednesday progress would require movement by both sides. but U.S. officials said they anticipated no major Soviet concessions.

Computer paraphrase: CYRUS VANCE MET WITH ANDREI GROMYKO IN THE UNITED STATES ABOUT THE SALT AGREEMENT.

Other approaches to this problem include Lehnert (1981) and Wilensky (1982).

This section has illustrated the importance of inference and the importance of the development of AI programs for helping us to recognize inferences. Two further aspects of inference remain to be discussed: the dependence of inferences on world knowledge and control of the inference application process. The solution to the problem of controlling inferences thus involves several topics yet to be discussed: memory organization, variable depth processing, and reminding-controlled reasoning.

KNOWLEDGE

We saw how early AI avoided knowledge in the interest of simplification – and in the end made the reasoning task harder than it need be. Handling large amounts of knowledge does introduce some hard problems of management, but problems caused by paucity of knowledge are far more significant. Lack of knowledge in a computer program can make performing the task much harder than it would be for humans because the program is then forced to figure out far more than the human needs to.

Further, there are cases in which prior knowledge is absolutely essential to intelligent behavior. Consider, for instance, the question of the point at which one pays for food in a restaurant. In traditional restaurants, of course, one pays after eating, just before leaving; in cafeterias, once one has possession of the food but before starting to eat it; in fast-food joints, after ordering but before receiving one's food; and in eat-all-you-want smorgasbords, before even selecting one's meal.

What is the general rule from which the answer could be computed? There really is none. The idea of payment could perhaps be derived from a more general idea of barter or exchange of goods and services, and some constraints on the sequence could perhaps be derived from general knowledge about dishonesty and distrust, but the problem is still greatly underconstrained. The question of when one pays in a restaurant simply cannot be answered from first principles. There are conventions and people learn to follow them. Such social conventions are called *scripts* (Schank & Abelson, 1977).

Thus AI has increasingly become concerned with defining the kind of knowledge people have and learning how it is stored, accessed, used, and acquired (Black, Wilkes-Gibbs, & Gibbs, 1982). The reason for this focus is the growing awareness of the extent of world knowledge on which people's ability to do anything requiring intelligence rests. An AI simulation of an expert chemist requires determining what that chemist *knows*. Similarly, a simulation of a 3-year-old's linguistic ability (Selfridge, 1980) requires discovering what the child knows (and other things). Even branches of AI not directly interested in human intelligence have entered the knowledge business in a big way in the last few years, partially because of the success of MYCIN, DENDRAL, and other such programs.

Even when a program omits only knowledge that is in principle inferable, consequences can be severe. The additional inferencing required is far more serious than it might at first appear, because the problem of combinatorial explosion can be avoided only by keeping inference chains relatively small. Further, the lack of knowledge eliminates clues as to which direction the problem solver would find most promising. The single most frustrating problem of machine intelligence that propelled the interest in human intelligence, in fact, was the control of exponential explosion. Exponential explosion was all-pervasive in machine approaches, yet people seemed to avoid it. If systematically trying everything does not work, and if a random search for a solution does not work, how did anyone ever find the right answer to anything?

Let us return to the idea of a problem tree. Heading straight for a leaf does not take us very long – the problem arises when we try to visit *every* leaf. So if we can somehow tell what direction to head in, we will reach the solution quickly enough. How does one *find* the right direction? Prior experience and prior knowledge tell us which way to go in mental space. This is why if we are in a restaurant and want something to eat we "realize" that we should try asking the waitress before drawing a gun and checking to see whether the cashier has an apple in his or her pants pocket. It is *possible* that the cashier has such an apple and that it would alleviate our hunger, but asking the waitress for something listed on the menu is the more promising approach.

For most forms of intelligent processing, both general and specific knowledge is required. General knowledge and general techniques (such as means–end analysis and Rieger inferences) are important because they help define the problem space; still, with nothing *but* general knowledge as a guide, one can wander forever without ever finding anything. Specific knowledge is important because it tells us which direction to take; still, with nothing *but* specific knowledge, we will not understand the problem space through which we are so purposefully striding. We might head east and become trapped in a local cul-de-sac. General knowledge is needed to give us a more global view, to increase robustness.

The observation that even stupid people have basic natural language capabilities and that even moderately bright people have problems with calculus and formal logic and chess caused early AI researchers to focus on the latter problems as more interesting. Still, one of the reasons why these and many academic subjects are so hard to learn may be that students try to master them in a knowledge-starved environment.

It is easy to underestimate all that goes into processing natural language because people seem to acquire it and use it so easily. Computer models have revealed the vast quantities of knowledge we actually have and use. For instance, in understanding the sentence "The policeman held up his hand and stopped the car," we are using knowledge about communication (the raising of a hand can be a signal meaning "halt"), authority (most motorists recognize traffic cops' right to direct traffic and comply with their directions), basic auto mechanics (brakes physically stop cars), basic anatomy and the spatial organization of a car (we know how the motorist reached the brake and used it), and much, much more.

Noam Chomsky has explained the ease with which children learn something as hard as language, although they labor so painfully to learn much simpler subject matter, such as mathematics, as being due to innate, special-purpose capabilities of the human brain. A natural extension of such an argument would be to grade all subject matter in terms of the amount of effort people *seem* to put into learning it, to derive the rest of the idiosyncratic human brain design! Alternatively, however, we could, with the help of AI programs, recognize the huge amount of knowledge that is required for most cognitive activities and could reexamine curricula in that light. For instance, most people find Newtonian mechanics easier to learn than Einsteinian relativity. Still, most people played with balls before formally studying physics, and even though they may never have realized that the flight of the ball they were running to catch was parabolic, they did have many opportunities to build up intuitions and to acquire relevant knowledge. Many of these people first encounter relativity, however, in a knowledge vacuum so great that their ability ever to understand it at all is amazing!

A child spends years acquiring his or her first language, undergoing massive learning and mental reorganization. This process does not *look* as hard as academic training because each step is eased by prior knowledge and memory organization. Some educators are already applying this realization in efforts to create similarly rich environments in other areas (Papert, 1973, 1980).

BELIEFS

Beliefs serve a role very similar to that of knowledge in an intelligent understander. For example, the simple sentence pair

> I was out until 2:00 A.M. yesterday.
> Boy, did my wife give it to me.

requires a set of beliefs about husband–wife relationships and normal times of arrival and departure. Surely all readers realize that the speaker came home too late, but this realization is in no way contained in the sentence. The speaker might just as well have come home too *early*. Still, we know something about normal times of arrival as well as about the nature of wives' usual complaints under normal circumstances. In addition, we need to make all sorts of inferences. Our hero came home, presumably, but the story says no such thing. What did his wife give to him? How do we know that the expression is an idiom? Why not attempt to find the referent of *it* somehow, as we normally would?

The answer to all these questions requires an adequate cognitive model of the world, complete with beliefs and expectations concerning the normal behavior of people within it. Even the dullest of people can make inferences such as those required here, and to do so they must rely on an available store of beliefs.

POLITICS (Carbonell, 1979a) is an AI program that could assume the political beliefs of either an American conservative or a liberal about the goals of the United States, Russia, and third-world nations and about their relative priority of the goals of each. All other knowledge and mechanisms were the same in both political variants of the program (including natural language capabilities sufficient for reading certain political stories and answering questions about them).

The effects of variation of beliefs were explored by giving each political variant of the program the same stories to read and then probing the understanding of each with a series of questions.

Below are examples of dialogues held with each of its two perspectives.

Input text: Russia massed troops on the Czech border.

Dialogue with conservative:
Q: Why did Russia do this?
A: BECAUSE RUSSIA THOUGHT THAT IT COULD TAKE POLITICAL CONTROL OF CZECHOSLOVAKIA BY SENDING TROOPS.
Q: What should the United States do?
A: THE UNITED STATES SHOULD INTERVENE MILITARILY.

[1979a, p. 67]

Dialogue with liberal:

Q: Why did Russia do this?

A: BECAUSE RUSSIA WANTED TO INCREASE ITS POLITICAL INFLUENCE OVER CZECHOSLOVAKIA.

Q: What should the United States do?

A: THE UNITED STATES SHOULD DENOUNCE THE RUSSIAN ACTION IN THE UNITED NATIONS.

[1979a, p. 72]

Input text: The U.S. Congress is expected to approve the Panama Canal Treaty.

Dialogue with conservative:

Q1: Should the U.S. approve the treaty?

A1: NO, THE TREATY IS BAD FOR THE UNITED STATES.

Q2: Why is the treaty bad for the U.S.?

A2: THE UNITED STATES WOULD LOSE THE CANAL TO PANAMA AND THE UNITED STATES WOULD BE WEAKER.

Q3: What might happen if the United States loses the Canal?

A3: RUSSIA WILL TRY TO CONTROL THE CANAL.

Q4: Why would Russia try to take over the Canal?

A4: RUSSIA WANTS TO EXPAND ITS MILITARY CONTROL. THE PANAMA CANAL HAS HIGH MILITARY VALUE.

Q5: How might this happen?

A5: THE UNITED STATES MAY NOT BE ABLE TO STOP ANYONE TAKING OVER THE PANAMA CANAL. TORRIJOS IS A COMMUNIST. TORRIJOS WILL LET RUSSIA CONTROL THE CANAL.

Q6: Why should the U.S. worry about Russia taking over the Canal?

A6: BECAUSE RUSSIA WANTS TO CONTROL THE WORLD.

Q7: What should the U.S. do to stop Russia from taking over the Canal?

A7: CONGRESS SHOULD VOTE AGAINST THE PANAMA CANAL TREATY.

[1979a, pp. 32–33]

Dialogue with liberal:

Q1: Should the U.S. approve the treaty?

A1: YES, THE PANAMA CANAL TREATY IS GOOD FOR THE UNITED STATES.

Q2: Why is the treaty good?

A2: THE PANAMA CANAL TREATY IMPROVES RELATIONS WITH LATIN AMERICAN COUNTRIES.

Q3: What happens if the U.S. keeps the Canal?

A3: THIS WILL CAUSE DISCONTENT AND CONFLICT IN PANAMA AND LATIN AMERICA.

Q4: Why would this lead to conflict?

A4: THE CANAL ZONE IS A UNITED STATES COLONY, LATIN AMERICA DOES NOT LIKE COLONIAL-ISM. THE UNITED STATES WOULD MAINTAIN COLONIALISM.

Q5: What if Russia tries to take over the Canal?

A5: RUSSIA DOES NOT WANT CONFLICT WITH THE U.S. RUSSIA WILL STAY OUT OF THE CANAL IF THE UNITED STATES DEFENDS IT. THE UNITED STATES DEFENDING THE CANAL IS PART OF THE TREATY.

[1979a, p. 36]

These examples illustrate the importance of beliefs in the ability to understand intelligently and to analyze a situation.

Beliefs also play an important role, of course, in political *arguments*. ABDUL/ILANA is a program with argumentation strategies and domain knowledge that enable it to argue about whether the Israelis or the Arabs were responsible for the 1967 war. Depending on whether it is run with "Arab" or with "Israeli" beliefs, it will take one side or the other. Its beliefs affect both how it understands the opponent's assertions and how it comes up with an effective reply – which turn out to be two very closely related issues (Flowers, McGuire, & Birnbaum, 1982).

MEMORY ORGANIZATION

We have already seen how machine intelligence evolved into human intelligence research. Central to simulation of human intelligence was a study of human memory mechanisms and the reasons why they coped with complexity so much better than mechanisms that had been developed so far for the computer.

Memory organization was not seen explicitly as a problem in early AI because more basic issues of computer representation and process demanded attention first. The native organization of memory in computers was substantially different, and its implications needed exploration.

Knowledge structures such as frames (Goldstein & Papert, 1976; Minsky, 1975; Winograd, 1975) and scripts (Cullingford, 1978; Schank & Abelson, 1977) were very valuable for AI programs in that they (a) provided a way of organizing the tremendous amounts of knowledge the need for which was becoming increasingly apparent and hence (b) allowed attention to be directed during processing of input. These structures were originally created to meet the need for *external* organization (for example, of visual input), but they were soon found also to be useful for internal organization (such as organizing one's information about birthday parties (see Charniak, 1972, 1977). As we have already seen, scripts provide a way of organizing knowledge about stereotypical situations.

Exploration of the potential of frames and scripts leads to a greater appreciation for reconstructive memory (Bartlett, 1932) and hence to MOPs (Kolodner, 1980; Lebowitz, 1980; Schank, 1979) and K-LINEs (Minsky, 1980). All of these serve both as computer data structures and as models, at an appropriate level of abstraction, of aspects of human memory.

By far the single most important issue within the natural language processing part of AI concerns memory (Norman & Schank, in press). Early work in natural language did not attempt to include memory in any serious way; for this reason, the systems that were built were inference-limited, that is, they had difficulty in drawing conclusions from statements and in tying statements together in an input. The role played by memory proves to be extremely important, as any given stream of sentences will not spell out all the references, entailments, implied propositions, and basic underlying assumptions that are an implicit part of the text they compose.

As the amount of knowledge in natural language processing systems grows, the importance of the organization of this knowledge in memory becomes increasingly critical. In a system that could easily be overwhelmed by the sheer amount of knowledge available to it, the ability to find the information one needs when one needs it is crucial. In order to do so, one's memory must be organized so as to be able to *find* what one "knows." For example, a system that placed information about "John's trip to Paris" under "trips" would not be able to answer questions about whether John flew or went sightseeing unless information relevant to these subjects was also indexed as being "trip related." Such indexing is easy enough, but how does a system attempt to answer the questions "has John climbed any tall buildings?" or "has John had any vacation time this year?" Questions such as these rely upon multiple indexing of inputs in memory at processing time. An intelligent processor needs to have stored the input about John's trip in a great many different places if it is to find what it needs efficiently. The consequences of inadequate filing can be perceived as lack of a "good memory" when in fact they are the result of poor memory *organization*. This poor organization depends on initially poor processing or, in the terms we have used above, on a failure to perceive accurately what will prove to be interesting and useful organization.

One effect of such poor organization can be seen in an inability to understand new inputs when that understanding depends on effective organization. The ability to understand an input crucially depends on one's original categorization of ideas and events to which those inputs refer. If one's categorization is "unintelligent," that is, if one has made insufficient multiple categorizations of prior events in memory as a guard against future needs, then one will find it hard to understand many statements that correspond only partially or abstractly to one's prior experience. The transmuting of an initial categorization into a categorization in a different domain is thus an important part of intelligence.

Some of the work on memory organization brought secondary benefits when many of the very hard problems from early AI finally became tractable. Let us consider some of these.

VARIABLE DEPTH PROCESSING: PRUNING REVISITED

As we have noted, early versions of AI programs had serious difficulties with combinatorial, or worse, exponential, explosion; we have also seen how this problem was represented by trees and the need to prune them. For instance, when a computer sought to understand a sentence, there were always many potentially matching Rieger inference patterns, and each of these generated more possible inferences. The potential for an explosion of relevant inferences was very great indeed, especially if inferences could possibly be in error, a capability that turned out to be crucial for real comprehension. From every input one could create myriad possible paths. For example, for the input "John hit Mary with a bat," we could begin an inference path that would describe why he might have done so, the consequences for him, the consequences for her, how he came to have the bat, the consequences for the bat, and so on. Each of these inferences would breed numerous potential others. For instance, following the path of possible consequences for John, we can imagine from the consequences for Mary that Mary might have died and John might be liable for arrest. This eventuality would cause John to want to hide, which might cause problems of conscience for his mother, and so on.

The problem for an intelligent understander is knowing which path to pursue when and how far. If *bat* had been *cat* or *rat* or *hat* or *pat*, we would have had very different stories. The stories would differ because of our ability to infer rather than simply because of the information directly present. Thus it might be more appropriate to focus on the consequences for Mary with *bat*, or the cat with *cat*, and John's emotions with *pat* and John's mental health with *rat*. Here, again, we are relying on available beliefs. More important for the present discussion, however, knowing where to focus and when is of crucial importance.

In the course of research on inference, the programs built tended to have one of two extremely different problems. The inference mechanisms we devised were either too general or too restrictive. For instance, the MARGIE program (Schank, 1975) used its inference mechanisms so that it simply inferred from everything. The basic mechanism worked, but controlling it was an unsolved problem. As part of the solution to that problem, two control mechanisms were developed. The first, causal chain construction, focused the inference process so that the only inferences made were those that tied events together by connecting them (a) to the states that permitted their occurrence or (b) to the resultant states that they affected. The second, embodied in the SAM program (Cullingford, 1978), was the use of scripts (Schank & Abelson, 1977) to supply packages of premade inferences in standard situations that the program knew about.

During research into the kind of high-level memory structures that guided inference, however, it was found that plans and goals were useful (Carbonell, 1979a; Meehan, 1976; Schank & Abelson, 1977; Wilensky, 1978) – and the job of inferring the plans and goals under which people operate proved as complex and uncontrolled a task as the original inference problem!

Two further mechanisms were then developed – those of *interestingness* and *partial parsing* of input – to help control the inference process (Schank, 1978b; Schank, Lebowitz, & Birnbaum, 1978). Simply stated, interestingness involves the idea that because people cannot pay attention to all possible inferences, they seek those inference paths that seem most likely to prove relevant and then pursue those paths that are found interesting. The partial parsing idea came into play as a method of controlling the unnecessary processing of new input that is not found to be interesting. This control allowed time to concentrate on processing in depth the input that *had* been determined to be interesting. One could thus buy extra processing time in one area at the expense of less processing time elsewhere. With the development of a theory of memory organization, the old problem of pruning, or of heuristically directed search, started becoming tractable.

Interestingness is an essential guide to intelligent processing of *any* complex problem. We have been implicitly discussing it in terms of story understanding, but it is equally important in such tasks as making discoveries (Simon, 1979). Major discoveries are always preceded by many that are minor, and one needs to know *which* of the preliminary observations are most likely to lead to something important – that is, which are worth further exploration. If one finds all minor discoveries equally interesting, or has a poor sense of which ones are interesting, one simply will never get far enough through the exponential search space to find anything worthwhile.

AM (Lenet, 1976) is a program that makes mathematical discoveries. On one especially inspired run, in which it started with no more of a mathematical knowledge base than the concepts of set theory, it discovered the integers, the four arithmetic operations, prime numbers, and an area of math dealing with maximal factors of prime numbers with which the program designer himself was completely unfamiliar (this area eventually proved to have been previously discovered by an obscure Indian mathematician). AM was able to make such progress from its rudimentary initial conceptions of mathematics by having a good sense of what was interesting, such as borderline cases.

BACON (Langley, 1979) is a program that discovers empirical laws from observational data. Its most impressive discoveries include versions of Coulomb's law, Galileo's laws for the pendulum and constant acceleration, the idea gas law, Kepler's third law, and Ohm's law. BACON finds such phenomena as regularities interesting and actively looks for them in the raw data.

REMINDING: REASONING AND PATTERN RECOGNITION REVISITED

We have seen that memory organization is central to intelligence. Reminding is an important phenomenon in that it gives us insight into how we have organized knowledge, beliefs, and experiences in our memories; as such, it has been used as a diagnostic by Freudians and other psychologists.

Reminding also has an important *function* in intelligence, however, as a way of finding solutions. Research in reminding has, in this sense, evolved from the early AI concern with *reasoning*. Early AI attempted to solve problems using formal reasoning, such as theorem proving. Later, natural language work encountered the problem of causal chain construction with more naturalistic inferencing. Both forms of inferencing suffered, however, from the problem of exponential explosion. Reminding is a way of bypassing the very hard problem of reasoning. It can serve the same function while avoiding the computational problems (Dehn, 1981b; McGuire, Birnbaum, & Flowers, 1981).

Reminding-based reasoning is, in fact, part of the understanding process. Depending on how one's attention is initially directed, one will notice different aspects of the input; the abstract representation of the input serves as an index into prior memories, which then become a source of predictions that in turn further direct one's attention. This theory explains, for instance, how a chess master can understand the implications of a move or position at a glance: He actually is *not* determining all possible consequences as chess programs have tried to do. Recognition at a glance, of course, is the old pattern-matching problem, but there is now available a memory organization serving as cognitive context to direct one's attention to the appropriate aspects. In this same chunk of memory was incorporated, plainly, the memory of a prior game. One may carefully check one's intuitions by a follow-up, more formal chain of reasoning, but inasmuch as one has determined the *direction* the reasoning will take, the decision tree has already been pruned down to a stalk.

How well this reminding-based reasoning method works depends on one's observations about the input in the first place, which depend on what one earlier sensed to be important. Experts tend to have very good memory organizations for representing the areas of their expertise and thus are very good at knowing where to direct their attention, a facility that in turn allows them to penetrate to the heart of a matter. Novices have very crude memory organizations and are likely to be distracted by irrelevancies, thrashing around for a long time without much success. Novices become experts by having experiences that build memory adequately. Teaching can greatly expedite the learning process, not by rote introduction of more examples, but by constructively directing the students' attention so that they start noticing the right things.

FORGETTING

The other side of reminding is forgetting. In explaining the drive from machine intelligence to human intelligence research, we claimed that certain characteristics that had at first seemed weaknesses began to be recognized as sources of strengths – fundamental to the robustness and generality of human intelligence. We have already seen a few examples, but yet another is the phenomenon of forgetting.

The data bases of traditional computers never forget anything. This characteristic can be very useful in keeping financial records and for other traditional computer applications. Humans, of course, do forget *nonmnemonic* details. Why is this the case, and how does it relate to intelligence? To discover the answer, we have to consider separately several different sources of forgetting.

1.   The item was never really noticed in the first place.
2.   The item was placed in memory but has since been overwhelmed by a generalization.
3.   The item is somewhere in memory but inaccessible (a) from current context and cues or (b) from anywhere else.

Not noticing everything in the first place is a virtue, necessary to keep processing within reasonable bounds. Discarding information once it has served its purposes helps minimize internal distractions (such as spurious inferences and considerations) and thus makes the job of intelligent ignoring a little easier. Masking items so that they are visible only when actually relevant is a yet more important means of eliminating distractions.

On the other hand, although the capacity to forget seems to be essential to intelligence, greatly reducing the time and space needed, an intelligent system should not forget things that it *needs* to remember. In fact, if one has made intelligent predictive generalizations during input, one should be able to find what one needs when one needs it. This phenomenon of predictive generalization, in fact, can help explain why people effortlessly remember things that they understand (have a good organization for) but have much difficulty memorizing things by rote, without a good place to put them or a good way to find them later.

ERRORS

Computers are popularly viewed as being very logical, accurate, and precise and as never making mistakes; the term *computer errors* generally actually refers to the *human* errors of programmers and data entry clerks. In the early days of computers, such characteristics were seen as indications that machine intelligence could *surpass* human intelligence. More recently it has become increasingly apparent that until computer programs start making *their own* mistakes, they will never approach the general intelligence of humans.

Errors prove vital to intelligence in ways that had not been anticipated. Part of the lack of foresight was due to inadequate discrimination between intelligent and unintelligent mistakes. In the context of testing, the former reflect cognitive techniques that usually work (i.e., good heuristics), the latter, grossly inadequate memory organization. An intelligent mistake can actually be a stronger positive predictor of competence or of intelligence than a correct answer, which may have been reached by mistake or by chance. Errors are important windows into the process by which the task is being accomplished. Optical illusions, for instance, reveal far more about the human vision process than do correct perceptions.

Even more important, however, is the role errors play in learning. The following three AI efforts have exploited the virtue of errors in the learning process.

1. LOGO was a pedagogical project that stemmed from an AI project largely centered around *learning by debugging* (Papert, 1973, 1980).

2. What was learned or confirmed by the LOGO experience was reintegrated into AI in a program called HACKER (Sussman, 1975), which developed successively better theories by doing the best it currently could, failing, discovering the bug, and then producing a new theory that took the newly discovered bug into account.

3. Most recently, errors have been hypothesized to be central to learning in the most basic sense, in a theory called Failure Driven Memory, or FDM (Schank,

1981). The role of errors in learning, according to this hypothesis, is threefold. First, errors detected during processing force one to shift one's attention, helping one to focus on what is important. Second, this focus and extra processing are reflected in altered memory organization, including a branch from the place in memory that was guiding processing when one made the error. Finally, future processing of similar situations takes this newly learned discrimination into account.

What is important about failure-driven memory is that it is a model of *integrated learning* – the all-pervasive evolution of one's memory organization that is happening all the time and is affecting all further processing that one ever does.

CREATIVITY

One of the areas of intelligence most difficult to investigate has been creativity – its source and its relation to other forms of intelligence. A particularly salient *superficial* characteristic of a creative solution is its difference from more "standard" ones. This characteristic has caused some researchers to be unduly concerned with introducing sources of variability, ignoring the motivation *behind* such variance. The processing power of computers allowed, in fact, experimentation with the theory of *random generate and test* as a source of creative solutions.

As in other generate-and-test paradigms (Nilsson, 1971), ideas would be proposed, evaluated, and then either used as a basis for further work or discarded. Thus, although an "intelligent" or "careful" approach consisted of systematically working through the tree of possibilities, a "creative" approach was hypothesized to proceed by random selection of branches to follow. This was a grossly inadequate model. Although it led to places different from those indicated by systematic approaches, the space of possible solutions was so large (in any problem for which a creative solution seemed possible and useful) that the probability of finding something good by that approach was vanishingly small. Further, it is dissatisfying as a process model of human creative thought.

An early machine intelligence program, for instance, attempted to compose music by random generate and test (Hiller & Isaacson, 1959): A random note generator proposed next notes, which would then be considered by evaluation functions, basically machine encodings of the prescriptive rules of species counterpoint. (Species counterpoint is a highly formalized form of counterpoint developed in the eighteenth century by J. J. Fux as a pedagogical technique for teaching human students freer counterpoint.) From a purely computational standpoint, relatively few tries were needed early in the cantus to find an acceptable note, but the task became very hard very fast. The method is analytically implausible even before it encounters computational difficulty because of the *nature* of the errors that were made. Although it is certainly true that a student writing a cantus firmus (the first voice, or line, of the counterpoint) makes many wrong decisions, each one is motivated by the student's current working hypotheses; errors should thus be fairly predictable, given a model of the student's hypotheses. Further, each failure should (according to the FDM hypothesis) modify the student's understanding of the problem and should hence spur a somewhat modified new assault.

According to old, machine intelligence AI, we see that intelligence meant systematicity, whereas creativity meant unexpected leaps. According to more recent human intelligence AI, however, we see that intelligence is the ability to abstract information from input that is relevant with respect to future processing needs, and creativity is an extremely general form of intelligence; a creative person is someone especially good at maintaining his or her own memory organization. The fundamental test of intelligence is the ability to organize input intelligently for future reference; the fundamental test of creativity is the ability to use input to diagnose problems of memory organization. Intelligence is understanding things in terms of what one already knows, with failure-driven memory as a source of memory growth; creativity entails a more fundamental mental reorganization motivated by anomalies. Thus, theory generation, story generation, and paper generation are all tests of creativity and hence, ultimately, of general intelligence.

We may now return to the question of how creative solutions are reached. Unique solutions involve basically the same mechanisms as less creative ones but work from a different memory organization. Thus, many "creative" solutions result not from actual *reorganization* but simply from a different *prior* organization. This could indicate a prior creative reorganization or merely reflect what one has been taught. In fact, the alienness of an individual coming from a different culture or paradigm can produce an illusion either of stupidity (because he or she misses what is "obvious") or of creativity (because of the different perspective he or she has).

Still, ideas that are different just to be different cannot, with any consistency, lead to creative solutions. By the same token, neither can randomly different memory organizations. The key to creative solutions is their extreme *appropriateness,* and this aspect depends largely on the adaptability of memory organization. Thus, if one were to order the intelligence required for various kinds of processing, the continuum would look as follows:

1.   special purpose program
2.   script processing
3.   intelligent, reminding-based FDM processing
4.   creative reorganizing of memory.

Creativity is, then, the most extreme form of general intelligence.

7.6.   IMPLICATIONS OF ARTIFICIAL INTELLIGENCE FOR ISSUES IN THE
       PSYCHOLOGY SUBFIELD OF INTELLIGENCE

Now that we have seen AI hypotheses concerning the characteristics and mechanisms of basic human intelligence, we can consider some implications of AI research for issues in the psychology subfield of intelligence.

GENERALITY OF INTELLIGENCE

AI, through its successes and failures, has revealed much, and has suggested yet more, about the nature of general intelligence: First, early machine intelligence efforts and more recent "expert systems" have produced some examples of truly nongeneral "intelligence" – programs that can achieve particular tasks usually thought to require intelligence yet lacking the ability or even enhanced potential for performing any other tasks. Such programs have helped clarify the meaning of intelligence (in motivating reformulations that would exclude them) and have also, by the contrast they provide, increased our sensitivity to the generality (in the sense of cross-domain transference) of human intelligence. Second, early AI work has shown that *ability to reason* is not the basis of general intelligence. If it were, theorem provers would, at least in principle, have been close to an embodiment of pure general intelligence. The flaw with this theory was found to be the amount of time needed to solve problems by pure reasoning – the complexity of most problems meant that the solution would be too long in coming to be of any practical use. Rather, general problem-solving ability called for the ability to deal with complexity – the ability to focus one's attention appropriately and to ignore irrelevancies, both in perceiving the original problem and in controlling inferences made on the way to the solution. This ability, in turn, was found to depend on memory *organization*: The original perception of a problem is controlled by prior expectations of what is likely to be important or interesting; finding the solution to the problem is greatly expedited if one reminds oneself of relevant similar prior experiences.

Then, too, it was observed that knowledge can be transferred from one domain to another if the right generalizations can be derived from memory. Analogies should not be viewed as a reasoning task but rather as a diagnostic probe of memory organization. *Specific knowledge* is thus essential to *general intelligence*. Its acquisition is necessary for the construction and reorganization of the kind of memory necessary for general problem solving. Its existence is necessary for the application of general intelligence capabilities to any given problem.

Early AI favored generality, but naively so – merely reflecting widely held beliefs. With the growing realization of the inadequacy of general reasoning and of the importance of specific knowledge, AI rejected generality and the theorem-proving paradigm and embraced such paradigms as expert systems, microworlds (Sussman, 1975; Winston, 1977), and scripts. Modern AI, with a growing understanding of the importance and role of memory organization, has once again (but this time with more of a basis) become a supporter of the theory of the generality of intelligence.

INDIVIDUAL DIFFERENCES

Recent AI has been concerned with common mechanisms of basic intelligence rather than with differences between more and less extraordinary individuals. Early AI was interested in the question of individual differences in the sense that it was concerned with the prerequisites needed to perform tasks that only especially smart people performed, but this concern was premature because there was no underlying theory of normal intelligence on which to base it. Thus very little worthwhile research within AI has directly addressed individual differences.

Nonetheless, AI serves as a source of suggestions about individual differences in intelligence, and of appearances of intelligence, in at least three ways.

1.   The historic evolution of AI programs from less to more intelligent, although not perfectly mirroring degrees of human intelligence, nonetheless supplies a series of examples of elements that do and do not account for varying degrees and types of intelligent behavior.
2.   AI models are sufficiently explicit in process and knowledge sources to be amenable to analysis and determination of places where variation *could* occur.
3.   AI programs could be used as apparatus with which to tinker with hypothesized variables of intelligence and to determine the differences they make.

One such source of variation is *beliefs*. To a large extent, the beliefs available to a cognitive system determine its ability to comprehend the world. In the example we saw earlier ("I was out until 2:00 A.M. yesterday. Boy, did my wife give it to me"), the belief that wives do not like their husbands to stay out late is crucial to understanding the story. The lack of such a belief will result in misunderstanding.

Beliefs do not vary because of the application process – people who have a belief in their memories *will* be able to find that belief – the variation lies, rather, in the nature of the beliefs that a person has acquired and the priority of each relative to others. Children's lack of reading comprehension ability can often be attributed to lack of available beliefs (or to lack of other knowledge). Exposure to the world is a factor in intelligence that is critical for comprehension of what people say to one or what one reads. Issues of intelligence relating to the ability to comprehend are thus liable to depend upon experience in the world.

In one sense, both the conservative and liberal variants of POLITICS were equally intelligent or unintelligent. Yet most people would feel that the "reasoning" of one was sounder than that of the other. We do not generally evaluate the reasoning of others by checking their step-by-step decisions as a mathematician might check a colleague's or student's proof but rather assume that others share our own beliefs and knowledge; indeed, the conclusions of either variant of the program would require a bizarre reasoning chain were it starting from the beliefs of the other.

Another source of individual difference is script usage. Scripts play both positive and negative roles in intelligence. One positive role is specifying intelligent or appropriate behavior – when a problem falls within scriptal bounds, one *should* take scriptal constraints into account. One may deliberately and intelligently override scriptal suggestions, but one's behavior will not be intelligent if one is oblivious to the fact that a script *is* being violated – one simply will not be understanding one's situation. Thus it is not generally intelligent for the hungry customer to concoct an elaborate scheme to bribe the waitress to bring food when all he or she needs to do is *ask* her to.

Scripts in intelligent processing also radically reduce the inferencing required to reach solutions. Further, use of standard solutions makes it easier to interface with other standard solutions. The customer who was violating the restaurant script with an innovative way of ordering was also making the rest of the problem (of getting fed) more difficult – surely an unintelligent approach! Knowledge of scripts and of other noninferable world knowledge is thus prerequisite to intelligent behavior.

Still, people who rely upon scripts *too* heavily will see no more than they have seen before. That is, an expectation-based theory of processing can at times rely exclusively on "top-down" predictions. Such a system will cope very well in worlds with which it is intimately familiar but will fall apart in an entirely new situation. The least intelligent inferencing system is therefore one that relies exclusively on scripts.

The most important source of individual differences, however, concerns the making of discriminations: The more intelligent understanders are, and the more properties of a situation they are interested in or attentive to, the more discriminations they will make. This trait is both a cause and an effect of intelligence and is both caused by and reflected in one's idiosyncratic memory organization; an intelligent concertgoer, for instance, will hear music in a much richer sense, noticing more about it, than a person with less developed musical intelligence. Discriminations form the basis of categorizations in terms of which the full concept of an entity in memory is formed.

Intelligent understanders must anticipate to some extent their future needs, though they cannot, of course, be expected to be prescient. The identification of those aspects of new experiences that will be relevant for making predictions later is one of the most formidable discrimination tasks facing an understander. Discriminations must be done at processing time; one cannot know beforehand where relevant similarities for future inputs might lie. Thus a very important part of understanding is the analysis of experience as it is acquired to judge how relevant the newly encountered events may be for predictive purposes when future inputs are encountered.

The total number of discriminations pointing to a concept indicates how well that concept has initially been categorized and understood. Undergoing an experience without discriminating much about it amounts to not really paying attention or not understanding. Intelligent people paying serious attention to events will create a large number of sometimes unique discriminations relating to what they have seen. The ability to abstract information from an input that will prove relevant to one's future processing needs is, in this sense, the ultimate determinant of intelligence.

7.7.   SUMMARY

AI, even human-intelligence-oriented AI, does not share the research goals of human intelligence research within psychology. Nonetheless, results of AI research, as we hope to have demonstrated, are relevant to human intelligence research within psychology.

We have paid some attention to the origins and methodology of current AI in order both to clarify the current goals and recent achievements of AI and to suggest the nature of AI's possible future contributions to our understanding of human intelligence. None of the programs discussed here, or indeed any of the programs that exist yet at all, is truly intelligent – despite any impressive-looking abilities some may have – even to the extent that a 3-year-old is intelligent. The major value of AI does not lie in the present or future capabilities of these programs, nor even in the precise mechanisms by which these programs perform such tasks; after all, we already *have* systems that can perform these tasks and that even use exactly the same mechanism as humans do – namely, humans themselves! Rather, AI's chief value relates to the insights we will gain into intelligence in the process of developing such models. As a methodology for studying intelligence, AI has already made substantial contributions to theories of intelligence, but its true value lies in the future refinement and revision of these theories.

NOTES

1 The best source for a comprehensive view of the complete field of artificial intelligence is the more recent volumes of the biennial *Proceedings of the International Joint Conference of Artificial Intelligence* (see 1975, 1977, 1979, 1981).
2 This statement is meant in the pragmatic sense. The theoretic limit of complexity (in the *mathematical* sense) of task that a computer was capable of achieving was, of course, unaffected (Church, 1936; Turing, 1936).

REFERENCES

Allport, G. W., & Postman, L. J. The basic psychology of rumor. In E. E. Maccoby, T. M. Newcomb, & E. L. Hartley (Eds.), *Readings in social psychology*. New York: Holt, Rinehart & Winston, 1958.

Automatic Language Processing Advisory Committee (ALPAC). *Language and machines: Computers in translation and linguistics* (Publication No. 1416). Washington, D.C.: National Academy of Sciences, 1966.

Baggett, P. Memory for explicit and implicit information. *Journal of Verbal Learning and Verbal Behavior*, 1975, *14*, 538–548.

Bamberger, J. Capturing intuitive knowledge in procedural description (Artificial Intelligence Memo No. 398; also LOGO Memo No. 42). Cambridge, Mass.: MIT, 1976. (a)

Bamberger, J. Development of musical intelligence II: Children's representation of pitch relations (Artificial Intelligence Memo No. 401; also LOGO Memo No. 43). Cambridge, Mass.: MIT, 1976. (b)

Bar-Hillel, Y. The present status of automatic translation of languages. In F. L. Alt (Ed.), *Advances in computers* (Vol. 1). New York: Academic Press, 1960.

Bartlett, F. C. *Remembering*. Cambridge, England: Cambridge University Press, 1932.

Bower, G. H., Black, J. B., & Turner, T. J. Scripts in text comprehension and memory. *Cognitive Psychology*, 1975, *11*, 177–220.

Bower, G. H., Karlin, M. B., & Dueck, A. Comprehension and memory for pictures. *Memory and Cognition*, 1975, *3*, 216–220.

Berliner, H. J. *Chess as problem solving: The development of a tactics analyzer*. Unpublished doctoral dissertation, Carnegie-Mellon University, 1974.

Berliner, H. J. Experiences in evaluation of with BKG – a program that plays backgammon. In *Proceedings of the Fifth International Joint Conference on Artificial Intelligence* (Vol. 1). Pittsburgh, Penna.: Carnegie-Mellon University Department of Computer Science, 1977.

Bernstein, M. I. Knowledge-based system: A tutorial (Rep. No. TM-(L)-5903/000/00A). Santa Monica, Calif.: Systems Development Corporation, 1977.

Bernstein, A., Roberts, M., Arbuckle, T., & Belsky, M. A. A chess-playing program for the IBM 704. *Proceedings of the Western Joint Computer Conference*, 1958, *13*, 157–159.

Black, J. B., Wilkes-Gibbs, D., & Gibbs, R. W., Jr. What writers need to know that they don't know they need to know. In Nystrand, M. (Ed.), *What writers know: Studies in the psychology of writing*. New York: Academic Press, 1982.

Bobrow, D., & Collins, A. *Representation and understanding: Studies in cognitive science*. New York: Academic Press, 1976.

Bransford, J. D., & Johnson, M. K. Contextual prerequisites for understanding: Some investigations of comprehension and recall. *Journal of Verbal Learning and Verbal Behavior*, 1972, *11*, 717–726.

Brewer, W. F., & Treyens, J. C. Role of schemata in memory for places. *Cognitive Psychology*, 1981, *13*, 207–230.

Buchanan, B. G., Sutherland, G., & Feigenbaum, E. Heuristic DENDRAL: A program for generating explanatory hypotheses in organic chemistry. In B. Meltzer & D. Mitchie (Eds.), *Machine intelligence 4*. New York: American Elsevier, 1969.

Carbonell, J. G. *Subjective understanding: Computer models of belief systems* (Computer Science Research Report No. 150). Unpublished doctoral dissertation, Yale University, 1979. (a)

Carbonell, J. G. The counterplanning process: A model of decision making in adverse conditions (Department of Computer Science Report). Pittsburgh, Penna.: Carnegie-Mellon University, 1979. (b)

Carbonell, J. G., Cullingford, R. E., & Gershman, A. V. Knowledge-based machine translation (Computer Science Research Report No. 146). New Haven, Conn.: Yale University, 1978.

Charniak, E. *Towards a model of children's story comprehension* (Artificial Intelligence Laboratory AI TR-266). Unpublished doctoral dissertation, MIT, 1972.

Charniak, E. Ms. Malaprop: A language comprehension program. In *Proceedings of the Fifth International Joint Conference on Artificial Intelligence* (Vol. 1). Pittsburgh, Penna.: Carnegie-Mellon University Department of Computer Science, 1977.

Charniak, E., Riesbeck, C., & McDermott, D. *Artificial intelligence programming*. Hillsdale, N.J.: Erlbaum, 1980.

Church, A. An unsolvable problem of elementary number theory. *American Journal of Mathematics*, 1936, *58*, 345–363.

Cullingford, R. E. *Script application: Computer understanding of newspaper stories* (Computer Science Research Report No. 116). Unpublished doctoral dissertation, Yale University, 1978.

Davis, R., & King, J. An overview of production systems (Artificial Intelligence Memo AIM-271). Stanford, Calif.: Stanford University, 1975.

Dehn, N. J. Story generation after Tale-spin. In *Proceedings of the Seventh International Joint Conference on Artificial Intelligence* (Vol. 1). Menlo Park, Calif.: American Association for Artificial Intelligence, 1981. (a)

Dehn, N. J. Memory in story invention. In *Proceedings of the Third Annual Conference of the Cognitive Science Society*. Berkeley, Calif.: Cognitive Science Society, 1981. (b)

Dejong, G. F. *Skimming stories in real time: An experiment in integrated understanding* (Computer Science Research Report No. 158). Unpublished doctoral dissertation, Yale University, 1979.

Duda, R., & Hart, P. *Pattern recognition and scene analysis*. New York: Wiley, 1973.

Dyer, M. G., & Lehnert, W. G. Memory organization and search processes for narration (Computer Science Research Report No. 175). New Haven, Conn.: Yale University, 1980.

Englemore, R., & Nii, H. P. A knowledge-based system for the interpretation of protein X-ray crystallographic data (Computer Science Department Memo HPP-77-2). Stanford, Calif.: Stanford University, 1977.

Evans, T. G. A program for the solution of a class of geometric-analogy intelligence-test questions. In M. Minsky (Ed.), *Semantic information processing*. Cambridge, Mass.: MIT Press, 1963.

Fahlman, S. A planning system for robot construction tasks. *Artificial Intelligence*, 1974, 5, 1–50.

Feigenbaum, E. The art of artificial intelligence: Themes and case studies of knowledge engineering. In *Proceedings of the Fifth International Joint Conference on Artificial Intelligence* (Vol. 2). Pittsburgh. Penn.: Carnegie-Mellon University Department of Computer Science, 1977.

Feigenbaum, E. A., & Feldman, J. (Eds.). *Computers and thought*. New York: McGraw-Hill, 1963.

Fikes, R. E., & Nilsson, N. J. STRIPS: A new approach to the application of theorem proving to problem solving. *Artificial Intelligence*, 1971, 2, 189–208.

Finkel, R. *Constructing and debugging manipulator programs* (Artificial Intelligence Memo AIM-284). Stanford, Calif.: Stanford University, 1976.

Flowers, M., McGuire, R., & Birnbaum, L. Adversary arguments and the logic of personal attacks. In W. Lehnert & M. Ringle (Eds.), *Strategies for natural language processing*. Hillsdale, N.J.: Erlbaum, 1982.

Galambos, J. A., & Rips, L. J. Memory for routines. *Journal of Verbal Learning and Verbal Behavior*, 1982, 21(4), in press.

Gibbs, R. W., & Tenney, Y. J. The concept of scripts in understanding stories. *Journal of Psycholinguistic Research*, 1980, 9 (3), 275–284.

Goldstein, I. P., & Papert, S. A. Artificial intelligence, language, and the study of knowledge (Artificial Intelligence Memo No. 337). Cambridge, Mass.: MIT, 1976.

Green, C. *The application of theorem-proving to question-answering systems* (Stanford Artificial Intelligence Project Memo AI-96). Unpublished doctoral dissertation, Stanford University, 1969.

Hayes-Roth, F., Mostow, D. J., & Fox, M. S. Understanding speech in the HEARSAY-II system. In L. Block (Ed.), *Speech communications with computers*. Berlin, West Germany: Springer, 1978.

Hiller, L. A., Jr., & Isaacson, L. M. *Experimental music*. New York: McGraw-Hill, 1959.

Horn, B. K. P. Obtaining shape from shading information. In P. H. Winston (Ed.), *The psychology of computer vision*. New York: McGraw-Hill, 1975.

International Joint Conference on Artificial Intelligence. *Proceedings of the Fourth International Joint Conference on Artificial Intelligence*. Ann Arbor, Mich.: University Microfilms, 1975.

International Joint Conference on Artificial Intelligence. *Proceedings of the Fifth International Joint Conference on Artificial Intelligence*. Pittsburgh, Penna.: Carnegie-Mellon University Department of Computer Science, 1977.

International Joint Conference on Artificial Intelligence. *Proceedings of the Sixth International Joint Conference on Artificial Intelligence*. Stanford, Calif.: Stanford University Computer Science Department, 1979.

International Joint Conference on Artificial Intelligence. *Proceedings of the Seventh International Joint Conference on Artificial Intelligence*. Menlo Park, Calif.: American Association for Artificial Intelligence, 1981.

Knuth, D. E. *Fundamental algorithms*. Reading, Mass.: Addison-Wesley, 1973.

Kolodner, J. L. *Retrieval and organizational strategies in conceptual memory: A computer model* (Computer Science Research Report No. 187). Unpublished doctoral dissertation, Yale University, 1980.

Langley, P. Rediscovering physics with BACON.3. In *Proceedings of the Sixth International Joint Conference on Artificial Intelligence*. Stanford, Calif.: Stanford University Computer Science Department, 1979, *1*, 505–507.

Laske, O. E. *Music, memory, and thought*. Ann Arbor: University Microfilms International, 1977.

Lea, W. (Ed.). *Trends in speech recognition*. Englewood Cliffs, N.J.: Prentice-Hall, 1980.

Lebowitz, M. Reading with a purpose. *17th Annual Meeting of the Association for Computational Linguistics: Proceedings of the Conference*. La Jolla, Calif.: University of California at San Diego, 1979.

Lebowitz, M. *Generalization and memory in an integrated understanding system* (Computer Science Research Report No. 186). Unpublished doctoral dissertation, Yale University, 1980.

Lehnert, W. G. *The process of question answering*. Hillsdale, N.J.: Erlbaum, 1978.

Lehnert, W. G. Affect and memory representation. *Proceedings of the Third Annual Conference of the Cognitive Science Society*. Berkeley, Calif.: Cognitive Science Society, 1981.

Lenet, D. *AM: An artificial intelligence approach to discovery in mathematics as heuristic search* (Stanford Artificial Intelligence Project Memo SAIL AIM-286). Stanford, Calif.: Stanford University, 1976.

Levy, D. *Computers and chess*. Potomac, Md.: Computer Science Press, 1976.

Locke, W. N., & Booth, A. D. (Eds.). *Machine translation of languages*. New York: The Technology Press of MIT and Wiley, 1955.

Marr, D. Representing visual information (Artificial Intelligence Memo No. 415). Cambridge, Mass.: MIT, 1978.

Marr, D. Visual information processing. In *Proceedings of the Sixth International Joint Conference on Artificial Intelligence* (Vol. 2). Stanford, Calif.: Stanford University Computer Science Department, 1979.

Martin, N., Friedland, P., King, J., & Stefik, M. Knowledge base management for experiment planning in molecular genetics. In *Proceedings of the Fifth International Joint Conference on Artificial Intelligence* (Vol. 2). Pittsburgh, Penna.: Carnegie-Mellon University Department of Computer Science, 1977.

McGuire, R., Birnbaum, L., & Flowers, M. Opportunistic processing in arguments. In *Proceedings of the Seventh International Joint Conference on Artificial Intelligence* (Vol. 1). Menlo Park, Calif.: American Association for Artificial Intelligence, 1981.

Meehan, J. R. *The metanovel: Writing stories by computer* (Computer Science Research Report No. 74). Unpublished doctoral dissertation, Yale University, 1976.

Meehan, J. R. An artificial intelligence approach to tonal music theory (Computer Science Technical Report No. 124). Irvine, Calif.: University of California at Irvine, 1978.

Miller, J. A. Autonomous guidance and control of a roving robot. In *Proceedings of the Fifth International Joint Conference on Artificial Intelligence* (Vol. 2). Pittsburgh, Penna.: Carnegie-Mellon University Department of Computer Science, 1977.

Minsky, M. (Ed.). *Semantic information processing*. Cambridge, Mass.: MIT Press, 1963.

Minsky, M. A framework for representing knowledge. In P. H. Winston (Ed.), *The psychology of computer vision*. New York: McGraw-Hill, 1975.

Minsky, M. Plain talk about neurodevelopmental epistemology. In *Proceedings of the Fifth International Joint Conference on Artificial Intelligence* (Vol. 2). Pittsburgh, Penna.: Carnegie-Mellon University Department of Computer Science, 1977.

Minsky, M. K-Lines. *Cognitive Science*, 1980, *4* (2), 117–133.

Minsky, M. Music, mind and meaning. *Computer Music Journal*, 1981, *5* (3), 28–44.

Moses, J. Symbolic integration (Project MAC Report MAC-TR47). Cambridge, Mass.: MIT, 1967.

Newell, A. Production systems: Models of control structures. In W. Chase (Ed.), *Visual information processing*. New York: Academic Press, 1973.

Newell, A., Shaw, J., & Simon, H. A. Chess-playing programs and the problem of complexity. *IBM Journal of Research and Development,* 1958, 2 (4), 320–335.

Newell, A., & Simon, H. A. GPS, a program that simulates human thought. In H. Billing (Ed.), *Lernende Automaten.* Munich, West Germany: Oldenbourg, 1961.

Newell, A., & Simon, H. A. *Human information processing.* Englewood Cliffs, N.J.: Prentice-Hall, 1972.

Nilsson, N. J. Searching problem-solving and game-playing trees for minimal cost solutions. In A. J. H. Morrell (Ed.), *Information processing 68* (Vol. 2). Amsterdam, The Netherlands: North-Holland, 1969.

Nilsson, N. J. *Problem-solving methods in artificial intelligence.* New York: McGraw-Hill, 1971.

Norman, D., & Schank, R. C. *Memory and cognitive science: A dialogue.* Hillsdale, N.J.: Erlbaum, in press.

Oettinger, A. G. *Automatic language translation.* Cambridge, Mass.: Harvard University Press, 1960.

Papert, S. A. Uses of technology to enhance education (Artificial Intelligence Memo No. 298). Cambridge, Mass.: MIT, 1973.

Papert, S. A. *Mindstorms,* New York: Basic Books, 1980.

Pople, H. E. The formation of composite hypotheses in diagnostic problem solving: An exercise in synthetic reasoning. In *Proceedings of the Fifth International Joint Conference on Artificial Intelligence* (Vol. 2). Pittsburgh, Penna.: Carnegie-Mellon University Department of Computer Science, 1977.

Pylyshyn, Z. W. Computation and cognition: Issues in the foundations of cognitive science. *Behavioral and Brain Sciences,* 1980, 3, 111–169.

Reddy, D. R. (Ed.). *Speech recognition: Invited papers of the IEEE symposium.* New York: Academic Press, 1975.

Reicher, G. M. Perceptual recognition as a function of meaningfulness of stimulus material. *Journal of Experimental Psychology,* 1969, 81, 275–280.

Reichman, R. Conversational coherency. *Cognitive Science,* 1978, 2 (4), 283–327.

Reiger, C. Conceptual memory. In R. C. Schank (Ed.), *Conceptual information processing.* Amsterdam, The Netherlands: North-Holland, 1975.

Sacerdoti, E. D. Planning in a hierarchy of abstraction spaces. *Artificial Intelligence,* 1974, 5 (3), 115–135.

Sacerdoti, E. D. *A structure for plans and behavior.* New York: Elsevier North-Holland, 1977.

Sacerdoti, E. D. Problem solving tactics. In *Proceedings of the Sixth International Joint Conference on Artificial Intelligence* (Vol. 2). Stanford, Calif.: Stanford University Computer Science Department, 1979.

Samuel, A. L. Some studies in machine learning using the game of checkers. *IBM Journal of Research and Development,* 1959,3(3), 210–229.

Samuel, A. L. Some studies in machine learning using the game of checkers II: Recent Progress. *IBM Journal of Research and Development,* 1967,11(6), 601–617.

Schank, R. C. *Conceptual information processing.* Amsterdam, The Netherlands: North-Holland, 1975.

Schank, R. C. Inference in the conceptual dependency paradigm: A personal history (Computer Science Research Report No. 141). New Haven, Conn.: Yale University, 1978. (a)

Schank, R. C. Interestingness: Controlling inferences (Computer Science Research Report No. 145). New Haven, Conn.: Yale University, 1978. (b)

Schank, R. C. Reminding and memory organization: An introduction to MOPs (Computer Science Research Report No. 170). New Haven, Conn.: Yale University, 1979.

Schank, R. C. Failure-driven memory. *Cognition and Brain Theory,* 1981, 1, 41–60.

Schank, R. C., & Abelson, R. P. *Scripts, plans, goals, and understanding.* Hillsdale, N.J.: Erlbaum, 1977.

Schank, R. C., Lebowitz, M., & Birnbaum, L. A. Integrated partial parsing (Computer Science Research Report No. 143). New Haven, Conn.: Yale University, 1978.

Schank, R. C., & Lehnert, W. G. The conceptual content of conversation (Computer Science Research Report No. 160). New Haven, Conn.: Yale University, 1979.

Schank, R. C., & Riesbeck, C. (Eds.). *Inside computer understanding: Five programs with miniatures.* Hillsdale, N.J.: Erlbaum, 1981.

Selfridge, M. *A process model of language acquisition* (Computer Science Research Report No. 172). Unpublished doctoral dissertation, Yale University, 1980.

Selfridge, O. Pandemonium: A paradigm for learning. In D. V. Blake & A. M. Uttley (Eds.), *Proceedings of the Symposium on Mechanisation of Thought Processes*. London, England: Her Majesty's Stationery Office, 1959.

Shortliffe, E. H. *Computer-based medical consultations: MYCIN*. New York: American Elsevier, 1976.

Simon, H. A. Artificial intelligence: Research strategies in the light of AI models of scientific discovery. In *Proceedings of the Sixth International Joint Conference on Artificial Intelligence* (Vol. 2). Stanford, Calif.: Stanford University Computer Science Department, 1979.

Slagle, J. A heuristic program that solves symbolic integration problems in freshman calculus. In E. A. Feigenbaum & J. Feldman (Eds.), *Computers and thought*. New York: McGraw-Hill, 1961.

Smoliar, S. W. *A parallel processing model of musical structures* (Artificial Intelligence Laboratory AI TR-242). Unpublished doctoral dissertation, MIT, 1971.

Sussman, G. J. *A computer model of skill acquisition*. New York: American Elsevier, 1975.

Sussman, G. J., & Stallman, S. R. M. Heuristic techniques in computer aided circuit analysis. *IEEE Transactions on Circuits & Systems*, 1975, *CAS-22* (11), 857–865.

Turing, A. M. On computable numbers, with an application to the Entscheidungsproblem. *Proceedings of the London Mathematical Society*, 1936, 2-42, 230–265.

Ullman, S. *The interpretation of visual motion*. Cambridge, Mass.: MIT Press, 1979.

Waltz, D. Understanding line drawings of scenes with shadows. In P. H. Winston (Ed.), *The psychology of computer vision*. New York: McGraw-Hill, 1975.

Weizenbaum, J. ELIZA – A computer program for the study of natural language communication between man and machine. *Communications of the ACM*, 1966, *9*(1), 36–45.

Wilensky, R. *Understanding goal-based stories* (Computer Science Research Report No. 140). Unpublished doctoral dissertation, Yale University, 1978.

Wilensky, R. Points: A theory of story content. In W. Lehnert & M. Ringle (Eds.), *Strategies for natural language processing*. Hillsdale, N.J.: Erlbaum, 1982.

Wilks, Y., & Charniak, E. *Computational semantics*. Amsterdam, The Netherlands: North Holland, 1976.

Winograd, T. Frame representations & the declarative/procedural controversy. In D. G. Bobrow & A. Collins (Eds.), *Representation and understanding: Studies in cognitive science*. New York: Academic Press, 1975.

Winston, P. H. *The psychology of computer vision*. New York: McGraw-Hill, 1975.

Winston, P. H. *Artificial intelligence*. Reading, Mass.: Addison-Wesley, 1977.

8 *Mental retardation and intelligence*

JOSEPH C. CAMPIONE, ANN L. BROWN,
AND ROBERTA A. FERRARA

8.1. INTRODUCTION

Our goal in this chapter is to describe how a research emphasis on exceptional persons can advance our understanding of human intelligence and facilitate the development of an adequate theory of intelligence. We will indicate what research of this type *might* tell us about intelligence, discuss what such research *has* provided, and then examine the directions that future research might take if the aim were to narrow the difference between what we have learned and what we could learn.

SUBJECT POPULATIONS AND TYPE OF INTELLIGENCE CONSIDERED

The overall goal is very general and could be pursued in a number of ways. This flexibility stems from the fact that the terms *exceptional* and *intelligence* have been underspecified. To illustrate, consider the term *intelligence*. As an initial statement, we might regard intelligence as the ability to adapt to some set or sets of tasks or the ability to perform acceptably in some domain. Note that the nature of *sets of tasks* or *domain* is not specified. This omission leaves open the possibility that there can be different types of intelligence, for example, academic, social, and everyday. The different types presumably are reflected in different sets of situations, and it can be argued that different theories would be needed to describe each different type. The questions here concern the kinds of situations that one would choose to investigate, given interest in a particular type of intelligence and in the extent to which the different types truly differ. How different would theories of, say, academic and everyday intelligence prove to be? Would reliable indexes of the two types tend to be correlated, or would academic and everyday intelligence be relatively independent of each other? Are people who perform poorly in school (an index of academic intelligence) likely to experience undue problems with everyday situations?

We will not deal with questions regarding the extent to which different types of intelligence can be specified. Although we believe that this is an extremely interesting and important area of inquiry, and that research with exceptional persons can be relevant to such questions, we simply do not believe that there are sufficient data upon which to base any strong claim. In section 8.6 we will return to this question and will describe some of the ways in which research involving exceptional persons could prove helpful.

This chapter will be concerned mainly with academic intelligence (Neisser, 1976), the ability to perform well in schoollike and testlike situations. This usage of the term *intelligence* has been dominant, and it has spawned the greatest amount of research and theorizing.

392

Our terminological restriction plainly indicates the form of exceptionality that we might choose to examine – individuals who are exceptional in their adaptation to academic or schoollike tasks. Thus we need to consider research on children who are having difficulties in school and test situations, mildly retarded and learning disabled children, and gifted children, those who do unusually well in such contexts. Although this statement of scope might hold in principle, in fact once again the choice is constrained, as the vast majority of the literature involves retarded children. Accordingly, we will focus here primarily on the implications of research with mildly retarded children for theories of academic intelligence,[1] although we will have occasion to refer to the learning disabilities literature.

We believe that the arguments concerning the importance of research with retarded children for theories of academic intelligence are general ones. In any area the study of the ways in which some process or ability breaks down will provide insights into "normal" functioning. The focus on mental retardation and academic intelligence is just one specific example of the more general approach. We turn now to a discussion of various ways of conceptualizing the role of exceptionality in terms of theories of intelligence.

ROLE OF EXCEPTIONALITY

We believe everyone would agree that research with retarded children can contribute to a theory of intelligence. How large that contribution might be, and the related question of whether such research is simply helpful or absolutely necessary, depends upon some metalevel assumptions about the nature of intelligence and intelligence theory. For example, one could assume that intelligence refers to the ability of individuals to perform acceptably on academic tasks and/or intelligence tests. In such a view, one type of theory of intelligence (Theory 1) would specify the knowledge and processes needed for adequate performance on the tests. Here work with poor performers is not necessary, although it could still be helpful. An analogy may be useful. We might wish to develop a theory of how the liver functions. Such a theory could in principle be developed by considering only normal livers; or, more importantly here, the theory need not contain any reference to faulty livers. Even in such a case, evidence from patients with liver problems would certainly provide important information about the liver's function and would thus contribute to the development of the overall theory. The essential point is that the theory would describe the role of a normal liver only.

An alternative view is that intelligence is primarily a relative term that serves to rank order individuals according to their ability to deal with those tests. That is, intelligence is an individual difference construct, and a theory of intelligence represents a specification of the ways in which individuals differ from each other. Given this orientation (Theory 2), important components of intelligence are those that serve to differentiate individuals or groups of individuals. Here comparative research is not only nice but necessary. It would be impossible to construct a theory of intelligence without considering individuals who have different "amounts" of it.

Suppose, for example, that we employed a homogeneous group of subjects in some task and were able to show analytically that successful performance required components $X_1, X_2, \ldots X_n$. In the case of Theory 1, we would conclude that intelligence consists of components X_1 through X_n. Theory 2, however, would remain unspecified. Suppose that we could show that without X_1 no one could succeed on the task; thus X_1 would certainly be an important component of that task. Suppose further that we could show that under normal circumstances all subjects could perform equally well with regard to X_1. Given Theory 1, X_1 would be a component of intelligence; but in Theory 2, X_1 would not appear. It is clear that Theory 2 represents a refinement of Theory 1 and may require Theory 1 as a first step. The general procedure is to analyze the target task(s) in terms of the processes necessary for successful completion (Construct Theory 1), to develop operations for evaluating the use or effectiveness of the various processes, and then to ascertain which are related to overall intellectual ability and how strong those relations are (Construct Theory 2). Adopting Theory 2, the importance or centrality of any process for a theory of intelligence is indexed by the extent to which it contributes to individual or comparative (group) differences in performance.

The way in which a person theorizes determines the way in which he or she interprets the existing literature and the extent to which that literature provides directly relevant information. For proponents of Theory 1, the existing literature can be extremely helpful. Given this theoretical preference, research with retarded children makes its contribution by highlighting sources of performance that may go unnoticed in more successful responders. That is, determinants of performance that run off smoothly and automatically for mature learners may not be detected readily by either the learner or the theorist. Those aspects may become "apparent" when they are either executed more poorly or not carried out at all. As an example, consider a case in which according to some theory, Processes A and B are required for solution of some problem. We might note that retarded children seem to carry out A and B reasonably well, but still "fail" the item. The implication is that performance requires more than A and B, that is, that the theory is incomplete. Ideally, of course, the specific way in which the retarded child performs differently from his more capable counterpart would provide information about the source of the difference. We will in fact be able to provide examples of such information in section 8.3.

A related but slightly different approach that is quite common is to instruct the retarded child in the use of A and B and then to observe his or her performance level. Improvement to the level of comparison subjects would reinforce the view that the theory adequately specifies the task components, whereas poorer performance on the part of the retarded child would suggest that the theory was incomplete or wrong.

In this view, work with slow-learning children can help by uncovering processes or skills overlooked by a focus on those who are more efficient. Such research proceeds in part by allowing a check on the completeness of existing task analyses. That is, a theory of intelligence of Type 1 would list the various components and their interactions that underlie successful performance. Work with retarded children is nice here, as it may help to indicate some additional components overlooked in other research. Such work is not necessary, however, as in principle a complete listing could be obtained by a consideration of only efficient performers. Work with retarded children could result, for example, in "simply" reinforcing the theories developed with faster learners.

For Theory 1 proponents, the literature as it stands is of fairly direct relevance to the theory construction goal. A consideration of the existing literature does highlight a number of component skills and processes that are necessary for efficient performance on a host of intellective tasks. Further, we believe that this research has isolated a number of factors not emphasized by those who work with average and above-average subjects. We stress here the fact that experiments of relevance to Theory 1 can involve only retarded subjects – comparisons among groups are not necessary or even of much importance.[2]

If we consider Theory 2, however, the picture changes in a number of ways. To arrive at Theory 2 we need to specify both the processes involved in intellectual functioning *and* the extent to which individuals differ with regard to those processes. We need both a listing of processes and methods for ranking them in terms of importance or centrality. In this view, both the importance of research with slow-learning children and the requirements for the research change. Obviously, given this view, research with the retarded acquires considerably greater importance. First and simply, increasing the range of performance variation that we observe makes it easier to identify sources of differences. Also, and more important, retarded performers may differ from average and gifted ones in ways that depart from those that distinguish more average performers from each other and average performers from above-average ones. (Again, a full picture does require research with gifted performers, for similar reasons.) We have taken this position previously in arguing that intelligence consists in good part of the processes lacking or weak in the retarded (Campione & Brown, 1978). To the extent that we document areas of exceptional weakness for the retarded, we are simultaneously specifying important components of intelligence. We prefer Theory 2, and this preference determines the way in which we evaluate the literature.

Research with retarded children is now both nice and necessary. Also, the type of research needed is somewhat different. If the centrality of some process to a theory of intelligence is defined in terms of its contribution to an explication of individual differences, we need to specify the extent to which retarded children experience *particular* problems with regard to that process, that is, how large, relative to more successful performers, is each problem or set of problems? Simply demonstrating that retarded children experience difficulty with respect to some process is not sufficient to document the importance of that process for the theory; nonretarded individuals could experience a problem of comparable severity. The implication is that to demonstrate a particular problem of the retarded, some kind of *comparative* work must be undertaken. In this regard, the literature is much weaker. Frequently, the necessary comparative research has not been done, and we are forced to make some cross-experiment comparisons to support our arguments regarding particular problem areas.

This theoretical orientation leads to one other immediate and serious problem. How can we determine how "severe" one problem is relative to another? We have no clear answer to this question but can suggest some ways of proceeding. The list is not exhaustive, nor is it clear which, if any, metric is preferable. Ideally, each could be assessed in some area, and the hope would be that they would converge on some set of processes. The candidates include: (a) the magnitude of the correlation between estimates of target processes and performance; (b) estimates of mental age (MA) or chronological age (CA) lag; (c) resistance to instruction; and (d) generality – other things equal, processes involved in more aspects of intellectual functioning are of greater importance.

To elaborate, we can obtain estimates of processing parameters on some set of tasks administered to subjects differing widely in intelligence or to groups differing in gross intelligence levels. Important components correlate most highly with intelligence test scores or with performance on some other criterion task or account for the largest portion of the variance in performance differentials. In some cases, it may be difficult to obtain reasonable quantitative indexes of the operation of some process. An alternative is to ask how far retarded children lag behind nonretarded children. For example, suppose some capability is shown by those of average intelligence at about 8 years of age; evidence for it in the retarded would appear slightly later, say at 9 years, if the underlying process is of some relevance to intelligence, but would be delayed further in appearance, say until age 12, if the capability were more central. Spitz (1981) has applied reasoning of this type to argue for the importance of the use of various problem-solving strategies to notions of intelligence.

Another possible metric, and one that we have emphasized in our own work, is resistance to instruction. The more difficult it is to teach some skill(s) to retarded individuals, the more central the target skill(s) to a theory of intelligence. This general assumption is of course at the heart of the control process–structural feature distinction (Atkinson & Shiffrin, 1968) and its application in the area of retardation (e.g., Brown, 1974, 1978; Campione & Brown, 1977, 1978; Fisher & Zeaman, 1973). Atkinson and Shiffrin, using the computer as a metaphor for human memory, distinguished between the hardware (structure) and software (control processes) of the system. The hardware is a permanent, unchanging set of components, whereas the software is optional and can be changed at the will of the user. Fisher and Zeaman (1973) borrowed the distinction and proposed, "since individual differences in intelligence are highly stable traits in our retardate population, only stable parameters, those representing structural features, are meaningfully relatable to intelligence" (p. 251). In the strongest statement of this view, structural features are not modifiable and are the major components of intelligence. We will adopt a slightly weakened position for a number of reasons. First, we can then avoid a discussion of whether intelligence can be trained; those readers interested in some additional observations on that topic are referred to Brown and Campione (in press) and the papers discussed there and to an upcoming volume based on the Conference on Learning and Thinking Skills held at the University of Pittsburgh and sponsored by the Learning Research and Development Center and the National Institute of Education. Second, it is difficult, if not impossible, to demonstrate that something is not trainable, given the problems of interpreting negative results. Lastly, the trainable–not trainable dichotomy is for our purposes better regarded as a continuum representing ease of instructibility. Some skills can be instructed easily; others are instructible, but only with considerable effort and ingenuity on the part of the teacher. To reiterate, all of these measures have problems associated with them, and the clearest evidence for the importance of any skill(s) would be obtained if the various measures could all be applied and all led to similar conclusions, that is, the importance here of converging operations is clear.

Finally, one other criterion can be applied. Retarded children do in fact perform poorly in many situations. Therefore one additional determinant of the importance of some component(s) to a theory of intelligence is the generality of the component(s). (This criterion is related to the first one mentioned above. To the extent that some component is involved in many different intellective tasks, it is likely to account for a greater proportion of the overall variance in intellectual functioning.) If two components are, according to the previous criteria, of approximately equal importance, for example, if they show the same developmental lag and/or are equally difficult to instruct, the one that is involved in the greater array of tasks would be of greater import. This statement is equivalent to the assertion that if they exist, general factors are more important components of intelligence than more specific factors. Differential effectiveness of general factors would account for performance variations across individuals in many situations.

To summarize, we will be concerned primarily with the performance of mildly retarded children on tasks related to academic intelligence. Our bias is to adopt Theory 2, which emphasizes that the importance of any component to a theory of intelligence depends upon the extent to which that component contributes to an account of individual differences. This latter bias strongly suggests the need for comparative research and indicates one major lack in the intelligence literature – a paucity of good comparative experimentation.

This emphasis also leads us to look for comparative research involving other groups of children with atypical learning skills, notably the learning disabled and gifted. Our searches of the literature did not lead us to much work that is relevant to a theory of intelligence; although some work with these groups is included in our review, there is considerably less than we would like to see. In section 8.6 we will outline in more detail the reasons for studying learning disabled and gifted children and the way(s) in which such research can advance theoretical development. We will also say why we feel that the current literature is less than satisfactory and will indicate the specific kind of research that in our opinion should be undertaken.

PLAN OF REMAINDER OF CHAPTER

In section 8.2 we will outline a broad framework useful in searching for and classifying intelligence-related processes. Comparative differences receive consideration in terms of the effects of differences in speed of processing, the knowledge base, the use of strategies and plans, and general metacognitive and executive functioning. In that section, our preferences will be apparent from the kind of research we include. Not surprisingly, these preferences lead us to ignore areas of literature that others might emphasize, for example, Piagetian research and an analysis of motivational determinants of performance.

Another area that we have chosen to exclude encompasses more traditional psychometric work. We have omitted it because our own approach to the area of exceptionality differs from that of traditional test builders and psychometrically oriented theorists in one important way. Our (eventual) aims are both improved diagnosis and remediation. The goal of reducing the problems encountered by slow learners requires a more detailed and elaborate process analysis than does the construction of standardized tests, a task in which the products of previous experience can provide all the information necessary. Thus we are concerned with the components of intelligent functioning rather than with its correlates or products.

In section 8.3 we will present a selective review of the experimental literature. That section has two major goals: first, to summarize our knowledge in the areas we have chosen to review, and second, to indicate areas where additional research is needed. We note that although a large amount of research has been concerned with the role of memory and with problem-solving strategies, as well as with the use and understanding thereof (metacognition) by retarded subjects, we know very little about speed-of-processing factors and the extent to which knowledge-base limitations are responsible for impaired performance on the part of retarded children. In addition to noting these "simple effects" we argue that we desperately need data on the ways in which the different factors interact (cf. Bransford, 1979; Brown, 1982a;

Brown, Bransford, Ferrara, & Campione, in press; Jenkins, 1979); such interactions have only infrequently been assessed.

In each area, we will present only a few examples of specific experiments. In some cases up-to-date reviews already exist, and we will refer the reader to those sources for additional details. We will try to illustrate the kind of data upon which claims about the nature of intelligence might be based. We will also describe the strengths and weaknesses of the existing literature in each area.

Readers familiar with the experimental literature may wish to turn directly to section 8.4, which is concerned with clinical and educational approaches to the study of retardation. Workers in these areas obviously share our concern with both diagnosis and remediation; they are also concerned, as we are, with the ways in which specific diagnoses can contribute to the development of instructional programs. Our main point in this section will be the happy one that the views on the retarded child emerging from research taking this approach converge very closely with those developed from a consideration of the experimental literature. Thus, although the experimental and clinical approaches exist quite independently of each other (there is almost no cross-referencing to be found), the dominant ideas in the two areas are extremely similar. Again, those who are aware of the clinical–educational literature could ignore this section and could proceed to section 8.5. Readers concerned primarily with speculations about a theory of intelligence could skip sections 8.3 and 8.4 and go to section 8.5.

Section 8.5 represents our attempt to package our knowledge about retarded (and other exceptional) children in a number of broad statements relevant to a theory of intelligence. In this section, we emphasize our view of intelligence as the efficiency of new learning, couched in terms of the ability to profit from incomplete instruction and of the intimately related ability to transfer old learning to new situations. This is certainly not a new view (we doubt that much in this area is or could be new), and we outline our current view in historical perspective. We reaffirm the old (original?) view of intelligence as the ability to learn, and we describe some reasons why this position seemed to fall into disrepute for a time. Finally, section 8.6 outlines a number of directions in which research should proceed in the future and indicates why we regard those directions as important.

8.2.   GENERAL FRAMEWORK

We do not intend to provide an exhaustive review of the literature; rather, our aim is to discuss some representative experiments in each of a number of areas of research and to indicate their importance for theories of intelligence. In this context, we will emphasize some of the major methodological issues that need to be considered. Some problems have been solved relatively well, but others still need resolution. The failure to find answers to some methodological questions means that a number of the conclusions we would like to draw cannot be supported as strongly as would be desirable. Our review is influenced by two sets of considerations, one pertaining to the specific types of studies selected and the second pertaining to the interpretation of these studies.

The selection of studies reflects a general information-processing approach to the study of the cognitive system. As we indicated above, we are concerned with both diagnosis and remediation. In some sense, diagnosis, or description of intellective functioning, may be seen as the primary theoretical aim; as will be seen, we regard instructional, or remediational, attempts as a major way of evaluating the status of existing theory. Thus, in addition to its practical importance, attempts at remediation do facilitate the development of theory. An information-processing framework does lend itself well to discussion and organization of both diagnosis and instruction and we chose it for this reason. Adoption of this framework means the exclusion of some literatures, a fact we are willing to live with. It does, however, lead to other problems that are more serious from our point of view, and we will address those problems later in this section.

Within this frame of reference, we will use the distinction between short-term, or working, memory (STM) and long-term memory (LTM). Working memory is conceived as a limited capacity system from which unattended information is rapidly lost. Space in working memory is used by both the information residing there and the operations used to identify, maintain, and operate upon those items. In contrast, long-term memory is a relatively permanent, large capacity system containing an individual's organized knowledge of the surrounding world. We will be concerned with the characteristics of those stores, with their contents, and with the operations and procedures by which individuals manipulate both the systems and their contents.

We shall deal briefly with the architecture of the system (Campione & Brown, 1978; Hunt, 1978) and shall then spend more time on four general determinants of performance on intellective tasks. This classification simplifies the discussion and should not be taken as an indication that we regard the four topics as independent or even separable. In fact, we will mention throughout our review that performance in almost any situation depends upon the interaction of two or more determinants. The four areas are: (a) the speed, or efficiency, with which elementary information-processing operations are carried out; (b) the subject's knowledge base; (c) the role of various strategies in dealing with memory and problem-solving situations; and (d) metacognition and executive decision making.

The first determinant of performance that we shall consider is speed, or efficiency, of processing, the rate at which elementary operations are carried out. Research in this area is best typified by the work of Hunt and his associates (see Hunt, 1978, for a recent statement). This factor is of potential importance for many reasons. As one example, it is likely that performance in many complex domains is interactive. In the area of reading, Rumelhart (1977) and Rumelhart and McClelland (1980) have outlined an interactive model in which the reader considers information from a variety of levels of analysis simultaneously, with information from each source influencing the interpretation of information from others. For such an interactive system to proceed smoothly, the different inputs need to be processed efficiently. A breakdown in one system results in a delay in the input to another, thereby minimizing the contribution of the second. If one or more of the component executions are somewhat slow or inefficient, the whole system must suffer. Thus the efficiency with which the components are executed represents a potential source of individual differences, where differences associated with relatively specific processes can have more widespread effects.

As another example, many learning and problem-solving situations place a heavy demand on working memory (e.g., Simon, 1976). As suggested earlier, "space" in working memory is taken up by both its contents and the maintenance and transformation operations carried out on them, that is, the amount of effort expended on any cognitive activity is one determinant of the amount of space required by that activity. The more efficiently those activities can be carried out, the less the strain on the system. Thus, rapid execution of component activities can result in an increase in *functional* memory capacity, making it less likely that capacity limits will be exceeded and more likely that the problem will be solved.

Our second factor is the knowledge base, the extent and organization of relevant knowledge available to the learner. On a simple level, it is obvious that performance in some domain will be influenced by the amount of knowledge an individual has about that domain. Of more interest to us is the way in which that knowledge influences other components of the system. We also need to consider the question of whether an inadequate knowledge base is better regarded as a cause of poorer learning on the part of the retarded or as a consequence of poor learning skills.

It is also clear that the knowledge base includes a variety of procedures and strategies for dealing with problem situations (our third factor) and knowledge about those strategies (part of our fourth factor). We will treat these latter two areas separately, not because we think they should be regarded as separate, but rather because they have received heavy emphasis in the literature, where they have tended to be regarded as separable.

The third factor we will discuss is the role of strategic activities. Although much learning may proceed incidentally or automatically, many more complex, schoollike problems require some planful, active processing for optimal performance. In this context, we will consider the extent to which poor performance by the retarded stems from a failure to employ task-appropriate strategies. The majority of the research in this area has been concerned with the use of memory strategies. The typical situation investigated is one in which a supraspan amount of material is presented, that is, the capacity of working memory is exceeded, and the experimental question concerns the extent to which the memory problem is "solved" by the application of some reasonable strategic ploy. Although there has been a preponderance of memory research in this area, we presume that laws and regularities regarding strategic behavior in the domain of "intentional memory" will be generalizable to other problem domains.

The fourth area of concentration is metacognition (Brown, 1978; Flavell, 1978). Within this area we will be concerned with two distinct classes of observations (for a more detailed discussion of this distinction and the separate roots of each class, see Brown & Campione, 1981, in press) – knowledge about cognition (metacognition) and regulation of cognitive activities (executive control). Of these two topics, the role of executive control, the choice, timing, sequencing, and monitoring of cognitive activities, is of particular relevance to a general information-processing approach.

One weakness of computer-based information processing approaches is that they tend to result in static models. They do not lead readily to a discussion of growth or change (e.g., Brown, 1979, 1982a). It is easy to talk about the organization and contents of memory in terms of factual (or declarative) and strategic (or procedural) knowledge and the various relations, but the models are likely to be silent regarding where and how that knowledge was acquired. They do not provide a good vehicle for discussing learning. Throughout the remainder of this chapter, we will supplement our discussion of the separate areas by considering the role of learning in the information-processing systems that have been noted in the research.

8.3.   SELECTIVE REVIEW OF THE EXPERIMENTAL LITERATURE

A survey of the recent experimental literature with retarded children indicates that the favorite topic has been the role of strategic factors in mediating performance.

This focus has been supplemented by a spurt of research emphasizing metacognitive functioning. During the heyday of strategy research (the early and middle 1970s), it is probably safe to say, the importance of strategies was overstated. It seemed on occasion that some believed that strategies accounted for everything. Most experimental tasks investigated did require the use of strategies for effective performance, and it was typically found that retarded children were less likely to employ those strategies than were nonretarded children. Further, as we will see, teaching retarded children to use the relevant strategies did result in enhanced performance.

Strategy deficits were ubiquitous and clearly important and led to further research aimed at understanding the sources of those deficits – research on metacognition and executive functioning. This research was exciting because of its educational implications as well as its theoretical component. If strategy use was the main determinant of performance on a wide variety of tasks, and if people could be taught to carry out those strategies, then worthwhile improvements in cognitive performance could be effected. This emphasis coupled with the failure to find comparative differences in some "nonstrategic" behaviors (see "Strategies") resulted in a tendency to distract attention from the effects of the knowledge-base and speed-of-processing parameters.

This same tendency has been present in the general developmental literature, although the imbalance is beginning to be redressed. A number of authors, most notably Chi (1981), have begun to demonstrate experimentally the role of the knowledge base in contributing to differences between younger and older children, a factor that was considered only theoretically by earlier writers (e.g., Brown, 1975). Speed-of-processing factors have also become the target of additional research, and there are now data indicating developmental and comparative differences in this area (Chi, 1977b; Huttenlocher & Burke, 1976; Keating & Bobbitt, 1978). One problem we see is that the interpretation of performance differences seems to be an either–or decision. As the effects of the knowledge-base and processing parameters become clarified, there is a tendency to downgrade the importance of strategies and metacognitive factors. An extreme illustration of this stance is to argue that the tendency to appear strategic is nothing more than an automatic consequence of a well-organized knowledge base. In our view, although the knowledge-base research is welcome and necessary, it appears that the earlier overemphasis on strategies is being replaced by an overemphasis on the knowledge base.

We will argue for the importance of both sets of factors and will indicate the need for research considering them simultaneously. Essentially we believe that the tendency to be strategic varies with intelligence and that the ability to execute a strategy efficiently in some domain depends upon the quantity and quality of the performer's knowledge of that domain. Without the appropriate knowledge, some strategies may be precluded; however, even when the knowledge is available, some individuals may not employ the strategies made possible by that knowledge.

In our review we will consider the effects of speed-of-processing parameters, followed by the role of knowledge-base variation, and finally the role of strategic behavior and metacognitive factors. In the first two areas, few data are available, and the discussion will be somewhat speculative. We will also try to indicate where we believe additional research is necessary. We will concentrate more on the strategy and metacognitive areas, where the vast majority of the work has been conducted.

Our major aim is to identify prominent sources of comparative differences, as our assumption is that such differences will contribute to a definition of intelligence. Implicit in such a statement is the belief that there exist areas in which retarded individuals differ only minimally or not at all from nonretarded individuals. Such an assumption is not universally shared, at least not in its strong form. For example, Ellis (1978) has stated that there are no commonalities: ". . . the concept of a deficiency in a process implies that other processes are intact. Few processes seem 'normal' in the retarded. Indeed, studies that find normal functioning in any task are suspect" (p. 52). Given the diversity of opinion, it seems worthwhile to ask whether some processes are efficient in the retarded, and it is to this question that we briefly turn.

AREAS OF STRENGTH

We introduce this section by noting that in many situations we acquire and maintain material without any pronounced attempt to do so. In such cases, the processing system appears to carry out its work automatically, or at least relatively effortless processing is involved (Brown, 1975; Hasher & Zacks, 1979; Schneider & Shiffrin, 1977). Information is constantly being perceived, identified, and retained for various periods of time with what is apparently only the passive involvement of the system. There is reason to believe that on many occasions of this sort the performance of retarded subjects is comparable to that of nonretarded subjects. Although the evidence is not overwhelming, in good part because the necessary comparative studies have not been done, there is sufficient work to invite the inference that in these areas of "automatic" cognitive functioning, retarded persons differ from average learners, if at all, by such small amounts that the variations are trivial.

Evidence for excellent performance comes from tasks that Brown (1975) has termed *nonstrategic, nonsemantic*. In these tasks strategies appear to be unnecessary, and subjects' performance is relatively unaffected by differences in their knowledge bases. The prototypical tasks here include recognition memory for *simple, unrelated* pictures and judgment of relative recency (Brown, 1975), along with judgments of frequency of occurrence (Hasher & Zacks, 1979). In each of these areas, there is some evidence that minimal developmental changes occur within the nonretarded population. With regard to recognition memory, preschoolers have achieved performance levels equal to those of adults in a number of studies (cf. Brown & Campione, 1972; Brown & Scott, 1971). Although ceiling effects are present when the retention intervals are relatively short, preschoolers' performance after 1 week is well short of perfect and is still comparable to adult levels reported by Nickerson (1968). When more complex stimuli are used in recognition studies (e.g., Mandler & Johnson, 1976; Dirks & Neisser, 1977), developmental differences emerge but appear related more to acquisition or to scanning strategies (Mackworth & Bruner, 1970) than to memory dynamics. In support of this latter notion, Wickelgren (1975) plotted recognition functions for delays of as much as 2 hours with groups of children ($9\frac{1}{2}$ years old), adults (college students), and the elderly (68 years old). Although group differences appeared in overall performance, they were attributable to acquisition dynamics; there were no retention differences.

Studies on retarded children's recognition memory have either shown high levels of performance, comparable to those of nonretarded children (Brown, 1972a; Martin, 1970), or have found differences reflecting acquisition rather than retention effects (Ellis et al., 1977). Although the conclusion rests on a weaker data base than we would like and requires in addition some cross-experiment comparisons, the assertion that retarded children's recognition memory dynamics are intact seems defensible. A more thorough evaluation of this contention would require a comparative study in which ceiling effects were absent.

Considering judgment of relative recency and the use of contextual cues to mediate such judgments, there is again strong evidence that developmental differences are of very small magnitude in a variant of the task where strategic intervention is precluded (Brown, 1973a; Brown, Campione, & Gilliard, 1974); however, when strategies could be used, developmental trends did appear. When retarded children were tested for their ability to make use of contextual and temporal cues to indicate a number of discriminative judgments, their performance was also excellent (Brown, 1973b), although strong conclusions are difficult because comparable data with nonretarded children were not collected. Thus there are again weak data indicating that in nonstrategic tasks (Brown, 1975) or in tasks requiring automatic operations (Hasher & Zacks, 1979), retarded adolescents perform quite well. Again, this conclusion could be more stringently tested in an appropriately designed comparative study. We should mention here that the students who performed so well in the Brown (1973a) study were the same ones who performed extremely poorly in a "strategic" short-term memory task, the "keeping track task," to which we will refer in a later section of this chapter. The point is that the same subjects seem to perform quite efficiently in tasks that involve the passive or automatic operation of the system but very poorly when additional effort is required.

Many of the short-term memory tasks examined in the experimental literature do require the use of strategies such as rehearsal for efficient performance, and it is here that clear developmental and comparative trends are found (Brown, 1974, 1975; Campione & Brown, 1977; Flavell, 1970). It is the magnitude as well as presence or absence of differences that is particularly diagnostic. Even in such tasks, however, in one area intelligence-related differences seem to be minimal, and that concerns the durability of information in working memory. Ellis (1963) hypothesized that low IQ subjects, compared with brighter ones, have diminished and more rapidly fading stimulus traces.[3] Thus, performance in a memory situation should drop off more steeply for less intelligent rememberers, and an IQ × Retention Interval interaction would be expected. In critically reviewing the literature that ensued, Belmont and Butterfield (1969) concluded that the weight of the evidence was clearly opposed to that prediction. In the majority of the studies they reviewed, there were no significant IQ × Retention Interval interactions; where such interactions were reported, it was possible to account for them in terms of differential strategy use, the more intelligent subjects being presumed to employ more sophisticated strategies. Belmont and Butterfield's conclusion, thus, was that the data indicated no intelligence-related differences in the durability of items in working, or short-term, memory.

To summarize, it appears that retarded subjects perform comparably to nonretarded ones when we try to assess the automatic, or passive, operation of the memory system uncontaminated by variations in the knowledge base. These conclusions remain weak, given the paucity of data and the even more severe restriction on the number of comparative studies. We should reemphasize that we find attempts to locate sources of processing efficiency as interesting as work addressed to finding sources of inefficiency. We hope that additional data will be collected in more appropriate experiments to allow a stronger test of the constancy hypothesis.

SPEED OF PROCESSING

In many ways, the relevance of speed-of-processing estimates to the problem of mental retardation is obvious. A traditional view of retarded children is that they can be characterized as having sluggish nervous systems. In fact, they are frequently described as "slow." A number of writers, most notably field theorists (Lewin, 1935; Spitz, 1963), have emphasized the general torpidity of the system. A problem with their approaches was that there were no good methods of estimating processing speed; as a result, more indirect methods had to be used, such as the frequency of shifts in the appearance of reversible or ambiguous figures (Spitz, 1963). This state of affairs has changed. A number of detailed analyses of experimental tasks have been made, and our ability to assess the speed with which various types of mental operations can be carried out has increased noticeably. Much of the chronometric work relevant to the topic of intelligence has been reviewed by Cooper (see chapter 3 in this volume), and the reader is referred to that chapter for a thorough discussion of the main issues. In the most detailed set of studies in this area, Hunt and his associates (Hunt, 1978; Hunt, Frost, & Lunneborg, 1973; Hunt, Lunneborg, & Lewis, 1975) have found that college students with high and low verbal ability differ from each other in the speed with which they carry out various mental operations. Examples include the rate of searching short-term memory, the rate at which over-learned LTM codes can be accessed, and the speed with which typical operations, such as negation, can be performed. This "cognitive correlates" approach (Pellegrino & Glaser, 1979) has been infrequent in the literature on exceptional children, and relatively few direct data are available. Indications from the extant literature are that educable mentally retarded (EMR) children may be less efficient in their processing than nonretarded children of the same age. Still, the studies raise more questions than they answer. Our goal here will be to review a few of the studies, to examine the significance and various interpretations of the available data, and to suggest some directions that future research might take.

The tasks we have chosen to consider are the Sternberg (1966) STM scanning task and the Posner, Boies, Eichelman, and Taylor (1969) method for estimating the facility with which individuals can locate familiar items in LTM (see chapter 3 in this volume for details). In the Sternberg task, the subjects memorize a set of n items and are then shown a simple probe item. Their task is to indicate whether that item was or was not in the memorized set, and the main dependent variable is reaction time. The typical finding is that reaction time increases as a linear function of n.

The two parameters of the line, relating reaction time and n, its slope and intercept, provide estimates of the efficiency of several component processes. The slope is taken as a measure of the rate at which the contents of memory can be searched, and the intercept reflects the combined duration of other component processes (identification, decision, responding, etc.). Several studies (e.g., Harris & Fleer, 1974) have found that slope values obtained with retarded children are larger, hence memory scanning rates slower, than those produced by nonretarded children. In an experiment reported by Keating and Bobbitt (1978), this relation was extended further along the intelligence continuum. They found that children of above-average ability searched memory more rapidly than those of average ability.

Another aspect of speed of processing that has received considerable attention is the speed with which incoming items can be identified and labeled. One fairly direct measure of encoding time, or the amount of time required to retrieve the name of an item from LTM, is based on a procedure developed by Posner. This procedure is described in detail by Cooper (chapter 3 in this volume). Briefly, the subjects are required to make same–different judgments to pairs of letters. In one variant of the task, they are required to respond "same" when the letters have the same name and "different" otherwise. Considering "same" responses, the comparison of interest concerns reaction time to pairs of letters that are the same only in name (NI, or not identical: e.g., *Aa*) and pairs that are also physically identical (PI, or physically identical: e.g., *AA*). As the PI decision can be made without the subject's having to go beyond the physical features of the letters, the difference between the NI and PI reaction times is taken as an index of how long it takes the subject to retrieve the name(s) of the letters from LTM. This difference does seem to correlate with a number of indexes of academic achievement. High-verbal college students have smaller difference scores, indicating more rapid encoding, than less-verbal students (Hunt et al., 1975); adult good readers have smaller difference scores than poorer readers (Jackson & McClelland, 1979); encoding is more rapid in above-average, as compared with average, ability children (Keating & Bobbitt, 1978) and retarded children take longer to encode familiar items than nonretarded subjects do (Hunt, 1977). The data thus do indicate a relationship between encoding rate and intelligence.

Finally, on a more general level, Jensen and Munro (1979) have demonstrated sizable correlations between intelligence scores and measures of choice reaction time. In a simple situation where the subject had to make some indicator response (typically button pressing) to indicate which of n possible stimuli had occurred, reaction times of less intelligent subjects increased more sharply with increases in n than did those of more intelligent students.

Although this area has not been a popular one, the data do indicate that retarded children may be less efficient in their execution of simple mental operations, and we anticipate an increase in the amount of research devoted to this topic. We would like to interject a few comments here, however, about the nature of that research. Specifically, we will consider three topics: (a) the need for reliability data, (b) demonstrations of the relation of these mental operations to more motor behaviors, and (c) the role of a developmental analysis.

With regard to reliability, although the efficiency measures are taken to represent important individual difference variables, there is typically no attempt to specify the within-subjects stability of these measures. This is a problem in itself, as Carroll (1978) has argued in a review of much of this research, but it is a particular problem in comparative research, where, for any of a number of reasons, the data from retarded (or young) children may be less reliable or stable than those from non-retarded (or older) children. Given this possibility, it would seem necessary to provide estimates of reliability for each group of subjects before embarking on any comparison. For example, some data with college students indicate that it may take several sessions before Sternberg slope values stabilize and produce acceptable levels of reliability (Chiang & Atkinson, 1976). The number of sessions needed for this stabilization could easily vary for subjects of varying intellectual maturity.

Our second comment concerns the extent to which these efficiency factors are "important" components of intelligence. What, and how widespread, are the sequelae to inefficient processing? The initial research was of necessity concerned with demonstrating the covariation between efficiency measures and measures of academic ability. It is as important to show how these differences affect other, more interesting performances. Such research is beginning to appear, and we will provide brief descriptions of two classes of it. It is interesting to note that these efforts have involved comparisons of individuals who vary in ability, and the aims have been both to use individual variation as a way of building theory (about reading) and to use extant theory to begin to understand more specific disabilities (e.g., language delay).

Slow or inefficient processing contributes to the problems faced by poor readers (e.g., Jackson & McClelland, 1975, 1979; McClelland & Jackson, 1978; Perfetti & Hogaboam, 1975; Perfetti & Lesgold, 1979). Some of this work is reviewed in more detail by Cooper (chapter 3 in this volume), and we will be brief here. Jackson and McClelland (1979) investigated a number of possible correlates of reading efficiency (efficiency here = Reading Speed × Comprehension Accuracy) in average and above-average readers (college students: Ability groups corresponded to the lower and upper 25% of their subjects). The ability to access letter names was a major correlate of reading efficiency, as it and accuracy-based listening comprehension scores accounted for almost all the variance in criterion reading task performance. Jackson and McClelland also included a test of auditory letter span. This correlated highly both with reading efficiency and with speed of name access. Thus, speed of encoding does relate to span performance as well as to reading performance.

The importance of encoding rate and working-memory limitations in affecting reading has also been emphasized by Perfetti and Lesgold (1977, 1979). They have outlined a model of discourse processing emphasizing certain processes involved in the short-term encoding of linguistic information and the retrieval and use of word names and meanings. They summarize some of their work with the following view of the unskilled reader: "The poor reader is slower at getting to the point in the comprehension process beyond which exact wording is not needed, but he is also poorer at retaining exact wording. Thus, he is confronted with a double whammy – slower processing and lower tolerance (in terms of working memory), both of which combine to create more processing needs than might otherwise exist" (1977, p. 178). Individual differences in efficiency parameters do relate to variations in reading ability.

One of the best examples of research involving speed-of-processing factors and exceptional children is the work of Tallal and Piercy (1973, 1978; Tallal, 1978). Their work is truly noteworthy because they demonstrate a close link between theory and experimentation. Whereas with most of the studies in the learning disabled (LD) literature the choice of experimental tasks and target processes appears random (the underlying rationale is presumably that LD children could experience problems almost anywhere), Tallal and Piercy were able to direct their attention to narrowly defined areas in which their subjects' particular limitations could be based. They were then able to identify specific deficiencies leading to a much more general and widespread problem. These investigators have worked with well-defined groups of children with specific language delay (developmental dysphasics). Although the idea underlying their research is an old one – that problems of language use may reflect hearing difficulties – they have shown how detailed analyses based on sophisticated theory can succeed in isolating the factors responsible for the delay. Children with developmental dysphasia pass a number of standard tests of auditory discrimination, but they can be shown to be impaired in a more specific area, the perception of the temporal sequence of rapidly presented acoustic stimuli. Research on speech perception employing synthesized speech stimuli has been able to identify some of the cues underlying discrimination of classes of sounds. Vowel discrimination is based on stable intensity patterns of relatively long duration (around 250 msec), whereas discrimination of stop consonants (/ba/, /da/, /ga/) depends upon rapid (50 msec) formant transitions (Liberman et al., 1967). Whereas language-delayed children did not differ from controls on tests of vowel discrimination, they were significantly inferior when they were required to discriminate stop consonants from each other. Subsequent experiments showed that the problem resulted from a failure to perceive the formant transitions. When the formant transitions were extended to 93 msec, the language-disordered children's discriminations were found to be unimpaired.

This work is unique in the LD literature in that a specific problem was delineated and a theoretical analysis of that disability pointed to sources of the weakness. Careful experimentation then led to identification of the locus of the problem. We find this work exemplary in that the theory led to specific expectations about the population's problems. This approach contrasts with the more typical procedure of simply looking for general differences between LD and control groups and represents a model for the kind of research that we would like to see in this area.

The examples cited show that efficiency variations do lead to performance differences in more molar, and important, areas; they thus lend support to the idea that efficiency differences can have widespread effects. They also indicate how research with groups of varying ability can facilitate theory development. We shall return to this point, and particularly to the Tallal data, in section 8.6.

Our final general point here concerns the importance of a developmental analysis. Given that retarded children differ from nonretarded children in, say, the speed of searching STM, we would still like to know the "history" of that difference. A strict structural feature interpretation would suggest that the differences emerge early and that the processes do not change with development or at least asymptote quickly. That is, individuals "come with" some scanning rate capability. That capability is invariant and serves to differentiate individuals. Alternatively, some aspects of efficiency could increase with development; individual differences could remain of constant magnitude or could show progressive increases or decreases (see Campione & Brown, 1978). Such pattern variations do seem to exist. For example, STM scanning efficiency may not vary appreciably with age (Harris & Fleer, 1974; Keating & Bobbitt, 1978; but see Herrmann & Landis, 1977), whereas encoding rate does increase developmentally (Keating & Bobbitt, 1978).

In summary, there do appear to be intelligence-related differences in the efficiency with which basic cognitive processes are carried out, although the comparative–developmental data base is still extremely weak. Attempts have been made to relate these efficiency differences to variations in performance on more complex tasks. We would hope that future research will complete our picture of the relationships among efficiency factors and that more work will be addressed to the interaction of those factors with other processing components.

A special case – memory span

One of the standard items found on intelligence tests is digit span, and a prime reason for its inclusion is that it is regarded as being particularly sensitive to low intelligence. The data are in accord with this belief. In reviewing the digit-span literature, Spitz (1972) noted that adults' immediate memory span for digits (*span* being the number of digits a subject could recall correctly 90% of the time) ranged from 5 to 7; but for retarded adolescents (CA = 14), the range was 3 to 4.

Although the existence of digit-span differences associated with variations in intelligence has been little disputed, there has been considerable disagreement about the way in which those differences should be interpreted. Alternative views hold that digit-span differences reflect variations in: (a) STM capacity; (b) the operation of rehearsal or chunking strategies; (c) speed of item identification; and (d) maintenance of item order information. Unfortunately for our purposes, not all of the hypotheses have been evaluated with retarded children, and our conclusions here are based in good part on work with nonretarded subjects.

A thorough review of this literature has recently been provided by Dempster (1981), and we will simply indicate some of the salient features that have emerged. We review this material in this section because memory-span differences appear to reflect differences in efficiency of item identification. Earlier work with retarded subjects was designed to show that part of their problem in digit-span tasks resulted from a failure to chunk the digits on input. Treating three one-digit numbers as one three-digit number is thought to increase the informational content of individual chunks, and because the number of chunks limits the contents of STM, such chunking should lead to increased recall. If so, then subjects who carry out this recoding would have larger digit spans than those who do not. Further, for subjects who do not impose this type of organization on the input, providing such organization for them should improve their span performance. A number of studies have in fact supported this notion. For example, presenting digits grouped (e.g., 25, 71, 48) rather than ungrouped (e.g., 2, 5, 7, 1, 4, 8) does result in increased digit spans for moderately retarded subjects (MacMillan, 1970; Spitz, 1966). Thus it appears that these subjects do not spontaneously chunk the input but can use such chunking if it is done for them. It is not clear, however, that this fact leads to a simple explanation of performance differences. If intelligence-related differences are due to differential tendencies to impose or use organization on a given task, highlighting the potential organization should reduce comparative differences in performance. The argument is that the external support will be of less help to the brighter subjects, because they are already carrying out the grouping operation and hence do not require help. Although Spitz (1966) obtained considerable data of this type, his findings are not unchallenged. For example, MacMillan (1970) found that grouping digits for his subjects was more beneficial to older retarded children (12 years) than to younger ones (9 years).

Huttenlocher and Burke (1976) administered digit-span tests to children of average intelligence who varied in age. In a standard condition, the auditory presentation was made at a constant rate, whereas in a second condition, the items were segmented into groups. This latter condition was presumed to induce the kind of chunking characteristic of the older subjects and thus to equate the various age groups in terms of the use of such a strategy. Further, the digits were presented very rapidly in an attempt to eliminate the use of rehearsal strategies. In the standard condition, developmental differences in memory span were obtained. Of more interest, although chunking items at input increased span performance, it did so equally for all groups. If differences in the standard condition had been due to differential use of the chunking strategy, and if the experimenter-imposed grouping had succeeded in equating the various groups with regard to the use of this strategy, developmental differences in span should have been eliminated or at least reduced. As they were not, Huttenlocher and Burke concluded that nonstrategic factors were responsible for the span differences. Their favorite candidate was the speed with which incoming items could be identified. Similar results, and a similar explanation, have been reported by Lyon (1977), using college students as subjects. (There is one potential problem with these studies. Although the digits were blocked on input, it is not clear that the subjects actually used the blocking in the way the authors assume. There is no independent evidence that a chunking strategy was employed. As we shall note in the strategy section, one requirement for a clear interpretation of strategy studies is some method for inferring strategy use, a method that is independent of simple amount recalled.)

Somewhat more direct evidence concerning the effects of encoding time on span performance has been reported by Chi (1977a). She found in a span task involving memory for faces that adults' span was approximately twice that of 5-year-olds. It was also true that it took the children twice as long as the adults to identify the faces. Reducing exposure time for adults in a fashion designed to counteract the identification time difference resulted in an elimination of age differences in span when recall was scored for accuracy without regard to order of report.

Although additional data with retarded subjects would be helpful, as would more demonstrations of direct links between efficiency and span, current research suggests that retarded children do have lower digit spans than nonretarded children and that these span differences may best be explained in terms of the efficiency with which stimulus identification and ordering take place; thus, the digit-span data also implicate efficiency factors as determinants of individual differences.

KNOWLEDGE BASE

It is amply clear that retarded children know less than nonretarded children of comparable CA. This leads to two broad types of questions. One very general kind is: Why do they know less? In some sense, the whole point of this chapter is to provide an answer to this query, that is, what are the factors limiting the amount of learning that seems to take place in retarded children? Do they process information slowly, thus increasing the scope of the bottleneck imposed by working-memory limitations? Do they lack the strategic devices and control of them necessary to overcome the limitations? Both of these possibilities may be true, leading to double danger. Inefficiency imposes constraints, and failure to employ clever devices to overcome any limitations makes the individual's plight that much worse; the consequence is impaired acquisition of knowledge.

There is, in addition, a more specific type of question, and that concerns the extent to which knowledge itself affects further learning. Differences in knowledge obviously affect what can be learned, and it is of considerable importance to ask how much variation in performance can be accounted for by knowledge differences and how much performance variance remains after knowledge differences have been partialed out.

Chi (1981), working with nonretarded children, has argued that many developmental differences in memory performance can be accounted for in terms of differential knowledge (older people have more, and better organized, knowledge than younger ones do) and without recourse to additional, relatively independent skills, such as the tendency to be strategic. To support this notion, Chi has arranged situations where the age–knowledge correlation is broken – by choosing groups of subjects where the children are the experts and adults the relative novices (using chess as a vehicle) or by looking at the performance of a single child in areas in which he had various amounts of expertise (dinosaurs). Her findings are as follows: Child chess experts remember more chess-related information than adult novices do, and the children are better able to predict how powerful their memory will be. Also, a child's recall of dinosaur names is twice as high for a well-known set of dinosaurs than for a less well-known set. Given these data, Chi would like to argue that strategy use and knowledge about memory are consequences of the extent of knowledge available (Chi, 1981). How much you know determines what you do with that information. The important individual difference variable concerns amount and quality of knowledge rather than the extent to which one can operate upon that knowledge, as the latter is determined by the former. Although Chi has criticized prior strategy-oriented studies on the grounds that they did not include independent assessments of possible confounding knowledge-base differences, it can also be argued that in her knowledge-base work, there is no independent assessment of possible strategy use (see Brown et al., in press, for further discussion).

We do not agree with this extreme view, as will become evident, but we do agree that knowledge-base factors are important and that they have been under-emphasized in past treatments. There are clear instances where retarded children do know much about certain subjects – sports, television shows, music, and so forth – and it is generally accepted that their memory for events within these spheres is much better than would normally be expected. There are, in addition, the traditional clinical findings regarding idiot savants (Hill, 1978), where isolated packages of knowledge are associated with extremely impressive performance levels. We do not, however, have the kind of comparative research necessary to evaluate any strong assertions. We need research investigating the performance of retarded and non-retarded children whose knowledge in some domain is equated.[4] It would then be possible to see where and how they differed within that domain, for example, in use of the information elsewhere, learning more about the topic, remembering informa-tion about the subject, and so forth. That is, certain things must be true. Subjects who do not know anything about certain categories, for example, that horses and dogs are animals or that Olympia, Salem, and Sacramento are state capitals (if they are) cannot use that information to organize their recall of lists including those items. It is less clear whether children of varying intelligence "equated" in such knowledge will be equally likely to use that organization to structure their recall.

The little evidence we do have suggests that retarded children are less likely to use information that they are known to have. Specifically, consider the area of recall of lists of words drawn from a small set of taxonomic categories. Retarded children do not recall such lists as well as nonretarded children do, nor do they give evidence of organizing their recall around those categories (see "Strategies" below). It is not the case, however, that they do not have information about the structure of the list items available to them. For example, if asked to recall the items by category, they do so, and recall improves. Also, attempts to assess the organization of their knowledge about these categories based on automatic processing reveal similarities, rather than differences, between retarded and nonretarded children. Examples here include research on semantic priming (Sperber, Ragain, & McCauley, 1976) and PI release (Winters & Cundari, 1979).

In the case of semantic priming, the speed of identifying the second word of a pair is greater if the two words are drawn from the same, as opposed to different, categories. The latency to identify *cat* is faster if the previous word was *horse* than if it was *house*. The presence of such priming effects does indicate that the within-category items are associated in memory. With PI release, the subject is given a series of trials on which he or she is to recall a small number of items. During a series of trials, the items are all drawn from the same category, and there follows a trial on which items from a new category are presented. The typical finding (Wickens, 1972) is that performance declines during the series of same-category items (proactive inter-ferences build up) and then increases when the category is changed (release from PI), this pattern indicating that the items drawn from the first category are in fact grouped in memory and are relatively distinct from those in the new category pre-sented on the final trial. In both cases, retarded children provide data indicating that their organization of those items in memory is similar to that of nonretarded children.

That comparative differences in clustering and recall exist can then be taken as evidence that knowledge is not sufficient to elicit strategic use of that knowledge. The problem with this conclusion, however, is fairly obvious. The priming and PI tasks may assess only the most rudimentary knowledge that subjects have about the items, and more detailed and sophisticated analyses may be needed to reveal the differences that do exist. In any event, the kind of research necessary to deal with the questions is clear, and we hope that such research will be forthcoming.

STRATEGIES

The logic of training studies

A large proportion of the recent research with retarded children has centered on the role of various strategies on determining task performance. The general finding to emerge from this work is that when confronted with tasks requiring strategic inter-vention, retarded children fail to produce the necessary activities and consequently perform quite poorly. We will review only a few of the many relevant studies here. Much of what we know about the retarded child's use of strategies comes from training studies. Given that subjects initially fail to produce a strategy when left to their own devices, training studies provide information about the type of deficit or weakness involved. The first question is whether the deficiency is one of production or one of mediation (Flavell, 1970), that is, whether the subject can employ the strategy effectively when he is induced to use it (production deficiency) or whether he cannot use it effectively even when instructed in its use (mediation deficiency). It generally turns out that the subjects can use the (relatively simple) strategies that have comprised the bulk of the literature, and further questions about the nature of the original problem can follow.

The use of training distinguishes the strategy research from that reviewed in the previous sections. Rather than looking simply at baseline performance, a general test–train–test procedure is employed, whereby the baseline information is supple-mented by data on the responsiveness of the subjects to training. (In this way, the strategy research is more similar to the clinical attempts to describe and remediate aberrant populations – see section 8.4). It should be emphasized here that the training studies we shall review were designed for theoretical reasons and did not have remediation as their goal. We believe that the emphasis on, and refinement of, the training study as a theoretical tool for investigating cognitive development is one of the major accomplishments of research in this area. As we shall note, training studies can be sorted into three types – blind, informed, and self-control (Brown, Campione, & Day, 1981). The order in which they are listed matches their order of appearance in the literature, with the later forms emerging as a direct result of the results obtained with the earlier ones. As we progress along this scale, we also refine our views about the nature of intelligence.

The general logic of training studies has been described in detail elsewhere (Brown & Campione, 1978; Butterfield, 1981; Campione & Brown, 1978), and we will be brief here. The endeavor begins with a theoretical analysis of some interesting task and a hypothesis about a source of individual differences within that task or a reason why retarded children perform poorly on that task. It might be assumed that Components A, B, and C are required to carry out Task X and that retarded children do poorly because of a weakness in A. To test this assertion, we might train retarded subjects in the use of A and then retest them on X. If performance improves, two benefits accrue: The task analysis is reinforced, and the hypothesis about the retarded subject's problem area also gains support. If A were not an important component of X, performance should not improve; and if the subjects were efficient with regard to A originally, training should likewise have no effect.

The training approach is an iterative one, and a failure to eliminate comparative differences indicates that there are other sources of individual differences to be identified. At this point, the procedure is repeated; a new hypothesis about the source of differences is formulated, new training is undertaken, and performance changes are observed. This process continues until we eliminate differences or give up.

There are two benefits to be derived from this procedure. It helps us evaluate our analyses of the processes involved in the target task. The argument is similar to that involved in generating computer simulations of particular activities. If we understand what is required to perform well in some domain, we should be able to instruct a computer to do so. The need to produce a program that can solve problems of some type forces the theorist to be extremely explicit about the steps involved in successful performance. Correspondingly, if we understand the domain well enough, we should be able to instruct a slow-learning child to perform adequately (more readily than a computer, some would think). To the extent that instructed performance leaves something to be desired, we would conclude that the theoretical analysis underlying the intervention was incomplete or that we had encountered a component of performance that cannot be instructed, that is, a structural feature of the learner's system (cf. Campione & Brown, 1978; Brown, 1974).[5] As we shall see, retarded children are very helpful in this aspect of the research, as their need for detailed and explicit instruction provides a fairly rigorous check on our theorizing. If we fail to specify some necessary activity, they let us know by not filling in the missing bit themselves.

The second result of training research, and possibly more relevant to this chapter, is that it provides a powerful way of specifying or identifying important components of intelligence. Retarded children are those who perform poorly on a class of academic and test items. A specification of what it is we need to train in order to reduce or eliminate comparative differences would greatly help us formulate a theoretically based definition of intelligence.

In research concerned with the effects of strategy use, one methodological point needs to be emphasized. An essential ingredient for a readily interpretable strategy training study is a measure of strategy use that is independent of simple performance level. If this condition is satisfied, we can make stronger tests of any hypotheses regarding the use and role of strategies. The better studies provide both multiple and more direct measures of strategy use (see Butterfield & Belmont, 1977, for a more detailed discussion). As a simple example of the problems possible, consider a case where some intervention designed to induce strategy use has little or no effect on performance. If there is no independent measure of strategy use, we do not know whether training was ineffective in inducing the strategy at all or whether the strategy was being attempted with no success. Although this requirement appears obvious enough, it is not easy to achieve and in fact is unsatisfied in much of the published work.

All strategy training studies include a common component – the subjects are taught how to use some systematic approach to a problem – but these studies differ in the amount of additional information afforded the trainee. By *blind training*, we mean to imply that the students are not active conspirators in the training process. They are induced to use the strategy, or tricked into carrying out the desired activities, without a concurrent understanding of the significance of that activity. For example, the child is taught to use a cumulative rehearsal strategy by initially copying an adult, but he is not told *explicitly* why he is acting this way, or that it helps performance, or that it is an activity appropriate to a certain class of memory situations (Brown, 1974). In the task of free recall of categorizable materials, the child can be tricked into using the categorical structure by clever incidental orienting instructions (Murphy & Brown, 1975), or the material can be blocked into categories for the learner (Gerjuoy & Spitz, 1966), or recall can be cued by category name (Green, 1974), but the child does not necessarily know why, or even if, use of the categories helps recall. All of these tricks lead to enhanced recall because the child is induced or tricked into using activities that facilitate learning. Such studies, however, fail to lead to maintenance or to generalization of the strategy – that is, the child neither uses the activity subsequently on his volition nor transfers the activity to similar learning situations. This fact is scarcely surprising, as the significance of the activity was never made clear to the learner. We shall return to this point.

At an intermediate level of instruction, *informed training,* the child is both induced to use a strategy and given some information concerning the significance of that activity. For example, children may be taught to rehearse and may be given feedback concerning their improved performance (Kennedy & Miller, 1976); or they might be taught to rehearse on more than one rehearsal task, that is, they might be trained in multiple contexts so that they can see the utility of the strategy (Belmont, Butterfield, & Borkowski, 1978). In a task requiring free recall of categorizable lists, students may be given practice in putting items into categories *and* may be informed that this procedure will help them remember *and* may be cued by category on retrieval failure – that is, a whole package designed to show children a learning strategy that works (Burger et al., 1978; Ringel & Springer, 1980).

In the third level of instruction, *self-control training,* the child is instructed not only in the use of a strategy but also (explicitly) in how to employ, monitor, check, and evaluate that strategy.

The number of relevant studies decreases with increasing level, with the vast majority being of the blind type. The informed and self-control types are also more recent and are becoming proportionately much more frequent. We believe that the shift in type of study reflects the changing nature of the questions dominating the area. In the early 1970s the questions were whether memory problems experienced by the retarded were attributable to strategy deficits and whether these difficulties could be overcome through strategy training. This inquiry was an essential first step; prior to the emphasis on strategies in mediating memory performance, memory was conceived as a more or less unitary faculty with regard to which some people were good and others poor. Essentially, older and brighter students were seen as having more bins into which to place incoming information (digit span was seen as a measure of the number of bins available in memory). This view explained differences in memory performance, and theorists were then interested in showing how memory problems affected performance in other domains. Thus memory was used as an explanatory concept rather than being itself something to be explained. The strategy training research succeeded in changing this view of memory and emphasized the importance of the learner's activity as a determinant of memory performance itself.

As data accumulated, it became clear that strategy deficits were widespread. Therefore, if one were interested in remediation efforts, it would be necessary to show that training had fairly widespread effects; the alternative would be to attempt to teach the specific strategies associated with each task that the subjects might encounter. It followed that the initial instructional effects should be tested in more detail – over time (maintenance) and over tasks (generalization). The results here were clear: Maintenance could be achieved, but tests for generalization remained discouragingly negative (cf. Campione & Brown, 1977). At this point the training emphasis shifted, and, we would add, the research became more directly addressed to questions about the nature of intelligence. The game became a matter of attempting to engineer transfer; doing so would require that we understand and specify some of the factors involved in promoting the effective use of information.

The implicit assumption here is that intellectually average or superior students would transfer the fruits of learning more broadly. That is, the tendency or ability to use old learning to facilitate new learning, to transfer, was assumed to be a major aspect of intelligence. In fact, for some, the failures of retarded subjects to engage in strategic attempts to learn and remember were themselves regarded as transfer failures (e.g., Campione & Brown, 1977, 1978). Given this presumed relation between intelligence and transfer, the modified theoretical question became one of elucidating the component skills involved in transfer. The training experiment approach to this problem thus became a matter of engineering transfer. What additional skills needed to be taught to retarded children to enable them to demonstrate transfer?

One popular hypothesis was that transfer failures were due in good part to the trainees' failure to understand the significance of the instructed activities, that is, the sources of many of their problems were metacognitive (Brown, 1978; Flavell, 1978) in nature. Thus, informed training was undertaken in an attempt to induce understanding of the effects of training. Because students given blind training did not appear to discover the utility of the instructed routines, they were explicitly provided with more information regarding them. Although this procedure had some beneficial effects, there remained room for improvement, and self-control training attempts were the result.

Types of training

An enormous number of studies have been concerned with strategic behavior in the retarded. Detailed reviews of these studies exist elsewhere (see particularily chapters by Borkowski & Cavanaugh, Bray, Detterman, & Glidden in Ellis, 1979), and will not be repeated here. We will describe only a few studies and will concentrate on two classes of strategies, namely, rehearsal and organization. We believe that similar patterns emerge from the two lines of research, suggesting generality of our conclusions, but that the target activities are sufficiently different to permit a discussion of some of the problems encountered in the strategy research. The areas differ in the ease with which we can draw conclusions confidently about the intentional use of strategic approaches to "solve" memory problems.

BLIND TRAINING.   Blind training studies, historically the earliest, were concerned with evaluating the extent to which strategic deficits were responsible for poorer performance by retarded children. The first step was to see if in fact nonretarded children were more likely to engage in strategic activities. It was therefore necessary to find a task likely to elicit such activities and a way to determine whether those activities were produced. On the presumption that there would be comparative differences in strategy use, the next question concerned the form of the difference, that is, does the retarded subjects' deficiency relate to production or to mediation? On the assumption that the response to training would be positive, the next question concerned the extent to which the strategic difference represented the whole story, that is, does instruction in strategy use eliminate comparative differences in that task? The clearest answers to these questions can be obtained from research on rehearsal strategies. There are many appropriate experimental tasks and good methods for assessing strategy use within them.

REHEARSAL PROCESSES.   We will illustrate this work by reference to two series of studies, the first reported by Brown, Campione, Bray, and Wilcox (1973). The task employed was the keeping-track task, which requires that the subject keep track of several things at once. In an early study of keeping-track performance with mildly retarded adolescents, Brown (1972b) presented sequences of 4 pictures, each representing a different category (e.g., animals, foods, vehicles, or clothing). In one sequence the participants might be shown pictures of a horse, a pie, a car, and a shirt. Following this sequence, they would be asked to recall the instance presented for 1 of the 4 categories (e.g., animals). On the next trial, they might see a cat, a boat, a tie, and a cake and might then be asked to indicate which food had occurred. Across trials the order and instances of each category changed, so that the subject was required to keep track of the changing states (instances) of 4 different variables (categories). Of interest here is the composition of the set of pictures used in the experiment. A total of 16 pictures consisted of 2 examples, or states, of 1 variable (e.g., foods: pie, cake), 4 states of each of 2 variables (e.g., vehicles: train, boat, plane, car), and 6 states of the final variable. Thus, specific pictures would recur frequently over the series of trials.

The most efficient strategy for this type of task is to rehearse the four items presented in the current set, keeping them available until the test occurs. Yntema and Mueser (1960) found that the keeping-track performance of nonretarded adults was not influenced by the number of states of each variable. The adults apparently used a rehearsal strategy to update the information on each trial and were able to disregard previously presented instances. They would consider only the items presented on the current trial and would determine which of those was an example of the category being probed. With retarded adolescent subjects, however, Brown

(1972b) found that accuracy decreased as the number of states per variable increased. These results suggested that all of the states of the variable were being considered at the time of the test. It appeared, then, that the retarded subjects were not using a rehearsal strategy to keep track of the states of the variables.

These accuracy data can be supplemented by some speed-of-responding data. Brown, Campione, Bray, and Wilcox (1973) also measured the amount of time elapsing between the presentation of the probe question ("What was the animal?") and the subject's response. The expectation was that latencies of rehearsing subjects would be independent of the number of states of the probed variable. They would simply refer to their rehearsal set (which would include the four items presented on that trial) and would choose the one that was the animal. Thus the number of states of the probed variable would make no difference, as those states would never be considered. In the absence of rehearsal, however, the items just presented would not be available in working memory, and the subject would have to check through all the possible states to determine which had been seen most recently. This task should be more difficult and more time consuming as the number of alternatives increases from two to six.

Given this analysis, it should be easy to determine whether subjects are rehearsing or not. If they are rehearsing, both their accuracy (corrected for guessing, see Brown, Campione, Bray, & Wilcox, 1973) and latency scores should be independent of the number of states of the probed variable. For nonrehearsing subjects, in contrast, accuracy should decrease and response times increase as the number of states of the probed variable increases. The essential point is that these "rehearsal indicators" are independent of simple accuracy; presumably, subjects could show a rehearsal pattern and poor overall recall or high accuracy and a nonrehearsal pattern.

In a pair of experiments, one involving retarded adolescents and a second an equal CA comparison group of average intelligence, the following observations were made: (a) When left to deal with the task as they saw fit, the retarded children performed poorly and showed a consistent nonrehearsal pattern, that is, accuracy decreased and latency increased as the number of states of the probed variable increased; (b) nonretarded adolescents performed excellently and showed consistent rehearsal patterns; (c) retarded students instructed to rehearse improved their accuracy dramatically and evinced patterns presumed to be indicative of rehearsal; and (d) nonretarded adolescents prevented from rehearsing showed reduced accuracy and patterns indicating nonrehearsal.

These data are all consistent with a production deficiency account of the initial comparative difference. Retarded children perform much more poorly than nonretarded children of comparable CA. The nonretarded children's accuracy and latency scores are independent of the number-of-states variable, indicating rehearsal; for retarded children, the number-of-states variable had a larger and predictable effect on both accuracy and latency, indicating a lack of rehearsal. Although these data are sufficient to highlight the importance of rehearsal processes, the additional data collected in these studies strengthen that claim further. Nonretarded children prevented from rehearsing showed accuracy and latency patterns similar to those of uninstructed retarded children, and retarded children instructed to rehearse generated patterns that were similar to nonretarded subjects allowed to proceed unimpeded. This overall set of results indicates that the retarded child's poor performance compared with that of nonretarded children on this task was due to differential rehearsal use. It also indicates that a production deficiency was operating, in that instruction did result in effective use of the strategy.

We believe that these experiments suggest several important points, some methodological and some theoretical. Methodologically, we would like to emphasize the multiple convergent measures of rehearsal; given that factor, there is no question about the interpretation in terms of strategy use. In fact, given a series of sessions, it is possible to determine whether individual subjects are, or are not, rehearsing (Brown, 1974). Without this feature, as we shall see, the interpretation of single studies becomes much more complicated.

At the theoretical level we would like to emphasize the magnitude of the baseline comparative differences obtained in this task and the amount of change obtained through instructing the retarded children. Let us first consider the initial differences. Retarded children performed at 58% correct on the first three (nonrecency) items. Nonretarded children *could not be run* on the same task; in some pilot sessions, they simply never made errors. To bring their performance down from the ceiling, we were forced to include a filled retention interval (counting backward by threes in Spanish because the subjects were drawn from a Spanish class); the retarded children were given immediate probes. Even with the filled retention interval, the nonretarded students averaged 90% correct. Second, we found it very difficult to prevent rehearsal in the nonretarded students. We had to force them to name repeatedly the available items during stimulus presentation (say "cat, cat, cat," etc., until the next item was presented), and we had to include a filled retention interval before rehearsal was reasonably suppressed. Even then, many of the subjects reported that they "snuck in" a little cumulative rehearsal; and almost all were observed continually moving their eyes from left to right, reviewing the earlier windows even while they were repetitively naming one of the later items. Thus, although it was necessary to provide detailed instruction in rehearsal use before retarded students would engage in it, it was exceedingly difficult to prevent nonretarded students from rehearsing. We see a large comparative difference in the "propensity" to use an intentional memory strategy.

We turn now to the magnitude of strategy-related improvement obtained with the retarded students. Prior to training, they averaged 58% correct on the initial three items. Use of rehearsal resulted in an accuracy level on those items of 85%, a proportionate increase of 47%. Although measures of processing efficiency seem to account for relatively small amounts of variance (see chapter 3 in this volume), variation in strategy use is associated with large variations in task performance.

Our second illustration of rehearsal use and training is a study reported by Butterfield, Wambold, and Belmont (1973). Mildly retarded adolescents were shown sequences of six letters, each appearing on separate projection screens arranged in a horizontal array. A subject-paced procedure was used in which the participant pressed a button to view each successive item. The exposure time was held constant at .5 sec per item, but the subject was allowed to pause as long as he or she wished before pressing the button to expose the next item. At the end of each sequence, one of the letters appeared in a "probe" window. The subject was then to indicate the location of the probe letter in the sequence.

Belmont and Butterfield (1971) had previously found that mentally retarded adolescents paused very briefly, if at all, between presses, whereas nonretarded adults used a systematic pause pattern. Adults rehearsed the early items in the sequence and then quickly exposed the last few items. The adult strategy is well adapted to the task requirements, because the last few items remain available in working memory for a short time without rehearsal. Rehearsal of the first few items in the list helps maintain these items until the recall test.

Butterfield and associates (1973) first trained their retarded subjects to use a three–three rehearsal strategy similar to that used by adults. The subjects were trained to view the first three letters, to pause following the third letter, to rehearse that group of three as a set, and then to expose the last three letters quickly in preparation for an immediate test. This strategy raised the level of performance, especially for the first three letters in the sequence, but recall of the last items was still poor, suggesting the need for continued training.

This finding illustrates one advantage of the instructional approach to comparative or developmental psychology: It includes a self-evaluation component. If instruction does not eliminate comparative differences, this fact affords a clear indication that sources of comparative differences remain and that the theory underlying the development of the instructional regime is incomplete. It may also be the case (and instruction is ideally designed with this in mind) that aspects of the data suggest some other possible sources of differences. In the study reported by Butterfield and associates, there were several indicators available. First, the correlation between a measure of strategy use, based on pause patterns during study, and accuracy in locating the probe letter was not as high as might be expected. Second, performance was lower than might be expected primarily on the second half of the list. The authors noted that effective use of the specific acquisition, or study, strategy that had been instructed demanded the use of an equally specific retrieval strategy. This retrieval plan required two parts. First, when the probe item was presented, the last three items in the inspection set should have been searched, taking advantage of the fact that these items would not yet have "faded" from working memory. Then, if this search were unsuccessful, the first three (rehearsed) items should have been searched. Note that reversing this order would reduce the utility of the study strategy, as the passively viewed items would be given time to fade from memory. The fact that performance on the last three items was poor suggested that this reversal may have occurred. That is, the subjects did not spontaneously devise the necessary retrieval strategy. To evaluate this hypothesis, further training attempts were undertaken.

Ignoring a number of intermediate attempts, we turn to the final training procedure used by Butterfield and associates (1973), which involved several steps. The subjects were initially trained to rehearse a sequence of three letters cumulatively and to count to 10 before recalling the position of the probe item in that set. This exercise gave the subject practice in searching a set of three rehearsed items following a delay between the termination of rehearsal and the test. Next the participants were given six letters and were instructed to use the three–three rehearsal strategy, rehearsing the first three and exposing the last three letters with very short pauses between each of the last three letters and between the last letter and the probe. During this phase the subjects were told that the test item would always come from the last three items. To aid performance, the subjects were instructed to point to Screen Numbers 4 through 6, in sequence, trying to identify the position of the probe letter by saying the names of the letters. After practice at this the subjects were told that a probe letter might be taken from any of the six positions. To deal with this problem, they were instructed to recall the letters, beginning with Letters 4 through 6 and then 1 through 3. The combined rehearsal training and retrieval strategy training resulted in a substantial increase in recall for all six items, where the rehearsal training alone facilitated recall only on the first three items. In fact, final performance was better than that of nonretarded adolescents of the same CA not given training in the task.

This work and the keeping-track experiments discussed previously share several features. These are assessments of rehearsal use independent of recall accuracy, namely, pause patterns. Latency data were also employed, to evaluate notions about retrieval schemes; for example, if subjects respond to a probe by searching the last three items first, response times should be faster to the second set of three items than to the first. These separate indexes simplify the problem of interpretation. Also, the improvement induced by training was impressive, raising the retarded adolescents' performance to the level of performance shown by untrained control students.

A more important conclusion should be drawn from this set of experiments, and that concerns the dramatic need for clear and explicit instruction before the performance increments could be obtained. Not only did retarded subjects fail to produce a reasonable study strategy; when they were taught one, they did not use it effectively. They did not adopt the retrieval strategy dictated by that study strategy. Even when they were provided with the retrieval strategy (in some intermediate phases that we have not described), they failed to exploit its "full potential." They had to be instructed explicitly in the sequencing and coordination of the separate routines. Optimal performance required that the instructor teach both the separate components *and* then coordination of those components.

These data are illustrative of two general claims. One is that the use of retarded learners can help in the evaluation of an existing task analysis. A beginning analysis of this task might emphasize the importance of the rehearsal strategy – the fact that it dictates a particular retrieval plan could go unnoticed if subjects who used the rehearsal strategy "automatically" adopted the correct retrieval routine. Going one additional step, teaching the rehearsal and retrieval plans separately could be sufficient for more mature "nonproducers," that is, given the two components, the coordination of them could be automatic. With retarded children, this "executive control" of instructed routines does not emerge without instruction, making it more visible.

The second claim is that these data are typical and reinforce the view that a particularly important feature of the retarded child's cognitive profile is an inability to profit from incomplete instruction. We shall return frequently to this point, which forms the basis of our theoretical biases about the nature of intelligence (see section 8.5). The argument is that individuals of higher intelligence who were nonproducers would need less instruction to reach a comparable level of proficiency. In section 8.4 we will review other relevant data provided by the clinical and educational literature and will relate them to Vygotsky's notion of a "zone of proximal development" (Vygotsky, 1978).

As a final comment, we emphasize that even in the work by Butterfield and associates, there is no evidence that comparative differences were eliminated. First, the initially proficient were never instructed, and it may well be the case that if all groups were given instruction, the initial differences would be reinstated. Second, there is a clear danger of ceiling effect contamination. With short lists and unlimited study time, 100% accuracy is easily achievable.

In this regard, we can emphasize one possible interaction among our factors that may be important in rehearsal situations. Specifically, the extent to which individuals can profit from the use of rehearsal strategies may depend upon the facility with which the items can be named or identified (cf. Spring, 1976; Spring & Capps, 1974). Further, this interaction might be seen most clearly in situations where more limited study time is available. The suggestion is that, in at least some rehearsal situations, comparative differences may be impossible to eliminate because of underlying speed-of-processing differences.

ORGANIZATIONAL PROCESSES.   Material presented for learning frequently involves some degree of inherent organization, and it is clear that capitalizing on that organization can facilitate both the learning and the remembering of the information. On some occasions, that organization may be clear, whereas on others, the learner may have to expend considerably more effort before discerning it. A number of investigators, most notably Spitz (1966, 1972), have argued that one characteristic of retarded children is their failure to seek for, or impose, organization on material to be learned, with the result that they acquire that material more slowly. As we shall see, research on organizational factors involves a number of complexities that do not arise in the case of rehearsal. Although the problems are real ones and do render interpretation of some experiments difficult, we believe that the same conclusions can be drawn from the literature as from the rehearsal case.

To study the role and use of organizational factors, investigators have resorted primarily to free-recall methodologies. The impetus for this work stems from Bousfield's (1953) classic demonstration that college students recalling a list of words drawn from a small set of taxonomic categories recall the words grouped by categories rather than randomly or as a function of the order in which they were presented. The tendency to recall words by category is known as clustering, and a variety of measures of clustering have been developed (see Murphy, 1979, for a discussion) to assess the strength of that tendency. Although nonretarded adolescents tend to show clear evidence of clustering in their free-recall protocols (Moely, 1977), retarded children do not. In one early experiment by Spitz and Gerjuoy (reported in Spitz, 1966), retarded adolescents for (CA, $M = 14.5$ years) were compared with subjects who included a group of nonretarded children (matched for CA) on the free recall of a 20-item list. This list consisted of 5 exemplars of each of 4 categories. Although the nonretarded group showed significant amounts of clustering, the retarded subjects' clustering scores did not significantly differ from chance; further, the nonretarded subjects recalled significantly more items. These data are consistent with the notion that the retarded students failed to use the organization inherent in the list to be remembered, whereas their nonretarded counterparts did do so.

To evaluate further the role of organizational factors in mediating the group recall differences, Spitz and Gerjuoy attempted to induce the use of organizational processes by retarded children to see if recall scores would increase. They did so in two ways, which they described as *presented clustering* and *requested clustering*. In the former, the list was presented blocked by category, that is, on each trial, all words belonging to each category were presented together rather than being distributed randomly throughout the list. In the requested clustering condition, the list was presented in the normal way, with the words randomly ordered, but at recall the subjects were instructed to recall the words by category, for example, "Tell me all the animals you can remember from the list." In either case, both clustering scores and amount recalled improved significantly. These findings support the notion that a deficiency in the use of organizational principles was one factor underlying the originally poor recall performance of the retarded students. Although the results of these studies have not always been replicated exactly (see Glidden, 1979, for a recent review), the general picture appears clear enough: Retarded subjects do not seem to use organization spontaneously but can be induced to do so.

Before accepting this conclusion, we need to consider a number of problems associated with the use of clustering paradigms to investigate the use of strategies. A major requirement for any research effort here is the availability of a measure of strategy use (use of organization) that is independent of amount recalled. To show the importance of strategy use, we need to be able to identify occasions when the strategy is used and to show that its use enhances recall. In much of the literature, clustering scores serve as the measure of strategy use. The problems are the following: First, clustering scores may not provide an estimate of intentional and strategic use of organization. For example, Chi (1981) has argued that the tendency to cluster in free recall represents the relatively automatic effect of a well-developed knowledge base. Differences in clustering would then be assigned to differential knowledge rather than to strategic differences. Second, the relation between clustering scores and recall is controversial. For example, in some research with retarded individuals, investigators have reported intervention-based increases in clustering scores without accompanying recall increments (e.g., Bilsky & Evans, 1970; Bilsky, Evans, & Gilbert, 1972). Third, even the presence of a correlation between clustering scores and recall does not necessarily support the hypothesized relation. Many measures of clustering are not independent of recall level when there is some organizational tendency present (Murphy, 1979). Thus, positive correlations could be an artifact of the measure employed.

Despite these problems, we regard the free-recall evidence as consistent with the notion of a strategy deficit in retarded children. This conclusion stems from a number of other considerations indicating that knowledge-base differences are not sufficient to account for recall differences in other, related situations and for the effects obtained in instructional research.

Presume, for example, that we attempt to account for the finding that retarded children cluster less, and recall fewer items, than nonretarded controls by assuming that recall in such situations reflects the automatic effects of a well-organized knowledge base and that retarded children simply have a poorer knowledge base. The objections to this interpretation are threefold. First, if sensitive indicators of the knowledge base are used, retarded children seem to possess the relevant knowledge. For example, using a semantic priming procedure, Sperber, Ragain, and McCauley (1976) found evidence indicating the presence of categorical relationships in the memory structure of retarded adolescents. A similar conclusion can be drawn from experiments by Winters and Cundari (1979) using the release from proactive interference paradigm developed by Wickens (1972). Although it might be argued that these procedures are not sensitive enough to reveal more subtle but important differences, the data do indicate the presence of some relevant organized knowledge. Second, if knowledge is really inadequate, it is not clear why instructional efforts that do not aim at enhancing knowledge can have large effects. Finally, other investigations of the use of organization in situations suggest that knowledge differences are unimportant. For example, Spitz, Goettler, and Webreck (1972) investigated the tendency of retarded and nonretarded children to detect and to use two types of redundancy in digit-recall situations. *Couplet redundancy* consisted of strings of successive sets of repeating items, for example, 2, 2, 1, 1, 5, 5, 4, 4, and *repetition redundancy,* where the second half of the series was identical to the first half, for example, 2, 1, 5, 4, 2, 1, 5, 4. In both cases, retarded adolescents were much less likely to make use of the redundancy than were nonretarded subjects, although the provision of external prompts, for example, underlining to emphasize the patterns, did result in improvements in performance. Again, the organization could readily be used once it was pointed out, but retarded subjects were less likely to use it without intervention. It seems unlikely here that knowledge-base limitations are involved in the comparative difference. The conclusion is that the tendency to seek and/or exploit such organization spontaneously is the important factor.

In the instructional experiments reviewed thus far, the goal was to reduce or eliminate comparative differences by providing the slow learners with the tools used by the more efficient. Retarded children taught to use task-appropriate strategies did show consistently large improvements, particularly in following explicit and detailed instruction. It is also the case, however, that strategies for learning are used flexibly by mature learners, that is, they can be adapted to the varying demands of a family of situations. In addition to reducing differences within a task, we might also aim for across-tasks effects. The question of interest, then, concerned the extent to which retarded subjects taught a particular strategy would be able to use it flexibly or would show signs of transfer. The argument here is that if training has had any general effect on intelligence, it should be possible to detect its sequelae in other situations. If there were no transfer, the instructional routines would need to be supplemented, and the supplements required would then indicate the kinds of input needed to obtain more widespread effects of training and would consequently suggest more about the components of intelligence.

Although Butterfield and associates (1973) were able to claim considerable success within a task, studies involving across-tasks investigations resulted in essentially negative findings. Maintenance could be achieved; that is, retarded children could be shown to continue using trained strategies in the absence of explicit prompts to do so, as long as the task remained the same. Training in multiple sessions seemed sufficient if this were the goal of training. For example, the subjects in the study by Brown, Campione, Bray, and Wilcox (1973) were brought back to the laboratory 6 months after the initial training experiment, which had involved 12 training sessions. They were told that they would again be asked to remember some pictures, but no mention was made of the rehearsal strategy that they had been taught to use. Analyses of individual subjects' data showed that 8 of the 10 instructed children continued to rehearse and were correct on 82% of the trials (Brown, Campione, & Murphy, 1974). This figure is comparable to that obtained during training, that is, the subjects who continued to rehearse did so with no appreciable dropoff in accuracy.

When transfer to other tasks was investigated, however, the data were less encouraging; there was no strong evidence for transfer to new tasks (Brown, 1978; Campione & Brown, 1977, 1978). These outcomes suggested that generalized effects of training would have to be programmed rather than simply hoped for. In retrospect, this finding is not at all surprising. In most cases, the strategies taught in these studies were fairly simple ones, and it is reasonable to assume that all their components were available to the trainees before the experiment began. If so, the failure of the subjects to employ the strategies spontaneously could be regarded as failures of transfer. Nothing in the blind training approach would help overcome this problem, and it is thus not surprising that it failed to do so. Viewed in this way, the transfer failures could be seen as simply a rediscovery of the subjects' original problem – a failure to access and assemble available components and routines to form a plan for dealing with a current problem.

Whether this identification of initial production deficiencies with transfer failures in the first place is correct or not, the data were clear. Training did not result in flexible use of the instructed activities. Attention was then turned to a determination of the conditions under which trainees might generalize the effects of instruction. Our own assumption was that transfer would be obtained to the extent that subjects understood the significance of the activities that they had been taught. Transfer would require that the subjects realize, among other things, that some strategy was necessary and that passive involvement would not work, that the use of the strategy did result in enhanced performance, that the choice of the specific strategy was determined by some properties of the target task, and that that strategy, or a close variant of it, would be useful on other tasks sharing many of those properties.

INFORMED TRAINING. As blind training attempts did not appear sufficient to lead retarded children to infer those features, it became necessary to provide the information more or less directly, and a series of what we have called informed training studies (Brown, Campione, & Day, 1981) were undertaken. The guiding question here is: What does a student need to know to generalize effectively? What do more intelligent individuals know about specific activities in context that results in broad use of those activities? We have outlined elsewhere (Campione & Brown, 1977) a series of steps involved in the choice and use of a strategy and have described the factors we need to consider in designing instructional routines in a follow-up paper (Brown & Campione, 1978). We will not reproduce those discussions here but will simply indicate some of the factors that do lead to more widespread use of instructed activities.

If we consider the long-term effects of training, the simplest case is that of maintenance (Campione & Brown, 1977), which involves having the subject continue to use the trained routine in the absence of prompts on the same task involved in training. The more complex process, generalization, refers to the adoption, and typically modification, of the instructed strategy on some task related to but different from that of the training situation. Some factors that might underlie continued and extended use of a strategy are the realization that it is effective and the knowledge that it can be modified to apply to a number of situations. Informed training goes beyond blind training by attempting to make such information available to the learner.

In a number of studies with nonretarded children (e.g., Borkowski, Levers, & Gruenenfelder, 1976; Kennedy & Miller, 1976), an instructed strategy was more likely to be maintained in the absence of experimenter prompts if it had been made clear that the use of the strategy did result in improved performance. Apparently, for these subjects, the utility of the strategy was not appreciated without explicit feedback, and simply providing that information resulted in increased transfer. In a pair of studies with nonretarded (Kestner & Borkowski, 1979) and retarded (Kendall, Borkowski, & Cavanaugh, 1980) children, training centered on the use of elaborative strategies to facilitate paired-associates learning. The training lasted 4 days and involved a number of features, including explicit feedback about the strategy's effectiveness. A near-generalization task was also employed; the difference here was that the children were required to learn triads, rather than pairs, of words. In both experiments, children given the elaboration training outperformed control children on both the training and near-generalization tasks. Thus, whereas subjects who simply execute the instructed activity are unlikely to continue use of that activity in either the same or similar situations, those told how effective the routine was are more likely to use it subsequently. The implication is that developmentally immature individuals do not spontaneously evaluate their performance to realize the utility of the strategy.

A more detailed training program that also provided information about the use and effectiveness of instruction has been developed by Burger, Blackman, Holmes, and Zetlin (1978). They showed mildly retarded adolescents 16 cards, each presenting a picture of a common object. The pictures were from 4 categories (e.g., clothing, foods, flowers, and tools), with 4 instances of each category. During the first session (baseline), the 16 cards were presented for approximately 2 min. and were then covered. The subject then attempted to recall the picture names. The categorization training given to one group of subjects during Sessions 2 through 4 consisted of several components. The subject was first asked to put the pictures that "go to-gether" in horizontal rows. Suggestions were given, if necessary, for arranging the cards by category. The subject was then asked to label each category represented in the sorting and to name and count the instances within each category. Next, the subject was told that the pictures could be remembered best if he or she would try to recall the pictures by the groupings. The pictures were then covered, and the subject was asked to recall the picture names. If all of the picture names were not recalled, the experimenter supplied the appropriate category name as a cue. Explicit feedback about the amount of recall was also given.

This training procedure was repeated three times with a different set of pictures each session. There were two follow-up tests, the first 2 or 3 days following training and the second 3 weeks later. Recall and clustering following training were significantly higher than for the baseline session. Performance was also higher than the recall and clustering of a group of mentally retarded adolescents who had received the same amount of practice on the same stimulus sets but were not trained to use the categorization strategy. Attempts to teach subjects the significance of a trained routine do seem to result in somewhat enhanced transfer.

Transferring a strategy beyond the training situation would seem to require that the subject be aware of the general utility of the trained routine. This awareness can be brought about simply by telling the subject that the strategy can and should be used in a variety of tasks. A less direct method would be to train the strategy in multiple contexts, thereby demonstrating that it, or some close variant of it, is useful in more than one situation. One recent study involving retarded subjects and investi-gating the role of training in multiple, rather than single, contexts has been reported by Belmont, Butterfield, and Borkowski (1978). They were concerned with the use of a family of rehearsal strategies on a number of short-term memory tasks. In each case, the subjects, 12–15-year-old retarded children, saw a series of 7 letters, one in each of a row of windows. They were allowed to view the list at their own rate. This study trial was then followed by one of the memory tests. In three of the test situations, the subjects were required to recall all 7 items, although in different orders. In the 3/4 (4/3, 2/5) condition, they were to recall the last 3 (4, 2) items of the set, followed by the first 4 (3, 5) items. In a probed recall task, the set of 7 items was followed by a test letter, and they were told to indicate the window in which that letter had appeared. The point is that rehearsal processes are useful on each of these tasks, although the exact form of the strategy must be modified to take into account the specific demands of each. For example, in the 3/4 case, the optimal strategy would be to view the first 4 items and then to pause and rehearse them as a group until they are learned. Following this the last 3 items should be viewed more rapidly, and the subjects should attempt recall of the set immediately. Going from a 3/4 recall to a 4/3 recall requires that the learner both recognize the continued need for rehearsal and modify the strategy to conform to the changing response requirement.

In the study by Belmont and associates, two groups of retarded children were involved; one received training on only the 3/4 task, and one was taught to deal with both the 3/4 and 4/3 tasks. Although the group trained on only the 3/4 case did not show evidence of generalization, the twice-trained group did continue to rehearse on the 2/5 and probed-recall task. In these tasks, they showed study patterns consistent with rehearsal usage, and their recall scores were about 170% of those of the singly trained group. Although the variations in the tasks employed here are small, and thus the amount of generalization demonstrated somewhat limited, the results are promising and indicate the potential gains to be achieved through training in multiple contexts. Of import here, information about the cross-situational utility of instructed activities must be provided during training – slow-learning children do not make the inference themselves.

SELF-CONTROL TRAINING. Although these results both indicate that some evidence for transfer can be obtained and help clarify the source of the original problem, the transfer tasks have been very similar to the training vehicles. In an attempt to identify the processes that are responsible for more flexible use of learning routines in average functioning individuals but are weak or absent in the retarded, self-control training attempts have begun to emerge. Here the child is instructed not only in the use of a strategy but also explicitly in how to employ, monitor, check, and evaluate that strategy. The idea is that the use of these higher-level, general overseeing functions that are routinely used by effective learners and that play a major role in strategy choice and execution, that is, in transfer performance, is determined in good part by metacognitive and executive functioning (Brown, 1978; Brown & Campione, 1978; Campione & Brown, 1977, 1978).

For a number of reasons we should expect some of these general control skills, such as *planning* one's next move, *monitoring* the effectiveness of any attempted action, *testing, revising,* and *evaluating* one's strategies for learning (Brown, 1978; Brown & DeLoache, 1978), to play a role in transfer, and they should be featured prominently in a theory of intelligence.

This emphasis on more general skills can be defended in a number of ways. First, given the pervasive nature of problems encountered by EMR children, it seems reasonable to assume that those problems are mediated in part by a set of general factors common to a wide variety of situations. Second, we already have impressive evidence of young children's general problems with self-regulation and control of their goal-directed activities (Brown, 1975, 1978; Brown & DeLoache, 1978; Meichenbaum, 1977; Mischel & Patterson, 1976). If it is true that slow-learning children in particular experience major problems when they are required to orchestrate and regulate their own attempts at strategic intervention (Campione & Brown, 1977, 1978), then an alternative or supplement to the training of specific skills would be the training of general "metacognitive" skills (Brown, 1975, 1978; Flavell,

1971, 1978) notably absent in the academic problem solving of these children (Brown, 1978). Positive outcomes from the training attempts would reinforce the argument concerning the importance of these skills. General metacognitive skills, such as checking, planning, asking questions, self-testing, and monitoring current activities, rarely appear in the protocols of slow-learning children but are very general skills applicable in a wide variety of situations.

On a slightly different level, the failure of learners to employ these general overseeing functions has been seen as a major reason for their failure to transfer learned information (Brown, 1974, 1978; Campione & Brown, 1977, 1978). Given this analysis, the logic for directing training at these skills seems strong. When we consider the targets of typical training studies, it becomes apparent that the task is made difficult for the subject because of the emphasis on specific skill training. One problem with such specific skills is that they are just that – specific to a very small class of situations. Before learners could generalize the effects of instruction in the use of specific routines, they would have to be able to discriminate between situations in which the routine would be appropriate and those in which it would not. Adequate generalization requires both extended use in novel situations and decisions not to use the trained routines in other situations where they would not be beneficial (Brown, 1978; Campione & Brown, 1974, 1978). In the case of truly general skills, this discrimination should not be necessary, as the skill or routine could simply be used in a whole battery of problem-solving situations without regard to any subtle analysis of the task being attempted. In this sense, "general metacognitive skills" might be regarded as easy ones to instruct, or at least as the ones most likely to lead to transfer across task boundaries, and it makes sense to begin training with the simplest skills.

In this view, general metacognitive and executive control processes are directly implicated in both training and transfer. The self-control mechanisms that are the targets of training are essential components of successful performance. They may also function in a more indirect fashion by acting as retrieval and motivational aids to successful performance. For example, we have presented data indicating that maintenance of trained routines can be enhanced by providing information about the effectiveness of the trained strategy. Presumably, this information would have to come after each training attempt. If, however, the learner does monitor his progress and performance, he may be led to draw the correct conclusion about a strategy's effectiveness without prompting; teaching these skills would then result at least in maintenance in a variety of training situations. Knowing that, say, rehearsal improves performance is of minor importance. Carrying out the operations needed to arrive at that conclusion is much more important. In the next section, we will emphasize a distinction between metacognition and executive control and will argue that the latter is the more important concept for theories of intelligence.

To illustrate the effects of self-control training, we turn to a series of studies conducted in our laboratories (Brown & Barclay, 1976; Brown, Campione, & Barclay, 1979; Day, 1980). We considered the effects of instructing a general stop-test-and-study routine in the context of teaching specific memory strategies. This checking skill is an essential prerequisite for effective studying and one that young children have difficulty understanding (Flavell, Friedrichs, & Hoyt, 1970). So we devised a simple task in which we could make the self-checking demands of such studying activities quite explicit. The hope was that with the essential elements made clear in a simple situation, we could look for transfer to more complex, school-like learning tasks.

The simple training task consisted of presenting the students with a list of pictures equal to one and one-half times their span for picture lists. The pictures were presented in a series of windows and could be viewed when each window was pressed. Only one picture was visible at a time, but the students could investigate the windows in any order and as frequently as they wished. (Note one important difference between this procedure and that of Belmont and Butterfield, who also allowed their subjects as much time as they wanted for study. In their situation, the subjects were restricted to one pass through the list. Here subjects could review the list as often as desired.) They were also told to ring a bell when they felt they were ready to be tested for recall. Performance was initially poor, even though the children were free to study for as long as they liked.

During the training portion of the study, children were taught strategies that could be used to facilitate their learning of the lists, along with the overseeing or monitoring of those strategies. The latter aspect of training was accomplished by employing strategies that included a self-testing component and by telling the children to monitor their state of learning. For example, in a rehearsal condition, the subjects were told to break the list down into manageable subsets (three items) and to rehearse those subsets separately. They were also instructed to continue rehearsing the subsets until they were sure they could recall all of the items. Note that one can only continue to rehearse all the items if one can remember them well enough to produce them for rehearsal. Thus in this situation, rehearsal serves both to facilitate learning and to provide a check on the state of that learning. Anticipation was another trained strategy that included self-testing features. Here the children were instructed to try to remember the name of a picture before they pressed the window. Children in a final condition, "labeling," served as a control group; they were told to go through the list, repeatedly labeling each item as they exposed it. In all conditions, the students were told to continue the trained activity until they were sure they were ready to recall all the picture names.

The data are presented in Figure 8.1. Consider the older children (MA = approximately 8 years, CA = approximately 11 years). Those taught the strategies involving a self-testing component improved their performance significantly, whereas those in the control condition did not. These effects were extremely durable, lasting over a series of posttests, the last test occurring 1 year after the training had ended.

The younger children (MA = 6 years, CA = 9 years) did not benefit so much from training. They improved their performance significantly above baseline only on the first posttest, which was prompted, that is, the experimenter told the children to continue using the strategy they had been taught. In the absence of such prompts, they did not differ significantly from baseline. Note that the younger and older children did not differ on original learning but did differ in how readily they responded to training. Tests of original competence provide only part of the picture, for the degree to which students can profit from training is also essential information for diagnosis of their zone of proximal development (Brown, 1980; Brown & French, 1979b; Vygotsky, 1978) – that is, how well they can operate in some domain given support. We shall return to this point shortly, for as we shall argue in sections 8.4 and 8.5, we feel that this ability to benefit from instruction is fundamental to any conceptions of intelligence and development.

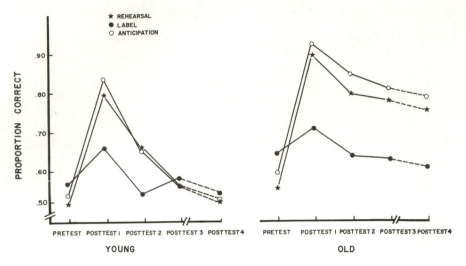

Figure 8.1. Proportion of items correctly recalled on recall-readiness pretest and posttest as a function of mental age and training condition. (From "Training Self-Checking Routines for Estimating Test Readiness: Generalization from List Learning to Prose Recall" by A. L. Brown, J. C. Campione, and C. R. Barclay, *Child Development* 1979, 50, 501–512. Copyright © 1979 by the Society for Research in Child Development, Inc. Reprinted by permission.)

The tendency for the younger children to abandon a trained strategy when not explicitly instructed to continue in its use is illustrated quite dramatically in the 1-year maintenance data shown in Table 8.1. On the first 2 days of testing, the children were not prompted to use a strategy, and they performed at baseline levels. On the 3rd day the experimenter told them: "Try to remember when we did this game before – remember that you said the picture names over and over [rehearsal], or remember that you tried to guess the picture names before you pressed the windows [anticipation]." These mild prompts resulted in significant improvements in performance on Day 3, improvements that were not maintained on the final, unprompted test (Day 4). This is a clear illustration of a common problem that bedevils would-be trainers of slow-learning children. Such children tend not to use even the skills they have available to them (Brown, 1980; Brown & Campione, 1981). Again, the distinction between the availability of routines and unprompted access to them is essential.

As Table 8.1 clearly shows, the picture was much more optimistic for the older children, and therefore we decided to investigate whether they had learned any general features about self-testing and monitoring on the simple laboratory task that they could transfer to a more schoollike situation, learning the gist of prose passages. The students (previously trained in gist-recall procedures) were seen for 6 days. On each day they studied two stories commensurate with their reading ability. When it was clear that the children could read all the words, they were instructed to continue studying until they were ready to attempt recall. The transfer data are shown in Figure 8.2. The trained students (in the anticipation and rehearsal groups) outperformed a pair of control groups (label and naive control) on four measures: (a) the

Table 8.1. *Mean proportion of correct recall as a function of groups, conditions, and test days: Maintenance phase*

Group and condition	Test days			
	Day 1 (unprompted)	Day 2 (unprompted)	Day 3 (prompted)	Day 4 (unprompted)
Young				
Anticipation	.50	.48	.81	.57
Rehearsal	.46	.50	.90	.63
Label	.46	.58	.78	.54
Old				
Anticipation	.80	.72	.95	.85
Rehearsal	.74	.73	.84	.83
Label	.60	.61	.67	.63

Source: Brown, Campione, and Barclay (1979).

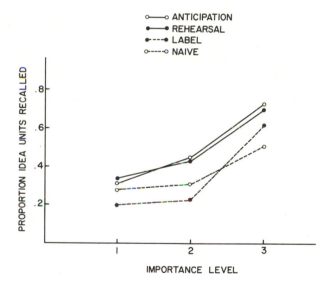

Figure 8.2.   Proportion of prose units recalled as a function of thematic importance of the units and treatment group. (From "Training Self-Checking Routines for Estimating Test Readiness: Generalization from List Learning to Prose Recall" by A. L. Brown, J. C. Campione, and C. R. Barclay, *Child Development* 1979, 50, 501–512. Copyright © 1979 by the Society for Research in Child Development, Inc. Reprinted by permission.)

total amount recalled, (b) pattern of recall as a function of textual importance, (c) time spent studying (although time on task was not the main determinant of efficiency), and (d) observations of overt strategy use (such as lip movement, looking away and self-testing, etc.). Training on a simple self-checking task did result in transfer to the schoollike task of studying texts, a result that reinforces the view that such skills are importantly involved in transfer and are major components of intelligent behavior. Our conclusion is that as a result of the self-control training, subjects had to realize the need for some strategy and had to notice the fact that its use was producing the desired effect. This awareness, in combination with the general nature of the skill being trained, increased the likelihood that generalization would be obtained.

Recall that the young and old subjects in this research did not differ significantly on baseline performance. Group differences emerged in response to instruction; thus the groups differed primarily in their ability to profit from instruction. We will argue later that this test–train–test procedure is particularly sensitive to comparative and developmental differences (see section 8.4).

One clear implication of these data is that groups equated on baseline performance may differ in terms of the amount of instruction necessary to effect improvement, either specific (within a task) or general (across tasks). Although this suggestion is not new, relatively little systematic comparative research is directly relevant. A recent doctoral dissertation prepared by Day (1980) is an exception. She was interested in the ability of junior-college students to summarize prose passages. The students were divided into two groups: "normal" students with no identified reading or writing problems (who were, however, reading at only the 7th grade level) and remedial students who, although considered normal in reading ability, were diagnosed as having writing problems.

Within each of the two groups, there were four instructional conditions that varied in degree of explicitness of training: (a) Self-management: the students were given general encouragement to write a good summary, to capture the main ideas, and to dispense with trivia and all unnecessary words – but they were not told rules for achieving this end. (b) Rules: the students were given explicit instructions and modeling in the use of the rules. For example, they were given various colored pencils and were shown how to delete redundant information in red, to delete trivial information in blue, to write in superordinates for any lists, to underline any topic sentences provided, and to write in a topic sentence if one was needed (see Day, 1980, for a more detailed discussion of the rules). Then they were to use the remaining information to write a summary. (c) Rules plus self-management: The students in the third group were given both the general self-management instructions of Group 1 and the rules instruction of Group 2, but they were left to integrate the two sets of information for themselves. (d) Control of the rules: The fourth and most explicit training condition involved training in the rules, as in Condition 2, and additional explicit training in the control of these rules – that is, the students were shown how to check that they had a topic sentence for each paragraph (either underlined or written in), that all redundancies had been deleted, all trivia erased, and so forth, and that all lists of items had been replaced with superordinates. The integration of the rules and appropriate self-control routines were explicitly modeled for the students. The amount of time spent in training and practice was the same for each condition.

We will give only a few selected outcomes here. The first main point is that on pretest measures the groups did not differ. Second, the type of instruction required to achieve a maximum result varied with both rule difficulty and ability level. With the select-topic-sentence rule, one of intermediate difficulty, the performance of the lower-ability subjects was maximized in the most explicit control-of-rules condition, where the rule and its management were explicitly taught. In the higher-ability

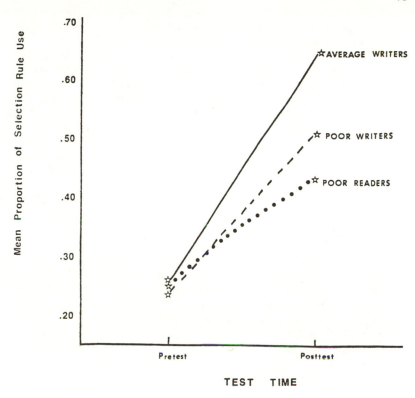

Figure 8.3. Mean proportion of rule use before and after instruction, as a function of ability group. (From *Training Summarization Skills: A Comparison of Teaching Methods* by J. D. Day, unpublished doctoral dissertation, University of Illinois, 1980. Reprinted by permission.)

subjects, the rules-plus-self-management condition was sufficient to lead to maximal performance levels. The poorer learners required more explicit instruction.

Considering only the more proficient group, we can investigate the effects of rule difficulty. Performance with the most difficult rule, "invent topic sentence," was maximal in the control-of-rules condition. In the select-topic-sentence condition, explicit instructions about rule management were not required; however, as the target rule became more difficult, the "power" of the instructional intervention required increased.

As a final point, recall that the groups did not differ in terms of baseline performance levels. We can also ask about group differences after instruction. In Figure 8.3 we show the pretest and posttest levels of three groups of subjects, the normal and poor writer groups already mentioned and an additional group of subjects whose learning problems were more severe – they were diagnosed as having both writing and reading problems (see Experiment 2 of Day, 1980). The subjects in this latter group received only the most explicit control-of-rules instruction. The posttest data in Figure 8.3 were all obtained following this type of instruction. The three groups of subjects do not differ prior to training; however, after training, large and significant differences are apparent. As in the recall-readiness study, the more competent students were better able to profit from instruction.

Although we will not review the many specific studies here, the statement that retarded individuals show a deficiency in the use of active, task-appropriate strategies receives support from research in many other areas. In a variety of problem-solving or gamelike situations, ranging from simplified versions of tic-tac-toe through a variety of question-asking situations (such as 20 questions) to variants of the Tower of Hanoi problem, retarded subjects do not appear to produce reasonable and systematic approaches to the problem (Spitz, 1978, and others). Our own view is that the "memory" area that has received so much attention in the literature (and here) is actually the more restricted domain of intentional memory. Accordingly, we see all of the work as research on problem solving. The subject is presented with a problem – committing some material to memory – and must develop some method for solving that problem. Thus we would expect many of the findings obtained in the "memory" area to be the same as those obtained from "more direct" (?) investigations of problem solving.

SUMMARY.   Much attention has been focused on the role and use of strategies by retarded children in problem-solving and memory problems, with the training study being the major vehicle for the research. The initial, or blind, attempts established the fact that retarded children were less likely than nonretarded comparative groups to employ strategies spontaneously, although they could readily be taught to do so. When tests for transfer were carried out, the results were consistently negative, so negative in fact that the failure to transfer learning was regarded as a major indicant of retardation (Campione & Brown, 1977, 1978). In this context, understanding the factors responsible for transfer would refine our views of intelligence, and the question became: What additional input is required, or what other aspects of thought must be instructed, to induce retarded children to generalize? This statement of the issue led to the more recent informed and self-control training packages, the outcomes of which have implicated metacognitive and executive decision-making functions as central to any conception of intelligence.

The two main findings in this area are the failure of the retarded child to acquire and produce strategies to meet the demands of a variety of problems and a failure to transfer instructed strategies beyond the original training context. These two breakdowns are not independent, and we have argued elsewhere that they reflect the same underlying processes (e.g., Campione & Brown, 1977). Both can be described as the failure to learn incidentally or the failure to profit from incomplete instruction. For example, many of the mnemonic strategies employed in a typical memory experiment do not appear to be taught explicitly anywhere, but individuals of average ability seem to educe them from their own experiences. Retarded children need, however, complete instruction before the strategies are employed. In the case of transfer performance, the same pattern appears. To obtain transfer, it is necessary to provide explicit instruction in each step of the overall process before retarded children begin to use information flexibly. They do not go beyond the initial instruction and begin to grasp the significance of the routine until it is pointed out, and this failure leads to restricted use.

It is clear from these data that lower-ability subjects require more explicit instruction before they begin to show improvement or to reach some criterion of effectiveness. In addition, they require still more input before they can transfer what they have learned. That is, even when routines are known to be available to them, there is no guarantee that they will use them spontaneously, even when the "transfer" task is the same as that of original learning (cf. Brown, Campione, & Barclay, 1979). We will return to the distinction between knowledge and use of knowledge in section 8.5. Of particular interest to a theory of intelligence is the type of additional training necessary to elicit transfer. In our view, the components that emerge without instruction in the intellectually average and above average but that required explicit instruction for those of below-average ability constitute the hallmark of intelligence. The indications here are that those components are of the general metacognitive variety, those attributed to the executive in many contemporary theories of memory or machine intelligence. Theorists have come to agree that an important requirement of any functioning system is that it include the capacity for self-awareness, or accurate knowledge and understanding of its own weaknesses and properties (Becker, 1975; Bobrow, 1975; Bobrow & Norman, 1975). In such a system, some specific executive responsibilities include recognizing its own limitations, being aware of the routines available, being able to characterize the current problem, planning and scheduling strategies, and monitoring the effectiveness of the chosen routine. Given the correspondence, an alternative statement of our conclusions is that intelligence differences are attributable to variations in the efficiency of the executive or in the quality of control that the executive exerts. It is interesting to note in this context that these executive functions are also the most difficult to instill in a computer.

METACOGNITION

In its most general sense, *metacognition* refers to the subjects' understanding of their cognitive systems. Two fairly distinct lines of research have appeared under this heading (Brown & Campione, 1981, in press). Metacognition is "knowledge or cognition that takes as its object or regulates any aspect of any cognitive endeavor" (Flavell, 1978, p. 4). The first line is concerned with people's knowledge of their own cognitive resources and their compatibility as learners with the learning situation. Prototypical of this category are questionnaire studies and confrontation experiments, the main purpose of which is to find out how much individual children know about certain pertinent features of thinking, including themselves as thinkers. The focus is on measuring the relatively stable and statable information that the child has concerning the cognitive processes involved in any academic task. This information is stable in that one would expect that a child who knows pertinent facts (e.g., that organized material is easier to learn than disorganized material, that passages containing familiar words and concepts are easier to read than those composed of unfamiliar elements) would continue to know these facts if interrogated properly. This information is also statable; the child is able to reflect on the processes and to discuss them with others.

  The ability to reflect on one's own cognitive processes, to be aware of one's own activities while reading, solving problems, and so forth, is a late-developing skill with important implications for the child's effectiveness as an active, planful learner. If the child is aware of what is needed to perform effectively, then that child can take steps to meet the demands of a learning situation more adequately. If, however, the child is not aware of his or her own limitations as a learner or of the complexity of the task at hand, then he or she can hardly be expected to take preventive actions in order to anticipate or recover from problems.

The second cluster of activities studied under the heading *metacognition* consists of the self-regulatory mechanisms used by an active learner during an ongoing attempt to solve problems. These indexes of metacognition include *checking* the outcome of any attempt to solve the problem, *planning* one's next move, *monitoring* the effectiveness of any attempted action, and *testing, revising,* and *evaluating* one's strategies for learning. These are not necessarily stable skills in the sense that although they are more often used by older children and adults, they are not always used by them, and quite young children may monitor their activities on a simple problem (Brown, 1978).

In section 8.2 we emphasized the interactive nature of our four major determinants of performance, and this interdependence is particularly clear here. In discussing the role and use of strategies, we have been unable to avoid frequent reference to the topic of metacognition. Strategies can be beneficial only to the extent that learners anticipate their need, select from among them, oversee their operation, and understand their significance. Similarly, high-level executive routines are not of much interest unless the learner possesses some more specific routines to control.

Of greater significance here is the distinction between the "two types" of metacognition; we will use *metacognition* to refer to knowledge about cognition and *executive control* to denote the overseeing, management functions. We wish to argue that the latter appears more central to notions of intelligence. Notice, for example, that the training attempts that have led to transfer have included explicit instruction in self-management, or monitoring, techniques. Inducing executive control does seem to lead to increased transfer or to more intelligent behavior.

The point is that although retarded children do demonstrate lags in the acquisition of knowledge about their own memory, for example, it is not the case that teaching them information about their memory leads to any general improvement in memory performance. Inducing executive control does facilitate both immediate response to training and transfer; enhancing knowledge about memory does not appear to do so, at least not to the same extent. Given this difference, we would infer that executive decision making is more central to intelligence than is metacognition – its effects are larger and more general.

Although we would like to make that claim, we would also admit that the data base for it is still weak. We will review here some of the available data that seem consistent with the assumed importance of executive functioning. There are four main points involved in the argument: (a) Retarded children manifest deficiencies in executive functioning; (b) executive functioning is a mediator of transfer; (c) retarded children manifest deficiencies in knowledge about cognition; and (d) knowledge about cognition is less likely to be a mediator of transfer. We believe that the first two statements are true, and we have reviewed that evidence in the previous section and will not repeat it here.

Statement C is certainly supported by existing data. For example, in a series of studies summarized in Brown (1978), we have found that educable retarded children are not as insightful about their memories as nonretarded children of comparable CA (based on across-experiments comparisons). They do not appear to be aware of the severity of working-memory limitations and seriously overestimate their memory span (Brown, Campione, & Murphy, 1977). They are also not as cognizant of the contents of their memory. In a study on the feeling-of-knowing phenomenon, Brown and Lawton (1977) found that mildly retarded subjects' ability to predict whether they would recognize a name they had previously been unable to recall was below levels expected on the basis of work with nonretarded children. Interestingly, although retarded subjects had some trouble predicting how good their recognition would be, they were quite good at evaluating the accuracy of their recognition choices *after* they had been made. As a final example, they do not appear to know as much as nonretarded children about the kinds of material that are easy or hard to remember. Tenney's (1975) method was used, whereby children are asked to generate lists of items that would be easy to remember. Retarded children were less likely than nonretarded ones to construct organized lists in response to this request, and even when they did include items from within a (taxonomic or thematic) category, their choices were more likely to be "broad" (1, 4, 2, 7) rather than "narrow" (1, 2, 3, 4) (Brown, 1978).

Now, consider Statement D, concerning the effects of teaching retarded children metamemorial knowledge. Brown, Campione, and Murphy (1977) taught mildly retarded children to evaluate their own memory span for pictures. Although the children originally overestimated the number of pictures that they would be able to recall – many predicted 10, the maximum allowable estimate – they eventually became realistic, predicting that their span was about 4. They showed some additional insights after the training, for example, they correctly predicted that they would recall more items from a blocked, categorized set than from a set of unrelated items, but the effects were extremely limited. When tested for their estimate of how many digits they could recall, they reverted to optimistic and unrealistic estimates. Similarly, when they were asked to predict their picture memory span using a slightly different "questioning" technique, they again significantly overestimated their ability. Instructing metacognitive knowledge per se results in limited transfer.

Although any conclusions must be tempered due to the restricted data base, the pattern is consistent with the argument regarding the importance of executive processes. To buttress this conclusion further, we would argue that executive processes and knowledge about cognition may be hierarchically related. For example, in many cases, metacognitive awareness can follow from self-management routines, and the absence of that knowledge can be regarded as reflecting a weakness in planning and monitoring proclivities. If one engages in some self-testing, for example, it becomes clear when capacity limitations are being exceeded. That is, when a person is shown 10 items and is asked how many he or she will be able to recall, it is possible to look away and to conduct a mock recall trial upon which to base the judgment. The knowledge need not be there; it can be readily generated. Given this orientation, the failure to engage appropriate self-management or executive routines is a source of the knowledge deficiencies.

The issue here is the same as that encountered when we consider the effects of the knowledge base. Retarded children have relatively impoverished knowledge bases. It is also true that the ease of learning and retaining information within some domain is related to the amount of knowledge the learner possesses regarding that domain (e.g., Chi, 1981). It is thus tempting to conclude that the learning problems demonstrated by retarded children are a result of inadequate prior knowledge. Our preference is to treat the deficient knowledge base as a symptom of the major underlying problems rather than as a source of them. As we have argued elsewhere (Brown, 1978; Brown & Campione, 1981; Campione & Brown, 1978), inculcating knowledge is not the main problem. The problem is that even when the relevant knowledge is known to be available to poor learners, they experience particular difficulties in accessing and operating upon it. As we argue in section 8.5, major components of intelligence are the learning and transfer skills responsible for the accretion and use of knowledge.

SUMMARY

In the first part of this section, we indicated some areas in which retarded children seem to perform at approximately the same level as nonretarded children. The architecture of the system seems intact, and in a variety of nonstrategic tasks, the performance of retarded children appears normal. Our main concern here is that these conclusions are in good part derived from cross-experiment comparisons, with all their attendant problems. Well-designed comparative work is needed before strong conclusions can be drawn.

In the next four sections, we reviewed data indicating that retarded children differ from nonretarded children in the efficiency with which they carry out some elementary mental operations, in the extent of their knowledge base, in the deployment of task-appropriate strategies, and in the development of metacognition and executive control. In general, these factors are treated separately, although we would argue that in almost any case, performance is determined by the interaction of several of them. Our picture would be much clearer if more attempts had been made to consider some of the potential interactions. Although there have been some attempts, for example, study of the relations between efficiency and strategy use, and between strategy use and metacognition, such endeavors are quite rare.

In addition to research aimed specifically at some of these interactions, we believe that more comparative research is necessary to complete our theories of intelligence. If intelligence is regarded as a relative term, and if important components of intelligence mediate large comparative differences, comparative studies are essential. Still, many of the comparative data we need are not available.

Given these limitations, strong conclusions may be unwarranted, but we will nonetheless offer our own interpretation of the literature to date. We do so briefly here and then proceed to a review of the educational and clinical literature. Following that review, we will argue that the conclusions we wish to draw from a consideration of the experimental literature are also consistent with the educational literature. In section 8.5 we consider the conclusions in more detail.

The most general conclusion we wish to draw is that retarded children are deficient in the abilities to acquire and use information, that is, we favor a definition of intelligence in terms of speed of learning and/or breadth of transfer. Although retarded children do have impoverished knowledge bases, we regard that characteristic as a symptom, rather than a cause, of their underlying problems. The major evidence for that view stems first from the retarded child's need for complete and explicit instruction before any routine is acquired (cf. Butterfield et al., 1973). Even after the routine is learned and is available to the retarded child, he or she still experiences major problems in accessing and using that routine effectively (cf. Brown, Campione, & Barclay, 1979). That is, although knowledge can be instilled, much instruction is necessary, and after it is instilled, the knowledge does not appear to be used flexibly.

This distinction between knowledge and the use of that knowledge also emerged in the metacognition section, where we reserved the term *metacognition* for knowledge about cognition (more specifically memory) and distinguished it from executive control, the process whereby we select, monitor, and generally oversee our own cognitive activities. We argued there that the executive routines underlying use of knowledge rather than metacognition, or the knowledge about aspects of the system, are central to theories of intelligence. The evidence here was that instructing meta-cognition did not seem to result in general improvements in performance, whereas training involving some self-management routines did appear to produce more wide-spread effects.

8.4.   CLINICAL ASSESSMENTS OF LEARNING POTENTIAL

We turn now to an area of investigation that has developed quite independently from the experimental research literature described in the previous section, as indeed the experimental literature developed without apparent knowledge of the clinical assess-ment programs that we will review in this section. Although the two areas of investi-gation did develop independently, they both reflect a concern with the academic performance of aberrant learners, both in order to inform remediation and in order to throw light on the nature of intelligence in general. As we will show, the conclusions reached in both areas are remarkably congruent, particularly given their differential and independent genesis. In this section we will consider three clinical assessment programs that have aimed to go beyond static IQ measures in diagnosing problem learners.

One of the traditional definitions of intelligence is the ability to learn. If this definition is correct, then "estimates of it [intelligence] are, or at least should be, estimates of the ability to learn. To be able to learn harder things, or to be able to learn the same things more quickly, would then be the single basis of evaluation" (Thorndike, 1926, pp. 17–18). Despite this early claim that intelligence tests should measure learning potential, static measures have in general been used to assess intellectual functioning, and there is considerable dissatisfaction with the use of traditional IQ measures to achieve this end. Such measures reflect the end result of prior learning, but they may not provide a sensitive index of the potential for im-provement over current performance levels. There are strong reasons to believe that for many people, particularly those from disadvantaged homes, the static test scores represent an underestimate of ability. In addition, static IQ measures do not provide direct information concerning the optimal level of performance of which the testee is capable, an optimal level that is of considerable interest for those who wish to design instruction.

We will begin this section by considering how static IQ tests are and will then consider three programs of research that have specifically addressed the problem of dynamic assessment and learning potential: Feuerstein's Learning Potential Assess-ment Device (LPAD), Budoff's Learning Potential and Educability Program, and recent advances in Soviet clinical assessments of the zone of proximal development (Brown & French, 1979b; Vygotsky, 1978), together with our own experimental examinations of their claims (Brown & Ferrara, in press).

Standardized test procedures used for measuring IQ or academic performance are explicitly designed so that they will provide the same environment for each testee. Examiners are specifically trained to remain neutral, not to question or to add to the child's response, not to help the child in any way. Still, recent work by Mehan (1973) and others has shown that the testing environment is by no means constant for each child. Testers inadvertently provide prompts, such as indicating, verbally or other-wise, that the answer is incomplete or that a correct answer has been given and the child may terminate his or her search. Testers also provide additional information and question a response so that the child knows to self-correct. Even the simple practice of just waiting for a response elaboration gives the child time to amend an inadequate first reply. Scoring the test protocols according to the strict criterion of considering only the child's unaided responses provides a picture of his or her ability quite different from that produced using the lenient criterion of accepting the child's responses as modified by the inadvertent aid; as much as a 27% difference has been reported between the strict and lenient criteria (Mehan, 1973). The effects due to tester–testee interactions are not trivial. Furthermore, considerable evidence suggests that such biasing effects are more likely to benefit the middle-class child. A self-fulfilling prophecy operates, whereby the tester expects the white, middle-class child to do well and therefore treats inadequate first responses as hasty mistakes rather than as indexes of stupidity – leeway is inadvertently given, and the child scores higher than strict procedures would permit. Such leeway is not usually afforded the lower-class child. The substantial improvement over initial response that is achieved via the interaction of the adult and child is precisely what learning-potential methods aim at measuring. By offering graded hints to all participants, the tester is able to evaluate if and how much the child can improve over initial performance.

THE ZONE OF PROXIMAL DEVELOPMENT

Vygotsky's theory of cognitive development rests heavily on the key concept of *internalization*. Vygotsky argues that all psychological processes are in genesis essentially social processes, initially shared between people, particularly between children and adults. Children first experience active problem-solving activities in the presence of others and slowly come to perform these functions for themselves. The process of internalization is gradual; first the adult, or knowledgeable peer, controls and guides the child's activity, but eventually the adult and the child come to share the problem-solving functions, with the child taking the initiative and the adult correcting and guiding when the child falters. Finally, the adult cedes control to the child and functions primarily as a supportive and sympathetic audience. This developmental progression from other-regulation to self-regulation is the essence of mother–child learning dyads (Wertsch, 1978), but age or the nature of the social agent is to some extent irrelevant. Teachers, tutors, and master craftsmen in traditional apprenticeship situations all function ideally as promoters of self-regulation by nurturing the emergence of personal planning as they gradually cede their own direction. In schools, effective teachers are those who engage in continual prompts to encourage children to plan and monitor their own activities. Four general strategies are used to facilitate children's learning (Schallert & Kleiman, 1979): (a) tailoring the message to the child's existing level of understanding, (b) activating relevant prior knowledge, (c) focusing attention on important facts, and (d) monitoring comprehension by means of such Socratic ploys as invidious generalizations, counterexamples, and reality testing (Collins, 1977). In short, the expert teacher models many forms of critical thinking for children, processes that they must internalize as part of their own problem-solving activities if they are to develop effective autocritical (Binet, 1911) skills of self-regulation.

Within this context of the gradual internalization of cognitive activities that were originally shared interactive processes Vygotsky introduced his concept of the zone of proximal development. Vygotsky's (1978) definition of the zone of proximal (or potential) development is "the distance between the actual developmental level as determined by individual problem solving and the level of potential development as determined through problem solving under adult guidance or in collaboration with more capable peers" (p. 86). For Vygotsky, the fundamental process of development is the gradual internalization and personalization of what was originally a social activity.

We propose that an essential feature of learning is that it creates the zone of proximal development; that is, learning awakens a variety of developmental processes that are able to operate only when the child is interacting with people in his environment and in cooperation with his peers. Once these processes are internalized, they become part of the child's independent developmental achievement. [Vygotsky, 1978, p. 90]

From Vygotsky's viewpoint it is essential to consider a child's problem-solving abilities in situations other than traditional testing milieus, situations such as mother–child dyads (Wertsch, 1978), children tutoring children (Allen, 1976), and group problem-solving situations (Bos, 1937; Kelley & Thibaut, 1954).

This essentially interactive theory of learning had an important effect on the development of clinical testing in the Soviet Union. For a variety of historical and social reasons standardized intelligence tests have been criticized and at times officially banned (Brozek, 1972; Wozniak, 1975); at the same time, however, an essential feature of Soviet social policy is a major commitment to special education (Vlasova, 1972). In recent years there has been a growing interest in the development of reliable methods for the differential diagnosis of learning disabilities, or temporary retardation, and more serious and permanent mental impairment (Vlasova & Pevzner, 1971; Zabramna, 1971). Given the unfavorable climate for the establishment of standardized testing, the Soviets have concentrated on the development of clinical batteries of diagnostic tasks to serve the purpose of evaluating differences in learning potential. Perhaps surprisingly, the clinical batteries do not seem to vary greatly in content from our standardized psychometric tests, but the methods of testing and the data of prime interest reflect different testing philosophies.

The method of clinical assessment is based on Vygotsky's theory of a zone of proximal development just described. The distinction is made between children's actual developmental level, that is, their completed development as might be measured on a standardized test, and their level of potential development, the degree of competence they can achieve with aid. Both measures are seen as essential for the diagnosis of learning disabilities and for the concomitant design of remedial programs (Egorova, 1973; Pevzner, 1972).

A child's standardized test performance is regarded as providing at best a quantitative index of current developmental status or actual developmental level. Although informative concerning what the child knows now, it provides only indirect evidence about how he arrived at this state. Vygotsky claims that such measures also fail to provide any information about

those functions that have not yet matured but are in the process of maturation, functions that will mature tomorrow but are in the embryonic static. These functions could be termed the "buds" or "flowers" rather than the "fruits" of development. The actual developmental level characterizes mental development retrospectively, while the zone of proximal development characterizes mental development prospectively. [Vygotsky, 1978, pp. 86–87]

The zone of proximal development is used as an indication of learning potential; children with the same current status on an IQ test item may vary quite widely in terms of their cognitive potential. For example, it is claimed that a major difference between learning disabled and truly retarded children lies in the width of their potential zone. Of prime importance for the diagnosis of the cause of school failure is the Soviet claim that whereas learning disabled (developmentally backward) and mildly retarded children tend not to differ greatly in terms of their starting competence on a variety of cognitive tasks, the two groups differ dramatically in terms of their ability to benefit from the additional cues provided by the tester. Learning disabled children need less aid than retarded children before they arrive at a satisfactory solution. They are also more proficient at transferring the result of their brief learning experience to new variations of the task within the testing situation and in subsequent independent class performance. In studies where comparisons with normal children were included, the average children were even more effective at initial learning and subsequent transfer than were the two clinical populations (Egorova, 1973; Lubovsky, 1978).

In support of these findings we have repeatedly found in our laboratory that baseline measures are insensitive to differences in cognitive ability (Brown & Campione, 1977; Brown & Barclay, 1976; Brown, Campione, & Day, 1981; Day, 1980) that are revealed when training is instigated. For example, in the recall-readiness study described in the previous section, educable retarded children (MA = 6 years and 8 years) did not differ in their original performance on the task, but they did differ dramatically in how readily they responded to training, in how long they maintained the effects of training, and in how far they transferred the skills they had acquired (Brown, Campione, & Barclay, 1979; Brown, Campione, & Day, 1981). Similarly, with a quite different population (junior-college students) and task (learning rules for summarizing texts), Day (1980) also found no pretraining performance differences between students who were or were not diagnosed as remedial writers, even though the results were not contaminated by floor or ceiling effects. After training, however, the groups differed significantly. For the more advanced students, instruction resulted in greater use of the trained rules, and this improvement was effected with less explicit intervention. For those students with more severe learning problems, however, training resulted in less improvement over baseline levels, and more explicit instruction was needed before there was any effect of intervention (Brown, Campione, & Day, 1981; Day, 1980). The extent of instruction needed to bring about improvement is a sensitive measure of the student's zone of potential development in the cognitive domain under consideration, and we learn much about a student's competence by assessing not only his starting level but also his readiness to benefit from instruction.

Let us return to the Soviet clinical assessment of the zone of proximal development and consider how the Soviets assess the child's potential. A typical testing session consists of the initial presentation of a test item exactly as it would occur in an American IQ test, with the child being asked to solve the problem independently. If the child fails to reach the correct solution, the adult progressively adds clues for solution and assesses how much additional information the child needs in order to solve the problem. The child's initial performance, when asked to solve the test item independently, provides information comparable to that gained with standardized American IQ testing procedures. The degree of aid needed before a child reaches solution is taken as an indication of the width of his or her proximal zone. Once solution on a particular test item is reached, another version of the original task is presented, and transfer to the novel item is considered by calculating whether or not the child requires fewer cues in order to reach solution.

The following is a concrete example of the testing materials and procedures. The problem presented to the child is a common IQ test item, usually referred to as pattern matching, or geometric design. Such items occur on many standard tests, including the Binet, the Wechsler Preschool and Primary Scale of Intelligence (WIP-PSI), and the Wechsler Intelligence Scale for Children (WISC). The child is given a model (picture) of a silhouette shape and must copy this model by combining a subset of wooden geometric forms. In the Soviet version of this task, however, there is an interesting trick; some of the requisite shapes are not included in the set of available wooden pieces but must be constructed by joining two wooden pieces together.

The first step in the testing procedure is to present a small model picture and ask the child to copy it using the wooden shapes; the child who fails next receives a life-sized representation of the shape to be copied. There is a series of additional prompts, including a model that has one of the composite geometric shapes (corresponding to one of the wooden pieces) clearly delineated in the picture. If this clue does not lead to solution, the child is given a further detailed model that explicitly shows the join (trick) necessary to create the missing form. If all else fails, the tester constructs the figure and then encourages the child to go through the construction with the tester's help.

Of particular interest are the transfer tests. Following solution of Problem 1 (provided by the tester if all else failed), the second problem is immediately presented, with the same series of aids if needed. Problem 2 is a new picture problem in which it is necessary to construct (by joining) two of the composite forms. One of the required joined shapes is identical to that required in Problem 1, the other is a new construction. It seemed to us that these features of Problem 2 tapped two kinds of transfer. Specific transfer would be measured by the recognition that the subpart constructed to solve Problem 1 was again required for Problem 2 solution. More general transfer would be the knowledge that joining shapes in general would be a requirement of the pattern-copying task, and this knowledge should be reflected in the facility with which the child attempts to construct the new joined subpart.

The Soviet diagnostic testing method provides invaluable information concerning the child's starting level of competence and an estimate of the width of his or her zone of potential development, the level of competence he or she can reach with aid. In addition we gain information concerning the child's ability to profit from adult assistance, speed of learning, and the facility with which the new skill is transferred across tasks.

Quite explicit in the Soviet description of their testing program is the role of Vygotsky's theory of a proximal zone of development; the Soviets emphasize the place of graduated aids in uncovering the readiness of children to perform competently in any task domain. This position also entails an implicit theory of task analysis and transfer of training, which is at least as important to contemporary theories of cognition. We would argue that testing the zone of proximal development as a means of diagnosis requires a detailed analysis of a suitable set of cognitive tasks and detailed task analysis of possible transfer probes (Brown, 1978; Campione & Brown, 1978). Without this information it would be difficult to select either the series of graduated aids for the original learning task or suitable methods for assessing the

Table 8.2. *Summary of design and examples of test items*

Pattern type	Problem	Answer
Original learning		
NN (Next relations between letters; period = 2)		
	N G O H P I Q J _ _ _ _	*R K S L*
NINI (Next and *I*dentity relations between letters; period = 4)		
	P Z U F Q Z V F _ _ _ _	*R Z W F*
Maintenance (Learned pattern types; see above)		
Near transfer (Learned relations and learned periodicities, but in different combinations)		
NI	*D V E V F V G V _ _ _ _*	*H V I V*
NNNN	*V H D P W I E Q _ _ _ _*	*X J F R*
Far transfer (Addition of *B*ackward Next relation, *B*, or a period of three letters)		
BN	*U C T D S E R F _ _ _ _*	*Q G P H*
NBNI	*J P B X K O C X _ _ _ _*	*L N D X*
NIN	*P A D Q A E R A _ _ _ _*	*F S A G*

Source: Adapted from Brown and Ferrara (in press).

speed and efficiency of transfer. The importance of this point should not be lost in the rhetoric surrounding Vygotsky's theory of cognitive potential. In the diagnostic sessions, what is being measured, or at least the factor that the Soviets claim is essential for differential diagnosis, is the efficiency of learning within any one task domain. The assessment of the width of a child's zone of proximal development actually translates into the assessment of how many prompts he or she needs to solve Problem 1, versus Problem 2, versus Problem 3, and so forth (i.e., how quickly children learn and how far they transfer). A child judged to have a wide zone of proximal development is one who reduces the number of prompts needed from trial to trial, that is, who shows effective transfer of a new solution across similar problems.

   Inspired by the Soviet approach to testing learning potential as a means of differential diagnosis, we have begun a series of studies in our laboratory to examine the experimental reliability of their clinical claims (Brown & Ferrara, in press). We have selected variants of two IQ test items: the letter series completion task and Raven's Progressive Matrices. We chose these tasks because of (a) their demand for active processing strategies that could be acquired in a learning session, (b) their frequency of occurrence on common IQ tests and (c) their similarity to the material used by the Soviets (Lubovsky, 1978).

   Our letter series completion task was based on Kotovsky and Simon's (1973) analysis. Using it as a starting point we developed an instrument to estimate the zone of proximal development. Basically, there are three alphabetic rules employed in these problems: *identity*, where a letter is repeated; *next*, where the adjacent letter in the alphabet occurs; and *backward next*, where the adjacent letter of the alphabet in reverse order is the solution. The period refers to the number of letters that occur prior to the appearance of regularities. For example, in the simple problem *A D A D A D _ _* (answer = *A D*) the period is two and the relationships are both identity. In the problem *A B A C A D _ _* (answer = *A E*), the period is again two and the relationships are identity for the first letter and next for the second. In

Series completion hints

1. "Is this problem like any other you've seen before?" IF SO: "How did you solve the other problem?"
2. "Read the letters in the problem out loud. . . . Did you hear a pattern in the letters?"
3. "Are any of the letters written more than once in the problem?" IF SO: "Which ones? . . . Does that give you any ideas about how to continue the pattern?"
4. "How many other letters are there between the two Z's? . . . Does that give you any ideas about how to complete the pattern?"
5. "Are any of the letters in the problem next to each other in the alphabet?" IF SO: "Which ones? . . . Does that help you to solve the problem?"
6. "How many other letters are there between the P and the Q in the problem? . . . And how many other letters are there between the U and the V? . . . Does that give you any ideas about the answer?"
7. "Point to the P and the Q in the alphabet . . . and to the U and the V. . . . Does that help at all?"
8. PUT FIRST TRANSPARENCY DOWN (THE BEE). "The *bee* is going from the *P*, skipping three letters, landing on the *Q*, skipping three more letters, and landing on the *first* blank. If he were going to *continue* that pattern, what letter do you think he'd put in the blank?" (see figure below.)
9. PUT SECOND TRANSPARENCY DOWN (THE RABBIT). Verbal accompaniment similar to that for the first transparency.
10. PUT THIRD TRANSPARENCY DOWN (THE BUTTERFLY). Verbal accompaniment similar to that for the first transparency.
11. PUT FOURTH TRANSPARENCY DOWN (THE BIRD). Verbal accompaniment similar to that for the first transparency.
12. FILL IN FIRST BLANK WITH CORRECT LETTER (*R*).
13. FILL IN SECOND BLANK WITH CORRECT LETTER (*Z*).
14. FILL IN THIRD BLANK WITH CORRECT LETTER (*W*).
15. FILL IN FOURTH BLANK WITH CORRECT LETTER (*F*).

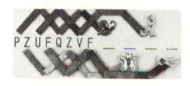

Superimposition of the four transparencies (hints 8–11)

Figure 8.4.   Example of series completion problem and sequence of hints. (From "Diagnosing Zones of Proximal Development" by A. L. Brown and R. A. Ferrara, in J. V. Wertsch [Ed.], *Culture, Communication, and Cognition: Vygotskian Perspectives* [New York: Academic Press, in press]. Reprinted by permission.)

the problem *E T D T C T* __ __ (answer = *B T*), the period remains two, and the relationships are backward next followed by identity.

We examined children's zones of proximal development for such problems. So far only third and fifth graders of average and above-average IQ have been tested. Briefly, the procedure was as follows. Each child was tested on 3 separate days, and the overall design of the experiment is illustrated in Table 8.2. On the 1st day, the child was given a number of series completion problems with prompts provided by an adult as needed to arrive at the solutions. The prompts, shown in Figure 8.4, were delivered in a graduated sequence of increasing explicitness. The initial learning problems included two patterns embodying the next and/or identity relations. The period was either two or four letters. For example, one of the problem types involved two next (N) relations and two identity (I) relations and had a period of four letters

(NINI problem, e.g., $P\ Z\ U\ F\ Q\ Z\ V\ F$ _ _ _ _; answer = $R\ Z\ W\ F$). The first session ended when the child had completed a total of three problems of each type without aid from the adult.

On the 2nd day, maintenance and transfer of learning were assessed in a standard paper-and-pencil test situation (i.e., the child worked alone and unassisted). Some of the problems were of the pattern types learned on the previous day, whereas others deviated in systematic ways. Breadth of transfer in this situation was indexed by the number of ways in which an item differed from the training problems. Maintenance items consisted of new examples of the problem types learned to criterion on Day 1. Near transfer items involved the relations (identity and next) and periodicities (two and four) already learned but displayed them in new combinations. Far transfer items incorporated either a new relation, backward next, or a new period of three letters. Examples of the maintenance and transfer items are shown in Table 8.2. In addition, very far transfer items required the child to finish coding a brief message. This task involved backward next as well as next relations that existed *between* rows of letters rather than within a row, for example:

$$S\ I\ X\ \ S\ H\ I\ P\ S\ \ G\ O\ N\ E$$
$$T\ H\ Y\ \ R\ I\ H\ Q\ R\ \_\ \_\ \_\ \_ \qquad \text{Answer} = H\ N\ O\ D.$$

On the 3rd day, a more sensitive measure of transfer was taken by reinstating the interactive situation. The child worked on the same set of problems attempted the day before, but this time the adult gave gradated hints if the child needed them to solve each problem.

The findings from this study do agree with expectations based on the Soviet work. First we must note that these problems are extremely difficult and that untrained performance levels are very low for all subjects. The data from Day 1 indicated that children of average ability (IQ M = 103) required more prompts to reach criterion than did above-average children (IQ M = 125). Further, on Day 3, the average and above-average subjects differed in interesting ways. They were equally facile with the maintenance and near transfer items but differed significantly on the far and very far transfer probes. Thus, the average children tended to take longer (to require more prompts) to master the initial problem types. In addition, although they continued to perform well on novel instances of those and similar problem types in subsequent sessions, they were less able than the above-average children to adapt to more pronounced task variations. Even in situations where initial performance is very poor, brighter children usually require less explicit instruction to show signs of learning and then transfer that learning more broadly than do subjects of lower ability. Given these findings, the dynamic assessment procedure does appear to be sensitive to ability-related differences.

Although brighter children in general learned more quickly and transferred more broadly than average children, the exceptions to this pattern are also of considerable importance. For example, we are particularly interested in the children who required many prompts to learn initially (slow learners) but who subsequently showed a wide zone of proximal development in that they transferred widely throughout the entire problem space. These children contrast with the more typical patterns of (a) slow learning, low transfer; and (b) fast learning, high transfer. In addition we are also interested in fast learners with only average IQ scores and generally poor performers with relatively high IQ scores.

That is, although IQ and our learning and transfer measures are related, the relation (not surprisingly) is less than perfect. Some average-ability children learn quickly and transfer broadly, whereas some above-average subjects perform less well. For these children, the static and dynamic assessments lead to different expectations about future performance, and the interesting question concerns which procedure will make possible more accurate predictions.

Before leaving this topic, we would like to mention one other set of data we have collected bearing on the across-tasks consistency of classifications obtained from these procedures (see Brown & Ferrara, in press, for more details). An analogous assessment procedure using a variant of Raven's Progressive Matrices has also been developed. The task consists of 3×3 matrices of geometric figures following certain transformational patterns across columns and/or rows – the testee's job is to figure out how the missing figure in the lower right corner should look. We have developed a computerized testing situation in which the child can construct the missing figure using a touch-sensitive panel and can receive animated hints from the computer with the touch of a button. An adult is present at all times to read the instructions and hints on the screen, to give verbal praise, and to provide general guidance if the child has problems interacting with the computer. We are using the same general paradigm developed for the letter series completions. Specifically, it entails a session in which the child learns three rules (superimposition, subtraction, and rotation of figures) with animated hints involving the rules for solution. Prompts are given as needed to reach a certain criterion. In subsequent sessions, maintenance and transfer are assessed again, with hints given when needed. Transfer matrices involve a combination of two of the rules initially learned in the context of separate matrix problems. For example, one such problem would involve rotating in a clockwise direction the left-most figure in each row 90° *and* superimposing that rotated figure on the one in the middle column to generate the right-most item.

Thirteen subjects were run on the series completion and matrix problems. In each situation, each subject was classified as a fast or slow learner and as a high or low transferrer – the classification was based on a simple median split. Of interest here, the reliability of those classifications was impressively high. Nine of the 13 were classed exactly the same on both tests (5 as slow learners/low transferrers and 4 as fast learners/high transferrers). Three subjects were in the fast, high category on one task and in the slow, high category on the other; they consistently showed high transfer. The final subject was a slow learner in both situations but once showed high transfer and once low. Thus, although more data are certainly needed, these initial indicators of reliability of classification are encouraging. We are currently extending this work by involving other populations, specifically mildly retarded and learning disabled children. If the Soviet claims continue to hold, we should be able to differentiate these groups via zone-of-proximal-development procedures.

We believe that two points emerge from this work, and they may appear to be contradictory. One is that the dynamic assessment procedures can be sensitive to differences that are not apparent in more static assessments. In this regard, the indication is that they can serve as useful supplements to more standard assessment vehicles. This point is emphasized by Budoff and Feuerstein.

The second point is that the dynamically based learning and transfer measures are significantly related to IQ scores, at least within the normal range. We believe the importance of this point should not be overlooked. As we noted at length in section 8.5, we believe this result indicates that learning speed and transfer proclivity are important components of intelligence. That is, if we use these procedures with children of varying intelligence, the data indicate that there is a strong relation between intelligence and the ability to learn. (According to the views espoused by

Budoff and more clearly emphasized by Feuerstein, the static–dynamic test relations might be expected to be weaker within the population of mildly retarded children. Whether or not this is true remains an open and interesting question. In any event, the rationale for this expectation is outlined in the upcoming sections.)

LEARNING POTENTIAL AND EDUCABILITY

During the 1960s and early 1970s, Milton Budoff of the Research Institute for Educational Problems in Cambridge, Massachusetts, developed a series of procedures for assessing the learning potential of educably retarded individuals. The rationale was essentially similar to Vygotsky's and, not surprisingly, the tasks developed bear some striking resemblances to those in the Soviet clinical battery. Budoff was also convinced of the unsuitability of static tests, particularly for low-achieving children, and as a result he added a basic test–train–test procedure to all his assessment measures. We were not aware of Budoff's program until recently, well after we had initiated our own work based on the Soviet zone-of-proximal-development assessments, and we were certainly struck by the similarity of Budoff's approach and that developed at the Institute of Defectology in Moscow. Budoff's theory also sounds reminiscent of Vygotsky. For example, Budoff regarded pretraining scores on any psychological test as reflecting the "present functioning ability of the child, and these scores correlate with verbal and performance IQs. Like IQ scores they correlate also with such socioeconomic indication as size of family, degree of intactness of family, race, English language competence, etc." (Budoff, 1974, p. 33).

Posttest scores are a composite measure reflecting the initial starting level of competence, an effect due to practice, and an effect due to specific training. Budoff reports that although low-IQ children tend to gain little from mere practice without specific training,

following suitable training, many low IQ children will function at a level similar to the child from more privileged circumstances. This posttraining score, regardless of pretraining level, represents the child's optimal level of performance following an optimizing procedure. It permits a comparison between his *presently* low level of functioning, as indicated by his IQ, and his *potential* level of functioning – the third score is the posttraining score adjusted for pretest level. This residual score indicates the child's responsiveness to training, and by extension to the classroom regardless of his pretraining level. It is hypothesized to indicate the student's amenability to training given suitable curricula and school experience. [Budoff, 1974, p. 33]

Budoff's learning-potential approach is based on a conceptualization of intelligence that stresses trainability, or the ability to profit from learning experiences directly related to the task at hand. Improved performance after training indicates problem-solving capability not evident when instruction is not provided as part of the test administration. Of interest is the way in which these training sessions were devised. Budoff, like the Soviet clinical testers, also concentrated on IQ-type tasks such as Raven's matrices and block building, and the similarity between the two approaches is particularly striking when one considers Budoff's work with Kohs Blocks, which we will describe in some detail to provide an example of the general approach.

Following a pretest on several block designs, the subjects enter into the training phase of the test–train–test assessment procedure. The initial stage consists of presenting the problem without aid and waiting until the children solve it or fail to solve it on their own. If a child fails, a series of more and more explicit prompts is given

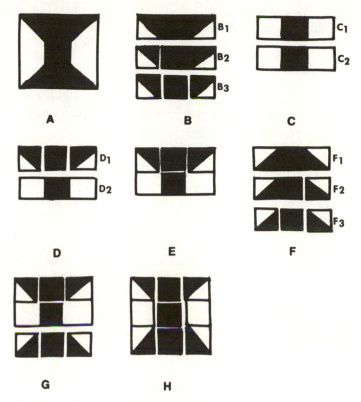

Figure 8.5.   Learning-potential assessment for Kohs blocks: illustration of coaching procedure. A, Initial design card; B, stimulus cards for top row of design; C, stimulus cards for middle row of design; D, card showing relationship of upper two rows of design; E, card showing the two rows placed together; F, stimulus cards for lowest row of design; G, cards showing the relationship of upper two rows and lowest row of design; H, final card with all blocks outlined. (From *Learning Potential and Educability among the Educable Mentally Retarded* by M. Budoff, Final Report Project No. 312312 [Cambridge, Mass.: Research Institute for Educational Problems, Cambridge Mental Health Association, 1979]. Reprinted by permission.)

until solution is reached. The series of prompts for Kohs Blocks problems is illustrated in Figure 8.5. The first prompt is a presentation of only one row of the design. Initially the blocks composing the row are not outlined. On succeeding presentations, if the subject fails to align the blocks correctly, the design is progressively outlined, for example, see the progression in Figure 8.5. On the prompt cards where the blocks are given in outline (B3, C2, F3) and on the final card (H), subjects are required to check whether each block in their designs corresponds exactly with the comparable block on the card. Throughout the training period the child is encouraged to check his or her construction block by block against the design card, to "actively point, block by block, to his constructed design and the corresponding blocks on the design card – it was hoped thereby to encourage a more planned and systematic work approach and to allow the subject to see concretely the success he is achieving" (Budoff, 1974, p. 7). The similarity to the structured hints approach demonstrated by our Soviet colleagues is indeed striking.

Following training such as this, on a variety of IQ-like test items, Budoff found three classes of children within his EMH population: (a) subjects who demonstrate little or no gain following instruction (*nongainers*), (b) subjects who show quite marked gain (*gainers*), and (c) *high scorers,* those who performed quite adequately on the pretest. There are some problems associated with Budoff's approach, notably the concentration on product rather than on process. For example, a gainer might be one who improved over pretest by four items, whereas a nongainer improved one item or less. Budoff was aware that this performance was difficult to interpret, as the child who solved no blocks on pretest and five on posttest is difficult to compare with a child who solved five on pretest and posttest. Despite the difficulties, Budoff reported interesting correlates of the gainer, nongainer status. For example, middle-class children in special education classes tend to be nongainers, whereas lower-class children have a high incidence of gainers. Learning-potential status also predicts performance on a variety of laboratory concept-learning tasks and a specially constructed math curriculum. It also predicts successful adaptation to mainstreaming, the ability to find and hold jobs during adolescence, the mother's perception of the child, and a variety of positive personality characteristics. Despite the vague specification of the specific effects of training, the importance of considering gainers and nongainers (within a task domain) seems to be well justified. Our own work described in the preceding section (Brown & Ferrara, in press) is aimed at providing just such information but is based on a more detailed process approach. In other words, we are interested in comparing gainers and nongainers in terms of the processes they gain and how far they transfer the results of learning within a suitable task domain.

FEUERSTEIN'S LEARNING POTENTIAL AND INSTRUMENTAL ENRICHMENT
PROGRAMS

Feuerstein's theory of cognitive development is very similar to Vygotsky's and Budoff's. According to Feuerstein, cognitive growth is the result of incidental and mediated learning. Incidental learning occurs as a result of the child's exposure to his changing environment, but mediated learning is the more important shaper of human growth. "Mediated learning is the training given to the human organism by an experienced adult who frames, selects, focuses and feeds back an environmental experience in such a way as to create appropriate learning sets" (Feuerstein, 1969, p. 6). Mediated learning refers to a learning experience where a supportive other (a parent, teacher, peer, etc.) is interposed between the organism and environment and intentionally influences the nature of the interaction. These mediated learning experiences are an essential aspect of development, beginning when the parent selects significant objects for the infant to focus on and proceeding throughout development, with the adult systematically shaping the child's learning experiences. This is the principal means by which children develop the cognitive operations necessary for learning independently. Thus Feuerstein's theory is also an internalization theory. By interacting with an adult, who guides problem-solving activity and structures the learning environment, the child gradually comes to adopt structuring and regulatory activities of his or her own.

Feuerstein believes that the principal reason for the poor performance of many disadvantaged adolescents is the lack of consistent mediated learning in their earlier developmental histories, because of parental apathy, ignorance, or overcommitment.

The resultant picture is poor performance on a wide range of academic tasks, and the level of performance displayed by retarded performers is an underestimation of the level they could achieve if subjected to intensive remedial mediated learning experiences. Like Budoff (1974) and Brown and Ferrara (in press) in America and Lubovsky and his colleagues in the USSR, Feuerstein is predicting that retarded performers, who do poorly because of inadequate early learning environments, will be gainers or will show a wide zone of potential development. By contrast, more severely retarded individuals and those with organic brain damage would be expected to show less benefit from intensive intervention aimed at supplying the missing mediated learning experience. Feuerstein's basic position seems to be that, to the extent that children's prior histories have been suboptimal, the static and dynamic assessment procedures will lead to less agreement.

In order to test his theory, Feuerstein developed two assessment packages that are now commercially available and are beginning to be used widely in America. The Learning Potential Assessment Device (LPAD) and the Instrumental Enrichment (IE) intervention program. In the LPAD, Feuerstein also adopted the now-familiar test–train–test procedure as a measure of the child's current status and potential for learning. In addition, similar to the other approaches, the LPAD tasks are variants of common IQ test items such as matrices problems, analytic perception, span tasks, and embedded-figure-type problems. Moreover, Feuerstein reports dramatic improvement as a function of brief training exposure to these items. We will not give further detail of the LPAD because it is essentially similar to the previously described approaches, although it lacks the systematic gradation of hints based on a process analysis. Furthermore, there are many existing descriptions of the device other than Feuerstein's own (Haywood et al., 1975; Hobbs, 1980; Narrol & Bachor, 1975).

Feuerstein differs from the other programs in that he has developed an intensive intervention curriculum, the IE program, to supplement his original diagnostic device. The IE program has been widely cited as a successful intervention program both in Israel (Feuerstein, 1980; Feuerstein et al., 1979) and in the United States (Haywood & Arbitman-Smith, 1981). An excellent analysis of the IE program has been provided by Bransford, Stein, Arbitman-Smith, and Vye (in press). From our point of view the IE program can be examined at three different levels: at the level of the actual materials, with respect to the actual training procedures or the use of the materials by the teacher and in relationship to Feuerstein's theory of cognitive development. We will discuss the second two levels in more detail because the actual materials themselves may have less to do with the success of this program than the training procedures. The IE materials in fact are very similar to IQ test items and achievement test batteries, consisting as they do of systematic easy-to-hard sequences of "content-free" (!) materials on analytic perception, comparisons, categorization, orientation in space, temporal relations, transitivity, and so forth. When systematic practice is provided on such tasks, it is not surprising that IQ gains have been reported on the very similar IQ test items.

Of more interest, perhaps, is how the materials are used in training, and this *how* reflects Feuerstein's characterization of the cognitive problems of retarded performers, which we will consider next. Feuerstein's description of the problem solving of disadvantaged Israeli adolescents is reminiscent of the type of cognitive deficit that we and others have termed *metacognitive* (Brown, 1975, 1978, 1980; Brown & Campione, 1978, 1981; Campione & Brown, 1977, 1978). These learners were described in section 8.3 as lacking a variety of systematic data-gathering, checking, monitoring, and self-regulatory mechanisms – in short, they are deficient in auto-critical skills (Binet, 1911). They tend to follow instructions blindly (Brown, 1978; Holt, 1964), lack adequate question-asking skills (Miyake & Norman, 1979), tolerate contradictions and inconsistencies happily (Markman, 1979), and do not seek to overcome comprehension problems with remedial strategies (Baker & Brown, in press-a; Brown, 1981). They have a tendency to treat each problem as a new prob-lem, regardless of relevant prior experiences, and generally develop learning sets slowly, transferring the effects of past learning reluctantly (Brown & Campione, 1981).

Feuerstein's terminology differs from that used in the previous section on experi-mental studies of learning efficiency, but the message is essentially the same. On the problem of comprehension monitoring, he claims, "Contradictions are not point-ed out; clarification is not sought; inconsistencies are swallowed without question" (Feuerstein, 1969, p. 9). Furthermore, on using prior knowledge and reasoning by analogies, Feuerstein claims:

The culturally deprived child does not internalize problems as they occur. . . . In his trial and error stabs at coming to grips with a situation, whichever resolution is finally hit upon is not insightfully incorporated into his behavioral schema with the result that upon a fresh recur-rence of the situation, he must start from scratch. Every problem is a new problem. Internaliza-tion leads to the building of learning sets which the culturally deprived notably lack in their conceptual repertoire. [Feuerstein, 1969, pp. 8–9]

Because of this diagnosis of executive or access problems in learning, it is not surprising that Feuerstein also concentrates on self-control and self-regulation in his IE training program. The essential aim is, via the mediation of a supportive teacher, to make children aware of the significance of their learning activities they will eventually, by internalization, perform cognitive regulatory functions for themselves that they have originally experienced in collaboration with an adult (Brown, 1980; Brown & French, 1979b). This aim is explicitly stated:

The salient characteristic in Instrumental Enrichment is its conscious, intentional, focused and volitional nature. The student is made aware that a certain concept is to be taught; he is made to focus on that concept and gradually to perfect his abilities with relationship to it. It is deemed of the utmost importance that his awareness and cooperation in this effort be enlisted and it will not be left to chance that perhaps he will come to understand the purposes and logic behind the disparate exercises. [Feuerstein, 1969, p. 18]

Again similar to the work described in the preceding section, the essential aim of insightful learning is transfer of training or access and use of information that is potentially available to the learner (Brown, 1980; Brown & Campione, 1981; Brown, Campione, & Day, 1981). In Feuerstein's words:

Transfer of training is most observable in instances where learning is based on insightful processes. In order to achieve such insights (e.g., to provide the learner with skills, attitude, problem solving behavior, category labels, etc.) the learner must be able to perceive the general characteristics and applicability of a given concept. Furthermore, one has to present the learner with a number of varied situations to which the newly acquired skills are applicable. [Feuerstein, 1969, p. 21]

The similarity to our experimental work is striking, and indeed we wish that we had become familiar with Feuerstein's work earlier. We differ from Feuerstein in two ways. First, we concentrate on process-oriented task analyses of the domains to be trained and on the transfer tasks that will assess the benefits of training. Feuerstein relies primarily on general improvement on standardized IQ and achievement test batteries (Feuerstein et al., 1979). Second, we disagree with Feuerstein's position that school subject matter learning "cannot be molded easily" into a suitable vehicle for training. We believe that the material of the IE intervention program is secondary to the training philosophy that underlies it and that it is possible to train monitoring and autocritical skills within the domain of actual school tasks. Programs such as our own with reading, writing, and studying strategies (Baker & Brown, in press-a; Brown, 1981; Brown & Campione, 1979; Brown, Campione, & Day, 1981; Brown & Smiley, 1978), Collins and Smith's (in press) comprehension monitoring training program, and Bransford's reading comprehension enrichment procedures (Bransford et al., 1981) all incorporate metacognitive training similar to that prescribed by Feuerstein without recourse to content-free materials such as those used in the IE battery. It remains to be seen which approach, if any, is more effective, but given the dramatic lack of evidence of ready transfer across disparate domains already documented for slow-learning children, training of self-regulatory skills in the target context of academic learning would seem to be indicated.

In summary, the three clinical programs of research concerned with the dynamic assessment of learning potential have many features in common and, furthermore, these features are not dissimilar to aspects of the current position of many experimental psychologists interested in training studies and a theory of intelligence. All agree that static measures of intelligence provide only an indication of current performance, which may be depressed for a variety of reasons. Accordingly, they agree that it may be necessary to supplement existing test procedures to obtain more refined diagnoses of academic potential. Their efforts to develop such procedures all lead them to the same kind of assessment device, one that provides a more direct assessment of learning than is obtainable from existing IQ tests. They also agree on the way in which such learning should be assessed. They reject situations involving simple reinforced practice in favor of a more interactive, instructional testing environment; they attempt to look specifically at the ability to profit from guided instruction. (It is interesting to note that this testing environment is more analogous to school learning situations than to other kinds of learning tasks. If the goal of the testing procedure is to predict school achievement, or the ability to profit from instruction, the use of such interactive assessment devices appears to possess clear face validity.)

On a more theoretical level, all of these researchers put forward, at least implicitly, an internalization theory of learning that follows a prototypic path from other-regulation to self-regulation. Finally, all pinpoint self-regulatory, or autocritical, skills as essential determinants of adequate initial learning and flexible transfer of training. Thus, whereas these programs have been developed independently, they agree in: (a) a need for supplemental diagnostic procedures; (b) the content of these procedures – relatively direct measures of learning and transfer; (c) the way in which learning should be assessed – responsiveness to guided instruction; (d) a general view of learning as internalization; and (e) the importance of self-regulatory skills.

This emergent literature, together with the previously described experimental studies of learning difficulties in aberrant populations, lends credence to traditional theories that identify intelligence as the speed and efficiency of learning in the absence of direct or complete instruction (Resnick & Glaser, 1976) and the extent to which wide lateral transfer or use of information is achieved (Gagné, 1970; Höffding, 1892; Thorndike & Woodworth, 1901). With methodologies such as those being developed to measure the zone of proximal development, we should be in a stronger position to uncover learning potential in children that is masked by their ineffectual static test performance.

8.5.   IMPLICATIONS FOR A THEORY OF INTELLIGENCE

In this section we consider the implications for a general theory of intelligence that can follow a consideration of the experimental and clinical literatures on exceptional children. The section is divided into three parts: The first part focuses on learning rate; the second centers on a discussion of transfer and generality of knowledge; and in the third we consider learning to learn via internalization. We hasten to add that we do not see these areas as separable. As we hope will become clear, transfer theories of intelligence such as ours treat learning and transfer as inevitably interrelated (Ferguson, 1954; Hebb, 1949). The separation is for convenience only.

Operationally, we can distinguish between initial learning of some new routine and subsequent transfer of that routine to related problems. The "original learning" problem, however, can never be entirely independent of prior knowledge, so the learning of that problem must involve some transfer (recall that in section 8.3 we had occasion to describe production deficiencies – failure to produce an appropriate strategy on a novel task – as a transfer failure). Also, the transfer problems must involve some new components, or they would be simple restatements of the original problem; hence there is room for learning effects in those situations. Finally, there are qualitative differences in the ways in which individuals can approach a "new" learning situation. The "way" in which learning takes place, or the "way" in which the learning environment is structured, will influence what is learned and how it is learned and thus will in turn influence subsequent transfer.

We chose to center our discussion on these issues because we would like to substantiate our claim that contemporary theories and methods, and particularly research with slow-learning children, lend credence to traditional views of intelligence as: the efficiency of learning in the absence of complete instruction (Resnick & Glaser, 1976), the extent of transfer (Ferguson, 1954) and the capacity to acquire capacity (Woodrow, 1921), or the capacity to learn or to profit by experience (Dearborn, 1921).

LEARNING IN THE ABSENCE OF COMPLETE INSTRUCTION

A consideration of the experimental and clinical data lends considerable support to the claim that the extent of instruction needed to effect learning is a prime index of intelligence. One of the consistent findings in the literature is that slow-learning children need direct and explicit instruction before they will behave strategically (Campione & Brown, 1977) and before they will transfer the benefits of prior learning to novel situations (Borkowski & Cavanaugh, 1979; Brown, Campione, & Barclay, 1979; Brown, Campione, & Day, 1981; Brown & French, 1979b). We have reviewed the considerable evidence to support the Soviet position that an extremely sensitive index of intelligence is a subject's learning potential, or his or her ability to profit from instruction. Retarded children profit from instruction, but the extent of the instruction required to achieve any lasting change is considerable. We do not mean to deny the point made eloquently by Feuerstein (1980) and Budoff (1974) that within a supposedly homogeneous group of EMR children there exist gainers and nongainers. Indeed, within a supposedly homogeneous group of adults, the test–train–test procedures reveal the same stratification of good solvers, gainers, and nongainers (Fattu, Mech, & Kapos, 1954). We would similarly not deny that in simple laboratory tasks, considerable improvement in the performance of retarded children follows relatively brief training exposure (Belmont & Butterfield, 1977; Brown, 1974, 1978). We do, however, emphatically disavow a position of radical environmentalism or antistructuralism, a charge that has repeatedly been made (Belmont & Butterfield, 1977) and that we have repeatedly denied (Brown, 1978; Brown & Campione, 1981). Admittedly we now possess a powerful technology for considerably enhancing the cognitive skills of poor learners in a variety of academic domains (Brown, Campione, & Day, 1981), but in order to effect these improvements it is necessary to make explicit, or even to deliberately train, a wide range of strategic processes that the normal child acquires incidentally or spontaneously. Furthermore, there is little evidence to suggest that individual differences will be easy to "train away," except in the simplistic sense of mastery learning (Bloom, 1976). In situations where a ceiling effect is not deliberately imposed, as in mastery learning, and when training is given to a wide range of learners, the evidence would suggest that the difference between good and poor learners will broaden, that is, the bright benefit even more from training than do the originally less scintillating thinkers (Anderson, 1967; Brown, Campione, & Day, 1981; Cronbach, 1967; Snow & Yalow, chapter 9 in this volume; Stolurow, 1964). The more mature need less explicit instruction initially and transfer the effects of that instruction further (see section 8.4). Because of the reliability of this general finding across a wide variety of tasks and students, we reaffirm the traditional position of intelligence as the ability to learn in the absence of direct or complete instruction (Dearborn, 1921).

This position is not to be confused with the notoriously unsuccessful attempts during the behaviorist heyday to link rate of learning with IQ. Based on evidence provided mainly by Woodrow (1938, 1946), it was concluded that "intelligence, far from being identical with the amount of improvement shown by practice, had practically nothing to do with the matter" (Woodrow, 1946, p. 151). Such a view remained popular through the 1960s (Gagné, 1967). Still, let us consider the evidence on which this conclusion was based. Learning was defined as a change measure obtained by simply subtracting initial and final scores. Even the obvious ploy of calculating the residual gain consisting of final status minus the proportion predictable from initial status (Lord, 1958) provided evidence for a direct link between IQ and learning rate, but this evidence tended to be ignored, as did Gulliksen's (1942) work suggesting that learning curves correlate with IQ measures, whereas simple measures of rate, time, and number of trials to reach criterion do not (see also Stake, 1961, and Duncanson, 1964).

In addition to the problem of the measure of change, there was also the problem of tasks. No process analyses of what was changing or how were attempted. The tasks on which practice was given, apparently randomly selected, included backward writing, reproduction of spot patterns, horizontal adding, canceling letters, estimating lengths, and our favorite – speed in making gates (making four horizontal lines and one diagonal line in each square of a page divided into 1,000 squares) – perhaps not the most fertile ground in which to hunt for an elusive *g* factor!

Furthermore, the conditions under which learning was to occur were simply those of reinforced practice, that is, practice unguided except for knowledge of results. Unguided practice on a miscellaneous assortment of tasks did not uncover a learning rate parameter related to intelligence. The problem, of course, lies in the definition of learning – here, improvement (unspecified) via unguided practice.

Even in elegantly specified process theories of performance, similar problems can be found. For example, the most detailed analysis of learning processes in the retarded has been provided by Zeaman and House (1963). They analyzed the performance of retarded children and adolescents in a variety of two-choice discrimination learning situations. That retarded or younger children would take longer to reach some criterion than brighter or older children was not really at issue; rather, the researchers were concerned with explaining the source of those differences. Their theory included both attentional (P_o) and learning rate (θ_o and θ_r) parameters. Based on the theoretical analysis of performance on the problems they chose to investigate, individual differences emerged in the attention, but not learning, parameters. One of the learning parameters (θ_r) referred to the efficiency of learning which of two cues (e.g., red or green) was correct, given that the relevant dimension (e.g., color) had been determined. Within this framework, θ_- invariance across a wide range of subjects or an inability to relate learning rate with intelligence is not so surprising.

We have no argument with the emphasis on the importance of attentional processes in determining performance levels. To the contrary, we believe that these analyses are extremely important and do provide important information about the nature of comparative or developmental differences. As will be clear below, experts and novices, as well as retarded and nonretarded children, do differ in terms of the way in which they encode sets of problems; in the terminology of Zeaman and House, more proficient performers are more likely to attend to relevant dimensions of the problems than are poorer performers. We can carry the analysis one step farther and ask why this might be the case. That is, the attention parameters presumably reflect, at least in part, the products of prior experience; differences in those products may reflect something else of at least equal importance – such as learning dynamics. As in previous cases (section 8.3), the distinction lies between knowledge or competence and the processes whereby that competence is achieved and used. It is within this context that we are concerned with the fact that these results have been interpreted as suggesting that *in general* learning rate is not related to intelligence. The conclusion is fine *within the context of the specific theoretical use* of the term *learning* and the *kinds of experiments* that have been the subject of analysis. The conclusion is inappropriate when generalized beyond those boundaries. The problem is that there is a tendency to make such generalizations, that is, to remember the conclusion of such enterprises but to forget the nature of the data base that supports those conclusions and the place of the term *learning* within the specific theories those data were generated to test. Different theories and/or different experiments may lead to different conclusions. For example, Zeaman (1978) has recently argued that some of the earlier experiments in their laboratory may have been conducted in a way which was insensitive to θ_o (rate of learning which dimension is relevant) differences and that different kinds of experiments may in fact succeed in demonstrating θ_o–intelligence covariation.

In linking learning efficiency with intelligence we stress that it is necessary to have a theory of the task, a theory of the person, and a theory of the interactive nature of the learning situation. Learning efficiency or potential can best be examined on tasks designed to uncover how much the learner already knows, how much he can benefit from guided practice via systematic prompts, and how far he will transfer the fruits of learning (see section 8.4). We have just described Vygotsky's (1978) theory of proximal distance or the zone of potential development. The similarity of our position and that of Vygotsky to very early concepts of intelligence as the potential for improvement (Dearborn, 1921) is also striking. Contemporary research provides the empirical support for traditional claims about the nature of intelligence and the course of cognitive growth.

We will conclude this section with an alternative statement of the approach favored here. The guiding question of interest concerns the relation between learning ability and intelligence. The typical method has been to begin with a measure of intelligence, typically an IQ score, and some index of learning proficiency. Then the relation between the two is investigated. Such an approach involves a number of implicit assumptions, specifically that we have a good measure of intelligence and a good measure of learning. The open question is: Are they related? More often than not, the answer is no, and the conclusion is that learning rate and intelligence are unrelated.

A different approach can be taken. We might again assume that we have an acceptable measure of intelligence; we could also assume that learning rate and intelligence *are* related. The open issue in this case concerns the nature of the theories and the resultant experimental tasks needed to demonstrate and explicate that relation. Views of learning that consistently lead to tasks that do not uncover correlations between learning and intelligence become suspect; they are unlikely to be interesting theories of learning. The experimental procedures that result in weak or no relations between learning and intelligence are regarded as not tapping the learning processes with which we are concerned. Here the data on learning–intelligence relations serve to constrain our theories of learning and the operations used to assess these hypothesized processes.

It is within this latter view that we are particularly impressed with the zone-of-proximal-development-type studies (see section 8.4) and the data they generate. The theoretical notions upon which such experiments are based include a view of learning as the internalization of knowledge and processes resulting from a guided, instructional interaction. From this position, we are likely to learn more about learning by situating our experiments in contexts in which we can observe responses to guided prompts than we are by analyzing, à la Woodrow, primarily situations involving "simpler" unguided practice. Again, if intelligence tests are designed to predict, or be related to, school success, then it would seem that the learning processes of which they are an indirect measure are likely to be schoollike ones. And school learning does involve response to guided instruction.

FLEXIBLE USE OF INFORMATION: ACCESS AND TRANSFER OF TRAINING

Clinical and experimental programs aimed at uncovering the primary source of inadequate intellective functioning converge on a prime culprit; children diagnosed as inefficient learners have particularly severe problems with the regulation of their own activities. In the developmental literature, the type of processing implicated as deficient in aberrant populations has been referred to as metacognitive (Brown, 1978; Campione & Brown, 1977; Flavell & Wellman, 1977) or executive control (Belmont & Butterfield, 1977; Brown, 1974). These terms are by no means free of controversy, either in their fashionable "meta" instantiation or in their more familiar information-processing homunculi guises. Much of the contention surrounding the terms reflects some of the persistent problems in psychology (e.g., the nature of consciousness, will, purpose, epistemic mediation, deus ex machina, etc.). Still, despite the undoubted epistemological problems associated with the terms, the general consensus in the developmental literature is that here lies a primary site of learning problems in the immature.

Similarly, in cognitive psychology in general, a revived interest in metacognitive issues is becoming apparent, particularly in the emerging fields of instructional psychology (Glaser, 1978) and cognitive science (Brown, Collins, & Larkin, 1980; Collins & Smith, in press; Norman, 1980; Simon, 1979). Specifically relating issues of executive control to individual differences in intelligence, Sternberg (1980, see also chapter 5 in this volume) has also placed heavy emphasis on metacomponents. Although the issues of executive control are by no means novel considerations within an information-processing model, less familiar is the realization of a close link between metacomponents and efficiency of learning (Sternberg, chapter 5 in this volume). Again, the convergence with the clinical and developmental literatures is impressive, especially since these bodies of inquiry usually proceed in blissful ignorance of each other.

In a series of recent papers (Brown, 1978, 1980; Brown et al., in press; Brown & Campione, 1978, 1981; Brown & DeLoache, 1978; Campione & Brown, 1978), we have been developing a theory of intellectual function based on the concept of accessibility, or the ability to use flexibly and appropriately the information and skills available to the system. We make no claims that this is a new theory (or amiable set of hypotheses); for example, witness the following quote from Feuerstein (1969): "Specific training in the awareness, selection and flexible use of probable cues is precisely the goal of Instrumental Enrichment training" (p. 26).

In this section we will examine the central place of the concept of access in theories of intelligence from quite disparate schools of thought. This will by no means be an exhaustive review; we have chosen a few examples representative of such fields as artificial intelligence (Moore & Newell, 1974; Simon, 1979), developmental psychology (Brown, 1980; Brown & Campione, 1981; Gardner, 1978; Gelman & Gallistel, 1978), cognitive ethology (Rozin, 1976), and cross-cultural psychology work by the Laboratory of Comparative Human Cognition, or LCHC (see chapter 11 in this volume). We will then consider the importance of such a concept for considering individual differences in intelligence in children. Finally we will raise some persistent difficulties with the theory, specifically concerning the nature of a domain of knowledge, active versus inactive organisms and vertical versus lateral transfer.

Developmental concerns with metacognition

Pylyshyn (1978b), in his commentary on the issue of conscious planning in nonhuman species, makes the distinction between multiple and reflective access. *Multiple access* refers to the ability to use knowledge flexibly, that is, a particular behavior is not delimited to a constrained set of circumstances. Knowledge is then "informationally plastic" to the extent that it can be "systematically varied" to fit a wide range of conditions (Pylyshyn, 1978b, p. 593). *Reflective access* refers to the ability to "mention as well as use" the components of the system. This distinction between multiple and reflective access we have applied recently (Brown, 1980; Brown & Campione, 1981) to the different activities that have come to be subsumed under the heading of metacognition in the developmental literature (see also section 8.3).

Two separate lines of inquiry (at least) are currently proceeding rather uneasily under the same rubric, that of metacognition. The first, and probably the most common area of study, is concerned with the problems of reflective access, that is, with the ability to mention, or consciously describe and discuss, one's own cognitive activities. A considerable emerging body of literature suggests that immature learners are less than well informed concerning the workings of their own mind (see section 8.3, also Baker & Brown, in press-a). Many of these data come from questionnaire studies or from confrontation experiments, the main purpose of which is to find out how much children know about certain pertinent features of learning, including themselves as learners (person variables), the task to be undertaken (task variables), and the strategies by which the learning goal might be reached (strategy variables) most effectively (Flavell & Wellman, 1977). There are nontrivial problems associated with self-report techniques (Brown et al., in press). Briefly, even adults are less able to introspect about their cognitive knowledge than one would like (Nisbett & Wilson, 1977; but cf. White, 1980), and the problems of eyewitness testimony are no less acute when the witness is asked to testify about the workings of his or her mind rather than the activities of the surrounding world. These difficulties notwithstanding, the systematic interrogation of children concerning their own learning processes has led to considerable insights into the problem of self-awareness with which the novice learner must contend (Baker & Brown, in press-b; Flavell, 1981).

The second line of investigation is more concerned with the issue of *multiple access*, or the flexible use of information available to the system (see section 8.3). Here the prime interest is in the self-regulatory mechanisms that are used by an efficient learner during an ongoing attempt to access and use available resources, by activating prior knowledge (Brown, Campione, & Day, 1981), reasoning by analogy (Brown, 1980), and seeking relationships (Baron, 1978) between what is already known and what is to be learned. The kind of activities examined by those interested in multiple access include attempts to *relate* a new problem to a similar class of problems, to imbue the unfamiliar with the familiar, engaging in *means–ends analyses* to identify effective strategies, *checking* the outcome of any attempt to solve the problem, *planning* one's next move, *monitoring* the effectiveness of any attempted action, *testing, revising,* and *evaluating* one's strategies for learning. These are not necessarily stable skills in the sense that although they are more often used by older children and adults, they are not always used by them, and quite young children may monitor their activities on a simple problem (Brown, 1978). Learners of any age are more likely to take active control of their own cognitive endeavors when they are faced with tasks of intermediate difficulty (if the task is too easy, they need not bother; if the task is too hard, they give up). Effective learning requires an active monitoring of one's own cognitive activities. Whether or not these activities are conscious and statable, that is, can be subjected to reflective access, they are important problem-solving activities intimately related to intelligence. We have made considerable use of the concepts of accessibility in our discussion of transfer of training in slow-learning children (Brown & Campione, 1981).

Gardner (1978) is another developmental psychologist who makes a distinction similar to the one of multiple and reflective access. He suggests that the hallmarks of intelligence are: (a) generative, inventive, and experimental use of knowledge rather than preprogrammed activities (multiple access) and (b) the ability to reflect upon one's own activity (reflective access).

Note, however, Gardner's point that no organism ever reaches a level of "total consciousness, full awareness, and constant intentionality," for these are "emergent capacities," useful as indexes for comparative purposes both within and between species but never perfectly instantiated even in the mature human. To the extent that organisms come to exhibit more and more of the qualities of reflective and multiple access, we tend to say that they exhibit intelligent behavior. Conversely, to the extent that behaviors "(1) appear only when elicited by strong training models, (2) recur in virtually identical form over many occasions, (3) display little experimental playfulness, (4) exhibit restricted coupling to a single symbolic system, or (5) fail ever to be used to refer in 'meta' fashion to one's own activities, we are inclined to minimize their significance (as indices of intelligent behavior)" (Gardner, 1978, p. 572).

Cognitive ethology and the concept of access

In developing our interest in the concept of access, we were greatly influenced by the work of Rozin (1976) concerned with the evolution of intelligence. Rozin considers intelligence a complex biological system, hierarchically organized, and consisting of a repertoire of adaptive specializations that are the components or subprograms of the system. Throughout the animal world there exist adaptive specializations related to intelligence that originate to satisfy specific problems of survival. Because they evolve as solutions to specific problems, these adaptive specializations are originally tightly wired to the narrow set of situations that called for their evolution. In lower organisms the adaptive specializations remain tightly constrained components of the system. Rozin quotes such widely known examples of prewired intelligence components as the navigational communication ability of bees that is totally restricted to the defined situation of food foraging (Von Frisch, 1967, but see also Gould, 1978), and the exceptionally accurate map memories of gobiid fish for their own tide pool (Aronson, 1951). This form of intelligence is tightly prewired; although it can sometimes be calibrated by environmental influences, it is largely preprogrammed. Rozin's theory is that in the course of evolution, cognitive programs become more accessible to other units of the system and can therefore be used flexibly in a variety of situations. This flexibility is the hallmark of higher intelligence, reaching its zenith at the level of conscious control that affords wide applicability over the full range of mental functioning.

Rozin (1976) refers to the tightly wired, limited-access components in the brain as the *cognitive unconscious* and suggests that

part of the progress in evolution toward more intelligent organisms could then be seen as gaining access to or emancipating the cognitive unconscious. Minimally, a program (adaptive specialization) could be wired into a new system or a few new systems. In the extreme, the program could be brought to the level of consciousness, which might serve the purpose of making it applicable to the full range of behaviors and problems. [Pp. 256–257]

Just as part of the progress in evolution toward more intelligent organisms can be seen as gaining access to the cognitive unconscious, so, too, the progress of development within higher species such as *Homo sapiens* can be characterized as one of gaining access. Intelligent behavior is first tightly wired to the narrow context in which it was acquired and only later becomes extended into other domains. Thus, cognitive development is the process of proceeding from the "specific inaccessible" nature of skill to the "general accessible."

There are two main points to Rozin's accessibility theory. First is the notion of welding (Brown, 1974, 1978; Shif, 1969). Intelligence components can be strictly welded to constrained domains; that is, skills available in one situation are not readily used in others, even though they are appropriate. We would refer to this as a problem of multiple access. Rozin uses the concept to explain the patchy nature of young children's early cognitive ability, which has been described as a composite of skills that are not necessarily covariant. Young children's programs are "not yet usable in all situations, available to consciousness or statable" (Rozin, 1976, p. 262). Development is the process of gradually *extending* and *connecting together* the isolated skills with a possible ultimate extension into consciousness.

Closely related is the second notion of awareness, or knowledge of the system that one can use, or reflective access. Even if skills are widely applicable rather than tightly welded, they need not necessarily be stable, statable, and conscious. Rozin would like to argue that much of formal education is the process of gaining access to the rule-based components already in the head, that is, the process of coming to understand explicitly a system already used implicitly. As Gelman and Gallistel (1978) point out, linguistic (and possibly natural number) concepts are acquired very easily, early, and universally, but the ability to talk and the ability to access the structure of the language are not synonymous. The ability to speak does not automatically lead to an awareness of the rules of grammar governing the language. Thus, although he does not use these terms, the twin concepts of multiple and reflective access are central to Rozin's theory of the evolution of intelligence.

Artificial intelligence and instructional psychology

Researchers concerned with the creation of intelligent behavior in machines are forced to make explicit exactly what they think constitutes intelligence, hence the fascinating controversies surrounding the problem of how intelligent machines are now (or could be in the future). The issues raised by these controversies are central to our conception of mind (Bobrow & Collins, 1975; Boden, 1977; Flores & Winograd, 1978; Pylyshyn and following commentaries, 1978a). Fascinating as such arguments are, we will restrict ourselves to the problems of accessibility.

Moore and Newell (1974) made a succinct statement of the multiple-access problem when they defined the essence of machine understanding in reference to two criteria. First, "S understands K if S uses K whenever appropriate"; second, this "understanding can be partial, both in extent (the class of appropriate situations in which the knowledge is used) and in immediacy (the time it takes before understanding can be exhibited)" (pp. 204–205). We judge as intelligent the flexible, appropriate, and rapid application of the available knowledge. The distinction is between knowledge and the understanding of that knowledge, where understanding is defined in terms of appropriate use or ready access.

Problems of multiple access are then isomorphic with problems of transfer of training, and it is when considering transfer issues that terms suspiciously like *metacognition* enter into the discussion. One current controversy in the field of instructional implications of artificial intelligence (AI) research is the problem of whether intelligent performance is influenced by the operation of some general, powerful, domain-independent problem-solving skills or whether problem-solving skills are idiosyncratic to a particular task or domain (Newell, 1979). This is an old issue. In its most well known form it is the question of whether learning Latin helps us to think better (Thorndike & Woodworth, 1901). Current instantiations of the general, specific-skills argument abound. On the one hand, Goldstein and Papert (1977) claim that "the fundamental problem of understanding intelligence is not the identification of a few powerful techniques, but rather the question of how to represent *large amounts of knowledge in a fashion that permits their effective use and interaction*" (p. 85).

In response, Simon (1979) claims that "bare facts, however they are stored in memory, do not solve problems" (p. 85). In addition to the large body of knowledge represented in semantically rich domains, there must be processes for "operating on that knowledge to solve problems and answer questions." Simon claims that incorporated in AI systems such as MYCIN and DENDRAL are indeed the "few powerful techniques" that Goldstein and Papert dismiss, that is, general problem-solving techniques of AI such as means–ends analysis, hypothesis and test methods, best–first search procedures, and so forth (Feigenbaum, 1977; Newell & Simon, 1972; Simon, 1979). "The evidence from close examination of AI programs that perform professional-level tasks, and the psychological evidence form human transfer experiments, indicate both that powerful general methods do exist and that they can be taught in such a way that they are relevant" (Simon, 1979, p. 86).

Precisely these powerful general methods of monitoring, self-instruction, questioning, relatedness seeking, reasoning by analogy, and so forth are the learning skills that provide multiple access or flexible and efficient use of knowledge.

Following the argument surrounding the existence of general strategies is the concern with whether they are amenable to instruction. Again, there seems to be some controversy as to whether one should aim to train general or specific strategies. Simon, involved in the development of "instructable production systems" (Simon, 1979), believes that general determinants of effective learning can be taught explicitly and that the aim of such training is "problem solving with awareness." The key is to make explicit the general rules. "Since we know that skills will be transferred only when the principles on which they rest are made explicit, these procedures (i.e., means–ends analysis) need to be made evident for students" (Simon, 1979, p. 93). Similarly, Brown, Collins, and Harris (1978) emphasize that a great deal of essential strategic knowledge is tacit not only to students but to the teachers, who neither explicitly train it or recognize that it could be trained. Making explicit that which is tacit is an essential first step for the design of training studies, for as Brown, Collins, and Harris (1978) note, without explicit awareness of the "largely tacit planning and strategic knowledge" inherent in a complex problem domain, it would be difficult for a teacher to accelerate the learning process.

In addition to the complexity added by the tacit–explicit dimension, there is also the complexity resulting from the essentially interactive nature of knowledge acquisition, amply documented by the recent spate of in-depth analyses of complex problem solving in scientific subject domains. Expert knowledge does not readily fit into separate boxes labeled procedural, declarative, factual, strategic, and so forth, for there is a complex interrelationship between knowledge of principles and concepts and knowledge of problem-solving procedures. "Regardless of the sophistication of a solver's procedural and strategic knowledge, deficiencies in knowledge of facts, concepts, and principles constrain the scope of that individual's problem solving ability" (Larkin, Heller, & Greeno, 1980, p. 12).

This interrelation between knowledge and strategy factors poses problems not only for theory development but also for the design of training studies, as we have seen in section 8.3, where we discussed some differences between the training of specific versus general strategies in simple learning tasks. The dilemma is also illustrated by this pair of seemingly contradictory quotations from the same laboratory:

In much of psychology, there has been a bias toward emphasizing highly general, domain-independent mechanisms that are supposedly central to the instructional process. Our work demonstrates that such a perspective is incomplete without a detailed consideration of domain-specific knowledge. [Stevens, Collins, & Goldin, 1979, p. 145]

We have begun to see some surprising similarities in the kinds of strategies and knowledge used in these different domains (story comprehension, solutions to mathematical problems and electronic circuits). This suggests that there may be general learning strategies that will enhance a student's comprehension over a wide range of content areas. Rigney (1976) has claimed that "The approach to teaching students cognitive strategies has been through content-based instruction and maybe this is wrong and should be reversed; that is, content independent instruction." [Brown, Collins, & Harris, 1978, p. 108]

Quite simply, the argument is whether to train domain-specific or task-independent strategies (Newell, 1979), a very familiar theme for developmental psychologists working with exceptional children (Brown, 1978, 1979; Brown & Campione, 1981; Belmont & Butterfield, 1977; Butterfield, 1981). The answer is clearly both or either one, depending on what you want to achieve – and this question brings us back to the traditional problems of access – "what is learned?" "what is flexible use?" "what is a domain?" – that is, to the problem of transfer of training.

Problems with theories of access and transfer

Although we are relatively confident, on the basis of the empirical evidence (see sections 8.3 and 8.4), that inflexible access is a major learning problem for the immature and inexperienced, we do not wish to claim that we have solved any of the major problems. On the contrary, theories of transfer of training have been the subject of continual dispute since the emergence of psychology as a scientific discipline (Höffding, 1892); many of the issues raised before this century are by no means resolved today (Newell, 1979). This is not the place to discuss the history of the controversy in detail, but we will mention here some of the problems inherent in an attempt to identify extent of transfer as a prime index of intelligence. Our list is by no means exhaustive, and we do not pretend to have answers. Here we merely want to observe that many terms used freely by many researchers (including ourselves) are somewhat lacking in explanatory precision. Indeed, many of the labels used by contemporary cognitive psychologists also formed the basic terminology of the behaviorist tradition. Confusion follows this collective use of terms that convey non-trivial distinctions in different schools of thought.

The primary problem is the use of the term *domain* as if it should convey some precise information. Access theories including our own speak glibly of connecting domains of knowledge (Rozin, 1976), transsituational skills (Brown, 1978), range of applicability across domains (Brown, 1980), domain-specific versus general skills (everybody), even content-independent (Feuerstein, 1980) and decontextualized knowledge (Bransford, 1979; Brown, 1977). Whereas the general idea behind these concepts is clear, if we are to discuss transfer of training, the concept of a domain needs to be described with far greater precision, for we should make some attempt to predict where and when we expect transfer to occur. There is an ever-present danger of determining a posteriori that since transfer was observed between two tasks, that transfer was then due to the set of shared features of the tasks in question.

The confusion concerning a domain can be quite gross if we do not specify our meaning with some precision. For example, during the 1950s there was a considerable interest in transfer across physical domains exemplified by studies where subjects were required to learn a list of items in Room A and were then tested for retention in Room A versus Room B. Similarly, in a great many of the cognitive behavior modification studies (Meichenbaum, 1977), extent of transfer has a suspiciously physical ring. For example, children taught to control their impulsive behavior in the clinic or the laboratory are said to transfer widely if they maintain this behavior in the classroom. There are no problems with this position as long as we do not combine studies that look at extent of transfer through a physical domain and extent of transfer in a cognitive domain (Belmont, Butterfield, & Ferretti, in press; Brown & Campione, in press). Throughout the rest of our discussion, when we speak of extent of transfer we are referring to improvement in Task B following training on Task A, not improvement in the classroom following instruction in the laboratory.

This clarification by no means circumvents the problem of a domain, for restricting ourselves to cognitive domains provides no binding constraints. The problem of a domain is an old one, intimately tied to the problem of general or specific factors in intelligence, to which we will return. First, however, we will focus on the traditional problems of lateral transfer. Gagné (1970) distinguished between *vertical transfer* and *lateral transfer*. Vertical transfer occurs when training in a subskill contributes directly to the acquisition of the superordinate skill of which it is a component. Gagné's (1968) own work is one of the more elegant instantiations of this approach, which is the essence of effective task analyses. The concept of vertical transfer is also subject to considerable controversy, a controversy that is central to discussions of stages in learning (Brainerd, 1978; Flavell, 1971; Markman, 1978; Siegler, 1981). Here we are more concerned with the problem of *lateral transfer*, which refers to generalization that spreads over a broad set of situations.

In the case of this kind of transfer, the question of how much appears to be a matter of how broadly the individual can generalize what he has learned to a new situation. Presumably, there are limits to the breadth of generalization, which vary with different individuals. One could perhaps think of a whole range of situations of potential applicability of (some learned rules) that display decreasing degrees of similarity to the situation in which the rule had originally been learned. At some point along this dimension of breadth of generalizability, a given individual will fail to transfer his previously learned knowledge. Another individual, however, may be able to exhibit transfer more broadly to a wider variety of differing situations. [Gagné, 1970, p. 336]

The key problem with such positions is how broad one would expect the generalization effect to be. What is the domain or context within which transfer is to be constrained? In essence, this is a restatement of the traditional educational question of formal discipline in learning, that is, does learning Latin help us think better in a wide variety of domains? In their landmark paper rejecting this position, Thorndike and Woodworth (1901) revived the *identical elements* theory of traditional associationism, when they suggested that transfer will occur across tasks only to the extent that they share identical elements. Some version of identical elements theories has persisted throughout the behaviorist period (Ellis, 1965; Osgood, 1949) and into contemporary cognitive science. Theories of transfer of training put forward by ourselves (Brown, 1978; Brown & Campione, 1981; Campione & Brown, 1974, 1977) and others (Belmont & Butterfield, 1977) are all versions of identical elements theory, the difference lying in the specification of *identicalness* and the processes whereby similarity is determined.

We should note that Thorndike and Woodworth were behaviorists and defined identical elements primarily in terms of physical features of the tasks. Still, as the original identical elements theorist, Höffding (1892), observed, the real problem with transfer lies not only in the physical dimensions of the task environment but also in the subjective similarity as constructed by the learner. In fact, to be more than usually cynical, Höffding's position is essentially isomorphic with contemporary theories of transfer of training. In addition to requiring physical similarities among task contexts to determine transfer, Höffding was concerned with perceived, or subjective, similarity between situations, how new situations elicit old responses, how we recognize problem isomorphs, and how a new situation comes to be connected with the stored trace of previous learning, that is, the infamous Höffding step (1892), which is still, in its many guises, our main problem today.

Identical elements theories have been favored, then, by both behavioral and cognitive psychologists. Element similarity, however, can be determined by person variables, task variables, or both. Within a strict behaviorist tradition, identical elements were determined predominantly by task parameters. Even in cases where elements of similarity were conceived in nonphysical ways, for example, in investigations of semantic generalization, the tasks and stimuli employed were the primary, if not the sole, determinants of similarity. Transfer effects resulted from processes such as primary stimulus generalization, which in turn was seen as an automatic mechanism whereby an indicator response learned to some stimulus configuration would be elicited by other, similar configurations. The magnitude of this effect was proportional to the similarity of the training and transfer situations. The quantitative problems were most easily investigated with physical continua, although it was assumed that the laws resulting from such research would also apply to more complex situations.

If transfer is defined as an automatic response to partial identity, and identical elements are determined by the properties of the stimulus environment, then it is not clear where one would predict that comparative differences would reside. Such theories did not confer special status to age or species differences (Brown, 1980), for the extent of task commonality determines transfer; nothing in such theories lends itself well to an account of individual differences. One could, and theorists did, assert that high-level organisms have different generalization gradients than lower species, but this is a simple restatement of the data. It explains neither where such differences come from nor how they might be altered. If we considerably oversimplify the issue, it might be said that behaviorist theories were characterized by a *reactive* organism dominated by environmental forces. Identical elements tended to be just that, identical, and similarity was defined primarily by measurable physical gradients. Again, this is an oversimplification, for learning theories in the behaviorist tradition did consider this problem (i.e., the acquired-distinctiveness-of-cues controversy), but they were severely constrained by the central notion of a reactive organism.

Central to cognitive theories is the *active* organism, no doubt buried in thought (Hull, 1943; on Tolman), as products of cryptophenomenology (Kohler, 1951; on Tolman, 1959) often are, but also imbued with extraordinary decision-making propensities, an alarming responsibility. Behaviorist man reacts to stimuli. In contrast, cognitive man does not simply respond to stimuli but rather constructs them. The primary shift in cognitive theories is away from task-determined factors to a heavy reliance on the interaction of person variables and task environments (Brown, 1980). Stimulus situations, or problem types, are not similar or dissimilar in general but are seen as related by some subjects and unrelated by others. As Garner (1962) has argued in another context, when a subject is responding to a set of patterns, the "properties" of those patterns, in his case their redundancy, vary across subjects, as the perceived or subjective redundancy is a function of the number of potential patterns that the *subject* could generate on the basis of *his or her* perception of the constraints involved. Although this reasoning does not simplify the analysis in any way, it does at least provide a framework within which individual differences can be investigated. Individuals can differ in the ways in which they search for and perceive similarity.

What does such a shift in emphasis do to theories of transfer? Identical elements now translate into perceived similarity, or subjective identity. (Note that the terms *perceived*, or *subjective, similarity* are meant to imply only that the similarity of two or more situations depends upon the subject's analysis of those situations. The underlying similarity metrics are objectively specifiable for each subject; they are simply different for different groups of subjects.) When speaking of the transfer of cognitive activities, one is dealing with the identification of dimensions of the problem space, or with the classification of problems into similar types, an identification and classification that may depend on physical or surface elements for novices in some domain but depend upon more abstract, "deep structure" analyses for experts (Chi & Glaser, 1980; Larkin et al., 1980). Here classifications based on surface features tend to lead to nonproductive classification, whereas deep structure analyses are associated with increased proficiency. The learner must determine what the elements are, that is, as Höffding (1892) noted, the problem now resides in seeing relationships that are not physically specified.

Such a shift brings with it as many epistemological problems as it bypasses, and many will not see it as an advance (Skinner, 1977). Still, for those who play the comparative game, it does provide a basis for individual differences in the locus of transfer failure. Whereas in some situations, the prime determinants of similarity are likely to be equally salient to all performers, in other situations that is not the case. The latter occasions are most likely to be those where the basis for similarity is not given directly by the physical, or surface, features of the situations involved, with the result that the basis for classification needs to be discovered. Under these conditions, individuals vary in the extent to which they employ such deliberate problem-solving activities as seeking relationships among problems, in reasoning by analogy, in deliberately activating prior knowledge to render novel phenomena more familiar, in accessing knowledge across domains (Brown, 1980; Brown, Campione, & Day, 1981). Children are more limited by the variety of possible worlds they can imagine (Brown, 1978; Johnson-Laird, 1980) and their propensity to treat each new problem as independent of prior learning, that is, by the range of applicability of a particular process (Brown, 1980, see also LCHC, chapter 11 in this volume). With Newell (1979), Bransford (1979), and Feuerstein (1980), we believe that general reasoning-by-analogy-processes are basic to intelligent functioning and can be taught (Brown, 1980; Brown, Campione, & Day, 1981). In addition, differences in the basis for recognizing problem isomorphs, from physical similarity (e.g., words in the problem) to underlying conceptual identity, do seem to characterize the progression from novice to expert problem solvers (Anzai & Simon, 1979; Chi & Glaser, 1980; Larkin et al., 1980; Simon, 1979).

Theoretically, are we any further ahead, or have we just restated the data in another way? The latter is probably true, but identical elements theory restated as a subjective process of construing underlying process similarity does seem to be a more fruitful metaphor. Instead of altering the slope of an organism's gradient, or aiming for acquired distinctiveness of cues, we can describe the differences between experts and novices in rich qualitative terms that permit the design of successful training studies (Larkin et al., 1980). Such training aims (a) to help students identify the dimensions of a problem; (b) to make explicit that trainees should be active organisms; (c) to show how one can map a novel situation into familiar terrain by processes of analogy and metaphor (Bransford et al., 1981; Brown, 1980; Brown et al., in press; Brown & Campione, 1981; Newell, 1979). Although such training is especially needed for the slow-learning child, it is prescribed not only for the imma-ture but also for the inexperienced of any age. For example, witness novice physi-cists sorting problems on the basis of similarity of problem wording rather than on that of underlying conceptual processes (Chi & Glaser, 1980), and indeed, the startling lack of problem solving by analogy shown by college students (Gick & Holyoak, 1980; Simon & Hayes, 1976). The metaphor seems to be a useful one that has spawned a great deal of creative work on transfer of training in semantically rich domains that was not generated by identical elements theories as interpreted in the behaviorist tradition.

The astute reader may have noticed that we are going to extraordinary lengths to avoid attacking head-on the central question of the meaning of *domain;* however, the entire problem of defining identity for elements is essentially a question of domain specification, and we now turn to the argument of *specific* versus *general* skills that again centers on domains and their specification.

In his role as concluding speaker at the Carnegie-Mellon Conference on Problem Solving and Education, Allan Newell stated:

If there is one dichotomy that permeated this conference, it concerned the basic nature of problem solving. Specifically the poles are

Domain-independence of Problem-Solving	vs.	Domain-specificity of Problem-Solving

The dichotomy is an old one. [Newell, 1979, p. 184]

Thus, the specific–general dichotomy is thriving today, at least in Pittsburgh, but it was also crucial in guiding the development of early theories of intelligence. Binet fluctuated from pole to pole, attempting on the one hand to specify the key to general ability, as when in 1903 he identified attention as the key (Binet, 1903), but on the other hand being convinced by 1908 of the "multiplicity and complexity of mental functions" (Binet & Simon, 1908). His concluding stance was a compromise between specific and general factors. Although attributing great powers to specific knowledge, Binet identified four general factors as common to all intellective activities. "Comprehension, invention, direction and criticism – intelligence is constrained in these four words" (Binet, 1911, p. 118). Three of Binet's four general factors, "direction and persistence of thought, autocriticism, and invention," are thus very similar to current metacognitive factors or metacomponents of intelligence (Brown, 1974, 1978; Brown & Campione, 1981; Sternberg, chapter 1 in this volume). Note particularly the concepts of direction and autocriticism. In describing the characteristic learning mode of the retarded child, Binet (1911) claims, "The child is unreflective and inconstant; he forgets what he is doing . . . . he lets himself be carried away by fantasy and caprice . . . . he lacks direction" (pp. 119–120). Similarly on autocriticism: "The power of criticism is as limited as the rest . . . . *he does not know that he does not understand*. The whys with which his curiosity hounds us are scarcely embarrassing, for he will be contented naively with the most absurd becauses" (p. 122; italics added).

Following his description of inadequate intellectual functioning in retarded children, Binet discusses his prescription for "mental orthopedics" for the retarded, also "useful for normal children" (Binet, 1911, pp. 150–161). His training procedures, which stress self-awareness and autocritical skills, are fascinating reading for contemporary psychologists interested in cognitive skills training. Binet obviously believed in general factors and, furthermore, believed that they could be taught.

Spearman (1904, 1923, 1927) had less internal conflict than Binet in deciding in favor of general factors. Although he does formally accord influences to specific, or *s*, factors, his heart lies with his general factor, the infamous *g*. In the ensuing arguments, prompted mainly by measurement issues with respect to *s* and *g*, we have tended to lose sight of Spearman's definition of *g*. Interestingly, Spearman's general factors are not unlike Binet's and even more like constructs of contemporary theories of metacognition. The three principal components of *g* were (a) educing relations, (b) educing correlates, and (c) self-recognition, or the "apprehension of one's own experience." Spearman claims that people have "more or less" the power to observe what goes on in their own minds. "A person cannot only feel, but also know that he can feel; not only strive, but know that he strives; not only know, but *know that he knows*" (Spearman, 1923, p. 342; italics added). Similarly: "Any active knowing process, no less than any passive feeling one, belongs to lived experience, so that it can equally well evoke an awareness of its own occurrence and character . . . . I can know, not only *that* I know, but also *what* I know" (Spearman, 1923, p. 52). Spearman does not claim scientific priority with such notions of metacognition. Indeed, he observes:

Such a cognizing of cognition itself was already announced by Plato. Aristotle likewise posited a separate power whereby, over and above actually seeing and hearing, the psyche becomes aware of doing so. Later authors, as Strato, Galen, Alexander of Aphrodisias, and in particular Plotinus, amplified the doctrine, designating the processes of cognizing one's own cognition by several specific names. Much later, especial stress was laid on this power of "reflection," as it was now called by Locke. [Spearman, 1923, pp. 52–53]

Spearman did, however, contribute the identification of such metacognitive elements as essential elements of *g*, agreeing with Binet that self-awareness and autocritical skills are fundamental learning processes.

The Europeans Binet and Spearman both seemed satisfied with a composite model of intelligence, allowing specific factors but placing heavy emphasis on general factors of intelligence. In contrast, the Americans Thorndike and Cattell were avid adherents of the specific abilities pole, dismissing Binet's "unitary concept of mind" and suggesting that "intelligences" consist of large numbers of relatively independent traits (Thorndike, 1904). The resultant influence of the Thorndikian position in American psychology has been well documented (Sternberg, 1977; Tuddenham, 1962).

Group factors theories such as Thurstone's (1938) primary mental abilities were seen in the thirties as the middle ground between the positions championed by Spearman and Thorndike for so many years. This was at best an uneasy compromise, for the controversy scarcely abated. Were *g* factors merely descriptions of related abilities (Burt, 1940) or essential basic controlling elements? Does development proceed from general factors that differentiate over time into increasingly more specific lower-order processes? Alternatively, are specific abilities primary and general factors derived from them via positive transfer effects (Ferguson, 1954, 1956)? The arguments for specific to the general, general to the specific, specific only, and general only are still with us (Newell, 1979).

Newell (1979) claims that although the basic dichotomy remains unresolved, considerable advances have taken place in our understanding, despite the apparent lack of resolution. Newell's (1979) taxonomy of existing positions on the specific–general issue is particularly illuminating; we will consider a pertinent subset. Newell distinguishes between four basic positions in the problem-solving field: the big switch, the big memory, weak methods, and weak-to-strong methods. Consider first the *big switch* position; here the knowledge base consists of a large number of specific procedures with a discrimination net (the big switch) for gaining access to them. "Tens of thousands of such procedures form a mosaic that covers the world of all tasks. Each procedure has a small penumbra of generality, so that in total a large area of novel tasks can be accomplished" (Newell, 1979, p. 185). Individual differences within such a theory would presumably be in the number of such procedures and the size of the penumbra of generality as suggested by Brown (1980) and Cole (see LCHC, chapter 11 in this volume). The *big memory* position is the "bare facts in memory" stance, in which a web of facts is laid down in some organized fashion. The problem of access structure is acute for such positions, and Newell obviously prefers the big switch version.

The second distinction made by Newell is between a weak methods only and a weak-to-strong-methods approach. By *weak methods*, Newell means general strategies, termed *weak* because they trade generality for power. Such approaches lean heavily on the general problem-solving methods of AI, such as the ubiquitous means–ends analyses but also including: generate and test, heuristic search, subgoal decomposition, match, hypothesize and match, constraint satisfaction, and so forth. *Weak-to-strong* positions are similar to big switch positions in that there exists an expanding cone of methods of ever greater specificity and power. At the base of the cone are the multitudes of specific expert procedures with their penumbra of generality. Still, in addition, at the apex of the cone, the "tip of the iceberg," are the general ways of responding to tasks that are quite different from any for which the problem solver could have developed expert procedures.[6]

Considering the positions along the specific–general pole, the big switch and big memory theories adhere to the specific abilities pole, and the weak methods position is at the other end. We prefer the weak-to-strong-method stance (Brown, 1980;

Brown & Campione, 1981), a compromise approach that permits both specific and general factors to coexist but places severe limits on the generality of the general.

How does this generality arise? Newell claims that mapping, planning, learning, and discipline are involved in the genesis of generality, processes not unlike Spearman's educing relations and correlates and self-recognition and Binet's autocritical skills, direction and persistence and invention. Consider mapping, the process of transforming the novel into the familiar via analogy and metaphor. Candidates for solution of any new task are preexisting methods, so that "the problem solver always has a repertoire of methods available; in the limit there never exists 'general methods' because one always analogizes from some concrete method" (Newell, 1979, p. 187). Such a position equates a great deal of what we call learning with transfer, a point to which we will return. Thus, according to Newell, "generality is located not in the ability to perform but in the ability to learn. In a hard problem, the problem solver must actually learn the pieces out of which a solution is to be fashioned. Search becomes not so much to solve a problem as to learn about the domain" (Newell, 1979, p. 187).

The weak-to-strong-method sequence via mapping and learning shares many common features with the functional use theory of LCHC (this volume) and our own developmental position (Brown, 1980). Changing back weak-to-strong to specific and general, and reversing the implied sequence, there seems to be considerable consensus. The knowledge base consists of a large number of specific rules with their own small penumbra of generality. Generality is extended via the mapping procedures of analogy and metaphor, which to some extent relieves the learner from the severe constraints of contextual binding, or "welding" (Brown, 1974, 1980). Such extended generality results in the genesis of general strategies suitable for wider domains (problem solving, academic tasks, test taking, etc.), but there are still strong limits to this generality, as admirably demonstrated in the functional use theory put forward by LCHC (chapter 11 in this volume). We would add that the extent of generality, the efficiency of mapping, or the efficiency of general rule use are diagnostic of intelligent behavior.

Development is the process of going from the specific context-bound to the general context-free. Note, however, Gardner's (1978) warning that truly general, context-free, stable laws may be a chimera, an idealized end point; blatant failure to recognize problem isomorphs occurs in adults as well as children (Simon & Hayes, 1976; Gick & Holyoak, Note 3 [1980]). Knowledge in some sense must always be context-bound. But contextual binding permits of degrees; generalization and flexibility are not all-or-none phenomena but continua. It is the range of applicability of any particular process by any particular learner that forms the diagnosis of expertise or cognitive maturity. The less mature, less experienced, less intelligent suffer from a greater degree of contextual binding, but even the expert is bound by contextual constraint to some degree. [Brown, 1982a]

Such a theory accords special status to transfer functions far more general than those usually dealt with in transfer-of-training discussions. Indeed, it leads us to a position very similar to that put forth by McGeoch and Irion (1952), Hebb (1949), and Ferguson (1954), that later learning is heavily loaded with transfer effects (of early learning we know little and understand less; Brown, 1980). All later learning occurs within the context of experience:

After small amounts of learning early in the life of the individual, every instance of learning is a function of the already existent learned organization of the subject; that is, all learning is influenced by transfer. . . . Where the subject "sees into" the fundamental relations of a problem, or has "insight," transfer seems to be a major contributing condition. It is, likewise, a basic factor in originality, the original or creative person having, among other things, *unusual sensitivity to the applicability of the already known to new problem situations.* [McGeoch & Irion, 1952, pp. 346–347; italics added]

The problem with such theories is that like current schema theories of learning, with which they share many features, learning is essentially assimilative. A complete learning theory must accommodate accommodation (Brown, 1979, 1980), as noted by Hebb:

If the learning we know and can study, in the mature animal, is heavily loaded with transfer effects, what are the properties of the original learning from which those effects came? How can it be possible even to consider making a theory of learning in general from the data of maturity only? There must be a serious risk that what seems to be learning is really half transfer. We cannot assume that we know what learning transfers and what does not: for our knowledge of the extent of transfer is also derived from behavior at maturity. [Hebb, 1949, p. 110]

We agree with Hebb's call for a developmental and comparative approach to learning. To delineate a transfer theory of intelligence fully, one must consider extent of transfer (McGeoch & Irion, 1952), the special nature of early learning (Brown, 1980; Hebb, 1949), and the accommodation process (Brown, 1979, 1980). Our hunch that the mapping procedures of analogy and metaphor (Newell, 1979) are the key, that the intelligent deliberately seek relationships and activate prior knowledge, and that these activities are fostered by mediated learning will be examined in the next section.

The astute reader who remains astute after this somewhat lengthy preamble will note that we still have not specified what we mean by *domain*. Nevertheless, we hope that at least we have made clear that cognitive theories of learning must eventually incorporate a theory of domain similarity if they are to avoid a posteriori (not to mention ad hoc) reasoning concerning transfer.

LEARNING TO LEARN

We turn now to our last instance of old theories in new bottles, learning to learn. Again the concept of deutero-learning is an old one. In his fascinating book, *Les idées modernes sur les enfants,* intended as a practical aid for parents and teachers, Binet (1911) laid heavy emphasis on methods of inculcating "learning how to learn" and "learning by doing" procedures, noting his debt to Rousseau, Spencer, Dewey, Hall, LeBon, and Froebel in so doing. Similarly, the concept was quite popular in the 1921 *Journal of Educational Psychology* Symposium on Intelligence and Its Measurement (Dearborn, 1921), even among those who would later retreat from the position (Woodrow, 1921).

The theory became unpopular during the rule of panassociationism learning theories, primarily because of the emphasis placed on identical elements theories of specific transfer across physical domains. It was revived by the neobehaviorists in the forties because of their concern with nonspecific transfer. Harlow's (1949, 1959) classic work on learning-set formation is the most elegant instantiation of the neobehaviorists' interest in nonspecific transfer – nonspecific because the physical aspects of the stimulus environment change over trials, but the underlying solution (Win-stay, Lose-shift) is general.

The work of Harlow, and of others who followed, provided impressive evidence that rate of learning-set formation was a sensitive index of cross-species comparisons (Harlow, 1953) and indeed of individual differences in children (Harter, 1965, but cf. Kappauf, 1973). The learning-set procedure was not sensitive to individual differences when the problem sets were too simple, that is, one-trial learning followed the acquisition of the first problem. Binet (Binet & Simon, 1908) made the cogent point that differences between retarded and normal children will only be revealed on tasks of sufficient complexity, a theme reiterated by Zeaman and House (1967) and Brown, Campione, and Day (1981). Despite some shortcomings, the learning-set literature was an important and lasting contribution of neobehaviorists (Harlow, 1959; Zeaman & House, 1963).

With the current liberalization and rehabilitation of the term *learning* (Brown, 1980; Bransford et al., 1981), there is also a concomitant revival of the learning-to-learn concept in a guise more similar to the original conceptions of Binet. The difference in "modern" instantiations is the same as in "modern" theories of transfer of training – current approaches place heavy emphasis on subjective similarity and on deliberate accessing of prior knowledge. The current emphasis is on learning to learn via awareness. Awareness was not a favorite concern of neobehaviorists, not surprisingly, as the term is not even one of cryptophenomenology (Tolman, 1959).

Harlow developed an elegant technology for structuring the learning environment so that learning sets would be formed. As noted by LCHC (chapter 11 in this volume), systematic structuring of the environment is often a feature of traditional apprenticeship systems. Novices are guided to mastery by experts who structure tasks in an easy-to-hard sequence. Novices rarely engage in tasks where they might fail, as the sequence is carefully calibrated to fit their level of competence.

Procedures of errorless learning are very successful at promoting competence on a specific task, and indeed they have been refined into elegant technologies for engineering learning by Skinnerians. For example, Touchette (1968) taught severely retarded subjects a very difficult (for them) discrimination task by providing cues during the initial trials that explicitly signaled the solution. The crutch was gradually faded out in such a way that errorless learning was achieved. We do not doubt that such procedures are extremely effective. We do, however, question whether errorless learning is the best means of promoting transfer.

Consider apprenticeship training. The interaction of teacher and student is often one to one, and the teacher, an expert, is more interested in directly transmitting the essential information or skills to the learner than in engaging the learner in a Socratic dialogue. In this situation, the expert monitors the learner's performance and can notice and correct any misunderstandings without there ever being any need for the learner to become aware that he has failed to understand. Formal schooling is assumed to be quite different, in that the aim is to inculcate general skills of flexible thinking that we include under the heading of metacognition; for it is a common stricture that schools should teach children how to think rather than deluge them with specific content that may soon become outdated. One way in which schooling may implicitly foster the ability to learn new information and solve novel problems is through instilling an awareness of whether information being presented is understood. If we "know we don't know," then this knowledge can in turn lead to self-questioning routines such as "What do I know that might help me figure it out?" "What specifically do I not understand?" "Where can I go to find out?" In schools, instruction is carried out in groups, and it is essential that students learn to monitor their own comprehension, because the teacher in a large classroom cannot perform this function for them. To receive assistance the students must realize that they need it and must know how to request it. Generally, after a few years of formal education, students are asked to acquire much of their information from books. Learning through reading makes it even more crucial that students be able to monitor their comprehension, because there is no chance that a book will notice that the student has failed to understand (Baker & Brown, in press-a; Brown, Campione, & Day, 1981; Brown & French, 1979a).

Errorless learning, where another makes the executive decisions, may not be an appropriate procedure for promoting insightful learning, for it is in response to errors, overgeneralizations, and so forth that we change our understanding. Inappropriate application of rules leads to conflicts that can induce a modification of the specific rule into a more powerful hypothesis accounting for a wider range of phenomena, hence transfer. The notion that conflict induces change is basic to dialectic theories (Wozniak, 1975; Youniss, 1974) as well as to Piagetian models (Inhelder, Sinclair, & Bovet, 1974; Smedslund, 1966). A serviceable hypothesis is maintained until a counterexample, an invidious generalization, or an incompatible outcome ensues. Conflict generated by such inconsistencies induces the formulation of a more powerful rule to account for a greater range of specific experiences – sometimes!

Contemporary approaches to the learning-to-learn theory are concerned with mechanisms that foster just such insight, that is, induce learners to become aware of their own cognitive processes while learning (Bransford et al., 1981; Brown, 1980; Brown, Campione, & Day, 1981; Brown et al., in press). The training mechanisms favored are those of mediated learning, that is, learning via the mediation of a helpful expert who provides hints, clues, counterexamples, and so forth. This is the essence of both the Feuerstein (1980) diagnostic and training programs and the very similar programs based on Vygotsky's theory of a zone of proximal development (Brown & French, 1979b). Although the supportive other in the laboratory is usually the experimenter, these interactive learning experiences are intended to mimic real-life learning. Mothers (Wertsch, 1978, in press), teachers (Schallert & Kleiman, 1979), and clinicians (Feuerstein, 1980) all function as the supportive other, the agent of change responsible for structuring the child's environment in such a way that he or she will experience a judicious mix of compatible and conflicting experiences. Note also that inadequate mediated learning, either mother–child or teacher–pupil, has been implicated as a potential cause of the poor academic performance of the culturally deprived (Brown, 1977, 1978, 1980; Brown & Ferrara, in press; Budoff, 1974; Feuerstein, 1969; see section 8.4). Initially the supportive other acts as the interrogator, leading the child to more powerful rules and generalizations. The interrogative, regulatory role, however, becomes internalized in the process of development, and children become able to fulfill some of these functions for themselves via self-regulation and self-interrogation. Mature thinkers are those who provide conflict trials for themselves, practice thought experiments, question their own basic assumptions, provide counterexamples to their own rules, and so forth. In short, although much thinking and learning may remain a social activity (Brown & French, 1979b; Cole, Hood, & McDermott, 1978), through the process of internalization, mature reasoners become capable of providing the supportive other role for themselves.

Development, then, is the gradual internalization of regulatory skills first experienced by the child in social settings (Vygotsky, 1978). Via repeated experience with experts who criticize, evaluate, and extend the limits of his or her experience, the child develops skills of self-regulation. The development of a battery of such auto-critical skills (Binet, 1911) is essential for intelligent function.

SUMMARY

We argued that the research with retarded children reviewed in sections 8.3 and 8.4 reinforces the view that speed or efficiency of learning and breadth of transfer are central to any notion of intelligence. We also contended that these ideas, which featured prominently in early theories of intelligence, decreased in popularity during the behaviorist period of American psychology. Our speculations were that this trend was due in part to the kinds of learning theories that generated the research literature, along with the types of tasks that were used to assess learning. Whether that reasoning is correct or not, it is the case that more recent work has provided clearer evidence for the link between learning–transfer and intelligence.

We believe that much of the information upon which a revised interest in learning and transfer performance has been based followed from work with retarded children, particularly research employing instructional methodologies. Sophisticated adult performers employ learning strategies flexibly and well, and the adult cognitive psychology literature concerned with intelligence has been concerned in good part with the efficiency with which basic components may be carried out (cf. Hunt, 1978; Sternberg, 1977). Although these factors are clearly important, they are not the whole story, and useful supplemental information has been gained by looking at the sources of poor learners' problems. The resultant emphasis on use of strategies has led to a spate of studies documenting (a) the relative lack of spontaneous strategy use by the retarded and (b) failures on their part to show any signs of transfer following strategy instruction. The reliability and generality of these findings has led to a reaffirmation of the importance of learning and transfer in the absence of complete instruction as essential components of intelligence.

The most prominent features of theory and research (in retardation and elsewhere) that have succeeded in relating learning to intelligence are the conception of the learner as an active organism, a view of learning that emphasizes response to guided instruction and attempts to specify some of the qualitative differences that appear to characterize efficient versus inefficient performers. It is not only the efficiency with which actions are carried out but also the way in which component actions are selected, sequenced, and modified. In this context, we emphasized the role of somewhat general executive control skills, including monitoring, checking, seeking relations, and so forth. Efficient learners employ such skills both to bring to bear relevant prior knowledge to facilitate learning and to prepare for transfer (cf. Bransford's, 1979, notion of transfer-appropriate processing). When confronted with new problems, they employ general search and problem-solving strategies that allow access to previously acquired information. At the same time, when new routines are being acquired, there are attempts to understand why a certain routine works in the given situation, attempts that form the basis for subsequent transfer of that routine. The flexibility with which these general executive–metacognitive skills are carried out characterizes the intelligent performer.

Beyond the experimental retardation literature, we also considered the clinical–educational literature in that area, along with some research in the fields of artificial intelligence, instructional psychology, cognitive ethology, and developmental psychology. Our conclusions were that in each of these areas, there is agreement that the more intelligent, the more phylogenetically advanced, or the more successful learner is the one who can manipulate his or her knowledge to achieve multiple access, or transfer. There also appears to be some consensus that the skills involved here are the general executive ones we emphasized in our treatment of the experimental retardation literature. Thus converging lines of evidence implicate learning and transfer mechanisms in general and executive decision making more specifically as central to views of intelligence.

8.6.   SUGGESTIONS FOR FUTURE RESEARCH

In this section, we will indicate some specific questions and areas of inquiry in which we believe further research is both necessary and likely to lead to advances in the development of intelligence theory and to more practical payoffs. Our choices here are of course influenced by our view of the current state of theory. Our emphasis has been on the importance of learning–transfer processes, and the research emphasis suggested here is motivated by an attempt to refine those analyses or to indicate ways in which they are lacking. In the treatment, we will emphasize one general methodological tool, the case study approach, along with a set of more theoretical, or process-oriented, questions.

CASE STUDY APPROACHES

A theory of intelligence must be a theory of individual differences. In by far the greater part of the experimental literature, inferences about individual differences are made from group studies. Although this approach is in many cases the option of choice and has certainly been fruitful, it does not necessarily lead to rich descriptions of individuals. Further, as we shall argue below, it does not allow the kind of detailed analysis of a number of important hypotheses that we think is essential. We will be more specific in this regard in ensuing sections, but here we will simply indicate one general consideration. In the retardation area, and even more in the LD literature, there has been a tendency to treat subjects within groups as relatively homogeneous. In part, this tendency occurs because we typically have little information about individuals that can be used to "sort" them more accurately. Our suggestion is that typical large-scale independent-groups designs can be supplemented by in-depth analyses, or case studies, of relatively small numbers of subjects. In many cases, we will be better off having a large amount of data on relatively few subjects than having fewer data on a larger N. If such case studies were done, it would be possible to make more accurate diagnoses of the problem(s) of individual subjects, a necessary first step for tests of a number of specific hypotheses.

COMPARATIVE RESEARCH

If we agree that *intelligence* is a relative term, then comparisons involving performers of varying proficiency are essential. In many cases we do not have the data necessary to justify strong claims about differences between retarded and non-retarded children. For example, it would be desirable to have a number of studies comparing these groups directly in terms of the amount of instruction necessary to achieve some degree of learning or transfer or in terms of their performance in nonstrategic tasks. Most frequently, our conclusions are based on cross-experiment comparisons or upon assumptions about how well nonretarded children would have done had they been included in the experiment. We believe that extant analyses have pinpointed a number of important components of intelligence; we would simply hope that future research would include more direct comparisons of groups of subjects differing in intellectual ability.

A special case – the learning disabled

Although comparisons of retarded and nonretarded children are of clear interest, we believe more interesting or specific tests of theory can come from comparisons of retarded and LD children. According to conventional wisdom frequently supported by clinical observations, LD children represent a group that is intermediate between retarded and nonretarded groups. That is, LD children are assumed to be of normal, or above normal, intelligence but suffer from *specific* clusters of learning problems that are revealed both in diagnostic patterns of subitem difficulty on standardized IQ tests (digit span, encoding, symbol substitution, etc.) and in their relative difficulty in coping with some but not all of the main academic pursuits: reading, writing, spelling, and calculating. The common assumption is that specific identifiable clusters of abilities are involved in the learning impairment. Beyond this idea there is considerable disagreement. Some authorities prefer many such clusters, for example, "if one were to evaluate 100 children with this condition [LD], he or she might find 30 or 40 different profiles of strengths and disabilities" (Silver, 1978). Other authorities prefer dichotomous clusters, for example, dyseidetic dyslexia (visual problems such as visual perception, visual integration, visual memory, fine motor, and/or visual motor impairment) versus dysphonetic dyslexia (auditory problems such as auditory perception, auditory integration, auditory memory, and language output disorders). Taking what might not be regarded as the strongest possible stand on this issue, Public Law 94-142 provides a definition generous enough to cover most eventualities when it describes LD as "a disorder in one or more of the basic psychological processes involved in understanding or using language, spoken or written, which may manifest itself in an imperfect ability to listen, think, speak, read, write, spell, or do mathematical calculation."

In principle, contrasts among sets of these diagnostic categories should permit more refined tests of intelligence theories. We can adopt the not exactly controversial view that performance on a variety of tasks involves both general and specific skills and that the more general ones are the prime indicants of intelligence. The specific components, of course, vary from task to task. If these two statements are true, we should be able to show that LD children suffer from specific areas of weakness and that these areas vary with the particular form of the learning disability. Further, when tested in hospitable circumstances for the more general skills (presumed to be the hallmark of intelligence), they should perform at a normal level. For example, if we could arrange situations where their specific problem(s) were not important, their learning–transfer performance should match that of unimpaired learners. Such findings, if obtainable, would reinforce our overall views of intelligence, provide convergent evidence for identifying the major components of intelligence, and feed into the development of theories dealing with the more specified domains in which the various LD children experience problems (recall the Tallal research mentioned in section 8.3). In this way, we regard LD research as extremely important for the achievement of the goal of developing a theory of intelligence.

Unfortunately, we were, for a number of reasons, not very successful in progressing toward this goal. The main reason is that, as shown in recent reviews of the psychometric, clinical, and academic performance literatures, conventional distinctions such as those indicated above are far from easy to instantiate in actual differential diagnosis. Children in LD programs can vary considerably. In a recent survey of the LD population in a large midwestern city, we found four distinct patterns of test scores. A sizable subgroup had both performance and verbal scores at or below 80 (i.e., comparable to those of an EMR sample). An even larger group showed no interesting diagnostic pattern in their IQ performance (i.e., both verbal and performance scores of about 100 and no interesting subitem problems). The remaining two groups were in the low normal range for composite score but showed at least a 15-point discrepancy between verbal and performance subscores. Interestingly, almost as many children had verbal scores higher than performance scores as vice versa, although one stereotype of LD implicates impaired verbal performance only. Similarly, although clinical research has been quite successful at identifying many forms (clusters) of LD, the state of the art is not such that there are agreed-upon standards about which specific factors at which degree of intensity warrant a diagnosis of LD (Lynn, Gluckin, & Kripke, 1979):

Indeed, of the hydraheaded conditions that are variously referred to not only as specific learning disabilities but also as perceptual handicaps, brain injuries, minimal brain damage, cerebral dysfunctions, developmental aphasia, dyscalculia, dysgraphia and dyslexia of the (to name a few) genetic, environmental, developmental, dysmetric, dysphonetic and dyseidetic varieties, only one thing seems reasonably clear . . . : children with specific learning disabilities can be accurately identified or diagnosed on the basis of a definition that, for all practical purposes, spelled out primarily what the condition is *not*. [Lynn, Gluckin, & Kripke, 1979, p. 9]

Because of the difficulty of finding distinct groups within the LD population, researchers have tended to regard them as a single group and have then compared them with nondisabled control groups. Given the heterogeneity that characterizes the population, it should not be surprising that precise characterizations have not emerged. In fact, an examination of the LD literature results in a description of these children that sounds remarkably like current descriptions of EMR students.

Despite the current problems, we believe comparisons of EMR and LD children can be extremely interesting. Before the comparisons can be useful for theoretical purposes, however, we need accurate descriptions of the subjects involved, that is, we want to be as sure as possible that the LD students do have specific problems. Here the case study approach seems an optimal way to proceed. Detailed analyses of individual subjects would allow us to determine if we in fact have "true" LD and "true" EMR subjects. Only then would it be possible to ask the more specific theoretical questions in which we might be interested.

If one adopts the case study approach to this issue, several major questions arise. The first concerns whether the analytic tools we as psychologists have developed for assessing basic intellective processes, such as those described in section 8.3, can be used to form the basis for a classification of children into different subgroups. Can we evaluate children in terms of their speed of processing, their tendency to be strategic, their ability to profit from instruction, and so forth and produce "cognitive profiles" that supplement existing clinical descriptions? If not, we need at least to wonder why that is the case.

Next, if the first phase of this effort is successful and we are able to identify sets of children with fairly specific problems, we can proceed to involve those children in research designed to ask further theoretical questions. As one example, suppose we had a group of children whose sole problems seemed to stem from limitations in the use of working memory. Then, if they were assessed in terms of general intellectual skills, they should perform well whenever working-memory efficiency was not crucial. In a different vein, observing their performance in a number of tasks could facilitate the development of appropriate task analyses. Suppose that we were able to show that a group of children had only working-memory problems and that they did perform extremely well in a number of situations that did not involve working-memory factors. Suppose, further, that in another task there was some question about the extent to which working-memory limitations were of particular importance. The children could be run on that task and their performance level could be used as one method of assessing the importance of working-memory limitations.

In summary, comparisons of retarded and LD children can serve our goals in a number of ways. First, they provide a test of general cognitive theory. Given that LD children do exist, our theories should be able to serve as the basis for a description of them while distinguishing them from children with either no learning problems or more severe learning problems. Second, the EMR–LD comparison can make possible more specific tests of our intelligence theories. Finally, the LD groups can play an important role in contributing to the development of more specific task analyses.

ANALYSES OF LEARNING–TRANSFER

As implied by our emphasis on the importance of learning and transfer for theories of intelligence, we would like to see additional analyses of their subcomponents. One avenue would include devoting more attention to the *qualitative* differences in the activities of good versus poor performers that underlie more rapid learning and more flexible transfer. To illustrate, one factor that is assumed to be involved in successful problem solving is analogical reasoning, the ability to retrieve similar problems that have occurred previously and then either to borrow directly the solution plan from that problem or to use the solution as a starting point upon which to build an answer to the current problem (cf. Gick & Holyoak, 1980). An understanding of the components of such activities would have consequences for both theory and remediation. Examples would include the general class of self-interrogation procedures that efficient learners employ, presumably similar to the kinds of questions employed by effective Socratic teachers (Collins & Stevens, in press). These activities, such as regarding problems as instances of general classes, searching for similarities, generating other examples and counterexamples, and so forth, can both lead to retrieval of previously encountered problem isomorphs and set the stage for retrieval of the "new" problem on subsequent occasions. That is, appropriate questioning during attempts at problem solving may both facilitate solution of the current problem and help prepare the learner to deal with upcoming ones.

We also believe more detailed analyses of the dynamic learning assessment devices is in order. Claims by Budoff, Feuerstein, and Vygotsky that the data generated via these procedures provide valuable supplements to static IQ tests, and that such supplements are particularly important for poor IQ performers, are important both practically and theoretically. Theoretically, these results could inform our theories of intelligence and constrain our theories of learning. Practically, they may allow more refined diagnoses of learning problems and may lead to suggestions regarding the design of remedial instructional programs. A considerable effort in this area would seem indicated.

As a final suggestion here, it would be of real interest to investigate the performance of retarded and nonretarded children in domains where they have equal, or nearly equal, knowledge. In section 8.3 we discussed the notion that many of the "strategy" differences that have been reported are better regarded as manifestations of differences in knowledge (cf. Chi, 1981; Siegler & Richards, chapter 14 in this volume). Most simply stated, individuals differ not in some overall propensity to be strategic but in the amount of relevant knowledge they have; the more knowledgeable one is within a domain, the more strategic he or she will appear. The best test of this argument would involve a comparison of individuals of differing ability but equated for knowledge.

Although such an experiment may be difficult to perform, it is not impossible. There are retarded children who know a great deal about selected topics: sports, music, television programs, and so forth. In addition, there are methods for assessing amount and organization of knowledge: semantic priming, PI release, constructed semantic networks, and others. It thus seems possible both to find subjects of differing abilities who are equated for knowledge within some domain and to employ objective, theoretically based measures of that knowledge. Comparisons involving such subjects would be relevant to many of the major issues we have discussed, such as the importance of access problems to theories of intelligence and the existence of general problem-solving skills.

EXTENSIONS TO YOUNGER CHILDREN

Of particular importance, we would like to see more attention devoted to early cognitive development and to attempts aimed at identifying early indicants of subsequent learning problems. This is true for both theoretical and practical reasons. Practically, Public Law 94-142 mandates special education for all children who are going to experience problems in school. Typically, that instruction is to begin within the first 3 years of life. The problem is that we have been unable to develop good predictive measures for use with young children. The development of useful screening devices would obviously have considerable importance.

Under some circumstances, success in this area would be difficult, if not impossible. It could be the case that current tests administered early in life do not correlate well with later test scores because intelligence is qualitatively different at varying points in development. Rank orderings within one type simply may not be related to orderings later. A more interesting possibility is that there is continuity in the components of intelligence but that the items appearing on the different tests are not assessing the same processes, not a surprising eventuality, given that there is little theoretical rationale underlying the test construction. If this were true, more accurate predictions could be obtained if there were available a better theory of intelligence, along with test items that provide fairly direct assessments of the theoretically determined target processes. Within the framework outlined in section 8.5, we might expect that more direct measures of learning and transfer would represent one way to proceed. An alternative, or supplementary, proposal might be that efficiency, or speed-of-processing, measures would be appropriate. In any event, if a successful theoretically based screening device could be developed, it would both help solve the important practical problem and contribute significantly to theories of intelligence and cognitive development. For example, if our views are correct, we would expect estimates of speed of learning and breadth of transfer derived from dynamic assessment procedures to provide early indicants of individual differences in intelligence.

EXTENSIONS TO EVERYDAY INTELLIGENCE

Our discussion has been concerned with academically marginal children and theories of academic intelligence. As we indicated in section 8.1, there may be different kinds of intelligence, each requiring a different theory. As one example, it may be argued that everyday intelligence is different in kind from academic intelligence. Research with retarded children would seem relevant to such an assertion. If it were true, it would seem to suggest that many EMR children would lose their "special" status when they leave the school environment, that is, the "6-hour retardate" syndrome. Assessments of retarded individuals in nonschool settings would provide an interesting test of the separability of everyday and academic intelligence.

Although the relevance of research with the retarded seems clear in this context, the interpretation of that research requires a specification and analysis of the kinds of nonschool settings that one would observe. (Presumably, everyday intelligence refers to the ability to adapt to a set of everyday tasks and demands – the utility of the theory would be assessed in part by the variety of tasks it was able to subsume.) For example, retarded individuals might be observed in on-the-job settings and in fairly standard social situations. On the basis of their actions, it might be impossible for a trained observer to identify any ways in which they differed from academically more capable peers. Does such a finding tell us something about the academic–everyday intelligence contrast, or does it indicate that environmental factors are operating in a way to minimize the need for intelligence? Many of the typical occurrences of everyday life may be heavily scripted. Retarded individuals may take longer to learn the necessary scripts, but once they have done so, they may be able to avoid future problems within a given area. Only when new problems are encountered would intelligence-related differences become apparent. That is, the skills of everyday intelligence may be very similar to those of academic intelligence. Any school–nonschool difference may reside in the fact that the frequency of "real" problems is lower in everyday settings than in school settings. When such problems do occur in everyday settings, retarded individuals may still experience considerable difficulties. As Schank (1980) has noted: "People who rely upon scripts most heavily will only see what they have seen before. . . . Such a system will cope very well in worlds with which it is intimately familiar and will fall apart when thrown into an entirely new situation. So the least-intelligent inferencing system is one that relies exclusively on scripts" (p. 8).

Keeping this complexity in mind, research involving retarded individuals in everyday settings would provide information about the separability of academic and everyday intelligence and/or about the structure of many everyday activities.

DOES INTELLIGENCE INCREASE WITH AGE?

As a final comment, we would like to indicate one area where there appears to be less agreement among theorists than might be expected. It is commonly assumed that intelligence increases with age (cf. Siegler & Richards, chapter 14 in this volume; Sternberg, 1980, also chapter 1 in this volume). It is, however, possible to take the opposite view, that intelligence does not increase with age. We would like to speculate briefly about some of the assumptions and views that might underlie this difference.

One fact is clear. Performance on schoollike and intelligence tests undergoes dramatic increases with age. As children age, they answer more items correctly; however, this progress may simply reflect the fact that children come to know more about the world around them. Intelligence tests assess this knowledge, which can be presumed to be an indirect measure of learning ability. Saying that older children are brighter than younger children seems to equate knowledge with intelligence and ignorance with stupidity (see Brown & Campione, in press, for a discussion). As an example, consider a 12-year-old with an IQ of 80 and a 4-year-old with an IQ of 120. Who is more intelligent? The older child may know more and would answer more items correctly on an intelligence test, but the younger child's performance relative to his age group is better; we can also predict with some confidence that by the time that child reaches 12, barring cerebral insult, he or she will score better than the older child did at 12.

We would propose that the two conclusions regarding the age–intelligence relation follow from the two kinds of theory we referred to in section 8.1. Theory 1, which can be regarded as an absolute theory, sees intelligence as the efficient operation of a set of skills and processes. A theory of this type would regard intelligence as the ability to deal effectively with academic tasks. As individuals age in our society, they become more proficient at a larger set of relevant tasks; they acquire more skills; they carry them out more efficiently; they approach some idealized final state; they become more intelligent. Such theories deal happily with ontogenetic improvements in academic performance but seem silent on some important aspects of individual differences, notably the relative constancy of the IQ. Within these theories, if intelligence is increasing ontogenetically, there is a need to specify the factors that constrain this growth in such a way as to maintain an individual's rank ordering over time.

A Theory 2 approach takes the stance that intelligence is a relative term; intelligence is the set of processes that together account for an individual's relative ability to excel in academic domains. For such theories one salient feature of IQ scores is that, although there are some clear exceptions (cf. Siegler & Richards, chapter 14 in this volume), they tend to remain fairly constant for extended periods of time (if this were not true, there would be less interest in, and controversy over, intelligence testing). Relative theories have no problems accounting for this constancy – they merely state it as a fact – but do in addition need to explain the underlying stable factors that can result in performance increases. Positing a theory that the ability to learn, or to operate upon available information, is stable over time and results in cumulative performance increases or decreases is at least testable; further, it does suggest broad areas of remediation. Tentatively, the theory would suggest that as one matures, increased resources become available, via learning, with more accruing to more efficient learners. As the more capable learners can operate on this information more efficiently to generate and acquire more knowledge, they continue to maintain their advantage and simultaneously become capable of dealing with a wider and wider variety of problem situations. By this view, estimates of learning rate should indicate that our younger child with high intelligence would be able to learn more quickly within a new domain than an older but duller child. Whether this turns out to be a reasonable view or not, our main point remains the same. Theorists should be sensitive to the potential differences and, to facilitate communication, should be explicit about their underlying assumptions.

NOTES

Preparation of this manuscript and portions of the research reported therein have been supported by PHS Grants HD-05951, HD-06864, and HD-00111 from the National Institute of Child Health and Human Development.
1 The reader might wonder why we restrict our attention to children. The answer is that there is very little research on individuals who have school-related problems after they leave school. The research that is available is certainly important to our conceptions of intelligence (e.g., Edgerton, 1967), and we will return to this point in section 8.6.
2 In this discussion and those that follow, we emphasize the importance of research with slow-learning children. This stress is due to the fact that we will be concerned here primarily with problem learners. It is obvious that a similar argument could be made for the relevance of research with the gifted. We would certainly agree with any such argument and believe that a complete theory of intelligence requires data on the gifted. To simplify the discussion and make it more directly relevant to the literature we will review, however, we couch our discussion here in terms of slow, rather than fast, learners.
3 In a subsequent paper, Ellis (1970) modified his view and took the position that intelligence-related differences in memory performance were primarily due to a deficiency in the use of rehearsal strategies.
4 Whether this is even possible depends in part on the way in which the knowledge base is conceptualized. It may be impossible to talk about knowledge "within some domain" without considering other factors, particularly if the knowledge base can include some domain-independent procedures (see section 8.5).
5 There is, of course, a major problem here. Failures of training need not be diagnostic, i.e., they may simply be due to poor instructional practices, rather than to faulty theory or to faulty learners. Two points can be made. One is that refinements in the form of instruction can be introduced in an attempt to evaluate that hypothesis. The larger the number of attempts that fail, the more certain we become that inadequate instruction is not at fault. The problems would obviously be lessened considerably if we had a theory of instruction available to guide the attempts.
6 As the metaphor of the expanding cone implies, there are degrees of generality. The most general (and weakest) skills might be the monitoring and checking activities that we discussed earlier. One of their functions could be to provide access to, or to indicate a need for, the more specific but still somewhat general skills, such as means–ends analysis and searching for analogies. The results of these activities could in turn be the identification of a specific (and strong) method that makes possible problem solution. The most general activity provides the information that a specific, powerful approach has not been located, and this determination then leads to attempts to employ the intermediate skills to help locate the necessary specific routines. Although we cannot treat the problem here, we would guess that the execution of those intermediate skills would be the most difficult to instruct and therefore of most interest for theories of intelligence.

REFERENCES

Allen, V. L. Children as teachers: Theory and research on tutoring. New York: Academic Press, 1976.
Anderson, R. C. Individual differences and problem solving. In R. M. Gagné (Ed.), Learning and individual differences. Columbus, Ohio: Merrill Books, 1967.
Anzai, Y., & Simon, H. A. The theory of learning by doing. Psychological Review, 1979, 86, 124–140.
Aronson, L. Orientation and jumping in the gobiid fish. Bathygobius Soporator: American Museum Novitates, 1951, 1486, 1–22.

Atkinson, R. C., & Shiffrin, R. M. Human memory: A proposed system and its control processes. In K. W. Spence & J. T. Spence (Eds.), *Advances in the psychology of learning and motivation research and theory* (Vol. 2). New York: Academic Press, 1968.

Baker, L., & Brown, A. L. Cognitive monitoring in reading. In J. Flood (Ed.), *Understanding reading comprehension*. Newark, Del.: International Reading Association, in press. (a)

Baker, L., & Brown, A. L. Metacognition and the reading process. In P. D. Pearson (Ed.), *Handbook of reading research*. New York: Longman, in press. (b)

Baron, J. Intelligence and general strategies. In G. Underwood (Ed.), *Strategies of information processing*. London: Academic Press, 1978.

Becker, J. D. Reflections on the formal description of behavior. In D. G. Bobrow & A. Collins (Eds.), *Representation and understanding: Studies in cognitive science*. New York: Academic Press, 1975.

Belmont, J. M., & Butterfield, E. C. The relation of short-term memory to development and intelligence. In L. P. Lipsitt & H. W. Reese (Eds.), *Advances in child development and behavior* (Vol. 4). New York: Academic Press, 1969.

Belmont, J. M., & Butterfield, E. C. Learning strategies as determinants of memory deficiencies. *Cognitive Psychology*, 1971, 2, 411–420.

Belmont, J. M., & Butterfield, E. C. The instructional approach to developmental cognitive research. In R. V. Kail, Jr., & J. W. Hagen (Eds.), *Perspectives on the development of memory and cognition*. Hillsdale, N.J.: Erlbaum, 1977.

Belmont, J. M., Butterfield, E. C., & Borkowski, J. G. Training retarded people to generalize memorization methods across memory tasks. In M. M. Gruneberg, P. E. Morris, & R. N. Sykes (Eds.), *Practical aspects of memory*. London: Academic Press, 1978.

Belmont, J. M., Butterfield, E. C., & Ferretti, R. P. To secure transfer of training, instruct self-management skills. In D. K. Detterman & R. J. Sternberg (Eds.), *How and how much can intelligence be increased?* Norwood, N.J.: Ablex, in press.

Bilsky, L., & Evans, R. A. The use of associative clustering technique in the study of reading disability: Effects of list organization. *American Journal of Mental Deficiency*, 1970, 74, 771–776.

Bilsky, L., Evans, R. A., & Gilbert, L. Generalization of associative clustering tendencies in mentally retarded adolescents: Effects of novel stimuli. *American Journal of Mental Deficiency*, 1972, 77, 77–84.

Binet, A., *L'étude expérimentale de l'intelligence*. Paris: Schleicher Frères, 1903.

Binet, A. *Les idées modernes sur les enfants*. Paris: Ernest Flammarion, 1911.

Binet, A., & Simon, T. Le développement de l'intelligence des enfants. *L'année psychologique*, 1908, 14, 1–94.

Bloom, B. S. *Human characteristics and school learning*. New York: McGraw-Hill, 1976.

Bobrow, D. G. Dimensions of representation. In D. G. Bobrow & A. Collins (Eds.), *Representation and understanding: Studies in cognitive science*. New York: Academic Press, 1975.

Bobrow, D. G., & Collins, A. (Eds.). *Representation and understanding*. New York: Academic Press, 1975.

Bobrow, D. G., & Norman, D. A. Some principles of memory schemata. In D. G. Bobrow & A. Collins (Eds.), *Representation and understanding: Studies in cognitive science*. New York: Academic Press, 1975.

Boden, M. A. *Artificial intelligence and natural man*. Sussex, England: Harvester Press, 1977.

Borkowski, J. G., & Cavanaugh, J. C. Maintenance and generalization of skills and strategies by the retarded. In N. R. Ellis (Ed.), *Handbook of mental deficiency: Psychological theory and research*. Hillsdale, N.J.: Erlbaum, 1979.

Borkowski, J. G., Levers, S. R., & Gruenenfelder, T. M. Transfer of mediational strategies in children: The role of activity and awareness during strategy acquisition. *Child Development*, 1976, 47, 779–786.

Bos, M. C. Experimental study of productive collaboration. *Acta Psychologica*, 1937, 3, 315–426.

Bousfield, W. A. The occurrence of clustering in the recall of randomly arranged associates. *Journal of General Psychology*, 1953, 49, 229–240.

Brainerd, C. J. The stage question in cognitive development theory. *Behavioral and Brain Sciences*, 1978, 1, 173–181.

Bransford, J. D. *Human cognition: Learning, understanding, and remembering*. Belmont, Calif.: Wadsworth, 1979.

Bransford, J. D., Stein, B. S., Arbitman-Smith, R., & Vye, N. J. Three approaches to improving thinking and learning skills. In Segal, J., Chipman, S., & Glaser, R. (Eds.), *Thinking and learning skills: Relating instruction to basic research*. Hillsdale, N.J.: Erlbaum, in press.

Bransford, J. D., Stein, B. S., Shelton, T. S., & Owings, R. A. Cognition and adaptation: The importance of learning to learn. In J. Harvey (Ed.), *Cognition, social behavior and the environment*. Hillsdale, N.J.: Erlbaum, 1981.

Bray, N. W. Strategy production in the retarded. In N. R. Ellis (Ed.), *Handbook of mental deficiency, psychological theory and research*. Hillsdale, N.J.: Erlbaum, 1979.

Brown, A. L. A rehearsal deficit in retardates' continuous short-term memory: Keeping track of variables that have few or many states. *Psychonomic Science, 1972, 29,* 373–376. (a)

Brown, A. L. Context and recency cues in retardate recognition memory. *American Journal of Mental Deficiency, 1972, 77,* 54–58. (b)

Brown, A. L. Judgments of recency for long sequences of pictures: The absence of a developmental trend. *Journal of Experimental Child Psychology, 1973, 15,* 473–480. (a)

Brown, A. L. Temporal and contextual cues as discriminative attributes in retardates' recognition memory. *Journal of Experimental Psychology, 1973, 98,* 1–13. (b)

Brown, A. L. The role of strategic behavior in retardate memory. In N. R. Ellis (Ed.), *International review of research in mental retardation* (Vol. 7). New York: Academic Press, 1974.

Brown, A. L. The development of memory: knowing about knowing, and knowing how to know. In H. W. Reese (Ed.), *Advances in child development and behavior* (Vol. 10). New York: Academic Press, 1975.

Brown, A. L. Development, schooling and the acquisition of knowing about knowledge. In R. C. Anderson, R. J. Spiro, & W. E. Montague (Eds.), *Schooling and the acquisition of knowledge*. Hillsdale, N.J.: Erlbaum, 1977.

Brown, A. L. Knowing when, where, and how to remember: A problem of metacognition. In R. Glaser (Ed.), *Advances in instructional psychology* (Vol. 1). Hillsdale, N.J.: Erlbaum, 1978.

Brown, A. L. Theories of memory and the problem of development: Activity, growth, and knowledge. In L. S. Cermak & F. I. M. Craik (Eds.), *Levels of processing in human memory*. Hillsdale, N.J.: Erlbaum, 1979.

Brown, A. L. Metacognitive development and reading. In R. J. Spiro, B. C. Bruce, & W. Brewer (Eds.), *Theoretical issues in reading comprehension*. Hillsdale, N.J.: Erlbaum, 1980.

Brown, A. L. Metacognition: The development of selective attention strategies for learning from texts. In M. L. Kamil (Ed.), *Directions in reading: Research and instruction. Thirtieth yearbook of the National Reading Conference*. Washington, D.C.: National Reading Conference, 1981.

Brown, A. L. Learning and development: The problem of compatibility, access and induction. *Human Development, 1982, 25,* 89–115. (a)

Brown, A. L. Learning how to learn from reading. In J. Langer & T. Smith-Burke (Eds.), *Reader meets author, bridging the gap: A psycholinguistic and social linguistic perspective*. Newark, N.J.: Dell, 1982. (b)

Brown, A. L., & Barclay, C. R. The effects of training specific mnemonics on the meta-mnemonic efficiency of retarded children. *Child Development, 1976, 47,* 71–80.

Brown, A. L., Bransford, J. D., Ferrara, R. A., & Campione, J. C. Learning, remembering, and understanding. In J. H. Flavell & E. M. Markman (Eds.), *Carmichael's manual of child psychology* (Vol. 1). New York: Wiley, in press.

Brown, A. L., & Campione, J. C. Recognition memory for perceptually similar pictures in preschool children. *Journal of Experimental Psychology, 1972, 95,* 55–62.

Brown, A. L., & Campione, J. C. Training strategic study time apportionment in educable retarded children. *Intelligence, 1977, 1,* 94–107.

Brown, A. L., & Campione, J. C. Memory strategies in learning: Training children to study strategically. In H. Pick, H. Lebowitz, J. Singer, A. Steinschneider, & H. Stevenson (Eds.), *Application of basic research in psychology*. New York: Plenum Press, 1978.

Brown, A. L., & Campione, J. C. The effects of knowledge and experience on the formation of retrieval plans for studying from texts. In M. M. Gruneberg, P. E. Morris, & R. N. Sykes (Eds.), *Practical aspects of memory*. London: Academic Press, 1979.

Brown, A. L., & Campione, J. C. Inducing flexible thinking: A problem of access. In M. Friedman, J. P. Das, & N. O'Connor (Eds.), *Intelligence and learning*. New York: Plenum Press, 1981.

Brown, A. L., & Campione, J. C. Modifying intelligence versus modifying cognitive skills: More than a semantic quibble. In D. K. Detterman & R. J. Sternberg (Eds.), *How and how much can intelligence be increased?* Norwood, N.J.: Ablex, in press.

Brown, A. L., Campione, J. C., & Barclay, C. R. Training self-checking routines for estimating test readiness: Generalization from list learning to prose recall. *Child Development,* 1979, 50, 501–512.

Brown, A. L., Campione, J. C., Bray, N. W., & Wilcox, B. L. Keeping track of changing variables: Effects of rehearsal training and rehearsal prevention in normal and retarded adolescents. *Journal of Experimental Psychology,* 1973, 101, 123–131.

Brown, A. L., Campione, J. C., & Day, J. D. Learning to learn: On training students to learn from texts. *Educational Researcher,* 1981, 10, 14–21.

Brown, A. L., Campione, J. C., & Gilliard, D. M. Recency judgments in children: A production deficiency in the use of redundant background cues. *Developmental Psychology,* 1974, 10, 303.

Brown, A. L., Campione, J. C., & Murphy, M. D. Keeping track of changing variables: Long-term retention of a trained rehearsal strategy by retarded adolescents. *American Journal of Mental Deficiency,* 1974, 78, 446–453.

Brown, A. L., Campione, J. C., & Murphy, M. D. Maintenance and generalization of trained metamnemonic awareness by educable retarded children: Span estimation. *Journal of Experimental Child Psychology,* 1977, 24, 191–211.

Brown, A. L., & DeLoache, J. S. Skills, plans and self-regulation. In R. Siegler (Ed.), *Children's thinking: What develops?* Hillsdale, N.J.: Erlbaum, 1978.

Brown, A. L., & Ferrara, R. A. Diagnosing zones of proximal development. In J. V. Wertsch (Ed.), *Culture, communication and cognition: Vygotskian perspectives.* New York: Academic Press, in press.

Brown, A. L., & French, L. A. The cognitive consequences of education: School experts or general problem solvers? Commentary on "Education and cognitive development: The evidence from experimental research" by Sharp, Cole, & Lave. *Monographs of the Society for Research in Child Development,* 1979, 44(1-2, Serial No. 178). (a)

Brown, A. L., & French, L. A. The zone of potential development: Implications for intelligence testing in the year 2000. *Intelligence,* 1979, 3, 253–271. (b)

Brown, A. L., & Lawton, S. Q. C. The feeling of knowing experience in educable retarded children. *Developmental Psychology,* 1977, 13, 364–370.

Brown, A. L., & Scott, M. S. Recognition memory for pictures in preschool children. *Journal of Experimental Child Psychology,* 1971, 11, 401–412.

Brown, A. L., & Smiley, S. S. The development of strategies for studying texts. *Child Development,* 1978, 49, 1076–1088.

Brown, J. S., Collins, A., & Harris, G. Artificial intelligence and learning strategies. In H. F. O'Neill (Ed.), *Learning strategies.* New York: Academic Press, 1978.

Brown, J. S., Collins, A., & Larkin, K. Inferences in text understanding. In R. J. Spiro, B. C. Bruce, & W. F. Brewer (Eds.), *Theoeretical issues in reading comprehension.* Hillsdale, N.J.: Erlbaum, 1980.

Brozek, J. To test or not to test: Trends in the Soviet views. *Behavioral Sciences,* 1972, 8, 243–248.

Budoff, M. *Learning potential and educability among the educable mentally retarded.* Final Report Project No. 312312. Cambridge, Mass.: Research Institute for Educational Problems, Cambridge Mental Health Association, 1974.

Burger, A. L., Blackman, L. S., Holmes, M., & Zetlin A. Use of active sorting and retrieval strategies as a facilitator of recall, clustering, and sorting by EMR and nonretarded children. *American Journal of Mental Deficiency,* 1978, 83, 253–261.

Burt, C. *The factors of the mind.* London: University of London Press, 1940.

Butterfield, E. C. Testing process theories of intelligence. In M. Friedman, J. P. Das, & N. O'Connor (Eds.), *Intelligence and learning.* New York: Plenum Press, 1981.

Butterfield, E. C., & Belmont, J. M. Assessing and improving the cognitive functions of mentally retarded people. In I. Bailer & M. Steinlicht (Eds.), *Psychological issues in mental retardation.* Chicago: Aldine Press, 1977.

Butterfield, E. C., Wambold, C., & Belmont, J. M. On the theory and practice of improving short-term memory. *American Journal of Mental Deficiency,* 1973, 77, 654–669.

Campione, J. C., & Brown, A. L. The effects of contextual changes and degree of component mastery in transfer of training. In H. W. Reese (Ed.), *Advances in child development and behavior* (Vol. 9). New York: Academic Press, 1974.

Campione, J. C., & Brown, A. L. Memory and metamemory development in educable retarded children. In R. V. Kail, Jr., & J. W. Hagen (Eds.), *Perspectives on the development of memory and cognition*. Hillsdale, N.J.: Erlbaum, 1977.

Campione, J. C., & Brown, A. L. Toward a theory of intelligence: Contributions from research with retarded children. *Intelligence*, 1978, *2*, 279–304.

Carroll, J. B. How shall we study individual differences in cognitive abilities? – Methodological and theoretical perspectives. *Intelligence*, 1978, *2*, 87–116.

Chi, M. T. H. Age differences in memory span. *Journal of Experimental Child Psychology*, 1977, *23*, 266–281. (a)

Chi, M. T. H. Age differences in the speed of processing: A critique. *Developmental Psychology*, 1977, *13*, 543–544. (b)

Chi, M. T. H. Knowledge development and memory performance. In M. Friedman, J. P. Das, & N. O'Connor (Eds.), *Intelligence and learning*. New York: Plenum Press, 1981.

Chi, M. T. H., & Glaser, R. The measurement of expertise: Analysis of the development of knowledge and skill as a basis for assessing achievement. In E. L. Baker & E. S. Quellmalz (Eds.), *Educational testing and evaluation: Design, analysis, and policy*. Beverly Hills, Calif.: Sage, 1980.

Chiang, A., & Atkinson, R. C. Individual differences and interrelationships among a selected set of cognitive skills. *Memory and Cognition*, 1976, *4*, 661–672.

Cole, M., Hood, L., & McDermott, R. *Ecological niche-picking: Ecological invalidity as an axiom of experimental cognitive psychology* (Working Paper No. 14). New York: Rockefeller University, Laboratory of Comparative Human Cognition and the Institute of Comparative Human Development, 1978.

Collins, A. Processes in acquiring knowledge. In R. C. Anderson, R. J. Spiro, & W. E. Montague (Eds.), *Schooling and the acquisition of knowledge*. Hillsdale, N.J.: Erlbaum, 1977.

Collins, A., & Smith, E. E. Teaching the process of reading comprehension. In D. K. Detterman & R. J. Sternberg (Eds.), *How and how much can intelligence be increased?* Norwood, N.J.: Ablex, in press.

Collins, A., & Stevens, A. *Goals and strategies of inquiring teachers*. Hillsdale, N.J.: Erlbaum, in press.

Cronbach, L. J. How can instruction be adapted to individual differences? In R. M. Gagné (Ed.), *Learning and individual differences*. Columbus, Ohio: Merrill Books, 1967.

Day, J. D. *Training summarization skills: A comparison of teaching methods*. Unpublished doctoral dissertation, University of Illinois, 1980.

Dearborn, W. F. Intelligence and its measurement: A symposium. *Journal of Educational Psychology*, 1921, *12*, 210–212.

Dempster, F. N. Memory span: Sources of individual and developmental differences. *Psychological Bulletin*, 1981, *89*, 63–100.

Detterman, D. K. Memory in the mentally retarded. In N. R. Ellis (Ed.), *Handbook of mental deficiency, psychological theory and research*. Hillsdale, N.J.: Erlbaum, 1979.

Dirks, J., & Neisser, U. Memory for objects in real scenes: The development of recognition and recall. *Journal of Experimental Child Psychology*, 1977, *23*, 315–328.

Duncanson, J. P. *Intelligence and the ability to learn*. Princeton, N.J.: Educational Testing Service, 1964.

Edgerton, R. *The cloak of competence*. Berkeley: University of California Press, 1967.

Egorova, T. V. *Peculiarities of memory and thinking in developmentally backward school children*. Moscow: Moscow University Press, 1973.

Ellis, H. C. *The transfer of learning*. New York: Macmillan, 1965.

Ellis, N. R. (Ed.). *The handbook of mental deficiency, psychological theory and research*. New York: McGraw-Hill, 1963.

Ellis, N. R. Memory processes in retardates and normals. In N. R. Ellis (Ed.), *International review of research in mental retardation*. New York: Academic Press, 1970.

Ellis, N. R. Do the mentally retarded have poor memory? *Intelligence*, 1978, *2*, 41–54.

Ellis, N. R. (Ed.). *Handbook of mental deficiency, psychological theory and research* (2nd ed.). Hillsdale, N.J.: Erlbaum, 1979.

Ellis, N. R., McCartney, J. R., Ferretti, R. P., & Cavalier, A. R. Recognition memory in mentally retarded persons. *Intelligence*, 1977, *1*, 310–317.

Fattu, N. A., Mech, E. V., & Kapos, E. Some statistical relationships between selected response dimensions and problem-solving proficiency. *Psychological Monographs*, 1954, 68(Whole No. 337).

Feigenbaum, E. A. The art of artificial intelligence: Themes and case studies of knowledge engineering. *Proceedings of the Fifth International Joint Conference on Artificial Intelligence*. Pittsburgh: Carnegie-Mellon, 1977.

Ferguson, G. A. On learning and human ability. *Canadian Journal of Psychology*, 1954, 8, 95–112.

Ferguson, G. A. On transfer and the abilities of man. *Canadian Journal of Psychology*, 1956, 10, 121–131.

Feuerstein, R. *The instrumental enrichment method: An outline of theory and technique*. Jerusalem: Hadassah-Wizo-Canada Research Institute, 1969.

Feuerstein, R. *Instrumental enrichment: An intervention program for cognitive modifiability*. Baltimore: University Park Press, 1980.

Feuerstein, R., Rand, Y., Hoffman, M., Hoffman, M., & Miller, R. Cognitive modifiability in retarded adolescents: Effects of instrumental enrichment. *American Journal of Mental Deficiency*, 1979, 83, 539–550.

Fisher, M. A., & Zeaman, D. An attention–retention theory of retardate discrimination learning. In N. R. Ellis (Ed.), *International review of research in mental retardation* (Vol. 6). New York: Academic Press, 1973.

Flavell, J. H. Developmental studies of mediated memory. In H. W. Reese and L. P. Lipsitt (Eds.), *Advances in child development and behavior* (Vol. 5). New York: Academic Press, 1970.

Flavell, J. H. First discussant's comments: What is memory development the development of? *Human Development*, 1971, 14, 272–278.

Flavell, J. H. *Cognitive monitoring*. Paper presented at the conference on Children's Oral Communication Skills, University of Wisconsin, Madison, October 1978.

Flavell, J. H. Cognitive monitoring. In W. P. Dickson (Ed.), *Children's oral communication skills*. New York: Academic Press, 1981.

Flavell, J. H., Friedrichs, A. G., & Hoyt, J. D. Developmental changes in memorization processes. *Cognitive Psychology*, 1970, 1, 324–340.

Flavell, J. H., & Wellman, H. M. Metamemory. In R. V. Kail, Jr., & J. W. Hagen (Eds.), *Perspectives on the development of memory and cognition*. Hillsdale, N.J.: Erlbaum, 1977.

Flores, C. F., & Winograd, T. Understanding cognition as understanding. Unpublished manuscript, Stanford University, 1978.

Gagné, R. M. (Ed.). *Learning and individual differences*. Columbus, Ohio: Merrill, 1967.

Gagné, R. M. Contribution of learning to human development. *Psychological Review*, 1968, 75, 177–191.

Gagné, R. M. *The conditions of learning* (2nd ed.). New York: Holt, Rinehart and Winston, 1970.

Gardner, H. Commentary on animal awareness papers. *Behavioral and Brain Sciences*, 1978, 4, 572.

Garner, W. R. *Uncertainty and structure in psychological concepts*. New York: Wiley, 1962.

Gelman, R., & Gallistel, C. R. *The child's understanding of number*. Cambridge, Mass.: Harvard University Press, 1978.

Gerjuoy, I. R., & Spitz, H. H. Associative clustering in free recall: Intellectual and developmental variables. *American Journal of Mental Deficiency*, 1966, 70, 918–927.

Gick, M. L., & Holyoak, K. J. Analogical problem solving. *Cognitive Psychology*, 1980, 12, 306–355.

Glaser, R. *Advances in instructional psychology* (Vol. 1). Hillsdale, N.J.: Erlbaum, 1978.

Glidden, L. M. Training of learning and memory in retarded persons: Strategies, techniques, and teaching tools. In N. R. Ellis (Ed.), *Handbook of mental deficiency, psychological theory and research*. Hillsdale, N.J.: Erlbaum, 1979.

Goldstein, I., & Papert, S. Artificial intelligence, language, and the study of knowledge. *Cognitive Science*, 1977, 1, 84–123.

Gould, J. L. Behavioral programming in honeybees. *Behavioral and Brain Sciences*, 1978, 4, 572–573.

Green, J. M. Category cues in free recall: Retarded adults of two vocabulary age levels. *American Journal of Mental Deficiency*, 1974, 78, 419–425.

Gulliksen, H. An analysis of learning data which distinguishes between initial preference and learning ability. *Psychometrika*, 1942, 7, 171–194.

Harlow, H. F. The formation of learning sets. *Psychological Review*, 1949, 56, 51–65.

Harlow, H. F. Mice, monkeys, men, and motives. *Psychological Review*, 1953, 60, 23–32.

Harlow, H. F. Learning set and error factor theory. In S. Koch (Ed.), *Psychology: A study of a science, Study I: Conceptual and systematic* (Vol. 2). New York: McGraw-Hill, 1959.

Harris, G. J., & Fleer, R. W. High speed memory scanning in mental retardates: Evidence for a central processing deficit. *Journal of Experimental Child Psychology*, 1974, 17, 452–459.

Harter, S. Discrimination learning set in children as a function of IQ and MA. *Journal of Experimental Child Psychology*, 1965, 2, 31–43.

Hasher, L., & Zacks, R. T. Automatic and effortful processes in memory. *Journal of Experimental Psychology: General*, 1979, 108, 356–388.

Haywood, H. C., & Arbitman-Smith, R. A. Modification of cognitive functions in slow learning adolescents. In P. Mittler (Ed.), *Frontiers of knowledge in mental retardation: Proceedings of the Fifth Congress of IASSMD* (Vol. 1). *Social, educational, and behavioral aspects*. Baltimore: University Park Press, 1981.

Haywood, H. C., Filler, J. W., Jr., Shifman, M. A., & Chatelanat, G. Behavioral assessment in mental retardation. In P. McReynolds (Ed.), *Advances in psychological assessment* (Vol. 3). Palo Alto, Calif.: Science and Behavior Books, 1975.

Hebb, D. O. *The organization of behavior*. New York: Wiley, 1949.

Herrmann, D. J., & Landis, T. Y. Differences in the search rate of children and adults in short-term memory. *Journal of Experimental Child Psychology*, 1977, 23, 151–161.

Hill, A. L. Savants: Mentally retarded individuals with special skills. In N. R. Ellis (Ed.), *International review of research in mental retardation* (Vol. 9). New York: Academic Press, 1978.

Hobbs, N. Feuerstein's instrumental enrichment: Teaching intelligence to adolescents. *Educational Leadership*, 1980, 37, 566–568.

Höffding, H. *Outlines of psychology* (M. E. Lowndes, Trans.). London: Macmillan, 1892.

Holt, J. H. *How children fail*. New York: Dell, 1964.

Hull, C. L. *Principles of behavior: An introduction to behavior theory*. New York: Appleton-Century-Crofts, 1943.

Hunt, E. We knows who knows, but why? In R. C. Anderson, R. J. Spiro, & W. E. Montague (Eds.), *Schooling and the acquisition of knowledge*. Hillsdale, N.J.: Erlbaum, 1977.

Hunt, E. B. Mechanics of verbal ability. *Psychological Review*, 1978, 85, 109–130.

Hunt, E. G., Frost, N., & Lunneborg, C. L. Individual differences in cognition: A new approach to intelligence. In G. Bower (Ed.), *Advances in learning and motivation* (Vol. 7). New York: Academic Press, 1973.

Hunt, E. B., Lunneborg, C., & Lewis, J. What does it mean to be high verbal? *Cognitive Psychology*, 1975, 7, 194–227.

Huttenlocher, J., & Burke, D. Why does memory span increase with age? *Cognitive Psychology*, 1976, 8, 1–31.

Inhelder, B., Sinclair, H., & Bovet, M. *Learning and the development of cognition*. Cambridge, Mass.: Harvard University Press, 1974.

Jackson, M. D., & McClelland, J. L. Sensory and cognitive determinants of reading speed. *Journal of Verbal Learning and Verbal Behavior*, 1975, 14, 565–574.

Jackson, M. D., & McClelland, J. L. Processing determinants of reading speed. *Journal of Experimental Psychology: General*, 1979, 108, 151–181.

Jenkins, J. J. Four points to remember: A tetrahedral model and memory experiments. In L. S. Cermak & F. I. M. Craik (Eds.), *Levels of processing in human memory*. Hillsdale, N.J.: Erlbaum, 1979.

Jensen, A. R., & Munro, E. Reaction time, movement time and intelligence. *Intelligence*, 1979, 3, 121–126.

Johnson-Laird, P. N. Mental models in cognitive science. *Cognitive Science*, 1980, 4, 71–115.

Kappauf, W. E. Studying the relation of task performance to the variables of chronological age, mental age, and IQ. In N. R. Ellis (Ed.), *International review of research in mental retardation* (Vol. 6). New York: Academic Press, 1973.

Keating, D. P., & Bobbitt, B. L. Individual and developmental differences in cognitive-processing components of mental ability. *Child Development*, 1978, 49, 155–167.

Kelley, H. H., & Thibaut, J. W. Experimental studies of group problem solving and process. In

G. Lindzey (Ed.), *Handbook of social psychology* (Vol. 2). Reading, Mass.: Addison-Wesley, 1954.

Kendall, C. R., Borkowski, J. G., & Cavanaugh, J. C. Metamemory and the transfer of an interrogative strategy by EMR children. *Intelligence,* 1980, *4,* 255–270.

Kennedy, B. A., & Miller, D. J. Persistent use of verbal rehearsal as a function of information about its value. *Child Development,* 1976, *47,* 566–569.

Kestner, J., & Borkowski, J. Children's maintenance and generalization of an interrogative learning strategy. *Child Development,* 1979, *50,* 485–494.

Kohler, W. *Mentality of apes.* New York: Humanities Press, 1951.

Kotovsky, K., & Simon, H. A. Empirical tests of a theory of human acquisition of concepts for sequential patterns. *Cognitive Psychology,* 1973, *4,* 399–424.

Larkin, J. H., Heller, J. I., & Greeno, J. G. Instructional implications of research on problem solving. In W. J. McKeachie (Ed.), *Cognition, college teaching, and student learning.* San Francisco, Calif.: Jossey-Bass, 1980.

Lewin, K. A. *A dynamic theory of personality.* New York: McGraw-Hill, 1935.

Liberman, A. M., Cooper, F. S., Shankweiler, D. P., & Studdert-Kennedy, M. Perception of the speech code. *Psychological Review,* 1967, *74,* 431–461.

Lord, F. M. Further problems in the measurement of growth. *Educational and Psychological measurement,* 1958, *18,* 437–451.

Lubovsky, V. I. Personal communication, December 1978.

Lynn, R., Gluckin, N. D., & Kripke, B. *Learning disabilities: An overview of theories, approaches, and politics.* New York: Free Press, 1979.

Lyon, D. R. Individual differences in immediate serial recall: A matter of mnemonics? *Cognitive Psychology,* 1977, *9,* 403–411.

Mackworth, N. H., & Bruner, J. S. How adults and children search and recognize pictures. *Human Development,* 1970, *13,* 149–177.

MacMillan, D. L. Effects of input organization on recall of digits by EMR children. *American Journal of Mental Deficiency,* 1970, *74,* 692–699.

Mandler, J. M., & Johnson, N. S. Some of the thousand words a picture is worth. *Journal of Experimental Psychology: Human Learning and Memory,* 1976, *2,* 529–540.

Markman, E. M. Problems of logic and evidence. *Behavioral and Brain Sciences,* 1978, *1,* 194–195.

Markman, E. M. Realizing that you don't understand: Elementary schoolchildren's awareness of inconsistencies. *Child Development,* 1979, *50,* 643–655.

Martin, A. S. *The effect of the novelty–familiarity dimension on discrimination learning by mental retardates.* Unpublished doctoral dissertation, University of Connecticut, 1970.

McClelland, J. L., & Jackson, M. D. Studying individual differences in reading. In A. Lesgold, J. Pellegrino, S. Fokkema, & R. Glaser (Eds.), *Cognitive psychology and instruction.* New York: Plenum Press, 1978.

McGeoch, J. A., & Irion, A. L. *The psychology of human learning* (2nd ed., rev. ed.). New York: Longmans, 1952.

Mehan, H. Assessing children's language using abilities: Methodological and cross cultural implications. In M. Armer & A. D. Grimshaw (Eds.), *Comparative social research: Methodological problems and strategies.* New York: Wiley, 1973.

Meichenbaum, D. *Cognitive behavior modification: An integrative approach.* New York: Plenum Press, 1977.

Mischel, W., & Patterson, C. J. Substantive and structural elements of effective plans for self-control. *Journal of Personality and Social Psychology,* 1976, *34,* 942–950.

Miyake, N., & Norman, D. A. To ask a question, one must know enough to know what is not known. *Journal of Verbal Learning and Verbal Behavior,* 1979, *18,* 357–364.

Moely, B. E. Organizational factors in the development of memory. In R. V. Kail, Jr., & J. W. Hagen (Eds.), *Perspectives on the development of memory and cognition.* Hillsdale, N.J.: Erlbaum, 1977.

Moore, J., & Newell, A. How can Merlin understand? In L. W. Gregg (Ed.), *Knowledge and cognition.* Hillsdale, N.J.: Erlbaum, 1974.

Murphy, M. D. Measurement of category clustering in free recall. In C. R. Puff (Ed.), *Memory organization and structure.* New York: Academic Press, 1979.

Murphy, M. D., & Brown, A. L. Incidental learning in preschool children as a function of level of cognitive analysis. *Journal of Experimental Child Psychology,* 1975, *19,* 509–523.

Narrol, H., & Bachor, D. G. An introduction to Feuerstein's approach to assessing and develop-
ing cognitive potential. *Interchange*, 1975, 6, 2–16.
Neisser, U. General academic and artificial intelligence. In L. B. Resnick (Ed.), *The nature of
intelligence*. Hillsdale, N.J.: Erlbaum, 1976.
Newell, A. One final word. In D. T. Tuma & F. Reif (Eds.), *Problem solving and education:
Issues in teaching and research*. Hillsdale, N.J.: Erlbaum, 1979.
Newell, A., & Simon, H. A. *Human problem solving*. Englewood Cliffs, N.J.: Prentice-Hall,
1972.
Nickerson, R. S. A note on long-term recognition memory for pictorial material. *Psychonomic
Science*, 1968, 11, 58.
Nisbett, R. E., & Wilson, D. Telling more than we know: Verbal reports on mental processes.
Psychological Review, 1977, 84, 231–279.
Norman, D. A. Twelve issues for cognitive science. *Cognitive Science*, 1980, 4, 1–32.
Osgood, C. E. The similarity paradox in human learning: A resolution. *Psychological Review*,
1949, 56, 132–143.
Pellegrino, J. W., & Glaser, R. Editorial: Cognitive correlates and components in the analysis of
individual differences. *Intelligence*, 1979, 3, 187–216.
Perfetti, C. A., & Hogaboam, T. The relationship between single word decoding and reading
comprehension skill. *Journal of Educational Psychology*, 1975, 67, 461–469.
Perfetti, C. A., & Lesgold, A. M. Discourse comprehension and sources of individual differences. In P. Carpenter & M. Just (Eds.), *Cognitive processes in comprehension*. Hillsdale, N.J.: Erlbaum, 1977.
Perfetti, C. A., & Lesgold, A. M. Coding and comprehension in skilled reading and implications
for reading instruction. In L. B. Resnick & P. A. Weaver (Eds.), *Theory and practice of
early reading* (Vol. 1). Hillsdale, N.J.: Erlbaum, 1979.
Pevzner, M. S. [Clinical characteristics of children with retarded development.] *Dejektologiin*,
1972, 3, 3–9.
Posner, M. I., Boies, S. J., Eichelman, W. H., & Taylor, R. L. Retention of visual and name
codes of single letters. *Journal of Experimental Psychology Monograph*, 1969, 79(1, Pt. 2).
Pylyshyn, Z. W. Computational models and empirical constraints. *The Behavioral and Brain
Sciences*, 1978, 1, 93–99. (a)
Pylyshyn, Z. W. When is attribution of beliefs justified? *Behavioral and Brain Sciences*, 1978,
1, 592–593. (b)
Resnick, L. B., & Glaser, R. Problem solving and intelligence. In L. B. Resnick (Ed.), *The
nature of intelligence*. Hillsdale, N.J.: Erlbaum, 1976.
Rigney, J. *On understanding strategies for facilitating acquisition, retention, and retrieval in
training and education* (Tech. Rep. No. 78). Los Angeles: University of Southern Califor-
nia, 1976.
Ringel, B. A., & Springer, C. On knowing how well one is remembering: The persistence of
strategy use during transfer. *Journal of Experimental Child Psychology*, 1980, 29,
322–333.
Rozin, P. The evolution of intelligence and access to the cognitive unconscious. *Progression in
Psychobiology and Physiological Psychology*, 1976, 6, 245–280.
Rumelhart, D. E. Understanding and summarizing brief stories. In D. LaBerge & J. Samuels
(Eds.), *Basic processes in reading: Perception and comprehension*. Hillsdale, N.J.:
Erlbaum, 1977.
Rumelhart, D. E., & McClelland, J. L. *An interactive activation model of the effect of context in
perception: Part III* (CHIP Tech. Rep. No. 95). La Jolla, Calif.: Center for Human Infor-
mation Processing, University of California, San Diego, August 1980.
Schallert, D. L., & Kleiman, G. M. *Some reasons why the teacher is easier to understand than
the text book* (Reading Education Report No. 9). Urbana: University of Illinois, Center for
the Study of Reading, June 1979. (ERIC Document Reproduction Service No. ED 172
189)
Schank, R. C. How much intelligence is there in Artificial Intelligence? *Intelligence*, 1980, 4,
1–14.
Schneider, W., & Shiffrin, R. M. Controlled and automatic human information processing: I.
Direction, search, and attention. *Psychological Review*, 1977, 84, 1–66.
Shif, Z. I. Development of children in schools for mentally retarded. In M. Cole & I. Maltzman
(Eds.), *A handbook of contemporary Soviet psychology*. New York: Basic Books, 1969.
Siegler, R. S. Information processing approaches to development. In W. Kessen (Ed.), *Car-
michael's manual of child psychology* (Vol. 9). New York: Wiley, 1981.

Silver, L. B. The minimal brain dysfunction syndrome. In J. Noshpitz (Ed.), *The basic handbook of child psychiatry* (Vol. 2). New York: Basic Books, 1978.

Simon, H. A. Identifying basic abilities underlying intelligent performance of complex tasks. In L. B. Resnick (Ed.), *The nature of intelligence.* Hillsdale, N.J.: Erlbaum, 1976.

Simon, H. A. Problem solving and education. In D. T. Tuma & F. Reif (Eds.), *Problem solving and education: Issues in teaching and research.* Hillsdale, N.J.: Erlbaum, 1979.

Simon, H. A., & Hayes, J. R. The understanding process: Problem isomorphs. *Cognitive Psychology*, 1976, *8*, 165–190.

Skinner, B. F. Why I am not a cognitive psychologist. *Behaviorism*, 1977, *5*, 1–10.

Smedslund, J. Microanalysis of concrete reasoning, I. The difficulty of some combinations of addition and subtraction of one unit. *Scandinavian Journal of Psychology*, 1966, *1*, 145–156.

Spearman, C. "General intelligence," objectively determined and measured. *American Journal of Psychology*, 1904, *15*, 206–219.

Spearman, C. *The nature of "intelligence" and principles of cognition.* London: Macmillan, 1923.

Spearman, C. *The abilities of man.* New York: Macmillan, 1927.

Sperber, R. D., Ragain, R. D., & McCauley, C. Reassessment of category knowledge in retarded individuals. *American Journal of Mental Deficiency*, 1976, *81*, 227–234.

Spitz, H. A. A note on general intelligence and the MA deviation concept. *Intelligence*, 1981, *5*, 77–83.

Spitz, H. H. Field theory in mental deficiency. In N. R. Ellis (Ed.), *Handbook of mental deficiency.* New York: McGraw-Hill, 1963.

Spitz, H. H. The role of input organization in the learning and memory of mental retardates. In N. R. Ellis (Ed.), *International review of research in mental retardation* (Vol. 2). New York: Academic Press, 1966.

Spitz, H. H. Note on immediate memory for digits: Invariance over the years. *Psychological Bulletin*, 1972, *78*, 183–185.

Spitz, H. H. The universal nature of human intelligence: Evidence from games. *Intelligence*, 1978, *2*, 322–342.

Spitz, H. H., Goettler, D. R., & Webreck, C. A. Effects of two types of redundancy on visual digit span performance of retardates and varying aged normals. *Developmental Psychology*, 1972, *6*, 92–103.

Spring, C. Encoding speed and memory span in dyslexic children. *Journal of Special Education*, 1976, *10*, 35–40.

Spring, C., & Capps, C. Encoding speed, rehearsal and probed recall of dyslexic boys. *Journal of Educational Psychology*, 1974, *66*, 780–786.

Stake, R. E. Learning parameters, aptitudes, and achievements. *Psychometric Monographs*, 1961, No. 9.

Sternberg, R. J. *Intelligence, information processing, and analogical reasoning: The componential analysis of human abilities.* Hillsdale, N.J.: Erlbaum, 1977.

Sternberg, R. J. Sketch of a componential subtheory of human intelligence. *Behavioral and Brain Sciences*, 1980, *3*, 573–584.

Sternberg, S. High-speed scanning in human memory. *Science*, 1966, *153*, 652–654.

Stevens, A., Collins, A., & Goldin, S. E. Misconceptions in students' understanding. *International Journal of Man–Machine Studies*, 1979, *11*, 145–156.

Stolurow, L. M. Social impact of programmed instruction: Aptitudes or abilities revisited. In J. P. DeCecco (Ed.), *Educational technology.* New York: Holt, Rinehart and Winston, 1964.

Tallal, P. Implications of speech perceptual research for clinical populations. In J. F. Kavanagh & W. Strange (Eds.), *Speech and language in the laboratory, school, and clinic.* Cambridge, Mass.: MIT Press, 1978.

Tallal, P., & Piercy, M. Developmental aphasia: Impaired rate of nonverbal processing as a function of sensory modality. *Neuropsychologia*, 1973, *11*, 389–398.

Tallal, P., & Piercy, M. Defects of auditory perception in children with developmental dysphasia. In M. Wyke (Ed.), *Developmental dysphasia.* New York: Academic Press, 1978.

Tenney, Y. J. The child's conception of organization and recall. *Journal of Experimental Child Psychology*, 1975, *19*, 100–114.

Thorndike, E. L. *Introduction to the theory of mental and social measurements.* New York: Teachers College, Columbia University, 1904.

Thorndike, E. L. *Measurement of intelligence.* New York: Teachers College Press, 1926.

Thorndike, E. L., & Woodworth, R. S. The influence of improvement in one mental function upon the efficiency of other functions. *Psychological Review*, 1901, *8*, 247–261, 384–395, 553–564.

Thurstone, L. L. Primary mental abilities. *Psychometric Monographs*, 1938, No. 1.

Tolman, E. C. Principles of purposive behavior. In S. Koch (Ed.), *Psychology: A study of a science* (Vol. 2). New York: McGraw-Hill, 1959.

Touchette, P. E. The effects of graduated stimulus change on the acquisition of a simple discrimination in overly retarded boys. *Journal of the Experimental Analysis of Behavior*, 1968, *11*, 38–48.

Tuddenham, R. D. The nature and measurement of intelligence. In L. Postman (Ed.), *Psychology in the making*. New York: Knopf, 1962.

Vlasova, T. A. New advances in Soviet defectology. *Soviet Education*, 1972, *14*, 20–39.

Vlasova, T. A., & Pevzner, M. S. (Eds.). *Children with temporary retardation in development*. Moscow: Pedagogika, 1971.

Von Frisch, K. *The dance language and orientation of bees*. Cambridge, Mass.: Belknap Press, 1967.

Vygotsky, L. S. [*Mind in society: The development of higher psychological processes*] (M. Cole, V. John-Steiner, S. Scribner, & E. Souberman, Eds. and trans.). Cambridge, Mass.: Harvard University Press, 1978.

Wertsch, J. V. Adult–child interaction and the roots of metacognition. *Quarterly Newsletter of the Institute for Comparative Human Development*, 1978, *1*, 15–18.

Wertsch, J. V. Adult–child interaction as a source of self-regulation in children. In S. R. Yussen (Ed.), *The development of reflection*. New York: Academic Press, in press.

White, P. Limitations on verbal reports of internal events: A refutation of Nisbett and Wilson and of Bem. *Psychological Review*, 1980, *87*, 105–112.

Wickelgren, W. A. Age and storage dynamics in continuous recognition memory. *Developmental Psychology*, 1975, *11*, 165–169.

Wickens, D. D. Characteristics of word encoding. In A. Melton & E. Martin (Eds.), *Coding processes in human memory*. Washington, D.C.: Winston, 1972.

Winters, J. J., Jr., & Cundari, L. Accumulation of and release from proactive inhibition in short-term memory by retarded and nonretarded persons. *American Journal of Mental Deficiency*, 1979, *83*, 595–600.

Woodrow, H. A. Intelligence and its measurement: A symposium. *Journal of Educational Psychology*, 1921, *12*, 207–210.

Woodrow, H. A. The effect of practice on groups of different initial ability. *Journal of Educational Psychology*, 1938, *29*, 268–278.

Woodrow, H. A. The ability to learn. *Psychological Review*, 1946, *53*, 147–158.

Wozniak, R. H. Psychology and education of the learning disabled child in the Soviet Union. In W. M. Cruickshank & D. P. Hallahan (Eds.), *Perceptual and learning disabilities in children*. Syracuse, N.Y.: Syracuse University Press, 1975.

Yntema, D. B., & Mueser, G. E. Remembering the present states of a number of variables. *Journal of Experimental Psychology*, 1960, *60*, 18–22.

Youniss, J. Operations and everyday thinking: A commentary on "dialectical operations." *Human Development*, 1974, *17*, 386–391.

Zabramna, S. D. (Ed.). [*The selection of children for schools for the mentally retarded*]. Moscow: Prosveshchenie, 1971.

Zeaman, D. Some relations of general intelligence and selective attention. *Intelligence*, 1978, *2*, 55–73.

Zeaman, D., & House, B. J. The role of attention in retardate discrimination learning. In N. R. Ellis (Ed.), *Handbook of mental deficiency*. New York: McGraw-Hill, 1963.

Zeaman, D., & House, B. J. The relation of IQ and learning. In R. M. Gagné (Ed.), *Learning and individual differences*. Columbus, Ohio: Merrill Books, 1967.

PART III

Society, culture, and intelligence

9   *Education and intelligence*

RICHARD E. SNOW
in collaboration with ELANNA YALOW

The concepts of intelligence and education are so often discussed and studied independently that they are conventionally assumed to be distinct, just as "nature" and "nurture" are considered distinct. Still, one can entertain the notion that intelligence and education cannot really exist independently – that the referents of these terms are not separable strands intertwined in human mental life but rather are fundamentally confounded. In other words, human intelligence is fundamentally a product of education, and education is fundamentally a product of the exercise of human intelligence. The present chapter entertains this possibility.

More directly, the chapter aims (a) to describe the relationships that have obtained between concepts of educational theory and practice and concepts of intelligence through history; (b) to clarify some conceptual and methodological issues that have limited research on these topics in the past; (c) to summarize the current state of evidence and research relating intelligence and education; and (d) to draw implications for educational theory, research, and practice from current research on intelligence and suggestions for research on intelligence from observations about education. Following an introductory review of the goals of education and of educational research, which also helps to organize later discussion, four main sections correspond to these four aims. The last serves also as a recapitulation of and challenge to future research. Given the vast domain of scholarship and scientific work identified by the union of the terms *intelligence* and *education,* this chapter can at best serve only as an outline to guide further and deeper reading.[1]

9.1.   THE GOALS OF EDUCATION AND OF EDUCATIONAL RESEARCH

EDUCATIONAL GOALS

Whatever else is said about education and educational goals, three themes can be discerned, with varying emphasis, in the writings of virtually all educational theorists and philosophers. As the place of intelligence in the concepts and practices of education is examined, these themes must be distinguished.

First, educational institutions have always served as selection systems, or as part of such systems, for the societies in which they are situated. Sociologists (e.g., Davis & Moore, 1970) have studied the persistent societal need to identify and allocate talent and note (e.g., J. Meyer, 1977) that educational institutions will likely always be centrally involved in serving this function. In a democracy, the public school system may even be the institution best equipped to provide this

493

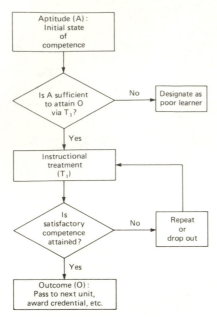

Figure 9.1. Glaser's Model I: Education as a selective system with limited instructional alternatives. (Adapted from *Adaptive Education: Individual Diversity and Learning* by R. Glaser [New York: Holt, Rinehart & Winston, 1977].)

function, so long as it is also equipped to provide equal opportunity for all to be selected.

Second, educational institutions exist to preserve and encourage the development of knowledge for its own sake. They are the institutions designated by society to maintain, exercise, and communicate the collective human intellect (that is, the culture, the civilization) of the past, and in the case of higher universities, to create new contributions to that collective.

Third, and perhaps most important for the purposes of this chapter, education aims at aptitude development. Since its earliest beginnings, education has always been concerned with human preparedness for further states of life. The term *aptitude* signifies some aspect of the present state of a human being that is propaedeutic to some future achievement, whether that achievement is defined as the attainment of heaven, good citizenship, socialization, vocational or marital satisfaction, higher education, or greater intelligence.

Intersecting these three themes, two broad categories of educational goals can be distinguished (Cronbach, 1967). There are individual goals, chosen by individuals themselves for their own purposes. The obvious examples, with their implied individual goals, are the elective courses available in most schools and colleges – music, art, home economics, foreign languages, volleyball, and so on. There are also common goals imposed on everyone by society – the minimal expectations in reading, writing, mathematics, citizenship, and physical education are examples. What is regarded as a common goal and what is left to indi-

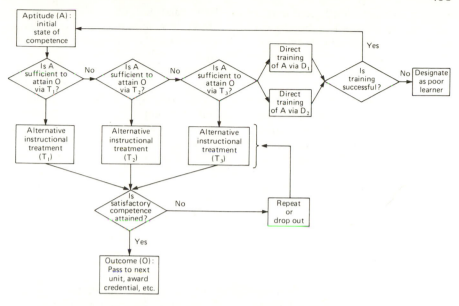

Figure 9.2.   Glaser's Model IV: Education as an adaptive system with instructional alternatives and direct training aimed at accommodating or removing aptitude differences. (Adapted from *Adaptive Education: Individual Diversity and Learning* by R. Glaser [New York: Holt, Rinehart & Winston, 1977].)

vidual choice varies across history and across locale, of course. The main concern here is with the common, aptitude development goals apparent in the educational programs of Western industrialized societies in this century, for this is where the concepts of intelligence and education intersect most substantially.

Figures 9.1 and 9.2 have been adapted from Glaser (1977) to depict schematically the contrast between a selective system and an aptitude development system aimed at common goals. Glaser also showed how a multiple version of Figure 9.2 could provide for individually chosen, divergent goals. The programs of most educational institutions, historically, would resemble Figure 9.1, where individuals must adapt to a fixed instructional treatment or drop out. Not many systems yet resemble Figure 9.2. Both systems provide a means of handling human intellectual diversity, but it is the realization of that shown in Figure 9.2 that sets the purpose of much modern research on intelligence and education. The educator's job today is to create and maintain a system that reconciles society's commitment to equal educational opportunity for all individuals with the fact that individuals differ in aptitudes relevant to learning at the start. As Cronbach (1967) and Glaser (1977) have both argued, to reach common educational goals the instructional system must be made adaptive to the diversity of human aptitudes. It must be geared either to adapt alternative instructional treatments (T_1, T_2, T_3) to fit persistent individual differences in prior aptitudes (A) or to train individual differences into irrelevance by developing the required aptitudes directly (D_1, D_2). The plan in Figure 9.2 includes provision for both kinds of individualization because in most educational enterprises there must be a trade-off between the two. The educator seeks directly to develop skill in reading because the ability to read is a common educational goal itself and because it is an aptitude for later learning in science and social studies, to name a few other common goal areas. If some individuals require many years to develop sufficient reading ability, then the educator must either adapt parallel instruction in science and social studies to fit the individual's present strengths and weaknesses or give up these other common goals. At any time, then, there is a compromise between direct aptitude development and adaptation of instruction to circumvent existing inaptitudes. One can think of direct aptitude training as remediation; but more is implied here. Training aims at transfer, not merely the building of competent performance on some task for its own sake. The adaptation of instruction seeks alternatives that capitalize on what strengths the individual has while compensating for persistent weaknesses. The outcome in either case is *transferable* competence, that is, aptitude. The credential is more a promise of future performance than it is a record of past performance.

RESEARCH GOALS

The current state of educational psychology attempts to cover all of the 2 × 3 table of educational goals formed by crossing individual versus common goal categories with selection versus knowledge for its own sake versus aptitude development, as well as many related topics. Interested readers can consult contemporary texts (e.g., Cronbach, 1977; Gage & Berliner, 1979) for a summary of much of what is now known on all these topics.

It may be said that educational psychology now recognizes intelligence as education's most important product, as well as its most important raw material. To be clear on what is meant by *intelligence* as both an aptitude and an outcome for education, however, we must demote the construct from the reified unity so often taken for granted in educational and other public discussions. Cronbach's (1977) definition seems to do this:

"Intelligence" is not a thing, it is a style of work. To say that one person is "more intelligent" than another means that he acts more intelligently, more of the time. "Efficiency" is a word of the same type. We cannot locate the efficiency of a factory in any one part of the operation. Rather, the purchasing division, the people who maintain the machines, and the operators, inspectors and shippers do their tasks with few errors and little lost time; efficiency is an index of how well the system functions as a whole. After Binet had observed excellent and inferior intellectual performance of children, he summed up the difference in this famous three-part description of intelligence:

> the tendency to take and maintain a definite direction;
> the capacity to make adaptations for the purpose of attaining a
> desired end;
> the power of auto-criticism. (Translation by Terman, 1916, p. 45.)

The first point has to do with accepting a task and keeping one's mind on it. The second point contrasts intelligent behavior with acting out of habit, with little analysis of the immediate situation. The third emphasizes that better performers prevent errors before they occur or catch them promptly when they are made. [P. 275]

The terms *intelligence, intellectual,* and the like are shorthand substitutes for this construction. We review research evidence that elaborates the construct primarily in its individual, cognitive, educational connection. Of most direct concern here, then, is the emerging agenda of "cognitive instructional psychology," in which intellectual functioning before, during, and after specified instructional treatments is increasingly a central topic (Glaser, 1978a; for detailed reviews, see Glaser & Resnick, 1972; McKeachie, 1974; Wittrock & Lumsdaine, 1977). The research seeks to understand in detail how individuals, and thus how different individuals, function psychologically to perform the kinds of tasks taken as indicators of intelligence, of learning from instruction, and of outcome from instruction. A principal question is how task characteristics moderate or modify this functioning. Resulting theory should be able to explain the chief empirical relations among intelligence, learning, and outcome indicators and to allow the design of the kinds of instructional treatments and measures needed to realize the educational system depicted in Figure 9.2.

9.2.   INTELLIGENCE IN EDUCATION THROUGH HISTORY

It is instructive to consider briefly some aspects of the history of ideas connecting intelligence and education. Some historical milestones and some modern and continuing themes in educational theory and research are reviewed.

HISTORICAL MILESTONES

Intelligence in educational philosophies. Thoughts about the relations between intelligence and education are nothing new. We do not know when, in the dawning of civilization, human beings generally became aware of their intellectual powers or of differences among themselves in these respects. Nor do we know when the teaching of the young was organized with aims beyond those of transmitting immediate survival skills, or when teachers became sensitive to the relevance of individual differences in this regard. We do know that the Chinese were using competitive performance tests – intelligence and educational achievement tests, one might say – in the selection of civil servants as early as 2357 B.C. (DuBois, 1970). An ancient Hebrew reference, in the Haggadah of Passover, concerns four sons – one wise, one wicked, one simpleminded, and one who asks no questions; the reader is instructed in ways to teach the meaning of Passover to each kind of child.[2] Certainly the Greeks also had much to say about intelligence and education, even though it remained for the Roman philosopher Cicero to coin the term *intelligentia* (Burt, 1955; Eysenck, 1979).

Formal education did emerge as one of the earliest social institutions, seemingly in parallel with the recognition that human intellect could and should be formally cultivated. Educational theorists, from antiquity to modern times, have recognized intelligence as relevant to education. Some made distinct assumptions about individual and group differences in intelligence, and some made provision for such differences in their educational designs.

Table 9.1 provides a sampling of major educational theorists through history to give some indication of the stance each took with respect to intelligence, differences in intelligence, and the role of education in intelligence. It reflects our inferences as to the major emphases of each theorist, though it obviously glosses over many lesser and sometimes apparently contradictory statements by each and many other major similarities and differences between them. The first section of

Table 9.1. *A checklist of educational theorists indicating their views on intelligence, human differences in intelligence, and the adaptation of education to such differences*

Column groupings:
- **Definitions of intelligence** — *Absolute and educable:* Single, Multiple; *Relative by:* Race, Social class, Sex, Individual; Differentially educable
- **Educational provisions for development of intelligence** — *Direct training:* Broad mental faculties, Special skills and habits, Special knowledge; *Indirect training:* Didactic experience, Discovery experience, Simplification, Tutoring, Knowledge of individual, Provision of explicit alternatives

Educational theorist	Single	Multiple	Race	Social class	Sex	Individual	Differentially educable	Broad mental faculties	Special skills and habits	Special knowledge	Didactic experience	Discovery experience	Simplification	Tutoring	Knowledge of individual	Provision of explicit alternatives	Other notes relevant to adaptive education
Socrates (470?–399 B.C.)	X							X									Socratic method implied some teacher adaptation
Isocrates (436–368 B.C.)	X						X	X									Emphasized the gymnastics of mind
Plato (427–347 B.C.)		X		X	O	X	X	X			X						Proposed state control of mandatory education and eugenics program for all
Aristotle (384–322 B.C.)		X	X	X	X	X	X	X	X				X				Allowed students to help form course of study
Quintilian (A.D. 35–95)		X				X	X	X							X	X	Initiated idea that teacher is crucial in adapting to student differences
Augustine (354–430)		X				X	X	X		X							Suggested that teachers make lecture summaries as extra help
Erasmus (1466–1536)		X			O	X	X		X	X				X			Stressed importance of early learning
Luther (1483–1546)	X				O	X	X			X			X				Stressed compulsory education for all
Ignatius Loyola (1491–1556)	X					X	X	X	X		O						Emphasized competition among class members
Comenius (1592–1670)		X			O	X	X	X	X	X	X	X			X	X	Proposed educational stages coordinated with intelligence development for graduated training and selection
Locke (1632–1704)		X		X		X	X	X	X			X		X	X		Proposed that learning requires readiness. Abilities develop through experience and exercise

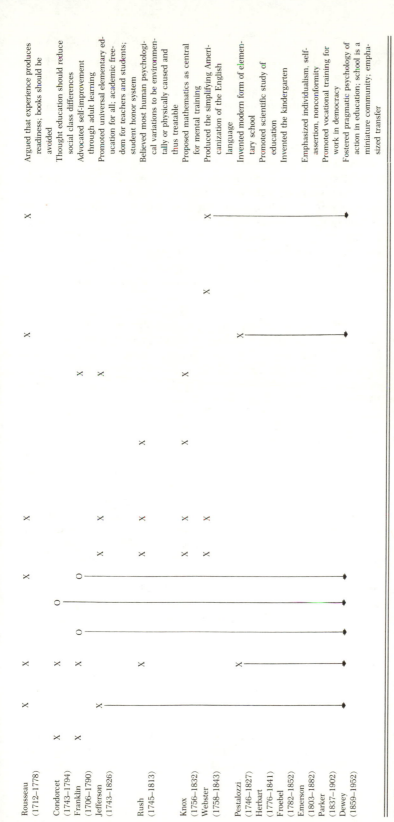

Note: X = a positive endorsement of the view indicated by the column heading; O = a contrary view, e.g., Plato regarded males and females as equal in intelligence and educability; blank = no strong view, or emphasis placed elsewhere; arrows = an unbroken consistency across theorists from that point.

the table notes whether each theorist tended to regard intelligence more simply as a single quality or more broadly as a multiple quality, as an educable quality in some absolute sense across humanity at large, and/or as a relative quality showing various group and individual differences, with or without the implication of differential educability. The second section then indicates some of the principal educational aims and means proposed by each theorist as relevant to the promotion of intellectual development. The last column includes other items about these theorists that relate to their views on adaptive education.[3]

Several trends seem notable. First, throughout most of Western history, human intellect has been regarded as multifaceted and educable, in either absolute or differential terms. The rare exceptions seem connected to emphases on religious doctrine (Luther and Ignatius Loyola) or to the brevity of the accounts of what may have been complex views (Socrates, Condorcet, and Franklin). For most early writers, observed differential educability *defined* differential intelligence. In other words, differences in intelligence were inferred from observed differences in ease of learning. Second, the view that education should and could reduce intellectual differences associated with race, social class, or gender had to wait for the Enlightenment and the American and French revolutions (Condorcet and Franklin), even though clear statements favoring equality of intelligence and education, between genders at least, had been part of several previous philosophies (Plato, Erasmus, Luther, and Comenius). Some theorists, who are regarded as intellectual giants of their times (Locke, Rousseau), were also clearly prisoners of their times with respect to social class or sex differences, and some proposals for the equalization of educational opportunity offered by later giants (Jefferson) were still relatively restrictive by today's standards. Third, a marked shift is evident in views on individuality and educability as educational history moved into progressivism (Pestalozzi to Dewey). The assumption of individual differences in educability resulting from prior individual differences in intelligence gave way to the assumption of mass educability without much regard to differential prior intelligence.

On the educational methods side of the table, emphasis on direct training of intelligence through the discipline of mental faculties, or its essence in some more specialized kinds of skill, habit, or knowledge, would appear to stretch from Socrates through Comenius. Although a softening of the old philosophies of innate ideas and mental disciplines had been apparent earlier (Quintilian, Erasmus, Comenius), a more drastic shift is associated with Locke.

Locke replaced the concept of innate ideas with a "blank slate," on which each individual's accumulating experience was recorded. Such a view led others to an extreme form of environmentalism, wherein anyone could be molded into anything by appropriate education. Still, Locke also acknowledged native faculties and powers and the importance of individual differences, although withholding judgment on their origins. These faculties were seen as potentials; they became specialized abilities and skills only through exercise in interaction with experience and were probably limited in transferability. Locke's views have had wide and divergent effects on up to the present (see, e.g., Cleverley & Phillips, 1976). They led to the practice of direct training of sensory and perceptual skills in early progressive education and to some modern forms of individualized instruction. They also, however, seem close to the psychology of differential abilities advanced in the first half of this century. Following Locke, some theorists continued to write of "improving minds" (Jefferson) or "training intellect" (Knox), but such references strike one as knowingly metaphorical rather than as implications that exercise develops general mental discipline directly. Both Jefferson and Knox laid more emphasis in their educational designs on indirect training of plural abilities through didactic diversity.

The progressive movement defined the modern elementary school and modern ideas about teacher training, beginning with Pestalozzi but with many echoes from Comenius and Rousseau. Froebel added the kindergarten and advocated special training in preschool education for mothers. The movement championed the education of the whole child through enriched sensory and perceptual experience, discovery learning, and learning by doing, preferably with natural objects and experiences rather than with books. This is termed *indirect training* in Table 9.1 to distinguish it from the mental discipline view, even though Pestalozzi, for example, believed in a psychology of mental faculties. One can then trace the elaboration of one or another aspect of progressive thought, from Herbart and Froebel to Parker and Dewey, up to World War II. Human beings, particularly children and the younger the better, are infinitely educable if treated humanely. Nevertheless, most progressives urged that subject matter be subordinated to the child's own activities and that book learning be delayed. Education should be child centered, using the educational values of the child's personal and social world, including the value of active, cooperative play. Education draws out the latent creative and esthetic qualities of personality much more than it puts knowledge in. The later progressives, and particularly Dewey, sought an integration of child and curriculum as an experiential medium for mental growth, but the aim of education was to be social morality and social progress, preparation for work and life in a democracy, not mastery of subject matter or knowledge for its own sake. Although new learning is interpreted and integrated in intellectual development by relating it to prior learning, interest and effort more than intelligence provide the keys.

A wealth of ideas in progressive theory suggest how teachers and parents might arrange early educational experiences to foster intellectual development, just as in Piagetian theory (see, e.g., Furth, 1970). The theories disregard or downplay, however, the growth of individual differences in intellect and the potential effects on this growth of formal teaching of the disciplines of later education. Dewey, and other modern writers in his wake, judged particular educational exercises according to their effectiveness in fostering higher cognitive processes, broader conceptual thinking, and social skills. By emphasizing transferable knowledge and skill rather than the immediate objectives of particular lessons, they were assuming generalizable aptitude development. The vehicle for transfer, however, was identical elements across experiences, because psychological experiments (Thorndike & Woodworth, 1901) had apparently written the end of the formal discipline hypothesis. Also, all of the progressives (from Pestalozzi to Dewey) did emphasize the individuality of learners in one way or another. Teachers were admonished to understand a child's nature so as to adapt teaching to the child. As Anastasi (1958) has noted, however, there was really no detailed concern for individual differences; *individual* in progressive writings often seems to refer more to the absolute qualities of "human nature."

Thus, the abstract idea of teaching adapted to intellectual differences among individual learners for the purpose of developing aptitude, directly or indirectly, has been carried along the whole stream of educational theory, but actual procedures for accomplishing this have never really been made explicit. One finds more relevant ideas in the older literature than in most of the progressive theories. Erasmus emphasized tutoring variations to fit individual differences. Comenius authored illustrated texts in multiple languages and advocated adjustment and staging of teaching to fit individual differences, though he used only one method himself. Aristotle and Luther, who had little else to say about adaptive education, produced alternative, simplified lectures and texts to fit "the masses." Ignatius Loyola, though he explicitly ruled out variation in teaching method, nonetheless counseled his Jesuit teachers to identify the talented for extra advanced help.

If one takes the primary premise of this chapter – namely, that education is an aptitude development program, that intelligence is an organization of aptitudes for learning and transfer, and that instruction must be designed both to remove inaptitudes directly where possible and to adapt alternative treatments to capitalize on or to compensate for persistent aptitude differences in order to develop other aptitudes – then the line of educational theory running from Quintilian through Erasmus and Comenius to Locke and the Enlightenment seems the most productive. Some selections from progressive theory can also be used (e.g., Dewey's concept of education for learning-to-learn and transfer), but they must be crossed with a modern interactional (i.e., Darwinian) view of individual differences. The 1st-century words of Quintilian, though the oldest in this line, may also be among the most suggestive:

It is generally and not unreasonably regarded as the sign of a good teacher that he should be able to differentiate between the abilities of his respective pupils and to know their natural bent. The gifts of nature are infinite in their variety, and mind differs from mind almost as much as body from body. . . . Many again think it useful to direct their instruction to the fostering of natural advantages and to guide the talents of their pupils along the lines which they instinctively tend to follow . . . . a teacher of oratory after careful observation of a boy's stylistic preferences, be they for terseness and polish, energy, dignity, charm, roughness, brilliance or wit, will so adapt his instructions to individual needs that each pupil will be pushed forward in the sphere for which his talents seem specially to design him; for nature, when cultivated, goes from strength to strength, while he who runs counter to her bent is ineffective in those branches of the art for which he is less suited and weakens the talents which he seemed born to employ . . . . to my thinking this view is only partially true. It is undoubtedly necessary to note the individual gifts of each boy, and no one would ever convince me that it is not desirable to differentiate courses of study with this in view. One boy will be better adapted for the study of history, another for poetry, another for law, while some perhaps had better be packed off to the country. The teacher of rhetoric will distinguish such special aptitudes, just as our gymnast will turn one pupil into a runner, another into a boxer or wrestler or an expert at some other of the athletic accomplishments for which prizes are awarded at the sacred games. But on the other hand, he who is destined for the bar must study not one department merely, but must perfect himself in all the accomplishments which his profession demands, even though some of them may seem too hard for him when he approaches them as a learner. For if natural talent alone were sufficient, education might be dispensed with. Suppose we are given a pupil who, like so many, is of depraved tastes and swollen with his own conceit; shall we suffer him to go his own sweet way? If a boy's disposition is naturally dry and jejune, ought we not to feed it up or at any rate clothe it in fairer apparel? For, if in some cases it is necessary to remove certain qualities, surely there are others where we may be permitted to add what is lacking. Not that I would set myself against the will of nature. No innate good quality should be neglected, but defects must be made good and weaknesses made strong. When Isocrates, the prince of instructors, whose works proclaim his eloquence no less than his pupils testify to his excellence as a teacher, gave his opinion of Ephorus and Theopompus to the effect that the former needed the spur and the latter the curb, what was his meaning? Surely not that the sluggish temperament of the one and the headlong ardour of the other alike required modification by instruction, but rather that each would gain from an admixture of the qualities of the other.

In the case of weaker understandings however some concession must be made and they should be directed merely to follow the call of their nature, since thus they will be more effective in doing the only thing that lies in their power. But if we are fortunate enough to meet with richer material, such as justifies us in the hope of producing a real orator, we must leave no oratorical virture uncared for. For though he will necessarily have a natural bent for some special department of oratory, he will not feel repelled by the others, and by sheer application will develop his other qualities until they equal those in which he naturally excels. [Butler, 1954, pp. 265–269]

Quintilian's five themes are clear, and as relevant to educational research and practice today as they were in 1st-century Rome.

1.   Identify apparent aptitudes and inaptitudes for each learner.
2.   Help to develop aptitudes by differentiating courses of instruction, allowing individual educational goals. Guide learners in choosing courses according to their aptitudes.
3.   Within a course of instruction toward a common goal, seek to develop all relevant aptitudes even if some are weak at the start; adapt alternative instructional treatments to the individual's aptitude pattern, so as to remove defects and to build up strengths where they are lacking.
4.   Use the individual's strengths to work on the weaknesses. Teaching that runs counter to an individual's aptitudes may actually weaken those aptitudes.
5.   Even if, below a certain level of general intelligence, little can be done other than to choose goals in keeping with special aptitudes, above that general level, appropriately adapted instruction can bring initially weak aptitudes up to equal other, prior, strengths.

Scientific beginnings. Unfortunately, early educational and psychological research did not address these hypotheses programmatically and, for the most part, still has not done so. Through the 19th and early 20th centuries, progressivism and pragmatism – and the social reform movement in general – mixed with two different misunderstandings of Darwin's then new theory. The mixture produced a framework for education that moved away from rather than toward the ideal of Figure 9.2. The traditional educational design of Figure 9.1 prevailed.

On the one hand, it was believed that universal education gave all persons the opportunity to show their natural talents, regardless of family background. Higher talents were thus selected for advanced development by the formal and informal tests of education. The "survival of the fittest" interpretation of Darwin's theory seemed consistent with this view. Galton (1869) demonstrated the link to heredity. Intelligence increasingly came to be regarded as the single rank ordering of people on general mental fitness, discoverable through differential educational progress. As in the centuries before, education defined intelligence.

On the other hand, the later wave of Social Darwinists turned Darwin's adaptation formula around; they saw environments as rank orderable from good to bad on a single continuum. The aim, therefore, was to design the best possible educational environment for all children, and this aim fit perfectly with progressive theory. The way to reduce the inequity of Figure 9.1 was not to change the design but to insert the optimum instructional treatment in the central box. Through this whole period, the basic idea of systematic adaptive instruction was missed. (Fuller discussion of these trends is available in Cronbach & Snow, 1977, pp. 6–12.)

Scientific psychology also moved in other directions at this time, owing partly to other transactions between intelligence and education. Systematic measurement of individual differences had begun early in the 19th century. Interest in the detailed anthropometric, psychomotor, and sensoripsychometric study of individual differences grew rapidly. The aim was to assess precisely all the elementary reactions associated with intelligence. The work of Galton and J. McKeen Cattell is notable, but Wundt, Ebbinghaus, and other luminaries in the history of psychology also made central contributions (see Boring, 1957). Jastrow (1901), in his presidential address to the American Psychological Association, summed up the hopes that this trend would illuminate the study of intelligence substantially.

The trend was dragged to a halt, however, by an educational study (Wissler, 1901). The detailed measurements of Galton and Cattell failed to correlate with college achievement, implying either that the measures did not represent intelligence or that the interpretation of intelligence as general learning or adaptation ability was wrong. Because academic achievements did correlate across subject areas, it was the Galton–Cattell measures that were questioned, not the theory of single rank ordering of intelligence and achievement. Spearman (1904) then identified intelligence with the central tendency apparent in intercorrelations among school achievement measures.

Meanwhile, Binet had been experimenting with some success, using measures of the more complex mental processes involved in judgment and reasoning. He was commissioned by the Paris schools to develop objective methods for distinguishing children who would be likely to profit from regular instruction from those who would not; the latter could then be removed to special schools for suitably simplified instruction. In effect, Binet was asked to study the interaction of intelligence and instructional treatment. The items found predictive of school achievement became the Binet–Simon scale and, through translation by Terman, the Stanford–Binet Intelligence Scale. The scale rapidly came into wide use in the United States, especially in education, in the hands of clinical, counseling, and school psychologists. The use of group mental tests, validated against the Stanford–Binet, also spread rapidly following the success of Otis's Army Alpha and Beta tests during World War I. Industrial use of such tests also became widespread. For a detailed historical review of the testing movement, see Linden and Linden (1968). Many original papers are conveniently collected in Jenkins and Paterson (1961). A biography of Binet was written by Wolf (1973).

Mental testing in the schools.   It was perhaps inevitable that educational systems would have to adopt some form of diagnostic assessment. As Tyler (1976) has noted, the passage of universal compulsory education laws placed before the schools the unprecedented problem of teaching to the full range of human diversity. With intelligence operationally and conceptually defined almost solely on educational criteria, and with the use of mental tests in schools proliferating rapidly, misinterpretation and misuses set in. The interpretation of intelligence as unidimensional native capacity lost sight of the fact that Binet, Terman, Otis, and their followers had put together fairly loose collections of empirically valid items, that many items reflected prior educational advantages, and that the original intent (of Binet, at least) had been to identify persons with special educational problems and needs. The tests were samples of scholastic ability, reflecting only a person's development to date of testing. To interpret them as measuring "general intelligence" was a flagrant overgeneralization. Yet, massive evidence accumulated to indicate that test-score differences were associated with educational progress all along the age scale. The results of comparisons among occupational, ethnic, socioeconomic, and other groups using the tests also fit with then current public attitudes. The prevailing interpretation produced the tendency to label children in schools according to arbitrarily defined levels along a single-rank-order continuum. Ability grouping became regular practice, and special education never really developed the truly *alternative* instructional treatments originally envisioned. Although controversy about the interpretation of mental tests continued in the public press, as well as in the scientific literature (see Cronbach, 1975), educational practice was unaffected; it solidified into a routine that remained virtually unchanged through World War II to the early 1960s, with minor exceptions. In the elementary schools, progressive ideas seeped in, but practical economics preserved the 30-child classroom. Learners were divided into faster and slower reading groups, mathematics groups, and so on, usually corresponding to measured or perceived ability levels, but not really into alternative instructional treatments still aimed at a common goal but adapted to different abilities. High schools developed the most obvious divisions based on scholastic aptitude, designated as "college preparatory," "regular," and "business" or "vocational" streams. The school systems of England and Western Europe employed similar organization, but the United States relied much more heavily on mental tests. The tests were deemed objective and thus fair; they could replace the socioeconomic, ethnic, religious, and familial privileges and prejudices that had influenced older educational systems, detrimentally, for centuries.

The influence of factor analysis. P. E. Vernon (1951) and other British psychologists, following Spearman (1923), used factor analytic studies of mental tests to evolve a hierarchical model of ability organization. Spearman's *g*, or general intelligence, was superordinate, but two clusters, called verbal–educational ability and spatial–mechanical ability, could be distinguished below it, at least in adolescence. These had obvious relation to different school subjects. Beneath these were the more minor, specialized abilities. In the United States, Thurstone (1938) and then Guilford (1967) concentrated on the special level, developing a long list of "primary" abilities, now organized into Guilford's structure-of-intellect model.

Educational practice was influenced by both these lines of work. For academic prediction and placement purposes, general ability measures yielding total IQ scores, and sometimes separating verbal and nonverbal subscores, were most often used. Attempts at developing diagnostic measures of more specific educational abilities, distinguishing vocabulary, reading comprehension, and the like, usually showed that the subdivisions were strongly correlated and thus not readily distinguishable. For counseling and guidance purposes among adolescents and adults, however, the multifactor aptitude batteries that emanated from the Thurstone–Guilford tradition were preferred because profile differences were thought to relate to success in different specialized educational programs and their associated subsequent occupations. The evidence tended to show that different abilities do correlate to some extent with success in learning different kinds of subject matter, and the patterns of correlations change over years of schooling as emphases in curricula change; differential ability tests can be useful in guiding individual choices (Cronbach, 1970). For some educational and many occupational prediction purposes, however, the differential measures have done no better than a general ability measure used alone (Ghiselli, 1966; McNemar, 1964).

Curriculum reform in the 1960s. General and special abilities had come to be regarded as fairly fixed, stable characteristics of persons. Differential development was thought to be predetermined by heredity. Education could make use of test-score information in various ways, but efforts to develop such abilities directly were expected to be fruitless, given psychology's denial of the doctrine of formal discipline, or even of transfer beyond identical elements. Educational rhetoric in these times, as often before, still included emphasis on general intellectual development – teaching students to think, to reason, to solve problems, and so on. Dewey and progressivism had changed the character of many elementary schools (Cremin, 1961), and ideas about cognitive structure and gestalt principles had come into favor in educational thinking (see Hilgard, 1964; McDonald, 1964). Much of educational practice, however, particularly in higher elementary levels and beyond, emphasized knowledge and skill acquisition, where the units were facts and fairly simple procedures. Associationism in psychology reinforced this orientation in education. If intelligence was simply "the sum of millions of situation-response connections" (E. L. Thorndike, 1921a, p. 4; see also 1921b, pp. 363–371), then education should concentrate on accumulating them.

A drastic change in theory and practice was then wrought by a combination of two strong forces. First, Sputnik ushered in the space era, bringing the implication that U.S. education had fallen behind in the development of scientific and mathematical talent. Scientists and mathematicians joined with educators to produce the "new curriculum" movement, which sought to correct this. "New math" and "new science" projects developed instructional materials aimed not at teaching the traditional facts and concepts but at developing aptitude. The new theory recognized that factual knowledge soon becomes obsolete, especially as technological advances accelerate. The educational requirement, then, was to equip students with the deep-structure understanding and flexible problem-solving ability they would need for later learning in a new and rapidly changing world. Teaching methods also changed to suit; the new emphasis was on the promotion of discovery learning.

Second, the civil rights movement and associated judicial decisions brought pressure and then federal programs to erase the educational disadvantages that stemmed from de facto and de jure inequities. Education was again seen as a principal vehicle for righting social wrongs. Head Start, Follow Through, Upward Bound, "Sesame Street," and many other attempts at compensatory education aimed frankly at developing intelligence.

This movement was fueled by the new awakening of psychology to the rich complexity of cognitive organization and development and to the role of experience in the production of intelligence. Major references, showing the direction of thought in cognitive and instructional psychology during this period, come from Miller, Galanter, and Pribram (1960) and from Bruner (1960, 1966). J. M. Hunt's (1961) early book presented the central hypothesis and its challenge for education. He combined ideas coming from research on learning-to-learn and transfer, factor analysis, Piaget's theory of development, Hebb's neuropsychological theory, and the then new work on computer simulation of cognition to conclude the following:

Intelligence . . . would appear to be a matter of the number of strategies for processing information that have been differentiated and have achieved the mobility which permits them to be available in a variety of situations. [P. 354]

Intelligence should be conceived as intellectual capacities based on central processes hierarchically arranged within the intrinsic portions of the cerebrum. These central processes are approximately analogous to the strategies for information processing and action with which electronic computers are programmed. With such a conception of intelligence, the assumptions that intelligence is fixed and that its development is predetermined by the genes are no longer tenable. [P. 362]

. . . it is no longer unreasonable to consider that it might be feasible to discover ways to govern the encounters that children have with their environments, especially during the early years of their development, to achieve a substantially faster rate of intellectual development and a substantially higher adult level of intellectual capacity. [P. 363]

The challenge was accepted, and a decade of educational and psychological research, development, and field evaluations ensued, fueled by unprecedented governmental support. The goal, simply put, was to improve the generalizable intellectual, learning, and problem-solving skills of students all across the public school years, particularly in reading, mathematics, and prescience. A primary focus was to provide enriched educational opportunities to young, disadvantaged children during their preschool and early-elementary-school years. Gains made during these early years were expected to carry over into later grades. Zigler and Valentine (1979) have produced a comprehensive history of Project Head Start, the focus of the movement.

Evaluation in the 1970s.   The 1960s ended in controversy. The massive study of equality of educational opportunity by Coleman and colleagues (1966), commissioned by the U.S. government following the Civil Rights Act of 1964, found that many American school districts were still largely segregated, with great regional and racial differences in school facilities, programs, and student characteristics. On average, disadvantaged, ethnic minority students scored lower on standardized ability and achievement measures than did middle-class white students; the gap increased with grade in school. Further, with student background characteristics such as ability and socioeconomic status controlled statistically, school characteristics accounted for only a small fraction of the differences in student achievement. Also, however, the achievement of majority students seemed less affected and that of minority students more affected by poor school quality. Reviewing the storm of reanalyses and adding data from other sources, Jencks and colleagues (1972) found the Coleman conclusions supportable, with some qualifications. Jencks's work also concerned the influence of educational opportunity on adult economic success, concluding that the relationship, though small, might well be underestimated (see also Jencks et al., 1979).

Results of evaluations of compensatory education programs also began to come in, suggesting limited success, if any. An early Head Start evaluation (Cicarelli, Cooper, & Granger, 1969) had compared participants and nonparticipants in full-year and summer programs. Although parents of Head Start children supported the program, the children's educational performance appeared not to differ appreciably from their non–Head Start peers. The Office of Economic Opportunity conducted a national experiment on performance contracting (Ray, 1972) that seemed to end in failure, despite some limited positive effects in some locations with some children. What gains there were in various compensatory programs seemed to dissipate in subsequent years. A study reported by Weikart (1972) had randomly assigned 3- and 4-year-old underprivileged children to either an untreated control group or to one of three enrichment programs. Treated children showed some initial gains in IQ relative to control children, but no differences were found 3 years after the children left the program. Similar findings came from other studies. The conclusion seemed to be that although preschool enrichment programs may produce modest, short-term increases in IQ scores, declines occur when children enter or return to regular public school. Even the modest increases might be attributable to practice on the tests rather than to basic intellectual advancement. The issue of heredity versus environment was again raised: How much substantive intellectual gain could be expected from compensatory education programs if individual differences were largely genetic in origin (Jensen, 1969, 1972)?

It was, however, also possible to discount some negative results, to find positive results, and even to begin to identify the characteristics of successful programs (White, 1973; Zigler, 1975). In the face of the mixed findings and the storm of public and scientific controversy, compensatory education programs were made more intense, more complex, and more experimental (Datta, 1975). The programs that followed, such as Head Start Planned Variation and Follow Through, sought to design and compare many alternative treatments systematically rather than to test the effectiveness of any one program against conventional practices.

Evaluation studies also necessarily became more important and more complex and thus less readily interpreted by both experts and educational decision makers. The effects of some programs were notable on relatively specific tasks that were closely linked to program goals. Direct instruction in reading and mathematics did seem to produce improvements in the specific skills taught. Long-term effects on general intelligence or achievement, or various affective outcomes, however, were still difficult to establish, and there was the implication that the programs producing the most immediate gains in special reading and math skills were not necessarily the ones that might promote more general, transferable intellectual development (Stallings, 1975; Stallings & Kaskowitz, 1974).

The evaluation of "Sesame Street" (Ball & Bogatz, 1970; Bogatz & Ball, 1971) suggested that children who viewed the programs most gained most on tests that had been developed to assess specific program goals. Small or no gains were associated with other cognitive tasks. Younger viewers (age 3) seemed to gain more than older viewers (age 5). Though Spanish-speaking children showed unusually large gains in the 1st-year evaluation, these findings were not verified in the 2nd year.

With the increasing complexity of field evaluations, serious questions began to be raised about how such studies were conducted. Summative evaluations (Scriven, 1967) had typically tried to apply conventional experimental paradigms in field settings, often with some difficulty. Program goals were identified and the study was then designed to determine the effectiveness of the program in achieving those goals. So, for example, the evaluations of "Sesame Street" attempted to establish random groups of viewers and control children in order to compare their performance on a series of cognitive posttests, designed to correspond to program objectives. However, random assignment to treatment is difficult to achieve or preserve in field studies. The parents and children determined the frequency with which they viewed "Sesame Street." Prior achievement level was confounded with amount of viewing; higher achievers viewed more. Differences at posttest could thus be attributed to preexisting differences between viewers and non-viewers. Other questions concerned the external validity of such evaluations: Did attempts to control the program, to the extent necessary for evaluation purposes, alter the nature of the program itself? In their reanalysis, Cook and colleagues (1975) cast "reasonable doubt about whether 'Sesame Street' was causing as large and generalized learning gains in 1970 and 1971 as were attributed to the program . . ." (p. 24–26).

The evaluations of compensatory education and of the quality of education in general, brought on by broad changes in desegregation patterns, television programming, and so on, have been filled with such inconsistencies from study to study and reanalysis to re-reanalysis. The implication is that educational results cannot be generalized in any event. Findings of positive or negative or no effect for a program in one study say little about what might be found for that program in another school or locale. As teaching personnel and students and settings vary, so do results. Thus, even apparently successful programs have to be monitored in new sites, and even in the same site over time (Cronbach, 1975; Snow, 1977a, 1977b). Longitudinal, locally based research and evaluation that is sensitive to multivariate outcomes, both anticipated and unanticipated, is required. It is striking to learn, for example, from Weikart's (see Epstein & Weikart, 1979) persistent follow-up that children who had not sustained measured intellectual advantages as a result of treatment nonetheless showed higher educational achievement, less high-school dropout, and more social and emotional maturity as young adults than did untreated controls. The implication of the Follow Through summary (Kennedy, 1978) is also sobering: programs that succeed in meeting short-term focused achievement goals may be particularly unsuccessful when judged on more general aptitude development criteria. The lessons learned in the growth of the educational evaluation movement are many – at the core of these is the clear demonstration that generalization in education, across people, places, tests, and time, is severely limited.

Searching discussions of educational goals and values have also been prompted. The "Sesame Street" results, for example, showed that advantaged children gained as much as, and perhaps more than, disadvantaged children from viewing the programs. If the effect was to widen the achievement gap, despite absolute gains, were such programs justified? The issue of the relative size of the "achievement gap" between advantaged and disadvantaged children questioned the basic goals of compensatory education. Was the educational problem of the disadvantaged a relative or an absolute one? As Cook and colleagues (1975) explain:

If "Sesame Street" had had larger effects in a single viewing season or if viewing for several seasons has larger effects than viewing for a single season, then one would be faced with the problem of deciding between an absolute and a relative conception of the educational problem of economically disadvantaged children. The problem would arise, because, under the conditions already outlined, the disadvantaged might absolutely gain from the show but might relatively lose by falling even further behind the advantaged. How can absolute gains be justified if there are relative losses? Which is more important to the disadvantaged or to the nation at large; that disadvantaged children know more than at present or that gaps between specific social groups be narrowed? Is the problem of the disadvantaged one of what they do not know or of what the advantaged know more than they? [P. 23–24]

The 1970s closed with these puzzles and with residual hopes in some quarters, and doubts in others, that intellect could in fact be directly or generally developed. The educators, left with mixed messages, continued to rely as always before on the kinds of handed-down educational practices that seemed to fit the demands of their everyday economic, social, and psychological realities.

MODERN THEMES

Two streams of educational research over recent decades aimed at studying systematically ideas that had been promoted by many prior educational theorists. One concerned the possibility of individualizing instruction to accommodate individual differences. The other concerned the educational value of guiding learners to discoveries in subject matter or in nature, rather than presenting concepts didactically. Each was a theme of one or another of the compensatory or new curriculum programs, but each has its own history distinct enough from other movements to be treated separately. Though not typically associated, the results of research on each connect in a potentially useful way. Beyond these is the new theme of modern cognitive psychology. This section takes up each of the three in turn, to bring the historical review up to the set of hypotheses addressed by current and continuing research.

Individualization of instruction.   Adaptation to individuals was a theme in the progressive education movement. The so-called Dalton plan and Winnetka plan of the 1920s were early attempts to realize this aim, reflecting also some of E. L. Thorndike's ideas about individual differences in intelligence (see Baker, 1973), and Pressey (1926) had developed educational tests geared to provide individualized feedback. In the 1950s, Skinner (1954; see also Glaser, 1978b) then opened an era of research on teaching machines and programmed instruction by drawing educational implications from his behavioral theory of learning; instruction was to be itemized into small steps in which correct responses could be shaped with immediate reinforcement. Students could control their own pace. Carroll (1963, 1965) also developed a conceptual model of school learning, based more on educational and cognitive theory than on behaviorism; it, too, identified aspects of time available for instruction and time needed by individual students as key focuses. From these bases grew much of the thinking behind computerized instruction (CAI) (Atkinson & Wilson, 1969), Individually Prescribed Instruction (IPI) (see Glaser, 1977; Weisgerber, 1971), Individually Guided Education (IGE) (see Klausmeier, Rossmiller & Saily, 1977), Programmed Learning According to Needs (PLAN) (see Weisgerber, 1971), mastery learning (see Block, 1971; Bloom, 1976; Block & Burns, 1977), and the Keller Plan (Keller, 1968; Kulik, Kulik, & Cohen, 1979).

The basic idea of all these programs is to provide for individual differences in pace of learning across an orderly sequence of instructional steps, on the assumption that intellectual differences among students are reflected mainly in differences in learning rate. There is little concern for qualitative or quantitative differences in intelligence that might predict substantive differences in the style or strategy of learning among individuals. However, the methods used to accomplish adaptation to learning rate differ in many details, including the roles assigned to teachers and learners. Some approaches allow far more flexibility in varying instruction to accommodate stylistic or other nonpace-connected student differences than do others. In mastery learning procedures, for example, learners who have not met established performance criteria for some instructional unit or topic can be led through a review by a teacher, who translates material into terms more likely to be understood by some individual students; alternative instructional treatments can be used when the first method of choice does not succeed and, as a last resort, individualized tutoring is possible. The advance of interactive computerized instruction also allows a variety of diagnostic and specialized help programs adapted to the needs of particular students; the computer can build up a unique learning history for each student and sequence further instruction accordingly. This is a far cry from the traditional Skinnerian linear program wherein pace variation is the only individualized feature of what is otherwise a uniform instructional treatment for all students.

Another feature of such instruction is its concentration, for the most part, on immediate specific instructional objectives. Both instruction and assessment measures tend to be criterion referenced (Glaser & Nitko, 1971). The generalization or extension of learning to other or more advanced material is not directly considered. Pacing variation is judged successful if more students reach the immediate criterion in such conditions, without regard for what faster learners do, or could do, beyond that criterion.

Research on programmed instruction has progressed to a point where an evaluation of the basic approach is fairly clear, but a solid research base for most of the later approaches is still being built and there are many methodological problems (see particularly Block & Burns, 1977; Kulik, Kulik, & Cohen, 1979; and Cronbach & Snow, 1977, for reviews and critiques of current research). The conclusion, so far, seems to be that no method of individualization yet invented removes all effects of prior differences in intellectual abilities. Even when some method appears to do so with respect to immediate achievement criteria, it is often found that aptitude differences reappear when retention or transfer is evaluated or when students move on to more advanced lessons. Individualization in the pace of instruction alone is clearly insufficient to overcome intellectual differences related to learning. This could suggest that there is more to the relation of intelligence to learning than simply individual differences in learning rate or mental speed. Qualitatively different alternative treatments are needed to adapt instruction to intellectual differences, and current research in several of the approaches mentioned is exploring such alternatives. Several of these approaches and alternatives might be made to fit the requirements of the truly adaptive system of Figure 9.2 in the future.

Learning by discovery. In contrast to research on individualization, work on discovery learning (or inductive teaching) has focused on cognitive outcomes beyond immediate achievement, such as the development of broader reasoning skills or deeper conceptual understanding. These were the objectives also of the new science and mathematics curriculum projects, whether the term *discovery*, or *induction*, was used explicitly or not. In research in either field, the pace of instruction was held more or less constant among contrasting treatments, whereas the style of teaching was varied. Teachers (or texts) give examples of phenomena or information about events, encouraging learners to ask questions about deeper meanings and structures. Often, the learner works directly with laboratory or demonstration materials as an active inquirer. In contrast, in didactic or expository instruction, examples follow rules and principles, all given explicitly by teacher or text; the learner here is a more passive receiver.

Curriculum evaluation studies and direct research on discovery learning reached no generalizable conclusion regarding the value of such instruction or the role of intelligence in it (Cronbach, 1977; Cronbach & Snow, 1977; Shulman & Keislar, 1966). The strongest implication runs counter to that of research on individualization by pace variation in two respects. Whereas individualized pacing can reduce the relation between prior intellectual differences and (usually) specific achievement criteria, inductive instruction often increases the relation between prior intellectual differences and (usually) more generalized achievement criteria. Thus, individualized didactic instruction may be helpful to less able learners but not to more able learners, and discovery-oriented, teacher-paced instruction may be helpful to more able learners but not to less able learners; the intellectual differences are less pronounced on immediate achievement and more pronounced on generalized achievement, retention, or transfer. This is a hypothesis for further research, not a grand conclusion. It displays, however, the type of complex hypothesis that has come out of educational research in recent decades. It suggests that intelligence comes into play in learning as a function of situational demand, that instructional situations vary in this respect, and that both individual intellectual differences and instructional situation differences are manifested in different kinds of cognitive outcome effects. In other words, as the learning situation demands higher-order cognitive functioning on the part of learners (i.e., as in typical inductive instruction as contrasted with typical programmed instruction) and/or as outcome measures reflect higher-order cognitive functioning (i.e., retention and transfer as contrasted with immediate achievement), intelligence differences become manifest in performance. What is needed, however, is a detailed understanding of these phenomena, expressed in psychological *process* terms: How do intelligence differences lead to differences in learning processes under different kinds of instructional treatments that lead in turn to different kinds of cognitive outcomes?

Modern cognitive psychology.   Here enters the modern psychology of cognition and instruction. World War II produced experimental psychologists who had had to apply what they knew about learning to the improvement of training. Assessment of this experience showed that the traditional psychology of learning had provided some semblance of an approach to education (Miller, 1957) but was in general woefully inadequate (Gagné & Bolles, 1959). Research then aimed toward an instructional psychology capable of meeting the problems of educational improvement (Ausubel, 1963; Gagné, 1965; Glaser, 1965, 1978a). At the same time, experimentalists had been induced by war necessities to examine the capabilities of humans as information processors (Broadbent, 1958; Sperling, 1960). The advent of information theory, cybernetics, and high-speed computers also helped to launch the revolution now called cognitive psychology (Neisser, 1967; Newell & Simon, 1972). Because of this development, psychology now has the opportunity to become more useful to education than it has ever been before. The theoretical machinery finally appears to be equal to the complexity of educational hypotheses, so there is new hope that such hypotheses can be addressed, unraveled, and understood. Conferences on the coordination of cognitive theory and instruction now appear with regularity (Anderson, Spiro, & Montague, 1977; Klahr, 1976; Lesgold et al., 1978). Though considerations regarding the role of intelligence in learning and education were not central early in this movement, they have come to the fore during its most recent years (Friedman, Das, & O'Connor, 1981; Resnick, 1976; Snow, Federico, & Montague, 1980). Thus the stage seems now finally set for the development of a cognitive psychology of intelligence and learning in education.

9.3. CONTINUING ISSUES AND A THEORETICAL FRAMEWORK

Several conceptual and methodological issues of importance to educational and psychological theory and practice emerge as one considers the history just reviewed. There are several lessons to be learned. These deserve fresh attention in the planning and the evaluation of future research on intelligence in education.

INTELLIGENCE AND LEARNING AS EDUCATIONAL CONCEPTS

The process of education, and the conduct of research, development, and evaluation in it, is seen to be complex: One does not simply apply the findings and methods of psychological science in educational settings, nor does one simply bring educational problems into the laboratory for systematic solution. Educational psychology is not psychology applied to education in any simple sense of the term *applied*. There is a two-way street, and the traffic consists of conceptual enrichment much more than it does of scientific laws, facts, or techniques. Concepts established in the laboratory enrich the thinking and observations of researchers, evaluators, and practitioners attempting to reach useful systematic analyses of educational phenomena where they occur. Concepts developed in educational research, evaluation, and practice, in turn, enrich the thinking of the laboratory researcher, for they show the ways in which provisional theoretical models are undercomplicated. This is the way it should be. Unfortunately for the psychology of intelligence and for the psychology of learning, it has not often been so.

The history shows that our concept of intelligence is, to a significant extent, an emergent property of education. Education exercises native faculties of intelligence already in place, or education produces intelligence, or both. Differences in intelligence are discoverable by observing differences in educability, or differences in education result in differences in intelligence, or both. In any case, education is fundamental to the definition of intelligence. When scientific psychology entered the historical scene, and since, its measures and its concepts of intelligence were sculpted to fit the educational criteria. Psychology has certainly contributed a measurement technology to education – perhaps psychology's major contribution to practical human affairs so far – but one can rightly complain that the resulting construct of intelligence is not fully representative of what one might wish to mean by use of the term (see Neisser, 1976, 1979). Nonetheless, a great deal of useful evidence has been accumulated in education by using the technology of mental testing. Educational theorists also have contributed a body

of useful thinking about intelligence and education. Some have thought of education as aptitude development and about adapting it to individual differences.
There are even some particular hypotheses about the psychological nature of
aptitudes in relation to alternative kinds of instruction. Still, the two-way connection was never really established. Educational thinking was not brought into the
laboratory. No psychological theory of mental-test performance has been developed to explain why individual differences in such performance relate so consistently and strongly to indexes of school learning. The call for such a theory has
appeared off and on throughout modern history (see, e.g., McNemar, 1964), but
the call has never really been answered.

Learning is also very much a construct rooted in education, and again educational thinkers have offered much of use. School learning tasks have long been
seen to involve the acquisition, adaptation, combination, and long-term storage,
retrieval, and use of complex cognitive structures that should be the prime focus
of learning theory. Reading James (1958) or Dewey (1900) or E. L. Thorndike
(1906), one might have expected that the development of learning theory would
never have strayed far from analyzing school learning as the most obvious instance of learning in life. Yet there has been little contact between education and
the psychology of learning since the 1920s. This is also not a new observation. As
Hilgard and Bower (1966, p. 424) observed:

> The argument has been made that more complex behaviors – thinking and problem solving –
> could be more easily understood once simple behaviors under especially simplified conditions
> were better understood. . . . After some 30 or 40 years without striking advances in our under-
> standing of the capabilities of the human mind, this argument has begun to have a hollow ring.

The emergent properties of learning, as seen in educational settings, were presumably lost in the laboratory.

Despite the failings of the past, it is clear that psychology and education have
never been better geared to contribute to mutual conceptual enrichment, and this
is now particularly true with respect to research on intelligence and learning.
Theoretical psychologists are now turning to the analysis of school learning tasks
because, as Greeno (1980) noted: "Basic principles of learning may be more easily
discerned by observing interactions between new information and existing knowledge structure than they have been in situations where the effect of prior knowledge has been minimized" (p. 38). Greeno went on to say that:

> it seems quite certain that instructional tasks constitute a domain of study and analysis that is
> potentially productive for psychological theory. Learning tasks in the school curriculum are
> complex enough to raise non-trivial theoretical questions. At the same time, the nature of the
> concepts and skills to be acquired has been shaped by a process of evolution in which materials
> that cannot be learned by most students and methods of instruction that are patently unsuc-
> cessful have been eliminated over the years. Cognitive psychologists can consider school
> learning tasks as species of learning that have adapted to the constraints of children's cognitive
> limitations and the normal abilities of teachers and authors of instructional materials. A deep
> theoretical understanding of the psychological processes involved in school learning could
> become the keystone of a significant new psychological theory of learning. [P. 39]

Much the same statement might be made about intelligence tests. They also
constitute a domain of study and analysis that is potentially productive for psychological theory. They are cognitive tasks more suitable than many others for use in

laboratory analyses of intellectual processes. They are complex enough to raise nontrivial theoretical questions. They, too, have evolved in such a way that materials and methods that are unsuccessful in predicting school learning performance have been eliminated. Thus, a deep theoretical understanding of the psychological processes involved in the role of intelligence in school learning could become the keystone of a significant new psychological theory of intelligence (see also Snow, 1980a).

Further, both mental tests and school learning tasks are convenient vehicles that might be used to ply the two-way street between laboratory and field, bringing the concepts arising from each kind of research into connection with one another. This thought comes at a time, too, when both conventional school curricula and mental-testing practices are under attack. There is demand for improvement on both fronts. The time is ripe for combined research, but a combined theoretical framework is needed. We first need to bring the threads of past thinking together.

Intelligence as learning ability. The early studies of Binet, Wissler, and Spearman seemed to equate intelligence with educational learning ability. Experimental psychologists expected, then, that mental tests should correlate with performance on the kinds of basic learning tasks they studied in the laboratory. Woodrow (1946), however, after a series of investigations, concluded that no such correlation could be found. Later studies conducted in the Thurstone tradition (Allison, 1960; Gulliksen, 1961; Stake, 1961) also failed to find substantial relationships. With the exception of a few (such as McGeogh & Irion, 1952), experimental psychologists thus largely ignored intellectual differences until the 1970s; learning, not intelligence, was the fundamental topic for scientific psychology. Unfortunately, research on the simple learning tasks of the laboratory had little to say to educators, beyond some suggestions about the organization of drill and practice and the value of reinforcement. Unfortunately also, Woodrow's early work was faulty on methodological as well as substantive grounds, and the later work missed what relations existed by concentrating on special abilities rather than on a more general ability construct. What evidence there is actually supports the view that general intelligence relates to conceptual learning and that a separable rote-memory ability relates to rote learning (Cronbach & Snow, 1977). Jensen's (1980) review also suggests that the characteristics of learning tasks that lead to high relations between intelligence and learning are those that also characterize school learning tasks, such as meaningfulness and complexity.

Educational psychology retained an interest in intellectual differences owing to the obvious relation of general mental tests to measures of learning in school, but efforts were bifurcated (Cronbach, 1957). Experimentally oriented research contrasted alternative instructional methods, seeking general improvements without regard to individual differences; initial intellectual differences among students were covaried out of instructional studies statistically or ignored altogether. Correlational research pursued individual prediction of achievement and factor analyses of aptitude and achievement without regard to the particular kinds of instructional programs within which students learned. Isolated hypotheses about the possibility of different kinds of learning abilities being more and less associated with what is called intelligence, such as Jensen's (1969) notion of Level I and Level II abilities, have been studied sporadically (e.g., Rohwer, 1970; Vernon, in press). In the continuing controversy over the heritability of intelligence, however, they have not been tested in sustained instructional research.

Recent research has sought to erase the bifurcation and to reaffirm the close conceptual relation between intelligence, interpreted as general scholastic ability, and learning, interpreted as complex knowledge and skill acquisition and organization. Renewed interest began with the Gagné (1967) symposium. Modern work stems most directly, however, from the development of cognitive psychology in the last decade, its new approaches to the analysis of intelligence (Friedman, Das, & O'Connor, 1981; Resnick, 1976) and of complex school learning (Klahr, 1976; Anderson, Spiro, and Montague, 1977), and its coalescence with research on aptitude × treatment interactions in educational settings (Cronbach, 1975; Cronbach & Snow, 1977; Snow, 1977a; Snow, Federico, & Montague, 1980). A new combination of these streams of research, and a new basis for thinking about intelligence and learning in education, seem to be at hand. Although it is too early to assess the products of this work, it is possible to sketch the outline of emerging theory. The outline goes back to some old ideas that now seem newly translatable and understandable in more detail than was previously possible.

First, intelligence and learning ability cannot be simply equated; school learning and intellectual development have to be thought of as a complex of interwoven multivariate progressions. One cannot assume, as some have done in the past (e.g., J. E. Anderson, 1939; Bloom, 1964), that intelligence measured at one point in time merely reflects experience to that point, whereas intellectual growth to a later point in time is an independent variable reflecting experience in the interim. The correlation between intelligence measures at the two points would in this view be simply understood as the overlap of earlier intelligence with later intelligence, plus a random increment. This "overlap hypothesis" has been discredited, partly on methodological grounds. Cronbach and Snow (1977) showed that estimated true mental age in any year is positively and substantially correlated with gain in mental age in subsequent years; they observed that "the semiconstancy of ranks in ability is rooted in part in the fact that, under ordinary conditions of development, the child who starts the period with an intellectual advantage is likely to improve his ability to answer test questions more rapidly than his age mates. Such increments in performance are certainly not random" (p. 149).

Second, to think of this improvement as a difference in simple learning rate is theoretically superficial as well as psychometrically unworkable. "Learning rate" has to be multivariate, because a person's rate will differ for different tasks and for different components within a task. Equating ability with learning rate provides merely an operational definition, not a substantive explanation. It has already been noted that attempts to individualize instruction based only on a notion of pace or learning rate fail to erase individual differences. There is more to ability differences than simple rate differences.

A more promising approach starts from J. M. Hunt's (1961) ideas and from Ferguson's (1954, 1956) early view that abilities develop as a function of learning-to-learn and transfer. These pick up some themes from Locke, but also from Dewey, that had been misunderstood or overgeneralized in the interim. Ability is attained through experience over time and consolidated through exercise. Skill in one kind of task performance transfers to performances on other tasks as a function of the similarity between tasks. Abilities thus develop as transfer relations within a class of tasks. Aptitude for learning, then, is readiness to transfer prior ability to new performances on similar tasks. In the new language, however, it is information processing skills and strategies rather than undifferentiated "powers" or "faculties" that transfer.

The application of information processing theory and computer simulation now makes it possible to extend this approach substantially. Simon (1976) set the new stage for interpreting intelligence as complex learning and transfer by suggesting that intelligence could be ". . . attributed to common processes among [various more specialized] performance programs, or to . . . individual differences in the efficacy of the learning programs that assemble the performance programs" (p. 96). In other words, there may be elementary information processes that are common to the performance programs for different tasks. These can account for some of the relations among tasks that we take as indicative of transferable ability. However, there may also be higher-order processes that learn to assemble and control the performance programs, and these also can account for some of the transfer relations among performance tasks.

Anderson (see Anderson, Kline, & Beasley, 1980) has now provided a detailed demonstration of how nonrandom increments in such ability might be realized and represented in a computer program. The program is, in effect, a general theory of learning, in which propositional networks represent factual–conceptual knowledge and production systems represent procedural knowledge. The production system model is used to show how generalizable ability might develop through exercise. The simulation assumes that a single set of learning processes underlies such development. It then provides for improvement of performance by learning, from the problems it faces, to extend or restrict the range of situations in which particular productions apply and to construct new productions, which then become strengthened and integrated into the system. Thus, the theory suggests how ability arises from learning and how such ability, once developed, is involved in further learning and thus in further ability development. The reciprocity can also be expressed in Simon's language: A learning program assembles and controls performance programs, the running and evaluation of which strengthens the learning program.

The theory is not yet complete (Norman, 1980), but both Greeno (1978, 1980) and now Anderson and colleagues (1980) have gone on to the important step of applying this kind of theory to the analysis of learning and instruction in high-school geometry. They suggest that conventional texts and classroom lessons are often *incomplete* with respect to some features that the theory considers crucial for learning. Anderson and colleagues (1980) note that important background features of geometry problems are often left implicit in presented diagrams. They also suggest that example exercises are often insufficient to provide students with the critical juxtapositions that build up the cognitive operations needed for learning and transfer. Both Anderson and Greeno emphasize the critical importance of strategic planning, that is, procedural knowledge. Greeno (1978) sums up his analysis with the observation that "strategic knowledge for setting goals and choosing plans is not a part of the explicit content of the course, although *it seems likely that many students acquire strategic knowledge by induction from example problems that present strategic principles implicitly*" (p. 72, emphasis added). Both the Anderson and the Greeno work prompt the hypothesis that some students learn the implicit yet essential strategic planning knowledge by induction from examples and some do not, and the difference would be predictable from intelligence tests. Learning from instruction that is incomplete in this way requires discovery learning whether it is called "learning by discovery" or not, and the ability involved is clearly what Spearman (1923) meant by "eduction of relations": given two or more examples, produce the rule that connects them. To the extent that the examples given are also insufficient, then the ability involved is also one of *eduction of correlates*, Spearman's term for producing connected examples given one example and a rule. Knowing how to produce and use the information of geometry, given that instruction is incomplete in these respects, constitutes intelligence in geometry. Knowing how to do this in school subjects generally constitutes scholastic intelligence. Learners who can elaborate their own cognitive structures and discover the necessary strategic knowledge by induction will show more facile transfer to new, different, and more difficult problems involved in learning from later instruction; this constitutes scholastic aptitude. Whether such ability transfers to task performances beyond the class of tasks represented by school learning depends on the similarity of those tasks to the tasks confronted in school. Thus, intelligence tests correlate most highly with success in school learning, somewhat less so with learning in job training situations, and much less so with indexes of later job success (Ghiselli, 1966; McNemar, 1964).

Another way to think about this phenomenon is to say that education is a medium of communication with both special form and special content. Scholastic aptitude represents skill in meeting the cognitive demands of this medium; effective performance in the medium both requires and produces transferable cognitive skills. As one moves from subject to subject, from grade to grade, and from high school to college, the messages change, sometimes gradually and sometimes abruptly, but the medium remains more or less the same. Transfer, both positive and negative, to other media depends on the degree to which the same or similar skills are functional or dysfunctional in the new medium. (For further discussion along this line, see Olson, 1974; Salomon, 1979; Snow, 1980b.)

Thus, knowing how to assemble and control performance programs for solving problems in geometry seems to involve the essence of what we call intelligence in education. This conception is close to that derived by Campione, Brown, and Ferrara (see Chapter 8, this volume). In education, at least, intelligence *is* learning ability, in the sense that it is the active organization of abilities needed to learn from incomplete instruction and to use what information may already be in the cognitive system, or can be induced therefrom, to help in doing this.

Learning as intellectual organization.   Much of the preceding discussion would also fit under the title of this section, to support a complex process, reciprocal, evolutionary–organizational view of learning and intelligence. The view is further strengthened by the results of many new cognitive psychological experiments.

Traditional laboratory learning tasks tended to be rote, repetitive, and cyclical; the student–subject could dump the contents of memory at the end of each experiment and was perhaps well advised to do just that. In contrast, school learning is cumulative, from week to week, month to month, and year to year. The student is engaged in building cognitive organizations that will be helpful in learning over the long haul. After one of many kinds of new experiments that suggest this view, Loftus and Loftus (1976, p. 152) noted: "In typical educational settings, the student is viewed as learning *facts*. . . . It seems reasonable, however, on intuitive, theoretical, and empirical grounds that 'what is learned' goes considerably beyond fact acquisition. . . . The process of learning involves a reorganization of semantic information and implementation of new retrieval schemes."

Based on their research, Rumelhart and Norman (1976) have characterized learning from instruction as composed of three overlapping stages – accretion, restructuring, and fine tuning – and much the same language can be used to describe the operations of computer-based theories such as Anderson's or Greeno's. There is a process of fact acquisition, but the masses of loosely and simply connected knowledge must also be organized and reorganized schematically as learning proceeds. Knowledge structures must become formalized for various purposes and sharpened into useful tools of thought and further learning. The organization thus produced integrates conceptual knowledge and procedural knowledge, and it is not hard to imagine the crystallization of such organization for educational purposes occurring over years of educational experience. Again, education can be seen as a medium that demands and produces certain kinds of cognitive organizations.

What is crystallized in this way can be called crystallized intelligence (Cattell, 1963, 1971; Horn, 1976) or verbal educational ability (Vernon, 1951). The product is reflected in performance on scholastic ability and achievement tests all along the line, and the basic learning processes involved may not be dissimilar to those categorized by Estes (see Chapter 4, this volume) as "fast" learning.

Estes, however, chose to form a separate category for "slow" learning, which may require a somewhat different theoretical language to explicate even if the same elementary processes are implicated. A theory such as Anderson's may also assume a single set of learning processes as the basis for developing a general ability, yet we might well hypothesize two or more developmental streams, at a more molar level of description, emanating from this base. Factor analytic research on ability tests has distinguished crystallized intelligence from fluid intelligence (Horn, 1976, 1978). The former is thought to be organized for and by learning in the formal educational medium. The latter is conceived of as an earlier developing organization geared, perhaps, more to reasoning and problem solving in the medium of the natural world before and outside of school. The two kinds of intelligence are separable in adolescence and adulthood, though perhaps not in childhood. In any event, they are interpreted as strongly related generalized abilities.

The two developmental streams can be labeled "crystallization" and "fluidation" to correspond to these two kinds of ability, respectively (see Snow, 1981). Applying again the combination of ideas from Ferguson, Simon, Anderson, and others, one can think of two constellations of ability appearing over long learning experience as a result of transfer functions. One, crystallized intelligence, represents the organization of more formal educational experience into functional cognitive systems applicable to aid further learning in educational situations. The transfer producing this coalescence need not be only of specific knowledge but also of organized processing strategies we think of as academic learning skills, which are in some sense crystallized as units for use in future learning whenever new learning conditions are similar to those in which these crystallized units have been useful in the past. Fluid ability, on the other hand, is thought of as analytic reasoning, particularly where flexible adaptation to novel situations is required and where, therefore, crystallized ability offers no particular advantage.

A summary hypothesis. The overall hypothesis, then, is that crystallized intelligence represents previously constructed assemblies of performance processes retrieved as a system and applied anew in instructional or other performance situations not unlike those experienced in the past, whereas fluid intelligence represents new assemblies, or the flexible reassembly, of performance processes needed for more extreme adaptations to novel situations. Both functions develop through exercise, and perhaps both can be understood as variations on a general production system development. It is possible, however, that the crystallized assemblies result from the accumulation of many "fast-process" intentional learning experiences, whereas the facility for fluid assembly and reassembly results more from the accumulation of "slow-process," incidental learning experiences. Both kinds of intelligence will be relevant to education. Fluid ability will pertain more to learning performance with new or unusual instructional methods or content. Crystallized ability will be more relevant in the progression of familiar situations and subject matters often characterized as conventional formal instruction.

CLASSIFICATION OF TESTS, TASKS, AND TREATMENTS

The guiding hypothesis just given distinguishes two kinds of intelligence – crystallized and fluid – and connects these to two kinds of educational environments – conventional and novel, respectively. Still, these two theoretical contrasts may gloss over what are really continuous dimensions. Moreover, in implementing research on intelligence in education, the investigator must choose to use actual tests and educational learning tasks that imperfectly represent these theoretical distinctions; any measure or situation will reflect some mixture or shade of gray along one or the other implied continuum. Thus, for conducting or reviewing research, and for the purposes of this chapter, a means of classifying tests and tasks with respect to these theoretical dimensions is needed.

There are many ways to classify the kinds of tests and tasks used to study intelligence and learning in education. Also, school learning tasks are organized into particular progressions, for presentation using particular teaching methods, in particular environmental contexts; these educational orchestrations (loosely called treatments) can themselves be classified to define treatment variables or contrasts. One can concentrate on taxonomies of different types of learning tasks (e.g., Gagné, 1970) or types of ability tests (e.g., Guilford, 1967). One can bring different types of educational objectives (e.g., Bloom, 1956) and different teaching methods into cross-classifications with these (Gage, 1964). For some purposes, these classifications can be aligned with one another (see Snow, 1973).

For this chapter, however, the classification must put the fluid–crystallized ability constructs and various possible educational treatments along similar continua. An expansion of Cronbach's spectrum of ability tests appears to be useful in this regard.

Figure 9.3 is adapted from Cronbach (1970, p. 282). The central column and left panel suggest a spectrum of tasks that are used to assess different kinds of

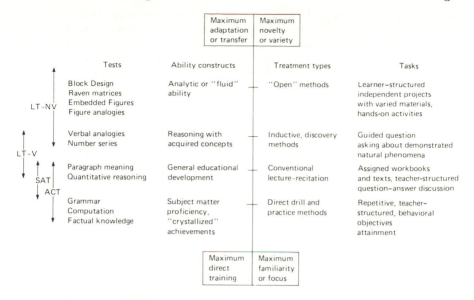

Figure 9.3.   A spectrum for comparing tests of ability, instructional tasks, and hypothesized relations between tests and tasks. (Adapted from *Essentials of Psychological Testing,* 3rd ed., by L. J. Cronbach [New York: Harper & Row, 1970].)

ability (whether ability here is thought of as aptitude for future learning or outcome from past learning). On the lower end of the continuum are tasks that sample directly from the explicit content of school work; they would tend to call for performances that have been directly taught, trained, or practiced, and thus would involve minimum transfer from general prior experience. At higher levels on the continuum are tasks that call for adaptation of prior experience; these performances are not directly trained in school. The tasks at higher levels are increasingly samples of unfamiliar, novel problems for which prior knowledge is of little help but flexible use of reasoning is required. On the far left, several well-known general ability tests and their sampling ranges are indicated. The Scholastic Aptitude Test (SAT) and the American College Testing Program (ACT) are both used as aptitude measures that sample educational development through high school to predict college-level achievement. The ACT samples more specific subject matter proficiencies, whereas the SAT avoids direct sampling from the school curriculum. Both would be interpreted largely as measures of crystallized intelligence, although, as their sampling range arrows suggest, neither can be regarded as exclusively representing a single narrow construct. The Lorge–Thorndike Verbal Intelligence (LT-V) score overlaps with these but includes abstract reasoning with concepts, whereas the Non-Verbal Intelligence (LT-NV) score moves further toward including abstract reasoning tasks that apparently require analytic ability, flexibility, or fluid intelligence. The Raven Progressive Matrices Test, and the Block Design Subtest of the Wechsler Intelligence Scales would in this view be the most direct measures of fluid–analytic ability.

Educational treatments can be arrayed along a similar continuum, as shown in the right panel of Figure 9.3. They range from treatments that focus teaching directly on mastery of a progression of familiar, structured, subject matter tasks to treatments that promote student-structured experience with a variety of novel problem-finding and problem-solving tasks. Although Figure 9.3 includes some suggestive labels for different treatment types, it is important to note that labels can be misleading, and perhaps more so on the right side of the figure than on the left. Just as tests may sample from different parts of the fluid–crystallized range, so too may educational treatments sample from different parts of the novelty–familiarity range. Any task can be novel for the inexperienced learner. A proper description of a treatment would need to indicate not only its central tendency on the spectrum but also its sampling range, as the arrows do for tests on the left side of the figure, and its departure in form or content from previous tasks in a series. To date, however, complex educational treatments have not been described systematically in this way, though it seems possible that a task-analysis technology could be developed for accomplishing this. In the meantime, the reader of educational research and the researcher as well must beware of treatment labels; "discovery" teaching may involve direct drill, and "rote" learning is rarely all rote.

The suggested parallel between ability constructs and types of treatment is meant to reflect some past hypotheses about connections between aptitude, treatment, and outcome, such as that noted in the individualized instruction and learning-by-discovery sections. Small-step programmed instruction, direct drill instruction, and presumably conventional lecture–recitation call most heavily upon previously crystallized achievement in the same or similar subject matter as aptitude, and they advance the development of crystallized ability, primarily, as outcome. Independent, learning-by-doing, and discovery methods call more upon flexible transfer and adaptive ability as aptitude and are more likely to promote the development of fluid ability as outcome. This relationship, however, is not suggested as being ironclad. It is conceivable that forms of direct training and practice might be invented to promote fluid-ability development and that experience with variety and novelty can be arranged to promote the formation of crystallized ability and knowledge.

The proposed spectrum oversimplifies the description of both tests and treatments, but it keeps the notion of sampling range in mind when one is considering the complex character of either. That both tests and treatments differ in sampling range, or scope, creates problems for reviews of educational research. Intellectual ability as aptitude (or outcome) might be represented in one study by a general factor based on tests such as the Stanford–Binet and the Wechsler Adult Intelligence Scale (WAIS), in another by a particular vocabulary or reading test, and in still another by a test of special ability such as perceptual scanning or memory span. Achievement tests (used to represent either aptitude or outcome) also differ in the scope or breadth of performance they are designed to assess; some are heterogeneous samples of broad content or skill domains, others focus on the specific facts included in a particular instructional unit. Educational treatments, also, can be composed of homogeneous samples of tasks aimed at a particular outcome or broadly heterogeneous collections of tasks aimed at many outcomes.

Any research study, then, represents a choice of aptitude measures, treatments, and outcome measures. Some studies may even contrast treatments or relate aptitude and outcome measures, chosen from quite different regions of the spectrum and with quite different sampling ranges. This situation complicates the problem of reviewing and summarizing the results of educational research immensely. Results will vary from region to region, and judgments about what regions particular studies represent often rest on subtle issues. Attempts at generalization of results often must gloss over some of these variations. Statements made earlier in this chapter about individualized instruction and immediate achievement and about inductive instruction and more generalized achievement are examples of this glossing over of details to reach gross summaries. Much educational research is necessarily of this character, because it is conducted in the real world of schools rather than in the laboratory. In subsequent sections of this chapter, an attempt is made to keep track of such variations from study to study, at least crudely.

Of note also for classification purposes is the view that general ability constructs and tests of the sort scaled on the continuum of Figure 9.3 can be placed near the top of a hierarchical model of ability organization. In such a model, general intelligence appears at the apex with the division of fluid and crystallized ability just beneath it. These are progressively differentiated into a variety of more specific or specialized skills and achievements (see, e.g., Snow, 1978, 1980b). The model is useful because it summarizes much of the data on ability-test correlations, gathered over decades of factor-analytic research, and because it organizes constructs and tests for different kinds of decisions. Broad ability constructs can be chosen for some analyses and decisions, in research or in educational practice, and for some curriculum evaluations. More finely differentiated abilities may be useful for some individual diagnosis or counseling decisions. A hierarchical view of cognitive processes may have similar value. Possibly, some such hierarchy or related multifaceted model could be worked out to expand the description of educational treatments as well. Variations on this classification scheme for both ability and situational constructs have been proposed over the years (see N. Frederiksen, 1972; Humphreys, 1962; Snow, 1979a). So far, however, a completely satisfactory scheme to elaborate the continuum of Figure 9.3 has not been worked out.

9.4.   CURRENT EVIDENCE AND CURRENT RESEARCH

With the relevant history, issues, and framework summarized, we can now add in the rest of the existing empirical evidence on various points of interest, drawing implications where possible for the future. First, the evidence from correlational research is summarized; some studies have correlated intelligence with amount of education obtained as well as with adult occupational and ability levels attained, whereas others are concerned with the relation of intelligence to educational achievement within a course or grade level. The correlational work is then used to define a context for examining research that focuses on the effects of educational interventions. Various categories of such interventions are reviewed. First, intelligence is examined as an aptitude for learning in different instructional treatments. Then intelligence is viewed as an outcome of instruction. Interventions aimed at influencing intelligence are discussed in descending order from those most likely to have an effect (e.g., broad educational programs) to those least likely to have an effect (e.g., simple coaching or teacher expectancy changes). Finally, current research on the analysis of intellectual processes in learning from instruction is discussed. It is impossible to review all of the empirical literature that bears on these topics. Rather, in each case, a representative summary of evidence is given and a few example studies are singled out to make important implications for future work at least somewhat more concrete.

CORRELATIONAL RESEARCH ON INTELLIGENCE IN EDUCATION

Correlations with amount of education. Early work on education and intelligence considered the relation between amount of schooling and mental-test scores. Anastasi (1958) cites studies during World War II that show substantial correlation between years in school and intelligence among army personnel. Longitudinal studies in the United States and Sweden have also shown relations between amount of education and intelligence, with higher intelligence associated with more years of schooling (Husen, 1951). Such studies, of course, cannot account adequately for the possible effects of preexisting differences in ability and such factors as family income or social class; they provide suggestive correlations, but they do not establish causal relations between years in school and intellectual growth.

More recent studies have used the method of path analysis to explore the linkages among intellectual, educational, and occupational variables at different points in time. Two such analyses are depicted in Figure 9.4. The first was produced by Li (1975) from data reported by Jencks and colleagues (1972); it is also discussed by Jensen (1980). The second comes from Duncan, Featherman, and Duncan (1972), as adapted and discussed by Cronbach (1977). In both parts of the figure, coefficients adjacent to curved connections represent the raw correlation between the two variables indicated. Coefficients adjacent to straight arrow connections represent standardized partial regression coefficients to indicate the unique direct influence of the earlier variable on the later variable.

The two analyses include slightly different variables and make slightly different assumptions, but they agree for the most part. Child ability contributes to the amount of education obtained by that child more than does father's education or occupation. Although child ability contributes most to the ability of that child at adulthood, amount of education obtained by the child also contributes to adult ability and to the level of occupation reached by the child as an adult. There are, however, other strong influences on child ability, adult ability, amount of education obtained, and level of occupation reached. This is to be expected; ability is only one of many factors influencing amount of education, and education is only one of many factors influencing adult ability and occupational level. Parental influence, also, must not be seen as just one push at the start; its effects are probably continuous throughout the development of the child (see the path analysis by Cronbach & Snow, 1977, p. 148, of the Bayley, 1954, longitudinal study of intelligence; see also chapter 14, by Siegler & Richards, this volume).

The issue is complex, because the characteristics of intellectual development, of ongoing education, and of ongoing parental influences are confounded. Formal schooling usually starts in the age range 5–7, a period during which psychological data show intellectual development to be in a state of transition. This transition is part of Piagetian theory (Flavell, 1963), but it is also suggested by other research (White, 1965). Another transition, from elementary to junior high school, occurs near puberty when various cognitive and social changes take place. High school is associated with the age range where formal operational thinking appears (Flavell,

A
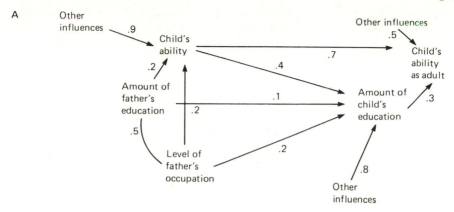

B
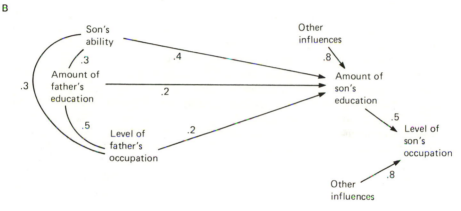

Figure 9.4. Two path analyses showing network of causal relations among parent and child intellectual, educational, and occupational characteristics. (*A*: adapted from *Path Analysis: A Primer* by C. C. Li [Pacific Grove, Calif.: Boxweed Press], 1975; *B*: adapted from *Socioeconomic Background and Achievement* by O. D. Duncan, D. L. Featherman, & B. Duncan [New York: Seminar Press, 1972]. Reprinted by permission.)

1963). Whether psychological development comes in distinct stage transitions or is better thought of as a more continuous stream (Flavell, 1979), it is not historical accident that educational transitions occur at these points; the latter seem to mark the significant stages of intellectual growth as perceived by educational theorists, without benefit of modern cognitive theory. The complex correlation between individual developmental and educational events undermines strong causal arguments running in either direction. It seems, therefore, most reasonable to think of intellectual and educational developments as reciprocal.

Correlations with educational achievement.   There is a vast correlational literature on intelligence measures as predictors of later measures of educational achievement, and several extensive reviews exist (Cattell & Butcher, 1968; Lavin, 1965; Tyler, 1965). Perhaps the most succinct and current summary is that given by Jensen (1980, pp. 316–337). The accumulated evidence supports five related points that need to be accounted for in further theory-oriented research.

First, the correlation of general mental tests with educational achievement measures is typically found to be about .50, on average. Higher correlations, with median values ranging around .60 to .70, are found at elementary-school levels. The typical median range is .50 to .60 in high school, .40 to .50 in college, and .30 to .40 in graduate school (Jensen, 1980). That is, there is substantial overlap in what is represented psychologically by the two kinds of measures, even though there is also considerable uniqueness; intelligence and achievement measures are closely related but not equivalent psychologically. As individuals grow and education progresses, the relation is reduced, presumably because increasingly differentiated experience involves other factors in the developmental process. Progressive restriction of the ability range due to drop out and selection as higher educational levels are reached also reduces the aptitude–achievement correlations obtained.

Second, general ability and achievement are thought to differentiate with age through childhood and adolescence. In other words, with increasing age general cognitive factors account for progressively less of the variance in mental task performances and relatively specialized cognitive factors account for more of the variance. Early views attributed this differentiation to maturational unfolding (Garrett, 1946). Later views emphasized the effects of learning and education, pointing to the increasing proliferation and specialization of transfer relations among tasks through this age range (Ferguson, 1954, 1956). Although the hypothesis has been controversial (see Guilford, 1967), the best evidence supports the view that ability and achievement differentiate as a result of education (Anastasi, 1970). There is some evidence that broad scholastic abilities may not continue to change during the college years, however, even while achievements do continue to expand and differentiate. Humphreys (1968; Humphreys & Taber, 1973) reported data showing that predictions from aptitude at high school and postdictions from aptitude measured near college graduation were similar; in either case, college freshman grade-point averages were most well predicted and senior grade-point averages were least well predicted. Thus, in this age range the college achievement measures may be changing more than the abilities involved. Nonetheless, evidence from adults suggests that education is a key variable; adults with less education show less ability differentiation than adults with more education (Anastasi, 1970).

Third, at least in the public school years, correlations between intelligence measures taken at one point in time and achievement measures taken at a later point in time tend to be higher than when the measures are taken in the reversed time-order (Crano, 1974; Crano, Denny, & Campbell, 1972). This fact has been interpreted to suggest that "intelligence differences cause achievement differences" rather than vice versa, although the methodology used in this reasoning has been seriously questioned (see Cook & Campbell, 1979; Rogosa, 1980). Other theoretical and empirical work, furthermore, provides a more subtle and complicated hypothesis. The theory of fluid and crystallized intelligence (Cattell, 1963, 1971; Horn, 1976, 1978) suggests that the presumably more native, fluid–analytic ability is invested by the individual in learning experiences, including formal education, to produce verbal-crystallized ability. The growth curve for fluid ability appears to precede that for crystallized ability across the childhood and young adult years, consistent with the theory. Crano (1974), however, has reported evidence suggesting different developmental patterns for different socioeconomic status (SES) groups. Among higher SES children, earlier verbal abstract abilities seem to operate as determinants in the acquisition of later concrete and culture-specific achievements. Among lower SES children, earlier spatial visualization abilities appear to determine later acquisition of verbal abilities, both concrete and abstract. One implication is that reliance on abstract verbal instruction in elementary schools may benefit higher SES children disproportionately. Improvements in methodology are now needed to explore these issues further.

Fourth, the more general mental tests, of both fluid and crystallized abilities, are highly correlated and apparently more centrally involved in the organization of human abilities than are the more specialized, peripheral skills and abilities (Guttman, 1965, 1969; Jensen, 1970; Snow, 1980b). It is the more general, central ability measures that correlate most highly with educational achievement measures, especially when the latter reflect more generalized achievement criteria rather than performance in specific or special subject matters. Although fluid and crystallized abilities are at times difficult to distinguish in this regard, there is reason to believe that verbal crystallized ability relates more to achievement in relatively conventional, familiar instructional settings (e.g., lecture, recitation, reading, discussion, etc.), whereas fluid–analytic ability relates to achievement in which novel problem solving or adaptation to unfamiliar instructional methods and materials is involved (Snow, 1981).

Finally, and in keeping with the fourth point, there appears to be marked variation in ability–achievement relations around the central tendencies usually obtained. This depends not only upon the ability and achievement measures used, the school level(s) and subject(s) in which achievement is assessed, and the heterogeneity of the population sampled but also upon the heterogeneity of the educational environments sampled, The last point can be illustrated from studies of the prediction of college achievement. Lavin (1965) reviewed many such studies and reported a range of .30 to .70 for validity coefficients in predicting college grade-point averages. Lenning (1975) obtained a range of .15 to over .64 in a similar study of ACT validity, for a sample of 120 institutions. Also, the manual of the General Aptitude Test Battery shows coefficients ranging from .10 to .64 in 48 college samples. Such variation suggests that the relation of intellectual aptitude measures to educational achievement is moderated by environmental variables. Potentially, greater understanding of ability–achievement relations could be gained by analyzing, perhaps even manipulating experimentally, the instructional environmental variables that influence such relations.

INTELLIGENCE AS APTITUDE FOR EDUCATIONAL TREATMENTS

Expectations about treatment effects. Correlational evidence from developmental studies and achievement prediction studies can be used to form a picture of the correlational network within which particular instructional treatments can then be evaluated and contrasted. To start from the evidence cited in the previous section, the typical expectation in research on instruction would be a correlation of about .50 between intelligence measured as aptitude at the start of instruction and achievement outcome measured at the end of instruction. In Figure 9.5A, this

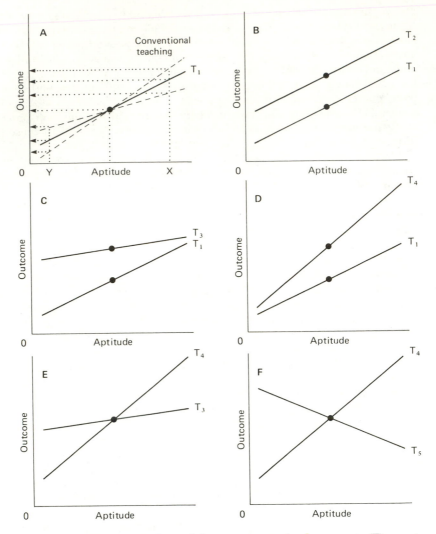

Figure 9.5.   Six possible effects of alternative instructional treatments (T) on outcome averages and outcome-on-aptitude regressions.

expectation is depicted as a solid line (called a regression slope) and labeled T_1, or
"conventional teaching," to suggest what happens under typical instructional
conditions in schools today. A regression slope is essentially a running average – a
line that shows the degree to which increases in scores on aptitude (the abscissa)
relate to increases in scores on outcome (the ordinate). Note that Person X, with a
high initial aptitude score is predicted to obtain a higher outcome score than is
Person Y, with a relatively low initial aptitude score. The heavy dot indicates the
average outcome score predicted from an average aptitude score. The dotted lines
can be used to trace these predictions. A range of dashed regression slopes is also
shown in Figure 9.5A, to suggest the range of correlations, varying between

about .30 and .70, often obtained in presumably comparable, conventional instructional environments. It should be clear that some environments are better than others for Person X and for Person Y, and some are worse than others for each person.

An important aim of research on educational-treatment effects is to improve upon this state of affairs by finding or devising treatments such as T_2 that raise the average outcome for everyone, as in Figure 9.5B, or treatments such as T_3 that improve outcome for less able students while preserving the high achievement of more able students, as in Figure 9.5C. Readers can trace the dotted projection lines for Persons X and Y onto these and other figures for themselves, to see the differences in predicted outcomes for different educational treatments.

Figure 9.5B suggests the goal of many treatment comparisons in traditional educational research, where it has often been assumed that class-average. achievement could be influenced by treatment variables but regression slopes on aptitude could not be. The aim was to find treatments like T_2. The pattern in Figure 9.5C schematizes the goal of special education (see chapter 8, by Campione, Brown, & Ferrara, this volume) and of much research on individualized instruction, which is to find treatments like T_3. This goal is sometimes achieved but usually only when fairly specific achievement measures geared directly to the content taught are used. In searching for generally improved teaching methods, however, the result shown in Figure 9.5D has also at times been obtained; some treatments, such as T_4, turn out to be particularly beneficial for more able students rather than for less able students. One could say that this is the goal of special programs for the gifted. Such a result also seems to be the most likely expectation for discovery or inductive treatments. This leads to the possibility of combined results such as those shown in Figure 9.5E; here, alternative treatments are found to produce improvements for different kinds of students. T_4 is best for higher-aptitude students, and T_3 is best for lower-aptitude students. This result suggests that students should be given the treatment most appropriate to their initial aptitude. In the extreme, if one designed alternative instructional treatments optimally for different aptitude groups, the result pictured in Figure 9.5F might be expected; regression slopes approximating that shown for treatment T_5 do sometimes occur, though negative slopes of this sort are more likely when personality measures rather than cognitive-ability measures are used as aptitude.

Figures 9.5B through 9.5F depict the possible kinds of relations one can expect regardless of what variables are entered as aptitude and outcome on the abscissa and ordinate, respectively. Thus, the same patterns serve to define the expectations when treatments that attempt to train intelligence directly are evaluated (i.e., when earlier and later ability scores are entered on the two axes) as when alternative treatments are compared using different kinds of aptitude and achievement measures on the two axes. Research results for either alternative treatment comparisons or direct training evaluations can therefore be examined in this way. In either case, the distance between the dots on each regression line indicates the average effect size or superiority of one treatment over another, and the nonparallelism of the regression slopes suggests the degree to which treatment effect size differs for students with different entering aptitude scores.

Intelligence × Treatment interactions. For much of this century, educational researchers have sought results like those in Figure 9.5B, an average treatment effect with parallel aptitude slopes. They could then recommend that educators adopt one kind of instructional method or program over another for all students. Occasionally, this end has been achieved. For example, studies comparing conventional teaching with the so-called Keller Plan (Keller, 1968), a structured form of individually paced and monitored instruction at the college level, have found average treatment effects favoring the Keller Plan with no change in the regression slope of achievement onto prior scholastic aptitude scores. (Kulik, Kulik, and Cohen, 1979). Thus, the more individualized, mastery-oriented Keller treatment benefited all students to more or less the same extent. It also, therefore, maintained the advantage accruing to those students who were more able to begin with, a point not often recognized in abstract discussions about what kind of instructional method is "best."

Often, comparative research of this sort has not measured student aptitudes at all, however, but checked *only* for average effect differences between instructional treatments. Such simple instructional contrasts often yield equivocal conclusions, and the summaries of this work often offer a confusing picture to educators, with no clear decision as to "best" treatments. For example, a review of experiments comparing teacher-centered (authoritarian) and learner-centered (democratic) modes of organizing classroom instruction showed that 8 studies favored the first mode, 11 studies favored the second, and 13 studies showed no difference between the two (R. C. Anderson, 1959). A review of comparisons of televised versus live classroom teaching yielded 83 studies favoring television, 55 favoring conventional teaching, and 255 with no significant difference between these two treatments (Schramm, 1962). In comparisons of college lecture versus discussion methods, 45 studies came out on one side, 43 on the other (Dubin & Taveggia, 1968). Such studies do not provide clear conclusions.

Suppose, however, that *different* instructional treatments are best for students at different levels of intelligence or other aptitudes. Suppose also that different research studies comparing two treatments include students of different intelligence levels. Then, confusing reversals of treatment effects from study to study could result. Patterns of results such as those shown in Figures 9.5E and 9.5F suggest that students at different aptitude levels need different kinds of instructional treatments. If such patterns exist in the population, and individual studies sample students from different parts of the aptitude range without actually measuring aptitude, the studies will reach different conclusions as the examples just mentioned did, without discovering why.

The patterns of Figures 9.5CDEF are all instances of interaction between aptitude differences and instructional treatment differences (i.e., Aptitude × Treatment interactions, or ATI for short). It is increasingly recognized that such regression patterns often occur even when they are not sought. Evidence of ATI is required to construct alternative treatments for the adaptive educational plan pictured in Figure 9.2, and hypothesized ATI patterns underlie much research and development on individualized instruction and on special educational programs for gifted or retarded students. Cronbach and Snow (1977) have concluded from a review of much of this literature that ATI are ubiquitous in education. No theories yet exist, however, that are adequate to explain why ATI occur.

Many different aptitude variables have been used in this research, including all manner of personality, motivational, and attitudinal characteristics, as well as general and specific cognitive abilities and relevant prior achievements. Research on ATI forms part of a movement toward an interactional psychology that ac-

Table 9.2. *A summary of ATI hypotheses relating general ability (G) to various instructional treatments (T)*

Description of T	Expected results[a]	
	Low G student	High G student
Placing burdens of information processing on learners	−	+
Using elaborate or unusual explanations	−	+
A "new" curriculum	−	+
Including discovery or inquiry methods	−	+
Encouraging learner self-direction	−	+
Relatively unstructured or permissive	−	+
Relying heavily on verbiage	−	+
Rapidly paced	−	+
Giving minimal essentials by PI[b] for learners to elaborate	−	+
Giving advance organizers on difficult material	−	+
Relieving learners of information processing burdens	+	0
Giving all essentials by PI[b]	+	0
Simplifying or breaking down the task	+	0
Providing redundant text	+	0
Substituting other media for verbiage	+	0
Using simplified demonstrations, models, or simulations	+	−
Varying the format of PI[b]	X	X
Including inserted questions	X	X
Using diagrammatic or pictorial presentation	X	X
Based on specialized film or TV	X	X

[a] − = poor; + = good; 0 = uncertain; X = inconsistent.
[b] PI = programmed instruction.
Source: Snow, 1977a, Table 2, p. 68.

counts for Person × Situation interaction generally (see, e.g., Endler & Magnusson, 1976; Magnusson & Endler, 1977; Pervin & Lewis, 1978). The concern here, however, is limited to research on general intellectual measures as aptitude in interaction with educational situation variables, in the service of finding or designing the alternative instructional treatments needed for the system suggested in Figure 9.2. Attempts at direct training of intellectual skills as aptitudes will be treated in a later section.

Table 9.2 provides a summary of the research literature on ATI relating to general intelligence. The literature supports the hypothesis, stated most generally as items 1 and 11 in Table 9.2, that intelligence measures relate more strongly to learning outcome as instructional treatments appear to place increased information processing burdens on learners, as opposed to relieving such burdens through structured aids, supports, or simplifications of the learning task.

It seems that as learners are required to puzzle things out for themselves, to organize their own study and build their own comprehension, the more able learners can capitalize on their strengths profitably. As instructional treatments are arranged to relieve learners from difficult reading, analyzing complex concepts, and building their own cognitive structures, such treatments seem to compensate for, or circumvent, less able learners' weaknesses and to reduce the regression slope. . . . [Snow, 1977a, p. 69]

Whereas less able students do poorly in some kinds of burdensome treatments, more able students often seem to do well no matter what instructional treatment is applied. Still, this is not always the case. Item 16 in Table 9.2 comes from research suggesting that some kinds of instructional devices may actually interfere with able students' learning.

Many newer studies lend further support to this account, but few yield a more analytic understanding of its underlying psychology, and there are inconsistencies. In much of this research, moreover, aptitude constructs are not well defined so that distinctions between fluid and crystallized intelligence or between general and specialized cognitive abilities are difficult or impossible to make. Also, the instructional treatment alternatives are not described in detail. Although in gross terms their central tendencies might be located on the treatment spectrum of Figure 9.3, little progress has been made in specifying what aspects of what kinds of treatments might constitute increases or decreases in the information processing burden placed on learners.

Two studies that attempted to distinguish fluid and crystallized ability and also used a fairly well described treatment can serve as an example of a replicated ATI pattern that approximates that shown in Figure 9.5E and is consistent with the hypothesis drawn from Table 9.2. Both Sharps (1973) and Crist-Whitzel and Hawley-Winne (1976) conducted year-long evaluations of Individually Prescribed Instruction (IPI), in fifth-grade reading and mathematics and in sixth-grade mathematics, respectively. IPI is a system of individually paced instruction that relies on a sequence of unit mastery tests, geared to specific instructional objectives and content, with frequent feedback to learners. It is more "directed" instruction, relative to conventional teaching, and may remove many of the organizational and strategic burdens that affect lower ability students adversely under ordinary school conditions. In both these studies, IPI was compared with conventional whole-class teaching using basal textbooks. A third treatment examined in one of the studies was relatively ineffective and can be ignored here. Using standardized ability and achievement tests as aptitude and outcome measures, the results of regression analyses in both studies showed that IPI was best for students low on crystallized ability initially, whereas conventional teaching was best for students high on crystallized ability initially. Thus, the structure provided by IPI helps less able learners, presumably by compensating for their relative weaknesses in conventional learning activities and strategies. At the same time, IPI seems to be dysfunctional for able learners; it holds them back in some sense or interferes with the conventional learning strategies in which they are already strong.

Fluid-ability measures yielded positive relations with outcome and no interaction in the Sharps study. The other study, however, used multiple regression procedures to reach the suggestion that fluid ability may interact in an opposite way, once crystallized ability differences have been removed. The implication is that IPI is best for students who are low in crystallized ability and high in fluid ability, that is, those who might be called "underachievers" in conventional instruction. The result makes sense, though it obviously needs further study. Students who have mastered the skills of conventional school learning do best in that medium; those who have not benefit from a different treatment that compensates for this inaptitude while capitalizing on what abilities they do possess.

Other research, contributed by Peterson and her colleagues, however, serves to exemplify some of the limits that must be placed on such generalizations. In one study, Peterson, Janicki, and Swing (1979) compared lecture–recitation, inquiry,

and public-issues discussion as alternative treatments in high-school social studies. Crystallized ability, though not fluid ability, was included as aptitude. Specific
achievement tests served as outcome measures. The interaction again resembled
Figure 9.5*E*, but the interpretation appears to conflict with the generalization
drawn from Table 9.2; the steepest regression slope occurred in the lecture–recitation treatment, with shallower slopes appearing in both inquiry and
public-issues treatments. The authors suggest that the lecture–recitation treatment was particularly burdensome, demanding careful listening, note taking, and
organization on the part of students. Thus, the treatments labeled "inquiry" and
"discussion," in this instance, may actually have placed less demand on
crystallized ability than more conventional teaching.

Understanding intelligence as an interacting aptitude in education will require
not only the analysis of fluid and crystallized functioning in particular treatments
of this sort but also study of the links between such functioning and aspects of
personality (see the chapter by Baron, this volume). It is suspected, for example,
that although there is little overall correlation between intellectual differences
and anxiousness, intelligence and anxiety interact multiplicatively with instructional treatment variables to affect learning outcome. In other words, anxiety has
different effects on learning at different ability levels, depending on the nature of
instructional treatment. Examples again come from Peterson's work. In one study
of a relatively unstructured treatment in high-school social studies (Peterson,
1977), crystallized ability differences were strongly and positively related to
achievement among students showing little anxiety but were negatively correlated with achievement among students high in anxiety. In other treatments
structured by the teacher or by student participation, relations between ability
and achievement were mildly positive at all anxiety levels. Research by Porteus
(1976; for discussion, see Snow, 1977a) has shown some similar trends in comparisons of teacher-centered (relatively structured) versus student-centered (relatively unstructured) treatments in high-school economics and educational philosophy. Yet Peterson (1979) has conducted a similar study at the college level and
found opposite trends; ability was particularly highly and positively related to
learning among high-anxiety students in an unstructured treatment. Such differences in findings, of course, can arise because high-school and college students are sampled from different parts of the intelligence range in the population
and because learning activities may differ at the two educational levels. This
underscores again the difficulties in reaching simple generalizations about intelligence as aptitude for learning.

The work in high-school social studies that contrasts lecture–recitation versus
inquiry versus public-issues treatments (Peterson, Janicki, and Swing, 1979)
does yield a replicated Ability × Anxiety interaction across two studies. In each
case, public-issues discussion worked best for low-ability students who were non-
anxious but was the worst treatment for those who showed high anxiety. Low-
ability students in the inquiry treatment showed the opposite trend. The ATI
pattern resembles Figure 9.5*F*. Anxiety differences did not appear to moderate the
performance of high-ability students appreciably in any treatment. The authors
suggested that public-issues discussion provided external demands that motivated low-ability–low-anxiety students and thus facilitated their learning, but
that might have increased the anxiousness of low-ability–high-anxiety students
to dysfunctional levels; the inquiry treatment required independent work and

thus had the reverse motivational effect. This hypothesis is similar to the implications of the earlier Peterson (1977) and Porteus (1976) results and is consistent with the theorizing of Spielberger and others (see Gaudry & Spielberger 1971; also see Sieber, O'Neil, and Tobias, 1977) regarding the relation of ability, anxiety, and task difficulty in learning from instruction.

Summary and implications. When intelligence is viewed as an aptitude input to educational treatments, it is often found that learning outcome depends not only on the student's initial ability level and on the overall effectiveness of the treatment but also on the interaction of ability level and treatment (ATI). In other words, the effects of given instruction vary as a function of student intelligence. It appears that some kinds of instruction impose information processing burdens that limit the learning of less able students while permitting more able students to excel. Some other kinds of instruction designed to help less able students may have deleterious effects on more able students. It appears also that individual differences in anxiety moderate and thus further complicate such Intelligence × Treatment interactions.

Current ATI research extends the observation made by Cronbach and Snow (1977, p. 391) that, often, one or another instructional variation ". . . was distinctly bad for a fraction of the learners. And some instructional treatments seemed to be beneficial to one subgroup while at the same time having negative effects for another subgroup." What aspects of instruction provide such negative effects for particular aptitude subgroups is an important question for further, more analytic research. Rohwer (1980) has reached a similar conclusion from a somewhat different perspective.

INTELLIGENCE AS OUTCOME OF EDUCATIONAL TREATMENTS

Whereas the research on intelligence as aptitude has tended to look only at crystallized ability and specific achievement as outcomes, other lines of work have studied more general intelligence measures and occasionally the fluid–crystallized distinction as outcomes of education. There are four categories of studies, which correspond to the effects of broad-scope educational programs, experiments aimed at direct training of particular abilities, studies of practice or coaching on the measures themselves, and studies of the effects of teacher expectations on student performance.

Educational programs for the development of intelligence. Studies of the effects of early childhood programs predate by several decades the evaluation studies of the compensatory education era. Anastasi (1958) and Tyler (1965) describe an extensive series of nursery-school studies during the 1930s and 1940s, many conducted by Beth Wellman and her associates. Some studies found average IQ gains of 6 to 7 points among children attending nursery school from fall to spring, with continued but diminishing gains over subsequent years. In another study, preschool children showed an average gain in IQ of 7 points from fall to spring, while over a similar period, matched control groups lost between 3 and 4 points, on average. Comparisons of the relation of initial ability to outcome ability within such groups were not made. Also, preschool and nonpreschool groups were not randomly assigned in this research nor were counterhypotheses explored. Thus, the question of the general intellectual effects of preschool attendance remained unresolved for the subsequent decades.

Studies of compensatory education in preschool and elementary-grade programs, such as Head Start and Follow Through, do not seem to change this picture appreciably. Thus, one can characterize all of this research by using the pattern of Figure 9.5B, if it is assumed that no Intelligence × Treatment interaction was involved. The figure would be drawn with parallel slopes and a modest average-effect size between regression lines that dissipates over time. Most of this research, however, did not bring initial intellectual differences among children into the statistical analysis in a way that lets us judge whether regression slopes remained parallel. The effects of some programs, such as "Sesame Street," which did study initial differences more directly, would probably look more like Figure 9.5D: increasing treatment-effect size as a function of higher initial ability. Similar results might be expected for the other kinds of intervention programs.

Different Follow Through programs also differed in the degree to which their treatments were focused directly on training particular cognitive outcomes, and the evaluation included multiple outcome measures. The results lead to an interesting hypothesis implied earlier in this chapter and clearly worth further research. Figure 9.6 was constructed from the summary data provided by Kennedy (1978). It shows the average treatment-effect size of each of nine different Follow Through programs, compared with control groups, on two kinds of educational outcome measures. As outcome criteria, the evaluation study had included the Metropolitan Achievement Test (with subscales for language skills, reading comprehension, math computation skills, and math problem solving) and the Raven Progressive Matrices Test. For our Figure 9.6, Kennedy's results for language, reading, and math computation were combined to represent effects on crystallized intelligence (G_c), and results for the Raven test were taken as effects on fluid intelligence (G_f). (Math problem solving was omitted because it probably reflects a mix of G_c and G_f abilities.) It seems that the programs showing the most positive effects on the development of crystallized ability (i.e., Direct Instruction and Behavior Analysis) also showed the most negative effects on the development of fluid–analytic ability. Three programs (Bilingual, Tucson Early Education, and Responsive Environment) apparently had modest positive effects on both outcome dimensions, whereas four programs (Bank Street, Education Development Center, Parent Education, and Cognitive Curriculum) had modest negative or no effects on both outcome dimensions. Thus, direct, intensively structured and focused instruction, concentrated on primary reading and mathematics skills, can help produce increases in crystallized intelligence but perhaps at a cost in the development of the nonverbal, flexible, and analytic reasoning skills that are taken to reflect fluid intelligence.

One cannot draw a hard conclusion from the Follow Through evaluation; the statistical analyses were complex and controversial, and the summary effects used to produce Figure 9.6 incorporate many assumptions and statistical aggregations of data from more detailed levels of analysis. Further research would need to examine in controlled studies the characteristics of instructional treatments that influence both kinds of educational outcome, and the correlation between them, for individual children. Still, the implication that direct training focused on the development of only one kind of aptitude may be detrimental to the development of another is striking. It suggests again the kinds of complex trade-offs that

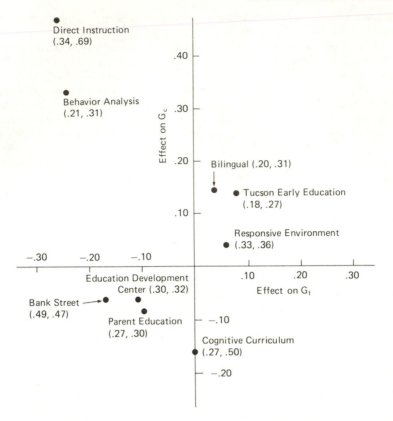

Figure 9.6.   Effect size on fluid (G_f) and crystallized (G_c) ability outcomes of nine alternative Follow Through Models, in adjusted standard deviation units. The standard deviations of effect sizes, for G_f and G_c, respectively, across sites within models are shown in parentheses. (Adapted from "Findings from the Follow Through Planned Variation Study" by M. M. Kennedy, *Educational Researcher*, 1978, 7, 3–11.)

educators must face and that psychologists must seek to understand. It harks back also to one implication of the old Brownell and Moser (1949) study. There it was found that children who were taught mathematics in the first and second grades by a rote drill procedure were unable to profit from explanation-oriented instruction in the third grade. Children who had experienced meaningful instruction were ready for the third-grade work. Thus some instructional methods may work well in one focused domain but produce inaptitude for other kinds of instruction in later or other domains.

More recently, even more massive attempts have been made to intervene both early and longitudinally to affect cognitive development than were made in the Head Start and Follow Through programs. McKay and colleagues (1978) developed a treatment that combined educational improvement with nutritional supplements and improved health care. The treatment was applied in graduated sequence to impoverished children in Colombia in such a way that length of

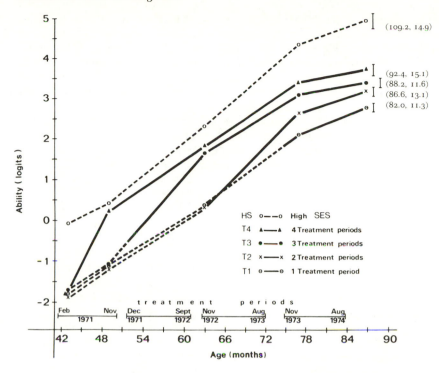

Figure 9.7. Growth of general cognitive ability of children from age 43 months to 87 months, the age at the beginning of primary school. Ability scores are scaled sums of test items correct among items common to proximate testing points. The solid lines represent periods of participation in a treatment sequence, and brackets to the right of the curves indicate one standard error of the corresponding group means at the fifth measurement point. At the fourth measurement point there are no overlapping standard errors; at earlier measurement points there is overlap only among obviously adjacent groups. Added in parentheses on the right are Stanford–Binet IQ means and standard deviations, respectively, for each group at age 8 years. (Adapted from "Improving Cognitive Ability in Chronically Deprived Children" by H. McKay et al., *Science*, 1978, 200, 270–278.)

treatment and age at onset could both be depicted. A stratified group randomization procedure was used to assign children to treatment lengths. An average treatment day consisted of six hours of health, nutritional, and educational activities; the latter included curriculum elements drawn from some of the more successful U.S. compensatory education programs, beginning with language, social, and psychomotor skills and eventually including work on reading, writing, arithmetic, and decision making. A variety of verbal, figural, numerical, memory, and reasoning tests provided a broad-gauge index of ability that combines fluid and crystallized intelligence. Unfortunately, assessment did not distinguish the two constructs.

Figure 9.7 shows the results. An untreated, high socioeconomic status group is shown for comparison purposes. An untreated, low SES control group is not shown, because its very low performance could be attributed in part to lack of testing experience. It is evident that the treatment had positive effects; the solid curves for each treatment group departed from the dashed curves as each group began its treatment. The effects were sustained over the duration of the study, and they were more pronounced the earlier the treatment was administered. Although treated children never equaled the intellectual performance of those untreated children favored by high social class conditions (the topmost dashed curve), treatment did substantially reduce the gap that would normally exist between socioeconomically privileged children and untreated impoverished children. The effects persisted and appeared on standardized intelligence measures at age 8 years. Also noteworthy was the difference in distributions (not shown here) of Stanford–Binet scores between treatment groups, which appeared increasingly bimodal from group to group as length of treatment increased. In other words, in each treatment group, some children showed more mental growth than did others; the longer (or earlier) the treatment, the sharper was the apparent distinction between those who showed more growth and those who showed less. Such a result suggests differential response to treatment among children within any one treatment group, with this difference becoming more marked with longer treatment. The further implication, then, is that the relation of ability at the start of treatment (age 3–5) to IQ at the end (age 8) would give a pattern like that in Figure 9.5D; Treatment T_4 would show a steeper slope than would Treatment T_1. McKay and colleagues (1978) did not report these relations, however.

It is at present impossible to disentangle the relative effects of educational, nutritional, and health care aspects of the treatment, but that should be possible in further research. In the meantime, the Colombian government is extending the treatment to rural and urban preschool children on a nationwide basis.

Venezuela, through a newly established ministry, has also begun to formulate broad-gauge, national programs aimed at the development of intelligence (Machado, 1980). In support of the Venezuelan project, Nickerson, Perkins, and Smith (1980) have reviewed research and theory on the nature and training of intelligence, problem solving, creativity, and the cognitive and metacognitive skills involved in thinking and reasoning. Pickett (1980) has added a review of previous attempts at compensatory educational intervention programs, and Collins and Smith (1980) have addressed directly one of the most central issues – the improvement of reading comprehension. The aim is to extract the best ideas from U.S. research and experience with compensatory education and from innovative developments elsewhere in the world and then to combine them into an integrated instructional program.

The work of Weikart and his associates, previously mentioned, is one such source (see Epstein & Weikart, 1979; Weikart, Bond, & McNeil, 1978; Weikart, et al., 1978). Other early intervention studies in the United States add important suggestions. Garber and Heber (1980), for example, have shown that preschool interventions, aimed at enriching the home intellectual environments of children judged to be at high risk of retarded development can be effective. Their procedure has been to identify newborn infants (without obvious pathology) whose mothers were seriously disadvantaged economically and also were shown to have an IQ score below 75 themselves. Remedial education and vocational and home management training were provided to the mothers, and early education experiences (starting at 3 months of age for the infants) in the form of language development and problem-solving skills were given to the infants and their siblings.

Follow-up comparisons of experimental with control children have shown an advantage due to treatment of 20 IQ points on average that is maintained through the fourth grade in school. Differences in social behavior and positive effects on siblings and on mother and child styles of problem solving have also been noted.

Feuerstein's (1979, 1980) work in Israel is another source. Feuerstein has developed extensive materials for assessing and promoting the cognitive development of retarded adolescents. His Instrumental Enrichment Program is based on a theory of mediated elaboration experiences in learning. Instructional exercises and teacher training focus on a variety of perceptual and cognitive skills interpreted as constituents of intelligence. (See chapter 5, by Sternberg, in this volume for discussion of some program effects on the development of analogical reasoning abilities.) As of 1979, 1,300 classes in Israel were using the approach, and experimental use has begun in North America as well. Evidence reported by Feuerstein suggests that such a program may be expected to promote substantially the intellectual development of low-achieving or retarded students.

Still another possible source is the work of Meeker (1969) and her associates in the International Society for Intelligence Education. They have developed curriculum materials based on Guilford's (1967) structure-of-intellect model. Their programs of diagnostic testing and ability training have been used in various school districts in the United States and have been incorporated also into special educational treatments for gifted students. A particularly extensive application is now under way in Japan.

Programs for gifted and specially talented individuals should serve as a source of ideas and instruments more generally. For a review of such programs, see Getzels and Dillon (1973). A particularly interesting recent program aimed at mathematically talented youth is the work of Stanley, Keating, and Fox (1974). Other approaches to direct development of intelligence in children and adolescents have been proposed and examined by Jacobs (1977), by Valett (1978), and also by Whimbey and Whimbey (1975). On yet another front, courses have been developed for high-school and college students, particularly those pursuing engineering and science, aimed at the development of problem-solving abilities. A review of current theory and research on problem solving and references to the major course development projects is available in Tuma and Reif (1980).

All of these educational programs attempt to train intellectual abilities directly in one way or another. As these attempts involve controlled experiments, they should provide a uniquely valuable means of improving our understanding of ability constructs and how they can be formed and developed. The best work in this line assesses the effects of carefully designed experimental treatments, not only on the task performances that are the focus of training but also on related retention and transfer tasks. The main criterion for ability training is, after all, aptitude transfer. Unfortunately, there have been relatively few such systematic and comprehensive evaluations of these approaches to date. In the next section, we review a selection of the research that exists.

Selected experiments on direct training. Attempts to train ability directly differ according to the choice of training task. We review first those studies that concentrated on fluid–analytic reasoning and spatial–visualization abilities and then move to work on the presumably more crystallized memory, verbal learning, and reading comprehension abilities. A third category includes some studies of metaphoric, inventive, and divergent thinking in complex problem solving and creativity, which presumably involves both fluid and crystallized intelligence. The studies in any category differ in the degree to which they emphasize the training of specific performance skills versus presumably more general strategic and executive processing skills. The studies also show differing interest in whether training benefits some kinds of students more than others, that is, whether ability-training treatments interact with initial status on the same or different abilities. We draw these threads together in a summary of the section.

A series of studies of the development of fluid–analytic ability was conducted with elementary-school students by Jacobs and his collaborators (Jacobs, 1966; Jacobs & Vandeventer, 1968, 1969, 1971a, 1971b, 1972; Jacobs & White, 1971). They investigated the effectiveness of training on the Raven Progressive Matrices and related figural classification and reasoning tasks, which can be considered measures of fluid intelligence. Early studies demonstrated measurable but temporary improvement on the Raven when students were trained specifically on it. Later studies, which were aimed at training classification skills, however, showed both an increment in performance on the trained task and transfer to related tasks, including in some cases the Raven. The effects of training were generally sustained over delays of 2 weeks to 3 months. It was also shown that the effectiveness of training depended heavily on the experience and skills of the trainer.

In another study of Raven performance, Guinagh (1971) trained black and white low SES third graders on the kinds of concepts used in the test. A digit-span test divided students into high and low performers on memory-span ability, which was considered an aptitude for the training. The treatment was found to be effective for all white students but only for those black students who were high in memory span. For the black students, then, there was an interaction of initial memory ability and training on Raven performance. Gains were still evident after a 1-month delay.

Piaget's developmental theory has also inspired direct attempts to accelerate the rate of development of fluid reasoning. These studies have had mixed results (Flavell, 1977). As one illustration, a study by Gelman (1969) gave discrimination training to 5-year-old children who had failed length, number, mass, and liquid conservation tasks. Both specific (length and number) and nonspecific (mass and liquid) transfers were assessed. Trained subjects were near-perfect on the specific conservation posttest; they also performed significantly better than controls on a nonspecific transfer test. A retention test administered 3 weeks later revealed no subsequent decline in performance. Gelman interpreted her findings as evidence that given appropriate training, including feedback, children could be taught to conserve. Other studies (e.g., Inhelder et al., 1966) have not been as successful but have found suggestions of differential progress as a function of the starting level of the child. For general discussions of Piagetian theory in relation to education, see Groen (1978), Murray (1980), and Biggs (1980). For an early review of training studies, see Beilin (1971a, 1971b). An important discussion of the role of training studies in research on cognitive development is available in Gelman and Gallistel (1978; see also Butterfield, 1981). It is extremely unfortunate that most Piagetian research, even today, includes no concern for individual differences in intelligence as psychometrically measured. Humphreys and Parsons (1979) have shown convincingly that performances on Piagetian tasks and on psychometric tests are closely related.

At the other end of the age scale, there have also been successful attempts to train fluid–analytic performance. An example comes from a study by Willis, Bliezner, and Baltes (1980). They trained a group of adults, averaging 70 years of age, to use verbal rule procedures in solving figural relations problems drawn from a commercially available fluid-ability test. A variety of fluid- and crystallized-ability measures were used to assess transfer of training after 1-week, 1-month, and 6-month delays. Compared with nontreated controls, the trained adults showed striking positive effects. These appeared to include both specific and more generalized transfer and were maintained across the 6-month period of the study.

Another analytic reasoning task is represented by Thurstone series-completion problems. Holzman, Glaser, and Pellegrino (1976) have successfully trained the performance of elementary-school children on such tasks. The training sought to teach children to recognize the basic kinds of relations and cycles used to generate letter-series problems, based on analyses conducted earlier (Kotovsky & Simon, 1973; Simon & Kotovsky, 1963). The treatment was clearly successful, relative to the performance of a control group, though retention and transfer were not tested. It is worth noting here, however, that the educational uses of these and other such findings may not be straightforward. Greene (1976), for example, used a similar training program for letter-series problems in elementary-classroom groups; the groups differed in the degree of choice the children could exercise over when and how they worked with the training materials. Outcome varied markedly among the groups. It appeared that free-choice conditions offered the best training for high-ability groups, whereas no-choice conditions (i.e., teacher controlled) were best for low-ability groups (see Snow, 1977a, for further discussion). In other words, the educational effectiveness of an ability-training program can be enhanced or limited by variables related to classroom use.

Research on analogical reasoning has begun to examine the possibility of training skills and strategies. This work has educational implications (see chapter 5, by Sternberg, this volume; Whitely & Dawis, 1973, 1974), but it also serves to advance the information processing analysis of intelligence. Whitely and Dawis (1974), for example, compared the effects of several different training treatments on high-school student performance with verbal analogies. It was shown that treatments involving only practice and feedback were ineffective, whereas treatments giving actual instruction in semantic categorization strategies were effective in improving performance.

Sternberg and Weil (1980) trained college students on linear syllogisms. Those in a visualization group were instructed to represent the problems mentally in a spatial array or series; those assigned to the algorithm group were taught a simplified rule procedure based on a linguistic model previously identified. A third group was given no special training. Apparently, the algorithm training resulted in more efficient performance; it reduced response latencies relative to the visualization strategy. Based on mathematical modeling of each individual's performance, Sternberg and Weil were then able to classify subjects into four homogeneous strategy groups, depending on whether a spatial or linguistic, or mixed spatial–linguistic, or algorithmic model best fit each performance. Correlations of performance with external measures of verbal and spatial ability showed strikingly different patterns for groups of subjects using different strategies. Success with a linguistic strategy depended on verbal but not spatial ability, performance with a spatial strategy showed an opposite correlation pattern, and the mixed strategy gave correlations with both abilities. As expected, the simplified algorithm strategy showed reduced involvement of verbal ability, relative to the full linguistic strategy. Sternberg (see Sternberg & Ketron, in press; Sternberg, Ketron, & Powell, in press) has also demonstrated that strategies for solving analogical reasoning problems can be effectively trained. Here, however, the aim was analysis of strategies on relatively simple figural analogies rather than performance improvements or relation to external ability measures; response latencies were affected by training, but error rates were low for all of the college subjects.

Attempts to train visual and spatial abilities have turned up some other implications. Older studies have yielded conflicting results on the trainability question (see McGee, 1979, for examples), and there is much new research on the biological and social bases of gender differences in spatial abilities (Wittig & Petersen, 1979). It is possible that training research can help clarify some issues in this field. Connor, Serbin, and Schackman (1977), for example, developed a brief training treatment for the Embedded Figures Test, with demonstrations of disembedding using transparent overlays. Performance on the test has been variously interpreted as indicating fluid–analytic or spatial ability or field independence (see Cronbach, 1970), and differences favoring males have often been reported (Witkin, 1976). The training treatment improved the performance of females to equal that of males, relative to control-group females; males were not improved by training.

A study by Frandsen and Holder (1969) investigated transfer of training on spatial–visualization skills to verbal problem solving. Earlier work by Gavurin (1967) had shown the role of spatial–visualization abilities in solving symbol–manipulation problems. Thus, Frandsen and Holder hypothesized that instruction in spatial–visualization techniques should improve verbal problem solving for those low in spatial–visualization ability. Students who were identified as either high or low on a test of space relations were pretested on verbal problems involving mental representation and manipulation of multiple pieces of information. Experimental subjects were then trained on the use of Venn diagrams, time lines, and other diagrammatic techniques of representing data. As predicted, students who were low in spatial ability profited from instruction and showed improved performance in verbal problem solving. Had Frandsen and Holder plotted regression slopes for their data, with initial spatial ability on the abscissa and verbal problem solving on the ordinate, a picture like that in Figure 9.5C would have been obtained; T_3 would represent the training result and T_1 the control group. No aptitude posttests were administered to determine if the specific skill changes would be reflected in performance on other spatial-ability tasks, nor was retention tested.

Another series of studies has added the contrast of strategy training with direct practice. In Salomon's (1974) research, film models of mental transformations thought to be useful in performing various spatial-scanning and visualization tasks were tested against several kinds of practice conditions. The hypothesis was that the models gave low-ability learners a cognitive operation to imitate. Results of several studies showed that the modeling treatment helped less able students and produced a decrement in performance for students who were high in ability initially, relative to the practice condition (i.e., something like the regression slope pattern pictured in Figure 9.5F was obtained, with T_4 representing the practice condition and T_5 the modeling condition).

In a recent study of this same type (Kyllonen, Lohman, & Snow, 1981), high-school students were trained on a paper-folding visualization task with films demonstrating either a folding–unfolding visualization strategy or a verbal coding strategy. These conditions were compared with practice and feedback. Students initially high in spatial ability performed best on both the trained task and a visualization transfer task when given the practice–feedback condition. This treatment, in essence, permitted them to practice, in their own idiosyncratic ways, skills that were already partially developed. Performance of low-spatial-ability students, however, depended on the level of their verbal ability as well as on the type of training they received. Students low in spatial ability and high in verbal ability made fewer errors on both the paper-folding and transfer tasks if exposed to either strategy training condition; their response time was also improved, specifically by the verbal-analytic training. Students low in both spatial and verbal ability were helped by the visualization training procedure, at least on transfer to the surface development task. The results were complex, but they clearly imply that strategy training alters performance, has different effects on students with different ability profiles, and may have different effects on transfer performance from those on primary task performances for some students.

The training of strategic activities of learners has been a central focus of recent research on learning and memory skills among retarded children and adolescents. This work is reviewed in detail by Campione, Brown, and Ferrara (see chapter 8, this volume), but it deserves note here as well because the training and transfer effects obtained so far appear by no means limited to memory abilities or to retarded populations. Research reviews by Brown (1978) and by Belmont, Butterfield, and Ferretti (1980) show clearly that methods for improving memory performance, such as using mnemonic strategies or apportioning study time appropriately, can be trained; that metaknowledge or self-awareness about one's own learning can be developed; and that transfer to different kinds of learning or problem-solving situations is possible if superordinate strategies for doing this are also trained. Self-monitoring and self-interrogation regarding the effects on learning of using more specific strategies, such as rehearsal, coupled with the development of awareness that effective strategies can be generalized and applied in new settings, are instrumental to transfer. As Brown (1978, p. 157–158) observes:

A particularly neglected research area has been the development of efficient training programs for the developmentally young, programs that concentrate on executive functioning such as predicting, planning, checking, and monitoring rather than the perfection of a specific skill. Training techniques to induce simple checking skills for example in those who would not introduce them spontaneously, at least in the context of school learning or traditional laboratory tasks, have not been developed. Although the problems entailed in devising such training programs cannot be overestimated, both the practical and theoretical benefits that would accrue warrant the expenditure of effort and ingenuity.

Corno (1980) has demonstrated how a training program on metalearning skills, designed to be used by parents and children at home, might influence classroom achievement. She found, however, that training was more effective for classes of more able students and also for students showing high-anxiety scores; the able students, particularly, seemed to have experienced more use of the program at home and consequently reaped more benefit in class.

In a related line of studies, Meichenbaum (1977) has investigated the use of instruction to modify inner speech and its effects on emotional behavior as well as on convergent and divergent thinking patterns. An instructor, for example, might model orally the pattern of inner speech used by effective problem solvers, including thoughts about self-checking, the use of imagery or analogy, or other heuristic devices. Meichenbaum has reported success in improving cognitive performance in a variety of instructional and therapeutic settings. Ideas about teacher modeling of this sort have been advocated in research on teaching for some time (see, e.g., Snow, 1970b), but systematic attempts to incorporate such techniques into classroom and teacher-training programs have not been forthcoming. Also it should be noted, for the benefit of further research, that some inner speech modification techniques may not always be helpful for all students. Ridberg, Parke, and Hetherington (1971) found that low-ability children were prompted to display more reflective strategies when film models both verbalized and demonstrated careful checking strategies, but high-ability children profited only from verbalization or demonstration; they were adversely affected by a combination of models. The Intelligence × Treatment interaction would look like Figure 9.5F; T_4 would represent a treatment using one or the other model, whereas T_5 would represent a combined model treatment.

Collins and Smith (1980) have proposed the use of a form of teacher modeling, similar to that studied by Meichenbaum, to improve reading comprehension ability. Their analysis identified two executive or control processes – called comprehension monitoring and hypothesis formation and testing – that appear to be crucial to reading ability and that might be demonstrated by teachers. The training technique would start with the teacher model reading aloud but would include an accompanying metalevel commentary. This would display both hypothesis generating and testing and monitoring for various kinds of identifiable comprehension failures. Questioning techniques would bring students into the process, and later stages of training would involve students in practicing the techniques during oral and eventually silent reading. It is hoped that such skills can be made relatively automatic with practice to reduce demands on conscious attention. The analysis is consistent with other empirical data on reading comprehension processes (J. R. Frederiksen, 1980) but has not yet been systematically evaluated in practice. Sternberg, Ketron, and Powell (in press) have also reported the beginnings of work on the training of word comprehension in the context of reading, but their evaluation has not been completed.

Beyond the training research that aims at relatively well defined intellectual ability and skill constructs, there are myriad studies concerned with the promotion of one or another kind of complex – and often not well defined – thinking skill. Descriptions of these skills have employed terms such as *productive, divergent, inventive, metaphoric,* or *creative* thinking. The research on such constructs has not progressed substantially compared with work on other general abilities, but it is clearly an important category. We have chosen three examples – one old, one new, and one long-term project – to suggest the bases that further research might build upon.

The old example comes from a series of studies by Maltzman (1960) and by Mednick (1963), based on the associationistic theoretical tradition in psychology. Maltzman sought to train abilities related to divergent thinking, using a repetitive remote associates procedure. Subjects practiced producing increasingly remote associations to standard lists of stimulus words. Performance was then seen to improve on independent transfer tests scored for degree of originality and fluency.

Mednick and Mednick (1967) have built the Remote Associates Test based on the associative view of creative thinking; there is evidence that the test relates to some real-world criteria of creative production and thus deserves attention in further research on thinking skills (Cronbach, 1970).

In a rather different line of new work, Kogan (1980) has begun to study individual and developmental differences in metaphoric thinking. The skills involved in sensitivity to and comprehension and use of visual metaphor, analogy, figurative language, and the like, may be centrally important in mediating transitions from old to new conceptual schemata in many areas and stages of science learning, as well as in the arts. Kogan's research shows that individual differences in metaphoric thinking are related inconsistently to various intelligence and school achievement measures and rather strongly to some indexes of analogical reasoning and divergent thinking abilities; it also shows that such thinking can be directly trained. A feedback–explanation condition was found to be effective in enhancing metaphoric thinking in children. Also effective was verbal encoding of stimulus features by the experimenter, which proved to be more effective than one in which students used their own verbal encoding. Interactions of training condition with other student abilities were not studied, however, nor was transfer to other tasks.

Finally, the Productive Thinking Program, produced by Covington and colleagues (1974), has been perhaps the most widely used and most evaluated of the instructional programs designed to develop thinking skills directly. It is examined in detail by Nickerson and colleagues (1980; for a list of references, see also Mansfield, Busse, & Krepelka, 1978). The program uses a series of self-instructional cartoon booklets to promote metacognitive thinking in children's own problem-solving processes. Evidence has been presented to show that the program enhances performance on problem-solving tasks similar to those dealt with in the booklets, relative to control groups. Results regarding transfer to other kinds of tests and tasks are mixed, however, so the generality of the program's effects is questionable. Nickerson and colleagues (1980) note that the program addresses a number of thinking skills judged as more generally important; the scope and length of the program might thus be expanded in further research to good effect or, at least, students might be taught to recognize when its particular approach might be applicable in more general problem-solving contexts.

Thus, there are many examples of training interventions designed to alter one or another kind of ability. Many more exist, but this is not the place for a comprehensive review. One of the lessons to be drawn from all this work should be noted in passing, however. The best attempts at training intellectual skills involved in more complex test performances seem to be derived in one way or another from detailed analyses of the process characteristics of task performance. This point has been emphasized also by Resnick (1976) and by Resnick and Glaser (1976) in their review of several other successful attempts at training. We will return to the topic of cognitive process analysis in a subsequent section of this chapter.

Practice, tuning, and coaching. Aside from direct training interventions, studies have been designed to test whether simple practice or feedback or coaching on test performance would have positive effects. Experienced and inexperienced students alike are thrown on their own at the onset of most ability tests and many instructional tasks. Individual differences in comprehending task instructions, in "warming up" to the task, in adopting efficient strategies for allocating time and effort, and so on, can affect performances on both tests and learning tasks and help produce a correlation between them. Thus, in test administration and in research on intelligence in education it is often recommended that initial instructions be complete and that students be "tuned" to the tasks at hand with sufficient initial practice (Cronbach & Snow, 1977). There have also been suggestions that the most valid assessment of ability would be one that includes practice, tuning, and coaching over repetitive testing until maximum performance is reached (Vygotsky, 1962). Beyond this, such effects would not be of educational interest but for two possibilities. One is that in the absence of appropriate preparation, differential bias related perhaps to ethnic or other social–cultural differences may be introduced into ability and learning assessments. The other concerns the psychological interpretation of ability and learning assessments if simple practice, tuning, and coaching on the tests have large positive effects.

Jensen (1980) has reviewed studies of practice on intelligence-test scores, concluding that practice effects can produce increases of from 2 to 8 IQ points. Such effects appear to be relatively lasting though not transferable to other tests; they are more pronounced for more able learners than for less able learners and on timed or nonverbal tests than on untimed or verbal tests. One recent line of work by Fleishman and his collaborators (Fleishman, 1976; Levine et al., 1979, Levine et al., 1980) used practice with feedback to train subjects on tasks such as flexibility of closure, spatial scanning, and spatial visualization, checking for transfer to more complex tasks presumed to require such abilities (e.g., troubleshooting of electronic circuits). Though practice continued for up to 15 hours, it was effective only for spatial scanning, not for closure flexibility or spatial visualization, and had no impact on performance on the criterion task. Prior practice on a fault-finding pretest, however, did decrease solution time at posttest. Subsequent analyses failed to confirm that practice was any more or less effective for students differing in the trained ability at the start.

Navarro (1980) and Jensen (1980) have both reviewed the earlier literature on tuning and coaching. The conclusion seems to be that attempts at specific coaching usually have relatively little effect over and above practice on the task. Some effects are obtained on some tasks; negative effects of tuning have even been obtained (e.g., by Navarro on the rod-and-frame task as a measure of analytic ability). It appears, however, that effects when obtained are highly specific and fade more rapidly than do practice effects.

On the other hand, there are studies showing notable effects when students are coached to use abilities they possess but do not recognize as relevant to the task at hand. This particular kind of effect has been called a "production deficiency" (Flavell, 1977) and is thought of as marking a transitional stage in strategy development for cognitive performances. It has been demonstrated most clearly in research on the use of memory strategies, such as rehearsal or mnemonic devices. Still, it is conceivable that individual differences in intelligence and performance on school learning tasks might involve such phenomena more generally. Research on this sort of strategic processing has only just begun, as noted by Brown (1978) and others previously discussed; the possibilities transcend the boundaries of this section and so will be taken up later.

The possibility that coaching has large effects for some students on such major scholastic aptitude tests as the SAT has recently fired substantial public controversy (Slack & Porter, 1980; Nairn & Associates, 1980). A review and reanalysis of both old and new research on SAT coaching (Messick, 1980) suggests several points worth further consideration. First, the average effect of coaching when compared with noncoached control treatments appeared to be approximately 10 points for the verbal subscore and 15 points for the quantitative subscore. These score changes are within the standard error of measurement of the test. In studies without control groups, in which coaching effects cannot be disentangled from the effects of student self-selection of a coaching treatment, the average treatment effect has been found to range up to 38 and 54 points for the verbal and quantitative scores, respectively. Second, and more important, effect size varied considerably across different kinds of coaching treatments. The treatments studied to date range from under 4 hours to upward of 300 hours of student contact time and from simple coaching in test taking to substantial instruction in verbal and quantitative comprehension and reasoning, with homework. The latter programs approximate the curriculum activities of conventional schooling. When effect size was correlated with student contact hours across all treatments studied, coefficients ranging from .60 to .80 were obtained. In other words, the more a coaching treatment approximated more extensive educational intervention, the more the score changed. Messick noted that the relationship actually appeared more logarithmic than linear. Thus, to obtain additive increases in SAT score, one would have to add student contact hours geometrically. An added observation was that treatment effects might be greater for some kinds of students than for others, but the research on coaching has not yet systematically addressed the possibility of Intelligence × Treatment interaction.

Teacher expectations. A celebrated study by Rosenthal and Jacobson (1968) raised the possibility that children's intellectual growth could be increased substantially simply by influencing their teachers' expectations about it. The claim was that teachers, given positive expectations about some children, behave in ways toward them that promote intellectual growth. The implied converse, which was not tested directly, was that negative teacher expectations would retard children's mental growth. The original Rosenthal and Jacobson data were rejected as methodologically deficient (Elashoff & Snow, 1971; Snow, 1969; Thorndike, 1968). The Elashoff and Snow review examined nine other attempts to demonstrate the effect of teacher expectancy on intelligence experimentally; all failed (see Baker & Crist, 1971). Mitman (1981) has now brought that review up to date, citing seven further attempts at replication, none of which counters the earlier trend. Teacher expectancy can be shown to influence teacher and student classroom behavior and, in some cases, measured student achievement, but there is no support for the view that teacher expectancy influences measured student intelligence as an outcome of instruction. If achievement can be affected, long-term changes in the development of crystallized intelligence might be expected, but the longitudinal research needed to examine this possibility has not been conducted.

Summary and implications. When intelligence, or one or another of the abilities or skills presumed to be constituents of intelligence, is viewed as an outcome of educational treatments, many different kinds of results are possible. Some broad educational programs (e.g., McKay et al., 1978) have shown marked positive effect on general ability measures. Others (e.g., the analysis of Follow Through by Kennedy, 1978) have suggested that programs showing positive effects on one kind of measured ability outcome may show negative effects on another kind of measured ability outcome. Still other programs have shown little effect either positive or negative.

More focused experiments aimed at direct training have also yielded mixed results, but some important successes (e.g., Holzman et al., 1976; Jacobs, 1977) have demonstrated the value of detailed process analysis for further work, and others (Frandsen & Holder, 1969; Kogan, 1980; Whitely & Dawis, 1974) have clear educational implications. The possibility of strategic training (e.g., Brown, 1978) is a particularly exciting idea.

The research to date leads to some generalizations and implications for the future. First, it is clear that attempts to train abilities must go well beyond simply manipulating practice and feedback, or coaching, or teacher expectations; they must provide substantive training on the component processes and skills involved in task performance, and they must also train directly the superordinate executive and control strategies involved in generalizing and transferring trained performance to new settings. Second, even with intensive interventions of this sort, the best effects of direct training are likely to come from treatments that are extensive, that is, that involve long-term regularized educational programs. Third, evaluation of such programs will need to examine the various delivery and situational variables in educational settings that can be expected to moderate training effects.

One generalization from the strategy training work appears to be that abilities and strategies interact. Attempts to train either component skills or strategies must fit training methods to an assessment of naturally occurring aptitude profiles. The study by Sternberg and Weil (1980) shows this most clearly. Another generalization appears to be that simple practice and feedback, although not effective on average, may provide the best training for students already somewhat proficient in the ability to be trained. Training that is cognitively more intrusive is often not helpful and seems sometimes actually to be harmful for able students; such intervention may disrupt effective idiosyncratic strategies. A further point related to both of these generalizations is that training to improve one kind of ability may work best when the treatment is designed to capitalize on some of the learner's other strengths. Several studies suggest this directly.

A demonstration of the kinds of complexities to be unraveled in further research comes from an old instructional study by Edgerton (1956). A 14-week course in weather observation was taught in two alternative sequences; theoretical explanations first, then computational techniques, or the opposite. The achievement posttest allowed a distinction between procedural *how* questions and conceptual *why* questions. On *how* questions, the theory-first treatment was especially good for students with low aptitude on numerical computation, presumably an aspect of crystallized intelligence. This treatment apparently gave these students a conceptual structure that helped them deal with the later material involving computation. On *why* questions, the techniques-first treatment was better for students low on a reasoning aptitude measure reflecting fluid intelligence. They were allowed to master computation first to facilitate later performance when conceptual reasoning was required. Each treatment sequence, then, first capitalized on learner strengths, then used them to build up learner weaknesses.

Here may be two instances of aptitude transfer running in opposite directions for learners with different ability profiles. Although the students' own learning strategies were not directly studied by Edgerton, one can imagine some individuals working out different sequences of this sort for themselves. Frederiksen (1969) has studied student choice of related learning strategies in a laboratory verbal learning task.

PROCESS-ANALYTIC RESEARCH

Training studies that improve upon the approaches just reviewed can contribute to a more detailed, process understanding of intelligence and education. Indeed, J. R. Anderson (1976, p. 16) proposed that ". . . we take 'understanding the nature of human intelligence' to mean possession of a theory that will enable us to *improve* human intelligence" (emphasis added). To evolve such a theory and thus to improve on the approaches discussed, research is needed that takes an experimental, task-analytic approach, emphasizing analysis of the cognitive processes involved in aptitude, outcome, and instructional task performance. Several other chapters in this volume examine aspects of recent progress along these lines. Other sources include Snow (1978) and many of the chapters in Snow, Federico, and Montague (1980). Thus, a detailed review need not be given here. It is important, however, to touch on the main implications of this work and to identify the areas that will need to be addressed by more detailed research if educationally relevant theory is to be advanced. Several foci within the broad theoretical framework outlined earlier especially need research attention.

Analyses of aptitude tasks. Aptitude and achievement tests should correlate, under given instructional conditions, because at least in part they both reflect individual differences in common or similar psychological functions called upon by those particular instructional conditions. Intelligence tests as indicants of aptitude have been designed with some such vague hypotheses in mind ever since Binet and Spearman.

In discussing the construction of one particular aptitude battery, Carroll (1974) described it as follows:

The tasks chosen for aptitude tests were those which were regarded as having *process structures* similar to, or even identical with, the process structures exemplified in actual learning tasks, even though the contents might be different. The tests were therefore measures of the individual's ability to perform the psychological functions embedded in . . . or . . . the information processing behaviors characteristic of the criterion learning tasks. The theoretical basis for assuming similarities between aptitude tasks and criterion tasks might be of the vaguest intuitive sort; what mattered was the empirical confirmation of one's intuitions by standard test validation procedures. An important aspect of this vague theory, however, was the assumption that there are stable individual differences in ability to perform specified information processing tasks, an assumption supported, however, by a tradition reaching back many years in the factor-analytic literature. [P. 294]

Goals of current research are to discover what these linking psychological functions are and how they are or can be influenced by different instructional conditions. Instructional treatments that are found to change such functions in a beneficial direction can be used to improve aptitude directly. The effects of functions that prove impervious to change may instead be moderated by the design of alternative instruction that relies less on, or compensates for, such functions.

In much prior research in education, however, both aptitude and achievement dimensions have been conceptualized as reflecting simply the "amount" of "ability" or "knowledge" that someone "possesses." The "process structures" had not been conceptualized explicitly until recently (see Carroll, 1976, 1978, and Carroll & Maxwell, 1979) nor have various possible "content structures" (Anderson, 1976; Norman, Rumelhart, & the LNR Research Group, 1975) been detailed.

There seem to be at least two levels of processes and the interaction between them that need to be examined in connection with the aptitude construct. These processes work on different kinds of cognitive content, which itself is structured, to produce achievement and aptitude development. Qualitative as well as quantitative aspects of these phenomena deserve attention.

In the new research on analyses of intelligence, however, early work focused rapidly on the search for "elementary" information processes, with narrow parameter measures of quite specific tasks. Rose (1980) has provided a summary of these in the form of a test battery, and Carroll (1980) has contributed an extensive review and reanalysis of the evidence on these elementary cognitive tasks. Several investigators have also shown that component processes can be identified in performance on the kinds of tasks that appear in intelligence tests. Sternberg (1977, 1981; Sternberg, Guyote, & Turner, 1980), Whitely (1976, 1979), and Pellegrino and Glaser (1979, 1980), for example, have analyzed various kinds of abstract reasoning tasks, such as analogies and letter or number series extrapolation, in this way. The kinds of components identified in analogies of the form "A is to B as C is to ?" for example, include encoding the terms of the analogy, inferring relationships between A and B, mapping these relationships between A and C, applying the results of inference and mapping to C in order to generate an ideal D, justifying an answer when no alternative exactly matches the ideal and producing a response (see chapter 5, by Sternberg, this volume). Other such analyses have examined the nature of verbal ability (Hunt, 1980a; Hunt, Frost, and Lunneborg, 1973; Hunt & Lansman, 1975), spatial ability (Cooper, 1980), and reading ability (J. R. Frederiksen, 1980).

Componential analyses of this sort have shown that it is possible to formulate and validate cognitive process theories of intellectual tasks, but early explorations have also suggested that individuals adapt processing strategies in such tasks and may shift strategies rather flexibly as their own self-monitoring dictates or as task characteristics change. Some initial indications of this phenomenon based on eye movement recording during task performance is summarized elsewhere by Snow (1980a). An experimental demonstration of the importance of strategies comes from Hunt and colleagues (see Hunt & MacLeod, 1978; MacLeod, Hunt, & Mathews, 1978; Mathews, Hunt, & MacLeod, in press). They showed that alternative linguistic and visual–spatial–imaginal strategies are possible in a standard sentence verification task, that different subjects choose different strategies, and that performance differences correlate with verbal or spatial-ability reference tests, respectively, depending on strategy choice. They further showed that college students, at least, can shift strategies if instructed to do so. The Sternberg–Weil and Kyllonen–Lohman–Snow experiments on strategy training also support this view, as does the work of Cooper (1980).

Thus, present evidence makes it necessary to posit a second, higher level of strategic processing concerned with the selection and organization of component processes to meet particular task demands. As tasks vary from item to item, trial to trial, or topic to topic, so must the collection of component processes; some kind of executive control must do this. The executive level has been conceptualized as "summation of strategic assembly and control" (Snow, 1978, 1980a), or as "meta-componential processes determining the components, representations, and strategies that will be applied, and at what rate of execution" (Sternberg, 1979), or as "higher level strategies controlling process integration and sequencing" (Glaser & Pellegrino, 1980). Current research is striving to explicate such processes in more detail, to fit the theoretical framework provided by the Anderson and Greeno computer models discussed earlier. An essential step in such research must be to explain in detail how the higher level processes come into existence, because that may be the educational question of most general importance. Furthermore, it seems possible that this higher, assembly process runs parallel to the elementary, component processes involved in reasoning within analogies, series extrapolation tasks, and the like.

Greeno (1978, p. 243) summed up the results of current research on reasoning in a way that lets us embellish his statement to bring out this parallel:

The psychological process of solving any analogy or series extrapolation problem [and of assembling a strategy for solving such problems in the future] involves identifying relations among components [of the analogy, but also of the problem-solving process, especially when used successfully] and fitting the relations together in a pattern [i.e., a storable and retrievable assembly]. These processes of apprehending relations and constructing [i.e., assembling, storing, and retrieving] an integrated representation are the main processes involved in understanding.

A closely related discussion of assembly functions in problem solving has been provided by Resnick and Glaser (1976). The further studies of Anderson and colleagues (1980) have added the important idea that assemblies, of either conceptual or procedural knowledge, can be acquired and retrieved as units; constructing and retrieving patterns of components can be unitized under certain conditions. Unitized, integrated, crystallized representations appear to be at the core of crystallized intelligence.

Glaser and Pellegrino (1980) have gone on to suggest that school learning skill (i.e., scholastic aptitude or crystallized intelligence) can be described in terms of three interrelated factors. Two of these are ". . . procedural knowledge of task constraints, and organization of an appropriate declarative (or conceptual) knowledge base" (p. 7). They conclude that

The improvement of the skills of learning will take place through the exercise and development of procedural (problem solving) knowledge in the context of specific knowledge domains. The suggestion is that learning skills are developed when we teach more than mechanisms of recall and recognition for a body of knowledge. Learning skill is acquired as the content and concepts of a knowledge domain are attained in learning situations that constrain that knowledge in the service of certain purposes and goals. The goals are defined by uses of that knowledge in procedural schemes such as those required in analogical reasoning and inductive inference. . . . Learning skills are probably developed through graded sequences of experience that combine conceptual and procedural knowledge. This is what must take place when a good instructor develops a series of examples that stimulate thinking." [Pp. 20–21]

The third factor identified by Glaser and Pellegrino is referred to as "management of memory load." E. Hunt (1974, 1980) has singled out a similar aspect of cognitive functioning related to intelligence, calling it "allocation of attentional resources." It appears that the reasoning required in tasks such as Raven Progressive Matrices, geometric analogies, or series extrapolation problems demands that individuals keep track of multiple dimensions of a stimulus series, in which the stimuli are usually designed *not* to connect with previously stored knowledge. "Management" and "allocation" both again imply "strategies," but here there is the added note that such strategies may have to be assembled *during* task performance, because relevant procedural assemblies have not been previously stored. Even with prior experience on similar tasks, retrieved procedural knowledge structures may have to be significantly adapted or reassembled to fit the novel task demands. This possibility links back to the fluid- versus crystallized-intelligence distinction noted in the theoretical framework section. We can expect flexible, adaptive learning to occur during novel task performance, and this should be linked more to fluid-intelligence differences.

There is now substantial interest in identifying the strategic, procedural knowledge aspects of school learning that may account for individual differences in the growth of crystallized ability and achievement. The Glaser and Pellegrino (1980) work points in this direction, as noted. Sternberg (1979) has defined metacomponents of acquisition, retention, and transfer and is pursuing research designed to investigate their character. Baron (1978) has also reviewed literature on strategic aspects of intellectual performance, emphasizing central strategies identified as "stimulus analysis," "relatedness search" (of stored memory), and "checking." Many new attempts to train learning strategies directly have also appeared (see Campione, Brown & Ferrara, Chapter 8, this volume; O'Neil, 1978; Rigney, 1980); some of these were noted in the earlier section on direct training. Task-analytic research and ability-training research will need to be closely linked in the future.

Analyses of instructional tasks for learning and transfer outcomes.   Viewing education as an aptitude development program makes all of what we have reviewed as relevant to the assessment of learning outcome as to the assessment of aptitude for learning. Indeed, in this view, the distinction between aptitude and achievement rests only on the point in time, before or after the instructional treatment, that is of primary interest. Still, the analysis of learning outcome is helped substantially by relating it directly to the analysis of instructional tasks and the learning activities they prompt. It is precisely because the prior (life experience) treatments that led to observable aptitude differences are unspecifiable that analyses of the nature of intelligence have been so difficult and controversial. Combined process analysis of learning outcome and instruction is best because, in Calfee's (1976, p. 24) terms, ". . . assessment is intimately interwoven with the development of substantive theories of instruction. A process-oriented assessment system should help us understand how a student thinks when he is learning something. This allows us to formulate reasonable hypotheses about the character of efficient instructional strategies, and to evaluate the effects of variation in instructional strategy." Finally, an examination of instruction and learning outcome separately from analyses of aptitude input allows some other old concepts of educational psychology to be brought back explicitly into the combined theoretical framework. These are the concepts of learning-to-learn and transfer.

Further research on these possibilities is only now under way. Even with a clear laboratory explication of the links between conceptual and procedural knowledge systems, strategic and component processes in task performance, and fluid and crystallized intelligence differences, the move to describing educational effects in these terms is a monumental effort. It is becoming possible, however, to imagine that the kinds of hypotheses derived from the Intelligence × Instructional Treatment interaction studies and from the evaluations of compensatory education can someday be given this kind of conceptual underpinning.

Gagné (1962, 1970) reestablished the importance of transfer in learning with his work in instructional task analysis. He distinguished vertical transfer, in which simpler learned components are incorporated directly in hierarchical fashion into the learning of more complex performances, from lateral transfer, in which a component learned in one task context is seen to be relevant and is thus carried over to performance in some other context. It was then possible to develop learning hierarchies for the promotion of vertical transfer and to design instructional sequences to accomplish this. Gagné and Briggs (1974) have discussed instructional design for the development of intellectual skills and strategies from this perspective.

Resnick (1976), however, has reported data suggesting that only some students profited on transfer measures from instruction arranged in hierarchical sequence. For other students who learned

... the more complex objectives without intervening instruction, however, "skipping" of pre-requisites was a faster way to learn. What these children apparently did was to acquire the prerequisites in the course of learning the more complex tasks. An important instructional question raised by these results is whether we can match instructional strategies to individuals' relative ability to learn on their own – that is, without going through direct instruction in all of the steps of the hierarchy. [Resnick, 1976, p. 68]

This point has also been made elsewhere (Cronbach & Snow, 1977); the hierarchical organizational sequences do not seem best for everyone.

A further point, as Royer (1979) has argued, is that emphasis on vertical hierarchy limits educational attention to the specific, literal, "identical elements" theory of transfer provided initially by Thorndike and Woodworth (1901). The possible roles of nonspecific, more "figural" transfer in intellectual and educational development have not been given substantial research attention. Yet it may be this latter kind of transfer that most needs to be understood in linking intelligence and educational learning. In Resnick's (1976) further research, it is reported that children transformed the mathematical algorithms originally taught to them into more efficient routines with fewer steps. That is, they discovered or invented efficient strategies for themselves, given what they were taught. As Resnick points out, a conclusion that these most efficient strategies should be taught directly does not follow; it may be that the best form of teaching is one that most promotes this kind of inventive transformation.

Such teaching might be direct for some learners and indirect for others. It is evident, however, that most conventional instruction is incomplete in some relevant sense for everyone. Based on her studies, Resnick (1976) drew out an implication much like Greeno's (1978, 1980). The same implication is supported by the research on Intelligence × Treatment interaction (Snow, 1977a, 1980b):

Differences in learning ability – often expressed as intelligence or aptitude – may in fact be differences in the amount of support individuals require in making the simplifying and organizing inventions that produce skilled performance. Some individuals will seek and find order in the most disordered presentations; most will do well if the presentations (i.e., the teaching routines) are good representations of underlying structures; still others may need explicit help in finding efficient strategies for performance. [Resnick, 1976, p. 78]

The processes by which learners can skip intermediate steps in a learning hierarchy or invent more efficient procedures in problem solving need much more intense study. Nevertheless, a workable hypothesis seems to be that these processes involve lateral nonspecific transfer, or what has been called learning-to-learn. Learners, at least some learners some of the time, are able to see connections between other learning experiences and the one presently faced. These connections may be based on identical common elements, as when conceptual or procedural knowledge acquired in a previous context is directly applicable without adaptation to a new context, but adaptation in some degree may often be required, and isomorphism between the new and the old may often not be. Learners may take advantage of analogies among situations that bear only "family resemblance" (Rosch & Mervis, 1975) to one another. A case can be made that analogical, metaphorical, and figurative thinking lies at the base of much scientific invention and discovery. It is not unreasonable to expect it at the base of intelligent learning and understanding at more elementary educational levels as well. Analogy and metaphor thus appear to be key concepts for research (Norman, 1980). This suggests that further task-analytic studies designed to understand these transferable, learning-to-learn strategies should examine how learners use their conceptual and procedural knowledge to assemble their attack on new learning tasks. Several other aspects of this process can be noted here.

First, as R. C. Anderson's (1977, 1978; Anderson and Freebody, 1979; Steffensen, Jogdeo, and Anderson, in press) research has shown, background knowledge is a critical factor in comprehending new material. It is not simply prior knowledge of the words used in the new material that is facilitative, however; it is the schemata or frames of reference and classification that background knowledge affords for interpreting and elaborating the new material and thus assimilating it into existing schemata while also accommodating them to it. Vocabulary tests representing crystallized intelligence will predict differences in learning the new material in part because they tap word knowledge directly, in part because they reflect breadth of background knowledge structure indirectly, and in part because they require reasoning from this background knowledge (Marshalek, 1981). Stevens and Collins (1980) have also shown how multiple conceptual models from prior knowledge are used to reason about new material in the process of tutoring. The mechanism appears to be analogical or metaphorical, and VanLehn and Brown (1980) have proposed a theory of analogy that is, in effect, a theory of learning by analogical reasoning.

Second, however, the learner must *engage* in this process of elaboration, assimilation, and accommodation. Rohwer (1980) has conducted a program of research on "elaborative propensity" – the degree to which individuals will construct mental events, such as associations, analogies, or images, that help encode and elaborate information for learning, given only implicit prompts to do so, or the degree of explicitness of prompts required to activate them to do so. This tendency to elaborate has been shown to facilitate learning and memory, to increase with age up to young adulthood, and also to vary widely among individuals within age groups. Apparently, then, individuals differ not only in the contents and structure of stored prior knowledge that can be used to construct elaborative mental events in new learning (Rohwer calls this their "event-repertoires") but also in the likelihood that they will use this background knowledge effectively in some literal or figurative way to facilitate the new learning. Elaborative propensity is presumably learned; as one learns to do this effectively, one is learning to learn.

Third, it appears that the characteristics of instruction can either facilitate or impede this process. Rohwer (1978) has provided a general discussion of this possibility. Wittrock (1977; Wittrock & Carter, 1975) has demonstrated it in related research on what he calls "generative" learning, wherein all learning with understanding is regarded as a form of discovery; individuals invent or construct organizational strategies for retrieving old information, relating it to new information, and storing the combined result. One line of studies, for example, examined individual differences in children's classification strategies, showing that instruction designed to complement or extend the individual's natural strategy produced positive transfer to other performances, whereas instruction that duplicated or reinforced the naturally developed strategy produced negative transfer. The implication is that instruction intended to promote learning-to-learn or lateral transfer must build on the individual's previously developed learning strategies and that it must be adapted for different individuals in this respect to avoid destructive effects. This harks back again to some of the findings from research on Intelligence × Treatment interaction and to attempts to train abilities directly. It also raises again Quintilian's hypothesis that instruction should build from strength to weakness.

Finally, research on aptitude, learning, and instruction in this vein must be sensitive to qualitative and context-specific aspects of learning outcome. The question What is learned? is often interpreted far too simply. Egan and Greeno (1973) demonstrated that particular instructional treatments will have effects on qualitative, interrelational aspects of the cognitive structures learned – that outcome cannot be simply characterized as more or less structured or more or less learned.

In research programs conducted by Marton and his colleagues (1975, 1976; Marton & Dahlgren, 1976; Marton & Saljo, 1976; Marton & Svensson, 1979; Svensson, 1977) and also by Biggs (1979), procedures have been developed whereby comprehension can be understood as sets of subjective meanings for individual learners. These can be examined as to their complexity and context specificity. Ordinal scales of "depth of processing" can be discerned, as can differing styles of learning and studying, but more important has been the emphasis, in Marton's group especially, on sensitivity to individual learners' perception and structuring of experience in instruction without the imposition of externally derived theoretical structures on student performance prematurely.

We can expect from all this work to reach more functional diagnostic descriptions of what is learned by whom under given instructional conditions. Further, we can expect that such process-oriented analyses of aptitude, learning, and instruction will transform our methods and our theories of intelligence and education.

Observations of intelligent behavior in learning activities. The direct observation of intelligent behavior in real-world situations has been neglected for decades in psychology with only a few exceptions (e.g., Barker, 1968). As Charlesworth (1976) describes it, the present research need is to observe how individuals cope with problematic situations in their environments, rather than to rely solely on standardized testing situations to assess and study intelligence. Furthermore, psychometric research on intelligence has not paid sufficient attention to the relation of test performance to the ways in which individuals apply their abilities outside of testing environments. Thus, there is a need to identify the cognitive activities involved in various kinds of real-world problem solving, to develop assessment procedures around these, and to study the network of relations across the different assessment domains. Goodnow (1976) has further questioned current definitions of intelligence and assessment procedures from a cross-cultural perspective. She urges caution in interpreting performance in other cultures on the basis of our conventional measurement indexes. Hence, cross-cultural measurement, whether it be intranational or international, should be sensitive to tacit cultural assumptions that may account, in part, for observed differences.

Thus, the ecological validity of traditional intelligence testing can be questioned, much as was the traditional laboratory learning task in an earlier section of this chapter. The difference, however, is that intelligence-test performance continues to be empirically connected in important ways to other kinds of observable performance in education, whereas performance on laboratory learning tasks was not. For educational research, the question remains one of improving our understanding and assessment of aptitudes, the linking of such assessments to observed learning activities in instruction, and the mapping of aptitude-learning transactions onto improved assessments of educational outcome. Observational techniques may be useful in enriching our description of these transactions and linkages and they may help check distortions in our theoretical accounts.

In recent years, observational studies of individual differences in ability and personality have been on the increase. New interest has been shown by clinical psychologists and child psychiatrists (see, e.g., Westman, 1973), by cognitive developmentalists (see, e.g., Carew, Chan, & Halfar, 1976), and by researchers interested in linking parent-child interaction patterns to educational performance (see, e.g., Hess, 1974). The program of research of Cole and Scribner (1974; see also Scribner & Cole, 1981) on cultural aspects of cognition has now extended to natural observations of intellectual interactions in educational settings. The use of classroom observation instruments, including more purely ethnographic methods, in educational research has been markedly expanded, but most of this work has not focused directly on intellectual ability displayed in learning activities. There are, however, selected examples of the potential value of this kind of approach at both group and individual levels and in both real instructional and laboratorylike settings.

Stallings's (1975; Stallings & Kaskowitz, 1974) evaluation of Follow Through Planned Variation used extensive classroom observations at both Follow Through and non–Follow Through sites. It was possible then to describe the degree to which each Follow Through model was observably implemented as planned and the major dimensions that distinguished one model from another. Further, it was possible to correlate initial ability with observed learning activities and various learning outcome measures at the classroom level. The Stallings–Kaskowitz report does not include all the needed correlations, but it was possible to construct Table 9.3 from their analysis to exemplify the kinds of findings that are possible (see also Berliner & Rosenshine, 1977).

For a total sample of 58 third-grade classrooms (both Follow Through and non–Follow Through), partial correlations were computed between classroom

Table 9.3. *Partial correlations between class means on selected classroom activities and learning outcome variables, with initial ability score partialed out*

Classroom activity variables	Tests of learning outcome[a]				
	Raven	Math comp.	Math concepts	Total reading	Language
Number of different material resources present over three days	.34	−.41	−.36	−.18	−.23
Academic activities with exploratory materials	.28	−.30	−.23	−.15	−.26
Child selection of own seating and work groups	.48	−.32	−.31	−.23	−.30
Amount of stories, music, dancing	.28	−.52	−.46	−.20	−.39
Variety of activities in one day	.35	−.44	−.42	−.20	−.36
Percent of checklisted academic activities occurring	−.31	.59	.47	.25	.42
Adult academic commands, requests or direct questions to children	−.41	.51	.36	.18	.30
Academic child responses	−.42	.52	.33	.15	.25
Academic activities with texts, workbooks	−.37	.38	.18	.11	.13
Reading, alphabet, language activity	−.44	.40	.26	.08	.23

Note: N = 58 3rd-grade classrooms. Initial ability measure was the Wide Range Achievement Test.
[a] For numbers in italics, $p < .05$.
Source: Stallings & Kaskowitz, 1974.

level indexes of learning activities and outcome measures, with initial ability partialed out. The pattern of coefficients shown in Table 9.3 suggests that activities associated positively with scores on the Raven test, a measure of fluid–analytic ability, are correlated negatively with crystallized-ability measures, and vice versa. Considering the kinds of activities associated with each pattern, the result repeats the implication of our plotting of effect sizes for alternative Follow Through models from Kennedy (1978; our Figure 9.6).

Some computerized instructional systems allow the collection of protocols on each student from which learning activity indexes can be constructed. In one study of this possibility (Snow, Wescourt, & Collins, 1980; see also Snow, 1980a), a sample of 28 college students spent 15 hours learning computer programming in an interactive instructional program called BIP. Figure 9.8 shows the pattern of obtained correlations among fluid- and crystallized-ability measures (G_f and G_c), a personality measure called independence-flexibility (I-F) (all administered more than a year before the course) and a program diagramming pretest (D), several learning activity indexes (help, success testing, etc.) and two outcome measures (learning curve slope, and posttest). Learning activities such as asking BIP for help or quitting problems frequently correlated negatively with fluid ability and with learning outcome but not with crystallized ability; the latter, although not correlated directly with outcome, did correlate positively with time spent implementing trial programs, which in turn correlated with outcome.

Although such studies of individuals or of groups in classrooms are hardly definitive, they do point to the possibility of observed learning activities serving as manifestations of intelligence–learning relationships. They nonetheless miss an

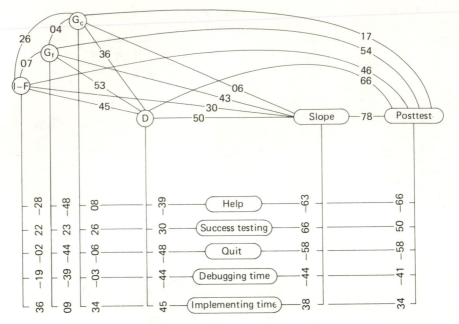

Figure 9.8. Correlations among selected aptitude, learning activity, learning summary, and outcome measures for the BIP course. N = 28; decimal points are omitted.
(From *Individual Differences in Aptitude and Learning from Interactive Computer-
based Instruction* by R. E. Snow, L. Westcourt, & J. Collins [Stanford, Calif.: Aptitude Research Project, School of Education, Stanford University, 1980]. Reprinted
by permission.)

aspect of the *relation* of individual to group that may be crucial to an understanding of the role of intelligence in educational learning and that also can be observed
in learning activities.

In education, individuals are often organized into groups for learning. Individuals bring their own intellect into the group, which then has a collective
intellect differing to some extent from that of each participant individual. There is
thus the character of individual ability, the character of the group's collective
ability, and the relation of individual to group ability, to examine. Observed personal or interpersonal behavior in learning may be conditioned by complex combinations of these sources of intelligence. Despite its importance, only a few
studies have specifically contrasted individual learning with learning in groups,
taking ability into account. Webb (1977) reviewed the literature and then conducted a study that can serve as an example of the kinds of effects that deserve
much further attention in educational research.

Students were given instruction and then asked to solve mathematical problems, both individually and working with a small group. For group work, they
were assigned to either a mixed-ability group or a uniform high-, medium-, or low-
ability group. Advantages in learning either individually or in groups varied as a
function of group composition as well as individual student ability. High-ability
students did equally well as individuals and in mixed-ability groups, but not as

well in uniform high-ability groups. Medium-ability students did best in uniform medium-ability groups and worst in mixed-ability groups. Low-ability students did best in mixed-ability groups, and worst in uniform low-ability groups.

Observations of group interaction indicated that high-ability students in mixed-ability groups tended to act as teachers, offering explanations to lower-ability students. Low-ability students in mixed-ability groups benefited from these explanations. In uniform-ability groups, those medium-ability students who offered explanations showed excellent performance; those who did not participate in this way performed worse than when learning alone. Thus, Webb concluded that active group members did better than those who did not participate and that they performed as well or better than in individual learning. The tendency to participate was a function of both individual ability and group composition.

Such phenomena complicate immensely the problems of research on intelligence and learning in education, for they show the importance of social contexts and social roles in determining the properties of ability–learning interrelationships. Virtually all research on ability and learning conducted in laboratories has assumed that an individual psychological level of analysis would be sufficient. Webb's data suggest that it is not sufficient.

9.5.   SUMMARY AND SPECULATIONS ABOUT THE FUTURE

Education is primarily an aptitude development program. Intelligence is both a primary aptitude for learning in education and a primary product of learning in education. The improvement of education in this regard requires two kinds of conceptual and technical assistance from scientific psychology. One concerns the means of adapting instruction so as to optimize learning outcome for all persons, despite intellectual differences among them that may be impervious to change. This requires improved methods of assessing individual intellectual strengths and weaknesses and improved methods of capitalizing on strengths to compensate for weaknesses. The second concerns the means of developing intellectual strengths directly. Both needs depend on improved content and process analyses of aptitude, learning, and instruction.

In turn, scientific psychology's commerce with education can be expected to lead to improved theories of intelligence and learning. Concentration on the understanding of performance tasks that display clearly nontrivial aspects of substantive intelligence and meaningful learning provides a kind of ecological validity to theory that may help extend it to service beyond the realm of education.

The history of interaction between education and the psychology of learning and intelligence shows many false starts toward an integrated theory. A confluence of old and new ideas now provides a framework for integrated research on intelligence and learning in education, within a modern cognitive instructional psychology. We can hope that a second *Handbook of Human Intelligence,* some years hence, will be able to expand substantially on this chapter's review of theory and research.

This final section summarizes the history of research on intelligence and education to date, as represented in the previous pages of this chapter. It takes the form of a list of hypotheses for further research and a list of admonitions designed to promote the advance of that research. Then follow some speculations about the future.

HYPOTHESES FOR FURTHER RESEARCH

Intelligence as learning from suboptimal instruction. All instruction is incomplete in some respects for someone. For that person, instruction can include errors of commission as well as errors of omission. It is hypothesized that the act of learning from some given instruction involves accessing, adapting, and applying whatever cognitive systems and structures one already has and inventing new systems and structures as necessary to overcome whatever instructional impediments one meets. Intelligence appears to represent the cognitive organizational facilities involved in doing this. Some kinds of instruction embody more gaps and snags than other kinds of instruction, and there are different kinds of gaps and snags. Some persons have become more facile at negotiating most of these impediments, most of the time, than have other persons. The degree to which individual differences in intelligence relate to learning outcome from instruction signifies the degree to which the given instruction places demands for these cognitive facilities on the persons involved. Analytic research is required to detail how prior intelligence differences are reflected as aptitude differences in meeting these demands.

Aptitudinal transfer. Intelligence acquired in prior learning situations transfers to learning from new instruction. Somewhere between the outmoded view of mental faculties and disciplines and the narrow psychological theory of transfer by identical elements there is room for the hypothesis that transfer can occur by analogy among instructional learning tasks sharing only family resemblance. What is transferred, then, may be a style of work, a mode of attack, a strategy, as much as a particular common concept, procedure, or fact. Again, individuals differ in the facility with which they do this, and research is needed to trace the details by which aptitudinal transfer, as well as the applicational transfer of common elements, is reflected in new learning.

Aptitude development. Over years of successful transfer, success breeds success, and the cognitive products of successful learning and transfer appear to become consolidated. Intelligence is manifested in consistent learning ability, and consistent learning is manifested in intellectual organization. It is possible, however, that different kinds of learning situations breed different kinds of aptitude for further learning as well as different kinds of inaptitude. The hypothesis that fluid–analytic and crystallized–synthetic intelligence, in particular, appear to derive from different streams of experience and to relate to different kinds of subsequent situational performances deserves longitudinal research attention. Such research will need to pay particular attention to the transfer relations among educational experiences that are hypothesized to result in ability formation and ability differentiation.

Aptitude × Aptitude interaction. Intelligence as aptitude for education is thus multivariate, and there are other "nonintellectual" aptitudes, such as anxiety, that can multiply or otherwise alter the effects of intelligence on learning. Research that seeks an account of aptitude for educational learning must look beyond intelligence, narrowly defined, to consider the multiplicity of personal attributes that condition response to instruction. There is evidence that verbal intelligence and anxiety interact in learning. There is also evidence that learners substitute aptitudes they possess for those they lack; in other words, there sometimes appears to be an intrapersonal trade-off between strengths and weaknesses. Such interactive effects cannot be unraveled without research that produces an account of the content and process structures involved in individual differences in aptitude for learning.

Aptitude × Instructional Treatment interaction.   There is also evidence of interaction between aptitude profiles and instructional treatment alternatives. The hypothesis is that treatments differ in the information processing demands they place on learners, following the implications of several of the hypotheses stated earlier. Process-analytic research is also required to understand interactive effects of this sort. The design of instruction adapted to fit aptitude differences, that is, to capitalize on learner strengths while compensating for weaknesses, requires the ATI paradigm to test such hypotheses and to evaluate the adequacy of attempts at such instructional adaptations.

Aptitude-training treatments.   General intellectual aptitudes have long been regarded as impervious to change through direct training interventions, even while being susceptible to long-term development through education. Present evidence supports the hypothesis that superficial interventions based on practice, coaching, expectancy changes, and the like, have little or no effect on ability development but that substantial educational interventions based on direct training of component skills and metacognitive strategies can sometimes have important positive effects. To the extent that further research can expose the cognitive components and metacomponents that are susceptible to training and can suggest how effective training can be designed, adaptive instruction that develops aptitude directly may be envisioned. It also appears that direct training can have negative as well as positive effects, depending on student aptitude profile, and thus the ATI paradigm is again required for training evaluation. In any event, the criterion for research of this sort is transfer to valued educational or other worldly performances, not direct training of ability itself.

Educational effects in context.   Evidence cited throughout this chapter suggests that research on intelligence and education must attend to the nature of educational contexts. Certain hypotheses propose that the effects of individual intelligence in learning depend on learning and teaching activities in the home and the school that are in turn context dependent. Other hypotheses claim that the mix of ability in groups and the social perceptions and transactions occurring in them condition learning outcome. Observation studies, field evaluation experiments, and social–psychological analyses are thus an indispensable bridge for the two-way street between laboratory and classroom.

ADMONITIONS FOR FURTHER RESEARCH

Theoretical frameworks and hypotheses that capture some significant amount of past thinking suggest further research possibilities, but the failings of past thinking and research must also be avoided. Many admonitions and suggestions, both conceptual and methodological can be distilled from the history of this field. Some of these have been treated elsewhere (Cronbach & Snow, 1977; Snow, 1978, 1980c). We touch here briefly only on the issues judged most generally important.

Choice of learning tasks.   If the cognitive organizational phenomena of school learning provide the primary medium in which intelligence and learning connect, then research on the connection must be based on school learning tasks. Early investigators were misled by the assumption that traditional laboratory learning tasks embodied all the essential features of learning.

Length of treatments.   If research is to examine the cognitive organizational phenomena connecting intelligence and school learning, then experiments must go on long enough for such phenomena to emerge. Short experiments on school learning are useless, save for displaying the role of prior aptitude or stored knowledge in the initial steps of new learning. Accretion, restructuring, and fine tuning as processes of complex learning can be expected to materialize over weeks and months, not over minutes. This point was also missed by early investigators.

Choice of tests.   The admonitions just cited apply as well to intelligence tests. Short, simple special ability tests do not necessarily embody all the features of intelligence that are essential for the study of its relation to school learning.

Multitrait–multimethod measurement.   If fluid–analytic and crystallized–synthetic intelligence reflect somewhat different aspects of prior learning history and apply to somewhat different aspects of a new learning task, then both constructs must be clearly assessed and distinguished in future research. If assessment of specific prior competence on the learning task itself is also necessary, then investigations of intelligence in educational learning can do with no fewer than six separate aptitude measures, two per construct. The logic of multitrait, multimethod thinking (Campbell & Fiske, 1959) is inescapable in this field, because two forms of aptitude transfer must be distinguished from task-specific competence as well as from each other.

Complexity of performance.   An individual's score on some test or tasks reflects neither a fixed nor a pure measure of ability. Measures are fallible, and scores reflect the combination of abilities and motivations brought to bear by a person for one performance at one point in time. Also, the same score can be achieved by two individuals who use different abilities and strategies and by the same individual who uses different abilities and strategies at different points in time. In any performance, human beings can be expected to use abilities they have to compensate for those they lack, regardless of what ability a test or task purports to represent.

Content and process diagnosis.   Instrumentation must be developed that provides both content and process diagnoses of aptitude input, instructional treatment, and learning outcome. These diagnoses will have to be made sensitive to the learning-to-learn and transfer phenomena that are presumed to mediate cognitive organizational change and, hence, aptitude development. This is the tallest order and is thus the prime topic for research in instructional psychology today. Several other chapters in this handbook, and several sections of the present one, address the need for analyses that will provide such instrumentation, at least for aptitude research, but comparable analyses of instructional tasks and learning outcome constructs are also required.

The lure of reductionism. Analysis conducted without persistent contact with the educational phenomena it will be used to address runs the risk of repeating history and missing the emergent properties once again. The tendency toward reductionism plagues science in general, and the psychology of intelligence and learning has not yet escaped it. Pellegrino and Glaser (1980) have lately suggested that "instructional tractability" should be regarded as an important criterion for choosing a level of analysis. What is needed are cognitive process constructs describing individual differences in aptitude for learning that are amenable to manipulation and modification by instructional interventions and that suggest new kinds of instructional procedures. If such a level can be defined, basic research on intelligence in learning can potentially reach both substantial and fundamentally useful theory for education.

Educational utility. It is appropriate to keep the criterion of educational utility in mind more generally by asking regularly what kinds of psychological concepts and distinctions are most useful to educators. Education is eclectic, pragmatic, and diverse; local usefulness more than general truthfulness is the criterion. There are two levels of use: A concept can be relevant at the level of instructional practice or at the level of school or state educational policy, or both. The criterion applies differently at the two levels.

One concept that is not useful at the practice level, for example, is the heredity–environment contrast. Educators are environmental engineers seeking to improve instruction for individuals and local groups so as to optimize outcomes. It helps not at all to decide that "environment" accounts for "only" 10% or 20% or 50% of the variance in some intellectual or educational index in some statistical population. Educators must work with students as given and know that the genetic potential of individuals cannot be estimated in any event.

On the other hand, Scarr and her associates (Scarr & Weinberg, 1978; Scarr & Yee, 1980) have shown how heritability analyses can inform educational and social policy. Results of this research suggest that although genetic variations and socioeconomic levels are similar in their effects on intelligence and school achievement test performance, the two types of tests differ markedly in variation owing to environmental influences. Achievement tests reflect environmental variation due to social class much more than do intelligence tests. Educational systems have lately been abandoning intelligence tests in favor of achievement tests for purposes of ability grouping, and they have been installing achievement tests, "minimum competency" tests, and the like, to evaluate schools and individuals for credentialing and graduation purposes. Scarr's analysis suggests that biases against students of working-class families will be increased by such practices. Thus, although achievement assessments are essential as guides to instructional practice, they may only exacerbate social problems when used as summary evaluations. The utility of concepts such as heritability applies differently at practice and policy levels.

The nature of research in education. As research is conducted *in* education, as opposed to *for* education, due respect must be paid to the complexities implied by several of the hypotheses and admonitions discussed here. Generalizations are often severely limited in education. What works in one locale may not work in another and it may not even work in the same locale in another decade because student and teacher populations, curricula, and various contextual factors vary so significantly from locale to locale and from era to era. Even if the same packaged treatment is used in all of them, it is embedded in a complex network of interactions among other factors. The implications of this limitation are substantial for the development of theory (Cronbach, 1975; Snow, 1977b). One cannot build theories of instruction from the top down. Rather, one aims at local theory, developing and describing in detail what works in a particular instance within a continuous longitudinal evaluation of that locale. Such theories can be extended as locales are found to be similar on key variables, but the theory-building process is from the bottom up.

Even aggregations of effects in the same place, as from individuals to classrooms to schools, are suspect, because the psychological meaning of measures may vary at different levels of aggregation. Each individual's intelligence-test score resides in a classroom distribution and also in a school distribution. Its meaning in relation to learning outcome will differ depending on the degree to which the individual's relative position in a group and absolute position in a group relate to learning differently (Cronbach, 1976). In other words, an individual's score may stand at the top of one classroom or school distribution, and at the bottom of another classroom or school distribution, while in an absolute sense it is the same score. Because of social factors, the aptitude–learning relationships may look quite different in these different absolute and relative distributions. In short, a social psychology and sociology of classrooms and schools must be combined with the cognitive psychology of intelligence and learning in education.

SPECULATIONS ABOUT THE FUTURE

Speculations about the future are tenuous at best, even when they are based on extrapolations from clear present trends. In this last section, we offer only a few such projections, relating to the major dimensions of education and educational research on intelligence. These are based on what we think will happen, but they incorporate to a significant degree what we think ought to happen. Identifying needs for future research in this way may help make a self-fulfilling prophecy.

Aptitude development and decline. The SAT is a measure of scholastic aptitude, or crystallized intelligence. The decline in national average SAT scores over the past two decades is taken by some as an index of decline in the effectiveness of education as an aptitude development program. It is feared that the expanding effects of television, drug abuse, the disintegration of the primary family, and other social problems, coupled with the continued proliferation of shallow or trendy elective courses in the public school curriculum, have undermined the scholastic ability of a whole generation of young people in the United States. This has led to predictions of continued SAT score decline. The military also continues to report decline in the mental-test scores and the observed educational learning skills of enlistees. As advancing technology requires increasingly skilled human performance, young adults as a whole seem increasingly less able to acquire it. Public concern has been rising. There is now a "back to basics" movement in elementary schools. Some colleges and universities are returning to "required" courses in the freshman year and a general tightening of "standards." Some high schools are joining this trend. These educational changes could presumably reverse the course of aptitude development in the United States, and the SAT curve as well.

Alternative theoretical explanations for the SAT score decline also lead to predictions of reverse trends. Zajonc's (1976) confluence model associates the intellectual level of generations to birth order, birth interval, and thus to birth rate. The intellectual climate of the home, he assumes, is more advantageous to firstborns, and less and less advantageous to children born later and later in order, in a family. Disadvantage is also greater with shorter intervals between births. The U.S. birth rate increased from World War II until the early 1960s, so there were more second and later children born in this period. Thus average birth order increased and average SAT scores declined in step (with a 17-year lag). Zajonc's projection of this relationship is shown in Figure 9.9. The lower part of the figure indicates the increase in average birth order due to increasing birth rate up to about 1960, and then a return to lower average birth orders for persons born after 1960 as the U.S. birth rate decreased. The upper part of the figure shows the declining SAT average in parallel with birth order but lagged by 17 years, the normal age at which the SAT is administered. Zajonc's SAT curve ran to 1974–1975. The shaded area shows his prediction. We have extended his curve up to 1979–1980 from data provided by the College Entrance Examination Board (see their annual reports, available to the public on request). Apparently no reversal is yet in sight, though there appears to be some leveling. A further study (Zajonc & Bargh, 1980) has suggested that rather little variance in the SAT data is accounted for by birth order and interval variables. One can imagine, however, intrafamily educational effects as hypothesized by Zajonc, multiplied by the formal educational effects of a tightened elementary and secondary curriculum, producing a substantial reversal of the SAT curve in future generations.

Scores on some general ability tests have apparently been going up, in some age groups. Thorndike (1975) reported that preschoolers, in particular, in 1972, averaged higher scores on the Stanford–Binet test than did comparable age groups tested in the norm sample of 1937. These differences were reduced by the age of 10, but reemerged to a lesser degree by adolescence. He credits the amount of verbal and visual stimulation available to modern children through such media as "Sesame Street" for this difference. Loehlin, Lindzey, and Spuhler (1975) have also noted that large-scale studies on IQ change have suggested either no difference between cohorts over a period of 10–20 years or increases in IQ scores. No studies have shown a decline in IQ across cohorts. Larger shifts have been noted in sites undergoing major educational change; stable educational institutions characterized the regions where no increase was noted. Zajonc and Bargh (1980) have also discussed recent apparent increases in ability scores among children.

It is unfortunate that the distinction between fluid and crystallized intelligence cannot be made in these data, because the two curves could conceivably show different trends. Following earlier hypotheses, one would expect crystallized-ability measures, such as SAT or school achievement tests, to show more pronounced effects owing to changes in the quality of formal education, with fluid-ability measures showing more the effects of expanded or diminished opportunities for "natural" problem-solving experiences in the home and in everyday life.

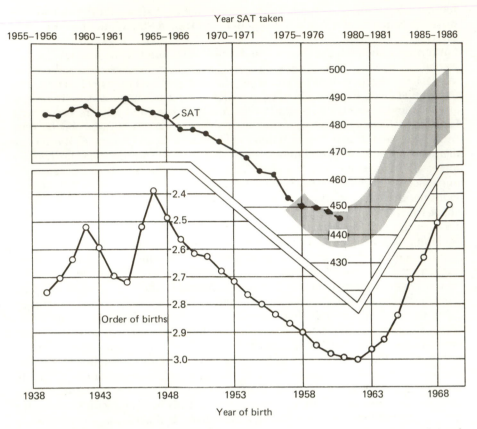

Figure 9.9. Average order of live births in the United States, 1939–1969, and average SAT scores for the first 18 cohorts. Future SAT averages are predicted to lie within the shaded area. (From "Family Configuration and Intelligence" by R. B. Zajonc, *Science*, 1976, *192*, 227–236. Reprinted by permission.)

Accountability and minimum competency testing.   Concern about the SAT score decline is part of a more general public apprehension about the quality of U.S. education today. The growth of the evaluation movement through the 1970s, noted earlier in this chapter, was in part a response to demands for accountability in public education (Atkin, 1979). A recent manifestation of this concern is the trend toward "minimum competency testing." The idea is to construct measurement devices that can be used to define and assess levels of competency in basic skills that all students must meet to graduate from high school, and thereby to pressure educational systems to focus on these skills as outcomes (Jaeger & Tittle, 1980).

  Minimum competency testing has come quickly into vogue. At this writing, more than 30 states now have mandated minimum competency testing programs (Shoemaker, 1980), and other states are likely to follow suit in the years to come. Great diversity exists, however, in the nature and scope of these programs; in

Florida, a statewide examination has been developed and administered, whereas in California, individual school districts have been encouraged to develop their own tests to fit local needs. Programs also differ as to the consequences of student failure to achieve specified performance levels, the frequency of assessment, the intended use of the test, and the specific skills being assessed (Baratz, 1980). In general, however, all such programs emphasize basic proficiency in reading, writing, and mathematics.

The consequences of this movement are still very much in doubt. Proponents argue that the potential of measurement for improving instruction has long been overlooked (Popham, in press). Carefully developed criterion tests, designed locally in collaboration with parents and teachers, should draw instruction toward important and teachable educational goals. Popham (1980) further asserts that such testing programs need not constrict education to training basic crystallized skills. Rather, by focusing directly on desired criteria such programs may lead to the development of tests that measure higher-order cognitive functions of the sort found in definitions of intelligence. This would in turn encourage efforts to develop such functions directly. Certainly, if educational tests can be designed to provide diagnoses of cognitive functioning at all levels and in sufficient detail to give direct help to teachers in planning instruction, then the movement could be beneficial. As with many earlier educational movements, however, changes are introduced in a rush without the needed concurrent research and evaluation. Psychological, psychometric, and legal problems exist and the social consequences may be substantial, as noted earlier in connection with Scarr's heritability analyses of intelligence and achievement tests.

Opponents fear that the competency tests will stigmatize failing students without providing effective remediation to improve performance (Cohen & Haney, 1980), and they argue that schools will substantially shift their attention to children in need of remediation, ignoring children who can easily achieve the minimum competencies. This, in turn, would lead to a "levelling downward of educational attainment" (Atkin, 1979). Greene (1980) suggests that education oriented toward specific achievements, rather than toward more general aptitude development and transfer, may not encourage the intellectual maturity that broader education should provide. Technical criticisms of the tests themselves and various legal issues have also been raised (Bardon & Robinette, 1980; Blau, 1980; Tractenberg, 1980). The critical issue for the purposes of this chapter is whether such tests can be made to serve the educational goal of aptitude development. To the extent that the tests are geared only to what is directly taught in schools, they cannot adequately assess the transfer objectives of education, whether these are stated in terms of aptitude for further learning or aptitude for problem solving in everyday life. Educational accountability would seem to demand assessments of aptitude all along the educational line. The substitution of minimum competency tests for such assessments seems not to be a step in this direction.

Research on intelligence and education.   The future of research in this area depends on economics for financial support and on the continued growth of cognitive psychological theory for substantive support. The latter at least can be predicted to expand, but the directions of expansion, chosen inevitably from among many possible alternatives, are critical for education. We have tried to emphasize in this chapter the importance of detailed process and content analyses of aptitude tests and instructional tasks, because this appears to be the most direct route to the construction of theoretically based instructional models patterned on Figure 9.2. These will be provisional models and it is to be hoped that more than one will be developed from this research, each embodying different sets of assumptions to permit evaluation of theoretically and practically important alternatives. They will undoubtedly have to vary also by subject matter as well as by the age range of learners to be served. Such models may be incorporated within existing systems of individualized instruction, such as IPI, or they may spawn new kinds of systems. We expect these systems to be variations on a theme, however, not monolithic, "one-best-way" designs set into place in educational settings without adaptation. They must be self-monitoring, and their evaluation in educational settings must be sensitive to local conditions, including the nature of teacher and student populations and classroom social contexts, and to change in these local conditions over time.

Research can provide important spinoffs for education even without the construction of anything that could be called an integrated instructional model or system. The analysis of performance on intellectual and learning tasks should produce assessment concepts, and perhaps technologies also, that expand and improve upon present intelligence tests. We thus would expect the intelligence tests of the future to provide diagnostic assessments of learning abilities and disabilities that link, at least conceptually, to direct training and instructional alternatives available to teachers. These instruments may look more like multifaceted within-subjects experiments administered by computer than like current tests. The analysis of instructional tasks, also, should provide insights and distinctions that enrich educators' views of the psychological effects of teaching methods and curriculum alternatives, whether or not they lead to specific instructional prescriptions. These should provide qualitative as well as quantitative characterizations of the cognitive structure of learning outcome linked back to particular instructional choices. For related views on the future of intelligence tests, see the symposium on this topic reprinted in Sternberg and Detterman (1979).

There is always the threat that cognitive psychology will again break up into many isolated camps, each with its own pet tests or tasks (Newell, 1973), and, further, that it will pay only lip service to the crucial importance of context (Neisser, 1976). One cannot take a series of items out of an intelligence test, or a series of exercises out of an instructional task, or either test or task out of the broader educational context, without running the risk of losing ecological validity. This is not an empty threat. What gets lost is not just "face" validity in the eyes of educators; it is the subtle emergent properties of intellectual and learning task performance that appear to be inexorably linked to aspects of the cognitive, motivational, and social contexts of educational processes. This was the message of the observational studies noted earlier, but it is a bigger problem than those studies suggest and its dimensions are not yet fully apprehended. New research that expects to enrich educational theory and practice will need to address this problem directly.

The new technologies. Any look into the future must note the advance of educational technology. Up to the present, the advance has usually been slower than predicted, but it is the case that miniaturization has now broken many of the economic barriers that kept technological innovations from widespread educational application. The hand calculator, the audiotape recorder, and the television receiver are already within the reach of virtually every student; the desk computer is close at hand for many. These instruments can and perhaps should become basic tools of education and of human intelligence. Furthermore, advances in computer technology and in the field of artificial intelligence have been instrumental in the advance of cognitive psychological theory generally. As the computer is made more intelligent, more intelligent use can be made of computers. Computerized interactive instruction, computerized adaptive testing, and computerized guidance systems now exist in several forms and have been installed in some high schools and colleges. Computerized reasoning and problem-solving games have been placed in some elementary schools. The potentials of word processing, videotape recording, and video discs for education are now on the horizon.

All this portends change in the medium of education. To the extent that intelligence is skill in this medium, changes in intelligence can also be expected. There has been speculation but rather little research, in education or out, concerning such changes. On the one hand, the new technologies can be used to capitalize on characteristics of human aptitudes, that is, to extend and exercise aspects of intelligence at new and higher levels, thereby strengthening and broadening the scope of intellectual skills already possessed by the individual. On the other hand, these technologies can also be used to compensate for characteristics of human inaptitudes, to do for individuals what they may not be able to do for themselves. Just as the writing tablet compensates for limits in human memory, the new technologies can be used to compensate for other information processing limitations of particular individuals or of all human beings.

We can sum up many of the ideas of this chapter by envisioning a computer system – call it QUINTILIAN, or QUINT, for short – designed along the lines of our Figure 9.2. It has five component programs with which students can interact, called aptitude profile assessment, counseling and guidance, direct aptitude development, adaptive instructional treatment, and outcome profile assessment. Also, it comes in three levels, QUINT I, II, and III, for primary, secondary, and tertiary educational usage, respectively. When a student signs on, QUINT administers an aptitude battery, using efficient adaptive testing methods to construct an aptitude profile for this particular individual. The aptitude battery includes tasks geared to provide detailed diagnoses of information processing strengths and weaknesses in various kinds of problem-solving situations, not merely total performance scores on a few dimensions. It also includes sample tests to assess stylistic and strategic processes in learning and to build up provisional representations of the individual's prior conceptual and procedural knowledge in a few broad and basic content domains. QUINT then asks the student questions concerned with counseling and guidance, assessing prior knowledge in particular domains in which the student expresses interest. It informs the student about the nature of instruction in the system and why certain common goals of the instruction to come are generally valued, asking also for student opinions about these. The student enters personal perceptions, preferences and values about personal talents, life goals, various occupations, and alternative courses of study. QUINT provides information on occupational characteristics and qualifications, types and levels of education required, distributions of the characteristics of people entering these courses and occupations, and so on. The student can explore alternatives interactively and iteratively, learning how to make educational career decisions intelligently in the process. Given the student's goal choices, preferences, and initial aptitude profile, the third and fourth components of the program work interchangeably to give instruction aimed directly at the development of relevant aptitudes and instruction adapted to fit the existing aptitude profile. Both common and individually chosen goals are included. One can imagine a whole bank of subprograms for different areas of knowledge and skill, constituting the curriculum upon which the executive program draws. The executive and/or the student may switch among direct aptitude training, common goal instruction, and individual goal instruction, as desired. The computer monitors knowledge and aptitude changes as the student progresses, builds up its representation of the student as it goes, and uses this to adjust its choices of succeeding items and tasks. This procession of minute-to-minute microadaptations occurs within broad alternative streams of treatment, chosen on the basis of the aptitude profile but updated month to month. There is thus both microadaptation and macroadaptation of instruction based on initial aptitude, goals, and subsequent learning history. Finally, the fifth component adds assessment of retention and transfer, provides intermediate advice and guidance, receives student suggestions and feeds back to adjust the representation of the student and various parameters of the program. Successive blocks of instruction run again through this cycle, with emphasis of different components depending on the stage and area of learning.

All this glosses over the complexities of producing such a system and the many nuances that might be built into it, but all of the components exist today in some form. Plans to create such a system are already on the drawing boards, and there are adaptations for military, government, and industrial use. It may not be long before a prototype, of the first and second components at least, will be found in some military recruiting offices. The first and fifth components exist for achievement measurements at least (Weiss, 1978). The second component is already available as a service in many colleges and universities, and in some high schools (Chapman et al., 1977; Katz, 1980). Special purpose CAI systems function somewhat like the third and fourth component (Atkinson, 1976). Such technology is no longer fanciful. It is the research program needed to develop such a system that remains behind.

Beyond tested intelligence. Intelligence tests were designed to allow systematic observation of intellectual performance in a controlled and standardized situation. The aim was to reduce subjectivity, bias, and various other sources of error. For assessment purposes, however, the skilled school psychologist uses direct observation while administering individual intelligence tests, as well as the resulting quantified measurements. Frequently also, the tester observes individuals interacting with teachers and other students in natural classroom and playground settings and consults with teachers about their mutual observations. Properly conducted educational assessments take a "whole child" view, as sensitive to emotional and social problems as to intellectual performance problems. The student's best interests are the prime concern.

With the mass production and mass use of group mental tests, some kinds of educational decision making and also research on intelligence in education came to rely heavily on the quantified score used alone. Much of the research summarized in previous sections of this chapter relied simply on total test scores. It is not clear at present to what degree educational decisions or our theoretical picture of the role of intelligence in education might be distorted or rendered unduly vague by reliance on group test scores. The issues of cultural bias in tests, or in decisions based on tests, are not dealt with in this chapter (see Jensen, 1980), but the accuracy, richness, and breadth of our present theoretical picture is a major concern here.

It is clear that although a cognitive psychological theory of tested academic intelligence and its role in educational learning would be a major triumph, it would not be sufficient. No one now believes that intelligence as aptitude for school learning is fully or adequately captured by performance scores on the Stanford–Binet or the Raven test, even though such scores bear strong relation to indexes of school learning. No one believes that the SAT and ACT tests represent fully or adequately the intellectual product of high-school education, even though as aptitude measures they are valid predictors of college success, as colleges are now constituted. Education as an aptitude development program must aim at much more than the development of academic intelligence. It must aim at producing aptitude for all the kinds of problem solving needed to advance and sustain human civilization. Research on intelligence will need to lead the way in this. At present, we have little understanding of what constitutes social intelligence or scientific creativity, or how conative and affective processes intersect with cognitive processes in learning and problem solving. We have virtually no concept of collective intellect with which to analyze the effectiveness of groups. The social, political, economic, and environmental problems surrounding us today seem to grow much faster than our ability to solve them. Many educators believe that H. G. Wells was right – we are in a race between education and catastrophe. We also believe that research on intelligence and education is centrally important in this race.

NOTES

This chapter was prepared while the senior author was in residence as Fellow at the Center for Advanced Study in the Behavioral Sciences, 1979–1980. He is grateful for financial support provided by the National Institute of Mental Health (2T32 MH14581–04); the Spencer Foundation; and the Personnel and Training Research Programs, Psychological Sciences Division, Office of Naval Research (Contract No. N00014–79–C–0171). The views and conclusions contained in this document are those of the authors and should not be interpreted as necessarily representing the official policies, either expressed or implied, of the Office of Naval Research, or the U.S. government. The authors thank Professors Lee J. Cronbach, Denis C. Phillips, and Robert J. Sternberg, and also Robert Curley, for helpful criticisms of portions of the manuscript but reserve responsibility for any errors contained herein to themselves.

1 To measure the size of this literature, a computer search of ERIC and *Psychological Abstracts* files identified 20,080 and 10,885 citations, respectively, that combine the terms *intelligence* or its synonyms and *education* or its synonyms in their titles or abstracts. We thank Dr. Carol Treanor, Center for Advanced Study in the Behavioral Sciences, for conducting this search.

2 This may be the earliest reference in history to adapting alternative instructional treatments to fit aptitude differences. We thank Professor Lee Shulman for bringing this passage to our attention.

3 This brief survey was constructed by first checking the helpful summaries provided by A. E. Meyer (1975), then looking to more detailed sources as needed. These sources included Archambault (1964), Best (1962), Butts and Cremin (1953), Cremin (1961), Garforth (1966), Gay (1964), Joncich (1962), Lee (1961), Nettleship (1968), Piaget (1967), Smail

(1966), and Woodward (1964). But the checklist is admittedly superficial, and our review was limited by time and resources. We hope that no gross errors have been allowed. It is notable that a great deal of scholarly effort has been devoted to the examination of educational philosophies over the centuries, without systematic attention to the psychology of individual differences in intelligence and other aptitudes presumed by these philosophies. At best, the present table may prompt specialists in the history and philosophy of education and psychology to a deeper analysis of original writings on these issues.

REFERENCES

Allison, R. B. *Learning parameters and human abilities.* Unpublished manuscript, Princeton, N.J.: Educational Testing Service, 1960. (NR 151–113)
Anastasi, A. *Differential psychology: Individual and group differences in behavior.* New York: Macmillan, 1958.
Anastasi, A. On the formation of psychological traits. *American Psychologist,* 1970, 25, 899–910.
Anderson, J. E. The limitations of infant and pre-school tests in the measurement of intelligence. *Journal of Psychology,* 1939, 8, 351–379.
Anderson, J. R. *Language, memory, and thought.* Hillsdale, N.J.: Erlbaum, 1976.
Anderson, J. R., Kline, P. J., & Beasley, C. M., Jr. Complex learning processes. In R. E. Snow, P.-A. Federico, & W. E. Montague (Eds.), *Aptitude, learning, and instruction: Vol. 2. Cognitive process analyses of learning and problem-solving.* Hillsdale, N.J.: Erlbaum, 1980.
Anderson, R. C. Learning in discussion: A resume of the authoritarian–democratic studies. *Harvard Educational Review,* 1959, 29, 201–215.
Anderson, R. C. The notion of schemata and the educational enterprise: General discussion of the conference. In R. C. Anderson, R. J. Spiro, & W. E. Montague (Eds.), *Schooling and the acquisition of knowledge.* Hillsdale, N.J.: Erlbaum, 1977.
Anderson, R. C. Schema directed processes in language comprehension. In A. Lesgold, J. Pellegrino, S. Fokkema, & R. Glaser (Eds.), *Cognitive psychology and instruction.* New York: Plenum, 1978.
Anderson, R. C., & Freebody, P. *Vocabulary knowledge* (Technical Report No. 136). Champaign, Ill.: University of Illinois, 1979.
Anderson, R. C., Spiro, R. J., & Montague, W. F. (Eds.), *Schooling and the acquisition of knowledge.* Hillsdale, N.J.: Erlbaum, 1977.
Archambault, R. D. *John Dewey on education.* Chicago: University of Chicago Press, 1964.
Atkin, J. M. Education accountability in the United States. *Educational Analysis,* 1979, 1, 5–21.
Atkinson, R. C. Adaptive instructional systems: Some attempts to optimize. In D. Klahr (Ed.), *Cognition and instruction.* Hillsdale, N.J.: Erlbaum, 1976.
Atkinson, R. C., & Wilson, H. A. (Eds.). *Computer-assisted instruction: A book of readings.* New York: Academic Press, 1969.
Ausubel, D. P. *The psychology of meaningful verbal learning.* New York: Grune & Stratton, 1963.
Baker, E. L. The technology of instructional development. In R. M. W. Travers (Ed.), *Second handbook of research on teaching.* Chicago: Rand McNally, 1973.
Baker, J. P., & Crist, J. L. Teacher expectancies: A review of the literature. In J. D. Elashoff & R. E. Snow (Eds.), *Pygmalion reconsidered.* Worthington, Ohio: Charles A. Jones, 1971.
Ball, S., & Bogatz, G. A. *The first year of "Sesame Street"; An evaluation.* Princeton, N.J.: Educational Testing Service, 1970.
Baratz, J. C. Policy implications of minimum competency testing. In R. M. Jaeger & C. K. Tittle (Eds.), *Minimum competency achievement testing: Motives, models, measures, and consequences.* Berkeley, Calif.: McCutchan Publishing, 1980.
Bardon, J. I., & Robinette, C. L. Minimum competency testing of pupils: Psychological implications for teachers. In R. M. Jaeger & C. K. Tittle (Eds.), *Minimum competency achievement testing: Motives, models, measures, and consequences.* Berkeley, Calif.: McCutchan Publishing, 1980.
Barker, R. G. *Ecological Psychology.* Stanford, Calif.: Stanford University Press, 1968.

Baron, J. Intelligence and general strategies. In G. Underwood (Ed.), *Strategies of information processing*. London: Academic Press, 1978.

Bayley, N. Some increasing parent–child similarities during the growth of children. *Journal of Educational Psychology*, 1954, 45, 1–21.

Beilin, H. Developmental stages and developmental processes. In D. R. Green, M. Ford, & G. B. Flamer, (Eds.), *Measurement and Piaget*. New York: McGraw-Hill, 1971. (a)

Beilin, H. The training and acquisitions of logical operations. In M. F. Rosskopf, L. P. Steffe, & S. Tarback, (Eds.), *Piagetian cognitive-development research and mathematical education*. Washington, D.C.: National Council of Teachers of Mathematics, 1971. (b)

Belmont, J. M., Butterfield, E. C., & Ferretti, R. P. *To secure transfer of training, instruct self-management skills*. Unpublished manuscript, University of Kansas Medical Center, 1980.

Berliner, D. C., & Rosenshine, B. The acquisition of knowledge in the classroom. In R. C. Anderson, R. J. Spiro, & W. E. Montague (Eds.), *Schooling and the acquisition of knowledge*. Hillsdale, N.J.: Erlbaum, 1977.

Best, J. H. (Ed.). *Benjamin Franklin on education*. (Classics in Education, No. 14). New York: Teachers College Press, 1962.

Biggs, J. Individual differences in study processes and the quality of learning outcomes. *Higher Education*, 1979, 4, 381–394.

Biggs, J. The relationship between developmental level and quality of school learning. In S. Modgil & C. Modgil (Eds.), *Toward a theory of psychological development*. Windsor, England: NFER Publishing, 1980.

Blau, T. H. Minimum competency testing: Psychological implications for students. In R. M. Jaeger & C. K. Tittle (Eds.), *Minimum competency achievement testing: Motives, models, measures, and consequences*. Berkeley, Calif.: McCutchan Publishing, 1980.

Block, J. H. *Mastery learning: Theory and practice*. New York: Holt, Rinehart & Winston, 1971.

Block, J. H., & Burns, R. B. Mastery learning. In L. S. Shulman (Ed.), *Review of research in education* (Vol. 4). Itasca, Ill.: Peacock, 1977.

Bloom, B. S. (Ed.). *Taxonomy of educational objectives: The classification of educational goals* (Handbook 1, Cognitive Domain). New York: David McKay, 1956.

Bloom, B. S. *Stability and change in human characteristics*. New York: Wiley, 1964.

Bloom, B. S. *Human characteristics and school learning*. New York: McGraw-Hill, 1976.

Bogatz, G. A., & Ball, S. *The second year of "Sesame Street": A continuing evaluation* (ETS PR-71-21). Princeton, N.J.: Educational Testing Service, 1971.

Boring, E. G. *A history of experimental psychology*. New York: Appleton-Century-Crofts, 1957.

Broadbent, D. C. *Perception and communication*. London: Pergamon Press, 1958.

Brown, A. L. Knowing when, where, and how to remember: A problem of metacognition, In R. Glaser (Ed.), *Advances in instructional psychology* (Vol. 1). Hillsdale, N.J.: Erlbaum, 1978.

Brownell, W. A., & Moser, A. G. *Meaningful versus mechanical learning: A study in grade 3 subtraction* (Duke University Research Studies in Education, No. 8). Durham, N.C.: Duke University Press, 1949.

Bruner, J. S. *The process of education*. Cambridge, Mass.: Harvard University Press, 1960.

Bruner, J. S. *Toward a theory of instruction*. Cambridge, Mass.: Belknap Press, 1966.

Burt, C. The evidence for the concept of intelligence, *British Journal of Educational Psychology*, 1955, 25, 158–177.

Butler, H. E. (Trans.). *The Institutio Oratoria of Quintilian* (Vol. 1). Cambridge, Mass.: Harvard University Press, 1954.

Butterfield, E. C. Testing process theories of intelligence. In M. Friedman, J. P. Das, & N. O'Connor (Eds.), *Intelligence and learning*. New York: Plenum Press, 1981.

Butts, R. F., & Cremin, L. A. *A history of education in American culture*. New York: Holt, 1953.

Calfee, R. C. Sources of dependency in cognitive processes. In D. Klahr (Ed.), *Cognition and Instruction*. Hillsdale, N.J.: Erlbaum, 1976.

Campbell, D. T., & Fiske, D. W. Convergent and discriminant validation by the multi-trait–multimethod matrix. *Psychological Bulletin*, 1959, 56, 81–105.

Carew, J. V., Chan, I., & Halfar, C. *Observing intelligence in young children*. Englewood Cliffs, N.J.: Prentice-Hall, 1976.

Carroll, J. B. A model of school learning. *Teachers College Record*, 1963, 64, 723–733.

Carroll, J. B. School learning over the long haul. In J. D. Krumboltz (Ed.), *Learning and the educational process*. Chicago: Rand McNally, 1965.

Carroll, J. B. The aptitude–achievement distinction. The case of foreign language aptitude and proficiency. In D. R. Green (Ed.), *The aptitude–achievement distinction*. Monterey, Calif.: CTB/McGraw-Hill, 1974.

Carroll, J. B. Psychometric tests as cognitive tasks: A new structure of intellect. In L. B. Resnick (Ed.), *The nature of intelligence*. Hillsdale, N.J.: Erlbaum, 1976.

Carroll, J. B. How shall we study individual differences in cognitive abilities? Methodological and theoretical perspectives. *Intelligence*, 1978, 2, 87–115.

Carroll, J. B. Discussion: Aptitude processes, theory, and the real world. In R. E. Snow, P-A Federico, & W. E. Montague (Eds.), *Aptitude, learning, and instruction:* Vol. 1. *Cognitive process analyses of aptitude*. Hillsdale, N.J.: Erlbaum, 1980.

Carroll, J. B., & Maxwell, S. E. Individual differences in cognitive abilities. *Annual Review of Psychology*, 1979, 30, 603–640.

Cattell, R. B. Theory of fluid and crystallized intelligence: A critical experiment. *Journal of Educational Psychology*, 1963, 54, 1–22.

Cattell, R. B. *Abilities: Their structure, growth, and action*. Boston: Houghton Mifflin, 1971.

Cattell, R. B., & Butcher, J. *The prediction of achievement and creativity*. Indianapolis, Ind.: Bobs-Merrill, 1968.

Chapman, W., Katz, M., Norris, L., & Pears, L. *SIGI: Field test and evaluation of a computer-based system of interactive guidance and information* (2 vols.). Princeton, N.J.: Educational Testing Service, 1977.

Charlesworth, W. R. Human intelligence as adaptation: An ethological approach. In L. B. Resnick (Ed.), *The nature of intelligence*. Hillsdale, N.J.: Erlbaum, 1976.

Cicarelli, V., Cooper, W., & Granger, R. *The impact of Head Start: An evaluation of the effects of Head Start on children's cognitive and affective development*. Athens, Ohio: Westinghouse Learning Corp., 1969.

Cleverley, J., & Phillips, D. C. *From Locke to Spock*. Melbourne: Melbourne University Press, 1976.

Cohen, D. K., & Haney, W. Minimums, competency testing, and social policy. In R. M. Jaeger & C. K. Tittle (Eds.), *Minimum competency achievement testing: Motives, models, measures, and consequences*. Berkeley, Calif.: McCutchan Publishing, 1980.

Cole, M. & Scribner, S. *Culture and thought*. New York: Wiley, 1974.

Coleman, J. S., Campbell, E. Q., Hobson, C. J., McPartland, J., Mood, A. M., Weinfeld, F. D., & York, R. L. *Equality of educational opportunity*. Washington, D.C.: U.S. Department of Health, Education, & Welfare, Office of Education, 1966.

Collins, A., & Smith, E. E. Teaching the process of reading comprehension. In *Project intelligence: The development of procedures to enhance thinking skills* (Final Report, Phase 1). Cambridge, Mass.: Harvard University, Bolt, Beranek & Newman, 1980.

Cook, T. D., Appleton, H., Conner, R. F., Shaffer, A., Tamkin, G., & Weber, S. J. *"Sesame Street" revisited*. Russell Sage Foundation, 1975.

Cook T. D., & Campbell, D. T. *Quasi-experimentation*. Chicago: Rand McNally, 1979.

Connor, J. M., Serbin, L. A., & Schackman, M. Sex differences in children's responses to training on a visual-spatial test. *Developmental Psychology*, 1977, 13, 293–294.

Cooper, L. A. Spatial information processing: Strategies for research. In R. E. Snow, P-A Federico, & W. E. Montague (Eds.), *Aptitude, learning, and instruction:* Vol. 1. *Cognitive process analyses of aptitude*. Hillsdale, N.J.: Erlbaum, 1980.

Corno, L. Individual and class level effects of parent-assisted instruction in classroom memory support strategies. *Journal of Educational Psychology*, 1980, 74, 278–292.

Covington, M. V., Crutchfield, R. S., Davies, L., & Olton, R. M. *The productive thinking program: A course in learning to think*. Columbus, Ohio: Merrill, 1974.

Crano, W. D. Causal analyses of the effects of socioeconomic status and initial intellectual endowment on patterns of cognitive development and academic achievement. In D. R. Green (Ed.), *The aptitude–achievement distinction*. Monterey, Calif.: CTB/McGraw-Hill, 1974.

Crano, W. D., Denny, D. A., & Campbell, D. T. Does intelligence cause achievement?: A cross-lagged panel analysis. *Journal of Educational Psychology*, 1972, 63, 258–275.

Cremin, L. A. *The transformation of the school: Progressivism in American education 1876–1957*. New York: Vantage, 1961.

Crist-Whitzel, J. L., & Hawley-Winne, B. J. Individual differences and mathematics achievement: An investigation of aptitude–treatment interactions in an evaluation of three instructional approaches. Paper presented at the meeting of the American Educational Research Association, San Francisco, April 1976.

Cronbach, L. J. The two disciplines of scientific psychology. *American Psychologist,* 1957, *12,* 671–684.

Cronbach, L. J. How can instruction be adapted to individual differences? In R. M. Gagné (Ed.), *Learning and individual differences.* Columbus, Ohio. Charles E. Merrill, 1967.

Cronbach, L. J. *Essentials of psychological testing* (3rd ed.). New York: Harper & Row, 1970.

Cronbach, L. J. Beyond the two disciplines of scientific psychology. *American Psychologist,* 1975, *30,* 116–127.

Cronbach, L. J. *Research on classrooms and schools: Formulation of questions, design, and analysis.* Stanford, Calif.: Stanford Evaluation Consortium, School of Education, Stanford University, 1976.

Cronbach, L. J. *Educational Psychology* (3rd Ed). New York: Harcourt Brace Jovanovich, 1977.

Cronbach, L. J., & Snow, R. E. *Aptitudes and instructional methods: A handbook for research on interactions.* New York: Irvington, 1977.

Datta, L. Design of the Head Start planned variation experiment. In A. M. Rivlin & P. M. Timpane (Eds.), *Planned variation in education: Should we give up or try harder?* Washington, D.C.: Brookings Institution, 1975.

Davis, K., & Moore, W. E. Some principles of stratification. In M. M. Tumin (Ed.), *Readings on social stratification.* Englewood Cliffs, N.J.: Prentice-Hall, 1970.

Dewey, J. Psychology and social practice. *Psychological Review,* 1900, *7,* 105–124.

Dubin, R., & Taveggia, T. C. *The teaching-learning paradox.* Eugene: University of Oregon Press, 1968.

DuBois, P. H. *A history of psychological testing.* Boston: Allyn & Bacon, 1970.

Duncan, O. D., Featherman, D. L., & Duncan, B. *Socioeconomic background and achievement.* New York: Seminar Press, 1972.

Edgerton, H. A. *Should theory precede or follow a "how-to-do-it" phase of training.* New York: Richardson, Bellows, Henry, 1966.

Egan, D. E., & Greeno, J. G. Acquiring cognitive structure by discovery and rule learning. *Journal of Educational Psychology,* 1973, *64,* 85–97.

Elashoff, J., & Snow, R. E. *Pygmalion reconsidered.* Worthington, Ohio: Charles A. Jones, 1971.

Endler, N. S., & Magnusson, D. (Eds.). *Interactional psychology and personality.* Washington, D.C.: Hemisphere, 1976.

Epstein, A. S., & Weikart, D. P. The Ypsilanti-Carnegie infant education project: Longitudinal follow-up. *Monographs of the High/Scope Educational Research Foundation,* 1979, No. 6.

Eysenck, H. J. *The structure and measurement of intelligence.* New York: Springer-Verlag, 1979.

Ferguson, G. A. On learning and human ability. *Canadian Journal of Psychology,* 1954, *8,* 95–112.

Ferguson, G. A. On transfer and the abilities of man. *Canadian Journal of Psychology,* 1956, *10,* 121–131.

Feuerstein, R. *The dynamic assessment of retarded performers: The learning potential assessment devise, theory, instruments, and techniques.* Baltimore, Md.: University Park Press, 1979.

Feuerstein, R. *Instrumental enrichment: An intervention program for cognitive modifiability.* Baltimore, Md.: University Park Press, 1980.

Flavell, J. H. *The developmental psychology of Jean Piaget.* Princeton, N.J.: Van Nostrand, 1963.

Flavell, J. H. *Cognitive development.* Englewood Cliffs, N.J.: Prentice-Hall, 1977.

Flavell, J. H. Monitoring social-cognitive enterprises: Something else that may develop in the area of social congition. Paper prepared for the Social Sciences Research Council Committee on Social and Affective Development during Childhood, 1979.

Fleishman, E. A. *Trainability of basic abilities.* Silver Springs, Md.: Advanced Research Resources Organization, 1976.

Frandsen, A. N., & Holder, J. R. Spatial visualization in solving complex problems. *Journal of Psychology*, 1969, 73, 229–233.

Frederiksen, C. H. Abilities, transfer, and information retrieval in verbal learning. *Multivariate Behavioral Research Monographs*, 1969, No. 2.

Frederiksen, J. R. Component skills in reading: Measurement of individual differences through chronometric analysis. In R. E. Snow, P-A Federico, & W. E. Montague (Eds.), *Aptitude, learning, and instruction:* Vol. 1. *Cognitive process analyses of aptitude*. Hillsdale, N.J.: Erlbaum, 1980.

Frederiksen, N. Toward a taxonomy of situations. *American Psychologist*, 1972, 27, 114–123.

Friedman, M., Das, J. P., & O'Connor, N. (Eds.). *Intelligence and learning*. New York: Plenum Press, 1981.

Furth, H. G. *Piaget for teachers*. Englewood Cliffs, N.J.: Prentice-Hall, 1970.

Gage, N. L. Theories of teaching. In E. R. Hilgard (Ed.), *Theories of learning and instruction*. Chicago: University of Chicago Press, 1964.

Gage, N. L., & Berliner, D. C. *Educational psychology* (2nd ed.). Chicago: Rand McNally, 1979.

Gagné, R. M. The acquisition of knowledge. *Psychological Review*, 1962, 69, 355–365.

Gagné, R. M. *The conditions of learning*. New York: Holt, Rinehart & Winston, 1965.

Gagné, R. M. (Ed.) *Learning and individual differences*. Columbus, Ohio: Charles E. Merrill, 1967.

Gagné, R. M. *The conditions of learning* (2nd ed.). New York: Holt, Rinehart & Winston, 1970.

Gagné, R. M., & Bolles, R. C. Review of factors in learning efficiency. In E. Galanter (Ed.), *Automatic teaching: The state of the art*. New York: Wiley, 1959.

Gagné, R. M., & Briggs, L. J. *Principles of instructional design*. New York: Holt, Rinehart & Winston, 1974.

Galton, F. *Hereditary genius: An inquiry into its laws and consequences*. London: Macmillan, 1869.

Garber, H., & Heber, R. *Modification of predicted cognitive development in high-risk children through early intervention*. Unpublished manuscript, University of Wisconsin, 1980.

Garforth, F. W. *John Locke's "Of the Conduct of the Understanding"* (Classics in Education, No. 31). New York: Teachers College Press, 1966.

Garrett, H. E. A developmental theory of intelligence. *American Psychologist*, 1946, 1, 372–378.

Gaudry, E., & Spielberger, C. D. *Anxiety and educational achievement*. Syndey, Australia: Wiley, 1971.

Gavurin, E. I. Anagram solving and spatial aptitude. *Journal of Psychology*, 1967, 65, 65–68.

Gay, P. (Ed.). *John Locke on education* (Classics in education, No. 20). New York: Teachers College Press, 1964.

Gelman, R. Conservation acquisition: A problem of learning to attend to relevant attributes. *Journal of Experimental Child Psychology*. 1969, 7, 167–187.

Gelman, R., & Gallistel, C. R. *The child's understanding of number*. Cambridge, Mass.: Harvard University Press, 1978.

Getzels, J. W., & Dillon, J. T. The nature of giftedness and the education of the gifted. In R. M. W. Travers (Ed.), *Second Handbook of Research on Teaching*. Chicago: Rand McNally, 1973.

Ghiselli, E. E. *The validity of occupational aptitude tests*. New York: Wiley, 1966.

Glaser, R. (Ed.). *Training research and education*. New York: Wiley, 1965.

Glaser, R. *Adaptive education: Individual diversity and learning*. New York: Holt, Rinehart & Winston, 1977.

Glaser, R. (Ed.). *Advances in instructional psychology* (Vol. 1). Hillsdale, N.J.: Erlbaum, 1978. (a)

Glaser, R. The contributions of B. F. Skinner to education and some counterinfluences. In P. Suppes. (Ed.), *Impact of research on education: Some case studies*. Washington D.C.: National Academy of Education, 1978. (b)

Glaser, R., & Nitko, A. J. Measurement in learning and instruction. In R. L. Thorndike (Ed.), *Educational Measurement* (2nd ed.). Washington, D.C.: American Council on Educaton, 1971.

Glaser, R., & Pellegrino, J. *Improving the skills of learning*. Unpublished manuscript, University of Pittsburgh, 1980.

Glaser, R., & Resnick, L. B. Instructional Psychology. *Annual Review of Psychology*, 1972, 23, 207–276.

Goodnow, J. J. The nature of intelligent behavior: Questions raised by cross-cultural studies. In L. B. Resnick (Ed.), *The nature of intelligence*. Hillsdale, N.J.: Erlbaum, 1976.

Greene, J. *Choice behavior and its consequences for learning: An ATI study*. Unpublished doctoral dissertation, Stanford Univeristy, 1976.

Greene, M. Response to "Competence and excellence: The search for an egalitarian standard, by the demand for a universal guarantee." In R. M. Jaeger & C. K. Tittle (Eds.), *Minimum competency achievement testing: Motives, models, measures and consequences*. Berkeley, Calif.: McCutchan Publishing, 1980.

Greeno, J. G. A study of problem solving. In R. Glaser (Ed.), *Advances in instructional psychology* (Vol. 1). Hillsdale, N.J.: Erlbaum, 1978.

Greeno, J. G. Some examples of cognitive task analysis with instructional implications. In R. E. Snow, P-A Federico, & W. E. Montague (Eds.), *Aptitude learning and instruction:* Vol. 2. *Cognitive process analyses of learning and problem solving*. Hillsdale, N.J.: Erlbaum, 1980.

Groen, G. J. The theoretical ideas of Piaget and educational practice. In P. Suppes (Ed.), *Impact of research on education*. Washington, D.C.: National Academy of Education, 1978.

Guilford, J. P. *The nature of human intelligence*. New York: McGraw-Hill, 1967.

Gulliksen, H. O. Measurement of learning and mental abilities. *Psychometrika*, 1961, 26, 93–107.

Guinagh, B. J. Social-class differentiation in cognitive development among black preschool children. *Child Development*, 1971, 42, 27–36.

Guttman, L. The structure of relations among intelligence tests. *Proceedings of the 1964 invitational conference on testing problems*. Princeton, N.J.: Educational Testing Service, 1965.

Guttman, L. Integration of test design and analysis. *Proceedings of the 1969 invitational conference on testing problems*. Princeton, N.J.: Educational Testing Service, 1969.

Hess, R. D. Social competence and the educational process. In K. Connolly & J. Bruner (Eds.), *The growth of competence*. New York: Academic Press, 1974.

Hilgard, E. R. The place of Gestalt psychology and field theories in contemporary learning theory. In E. R. Hilgard (Ed.), *Theories of learning and instruction*. Chicago: University of Chicago Press, 1964.

Hilgard, E. R., & Bower, G. H. *Theories of learning* (3rd ed.). New York: Appleton-Century-Crofts, 1966.

Holzman, T. G., Glaser, R., & Pellegrino, J. W. Process training derived from a computer simulation theory. *Memory and Cognition*, 1976, 4, 349–356.

Horn, J. L. Human abilities: A review of research and theory in the early 1970's. *Annual Review of Psychology*, 1976, 27, 437–485.

Horn, J. L. Human ability systems. In P. B. Baltes (Ed.), *Life-span development and behavior* (Vol. 1). New York: Academic Press, 1978.

Humphreys L. G. The organization of human abilities. *American Psychologist*, 1962, 17, 475–483.

Humphreys, L. G. The fleeting nature of the prediction of college academic success. *Journal of Educational Psychology*, 1968, 59, 375–380.

Humphreys, L. G., & Parsons, C. A. A simplex model to describe differences between cross-lagged correlations. *Psychological Bulletin*, 1979, 86, 325–334.

Humphreys, L. G., & Taber, T. Postdiction study of the graduate record examination and eight semesters of college grades. *Journal of Educational Measurement*, 1973, 10, 179–184.

Hunt, E. Quote the Raven? Nevermore! In L. Gregg (Ed.), *Knowledge and Cognition*. Hillsdale, N.J.: Erlbaum, 1974.

Hunt, E. The foundations of verbal comprehension. In R. E. Snow, P-A Federico, & W. E. Montague (Eds.), *Aptitude, learning, and instruction:* Vol. 1: *Cognitive process analyses of aptitude*. Hillsdale, N.J.: Erlbaum, 1980. (a)

Hunt, E. Intelligence as an information processing concept. *British Journal of Psychology*, 1980, 71, 449–474. (b)

Hunt, E., Frost, N., & Lunneborg, C. Individual differences in cognition: A new approach to intelligence. In G. H. Bower (Ed.), *The psychology of learning and motivation*. New York: Academic Press, 1973.

Hunt, E. & Lansman, M. Cognitive theory applied to individual differences. In W. K. Estes (Ed.), *Handbook of learning and cognitive processes: Introduction to concepts and issues* (Vol. 1). Hillsdale, N.J.: Erlbaum, 1975.

Hunt, E., & MacLeod, C. M. The sentence-verification paradigm: A case study of two conflicting approaches to individual differences. *Intelligence*, 1978, 2, 129–144.

Hunt, J. M. *Intelligence and experience*. New York: Ronald Press, 1961.

Husen, J. The influence of schooling upon IQ. *Theoria*, 1951, 17, 61–68.

Inhelder, B., Bovet, M., Sinclair, H., and Smock, C. D. On cognitive development. *American Psychologist*, 1966, 21, 160–164.

Jacobs, P. I. Programmed progressive matrices. In *Proceedings of the 74th Annual Convention of the American Psychological Association*. New York: American Psychological Association, 1966.

Jacobs, P. I. *Up the IQ!: How to raise your child's intelligence*. New York: Wyden Books, 1977.

Jacobs, P. I., & Vandeventer, M. Progressive matrices: An experimental developmental, nonfactoral analysis. *Perceptual and Motor Skills*, 1968, 27, 759–766.

Jacobs, P. I., & Vandeventer, M. *Evaluating the teaching of intelligence* (Research Bulletin 69–20). Princeton, N.J.: Educational Testing Service, 1969.

Jacobs, P. I., & Vandeventer, M. The learning and transfer of double-classification skills by first graders. *Child Development*, 1971, 42, 149–159. (a)

Jacobs, P. I., & Vandeventer, M. The learning and transfer of double-classification skills: A replication and extension. *Journal of Experimental Child Psychology*, 1971, 12, 240–257. (b)

Jacobs, P. I., & Vandeventer, M. Evaluating the teaching of intelligence. *Educational and Psychological Measurement*, 1972, 32, 235–248.

Jacobs, P. I., & White, M. N. *Transfer of training in double classification skills across operations in Guilford's structure-of-intellect model* (Research Bulletin 71–64). Princeton, N.J.: Educational Testing Service, 1971.

Jaeger, R. M., & Tittle, C. K. (Eds.). *Minimum competency achievement testing: Motives, models, measures, & consequences*. Berkeley, Calif.: McCutchan Publishing, 1980.

James, W. *Talks to teachers*. New York: Norton, 1958.

Jastrow, J. Some currents and undercurrents in psychology. *Psychological Review*, 1901, 8, 1–26.

Jencks, C., Smith, M., Acland, H., Bane, M. J., Cohen, D., Gintis, H., Heyns, B., & Michelson, S. *Inequality: A reassessment of the effect of family and schooling in America*. New York: Harper & Row, 1972.

Jencks, C., Bartlett, S., Corcoran, M., Crouse, J., Eaglesfield, D., Jackson, G., McClelland, K., Mueser, P., Olneck, M., Schwartz, J., Ward, S., & Williams, J. *Who gets ahead? The determinants of economic success in America*. New York: Basic Books, 1979.

Jenkins, J. J., & Paterson, D. G. (Eds.), *Studies in individual differences*. New York: Appleton-Century-Crofts, 1961.

Jensen, A. R. How much can we boost intelligence and academic achievement? *Harvard Educational Review*, 1969, 39, 1–123.

Jensen, A. R. Hierarchical theories of mental ability. In W. B. Dockrell (Ed.), *On intelligence*. London: Methuen, 1970.

Jensen, A. R. *Genetics and education*. London: Methuen, 1972.

Jensen, A. R. *Bias in mental testing*. New York: Free Press, 1980.

Joncich, G. M. (Ed.). *Psychology and the science of education: Selected writings of Edward L. Thorndike* (Classics in Education, No. 12). New York: Teachers College Press, 1962.

Katz, M. R. SIGI: An interactive aid to career decision making. *Journal of College Student Personnel*, 1980. 21, 34–40.

Keller, F. S. Goodbye teacher . . . *Journal of Applied Behavior Analysis*, 1968, 1, 79–89.

Kennedy, M. M. Findings from the Follow Through Planned Variation study. *Educational Researcher*, 1978, 7, 3–11.

Klahr, D. (Ed.). *Cognition and instruction*. Hillsdale, N.J.: Erlbaum, 1976.

Klausmeier, H. J., Rossmiller, R. A., & Sally, M. *Individually guided elementary education: Concepts and practices*. New York: Academic Press, 1977.

Kogan, N. A cognitive-style approach to metaphoric thinking. In R. E. Snow, P-A Federico, &

W. E. Montague (Eds.), *Aptitude, learning, and instruction:* Vol. 1. *Cognitive process analyses of aptitude.* Hillsdale, N.J.: Erlbaum, 1980.

Kotovsky, K., & Simon, H. A. Empirical tests of a theory of human acquisition of concepts for sequential patterns. *Cognitive Psychology,* 1973, *4,* 399–424.

Kulik, J. A., Kulik, C-L C., & Cohen, P. A. A meta-analysis of outcome studies of Keller's Personalized System of Instruction. *American Psychologist,* 1979, *34,* 307–318.

Kyllonen, P. C., Lohman, D. F., & Snow, R. E. *Effects of task facets and strategy training on spatial task performance* (Technical Report No. 14). Stanford, Calif.: Aptitude Research Project, School of Education, Stanford University, 1981.

Lavin, D. E. *The prediction of academic performance.* New York: Wiley, 1965.

Lee, G. C. (Ed.). *Crusade against ignorance: Thomas Jefferson on education* (Classics in Education, No. 6). New York: Teachers College Press, 1961.

Lenning, O. T. *Predictive validity of the ACT tests at selective colleges* (ACT Research Report No. 69). Iowa City: Research and Development Division, American College Testing Program 1975.

Lesgold, A. M., Pellegrino, J. W., Fokkema, S. D., & Glaser, R. (Eds.). *Cognitive psychology and instruction.* New York: Plenum, 1978.

Levine, J. M., Brahlek, R. E., Eisner, E. J., & Fleishman, E. A. *Trainability of abilities: Training and transfer of abilities related to electronic fault-finding* (ARRO Technical Report). Washington, D.C.: Advanced Research Resources Organization, March 1979.

Levine, J. M., Schulman, D., Buahlek, R. E., & Fleishman, E. A. *Trainability of abilities: Training and transfer of spatial visualization* (ARRO Technical Report). Washington, D.C.: Advanced Research Resources Organization, April, 1980.

Li, C. C. *Path analysis: A primer.* Pacific Grove, Calif.: Boxweed Press, 1975.

Linden, K. W., & Linden, J. D. *Modern mental measurement: A historical perspective.* Boston: Houghton Mifflin, 1968.

Loehlin, J. C., Lindzey, G., & Spuhler, J. N. *Race differences in intelligence.* San Francisco: Freeman, 1975.

Loftus, G. R., & Loftus, E. F., *Human memory: The processing of information.* Hillsdale, N.J.: Erlbaum, 1976.

Machado, L. A. *The development of intelligence.* Caracas, Venezuela: Projects in Progress, 1980.

MacLeod, C. M., Hunt, E. B., & Mathews, N. N. Individual differences in the verification of sentence-structure relationships. *Journal of Verbal Learning and Verbal Behavior,* 1978, *17,* 493–507.

Magnusson, D. & Endler, N. S. (Eds.). *Personality at the crossroads: Current issues in interactional psychology.* Hillsdale, N.J.: Erlbaum, 1977.

Maltzman, I. On the training of originality. *Psychological Review,* 1960, *67,* 229–242.

Mansfield, R. S., Busse, T. V., & Krepelka, E. J. The effectiveness of creativity training. *Review of Educational Research,* 1978, *48,* 517–536.

Marshalek, B. *Trait and process aspects of vocabulary knowledge and verbal ability.* Unpublished doctoral dissertation, Stanford University, 1981.

Marton, F. On non-verbatim learning: I. Level of processing and level of outcome. *Scandinavian Journal of Psychology,* 1975, *16,* 273–279.

Marton, F. On non-verbatim learning: II. The erosion effect of a task-induced learning algorithm. *Scandinavian Journal of Psychology,* 1976, *17,* 41–48.

Marton, F., & Dahlgren, L. O. On non-verbatim learning: III. The outcome space of some basic concepts in economics. *Scandinavian Journal of Psychology,* 1976, *17,* 49–55.

Marton, F., & Saljo, R. On qualitative differences in learning. I. Outcome and process. *British Journal of Educational Psychology,* 1976, *46,* 4–11.

Marton, F., & Svensson, L. Conceptions of research in student learning. *Higher Education,* Amsterdam: Elsevier, 1979, 471–486.

Mathews, N. M., Hunt, E., & MacLeod, C. Strategy choice and strategy training in sentence-picture verification. *Journal of Verbal Learning and Verbal Behavior,* in press.

McDonald, F. J. The influence of learning theories on education (1900–1950). In E. R. Hilgard (Ed.), *Theories of learning and instruction.* Chicago: University of Chicago Press, 1964.

McGee, M. G. *Human spatial abilities: Sources of sex differences.* New York: Praeger, 1979.

McGeogh, J. A., & Irion, A. L. *The psychology of human learning.* Toronto: Longmans Green, 1952.

McKay, H., Sinisterra, L., McKay, A., Gomez, H., & Lloreda, P. Improving cognitive ability in chronically deprived children. *Science,* 1978, *200,* 270–278.

McKeachie, W. J. Instructional psychology. *Annual Review of Psychology,* 1974, *25,* 161–193.

McNemar, Q. Lost: Our intelligence? Why? *American Psychologist,* 1964, *19,* 871–882.

Mednick, S. A. The associative basis of the creative process. In M. T. Mednick & S. A. Mednick (Eds.), *Research in personality.* New York: Holt, Rinehart & Winston, 1963.

Mednick, S. A., & Mednick, M. *Remote associates test manual.* New York: Psychological Corp., 1967.

Meeker, M. N. *The structure of intellect: Its interpretation and uses.* Columbus, Ohio: Charles E. Merrill, 1969.

Meichenbaum, D. *Cognitive-behavior modification.* New York: Plenum, 1977.

Messick, S. *The effectiveness of coaching for the SAT: Review and reanalysis of research from the fifties to the FTC.* Princeton, N.J.: Educational Testing Service, 1980.

Meyer, A. E. *Grandmasters of educational thought.* New York: McGraw-Hill, 1975.

Meyer, J. W. The effects of education as an institution. *American Journal of Sociology,* 1977, *83,* 55–77.

Miller, G. A., Galanter, E. & Pribram, K. H. *Plans and the structure of behavior.* New York: Holt, Rinehart & Winston, 1960.

Miller, N. E. *Graphic communication and the crisis in education.* Washington, D.C.: National Education Association, 1957.

Mitman, A. *Effects of teachers' naturally occurring expectations and a feedback treatment on teachers and students.* Unpublished doctoral dissertation, Stanford University, 1981.

Murray, F. The generation of educational practice from developmental theory. In S. Modgil, & C. Modgil (Eds.), *Toward a theory of psychological development.* Windsor, England: NFER Publishing, 1980.

Nairn, A., & Associates *The reign of ETS: The corporation that makes up minds.* Washington, D.C.: Ralph Nader, 1980.

Navarro, M. S. *The effect of test tuning on Chicano and Anglo children's performance on field dependence/independence measures.* Unpublished doctoral dissertation, Stanford University, 1980.

Neisser, U. *Cognitive psychology.* New York: Appleton-Century-Crofts, 1967.

Neisser, U. General, academic, and artificial intelligences. In L. B. Resnick (Ed.), *The nature of intelligence.* Hillsdale, N.J.: Erlbaum, 1976.

Neisser, U. The concept of intelligence. In R. J. Sternberg & D. K. Detterman (Eds.), *Human intelligence: Perspectives on its theory and measurement.* Norwood, N.J.: Ablex, 1979.

Nettleship, R. L. *The theory of education in the republic of Plato* (Classics in Education, No. 36). New York: Teachers College Press, 1968.

Newell, A. You can't play 20 questions with nature and win: Comments on the papers of this symposium. In W. G. Chase (Ed.), *Visual information processing.* New York: Academic Press, 1973.

Newell, A., & Simon, H. A. *Human problem solving.* Englewood Cliffs, N.J.: Prentice-Hall, 1972.

Nickerson, R. S., Perkins, D. N., & Smith, E. E. Teaching thinking. In *Project intelligence. The development of procedures to enhance thinking skills* (Final Report, Phase 1). Cambridge, Mass.: Harvard University, Bolt, Beranek & Newman, 1980.

Norman, D. A. Discussion: Teaching, learning, and the representation of knowledge. In R. E. Snow, P-A Federico, and W. E. Montague (Eds.), *Aptitude, learning, and instruction:* Vol. 2. *Cognitive process analyses of learning and problem solving.* Hillsdale, N.J.: Erlbaum, 1980.

Norman, D. A., Rumelhart, D. E., and the LNR Research Group, *Explorations in cognition.* San Francisco: Freeman, 1975.

Olson, D. R. (Ed.). *Media and symbols: The forms of expression, communication, and education.* Chicago: University of Chicago Press, 1974.

O'Neil, H. F., Jr. (Ed.). *Learning strategies.* New York: Academic Press, 1978.

Pellegrino, J. W. & Glaser, R. Cognitive correlates and components in the analysis of individual differences. *Intelligence* 1979, *3,* 187–214.

Pellegrino, J. W., & Glaser, R. Components of inductive reasoning. In R. E. Snow, P-A Federico, & W. E. Montague (Eds.), *Aptitude, learning, and instruction:* Vol. 1. *Cognitive process analyses of aptitude.* Hillsdale, N.J.: Erlbaum, 1980.

Pervin, L. A., & Lewis, M. (Eds.). *Perspectives in interactional psychology*. New York: Plenum, 1978.

Peterson, P. L. Interactive effects of student anxiety, achievement orientation, and teacher behavior on student achievement and attitude. *Journal of Educational Psychology*, 1977, *69*, 779–792.

Peterson, P. L. Aptitude × treatment interaction effects of teacher structuring and student participation in college instruction. *Journal of Educational Psychology*, 1979, *71*, 521–533.

Peterson, P. L., Janicki, T. C., & Swing, S. R. *Aptitude–treatment interaction effects of three teaching approaches: Lecture–recitation, inquiry, and public issues discussion* (Technical Report No. 517). Madison: Wisconsin Research and Development Center for Individualized Schooling, University of Wisconsin, 1979.

Piaget, J. *John Amos Comenius on education (Classics in Education*, No. 33). New York: Teachers College Press, 1967.

Pickett, R. M. Review of educational interventions. In *Project Intelligence: The development of procedures to enhance thinking skills* (Final Report, Phase 1). Cambridge, Mass.: Harvard University, Bolt, Beranek & Newman, 1980.

Popham, W. J. Curriculum and minimum competency: A reaction to the remarks of H. S. Broudy. In R. M. Jaeger & C. K. Tittle (Eds.), *Minimum competency achievement testing: Motives, models, measures, and consequences*. Berkeley, Calif.: McCutchan Publishing, 1980.

Popham, W. J. A modern conception of educational measurement. *Phi Delta Kappan*, in press.

Porteus, A. *Teacher-centered vs. student-centered instruction: Interactions with cognitive and motivational aptitudes*. Unpublished doctoral dissertation, Stanford University, 1976.

Pressey, S. L. A simple apparatus which gives tests and scores – and teaches. *School and Society*, 1926, *23*, 373–376.

Ray, H. W. *Final report on the Office of Economic Opportunity experiment in educational performance contracting*. Unpublished manuscript, Columbus, Ohio: Battelle Laboratories, 1972.

Resnick, L. B. (Ed.). *The nature of intelligence*. Hillsdale, N.J.: Erlbaum, 1976.

Resnick, L. B., & Glaser, R. Problem solving and intelligence. In L. B. Resnick (Ed.), *The nature of intelligence*. Hillsdale, N.J.: Erlbaum, 1976.

Ridberg, E., Parke, R., & Hetherington, E. Modification of impulsive and reflective cognitive styles through observation of film mediated models, *Developmental Psychology*, 1971, *5*, 369–377.

Rigney, J. W. Cognitive learning strategies and dualities in information processing. In R. E. Snow, P-A Federico, & W. E. Montague (Eds.), *Aptitude, learning, and instruction:* Vol. 1. *Cognitive process analyses of aptitude*. Hillsdale, N.J.: Erlbaum, 1980.

Rogosa, D. A critique of cross-lagged correlation. *Psychological Bulletin*, 1980, *88*, 245–258.

Rohwer, W. D., Jr. Mental elaboration and proficient learning. In T. P. Hill (Ed.), *Minnesota symposia on child psychology* (Vol. 4). Minneapolis: University of Minnesota Press, 1970.

Rohwer, W. D., Jr. How the smart get smarter. Paper presented at the meeting of the American Psychological Association, Toronto, August 1978.

Rohwer, W. D., Jr. An elaborative conception of learner differences. In R. E. Snow, P-A Federico, & W. E. Montague (Eds.), *Aptitude, learning and instruction:* Vol. 2. *Cognitive process analyses of learning and problem-solving*. Hillsdale, N.J.: Erlbaum, 1980.

Rosch, E. R., & Mervis, C. B. Family resemblances: Studies in the internal structure of categories. *Cognitive Psychology*, 1975, *7*, 573–605.

Rose, A. M. Information-processing abilities. In R. E. Snow, P-A Federico, & W. E. Montague (Eds.), *Aptitude, learning, and instruction:* Vol. 1. *Cognitive process analyses of aptitude*. Hillsdale, N.J.: Erlbaum, 1980.

Rosenthal, R., & Jacobson L. *Pygmalion in the classroom*. New York: Holt, Rinehart & Winston, 1968.

Royer, J. M. Theories of the transfer of learning. *Educational Psychologist*, 1979, *14*, 53–69.

Rumelhart, D. E., & Norman, D. A. *Accretion, tuning, and restructuring: Three modes of learning* (Report No. 7602). San Diego: Center for Human Information Processing, University of California, August 1976.

Salomon, G. Internalization of filmic operations in relation to individual differences. *Journal of Educational Psychology*, 1974, *66*, 499–511.

Salomon, G. *Interaction of media, cognition and learning.* San Francisco: Jossey-Bass, 1979.

Scarr, S., & Weinberg, R. A. The influence of "family background" on intellectual attainment: The unique contribution of adoptive studies to estimate environmental effects. *American Sociological Review,* 1978, *43,* 674–692.

Scarr, S., & Yee, D. Heritability and educational policy: Genetic and environmental effects on IQ, aptitude and achievement. *Educational Psychologist,* 1980, *15,* 1–22.

Schramm, W. Learning from instructional television. *Review of Educational Research,* 1962, *32,* 156–157.

Scribner, S. & Cole, M. *The psychology of literacy.* Cambridge, Mass.: Harvard University Press, 1981.

Scriven, M. The methodology of evaluation. In R. W. Tyler, R. M. Gagné, & M. Scriven (Eds.), *Perspectives of Curriculum Evaluation.* Chicago: Rand McNally, 1967.

Sharps, R. *A study of interactions between fluid and crystallized abilities and two methods of teaching reading and arithmetic.* Unpublished doctoral dissertation, Pennsylvania State University, 1973.

Shoemaker, J. S. Minimum competency testing: The view from Capitol Hill. In R. M. Jaeger & C. K. Tittle (Eds.), *Minimum competency achievement testing: Motives, models, measures, and consequences.* Berkeley, Calif.: McCutchan Publishing, 1980.

Shulman, L. S., & Keislar, E. (Eds.). *Learning by discovery.* Chicago: Rand McNally, 1966.

Sieber, J. E., O'Neil, H. F., Jr., & Tobias, S. *Anxiety, learning, and instruction.* Hillsdale, N.J.: Erlbaum, 1977.

Simon, H. A. Identifying basic abilities underlying intelligent performance of complex tasks. In L. B. Resnick (Ed.), *The nature of human intelligence.* Hillsdale, N.J.: Erlbaum, 1976.

Simon, H. A., & Kotovsky, K. Human acquisition of concepts for sequential patterns. *Psychological Review,* 1963, *70,* 534–546.

Skinner, B. F. The science of learning and the art of teaching. *Harvard Educational Review,* 1954, *24,* 86–97.

Slack, W. V., & Porter, D. The scholastic aptitude test: A critical appraisal. *Harvard Educational Review,* 1980, *50,* 154–175.

Smail, W. M. *Quintilian on education* (Classics in education, No. 28). New York: Teachers College Press, 1966.

Snow, R. E. Unfinished Pygmalion. *Contemporary Psychology,* 1969, *14,* 197–200.

Snow, R. E. Research on media and aptitudes. In G. Salomon & R. E. Snow (Eds.), *Commentaries on research in instructional media.* Bloomington, Indiana, Indiana University, 1970. (a)

Snow, R. E. (Ed.). *A symposium on heuristic teaching* (Technical Report No. 18). Stanford, Calif.: Center for Research & Development in Teaching, Stanford University, 1970. (b)

Snow, R. E. Theory construction for research on teaching. In R. M. W. Travers (Ed.), *Second handbook of research on teaching.* Chicago: Rand McNally, 1973.

Snow, R. E. Research on aptitudes: A progress report. In L. S. Shulman (Ed.), *Review of research in education* (Vol. 4). Itasca, Ill.: Peacock, 1977. (a)

Snow, R. E. Individual differences and instructional theory. *Educational Researcher* 1977, *6,* (10), 11–15. (b)

Snow, R. E. Theory and method for research on aptitude processes. *Intelligence,* 1978, *2,* 225–278.

Snow, R. E. Aptitude processes. In R. E. Snow, P-A Federico, & W. E. Montague (Eds.), *Aptitude, learning and instruction:* Vol. 1. *Cognitive process analyses of aptitude.* Hillsdale, N.J.: Erlbaum, 1980. (a)

Snow, R. E. Aptitude and achievement. *New directions for testing and measurement,* 1980, No. 5, 39–59. (b)

Snow, R. E. Intelligence for the year 2001. *Intelligence,* 1980, *4,* 185–199. (c)

Snow, R. E. Toward a theory of aptitude for learning: I. Fluid and crystallized abilities and their correlates. In M. Friedman, J. P. Das, & N. O'Connor (Eds.), *Intelligence and learning.* New York: Plenum Press, 1981.

Snow, R. E., Federico, P-A, & Montague, W. E. (Eds.). *Aptitude, learning, and instruction:* Vol. 1. *Cognitive process analyses of aptitude.* Vol. 2. *Cognitive process analyses of learning and problem-solving.* Hillsdale, N.J.: Erlbaum, 1980.

Snow, R. E., Wescourt, K., & Collins, J. *Individual differences in aptitude and learning from interactive computer-based instruction* (Technical Report No. 10). Stanford, Calif.: Aptitude Research Project, School of Education, Stanford University, 1980.

Spearman, C. "General intelligence" objectively determined and measured. *American Journal of Psychology*, 1904, *15*, 201–293.

Spearman, C. *The nature of intelligence and the principles of cognition*. London: Macmillan, 1923.

Sperling, G. A. The information available in brief visual presentation. *Psychological Monographs*, 1960, *74* (Whole No. 498).

Stake, R. E. Learning parameters: aptitudes and achievement. *Psychometric Monographs*, 1961 (Whole No. 9).

Stallings, J. Implementation and child effects of teaching practices in Follow Through classrooms. *Monographs of the Society for Research in Child Development*, 1975, No. 40.

Stallings, J., & Kaskowitz, D. Follow Through classroom observation evaluation 1972–1973 (SRI Project URU-7370). Stanford, Calif.: Stanford Research Institute, August 1974.

Stanley, J. C., Keating, D. P., & Fox, L. H. (Eds.). *Mathematical talent: Discovery, description, and development*. Baltimore, Md.: Johns Hopkins University Press, 1974.

Steffensen, N. S., Jogdeo, C., & Anderson, R. C. A cross-cultural perspective on reading comprehension. *Reading Research Quarterly*, in press.

Sternberg, R. *Intelligence, information processing, and analogical reasoning*. Hillsdale, N.J.: Erlbaum, 1977.

Sternberg, R. J. The nature of mental abilities. *American Psychologist*, 1979, *34*, 214–230.

Sternberg, R. J. Toward an unified componential theory of human intelligence: I. Fluid abilities. In M. Friedman, J. P. Das, & N. O'Connor (Eds.), *Intelligence and learning*. New York: Plenum Press, 1981.

Sternberg, R. J., & Detterman, D. K. *Human intelligence: Perspectives on its theory and measurement*. Norwood, N.J.: Ablex, 1979.

Sternberg, R. J., Guyote, M. J., & Turner, M. E. Deductive reasoning. In R. E. Snow, P-A Federico, & W. E. Montague (Eds.), *Aptitude, learning, and instruction: Vol. 1. Cognitive process analyses of aptitude*. Hillsdale, N.J.: Erlbaum, 1980.

Sternberg, R. J., & Ketron, J. L. Selection and implementation of strategies in analogical reasoning. *Journal of Educational Psychology*, in press.

Sternberg, R. J., Ketron, J. L., & Powell, J. S. Componential approaches to the training of intelligence. *Intelligence*, in press.

Sternberg, R. J., & Weil, E. M. An aptitude-strategy interaction in linear syllogistic reasoning. *Journal of Educational Psychology*, 1980, *72*, 226–234.

Stevens, A. L., & Collins, A. Multiple conceptual models of a complex system. In R. E. Snow, P-A Federico, & W. E. Montague (Eds.), *Aptitude, learning, and instruction: Vol. 2. Cognitive process analyses of learning and problem solving*. Hillsdale, N.J.: Erlbaum, 1980.

Svensson, L. On qualitative differences in learning III: Study skill and learning. *British Journal of Educational Psychology*, 1977, *47*, 233–243.

Terman, L. M. *The measurement of intelligence*. Boston: Houghton Mifflin, 1916.

Thorndike, E. L. *The principles of teaching based on psychology*. New York: Seiler, 1906.

Thorndike, E. L. *The psychology of learning*. Educational Psychology (Vol. 2). New York: Teachers College, Columbia University, 1921. (a)

Thorndike, E. L. *Mental work and fatigue and individual differences and their causes*. *Educational Psychology* (Vol. 3). New York: Teachers College, Columbia University, 1921. (b)

Thorndike, E. L., & Woodworth, R. S. The influence of improvement in one mental function upon the efficiency of other functions. *Psychological Review*, 1901, *8*, 247–261.

Thorndike, R. L. Review of "Pygmalion in the classroom." *American Educational Research Journal*, 1968, *5*, 708–711.

Thorndike, R. L. Mr. Binet's test 70 years later. *Educational Researcher*, 1975, *4*, 3–7.

Thurstone, L. L. *Primary mental abilities*. Chicago: University of Chicago Press, 1938.

Tractenberg, P. L. Testing for minimum competency: A legal analysis. In R. M. Jaeger & C. K. Tittle (Eds.), *Minimum competency achievement testing: Motives, models, measures, and consequences*. Berkeley, Calif.: McCutchan, 1980.

Tuma, D. T., & Reif, F. (Eds.). *Problem solving and education: Issues in teaching and research*. Hillsdale, N.J.: Erlbaum, 1980.

Tyler, L. *The psychology of human differences*. New York: Appleton-Century-Crofts, 1965.

Tyler, L. E. The intelligence we test – an evolving concept. In L. B. Resnick (Ed.), *The nature of intelligence*. Hillsdale, N.J.: Erlbaum, 1976.

Valett, R. E. *Developing cognitive abilities: Teaching children to think.* St. Louis, Mo.: Mosby, 1978.

VanLehn, K., & Brown, J. S. Planning nets: A representation for formalizing analogies and semantic models of procedural skills. In R. E. Snow, P-A Federico, & W. E. Montague (Eds.), *Aptitude, learning, and instruction:* Vol. 2. *Cognitive process analyses of learning and problem solving.* Hillsdale, N.J.: Erlbaum, 1980.

Vernon, P. A. Level I and level II: A review. *Educational Psychologist,* in press.

Vernon, P. E. *The structure of human abilities.* London: Methuen, 1951.

Vygotsky, L. S. *Thought and language* (E. Hanfmann & G. Vakar, Ed. and trans.). Cambridge, Mass: MIT Press, 1962.

Webb, N. M. *Learning in individual and small group settings* (Technical Report No. 7). Stanford, Calif.: Aptitude Research Project, School of Education, Stanford University, 1977.

Weikart, D. P. Relationship of curriculum, teaching, and learning in preschool education. In J. C. Stanley (Ed.), *Preschool programs for the disadvantaged.* Baltimore, Md.: Johns Hopkins University Press, 1972.

Weikart, D. P., Bond, J. T., & McNeil, J. T. The Ypsilanti Perry preschool project: Preschool years and longitudinal results through fourth grade. *Monographs of the High/Scope Educational Research Foundation,* 1978, No. 3.

Weikart, D. P., Epstein, A. S., Schweinhart, L., & Bond, J. T. The Ypsilanti preschool curriculum demonstration project: Preschool years and longitudinal results. *Monographs of the High/Scope Educational Research Foundation,* 1978, No. 4.

Weisgerber, R. A. (Ed.). *Developmental efforts in individualized learning.* Itasca, Ill.: Peacock, 1971.

Weiss, D. J. (Ed.). *Proceedings of the computerized adaptive testing conference.* Minneapolis: University of Minnesota, 1978.

Westman, J. C. (Ed.). *Individual differences in children.* New York: Wiley, 1973.

Whimbey, A., & Whimbey, L. S. *Intelligence can be taught.* New York: Dutton, 1975.

White, S. H. Evidence for a hierarchical arrangement of learning processes. In L. P. Lipsitt & C. C. Spiker (Eds.), *Advances in child development and behavior* (Vol. 2). New York: Academic Press, 1965.

White, S. H. *Federal programs for young children: Review and recommendations.* Vol. 1. *Goals and standards of public programs for children.* Cambridge, Mass.: Huron Institute, 1973.

Whitely, S. E. Solving verbal analogies: Some cognitive components of intelligence test items. *Journal of Educational Psychology,* 1976, *68,* 234–242.

Whitely, S. E. *Modeling aptitude test validity from cognitive components* (Technical Report No. NIE 79-2). Lawrence: Department of Psychology, University of Kansas, 1979.

Whitely, S. E., & Dawis, R. *A cognitive intervention for improving the estimate of latent ability measured from analogy items* (Technical Report No. 3010). Minneapolis: Center for the Study of Organizational Performance and Human Effectiveness, University of Minnesota, 1973.

Whitely, S. E. & Dawis, R. V. The effects of cognitive intervention on latent ability measured from analogy items. *Journal of Educational Psychology,* 1974, *66,* 710–717.

Willis, S. L., Blieszner, R., & Baltes, P. B. *Training research in aging: Modification of intellectual performance on a fluid ability component.* University Park: College of Human Development, Pennsylvania State University, 1980.

Wissler, C. The correlation of mental and physical tests. *Psychological Review Monograph,* 1901, *6,*(3).

Witkin, H. A. Cognitive style in academic performance and in teacher–student relations. In S. Messick & Associates (Eds.), *Individuality in learning.* San Francisco: Jossey-Bass, 1976.

Wittig, M. A., & Petersen, A. C., (Eds.). *Sex-related differences in cognitive functioning: Developmental issues.* New York: Academic Press, 1979.

Wittrock, M. C. A model of human generative learning. Paper presented at the meeting of the American Educational Research Association, New York, April, 1977.

Wittrock, M. C., & Carter, J. F. Generative processing of hierarchically organized words. *American Journal of Psychology,* 1975, *88,* 489–501.

Wittrock, M. C., & Lumsdaine, A. A. Instructional psychology. *Annual Review of Psychology,* 1977, *28,* 417–459.

Wolf, T. H. *Alfred Binet.* Chicago: University of Chicago Press, 1973.

Woodrow, H. The ability to learn. *Psychological Review,* 1946, *53,* 147–158.

Woodward, W. H. *Desiderius Erasmus concerning the aim and method of education* (Classics in education, No. 19). New York: Teachers College Press, 1964.

Zajonc, R. B. Family configuration and intelligence. *Science,* 1976, *192,* 227–236.

Zajonc, R. B., & Bargh, J. Birth order, family size, and decline of SAT scores. *American Psychologist,* 1980, *35,* 662–668.

Zigler, E. Has it really been demonstrated that compensatory education is without value? *American Psychologist,* 1975, *30,* 935–937.

Zigler, E., & Valentine, J. *Project Head Start: A legacy of the war on poverty.* New York: Free Press, 1979.

10   *Social policy and intelligence*

EDWARD ZIGLER AND VICTORIA SEITZ

People are interested in intelligence. Although many psychologists may disagree that "the measurement of intelligence is psychology's most telling accomplishment to date" (Herrnstein, 1971, p. 45), the IQ test is unquestionably a product that has had great social impact. At the peak of their popularity, IQ tests were administered to most American schoolchildren, and nearly everyone has taken an IQ test at one time or another. The definition of intelligence and the appropriate means of assessing it have always been subjects of controversy and will probably remain so. But psychologists can at least be certain that their research on intelligence is regarded as socially meaningful.

It is precisely because intelligence has relevance to problems of everyday life that researchers in this area find themselves entangled with social policy issues. If a research topic is sufficiently esoteric, a scientist can expect to be left in peace – say, to ascertain differences between yellow- and brown-bellied snails – without concern that premature, erroneous interpretation of any findings might adversely affect the happiness and well-being of others. However, most research areas relevant to intelligence have inescapable policy ramifications. To complicate matters further, the breadth of such topics is astonishing. Intelligence-related research not only includes studies of formal cognition, but can also involve those of malnutrition, substitute parental care, educational intervention, family support systems, and effects of income maintenance, to name a few. Should what appears to be a useful discovery emerge in any of these areas, the researcher must decide whether, when, and how it should be translated into widespread practice.

To take one example, suppose that an intervention project results in large IQ-score gains in children who were at risk of becoming mentally retarded. Suppose also that the project is very expensive and involves separating children from their families for most of their preschool years. Should psychologists recommend that the intervention be implemented on a large scale to prevent mental retardation? Should they insist upon further research involving both replication and systematic variation to determine whether some lesser form of intervention would be equally effective? Or is there a middle ground? The dilemma is a serious one. If a complex intervention is indeed necessary, then society is not doing what it could to save many children from mental retardation. Even so, what is the harm that may result both to parents and to children when such a disruptive interference in their lives is recommended as beneficial? And what happens should a measure this drastic eventually prove to be unnecessary? Weighing social policy alternatives can be a distasteful task for scientists who prefer the isolation of the laboratory, but as this example illustrates, doing so has become a responsibility thrust upon us by the social significance of our findings.

Just as "pure" psychological research often has implications for social programs, social programs in turn provide an impressive data base that can enhance psychological theory. A number of sizable and expensive governmental programs fill this bill. For example, at the close of the 1970s, Title I funds allocated under the Elementary and Secondary Education Act were expended at a cost of approximately $1.5 billion annually. These moneys have made possible numerous educational intervention programs at the local level across the country. Perhaps the best known of these is Head Start, a large-scale program for preschool children that is funded at over $400 million a year. Hundreds of thousands of children attend day-care programs subsidized by federal and state expenditures in excess of $2 billion annually. In the Women, Infants, and Children (WIC) program, more than $200 million a year are spent to improve the nutrition of pregnant women and very young children.

The existence of such programs generates a legitimate interest regarding their effectiveness among both taxpayers and social theorists. In governmental agencies concerned with taxpayer sentiment, the slang word for this interest is *accountability*. Among psychologists, interest has typically focused on how such programs can bolster our knowledge about development – especially intellectual development – and the factors that affect it. Whereas the government may be concerned with whether Project Head Start is worth the cost of supporting it, psychologists have been more interested in what the project can tell us about such issues as the relative plasticity of intellect and whether there are "critical periods" for intellectual development.

Despite the differences in focus between governmental accountants and psychologists, the two groups have developed an important working relationship. Like economic theorists, researchers who study intelligence have found themselves taken seriously by politicians and social planners. And like economists, psychologists have been forced to recognize that they possess an important, albeit incomplete, body of knowledge, some of which is of great immediate value to society. The 1960s and 1970s marked a coming-of-age for psychologists in ability to influence social policies in a substantial manner. In particular, Project Head Start was an educational experience for us, yielding firsthand information about the benefits and pitfalls of attempting to translate psychological knowledge into social action. (See Zigler & Valentine, 1979, for an edited history and commentary on this immense social experiment.) From this and other involvements, psychologists have learned a great deal about designing and evaluating social programs and are far better prepared to bridge the gap between psychological theory and societal needs than they were only a decade ago. The time has come for us to take our responsibilities seriously, to assess what we have learned from our early forays into social policy, and to make recommendations for the future.

10.1.   PRELIMINARY CONSIDERATIONS

USES OF RESEARCH IN SOCIAL POLICY

As Weiss (1978) has pointed out, there are many possible uses of psychological research in the construction of social policy. Ideally, research could be used directly for solving societal problems. More and more policy makers have adopted this view, for within the last decade there has been a dramatic increase in the amount of funding for research with perceived potential for meeting social needs. In 1977 the federal government spent nearly $2 billion on the gathering and application of social knowledge, a majority of which went to research (Weiss, 1978). In addition, evaluation requirements are written into many new social programs so that researchers conducting an applied project are required to provide generalizable statements of its effects. Clearly, the federal government is looking toward social scientists for some answers to societal problems.

The notion that research leads to solutions that lead to effective policy is actually an ideal belief. In the case of social research into subjects such as intelligence or community betterment, in reality it is the link least likely to occur. Many times the problem to be solved is not clearly delineated and there is no consensus among decision makers on the goals they wish to achieve. Consider, for example, two programs aimed at reducing malnutrition – the Food Stamp Program and the WIC program mentioned earlier. Solkoff (1977) noted that over the past decade the United States has made enormous strides in reducing hunger and malnutrition. Physicians who visited rural poverty areas 10 years ago and again very recently report a difference so great that it requires no statistical tests to prove that there are clearly visible benefits resulting from better nourishment. Yet formal outcome evaluations of these food programs have been impeded because of the vagueness of goals such as "reducing poverty" or "reducing malnutrition" and because of the inevitable variability among programs implemented in very different communities and populations. Similarly, part of the difficulty in evaluating the Head Start program has stemmed from the facts that its goals were initially presented rather vaguely and that the project varies widely at the local level.

Research can also be used as political ammunition. Even after policy makers have reached decisions and are unlikely to change their minds, they may use social science knowledge to bolster their arguments. This is a perfectly acceptable use of research, as long as the information is not distorted and is accessible to all sides. Sometimes, however, research is used in this way to advance self-interest. A politician may cite results that support his or her point of view and ignore those which do not. In other cases policy makers can delay taking an action they really do not favor by arguing that the needed evidence is not available. This was the case in the four-year moratorium on staffing regulations in the federal day-care standards, pending the results from the ABT National Day Care Study and the "Appropriateness Report" from HEW to Congress.

The last use of social science research to be discussed is the most amorphous, but perhaps the most important: "research as conceptualization" (Weiss, 1977). This definition of use encompasses sensitizing policy makers to new issues, turning research problems into policy issues, clarifying alternatives, and supplying a common language. This form of impact appears to be a common one. Caplan and his colleagues (Caplan, 1975; Caplan & Rich, 1977; Rich & Caplan, 1976) interviewed 204 policy makers in the executive branch of the federal government and asked them if, on the basis of their experience, they could "think of instances where a new program, a major program alternative, a new social or administrative policy, legislative proposal, or a technical innovation could be traced to the social sciences" (Caplan, 1975, p. 205). Although 82 percent of the respondents replied yes to this question, the examples they gave were not empirical studies. Rather, they most often cited general ideas and principles garnered from social science knowledge.

Although this is a "softer" use of research than is ideally desired, it can have far-reaching implications. Generalizations from the accumulation of research in an area can, over time, change the climate of ideas and become a part of the social consciousness. The negative aspect of this way of using research in policy is that not only hard facts, but myths and social fads, may be so publicized that they too become part of public "knowledge." Unfortunately, these myths often remain unquestioned and become the basis for new policy and further research. Examples of this problem include sentiments in favor of mainstreaming, deinstitutionalization, and the belief that "fade-out" is an inevitable fate of any positive effects of preschool intervention programs – all areas where our current policies and views are based more on popular opinion than on pure scientific evidence (Darlington, Royce, Snipper, Murray, & Lazar, 1980; Zigler & Balla, 1977a; Zigler & Muenchow, 1979).

A more positive use of generalities derived from social science research can be seen in the formation of Project Head Start. At the time, prevailing social science theories showed a revival of interest in the role of the environment in human development, and there were efforts to design educational intervention plans for disadvantaged children. On the political front, the nation was in the Civil Rights era and had waged the War on Poverty. These forces converged in the mid-1960s when a novel alliance between child development experts and social policy makers was created. From their combined efforts Head Start was born. Thus the use of broad principles based on social science knowledge can and does affect social policy.

VALUE ISSUES AND THE USE OF RESEARCH

One reason commonly cited for the inadequate use of social science knowledge is a conflict in values between social scientists and policy makers (Mayntz, 1977; Weiss, 1978; Weiss & Bucuvalas, 1977). Social science is presumably value-free, whereas policy decisions are made in a value-laden context. This dichotomy is certainly misleading. Research in the social sciences is not value-free, and even the most basic research takes on the values of the investigators. These are evident in the questions that are asked, the methodologies used, the presentation of results, and the interpretation of the data. For example, much research in early childhood intervention has been undertaken with the assumption that disadvantaged children have a deficit that needs correcting (see Baratz & Baratz, 1970; Yando, Seitz, & Zigler, 1979). Adopting this assumption certifies that the problems to be studied will concern the child rather than the school, home, or larger aspects of the environment. Buried deep in evaluations of early education programs are many other hidden value judgments – not only that the defect is in the child, but that schools routinely recognize and reward children's intellectual abilities, that higher IQs will enable children to perform better in school, and that education will actually change the children and make them better able to adapt to society than were their parents.

In addition to affecting the conduct of research, values enter into the utilization of knowledge. It might seem an unarguable goal to wish to reduce the incidence of severe mental retardation. However, a society may legitimately have financial and ethical values in conflict with this aim. A particularly good example of how conflicting values can be problematic in utilizing knowledge is provided in the area of genetic counseling and prenatal diagnosis of severe intellectual retardation.

Genetic counseling and prenatal diagnosis

Congenital defects are estimated to be present in approximately 4% of live births (A. Smith, 1975). Many of these defects are hereditary; many of them affect intelligence. Genetic counseling is one means of reducing the incidence of some of these disorders. Often persons who seek genetic counseling have already borne one afflicted child or know they have afflicted relatives. As screening for carriers of deleterious recessive genes becomes more feasible – as it presently is for Tay-Sachs disease – many more people may seek counseling, even if they have no indicative family history. Genetic counselors can usually provide accurate odds of a particular couple's bearing a defective child, but the chief shortcoming is that the advice is probabilistic rather than certain. Prospective parents are usually interested in whether they can *safely* have children; genetic counselors can only tell them what their odds are. Avoiding pregnancy thus becomes a difficult choice, a high price to pay, to be weighed against the also forbidding alternative of producing a seriously affected child. Both the involved couple and society as a whole have value judgments to make. Should societies make premarital screening for carriers of deleterious genes a standard practice? As more and more genetic disorders are identified and studied, the unwelcome conclusion has emerged that most of us are probably carriers of a few rare, abnormal, recessive genes. A consequence of putting present genetic knowledge into full use to reduce severe retardation would conflict with our present policy of relative freedom of choice in parenthood, at least to the extent of voluntary abstention from parenthood by certain couples.

The past decade has brought a far more accurate means of counseling parents – prenatal detection of genetic disorders through amniocentesis and sophisticated analysis of fetal and/or maternal blood during pregnancy. Amniocentesis is the best-known prenatal detection method. In this procedure a needle is inserted into the womb, and a small amount of the amniotic fluid surrounding the fetus is withdrawn. This fluid is then examined microscopically and biochemically to detect the presence of any abnormality in the fetal cells it contains. Amniocentesis is now known to be safe when performed under suitable medical circumstances. A careful study of 1,040 women who received amniocentesis showed they did not differ significantly from a control group in the rate of miscarriages, stillbirths, prematurity, fetal injury, or other fetal or maternal complications. At 1 year of age their infants also were comparable to the control infants (Milunsky, 1975). The procedure has an impressive accuracy rate of better than 99% in detecting some 100 disorders, including all the major chromosomal abnormalities and many biochemical disorders. The presence of Down's syndrome, Tay-Sachs disease, thyroid deficiency (responsible for cretinism), maple-syrup-urine disease, and phenylketonuria (PKU) are a few examples of disorders that can cause severe intellectual retardation but can be detected through amniocentesis.

Though amniocentesis is relatively safe and accurate, it is also expensive (costing several hundred dollars per test), and it must be performed relatively late, usually not until the fourth month of pregnancy. The lateness poses a severe psychological stress on the uncertain and anxious pregnant woman, and, should she elect an abortion, it is physically more dangerous than during the first trimester. The issue of abortion is one of the most value-laden of all topics affected by scientific knowledge and research. Amniocentesis also cannot detect all disorders. Sickle-cell anemia, for example, requires taking blood cells directly from the fetus, a riskier – though now feasible – procedure. Because both procedures are physically and personally intrusive, it seems unlikely that either will be adopted as standard practice in this country.

The technological door has been opened, however, and better prenatal detection techniques will almost certainly be developed. It is already common practice in England, for example, to perform AFP (alpha-feto-protein) tests on a mother's blood early in pregnancy to detect the presence of certain severe deformities, such as anencephaly in the fetus. Presumably the day will come when safe, early, inexpensive prenatal diagnosis will be available for the majority of genetic forms of severe retardation. Such tests would have an advantage over genetic counseling in that they would provide parents with certain answers instead of probabilistic statements. All the tests have the disadvantage of giving after-the-fact information, and thus requiring that abortion be accessible to parents who wish to discontinue a pregnancy in which the fetus is found to be affected. The technology will probably soon be available to reduce greatly the incidence of severe retardation. The decisions regarding societal usage of the technology will be affected by financial and ethical considerations.

In some cases, prenatal or early postnatal treatment may be an alternative to abortion. The technology is rapidly growing to prevent or reduce the severity of some forms of retardation by beginning this early in life. Blood transfusions can be given in utero; injections can be administered directly to the fetus. Treatment may also begin soon after birth, as is the case for PKU victims. By giving babies with PKU a diet without phenylalanine, they can be saved from the brain damage that would result from their inability to metabolize this amino acid fully. Unfortunately, this treatment is much less pleasant to live with than it is easy to describe. Because phenylalanine is extremely common, the diet is very restrictive: It must be adhered to for at least five to six years, during the very time it is most difficult to explain to the child. Sharing food is an important part of human social activity, yet the PKU child must remain on a private, boring diet and be constantly reminded of his or her differentness. The treatment is also not foolproof. The average IQ of treated PKU children is below 100, reflecting, perhaps, a too-late start of the treatment for some and occasional lapses for others. A treated PKU woman who becomes pregnant may also place her unborn child at risk because of excess phenylalanine in her bloodstream. In short, the availability of a treatment does not guarantee a good life for the affected individual. A society needs to give consideration to quality of life, not just to IQ scores, in formulating its policies. And as these examples illustrate, we cannot expect to avoid issues of values in considering social policies related to intelligence.

EVALUATION AND ACCOUNTABILITY

Psychologists have grown considerably in methodological expertise from their immersion in intervention research over the past two decades. Campbell and Stanley (1966) and a number of other evaluation specialists (see Guttentag & Struening, 1975; Struening & Guttentag, 1975) have so thoroughly documented the essentials of adequate evaluation research that we need not enumerate them here. Instead we will comment on several principles that have gained widespread recognition as a result of studies on intervention. One principle that has emerged is the necessity of evaluating programs broadly rather than in terms of laboratory measures alone. This approach can be seen in the increasing concern with ecological validity (Bronfenbrenner, 1977) and with establishing transcontextual validity of measures (Weisz, 1978). In intervention research, we see it spelled out in increasing demands that IQ-test data be supplemented by observations of children in their real-life pursuits, by information obtained from teachers about their adjustments to school, and by comments from their parents on the larger effects of the programs.

A second principle has been a growing awareness of the complexity of intervention effects and a willingness to avoid oversimplifications. Ten years ago we could accept a scientist's right to conclude categorically, "Compensatory education has been tried, and it apparently has failed" (Jensen, 1969, p. 2). In the 1980s we know that answers concerning the effectiveness of interventions will not be so simply given. As Ricciuti (1981) pointed out of his discussion of nutritional interventions, researchers are learning to specify particular populations, particular ages, and particular forms of nutritional supplements, rather than expecting to find that this type of intervention categorically either "succeeds" or "fails."

A third principle has been an acceptance of the need for both process and outcome evaluations. In process evaluation, the aim is to ascertain whether a program is being implemented in the manner originally intended (and, in federal programs, required by law). For example, Head Start centers are required to provide specific services such as medical evaluations and nutritious meals. A process evaluation is a straightforward check to determine whether these services are indeed available. Where the intended provisions of a program are less concretely specified, it is more difficult to ascertain whether the implementation of the program coincides with its description on paper. Outcome evaluation can be even more difficult, as it is an assessment of the verifiable impact of the program or services.

Until recently, governmental agencies tended to restrict themselves to process evaluations, whereas psychologists focused mostly on outcomes. It is easy to see that a process evaluations alone yields relatively unsatisfying results, but this is equally true for outcome evaluations alone. For example, despite the fact that Head Start programs vary enormously from one locale to another, researchers in an early, influential evaluation study compared on a nationwide basis graduates of Head Start with children who had not attended Head Start (Cicirelli, 1969). There was undoubtedly as much variability within groups as there was between them. As we have gained sophistication, it has become common practice to monitor the activities that actually occur in intervention programs. Occasionally attention is also given to documenting the experiences of control children who are being compared with the intervention group. One example of program monitoring is provided by Huston-Stein, Friedrich-Cofer, and Susman (1977), who documented differences among several Head Start centers within a single city and also determined the variations in children's behavior associated with the program differences. In another excellent study, Miller and Dyer (1975) documented a number of measurable classroom differences among preschool programs purporting to have different educational rationales. The investigators were able to ascertain, for example, that Bereiter–Engelmann classrooms were in fact as different from Montessori classrooms as their description would lead one to expect, and that children exposed to these different experiences came to behave differently.

Under the rubric of outcome evaluation we encounter the government's beloved concept "cost–benefit analysis." This elegant phrase, a creation originally of the Department of Defense, is usually translated as "How much bang do you buy per buck?" The cost–benefit analysis concept has been adopted with enthusiasm by government officials in the social services area, where the question they are asking is, What is being accomplished as a result of the expenditure of hundreds of millions of dollars?

Cost–benefit analysis presents at least two major problems. First, it is not easy to decide which variables to include and which to exclude in a cost–benefit equation. For example, should the equation count the career development of Head Start teachers or the health and education improvements in a community that are the result of Head Start's being there (Kirschner Associates, 1970)? The second problem with cost–benefit analysis is that it is often difficult to determine the exact dollar amount to attribute to particular outcomes. As has been asked before (Zigler, 1973), what dollar value do we assign to warding off a case of measles or raising a child's IQ-test performance by 10 points? For the present at least, we will be forced to live with these problems. If resources were unlimited, we could afford to be relatively unconcerned about outcome evaluations. However, given the realities not only of limited funds but also of the many unmet needs of American children and families, we must champion the value of outcome evaluation so that decision makers can be informed about whether they should perpetuate current programs or reallocate funds to other programs holding greater promise of achieving desired and explicit goals.

As Gallagher, Haskins, and Farran (in press) have pointed out, our current research knowledge about the causes of poverty could support recommendations for implementing at least seven different kinds of programs intended to reduce poverty. Because many of these proposals are also relevant to reducing the incidence of mental retardation, they have importance as social policies related to intelligence. They include (a) genetic counseling, (b) nutritional programs for pregnant women and young children, (c) health-care programs designed to reduce early brain damage and biological trauma, (d) early childhood educational intervention, (e) parent training to improve child rearing, (f) job training for adolescents and adults, and (g) a guaranteed income for all families. Each approach has evidence to show some usefulness in reducing poverty and its sequelae, such as poor intellectual performance. What we do not know is whether any one of these alone would be effective, whether any can be safely ignored, or whether some particular combination would provide the optimal societal strategy. Given this complexity, the need for highly skilled social scientists and for adequate outcome evaluations is obvious. Decision makers must depend on social science to provide some badly needed direction in how to spread a finite number of public dollars across what often appears to be an infinite number of possibilities.

10.2.   RECOMMENDATIONS

The translation of knowledge into policy is obviously most difficult when the knowledge base is weak. If we had reason to believe that a few more years of research would yield definitive answers to pressing problems, we might counsel waiting for such research to be completed. However, it is unlikely that this will occur for such complex societal problems as moderate intellectual retardation. We are unlikely soon to reach a consensus on defining it, on agreeing on its causes, or on prescribing efficacious remedies.

What the absence of a firm data base implies is the need for special expertise in examining existing data and for special care in making responsible recommendations. Researchers are in a better position than are nonresearchers to gauge the usefulness of incomplete psychological findings. However, the implications of research on intelligence are often publicized even when the investigator would prefer to wait for additional data. Thus, like it or not, we have a difficult but ineluctable responsibility to draw the best conclusions trained scientists can draw from a complicated, imperfect data base.

Despite the gaps in our current knowledge, several recommendations can nevertheless be made with confidence. First, we must distinguish between severe intellectual retardation with known causes and mild retardation, usually of unknown etiology. Policy provisions should be different for these two diagnostic classes. Second, societal interventions should focus on improving social competence rather than on attempting to alter cognitive abilities directly. As we will discuss shortly, at any given intellectual level there is considerable variance in how adequately individuals adjust to society. We know better how to increase social competence than how to influence cognitive abilities. Thus our efforts will be most successful if we promote policies and programs that attempt to raise the level of functional intelligence – that is, the socially competent behavior that people emit, regardless of their formal intellectual capacities.

Third, sound social policy should reflect an appreciation for the continuity of development. We have paid a high price for committing ourselves to a search for magic periods where we concentrate interventions at the expense of other periods in development. The fourth recommendation is related. Social policy must respect the fact of biological heterogeneity by recognizing that no single intervention will be best for all groups of individuals at risk. Fifth, we have learned the dangers of attempting to base social policy on extreme positions; future policies should reflect the moderate, defensible stances that can be justified by the actual state of knowledge.

Finally, it now appears that effective interventions will be family support systems, not single programs designed to aid children alone or to remediate any one particular problem known to be correlated with low social competence. As we shall see, there is evidence that thoughtfully designed family support systems work at least as well as and are less expensive than many other forms of intervention. We will now discuss each of these recommendations in greater detail.

ORGANIC VERSUS FAMILIAL RETARDATION – A CRITICAL DISTINCTION

If intelligence could be defined clearly and to the satisfaction of all, social policy related to intelligence would be far easier to develop than it presently is. We are not going to attempt such a definition here; the task may well be a Sisyphean one. But it is not necessary to understand fully what intelligence is in order to make some reasonable social policy recommendations. First, present knowledge both justifies and requires making a distinction between intellectual retardation with a known organic cause and retardation of unknown etiology. The problems of implementing scientific knowledge concerning retardation are not identical for the two classes of victims.

Organic retardation

Although there are several classification systems of mental retardation (e.g., American Association on Mental Deficiency, 1977; American Psychiatric Association, 1968; Group for the Advancement of Psychiatry, 1967), all of them separate cases in which there is known organic impairment from those in which none is evident. To a considerable extent, this distinction overlaps with a classification based on IQ scores. Severe intellectual handicap is often accompanied by gross physical handicaps. As Work (1979) observed, "Many of the categories of severe retardation occur in relation to biologic syndromes that involve and disfigure the entire body" (p. 403). Hydrocephaly, microcephaly, and gargoylism are examples, as are many types of brain damage resulting from such adverse prenatal influences as radiation, lead poisoning, or maternal infection with syphilis or rubella. Most persons affected by such disorders have IQs below 50 (American Psychiatric Association, 1968; Work, 1979; Zigler, 1978). By any definition they are mentally impaired. "Organic" or "clinical" cases of retardation occur with approximately equal frequency in all social classes and constitute about one-quarter of the mentally retarded population (A. D. B. Clarke & Clarke, 1977; Work, 1979; Zigler, 1978).

Severely low intelligence is a problem that warrants serious preventive efforts and humane treatment policies. (Excellent reviews of the status of prevention and treatment methods have been written by Begab, 1974, and by A. D. B. Clarke & Clarke, 1977.) If we used every technique now known to be effective in reducing the incidence of mental retardation (e.g., genetic counseling, amniocentesis, neonatal screening, prenatal and neonatal health care, and nutritional services for pregnant women and young children), we could all but eliminate certain organic disorders. Had these procedures been in full use for the past generation, the number of organic retarded persons in our society could have been reduced from approximately 2 million to 1 million (Zigler, 1978). A thought-provoking note is that in some cases, advances in medical technology can also *increase* the incidence of severe retardation, as by saving the lives of some infants born very prematurely.

In addition to prevention, much can be done to ease the family strains created by severe retardation. The child who has phenylketonuria, or any of a number of other organic conditions often associated with very low intelligence, requires demanding daily care. Uninformed social policy can result in miserable lives for such persons and their relatives. On the other hand, there are many relatively simple ways to ease the burdens of these families and to encourage conditions that allow caretakers to provide affection and concern rather than impersonal ministrations. Services to families such as homemaking assistance or an occasional trained babysitter can make an enormous difference in quality of life and can enable some families to keep their retarded children at home. The availability of institutions is also essential for those cases in which a severely retarded child (or adult) cannot be cared for at home. Though it has become somewhat fashionable to argue that institutions are inherently dehumanizing and should be abolished, the senior author and his colleagues have argued that families must continue to have the option of institutionalization open to them (Zigler & Balla, 1977a, 1977b). After years of research on institutions both in this country and elsewhere (see Balla, 1976; Balla, Butterfield, & Zigler, 1974; Balla & Zigler, 1975; Butterfield, 1967; Butterfield, Barnett, & Bensberg, 1968; Dentler & Mackler, 1961; King, Raynes, & Tizard, 1971; McCormick, Balla, & Zigler, 1975; Zigler & Balla, 1977a, 1977b; Zigler, Balla, & Butterfield, 1968; Zigler, Balla, & Watson, 1972; Zigler, Butterfield, & Capobianco, 1970; Zigler, Butterfield, & Goff, 1966; Zigler & Williams, 1963), we have gained considerable knowledge about the factors that make institutions good or bad. So long as we have severely retarded persons in our society we will need institutions to care for at least some of them. We should use our knowledge to make these institutions better.

Familial retardation

In the majority of cases of mental retardation, there is no known biological damage and the level of functioning is only moderately impaired. Social policy related to such retardation is far more difficult to formulate than is policy related to severe retardation, partially because there is no consensus on whether such persons should be labeled "retarded" by society and partially because the etiology of the condition is not clearly understood.

The number of persons considered to be just mildly retarded is substantial. In the nomenclature of the American Psychiatric Association's diagnostic manual (1968), "borderline mental retardation" describes a large group of persons with IQs between 68 and 85, many of whom function adequately in society. "Mild mental retardation" describes a smaller but still numerically large group of persons with IQs between 52 and 67 who are also not necessarily considered retarded unless they are confronted with tasks requiring complex learning. Given the Gaussian distribution of IQ scores between 50 and 150, about 15–16% of the population can be expected to fall into these two categories of mild to borderline mental retardation.

The cause of retardation where no organic cause is apparent remains the most perplexing problem in research on intellectual deficit (A. D. B. Clarke & Clarke, 1977; Zigler, 1967). The point on which investigators come closest to consensus is that this form of mental retardation reflects some complex interaction between genetic and environmental factors. The lack of agreement is reflected in the varying labels assigned to this classification. Until about a decade ago, the most common term was "cultural familial retardation." Because such persons are primarily from the lower social classes, many theorists have assumed that an impoverished home environment contributes to their intellectual deficit. Considerable research has been conducted in an attempt to ascertain whether certain child-rearing practices, maternal–child interactional styles, and other aspects of the underprivileged environment are possible psychosocial contributors to intellectual retardation. The "familial" portion of the label reflects the fact that this form of retardation typically occurs in close relatives. More recently, this diagnostic category has been relabeled "environmental," "sociocultural," or "retardation owing to psychosocial deprivation" (see Work, 1979). Because all these terms presuppose a known etiology, whereas in fact the etiology is very much in dispute, we will refer to this group just as "familial" – the only portion of the many labels that is purely descriptive.

Progress in our understanding of familial retardation will require an approach different from that which has advanced our knowledge in regard to the organic types of retardation. One need know only some of the most striking facts about familial retardation to realize that a behavioral approach will be required. Why is familial retardation so related to family income and parental occupation? Why is the prevalence of this disorder so much higher during the school years than in the postschool years? Why is IQ such a poor predictor of life outcome for this group of retarded individuals? These phenomena clearly have much more to do with behavior emitted, socialization, and social interaction than with defective physiological functioning.

There has been some impressive intervention research (discussed subsequently) directed toward raising the IQ-test performance of mildly retarded persons. However, we believe that the state of present knowledge makes recommending such programs a serious social policy error. Even if we were able to raise IQs, it does not necessarily follow that the consequences would benefit either the individuals or society. Considerable research now shows that the mildly retarded person can make either a good or a poor adjustment to society depending upon the quality of education received, the kinds of jobs available, and the nature of family and societal support systems. It is not at all uncommon to find one retarded person who is married, raising a family, employed, and participating in community events, whereas another retarded person whose IQ score is 20 points higher lives a life requiring constant supervision. Societies can do a great deal to ease the adjustment of mildly retarded individuals; and, as we will show later, policies directed toward this aim are less intrusive, less expensive, and less difficult to justify in a democracy than are efforts to raise IQ scores.

THE SOCIAL COMPETENCE ALTERNATIVE

Despite decades of progress in defining and measuring intelligence, we propose that intelligence should be replaced by social competence as the major indicator of the success or failure of social intervention programs. To develop this argument, we will review what has been learned about the advantages and disadvantages of employing IQ scores in evaluations of intervention efforts.

The IQ solution

Over the 20-year history of childhood intervention programs, the most often utilized outcome measure has been the IQ score or, more typically, the magnitude of change in children's IQ scores. One reason for this is historic. As part of psychologists' long-standing interest in the nature of intelligence, many intervention programs were initiated with the specific purpose of studying how much IQ scores can be influenced by life experiences (e.g., Garber & Heber, 1977; Gordon, 1973; Gray & Klaus, 1965; Karnes, Teska, Hodgins, & Badger, 1970; Levenstein & Sunley, 1968; Ramey, Collier, Sparling, Loda, Campbell, Ingram, & Finkelstein, 1976; Skeels, 1966; Skodak & Skeels, 1945, 1949; B. White, 1975). In addition, such theoretical godfathers of early childhood intervention as Hunt in his book *Intelligence and Experience* (1961) and Bloom in *Stability and Change* (1964) convincingly argued that the level of intellectual functioning is relatively plastic. This position was popularized by the mass media, and soon American parents were rushing to hang mobiles over their infants' cribs and to purchase "educational" toys in the hopes of raising their children's IQs to the genius level. Because this was about the time that large-scale education intervention programs were mounted, it is not surprising that researchers were concerned about the effects of such programs on IQ scores.

Another reason why the IQ became so popular an outcome measure is that standard IQ tests are highly refined instruments. Their psychometric properties are well documented and thus permit the user to avoid difficult measurement problems. Their ready availability makes them more attractive to researchers than are tests that must be requested from clearinghouses or from other researchers. Another plus is that standard IQ tests need little description in written reports, and the results are readily compared across studies. Ease of administration adds to the attractiveness of IQ tests, especially if one employs the Peabody Picture Vocabulary Test, the Ammons Full Range Vocabulary Test, or the Otis–Lennon Mental Ability Test, justifying the use of such 10-min measures on the basis of their relatively high correlations with the longer Stanford–Binet Intelligence Scale or the Wechsler Intelligence Scale for Children.

Another advantage is the presumed generalizability of IQ-test performance. Despite the many shortcomings of an IQ score, no other measure has been found to be related to so many other behaviors of theoretical and practical significance (Kohlberg & Zigler, 1967; Mischel, 1968). Because early childhood intervention programs are popularly regarded as efforts to prepare children for school, the fact that the IQ is the best available predictor of school performance is a particularly compelling rationale for its use as an assessment criterion. Beyond the school issue, if compensatory education programs are directed at correcting deficiencies across a broad array of cognitive abilities, the best single measure of the success of such programs is improvement on a measure reflecting a broad spectrum of such abilities – namely, an IQ test.

Paradoxically, a final reason why the IQ became a popular outcome measure was that those who mounted intervention programs of course wanted to demonstrate their effectiveness. The IQ was an instant hit once it became obvious that the most common outcome of just about any intervention effort (even a hastily mounted 8-week summer program) was a 10-point increase in IQ (see Eisenberg & Conners, 1966). We now have greater insight into the cause of these IQ increases. Considerable empirical evidence has shown that IQ changes resulting from preschool intervention programs such as Head Start reflect motivational changes that influence the children's test performance rather than changes in the actual quality of cognitive functioning (Seitz, Abelson, Levine, & Zigler, 1975; Zigler, Abelson, & Seitz, 1973; Zigler, Abelson, Trickett, & Seitz, in press; Zigler & Butterfield, 1968). But in the 1960s the IQ gains were narrowly interpreted as a dramatic demonstration of the effectiveness of intervention. Indeed, with such leading figures as Hunt (1971) reporting IQ improvements of 50 to 70 points as a result of early intervention, it became increasingly seductive to bet on improvement in the IQ as the bedrock outcome measure.

Disadvantages of using IQ. Despite the assets that make the IQ test an attractive evaluation measure, the IQ alone is an inadequate indicator of outcome. There are a myriad of factors that determine the quality and character of human functioning, and one can obtain a very high IQ score and still not behave admirably in the real world that exists beyond the confines of the psychologist's testing room. This fact is brought home in striking empirical fashion in the very modest relation that has been found between IQ scores obtained in childhood and measures of everyday performance in life in the postschool period. McClelland (1973) estimates this correlation to be around .20.

Just as a high IQ need not imply well-adjusted behavior, neither does a low IQ necessarily predict poor adjustment to societal demands. Several early workers in the mental retardation field, such as Fernald and Potter, felt that the difference between social adequacy and inadequacy in the large group of borderline retarded persons was a matter of personality rather than intelligence. Many workers adopted this position (e.g., Penrose, 1963; Sarason, 1953; Tizard, 1953), and a number of studies have confirmed their viewpoint (see Windle, 1962). One of the most persuasive of these was the comprehensive study by T. R. Weaver (1946) of the adjustment of 8,000 retarded persons, most of whom had IQs below 75, inducted into the U.S. Army. Of the total group, 56% of the males and 62% of the females made a satisfactory adjustment to military life. The median IQs of the successful and unsuccessful groups were 72 and 68, respectively. Weaver concluded that "personality factors far overshadowed the factor of intelligence in the adjustment of the retarded to military service" (p. 245).

The tendency to overemphasize the importance of intellect in the adjustment of moderately retarded persons was exposed in a survey by Windle (1962). He found that in most institutions for retarded persons, intelligence was presumed to be the critical factor in adjustment after release. However, the vast majority (over 20) of the studies he reviewed reported no relation between intellectual level and postinstitutional adjustment. Rather, this literature showed that the factors associated with poor social adjustment included anxiety, jealousy, overdependency, poor self-evaluation, hostility, hyperactivity, and failure to follow orders even when requests were well within the range of intellectual competence.

Although the IQ score fails as an indicator of life performance, it has much better efficiency as a predictor of school performance. As McClelland (1973) noted, it is not surprising that the correlation is approximately .70, inasmuch as good test performance and good school performance require superiority in playing similar "little games," the relevance of which to the person's needs is not always obvious. However, in comparison with psychology's usual correlations in the .30–.50 range, a .70 correlation seems so impressive that the IQ score is often given a primacy it does not deserve. Consider, for example, the meaning of the IQ in those popular labels *underachiever* and *overachiever* (see Thorndike, 1963). These labels operationally signify only that there is a disparity between the IQ score and school achievement, with the IQ score serving as the benchmark against which to assess school achievement. However, in everyday school practice, the specific operations utilized to define the constructs are often conveniently forgotten, and unfortunate labels take their place. Thus, if a middle-class child does not do very well in school, both the school and the family appear more comfortable if we call the child an underachiever. If an economically disadvantaged child does poorly in school, we are tempted to call him or her stupid, using the school performance itself as the ultimate gauge of intellectual potential. This situation becomes even more ridiculous when we consider the nonsensical label "overachiever." This peculiar title essentially asserts that some persons achieve more than they are capable of achieving. Do psychologists really wish to argue that human capacity is reflected better in the IQ score than in the child's everyday school performance? Only by adopting such a questionable assumption could we continue to employ this label.

Our unswerving faith in the IQ has led us to be nearsighted in other respects as well. One crucial but common oversight is that even where there are relatively high correlations between IQ scores and behavior in other contexts, a great deal of variance is attributable to other predictive factors. In a science that appears overly concerned with significance levels, we have allowed ourselves to be dazzled by a correlation of .70. What does not receive sufficient attention is the fact that this correlation indicates that only *half* of the variance in school performance is accounted for by children's IQ scores. What then is influencing the other half of the variance? Clearly – as is known to be true in the adjustment of retarded persons to society – it must include some collection of personal attributes or characteristics not very well assessed by our standard IQ test.

What the IQ test measures.   Given the advantages and disadvantages just discussed, how can we continue to benefit from the IQ test's better properties while avoiding the pitfalls in its usage? Paradoxically, for the very reason that the IQ is not a pure measure of cognition, it can be a useful part of a larger battery of social competence measures. This becomes evident when we consider what it is that IQ tests measure.

First, there is no question that IQ tests tap at least some abilities that are an important part of human cognition. For example, responses on an IQ test require abstracting ability, reasoning, speed of visual information processing, and many other formal cognitive processes that appear and reappear with regularity in factor-analytic studies of human intelligence-test performance. In keeping with the well-known process–content distinction, however, the standard intelligence test is also an *achievement* test. Individuals' experiences determine whether they have acquired particular knowledge, without which they cannot pass the item in question. If we ask a child what a gown is, and the reply is that he or she does not know, it is possible that there is something inadequate about the memory storage and/or retrieval systems, which are aspects of formal cognition. On the other hand, if in the child's experience the word *gown* has never been encountered, he or she will fail the item even though the storage and retrieval systems are perfectly adequate.

Intelligence-test performance is also greatly influenced by a variety of motivational and/or personality variables that have little to do with either formal cognition or achievement variables. Again, perhaps some simple but compelling examples might be helpful. While testing a child the senior author once asked, "What is an orange?" Because the child professed not to know, one might conclude either that this child (diagnosed as retarded) had low formal processing abilities, or (because he resided in an institution) that his experiences had been particularly impoverished. A third explanation, later verified through observation as correct, was that this child knew perfectly well what an orange was but preferred not to answer the question because to do so might terminate the test. The child's efforts during testing were concentrated on maximizing the social relationship with the examiner. This was a lonely child in a lonely place. What his behavior conveyed was that he was much more interested in obtaining a warm human interaction than he was in answering questions about oranges.

A related phenomenon is often encountered among the economically disadvantaged children whose performance is assessed in early childhood intervention programs. Many of these children typically reply "I don't know" to the simplest of questions, including such basic queries as "What is your name?" This phenomenon does not arise from a lack of cognitive ability or knowledge but rather reflects motivational factors, in this case, the child's strong desire to minimize the interaction with the examiner. Why exactly do children insist on engaging in what our value system tells us to be such self-defeating behavior? Do they dislike the adult examiner or do they dislike the testing situation? Our best hunch is that they are fearful of both and therefore behave in an adaptive manner having as its goal the termination of an unpleasant experience. Clearly, given the demands of our society, children who have adopted the "I don't know" strategy are not very likely to utilize their cognitive systems optimally or, if they keep up their behavior, to obtain those rewards (e.g., high grades in school, high salaries, and attractive jobs) that society dispenses for behaving in the manner it prefers.

It is this tripartite conception of IQ-test performance that explains why the IQ score is a relatively successful predictor of such a wide variety of behaviors. If one examines closely many of the criterion behaviors for which we would like the IQ to be a predictor, one discovers that they are themselves complex measures clearly influenced by the set of factors that influence the IQ score. Does anyone seriously question that the child with superior formal cognitive abilities, rich experience in the middle-class world, and a high motivation to do well in school will display better school performance than the child who may have had more restricted or at least less middle-class-relevant experiences and who may view the school as an alien and/or hostile place which demands behavior that has little relevance? It is safe to conclude that the IQ test will always be a predictor of other variables, provided these variables are influenced by the three factors that influence the IQ test. In fact, to the extent that psychologists are successful in developing relatively purer measures of cognition that are less affected by achievement and motivation, such measures can be expected to have less predictive value than existing intelligence tests.

Defining social competence

The foregoing discussion has doubtless made clear that we do not believe that IQ and social competence are one and the same. However, we must also reject the inference that could be drawn from McClelland's (1973) paper that IQ and competence are very minimally related. Our position is that because both concepts are influenced by some of the same variables, the IQ can profitably be employed as one index in the measurement of social competence. We do not wish to propose a standardized test of social competence in this chapter. Defining social competence has proved to be as complex a problem as defining intelligence, and the subject could easily merit a separate handbook of its own. We do wish to suggest some guidelines for what a useful social competence battery should include in the context of evaluating social intervention programs.

First, there should be measures of physical health and well-being. We list physical factors first precisely because psychologists have tended to overlook their significance as a determinant of a child's social competence. The child who is malnourished, who is ill much of the time, or who suffers handicaps of vision or hearing is clearly at a disadvantage in establishing a competent, happy relationship with adults and peers. However we may choose to define social competence, physical well-being is likely to contribute at least as much as any other single factor.

Psychologists may or may not choose to invest much research energy in attempting to define and measure physical factors. Understandably, they may view this as the province of other disciplines – although some remarkably productive research has been done by psychologists exploring the consequences of such events as premature birth or late versus early sexual maturation. Our argument here is only that psychologists must be willing to accord the same respect to physical as to intellectual factors. It should become routine practice to obtain and report at least minimal health information in any intervention evaluation. There are numerous physical health measures (reviewed by North, 1979) that can be used in assessments of early childhood intervention programs, including such pediatric standbys as height and weight for age and whether a child has received inoculations against preventable childhood diseases. Other valuable gauges to general health status include school attendance records and reports from teachers and parents that can disclose instances of chronically poor health. Physical health will not guarantee social competence, but we should take advantage of the certain positive correlation between the two to employ it as one of our measures.

A second social competence measure should be an index of cognitive ability. This might be a standard IQ test, a Piagetian measure of cognitive functioning, or some other measure arising from the productive endeavors in research on intelligence exemplified in this handbook. (As we have just discussed the use of IQ tests in detail, we will not repeat our reasons here.) Third, there should be at least one achievement measure to indicate how well a child is satisfying societal demands. There are many good candidates for inclusion, such as the Caldwell Preschool Inventory, the Peabody Individual Achievement Test, and a variety of well-standardized school achievement tests. At various ages there could also be ratings of behavior related to social expectancies, such as whether the child is involved in juvenile delinquency, teenage pregnancy, or child abuse (as either a victim or a perpetrator); and whether the child is in school rather than a dropout, in the appropriate grade for his or her age, in a regular rather than special-education classroom, or self-supporting rather than on welfare. All these measures are molar indexes and not fine-grained analyses of psychological development. But they are meaningful and have the advantage of being fully comprehensible and of mutual interest to taxpayers and decision makers.

As the reader may have noticed, we have presented the first three components of social competence in order of decreasing universality of agreement on their values. Virtually everyone can agree on the desirability of health and physical well-being. Though there is disagreement on what is meant by intellectual competence, in the abstract the trait is viewed positively. As the variable list of achievement tests and ratings just listed illustrates, the third area is a potentially more controversial one. The fourth area is still more so and adds the complication of being particularly hard to measure: That is, the final component of a social competence index should be the measurement of motivational and emotional attributes.

Highly intangible personality factors, held in different degrees and manifested in different ways by each person, would seem by far the most difficult area in which to suggest specific measures. However, the growing body of literature is rich with possibilities. For example, in a study of effects of institutionalization on retarded children, Harter and Zigler (1974) employed a battery of measures of "effectance motivation" based largely on the work of Robert White (1959). The investigators found that the effects of institutional life were mixed, in some ways helping retarded children utilize their abilities and in other ways hindering them. Specifically, noninstitutionalized children showed more curiosity and exploratory behavior than did institutionalized children – as might be expected from the stereotypic view of institutions as places with rigid routines that depress individuality and spontaneity. But noninstitutionalized retarded children were also less confident of their ability to solve problems, and they tended to settle for tasks that were too easy for them rather than risk failure. Evidently, one cost of life in the "mainstream" for retarded children is that they are frequently confronted with situations in which they are at a disadvantage and consequently adopt an overcautious problem-solving style.

We have chosen this particular example because there is currently so much debate about the merits of deinstitutionalization and mainstreaming. It is our belief that, as with any social policy, these recommendations intended to improve the life of retarded persons may eventually have the opposite effect if they are based on a too-restricted set of outcome measures. Institutions do not have simple, unidirectional effects. Certain kinds of institutions may be right for certain persons at certain times. In order to decide how best to humanize the treatment of retarded persons, we need information that captures the complexity of reality. We can take a necessary step toward understanding the multidimensional consequences of social programs – such as institutions and short-term interventions – by including measures of their motivational and emotional effects.

Among many other examples of research that sheds light on the personality effects of intervention is a study by Ramey and his colleagues (Ramey et al., 1976; Ramey & Haskins, 1981). These investigators found that children who had received several years of intensive preschool intervention were more aggressive than control children when they entered public elementary schools. A related finding is that children who received an early school-aged intervention program were more likely than were control children to report disliking their later school experiences (Seitz, Apfel, & Efron, 1978; Seitz, Apfel, & Rosenbaum, 1981). As we will discuss later, accounts such as these go far beyond information about cognitive abilities or achievement data alone in enriching our ability to interpret the effects of early intervention.

Numerous other motivational and emotional variables have been employed as outcome measures in intervention research. (See Zigler and Trickett, 1978, for a description of those listed here.) Such variables include (a) children's positive responsiveness to social reinforcement (Robertson, 1978; Zigler, 1961; Zigler & Balla, 1972); (b) locus of control measured for both the children in the program and their parents (Coleman, Campbell, Hobson, McPartland, Mood, Weinfeld, & York, 1966; Stipek, 1977); (c) expectancy of success (Gruen & Zigler, 1968; Ollendick, Balla, & Zigler, 1971); (d) wariness of adults (S. Weaver, Balla, & Zigler, 1971; Zigler et al., 1980); (e) verbal attention-seeking behavior (Kohlberg & Zigler, 1967; Robertson, 1978); (f) outer-directedness and degree of imitation in problem solving (Balla & Zigler, 1968; Turnure & Zigler, 1964; Zigler et al., 1980); (g) aspects of self-image (DeMott, 1978; Katz & Zigler, 1967; Katz, Zigler, & Zalk, 1975); (h) measures of learned helplessness (Achenbach & Weisz, 1975;

Weisz, 1975); (i) attitude toward school (Stipek, 1977); and (j) creativity (Yando et al., 1979). This list focuses on measures from our own research because of our close familiarity with such measures, but many further examples can be found in the research of others (e.g., Anderson & Messick, 1974; Begab & Richardson, 1976; Greenspan, 1981; Kohn, 1977; Mercer, 1973; O'Malley, 1977; Schaefer, 1976; Simeonsson, 1978; Sundberg, Snowden, & Reynolds, 1978). Our point here is not to prescribe particular measures but rather to promote the principle of including this class of variables in outcome evaluations.

Raising social competence. A principal advantage of focusing on social competence for social policy purposes is that we have already learned much about how to increase competence through such means as educational and training procedures. Even in the case of relatively severe retardation, skilled training can provide people with self-help abilities as well as socially useful competencies. To illustrate with a rather dramatic example of improving social competence, the senior author once encountered a retarded man in a sheltered workshop who was working with a highly complex piece of machinery. His ability to operate this machine far exceeded what would be predicted from his overall cognitive capabilities. The director of the workshop explained that the man had been taught through a shaping process not unlike that employed by Skinner in training pigeons. The effects of the training were very specific: This man could handle the machine quite adequately, but only if conditions were identical to those in which he originally learned. To emphasize this, the director rotated the machine approximately 90°, at which point the operator become somewhat agitated and was no longer able to run the equipment. (Piaget also noted that remarkable intellectual feats performed by young children on some task or other cannot be repeated following relatively minor alterations in the task stimuli.) In terms of the finished product, the retarded adult was performing just as competently as an operator with a normal IQ. But this accomplishment obviously did not indicate that the man had become normal in intelligence. Rather, he was using a different type of cognitive process to achieve his intelligent behavior. More important, the man had acquired a useful skill in which he clearly took pride. This accomplishment should be viewed as no less interesting or significant than an actual IQ-score increase would have been.

The notion of increasing social competence is based in large part on the concept of a capacity–performance difference. The existence of this difference is particularly well documented for retarded persons, who often perform more poorly on a wide variety of tasks than would be predicted from their general level of cognitive ability, typically defined by their mental ages. There is experimental evidence suggesting that much of this mental age deficit in performance is due to the attenuating effects of motivational factors (see Zigler, 1966; Zigler & Balla, 1979; Zigler & Harter, 1969), including many of those mentioned before as indicators of social competence.

Disadvantaged children are another group who may perform poorly on tests of cognitive abilities for reasons that are at least partially motivational. The fact that children from lower-class homes generally perform relatively poorly on measures of intellectual competence and academic achievement is now well documented (e.g., Armor, 1972a, 1972b; Coleman, 1972; Coleman et al., 1966; Jencks, Smith, Acland, Bane, Cohen, Gintis, Heyns, & Michelson, 1972; Jensen, 1969, 1973,

1979; St. John, 1970; Thorndike, 1973; Venezsky, 1970). But there is also sub-stantial evidence that disadvantaged children possess greater abilities than they usually reveal (Cole & Bruner, 1971; Havighurst, 1970; Seitz et al., 1975; Zigler et al., 1973, in press). Both schools and society appear routinely to underutilize the talents of disadvantaged children, many of whom are also members of ethnic minority groups.

The tendency for children from disadvantaged, castelike minority groups to do poorly in school is worldwide. For example, the Untouchables in India, the Maori in New Zealand, Oriental Jews in Israel, and the Buraku in Japan do not meet the achievement standards set by the majority-group children in their societies' schools (Ogbu, 1978). Although the reasons for the poorer performance are not fully understood, at least two studies suggest that the educational problems of minorities do not inhere in the children themselves. In one of these studies, Ito (1967) examined the school performance of Japanese immigrant children, includ-ing those of the Buraku subculture. In Japan, the Buraku is a lower-class minority group whose children have had a discouraging history of greater truancy and dropout rates and poorer school achievement than their peers. As adults, the Buraku tend to be employed in relatively low-level jobs. In the United States, however, Ito's study revealed that the Buraku immigrant children achieved as well as did other Japanese children within the American school system. Of course, such results could be caused by differential patterns of selective migration in the two groups. It seems more probable, however, that these data illustrate the effect of discrimination in occupational opportunities upon educational attainment. In another study, Weber (1973) reported data from four American schools located in urban black ghetto areas where the students' reading levels averaged at or above national norms. If disadvantaged minority children were less educable for reasons of health, culture, or genetics, it should not be possible to find entire school districts full of such children achieving at grade level on nationally standardized tests.

Another example of the underutilization of disadvantaged children's abilities is worth considering because it provides a longitudinal perspective on the problem (Seitz et al., 1978, 1981). In this study a group of inner-city boys participated in an experimental, socioeconomically integrated, educational intervention program from kindergarten through third grade. The curriculum emphasized mathematics and was unusual in that it was designed by a Chinese consultant to include many traditional oriental activities, such as paper folding and the creation of complex geometrical string designs. The children also cooked in the classrooms and were required to manipulate fractions within such practical contexts as increasing and decreasing recipe quantities for cookies and pies. The teaching of geometrical and quantitative concepts was thus perhaps more concrete and practical – as well as more playful – than is usually the case.

Not surprisingly, at the end of 3rd grade the intervention-group boys scored significantly higher in mathematical achievement than did a control group of boys, also studied longitudinally from kindergarten on. Specifically, the interven-tion group scored at grade level, whereas the control group scored a year below grade level. When these children were tested repeatedly during the following 7 years, the difference between the two groups diminished and became nonsignifi-cant. In 10th grade, the intervention-group boys were scoring 2 years, and the control boys 3 years, below national norms. The decline in achievement for the intervention children appeared to be a genuine one. There was no evidence of selective attrition, and because the same test was administered over the 7-year span, the interpretation of results was not muddied by the common problem of trying to compare scores from different tests administered under variable conditions at different grades and times of the year. In short, the dissipation of the intervention group's initial advantage represents a classic textbook case of fade-out.

The reason for the fade-out, however, did not appear to be an authentic loss of mathematical reasoning ability. Rather it appeared to reflect a surprising lack of exposure to appropriate high-school mathematics courses. To score at the 10th-grade level on the achievement test employed requires knowledge of algebra and geometry. Yet, whereas approximately 90% of the middle-class boys who had attended the early intervention program were taking these subjects in high school, only 43% of the disadvantaged intervention-group boys were doing so. (The proportion was similar for the control-group boys.) It is hardly surprising that as a group the boys from the intervention program were no longer performing at grade level, although it is not clear why some were not receiving the same level of mathematical instruction as their former classmates. At an individual rather than group level, the failure to utilize probable talent in these adolescents was striking. Two intervention-group boys with 10th-grade IQs of 110 and 120 and scores in mathematics near grade level were taking "business math" rather than algebra. Two other boys who scored well above grade level on the achievement test received marks of D and F in their algebra courses because of chronic truancy. Evidently they were managing to learn enough, despite infrequent class attendance, to continue to perform above national norms for students in their grade. The picture is not one of fading talent but of diminishing use of talent.

To the extent that deficits in performance occur for motivational reasons, practices aimed at reducing motivational problems will increase social competence. There is some evidence to indicate that Project Head Start has had this kind of motivational effect. In one study (Zigler & Butterfield, 1968), children attending Head Start were compared with children of similar backgrounds who were on Head Start waiting lists. Both at the beginning and at the end of the school year, the children received the Stanford–Binet IQ test twice, once under standard testing conditions and once under altered conditions designed to put them more at ease and thus to "optimize" their performance. At the fall testing, both groups of children performed comparably, and much better (about 10 points higher) under optimizing than under standard test conditions. Zigler and Butterfield argued that the children's optimal-condition IQ scores (averaging approximately 97 for the two groups) probably reflected their actual abilities better than did their standard-condition IQs. In the spring the Head Start children's optimal-condition IQs remained at the same level, whereas their average standard-condition IQ rose to 92. The non–Head Start children exhibited no significant gain in standard-condition IQs, and their optimal-condition IQs declined significantly by 5 points. As the authors noted, the demonstrated improvement in the Head Start children's standard IQs indicates that children were generally more competent by the end of the school year. They concluded: "In trying to improve the deprived child's general level of performance, it would appear at least as important to attempt to correct his motivational inadequacies by developing nursery programs geared specifically toward changing his adverse motivational patterns as it is to concentrate on teaching cognitive skills and factual knowledge" (Zigler & Butterfield, 1968, p. 12).

Jacobson and his colleagues (Jacobson, Berger, Bergman, Millham, & Greeson, 1971) tested this proposition directly. They found that negative motivational factors affecting test performance were reduced after disadvantaged children received a one-to-one social interaction program with a middle-class adult. Children in this experimental program exhibited gains in their Stanford–Binet IQ scores comparable to the gains shown by children in two or three cognitive-training programs also designed by the investigators.

Although Jacobson's study involved experimental laboratory conditions, it is reassuring to find similar evidence of the effectiveness of programs existing in the real world. Such evidence is provided by two studies conducted by the authors to follow up the Zigler and Butterfield study (Seitz et al., 1975; Zigler et al., in press). In both investigations, control-group children were selected by canvassing neighborhoods in which Head Start programs were not yet in existence to find Head Start–eligible children. As with the Zigler and Butterfield study, therefore, there is reason to believe that the preschool and control groups were comparable enough to permit any eventual differences between them to be attributed to the effects of the Head Start program.

In the first of these studies (Seitz et al., 1975), a situation roughly analogous to optimized versus standard testing was designed in which children were tested either at home or in a classroom away from home. Whereas the investigators had expected home testing to put children at their ease, in fact the reverse was true: Children tested at home tended to perform more poorly than did children tested away from home. In-home observations suggested that maternal anxiety over the children's performance was one reason for their apprehensiveness in the testing situation. Regardless of the exact cause, the problem was almost certainly motivational, because children had been randomly assigned to the two testing conditions and were unlikely to differ in cognitive ability. Head Start children were less susceptible to the place-of-testing effect than were control-group children. Averaged across two testing occasions, Head Start children tested at school scored 1 point higher than did their classmates tested at home; for the non–Head Start children the difference was 13 points.

In the second study (Zigler et al., in press), motivational characteristics were measured directly rather than inferred from the children's test performance. Children were tested prior to the beginning of the school year, soon after the Head Start program began, and near the end of the school year. The measures included the Stanford–Binet IQ test, an index of interpersonal distance maintained by the child from the examiner, and a measure of the child's willingness to imitate the examiner. On both the pretest and the retest 2 months later the Head Start and non–Head Start groups were comparable on all measures. (This design thus has the advantage of Campbell and Stanley's [1966] multiple-time-series approach in which the comparability of two groups is established on more than one occasion.) Although both groups showed a gain in IQ from pretest to retest, by the end of the school year the Head Start children's scores had risen still further, whereas the control group's scores had declined significantly. There were no significant group differences in imitation, but on interpersonal distance the non–Head Start children positioned themselves farther away at the posttest than they had at the retest, whereas the Head Start children maintained the same distance. Apparently this increase in wariness had been warded off by the Head Start program.

We belabor this point in such detail because critics have been quick to dismiss evidence of the benefits of Head Start as disappointingly small or as untrustwor-

thy for methodological reasons. In fact, as we hope we have convincingly documented, there is hard evidence that Head Start programs have positive effects on
children's functional intelligence as assessed by their ability to perform more
adequately under conditions that their compatriots find difficult. The still more
general point is that we know that we can affect children's social competence
through a variety of programs, including Head Start. We should not fail to capitalize upon this capability in formulating future social policy.

Having argued that the motivational route is a productive one, we should add
the caution that changes in motivation do not affect changes in intellectual competence itself. This point can be made especially clear in the case of persons who
are mentally retarded. Motivational problems aside, the essential difference between retarded and nonretarded individuals is cognitive. No amount of change in
motivational structure will enable retarded persons to become intellectually normal. But although a motivational approach holds no promise of a dramatic cure for
mental retardation, it can provide us with the means of helping retarded persons
use their intellectual capacities optimally. Although not especially sensational,
such a goal is realistic, and it is of the utmost social importance in light of the
evidence we have cited that the everyday adjustment and/or competence of retarded persons is a function more of personality than of cognitive factors.

It is also worth reflecting on how much cognitive ability is actually required to
meet the complex demands of our society. Most retarded persons have mental
ages in the 9–12 range. (Remember that on most tests a mental age of 16 is the
upper limit for an individual of average IQ.) Though these mental ages do not
predict success in college or the literary arts, they do indicate the intellectual
wherewithal to meet many requirements of everyday life. This becomes apparent
if one thinks about how much intellectual ability is really required to arise in the
morning, dress oneself, catch a bus or walk to a single location, perform some
undemanding sort of labor, and return home. Indeed, in the 1920s and 1930s
investigators found no fewer than 118 occupations in our society suitable for
individuals with mental ages from 5 to 12 (Beckham, 1930; Burr, 1925). This
figure may drop as society becomes more technological; but even in 1956, De-
Prospo noted that 54% of jobs required no schooling beyond the elementary level
(cited in Whitney, 1956).

Another major aspect of social competence is the individual's ability to abide by
the values of the society – for example, to obey laws. Again, retarded persons
commonly satisfy this requirement. Though the incidence of crime may be higher
among retarded than nonretarded persons, the difference is not great, especially if
one controls for the social class factor. There is thus no good reason to view
obedience to the law as somehow beyond the ability of retarded citizens. To
counter this notion, one can apply the concept of the stages of moral development
investigated by Piaget (1948) and Kohlberg (1966). These investigators have
argued that fairly young children are capable of a morality based on absolutism,
that is, one in which the rules inhere in the very fabric of existence and are not to
be broken under any circumstances. People who never achieve a higher stage of
moral development are certainly not candidates for Supreme Court justiceships,
but neither are they likely to break many laws.

In short, raising social competence is a practical, useful, and humane goal of
intervention programs. We can confidently make this goal one of our strongest
recommendations for social policies related to intelligence.

DEVELOPMENTAL CONTINUITY

A third recommendation is that social policy should be based on the principle of developmental continuity. All stages in development are important; none can be neglected.

For much of the history of developmental psychology, theorists have sought some magic time in a child's life at which to optimize development. To some extent this search was a legacy from the psychoanalytic assumption that "the child is father to the man." In this vein Kagan (1979) noted that "one of the dominant hypotheses of contemporary psychology, pediatrics, and psychiatry" is that "frequent, salient, and affectively pleasant interactions between infant and mother during the first two years of life produce dispositions that protect the older child against future anxiety and promote cognitive development for an indefinite period" (p. 886). Biological studies of development – especially in embryology – also inspired theorists to seek critical periods in psychological development during which environmental intervention could be expected to have maximal effects.

The issue of whether critical periods indeed exist for children's intellectual and emotional development has become controversial. For example, Ainsworth and her colleagues (Ainsworth, Blehar, Waters, & Wall, 1978) and Bowlby (1969, 1973) recently presented evidence supporting their existence, whereas Kagan, Kearsley, and Zelazo (1978) presented research suggesting their nonexistence. However – or even whether – this issue is resolved, social policy based on the notion of critical periods has had negative implications. We are certainly not at a stage of knowledge that justifies putting all our policy eggs in one critical-period basket. The efforts of the past decade to make a choice of this sort by investing heavily in preschool intervention unquestionably have had many ill effects. Many excellent preschool programs have fallen victim to a pessimistic backlash effect when unrealistic initial expectations were not met.

In the 1980s we run the risk of repeating the error of the 1960s by shifting our attention from the preschool years to adolescence. Nicholas Hobbs (1979, 1980) pointed out that more and more researchers, including the Clarkes (A. M. Clarke & Clarke, 1976) in England and Feuerstein and his colleagues (Feuerstein, 1980; Feuerstein, Krasilowsky, & Rand, 1974; Rand, Feuerstein, Hoffman, Hoffman, & Miller, 1979) in Israel, are urging that we do so. There are certainly good empirical and theoretical reasons to support the argument that adolescence is a particularly significant age. This is a time of rapid growth, and such periods are usually considered good candidates for critical periods. In Piaget's theory, the stage of formal operations begins at about age 11, ushering in a capability for many intellectual feats impossible to the young child (Piaget, 1970); programs for adolescents could therefore capitalize upon their expanded range of abilities. Some of these programs, such as the often effective instructional courses developed by the U.S. Army, have reported relatively dramatic success.

Nevertheless, we must take care not to recommend a full-scale set of societal interventions for adolescents at the expense of programs for people at other ages. The present-day enthusiasm for adolescence has a curiously familiar ring to those who recall yesterday's equally compelling cries that we put stock in the preschool years. The problem with critical periods is that there are too many of them. There are excellent arguments for, as critical periods, the prenatal period, the first few hours after birth (Klaus, Jerauld, Kreger, McAlpine, Steffa, & Kennell, 1972), the first few months of life (Ainsworth et al., 1978; Bowlby, 1969, 1973), the first 3 years of life (B. White, 1975), the preschool years in general (Bloom, 1964; Hunt, 1961), the first few years of school, and so forth. A policy maker who took the trouble to examine psychology's findings on critical periods might well decide never again to expose him- or herself to the trauma of digesting this too-rich literature.

Our recommendation is that psychologists and policy makers commit themselves to the principle of the continuity of human development. The task is to find not the right age at which to intervene, but rather the right intervention for each age. Genetic counseling and good prenatal care have their significant place at one stage in the life cycle; good educational programs have theirs at another. We should now recognize the dangers of trying to provide societal supports at one stage only, as if that time were magically less expensive and would absolve us from the need to be concerned with other ages as well.

The best example of an "intervention program" in nature is a good secure family – whatever the specific form it takes. It is noteworthy that families do not decide to care for children only during the preschool years, or only during adolescence, or for any other short, fixed period, with the assumption that a brief dose of parenting will suffice to meet the child's developmental needs. Instead, a family is permanently committed to a child and is flexible enough to modify its supportive style to meet the changes that occur during normal growth. Society should be ready to do likewise, by providing a different kind of safety net at different stages of a person's development from cradle to grave.

HETEROGENEITY

Only a society of mechanical robots could be physically and intellectually alike. Biological creatures reliably vary. Therefore, no matter how intelligence is defined, we may expect people to differ in the degree to which they possess it. Unless we build social policy that acknowledges normal biological variability, we are likely to create policies that fail.

One implication of this heterogeneity principle is that programs should not attempt to change children to fit into a uniform mold. All too often the behavior of white middle-class children has been taken as a standard against which the performance of all children is assessed. A number of investigators have now argued that research based upon this approach has yielded a biased picture of the abilities of other groups of children in our society (Baratz & Baratz, 1970; Cole & Bruner, 1971; Labov, 1970, 1972; Lesser, Fifer, & Clark, 1965; Loehlin, Lindzey, & Spuhler, 1975; Stodolsky & Lesser, 1967; Tulkin & Konner, 1973; Yando et al., 1979). For example, it may surprise some to learn that in a study of over 300 children (Yando et al., 1979), those who were very disadvantaged still showed certain strengths in comparison with middle-class white children. On a broad battery of tasks, each socioeconomic group showed a different profile of abilities and weaknesses; no group was uniformly superior or inferior. Clearly, a respect for cultural variation and diversity is a societal ideal that also makes good scientific sense.

Another implication of heterogeneity is that no single program or treatment is necessarily the best solution for all persons with a particular problem. As an example, we consider in some detail the dilemma regarding the best way to educate retarded children. These children are almost certain to face difficulties in school, as their disadvantage in a competitive formal learning situation is enormous. Yet there is no clear recommendation for reduction of these difficulties that can be made universally.

One potential solution is to place retarded children in special classes geared to their special needs. This arrangement, however, has proven to be less than ideal. Among the most serious problems associated with special placements has been stigmatization through formal, institutional labels. As some critics have pointed out, special placements are often made in a racist manner, in that minority-group children are more readily labeled "retarded" than nonminority-group children of the same measured ability (Mercer, 1973, 1975). Studies in Riverside, California, led Jane Mercer and her colleagues to conclude that many special-class students should be considered "6-hour" retarded children because their behavior and abilities are perceived as perfectly adequate outside the school environment (Mercer, 1973, 1975; Mercer, Butler, & Dingman, 1964). The fact that economically disadvantaged children tend to score lower on IQ tests than their abilities permit (Seitz et al., 1975; Zigler et al., 1973, in press) may also contribute to the misguided labeling of many minority children as retarded.

On the other hand, even if retarded children are correctly diagnosed and placed in high-quality special classes, such an environment may tend to reinforce their overdependence (Work, 1979). When school ends, adolescents may have difficulty adjusting to a world that does not provide them with special, kid-glove treatment. It is difficult to balance the short-term benefits against possible long-term drawbacks.

Given the pitfalls of special education, another potential way to educate retarded children is to place them with children of average and above-average intelligence. Yet if mildly to moderately retarded children are placed in regular classrooms, they are apt to experience stress and frustration; their tendency to avoid new tasks and to settle for low levels of accomplishment is likely to be exacerbated. There is also the danger that other children will shun the retarded child and make him or her feel different, unworthy, and unwanted. As one reviewer commented, "It is not surprising that [mainstreamed children] become truant, develop psychosomatic conditions, and often end up as runaways to avoid the stress of the learning situation" (Work, 1979, p. 413). Furthermore, where there is a genuine need for special educational treatment, attempts to mainstream some children in school may ironically reduce their chances to live and work in the mainstream as adults. As one deaf teacher put it, "The paradox is that without the education I got in *deaf* schools I would be hopelessly lost in the hearing world now" (Greenberg & Doolittle, 1977). The most critical question – and one to which we have few answers – is, How does mainstreaming affect a handicapped person's functioning in the adult world after graduation?

In short, there is no simple, general solution to the problem of how best to educate mentally retarded children. In principle Congress has taken a step in the right direction in passing the Education for All Handicapped Children Act of 1975 (P.L. 94–142), which mandates a "free appropriate public education" in the "least restrictive environment" for all handicapped children. This legislation also guarantees parents of handicapped children the right to participate in developing an "individualized education program" tailored to their children's particular abilities and needs. As Zigler and Muenchow (1979) observed, "This provision, if implemented, is a step toward parental involvement in the education of their children to be envied by many parents of normal children" (p. 993).

We must caution, however, that mandating respect for individual needs does not necessarily mean that the law will make this come true. Without adequate funding, laws can have effects entirely different from the intentions of the law-makers. In the case of P.L. 94–142, the cost of implementing the law could far exceed the moneys made available by Congress. As one Connecticut school super-intendent wryly commented, the federal government is "better at mandating than at allocating." Faced with local budget cutbacks, many school districts are likely to interpret "least restrictive environment" as "least expensive" and may abolish special-education facilities entirely so that handicapped children are routinely placed in regular classrooms. We will thus have heterogeneity in principle, but homogeneity – "dumping" vulnerable children into already overcrowded classes without necessary support services – in practice. This does not mean we cannot design and implement good laws that respect individuality and are affordable (we will discuss one model program later), and this should remain our social policy goal.

MODERATE POSITIONS

In the search for scientific truth it is common to aim for a clear, elegant, simple theory that brings order from chaos. Perhaps this ideal explains the popularity of extreme positions in theories about intelligence. It is more elegant to argue that intellectual potential is a simple function of environmental input, or, conversely, that intelligence is fixed by the genes at the moment of conception, than to argue that it is the result of some complex, unspecified interaction. If a strong position also fits well into the prevailing social philosophy, it is often easy to promote social policy based on that view. There are many instances to prove, however, that extreme positions breed extreme reactions. Further, there is a significant cost in public disillusionment and a loss of public credibility for scientists. For these reasons we argue that social policies relating to intelligence should be based on moderate positions that are at least defensible and most likely closer to the truth.

An excellent example of the dangers of extremism in public policy can be seen in the recent history of the treatment of retarded persons. During the past cen-tury, there was a period in which many workers believed in "mental orthopedics" – the idea that if retarded children were given the proper training, they could be made "normal." The state institutions that so many now decry as relics of an inhumane, unenlightened past were actually established with the goal of provid-ing the newest and best mental orthopedic experiences and thus guaranteeing retarded persons a self-sufficient future. But retarded residents did not become normal, and disillusioned professionals were surprisingly quick to adopt the op-posite belief that nothing could be done to alleviate mental retardation. The train-ing schools became human warehouses, and the treatment of retarded people entered a dark era.

The value of special training was subsequently rediscovered, but again it was oversold as being the best answer for all retarded children. In the 1960s school psychologists were arguing that "regardless of the outcome, special-class place-ment is important from a humanitarian point of view" for "preventing frustration and feelings of inferiority derived from undue competition" (Quay, 1963, p. 672).

Less than a decade later, special education was attacked on the same human-itarian grounds as being inherently stigmatizing, and today many professionals are arguing for the wholesale abolition of institutions and special-education class-es. As this brief history illustrates, the problem with basing social policy on strong slogans and good intentions is that the pendulum can shift very quickly in the opposite direction.

Another example of unproductive extremism is provided by the history of inter-vention programs for disadvantaged children. Many of the educational interven-tions initiated in the 1960s were the product of an extreme faith in the mal-leability of intelligence. This was the heyday of the "environmental mystique" – the belief that young children's intellects were enormously influenced by their experiences (see Zigler, 1970). The scientist's task was to uncover those stimula-tions which many middle-class parents provided as a matter of course – reading to the child, responding contingently to early language, finding age-appropriate toys to keep curiosity stimulated – and to extend them to economically deprived chil-dren whose parents were presumably less competent. The infant with nothing to do was in danger of intellectual stagnation: Babies needed lively, colorful mobiles to watch from their earliest days in the crib. The prescription for disadvantaged preschoolers was a heavy dose of concepts presumably missing from their life-style – colors, numbers, sizes – so that they would be ready to profit from school when they entered.

Numerous laboratory studies with animals seemed to support the view that an adequate environment was necessary for normal growth (e.g., Bennett, Diamond, Krech, & Rosenzweig, 1964; Denenberg, 1962; Harlow, 1959; Riesen, 1958; Scott, 1962). However, the translation from extremely deprived laboratory condi-tions to the real-life environments of disadvantaged children was not straightfor-ward. In the laboratory, an animal may be raised in darkness, deprived of han-dling, or kept in a barren cage with demonstrably negative effects. But although some disadvantaged children have exceptionally depriving environments, the ma-jority do not. Pavenstedt (1965) convincingly documented that most disadvan-taged children come from families who are not impoverished in warmth and love but only in the material goods that their low incomes cannot furnish. The belief that low-income parents necessarily provide a poorer environment than do mid-dle-income parents today strikes many as a quaint prejudice. Few people now believe that children's intelligence is mostly determined by the environment and that "experts" should contribute the training that parents cannot, in order to raise children's IQs. But this extreme environmentalism was itself a reaction to an earlier extreme position – that of fixed intelligence revealed through maturation.

Probably the best-known exponents of the maturational point of view were the workers at the Gesell Institute (Gesell, 1928, 1937; Gesell & Ilg, 1943, 1946; Gesell, Ilg, & Ames, 1956), who for many years documented the regularities of growth. Three-year-olds were found to be reliably different from 1-year-olds, who in turn could be counted on to differ from 2-year-olds, regardless of any expecta-tions of their parents or intervention efforts to the contrary. These findings were interpreted as support for the belief that normal development is a simple unfold-ing of the child's genetic potential. There are enough clear exceptions to have made pure maturationism ripe for the later assaults of extreme environmentalists. In particular, it is difficult to account for the behavior of young adolescents, some of whom have reached puberty while others are prepubertal, on the basis of age alone. The overall regularity of development explains why a maturational theory survived as well as it did, but pure maturationism was nevertheless a straw-man position, vulnerable to attack.

Just as environmentalism was a reaction to maturationism, we now find a maturationist stance returning to counter extreme environmentalism. Jensen (1969, 1973, 1979), Herrnstein (1971), and Kagan and his colleagues (Kagan, 1979; Kagan et al., 1978; Kagan & Klein, 1973) have espoused a neomaturationist position, arguing that early experiences have little if any lasting significance for later intelligence. It is difficult to view this development without a feeling of déjà vu. No matter how scientists may resolve the issue, the implications of neomaturationism for social policy are likely to be as negative as were the implications of pure environmentalism. We should have enough experience by now to realize that adopting a moderate position will lead to better social policy than will espousing either extreme. (We will elaborate on this theme in our final recommendation.)

Reaction range for intelligence.   Consonant with our view about taking a moderate position, we recommend rephrasing the "nature–nurture" issue to focus on the *reaction range* for intelligence. Decades of scientific inquiry and debate over whether nature or nurture determines intelligence have gotten us nowhere, so the time has come to rephrase the question. Given that the expression of any trait varies somewhat depending upon the environment the organism experiences, the question of most interest is, How large is this normal variability for any given trait? This question has provided a most productive strategy in the study of physical development. For example, the normal reaction range for adult stature has been found to be at least several inches; for bodily proportion, on the other hand, the reaction range appears to be very small (Tanner, 1978). Thus we may expect malnutrition to affect adult height but to have much less effect on whether, for example, people have relatively long or short legs for their overall height. Given the usefulness of the reaction range concept for physical development, it may well be useful for understanding intellectual development as well.

Stances on the reaction range issue can be divided into three identifiable positions. To one group, the reaction range for intelligence is thought to be very small. Kagan's (1979) recent work is a clear statement of this view. Jensen (1969, 1973, 1979) and Herrnstein (1971) take a related position, arguing that as environmental conditions improve through such means as nutritional and educational interventions, IQ scores increasingly come to reflect their true genetic value. To clarify this argument we will use the analogy of the secular trend for physical stature. Average adult stature has been gradually increasing among Americans; over the past few generations, sons have tended to be taller than their fathers and daughters taller than their mothers. This trend has almost certainly been the result of improved environmental conditions, especially in health care and nutrition (Tanner, 1978). It thus appears that many of our ancestors did not attain the full stature permitted by their genes. It is interesting, however, that this trend seems to have leveled out in the past decade. Apparently we are not destined to keep on growing into a nation of giants. Rather, environmental conditions now seem adequate for most of the population to attain full growth. Under these relatively good conditions, we can infer from a difference in two people's heights that they probably have different genotypes for stature.

What Jensen and Herrnstein have argued is that as environments improve the same thing will be true of intelligence. Whether it is worth intervening to change IQ, therefore, would hinge on whether the environment was considered adequate to permit the full development of a child's native abilities. To return to the example of stature, a special intervention to try to increase the eventual adult height of a healthy, well-fed child would be a waste of time and money. The effective reaction range of the trait, given existing environments, is near zero. The key question, of course, is whether most children with moderately subaverage IQ scores have been deprived of the necessary environmental stimulants. If their environments have been nourishing enough, intervention would be ineffective. This is essentially the modified, low-reaction-range-under-existing-circumstances position.

An opposite view is that intelligence has an almost limitless reaction range. A particularly articulate statement of this position is given by Hunt (1961, 1971). Although this viewpoint appears optimistic, the notion that IQ can be radically modified by such simple procedures as hanging mobiles over cribs is more disturbing than reassuring. If children's intellects were really so malleable, we would have great cause for concern over the many negative occurrences in life that are hard to control, such as illness, separation from parents, or war. For physical development, nature has built in an amazing capacity for "catch-up" growth following periods of stress. One common example occurs when physically small women give birth to infants destined to be physically large adults (Tanner, 1978). Because birth size is largely constrained by uterine size, such fetuses grow more slowly than they are capable of growing during the final trimester of pregnancy. Following birth, however, they exhibit a relatively rapid growth spurt. Similarly, children who experience brief periods of reduced food intake will respond to renewed food availability with very rapid growth. As Tanner commented: "The undernourished child slows down and waits for better times. All young animals have the capacity to do this; in a world where nutrition is never assured, any species unable to regulate its growth in this way would long since have been eliminated" (pp. 128–129). If intellectual growth were as markedly influenced by environmental conditions as is physical development, one would expect some similar catch-up mechanism to exist. Extreme pliability of intellect is presently a minority view.

A middle ground is that the practical reaction range of IQ under present conditions is probably at most 20–25 points (Cronbach, 1971; Zigler, 1970). Such a view is consonant with the results of certain intensive intervention studies in which disadvantaged children have been reared under highly advantageous conditions (Scarr & Weinberg, 1976; Schiff, Duyme, Dumaret, Stewart, Tomkiewicz, & Feingold, 1978) or have received other extensive programs (Garber & Heber, 1977; Skeels, 1966). This position has the advantage of generating energetic willingness to attempt interventions without unrealistic expectations about what they can accomplish.

One might well ask whether it is worth the effort to change IQs by this relatively modest amount. In our opinion, even a 10-point change would be of practical significance. By an increasingly common evaluation yardstick, a change of half a standard deviation in a group's performance is a respectable and useful outcome. Because the standard deviation of existing IQ tests is 15–16 points, a change of 8 points in a group's scores would represent such an accomplishment. Consider a

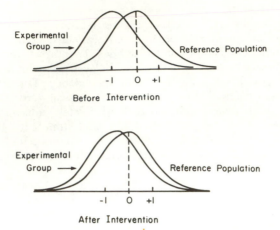

Figure 10.1.   A pictorial representation of the consequences of moderate improvement owing to intervention.

hypothetical case in which, before treatment, a group averages a full standard deviation below the mean of a comparison group, whereas after intervention, the groups differ by only half a standard deviation. As Figure 10.1 shows, the number of people in the intervention group scoring above the comparison group's mean would rise from 16% to 31%, and the overlap between the lower and higher groups would increase from 45% to 67%. This is less exciting stuff than gains of 3–4 standard deviations. Yet it is more significant than some critics seem to recognize (e.g., A. M. Clarke & Clarke, 1976), and it is a reasonable and defensible expectation of what existing preschool interventions can in fact accomplish.

FAMILY SUPPORT SYSTEMS

Our final and perhaps broadest recommendation is a relative newcomer to the social policy scene and therefore may seem less familiar and more controversial than the goals already detailed. However, we intend to argue forcefully that social intervention programs should be designed to be family support systems rather than efforts to aid children alone or to remediate any one problem. To some extent, this principle is based on the medical dictum *primum non nocere* – first do no harm. Where there is doubt about the best solution to the problem of retardation (as there is), we should not prescribe programs that have even the remotest possibility of being harmful. For example, taking children from their families through adoption into higher-income families or placement in intensive preschool education programs has obvious potential to damage family ties. If one must err in one direction rather than the other, we should err in the direction of believing that a supportive family is ultimately more important to a child than having a somewhat higher IQ.

A second rationale for advocating family support systems is that this course of action is consonant with our earlier recommendations. As we will show, family support systems focus on raising social competence, they are necessarily heterogeneous in approach, they allow an emphasis on developmental continuity, and they are based on moderate, defensible expectations.

Perhaps the best model for an effective family support system exists in the Child and Family Resource Programs (CFRPs) that have been experimentally implemented in several locales by the Administration for Children, Youth, and Families (Comptroller General of the United States, 1979). Before describing these CFRPs we will consider a number of specific interventions that have been tried and the evidence concerning their effectiveness. These include nutritional intervention, health-care programs, income maintenance, and intensive pre-school education – all approaches that have shown promise for reducing mental retardation. (We discussed another valuable approach, genetic counseling, earlier.) To anticipate our argument somewhat, we believe that the most effective program will be one that allows flexible choice among alternatives such as these on a family-by-family basis, in a manner that strengthens each family in the areas of its own particular vulnerabilities. If implemented carefully, such an approach can be actually less costly than are the other alternatives, including taking no action at all.

Nutritional programs

Many theorists suspect that the incidence of mental retardation could be reduced by correcting malnutrition among pregnant women and young children. This expectation is partially based on animal studies: Among laboratory animals, severe undernourishment has been shown to cause retardation both in physical growth and in learning ability. Among humans, evidence of a direct link between malnutrition and mental retardation remains inconclusive (Pollitt & Thomson, 1977). The value of nutrition in improving the intellectual adequacy of children is one of those commonsensical notions which is difficult to document with hard facts.

The impact of nutrition intervention is easier to document if we broaden the outcome measures to encompass social competence instead of the single component of intelligence. There is no question that nutritional supplements containing added protein and calories confer health benefits on both pregnant women and their offspring (Habicht, Yarbrough, Lechtig, & Klein, 1974). In the United States, the WIC program enacted in the early 1970s has provided milk, fruit juice, fortified cereals, infant formulas, and other high-quality food to about a million pregnant and nursing mothers and their preschool children each year. Existing evidence suggests that the program has been very effective in improving maternal and infant health and in reducing specific health problems such as iron-deficiency anemia. When the WIC program and similar nutritional therapy efforts in other countries have been made part of a large effort to provide quality prenatal care for poor women, there has been evidence of increased birth weights and decreased infant mortality (U.S. Department of Health, Education, and Welfare, 1975; Winick, 1976).

As Ricciuti (1970, 1981) has cogently argued, societal programs to improve the nutritional status of the poor are significant for humanitarian reasons alone. Attempts to justify such programs by their potential for reducing mental retardation are both misguided and dangerous, in that they may jeopardize the existence of these programs if effects on IQ cannot be documented. But societal policies to provide adequate nutrition can almost certainly improve the everyday functioning of its members – that is, their social competence – whether or not this effect shows up in measured IQ.

Health care

In a more general sense, adequate health care might also reduce the incidence of lowered intellectual functioning in a society. In the mid-1960s a number of Maternal and Infant Care projects were established in areas where infant mortality was especially high. By providing high-quality prenatal care, these programs have effectively reduced both maternal and infant mortality in the poor populations they serve (U.S. Department of Health, Education, and Welfare, 1975). There is good reason to believe that other special programs designed for pregnant teenagers can help reduce the risks of prematurity, low birth weight, and poor health among their infants (Mednick, Baker, & Sutton-Smith, 1979). As with malnutrition, however, the linkage between factors such as prematurity and later intellectual functioning is somewhat unclear. A careful analysis by Sameroff and Chandler (1975) indicated that factors which place a child at risk appear to be particularly harmful when they occur in conjunction with low socioeconomic status. Evidently, if a family can afford to buy adequate services and health care, it can often compensate for conditions, such as prematurity, that place a severe temporary strain on the infant and family. That is, no single negative event in itself tends to be predictive of an inevitably poor future for an infant. Rather, events operate in a probabilistic manner, and the general resource level of a family is an important factor in raising or lowering the probability that a potentially negative event will result in a negative outcome. Paradoxically, as health-care technology improves, we face the danger of creating retardation as a by-product of the ability to preserve the lives of infants born very prematurely. Newborn intensive care often permits premature infants to survive and to lead normal lives. In some cases, however, especially when infants are severely premature and weigh only somewhat more than a pound, medical care may save their lives but at the cost of their general health, hearing, eyesight, and intellect. Concern is rising over the ethical issues involved in choosing to direct the full arsenal of medical techniques toward keeping alive infants born very prematurely. Social policies related to this issue will definitely have a bearing upon the incidence of mental retardation in the society. In short, health-care programs may have a significant impact on functional intelligence in both positive and negative ways.

Educational intervention

Several comprehensive reviews of the many educational intervention programs have been written (e.g., Bronfenbrenner, 1975; A. M. Clarke & Clarke, 1976; Golden & Birns, 1976; Gordon, 1975; Palmer & Anderson, 1979). For our purposes, we have selected only a few programs to discuss specifically in terms of social policy implications. On the basis of sheer numbers, Head Start is by far the largest preschool intervention program. However, its very size and diversity have made it difficult to evaluate. Each Head Start center is mandated to respond to the needs of the community it serves, so the programs offered can vary as widely as do neighborhoods. In addition, as might be expected from a project that has so many outlets, there is considerable variability in implementation of programs. Some centers are well-run and deliver all the mandated services, but this is not true of all of them. As Huston-Stein and her colleagues (1977) have shown, even within a single city there may be substantial differences in Head Start centers.

Despite the variability, some overall effects of Head Start are discernible. The consequences for children's health have been demonstrably positive (Kirschner Associates, 1970; North, 1979). Physical problems have been diagnosed in approximately one-third of the children attending Head Start, and about 75% of these cases have been treated. Although the fact is not widely recognized, Head Start is one of our nation's largest deliverers of health services to poor children. Another outcome of the Head Start program has been career development for poor adults. Well over 10,000 unemployed or underemployed persons have been placed in college programs to prepare for professional roles in child care. This accomplishment is especially significant in view of the pressing need for high-quality child-care services as maternal employment in our nation increases.

More generally, Head Start has been a successful experimental program that demonstrates how society can tackle the problems of its citizens. To quote briefly from Donald Campbell (1969):

The United States and other modern nations should be ready for an experimental approach to social reform, an approach in which we try out new programs designed to cure specific social problems, in which we learn whether or not these programs are effective, and in which we retain, imitate, modify, or discard them on the basis of apparent effectiveness on the multiple imperfect criteria available. [P. 409]

In our opinion, Head Start has been a model of the way Campbell feels society should proceed. It has given rise to numerous refinements, including all of the following: (a) Parent and Child Centers; (b) Parent and Child Advocacy Centers; (c) Follow Through Programs; (d) Planned Variation Programs; (e) Head Start handicapped children's efforts; (f) Health Start; (g) Home Start; (h) Head Start Improvement and Innovation Efforts; (i) Head Start Developmental Continuity Efforts; (j) CFRPs; (k) Child Development Associate Programs; (l) Education for Parenthood Programs. We do not have space to comment on all these programs here, but we will discuss one – the CFRPs – later.

Though there is little question that Head Start has had positive effects on the health and social resources of poor American families, there are heated disagreements over whether it has had a significant impact on children's IQ scores. A fairly common finding is that IQ-test performance increases an average of about 10 points following Head Start. As we discussed earlier, there is reason to interpret such gains as reflecting motivational effects rather than true cognitive improvement. IQ gains of such magnitude are also not specifically associated with Head Start; they commonly are found when disadvantaged children attend any high-quality preschool program (Bronfenbrenner, 1975; Ryan, 1974).

The permanence of these IQ gains has been a controversial topic (Bronfenbrenner, 1975; Cicirelli, 1969; A. M. Clarke & Clarke, 1976). The most common position is that the advantage of Head Start children over non–Head Start children fades out by second or third grade. This finding was first reported in a study by the Westinghouse Learning Corporation in conjunction with researchers at Ohio University (see Cicirelli, 1969) and has somehow come to represent conventional wisdom on the issue.

In the Westinghouse–Ohio University study, first-, second-, and third-grade children who had attended Head Start programs were compared with carefully matched classmates from similar backgrounds who had not attended Head Start. Among the younger children, Head Start graduates tended to have higher IQ scores than did their non-Head Start peers. Among the older children, Head Start graduates were not superior to the matched comparison group.

There were numerous methodological problems in this study (see M. Smith & Bissell, 1970; S. White, 1970). No information was available concerning possible selection biases, and the matching procedures employed to choose control groups may have led to regression artifacts in a direction that would underestimate the true effects of Head Start programs (see Campbell & Erlebacher, 1970). Further, because the study was cross-sectional, and because it was performed soon after Head Start was mounted, the children who were evaluated probably had received quite different program experiences. Yet the study collapsed good, bad, and indifferent Head Start programs together as if all children who had attended "Head Start" had received one single, uniform kind of experience.

The meaning of fade-out. Despite these flaws, the Westinghouse study had immediate impact upon Washington decision makers and almost resulted in the early dismantling of the Head Start program. Even among scientists, who presumably should be well able to discern problems in research design, the Westinghouse study has left a legacy of general pessimism regarding long-term effects. First impressions do last the longest, and the concept of fade-out has evidently been too easily remembered and too compelling a notion to have received the full criticism it deserves. We therefore choose to criticize it here.

To begin with, there is one possible artifactual basis for fade-out that has not been widely appreciated. Most simply put, the average 8-year-old knows much more in absolute terms than does an average 4-year-old. Therefore, there is less difference in absolute knowledge between a 4-year-old who is slightly below average and one who is average than there is with a similar pair of 8-year-olds. For this reason it is probably relatively easier to raise a 4-year-old's than an 8-year-old's store of information to the average level. A large-scale example of such artifactual fade-out can be found in the normative tables for the 1972 revision of the Stanford–Binet test. Table 10.1 shows the average IQ, based on the 1930 norms, of children who were tested in the 1972 standardization. Relative to preschoolers half a century ago, preschoolers today appear to be much brighter. Children in the middle school years, however, are approximately comparable to their age-mates of the 1930s. Terman and Merrill (1973) interpreted the difference as a real one and attempted to explain it as follows:

In the 1930's, radio was new and relatively limited in its impact on small children, whereas in the 1970's television is omnipresent and viewed for hours each day by the typical preschooler. The impact of television and radio, the increase in literacy and education of parents, and the many other cultural changes of almost 40 years would appear to have had their most impressive impact on the preschool group. [P. 360]

The test constructors also interpreted the higher scores of present-day adolescents as the result of increased education, as teenagers typically remain in school longer today than they did in the 1930s.

Viewing Table 10.1, one might be tempted to label the great changes in Ameri-

Table 10.1. *1972 Stanford–Binet IQ-test performance relative to 1930 norms*

Age (years–months)	Mean	SD
2–0	110.4	15.7
2–6	110.6	15.9
3–0	110.7	16.0
3–6	110.8	16.1
4–0	110.7	16.2
4–6	110.4	16.3
5–0	109.7	16.4
5–6	108.4	16.6
6–0	107.1	16.7
7–0	105.0	17.0
8–0	103.3	17.2
9–0	102.1	17.2
10–0	101.9	16.9
11–0	102.2	16.6
12–0	102.5	16.4
13–0	102.9	16.5
14–0	103.3	16.8
15–0	103.9	17.2
16–0	104.7	17.6
17–0	105.7	17.9
18–0	106.9	18.0

Source: Terman & Merrill (1973).

can society from the 1930s to the 1970s as a massive cultural intervention for preschoolers that has resulted in impressive gains. After several years in school, however, these gains have faded away with numbers reminiscent of the results of studies of special intervention programs.

We do not mean to suggest that all fade-out is artifactual. Sometimes there may be a genuine difference between an intervention and a control group that exists at one point in time but disappears later. We discussed in an earlier section one example of boys whose early advantage in mathematics achievement dissipated in their high-school years. As we noted earlier, this loss was most likely due to the children's failing to receive the appropriate instruction in school; there was probably no true loss of ability. This interpretation may be confirmed by examining the scores of these same groups of boys on the general information subtest of a nationally standardized exam. Much like the information portion of the Wechsler IQ test, this subtest gauges knowledge of everyday facts. At the end of the intervention, the scores of the experimental-group boys were at the national average, whereas the control boys scored 4 months lower. Seven years later the intervention graduates were still scoring close to national norms, whereas the controls were scoring 3 years lower.

This pattern of results is important, because one implication of the fade-out hypothesis – especially when gauged by IQ-test performance – is that a decrease in scores over time represents a generalized loss of cognitive abilities. That is, it is usually assumed that all gains from intervention eventually disappear. What a careful longitudinal study showed, however, was a mixed picture: fade-out in one

Table 10.2. *Mathematics and general information test performance of intervention- and control-group girls*

	Intervention group (N = 10)			Control group (N = 18)		
Grade[a]	Mean raw score deviation[b]	SD	Grade equiv.[b]	Mean raw score deviation[b]	SD	Grade equiv.[b]
Mathematics						
3rd	−3.6	8.3	3–3	−9.2	7.2	2–9
4th	−0.7	6.4	4–6	−5.9	7.4	3–7
5th	+0.5	8.2	5–9	−4.0	5.8	4–9
7th	+1.9	7.5	8–4	−3.3	7.6	7–0
9th	−1.3	9.6	9–6	−10.2	7.2	6–7
General information						
3rd	−1.4	6.6	3–7	−7.6	6.2	2–9
4th	−2.9	6.9	4–6	−12.3	10.8	3–9
5th	−3.6	7.3	5–0	−16.2	12.7	4–0
7th	−3.8	8.3	6–8	−11.8	14.0	5–0
9th	−2.9	7.2	8–4	−14.1	15.1	5–6

[a]All tests were administered near the end of the school year.
[b]Analyses were performed on raw score differences between the child's actual performance and the performance expected for the child's age. The approximate grade equivalents are provided for ease of interpretation. The figure after the dash is the month of the school year; e.g., 5–0 is September of the fifth-grade year.
Source: Seitz, Apfel, & Rosenbaum (1981, p. 24).

area, continued maintenance of advantage in another, and evidence that the intervention was ineffective in two others. In the latter case, the two groups performed relatively poorly on reading and spelling achievement and did not significantly differ from each other at any time. (Thus the intervention boys were not simply a group of high achievers in general.) The issue of fade-out is obviously too simplistic to do credit to the true range of intervention effects.

A replication and extension of these results can be seen in the performance of a group of girls who later received the intervention (Seitz et al., 1981). Again the effects of the program were limited to mathematics and general information. Table 10.2 presents test results at the end of the intervention and for 6 years afterwards. As can be seen, there was considerable fluctuation in the control group's performance, so that any one time the difference between groups might or might not appear significant. This sort of borderline significance also contributes to reports of fade-out (e.g., note that differences in mathematics were insignificant in seventh grade but were again significant by ninth grade). Yet overall, the intervention girls were clearly superior in the two areas shown, averaging about 3 years ahead of control girls at the final testing.

Fortunately, several other evaluations of preschool intervention programs have been continued, and longitudinal results are now appearing to supplement initial reports. For example, data have become available regarding the long-term effects of 14 different preschool intervention programs involving a total of over 1,000 children. (For summaries, see Darlington et al., 1980; Lazar, Royce, Murray, Snipper, & Darlington, in press. For individual projects see Beller, 1973; Deutsch, Taleporos, & Victor, 1974; Gordon, 1973; Gordon, Guinagh, & Jester, 1977; Gray

& Klaus, 1970; Karnes et al., 1970; Karnes, Zehrback, & Teska, 1977; Levenstein, 1977; Madden, Levenstein, & Levenstein, 1976; Miller & Dyer, 1975; Palmer & Semlear, 1976; Palmer & Siegel, 1977; Seitz et al., 1981; Weikart, Delona, Lawser, & Wiegerink, 1970; Woolman, 1971.) Although there was no overall increase in IQs as a function of early intervention, the investigators discovered a significant difference in school performance. By late adolescence, children who had received early intervention were more likely to be in the school grade appropriate for their age; control children, on the other hand, were more likely to have been placed in special-education classes or to have repeated one or more grades. Thus, despite the absence of IQ effects, there were indications of increased overall competence as a function of early intervention.

Later intervention. Later educational intervention may also have beneficial practical consequences. This type of intervention need not be some special experimental program but can occur in the regular school milieu. For example, in an investigation in England, Michael Rutter and his colleagues (Rutter, Maughan, Martimore, & Ouston, 1979) examined the effects of different high schools on adolescents' social behavior and academic achievement. Contrary to the earlier pessimistic conclusions of the Coleman report (Coleman et al., 1966) and of the study by Jencks and his associates (1972), Rutter and his colleagues found that schools have substantial measurable effects. Even with the nature of the student population equated, different high schools had markedly different average scholastic achievement levels, truancy rates, and incidences of antisocial behavior such as vandalism and personal violence. (These results are consistent with Weber's [1973] report, discussed earlier, in which he countered the stereotype of the urban ghetto elementary school by finding several that were most effective in terms of their students' achievements.) The earlier belief that schools make little difference once family status has been taken into account appears to have resulted from considering the wrong kinds of data, such as performance on standardized tests only distantly related to the materials actually being taught in the schools under evaluation (Rutter et al., 1979). By concentrating on IQ scores and grade-level norms, we have overlooked the neighborhood schools' potential for affecting the social competence of their students. As James Comer (in press) argued persuasively, we now know a great deal about improving the general effectiveness of schools, even in impoverished neighborhoods. It is potentially very cost effective to do so.

Milwaukee Project. Several educational interventions seem relatively radical, in the sense that parents are replaced for most or all of the child's day from a very early age. One such intervention is the Milwaukee Project (see Garber, 1975; Garber & Heber, 1977; Heber & Garber, 1975), which involved 20 children whose families resided in one of the poorest sections of the inner city and whose mothers scored lower than 80 on a standardized IQ test. Twenty similar children were randomly assigned to a control condition in which no services were provided. Both groups of children were black. The intervention consisted of a 7-hour-per-day program given 5 days a week from the time the children were approximately 3 months old until they entered first grade. For the first few months of the program each infant was cared for by a "substitute mother," who dressed, fed, played with, and stimulated her charge. Gradually, infants were phased into small-group care, and by late preschool they were receiving special educational enrichment in groups of four to five. Medical care and good nutrition were provided for the children; their mothers also received a special educational program including vocational training and information about homemaking and parenting skills.

Both experimental- and control-group children were tested frequently and on a comparable time schedule. For the first year the two groups performed equivalently on the Gesell test; at about 18 months of age, the control group's performance began to decline. By age 4½, the difference in mean IQs was dramatic, with experimental-group children averaging approximately 120 and controls approximately 95. Both groups have shown declines since then, but a mean difference of over 20 points has remained. By age 8–9, the average IQ was about 104 in the experimental group and only about 80 in the control group. There was also substantial difference in academic achievement, with the experimental group's performance superior to that of the controls.

Concern has been expressed about whether the two groups of children were originally equivalent, and the program has been criticized for vagueness in descriptions of the actual everyday procedures. The results of this intervention, however, taken in conjunction with those of the other studies we will discuss, make it seem probable that extensive early intervention of the kind provided by the Milwaukee Project can in fact enable at-risk, disadvantaged children to succeed in performing at national norms on achievement and IQ tests. Yet there are many reasons to question whether such an intrusive, expensive program is either necessary or wise. We will return to this point after considering results from several other intervention efforts.

Abecedarian Project.   A program with many similarities to the Milwaukee Project is the Abecedarian Project being conducted in North Carolina by researchers at the Frank Porter Graham Child Development Center (see Finkelstein, Dent, Gallagher, & Ramey, 1978; Ramey et al., 1976; Ramey & Haskins, 1981). This study was begun in 1972 by identifying women in their last trimester of pregnancy whose expected children were likely to be at high risk of eventual school failure. The risk index was based on information on maternal IQ, family income, parental education, intactness of family, and other variables known to be correlated with children's school performance. Between 1972 and 1977, 121 families were admitted to the project; 64 of the families were randomly assigned to the experimental condition, and the remaining 57 (assigned evenly across time) formed the control group. The mothers in each group had an average IQ of approximately 84 and had received about 10 years of education. The average annual family income was about $1,100, and in approximately 80% of the cases the mother was the head of the family.

The experimental program provided day care in conjunction with a specialized educational curriculum, pediatric care, iron-fortified formula during the infancy period, and some family support services if the family requested them. (The control program was similar except that the children did not receive the day care and educational curriculum.) The day care was much like that in the Milwaukee Project, except that during infancy the teacher–infant ratio was 1:3 instead of 1:1. The children attended day care for 6 or more hours a day, 5 days a week, until they were of school age. The curriculum was designed to teach concepts and learning styles that would later facilitate their school performance (Sparling, 1975; Sparling & Lewis, 1978). In addition to the formal curriculum, routines were established to permit using everyday activities as educational opportunities. Setting the table, for example, became an occasion for children to practice counting places and napkins, and children were encouraged to name the shapes and colors of objects while playing with them. There was also daily language stimulation through questioning and discussion of play activities.

The effects of the preschool intervention have been evaluated on many measures, and we have room to summarize only a few of the results. During the first year, the experimental- and control-group children performed comparably on the Bayley test, with average development quotients (DQs) of about 105. From 18 months through the final preschool testing at 48 months, experimental-group children scored significantly higher than did the controls, both on the Bayley test and subsequently on the Stanford–Binet. By 4 years of age, the experimental group's mean Stanford–Binet IQ was 96, compared to 84 in the control group. As Ramey and Haskins (in press) noted, "Children who attended our preschool program enter the public schools with nearly normal IQ, and with about a 12-point IQ advantage over their peers from similar high-risk families."

The amount of stimulation provided by the children's home environments was also evaluated. The measure employed (Caldwell, Heider, & Kaplan, 1966) assesses the degree to which a child's mother is involved with, stimulates, and responds sensitively to the child, and also the extent to which educational and play materials suitable for the child's age are available in the home. The Abecedarian researchers administered this scale several times but found no significant differences between experimental and control groups at any age. On experimental measures of mother–child interaction in the laboratory, however, intervention-group mothers and children both were found to initiate more mutual play episodes than did control-group families. Experimental-group children also asked for and obtained their mothers' attention more often, as in asking their mothers to watch them build block towers or color pictures.

In school, the intervention-group children were rated by their teachers as more intelligent than the control children. They were also rated as being more aggressive. Observations of the children's behavior during school recess periods were consistent with their teachers' reports: The preschool intervention children were observed to emit nine times as many aggressive acts as either the control group or a sample of nondisadvantaged classmates. Observations outside school, in the children's neighborhoods, did not confirm the picture of general aggressiveness. Thus the response seemed to be school-specific.

Despite their nearly normal IQ scores, nearly all the intervention-group children were assigned to the lowest academic group in their classrooms, as were all of the control-group children. Although there are as yet relatively few graduates of the preschool program whose performance in school has been evaluated, their achievement does not appear especially promising. (A few of the children have received school-aged intervention, but the number is too small for us to comment on the results.) Because these children attend school with economically advantaged classmates, the researchers speculated that "the academic grouping practices of the public schools seem to pose a threat to any advantage enjoyed by children who attended the preschool program" (Ramey & Haskins, 1981, p. 108). In this, as in many other studies, we see that a higher IQ score has no necessary relation to a disadvantaged child's performance in school.

Adoption studies. Certain types of adoption can be conceptualized as an even more intensive preschool intervention than were the Milwaukee and Abecedarian projects. For example, Scarr and Weinberg (1976) studied 130 black children who were raised in white, middle-class homes. By late preschool and early school age, the mean IQ of these children was 106.3, and available school achievement data indicated that their performance was above average in reading, mathematics, and vocabulary. A comparison with white children adopted into some of the same families showed that they too were somewhat above average in IQ and school achievement.

Although there was no formal control group in this study, an implicit control value is provided by IQ data obtained in other investigations of lower-socioeconomic-status children. In numerous studies, the mean IQ of disadvantaged black children is below 100, often by a full standard deviation. Unless some marked bias in selective placement by adoption agencies was operative, the Scarr and Weinberg data suggest that being raised by white, middle-class families has approximately the same effect on disadvantaged black children's IQ-test performance as does attending years of an intensive preschool education program.

Another adoption study conducted in France by Schiff and his colleagues (1978) also suggests a marked effect on IQ and achievement when disadvantaged children are reared in economically advantaged homes. The investigators located 32 children of working-class parents who had been placed in high-SES homes before they were 6 months old; in 28 cases, the child had a full or half sibling who had not been placed for adoption. By the school years the mean IQ of the children who had been reared in upper-class homes was 111.5, whereas the mean IQ of the siblings raised by their biological mothers was 94.8. There were also marked school achievement differences: Of the 28 "control" children, 7 had been placed in special-education classes, compared to only 1 of the adopted children.

Studies such as these have significant theoretical implications for our knowledge concerning the reaction range of IQ. One policy implication of such studies is that our society could in fact substantially raise the IQ and school achievement performance of disadvantaged children by suitable interventions. That is, intervention in principle is not a mistaken policy. However, the specific form that intervention should take is not so clearly indicated by the studies we have discussed. Obviously, few people would believe it is ever in a child's best interests to be raised by adoptive parents simply because his or her biological parents are poor. But we must question whether effective intervention need be as expensive as was the Milwaukee Project, and whether the benefits might be obtained just as readily if the money is spent directly on improving the poor family's standard of living rather than indirectly on educational programs.

Yale Project. It is reassuring, therefore, to discover other interventions that seem to have produced substantial gains without removing children from their families or subjecting them to unnatural years of preschool education. One such effort was the Yale Project, conducted by staff at the Yale University Child Study Center (Provence, Naylor, & Patterson, 1977). The experimental sample consisted of 20 children from 19 low-income families residing in a disadvantaged inner-city neighborhood. Most of the children were black. The families were recruited from participants in the Women's Clinic of the Yale–New Haven Medical Center. Over several months all women who attended this clinic were interviewed and accepted into the project if (a) the pregnancy would result in their first-born child; (b) there were no complications of pregnancy, and the infant was expected to be full-term and healthy; (c) they resided in the inner city and had family incomes below the poverty level; (d) they were not markedly retarded or psychotic; (e) they were not planning to move from New Haven in the foreseeable future; and (f) they were willing to receive the project's services in return for promising to bring their infants to a nearby center for regular testing and to permit frequent home assessments and interviews by project staff.

Intervention began prenatally with physical care and nutritional supplements for the mother. Following the child's birth, medical and other services were provided for the entire family. Day care was given at the Yale Child Development Unit for approximately half the children as the families desired or the staff deemed necessary (as for one child who was physically abused). Mothers received nutritional advice, and staff social workers assisted many of them in obtaining job training, additional education, and/or better housing. The program thus entailed a variety of services delivered by trained professionals on the basis of each family's needs or desires. The intervention effort involving the services of physicians, social workers, and day-care supervisors continued until the children were 2½ years old. Approximately half of the children later attended Head Start or other early childhood programs.

There were a few changes in the initial sample, so initial evaluations of the project were based on 18 children from 17 families. Children were given regular diagnostic testing for both physical and psychological functioning. To assess the effects of the program at its end, a control group of 18 children – very carefully matched with the experimental sample on even such factors as parental education and events of birth – was located and tested. At 30 months, the two groups did not differ significantly in their overall scores on the Yale Developmental Schedule, but the experimental group scored significantly higher on the language subtest (Provence et al., 1977).

Five years later, follow-up testing was conducted for 17 of the 18 experimental-group children (see Rescorla, Provence, & Naylor, 1979; Trickett, Apfel, Rosenbaum, & Zigler, 1979). Sixty-four comparison children of the same age were also tested. Half of these children were from the inner-city neighborhood in which the experimental group had originally resided. The remaining half were from a lower-middle-class, predominantly black neighborhood to which many of the original families had moved. All of the comparison children were black and English-speaking.

The children were tested on intelligence and academic achievement scales, and on a number of motivational measures. Mothers of the experimental-group children and of a sample of the comparison children were also interviewed. Information about school functioning was collected, including data on academic grades, grade placement, and attendance. Results showed that the experimental-group children achieved significantly higher Peabody Picture Vocabulary Test IQs ($\bar{X}$ = 104) than did comparison children from either the better ($\bar{X}$ = 92) or original ($\bar{X}$ = 75) neighborhood control groups. Their Wechsler Intelligence Scale for Children IQs were lower ($\bar{X}$ = 92), but there was no control-group comparison for this score. The experimental-group children scored at grade level compared with national norms on the school achievement test; this score was higher than that achieved in either control group, but the difference was significant only in comparison with the original neighborhood children, who were approximately half a year below national norms. School attendance for the intervention group was excellent, averaging only 5 days absence per year compared with means of 10 and 25 days absence in the other two groups.

The most important finding was evidence of an improved quality of life for the experimental-group families. Fourteen of the 17 families studied had shown improvement in such areas as housing, medical care, socioeconomic status, educational or training status, social life, and engagement in community life. For example, family income had increased, and many families were able to relocate in a better neighborhood. Subsequent fertility was amazingly low. One-third of mothers had had no additional children, and another one-third had two-child families at the follow-up. This was markedly different from the fertility of the comparison samples.

Though the criteria for participation might suggest that the mothers were a select group of highly motivated individuals, there are indications that this was not the case. As described in the book by Provence and her associates, at least one of the mothers physically abused her infant. (For this family the project served – apparently successfully – as a crisis intervention center.) Other mothers had lengthy periods of depression, and/or were obese and required nutritional education, and/or required substantial assistance to find more adequate living quarters. In short, the case records give the impression of a fairly typical group of mothers for the area, although they were obviously not the most severely deprived women in their inner-city neighborhood. Most of the mothers were high-school graduates, they were in sufficiently good health to deliver healthy babies, and they were sufficiently well informed to attend the local hospital maternity clinic.

One could wish that the psychiatric team which mounted this high-quality intervention had also recruited a comparable control sample, but for both ethical and practical reasons this was insurmountably difficult to do. Despite the absence of an original control group, the 30-month controls were very carefully matched and probably provided a conservative estimate of the project's actual effects (Campbell & Erlebacher, 1970). The randomly selected 7-year-olds from a neighborhood not in the inner city also provided a conservative control, yet the experimental group exceeded their scores on several measures. In comparison with the nonconservative control group of children from their original neighborhood, the intervention-group children were strikingly superior in every cognitive measure.

The Yale Project differed in at least three significant ways from the Abecedarian and the Milwaukee projects: The active intervention began earlier (during pregnancy), it ended earlier (at age 2½), and it did not involve any specific educational curriculum. It is therefore of interest to compare the long-term gains from the Yale Project with the results from the other projects. Although the children's WISC IQs were not as high as those of children in the other projects, their vocabulary as assessed by the PPVT IQ, their school achievement and attendance, and their families' quality of life appear to have been very positively affected.

There is no airtight case to be made in summarizing results of educational intervention studies. Any single study has flaws that would permit a skeptic to discount the results. But there is a plausibility argument when the results of the intervention studies are considered together. Some of the possible errors tend to cancel each other. For example, in the Garber and Heber (1977) study, maternal IQs were 80 or below. In the Scarr and Weinberg (1976) study, parental IQs were probably substantially higher. The comparability of the IQs of the children in the two studies is therefore provocative. Although no intervention has turned groups of children into geniuses, several seem to have placed disadvantaged children's IQ scores in the normal range and to have improved their expected school performance. More important, multifaceted programs offered for extended periods seem capable of improving the overall quality of life for disadvantaged children and their families.

Income maintenance

A central conclusion of the Carnegie Council's Report on Children (Keniston, 1977) was that the most effective means of permanently reducing poverty and its sequelae would be to provide families with adequate incomes, rather than to offer them specific services such as Medicare, Head Start, or WIC. The theoretical implications of the money-versus-services debate for policy on intelligence are significant, but empirical evidence is almost nonexistent. There have been few social experiments on income maintenance, and the results usually have been reported in terms of sociological and economic variables rather than of psychological impact. For example, in the New Jersey Negative Income Tax Experiment (Kershaw, 1972; Pechman & Timpane, 1975; Watts & Rees, 1973), an important finding was that guaranteed family income did not have a negative effect on work incentive. There was no tendency for male heads of household to stop working in favor of living on the experimental payments. It would be interesting to know the long-term effects of income maintenance and, particularly, whether having a middle-class standard of living would lead children to perform in school more as their middle-class peers do. This appealing possibility has not yet been adequately assessed.

A study that comes somewhat closer to answering this question is a rural income-maintenance experiment involving about 800 families in North Carolina and Iowa (U.S. Department of Health, Education, and Welfare, 1976). The investigators – at the Institute for Research on Poverty at the University of Wisconsin – employed a broad variety of outcome measures, including information on housing, consumer purchases, health care, psychological well-being, and school performance. Although the families were studied for only 3 years, a number of significant differences were found between experimental and control groups. For example, family nutrition improved noticeably, as did the school performance of both black and white children in the experimental-group families. These families also were more likely to buy their own homes and – as in the New Jersey experiment – the fathers did not quit their jobs. Gallagher and his associates (in press) concluded:

There is at least a suggestion in these findings that the primary need of poor people is money. . . . When given the chance – which is to say when given adequate resources – the poor tend to behave much like middle-income people: they continue to work, they want to buy a house, they buy better food for their families, and perhaps they even encourage school achievement by their children.

The money-versus-services debate is far from over. There is no airtight proof that guaranteed income can eradicate the many negative events, such as juvenile delinquency, malnutrition, poor health, low achievement, and low measured intelligence, that are significantly correlated with poverty. We should now recognize the dangers of claiming too much on the basis of too little data in advocating particular social changes. Guaranteed income alone is probably no more a panacea than early childhood educational intervention has proved to be. We should also recognize that it is politically easier to support programs such as Medicare, food stamps, and housing allowances, which direct the way money is to be spent, than to advocate direct payment of moneys – however strong the evidence that the poor use those moneys for their children's shoes and lunches, and not for televisions and luxury cars. But, like the encouraging findings from nutritional and health-care programs, the results of the income-maintenance experiments do point favorably in the direction of a policy of family support rather than family replacement strategies.

Child and Family Resource Programs

The wave of the future may well be a variety of available services among which families can choose according to their actual needs. A model of this approach is the Child and Family Resource Program – CFRP for short – which has been experimentally implemented in 11 locales across the United States. The accomplishments of these centers have pleased government accountants – a group notoriously hardheaded when it comes to accountability (Comptroller General, 1979). We must emphasize that we do not wish to imply that CFRPs are the only form family support services could or should take. But we describe them in some detail to make the case that our recommendation of family support services is both feasible and economical, and that this approach can capitalize upon the strengths of the other forms of intervention already discussed.

CFRPs are centers designed to offer a variety of services tailored to the unique developmental needs of children in each enrolled family. The services are provided from the prenatal period through the time the child is 8 years old. The backbone of the program is several home visitors or "family advocates," who work to establish a close, trusting relationship with each family and to serve as resource persons who can advise families of services available both from the CFRP and from the larger community. As noted in the comptroller general's report (1979): "A problem that many families have is that they are either unaware of or unable to obtain access to existing community services. CFRP serves as a focal point for families who need assistance in effectively obtaining services and benefits for which they are eligible" (p. 55).

The services provided directly by CFRP, listed in Table 10.3, are thus designed to supplement rather than replace existing community resources. Many of these services are based on the premise that children's development cannot be optimal in the presence of serious unresolved family problems. Difficulties such as alcoholism, severe marital discord, unemployment, and substandard housing can easily cancel any positive effects of efforts to benefit the children. CFRPs therefore attempt to assist children in the context of their families.

The early education component of CFRP also builds on existing resources as much as possible. Infant programs are conducted at the children's homes and/or at CFRP centers, depending upon the preferences of the parents and staff. Head Start programs are part of the services for 3- to 5-year-olds. School linkage is provided in different ways in different CFRP programs, but always involves a staff

Table 10.3. *List of CFRP services to families*

Family services	Early childhood education services	Parent-involvement services	Health and nutrition services
Crisis intervention Referrals to community agencies Direct family counseling and assistance	Infant-toddler (ages 0–3) home-based–center-based combination Head Start (ages 3–5) School linkage (ages 5–8) Tutoring	Parent policy council Parent participation in the early childhood education component Parent education in a wide variety of subjects Social activities designed to promote family togetherness	Prenatal counseling and services Postnatal counseling and services Early and periodic screening, referral, and follow-up for all health needs of young children Meals for children

person who seeks to maximize parental involvement in the child's academic development. One example of school-linkage activities is CFRP-sponsored meetings in which school personnel, Head Start teachers, and parents share information and increase their awareness of one another's interests. For a more specific example, a Gering, Nebraska, school presented a slide show on a new reading series, and CFRP staff presented a session describing the CFRP. About 300 *parents* attended. Another form of involvement is exemplified by a school-linkage coordinator in Bismark, North Dakota, who sent a questionnaire to first-grade teachers with CFRP children in their classrooms. The information obtained helped the CFRP staff determine which children needed tutoring or other forms of assistance to resolve early school-adjustment problems. Given Rist's (1970) documentation of how the child's first few months in school can establish a negative pattern that persists for years, the attempt of CFRP to ease the transition of at-risk children into the public schools and to increase parents' interest and involvement in their education has good theoretical rationale.

The parent-involvement component of CFRP both involves parents as fully as possible in all decisions that affect their children and also provides certain services designed for the parents themselves. Specifically, CFRPs offer courses on parenting, early childhood education, use of community resources, sewing, cooking, nutrition, and exercise. Parents are encouraged to continue their formal education, and many have been motivated to complete high-school equivalency programs and/or to enroll in local community colleges. Most CFRPs also provide classes in the prevention, treatment, and identification of child abuse and neglect. Finally, CFRPs schedule social activities for their community of families, including parties, picnics, and outings to popular attractions.

The fourth component, health care and nutrition, is provided from the prenatal period onward. The services include medical and dental screening and free immunizations against a number of diseases. CFRP also provides free transportation to families who cannot get to their appointments. Home visitors help coordinate the needed health services.

The approximate annual cost per family has been estimated at $1,900 for the CFRPs directly and $1,150 in costs incurred by outside agencies that provide services to families referred by the program. The total cost (in 1979 dollars) is therefore approximately $3,000 per family per year. The documented benefits of the program include better preventive health care and nutrition for young children, rapid assistance to families during crises, correction of problems such as inadequate housing through appropriate referrals to existing agencies, and a general improvement in overall quality of life (Comptroller General, 1979). The CFRPs have not been evaluated for effects on children's IQ scores and school performance, or on parent's education and involvement in the larger community, but positive results would likely be found if such factors were examined. Despite these gaps in evaluation, CFRPs look most promising against the backdrop of studies of other intervention programs. The Yale Project, in particular, was essentially a short-term CFRP that resulted in children's surpassing their expected school achievement, in improved family living conditions, and in apparently decreased fertility.

The relative nonintrusiveness of CFRPs is a factor that recommends them over other types of program. Some forms of intervention, for example, apply a standard treatment to children without regard to parental input or desires. Yet parental involvement in intervention is probably a critical factor in determining its success (Bronfenbrenner, 1975). Another plus is the tailor-made nature of the programs, which common sense tells us is a better way to solve individual problems than is administering some fixed form of intervention to all families simply because they are broadly defined as being at risk. It is also in favor of CFRPs that their multi-faceted nature and long-term commitment are desiderata that most successful intervention programs have satisfied. Last but hardly least is the fact that parents like CFRPs. Parental interviews have revealed considerable enthusiasm for the CFRPs and their effects on the families' lives and the children's development.

10.3.   CONCLUSIONS

It may seem undramatic to end a discussion of social policy implications of research on intelligence with a recommendation of family support programs. It would certainly be more eye-catching to point to new cures for retardation or training procedures that create geniuses. But as we have argued in this chapter, our knowledge base generally does not support expectations that changes in societal practices will effect drastic changes in intelligence. Even in those cases where knowledge is secure (e.g., genetic counseling and amniocentesis to reduce the incidence of severe retardation), there are complex human and financial considerations to be weighed.

Despite these difficulties, psychological research on intelligence does have social policy implications, and we as members of the society have a responsibility to make the most we can of existing knowledge. As we have shown, there is good reason to believe that several kinds of intervention can raise functional levels of intelligence for persons whose measured IQ is commonly low. There is further evidence that a thoughtful coordination of these various interventions could help many children and their families to adapt better to society and to achieve a better quality of daily existence. In our opinion, this level of knowledge is definitely significant. Considerable research has been expended to show that we need not penalize people for being poor by raising their children for them, by abandoning them with the assumption of their probable inherent inferiority, or by recommending an identical regimen for all to improve their children's collective intellectual performance. In its own way, this is a very meaningful result of psychology's extensive research on intelligence.

REFERENCES

Achenbach, T., & Weisz, J. R. A longitudinal study of relations between outer-directedness and IQ changes in preschoolers. *Child Development*, 1975, *46*, 650–657.

Ainsworth, M. D. S., Blehar, M. C., Waters, E., & Wall, S. *Patterns of attachment: A psychological study of the strange situation*. Hillsdale, N.J.: Erlbaum, 1978.

American Association on Mental Deficiency. *Manual on terminology and classification in mental retardation*. Washington, D.C.: Author, 1977.

American Psychiatric Association, Committee on Nomenclature and Statistics. *Diagnostic and statistical manual of mental disorders* (2nd ed.) (DSM-11). Washington, D.C.: Author, 1968.

Anderson, S., & Messick, S. Social competency in young children. *Developmental Psychology*, 1974, *10*, 282–293.

Armor, D. J. School and family effects on black and white achievement. In F. Mosteller & D. P. Moynihan (Eds.), *On equality of educational opportunity*. New York: Random House, 1972. (a)

Armor, D. J. The evidence on busing. *Public Interest*, 1972 (Serial No. 28), 90–126. (b)

Balla, D. Relationship between institution size and quality of care: A review of the literature. *American Journal of Mental Deficiency*, 1976, *81*, 117–124.

Balla, D., Butterfield, E. C., & Zigler, E. Effects of institutionalization on retarded children. *American Journal of Mental Deficiency*, 1974, *78*, 530–549.

Balla, D., & Zigler, E. Cue-learning and problem learning strategies in normal and retarded children. *Child Development*, 1968, *3*, 827–848.

Balla, D., & Zigler, E. Preinstitutional social deprivation and responsiveness to social reinforcement in institutionalized retarded individuals: A six-year follow-up study. *American Journal of Mental Deficiency*, 1975, *80*, 228–230.

Baratz, S. S., & Baratz, J. S. Early childhood intervention: The social science base of institutional racism. *Harvard Educational Review*, 1970, *40*, 29–50.

Beckham, A. S. Minimum intelligence levels for several occupations. *Personnel Journal*, 1930, *9*, 309–313.

Begab, M. J. The major dilemma of mental retardation: Shall we prevent it? (Some social implications of research in mental retardation). *American Journal of Mental Deficiency*, 1974, *78*, 519–529.

Begab, M. J., & Richardson, S. A. (Eds.). *The mentally retarded and society: A social science perspective*. Baltimore: University Park Press, 1976.

Beller, E. K. Research on organized programs of early education. In R. Travers (Ed.), *Handbook of research on teaching*. Chicago: Rand McNally, 1973.

Bennett, E. L., Diamond, M. C., Krech, D., & Rosenzweig, M. R. Chemical and anatomical plasticity of the brain. *Science*, 1964, *146*, 610–619.

Bloom, B. *Stability and change in human characteristics*. New York: Wiley, 1964.

Bowlby, J. *Attachment and loss*. Vol. 1: *Attachment*. New York: Basic Books, 1969.

Bowlby, J. *Attachment and loss*. Vol. 2: *Separation: Anxiety and anger*. New York: Basic Books, 1973.

Bronfenbrenner, U. Is early intervention effective? In M. Guttentag & E. L. Struening (Eds.), *Handbook of evaluation research* (Vol. 2). Beverly Hills, Calif. Sage Publications, 1975.

Bronfenbrenner, U. Toward an experimental ecology of human development. *American Psychologist*, 1977, *32*, 513–531.

Burr, E. T. Minimum intellectual levels of accomplishment in industry. *Personnel Journal*, 1925, *3*, 207–212.

Butterfield, E. C. The role of environmental factors in the treatment of institutionalized mental retardates. In A. A. Baumeister (Ed.), *Mental retardation*. Chicago: Aldine, 1967.

Butterfield, E. C., Barnett, C. D., & Bensberg, G. J. A measure of attitudes which differentiate attendants from separate institutions. *American Journal of Mental Deficiency*, 1968, *72*, 890–899.

Caldwell, B. M., Heider, J., & Kaplan, B. *The inventory of home stimulation*. Paper presented at the annual meeting of the American Psychological Association, New York, September 1966.

Campbell, D. T. Reforms as experiments. *American Psychologist*, 1969, *24*, 409–429.

Campbell, D. T., & Erlebacher, A. How regression artifacts in quasi-experimental evaluations can mistakenly make compensatory education look harmful. In J. Hellmuth (Ed.), *The disadvantaged child*. Vol. 3: *Compensatory education: A national debate*. New York: Brunner/Mazel, 1970.

Campbell, D. T., & Stanley, J. C. *Experimental and quasi-experimental designs for research*. Chicago: Rand McNally, 1966.

Caplan, N. S. The use of social science information by federal executives. In G. Lyons (Ed.), *Social research and public policies*. Hanover, N.H.: Dartmouth College, 1975.

Caplan, N. S., & Rich, R. F. *Open and closed knowledge inquiry systems: The process and consequences of bureaucratization of information policy at the national level*. Unpublished manuscript, University of Michigan, 1977.

Cicirelli, V. G. *The impact of Head Start: An evaluation of the effects of Head Start on children's cognitive and affective development*. Washington, D.C.: National Bureau of Standards, Institute for Applied Technology, 1969.

Clarke, A. D. B., & Clarke, A. M. Prospects for prevention and amelioration of mental retardation: A guest editorial. *American Journal of Mental Deficiency*, 1977, *81*, 523–533.

Clarke, A. M., & Clarke, A. D. B. *Early experience: Myth and evidence*. London: Open Books, 1976.

Cole, M., & Bruner, J. S. Cultural differences and inferences about psychological processes. *American Psychologist*, 1971, *26*, 867–876.

Coleman, J. S. The evaluation of *Equality of educational opportunity*. In F. Mosteller & D. P. Moynihan (Eds.), *On equality of educational opportunity*. New York: Random House, 1972.

Coleman, J. S., Campbell, E. Q., Hobson, C. J., McPartland, J., Mood, A. M., Weinfeld, F. D., & York, R. L. *Equality of educational opportunity*. Washington, D.C.: U.S. Department of Health, Education, and Welfare, U.S. Government Printing Office, 1966.

Comer, J. *School power*. New York: Free Press, in press.

Comptroller General of the United States. *Report to the Congress: Early childhood and family development programs improve the quality of life for low-income families* (Document No. [HRD] 79-40). Washington, D. C.: U. S. Government Accounting Office, February 6, 1979.

Cronbach, L. J. Five decades of public controversy over mental testing. *American Psychologist*, 1971, *30*, 1–14.

Darlington, R. B., Royce, J. M., Snipper, A. S., Murray, H. W., & Lazar, I. Preschool programs and later school competence of children from low-income families. *Science*, 1980, *208*, 202–204.

DeMott, D. P. *Children's self-concept disparity: Effects of age, race, social class, and gender*. Unpublished master's thesis, Yale University, 1978.

Denenberg, V. H. The effects of early experience. In E. S. E. Hafez (Ed.), *The behaviour of domestic animals*. London: Baillière, 1962.

Dentler, R. A., & Mackler, B. The socialization of retarded children in an institution. *Journal of Health and Human Behavior*, 1961, *2*, 243–252.

Deutsch, M., Taleporos, E., & Victor, J. A brief synopsis of an initial enrichment program in early childhood. In S. Ryan (Ed.), *A report on longitudinal evaluations* (Vol. 1) (DHEW Publication No. [OHD] 74–24). Washington, D.C.: U.S. Office of Child Development, 1974.

Eisenberg, L., & Conners, C. K. *The effect of Head Start on developmental process*. Paper presented at the 1966 Joseph P. Kennedy, Jr. Foundation Scientific Symposium on Mental Retardation, Boston, April 11, 1966.

Feuerstein, R. *Instrumental enrichment: An intervention program for cognitive modifiability*. Baltimore: University Park Press, 1980.

Feuerstein, R., Krasilowsky, D., & Rand, Y. Innovative educational strategies for the integration of high-risk adolescents in Israel. *Phi Delta Kappan*, 1974, *55*, 1–6.

Finkelstein, N. W., Dent, C., Gallagher, K., & Ramey, C. T. Social interaction of infants and toddlers in a daycare setting. *Developmental Psychology*, 1978, *14*, 257–262.

Gallagher, J. J., Haskins, R., & Farran, D. C. Poverty and public policy. In T. B. Brazelton & V.

C. Vaughn (Eds.), *The family: Setting priorities*. New York: Science and Medicine Publishing Co., in press.

Garber, H. Intervention in infancy: A developmental approach. In M. Begab & S. Richardson (Eds.), *The mentally retarded and society: A social science perspective*. Baltimore: University Park Press, 1975.

Garber, H., & Heber, R. The Milwaukee Project. In P. Mittler (Ed.), *Research to practice in mental retardation*. Baltimore: University Park Press, 1977.

Gesell, A. *Infancy and human growth*. New York: Macmillan, 1928.

Gesell, A. Early evidences of individuality in the human infant. *Scientific Monthly*, 1937, 45, 217–225.

Gesell, A., & Ilg, F. L. *Infant and child in the culture of today*. New York: Harper & Row, 1943.

Gesell, A., & Ilg, F. L. *The child from five to ten*. New York: Harper & Row, 1946.

Gesell, A., Ilg, F. L., & Ames, L. *Youth: The years from ten to sixteen*. New York: Harper & Row, 1956.

Golden, M., & Birns, B. Social class and infant intelligence. In M. Lewis (Ed.), *Origins of intelligence*. New York: Plenum, 1976.

Gordon, I. J. *An early intervention project: A longitudinal look*. Gainesville: University of Florida, Institute for Development of Human Resources, 1973.

Gordon, I. J. *The infant experience*. Columbus, Ohio: Merrill, 1975.

Gordon, I. J., Guinagh, B., & Jester, R. E. The Florida parent education infant and toddler programs. In M. C. Day & R. K. Parker (Eds.), *The preschool in action: Exploring early childhood programs* (2nd ed.). Boston: Allyn & Bacon, 1977.

Gray, S. W., & Klaus, R. A. An experimental preschool program for culturally deprived children. *Child Development*, 1965, 36, 887–898.

Gray, S. W., & Klaus, R. A. The Early Training Project: A seventh-year report. *Child Development*, 1970, 41, 909–924.

Greenberg, J., & Doolittle, G. Can the schools speak the language of the deaf? *New York Times Magazine*, December 11, 1977, pp. 50;102.

Greenspan, S. A model of social competence: Implications for special education. In B. K. Keogh (Ed.), *Advances in special education* (Vol. 3). Greenwich, Conn.: JAI Press, 1981.

Group for the Advancement of Psychiatry, Committee on Mental Retardation. *Mild mental retardation: A growing challenge to the physician* (Report No. 66). New York: Author, 1967.

Gruen, G., & Zigler, E. Expectancy of success and the probability learning of middle-class, lower-class and retarded children. *Journal of Abnormal Psychology*, 1968, 73, 343–352.

Guttentag, M., & Struening, E. L. *Handbook of evaluation research* (Vol. 2). Beverly Hills, Calif.: Sage Publications, 1975.

Habicht, J.-P., Yarbrough, C., Lechtig, A., & Klein, R. E. Relation of maternal supplementary feeding during pregnancy to birth weight. In M. Winick (Ed.), *Current concepts in nutrition. Vol. 2: Nutrition and fetal development*. New York: Wiley, 1974.

Harlow, H. F. Love in infant monkeys. *Scientific American*, 1959, 200, 68–74.

Harter, S., & Zigler, E. The assessment of effectance motivation in normal and retarded children. *Developmental Psychology*, 1974, 10, 169–180.

Havighurst, R. J. Minority subcultures and the law of effect. *American Psychologist*, 1970, 25, 313–322.

Heber, R., & Garber, H. The Milwaukee Project: A study of the use of family intervention to prevent cultural-familial mental retardation. In B. Z. Friedlander, G. Sternitt, & G. Kirk (Eds.), *Exceptional infant: Assessment and intervention* (Vol. 3). New York: Brunner/Mazel, 1975.

Herrnstein, R. J. I.Q. *Atlantic Monthly*, 1971, 228, 43–64.

Hobbs, N. Families, schools, and communities: An ecosystem for children. In H. J. Leighter (Ed.), *Families and communities as educators*. New York: Teachers College Press, 1979.

Hobbs, N. Knowledge transfer and the policy process. In G. Gerbner, C. Ross, & E. Zigler (Eds.), *Child abuse: An agenda for action*. New York: Oxford University Press, 1980.

Hunt, J. McV. *Intelligence and experience*. New York: Ronald Press, 1961.

Hunt, J. McV. Parent and child centers: Their basis in the behavioral and educational sciences. *American Journal of Orthopsychiatry*, 1971, 41, 13–38.

Huston-Stein, A., Friedrich-Cofer, L., & Susman, E. J. The relation of classroom structure to social behavior, imaginative play, and self-regulation of economically disadvantaged children. *Child Development*, 1977, 48, 908–916.

Ito, H. Japan's outcastes in the United States. In G. DeVos & H. Wagatasuma (Eds.), *Japan's invisible race: Caste in culture and personality*. Berkeley and Los Angeles: University of California Press, 1967.

Jacobson, L. I., Berger, S. E., Bergman, R. L., Millham, J., & Greeson, L. E. Effects of age, sex, systematic conceptual learning, acquisition of learning sets, and programmed social interaction on the intellectual and conceptual development of preschool children from poverty backgrounds. *Child Development*, 1971, 42, 1399–1415.

Jencks, C., Smith, M., Acland, H., Bane, M. J., Cohen, D., Gintis, H., Heyns, B., & Michelson, S. *Inequality: A reassessment of the effect of family and schooling in America*. New York: Basic Books, 1972.

Jensen, A. R. How much can we boost IQ and scholastic achievement? *Harvard Educational Review*, 1969, 39, 1–123.

Jensen, A. R. *Educability and group differences*. New York: Harper & Row, 1973.

Jensen, A. R. *Educational differences*. London: Methuen, 1979.

Kagan, J. Family experience and the child's development. *American Psychologist*, 1979, 34, 886–891.

Kagan, J., Kearsley, R. B., & Zelazo, P. R. *Infancy: Its place in human development*. Cambridge, Mass.: Harvard University Press, 1978.

Kagan, J., & Klein, R. E. Cross-cultural perspectives on early development. *American Psychologist*, 1973, 28, 947–961.

Karnes, M. B., Teska, J. A., Hodgins, A., & Badger, E. Educational intervention at home by mothers of disadvantaged infants. *Child Development*, 1970, 41, 925–935.

Karnes, M. B., Zehrback, R. R., & Teska, J. A. Conceptualization of the GOAL (game-oriented activities for learning) curriculum. In M. C. Day & R. K. Parker (Eds.), *The preschool in action: Exploring early childhood programs* (2nd ed.). Boston: Allyn & Bacon, 1977.

Katz, P., & Zigler, E. Self-image disparity: A developmental approach. *Journal of Personality and Social Psychology*, 1967, 5, 186–195.

Katz, P., Zigler, E., & Zalk, S. Children's self-image disparity: The effects of age, maladjustment, and action-thought orientation. *Developmental Psychology*, 1975, 11, 546–550.

Keniston, K. *All our children*. New York: Harcourt Brace Jovanovich, 1977.

Kershaw, D. N. A negative-income-tax experiment. *Scientific American*, 1972, 227, 19–25.

King, R. D., Raynes, N. V., & Tizard, J. *Patterns of residential care: Sociological studies in institutions for handicapped children*. London: Routledge & Kegan Paul, 1971.

Kirschner Associates, Albuquerque, N.M. *A national survey of the impacts of Head Start centers on community institutions* (ED045195). Washington, D.C.: Office of Economic Opportunity, May 1970.

Klaus, M. H., Jerauld, R., Kreger, N. C., McAlpine, W., Steffa, M., & Kennell, J. H. Maternal attachment: Importance of the first postpartum days. *New England Journal of Medicine*, 1972, 286, 460–463.

Kohlberg, L. Sex differences in morality. In E. E. Maccoby (Ed.), *The development of sex differences*. Stanford, Calif.: Stanford University Press, 1966.

Kohlberg, L., & Zigler, E. The impact of cognitive maturity on the development of sex-role attitudes in the years four to eight. *Genetic Psychology Monographs*, 1967, 75, 89–165.

Kohn, M. *Social competence, symptoms, and underachievement in childhood: A longitudinal perspective*. New York: Halstead/Wiley, 1977.

Labov, W. The logic of nonstandard English. In F. Williams (Ed.), *Language and poverty*. Chicago: Markham, 1970.

Labov, W. *Language in the inner city: Studies in the black English vernacular*. Philadelphia: University of Pennsylvania Press, 1972.

Lazar, I., Royce, J., Murray, H., Snipper, A., & Darlington, R. Lasting effects after preschool. *Monographs of the Society for Research in Child Development*, in press.

Lesser, G. S., Fifer, G., & Clark, D. H. Mental abilities of children in different social class and cultural groups. *Monographs of the Society for Research in Child Development*, 1965, 30(4, Serial No. 102).

Levenstein, P. The mother–child home program. In M. C. Day & R. C. Parker (Eds.), *The preschool in action: Exploring early childhood programs*. Boston: Allyn & Bacon, 1977.

Levenstein, P., & Sunley, R. Stimulation of verbal interaction between disadvantaged mothers and children. *American Journal of Orthopsychiatry*, 1968, 38, 116–121.

Loehlin, J. C., Lindzey, G., & Spuhler, J. N. *Race differences in intelligence*. San Francisco: W. H. Freeman, 1975.

Madden, J., Levenstein, P., & Levenstein, S. Longitudinal IQ outcomes of the Mother–Child Home Program. *Child Development*, 1976, 47, 1015–1025.

Mayntz, R. Sociology, value freedom, and the problems of political counseling. In C. H. Weiss (Ed.), *Using social research in public policy making*. Lexington, Mass.: Lexington Books, 1977.

McClelland, D. C. Testing for competence rather than for "intelligence." *American Psychologist*, 1973, 28, 1–14.

McCormick, M., Balla, D., & Zigler, E. Resident-care practices in institutions for retarded persons: A cross-institutional, cross-cultural study. *American Journal of Mental Deficiency*, 1975, 80, 1–17.

Mednick, B. R., Baker, R. L., & Sutton-Smith, B. *Teenage pregnancy and perinatal mortality*. Unpublished manuscript, study supported by the National Institute of Child Health and Human Development of the Department of Health, Education, and Welfare, Grant No. 75-7-060, 1979.

Mercer, J. R. *Labeling the mentally retarded*. Berkeley and Los Angeles: University of California Press, 1973.

Mercer, J. R. Psychological assessment and the rights of children. In N. Hobbs (Ed.), *Issues in the classification of children* (Vol. 1). San Francisco: Jossey-Bass, 1975.

Mercer, J. R., Butler, E. W., & Dingman, H. F. The relationship between social developmental performance and mental ability. *American Journal of Mental Deficiency*, 1964, 69, 195–203.

Miller, L. B., & Dyer, J. L. Four preschool programs: Their dimensions and effects. *Monographs of the Society for Research in Child Development*, 1975, 40(5–6, Serial No. 162).

Milunsky, A. Risk of amniocentesis for prenatal diagnosis. *New England Journal of Medicine*, 1975, 293, 932–933.

Mischel, W. *Personality and assessment*. New York: Wiley, 1968.

North, A. F., Jr. Health services in Head Start. In E. Zigler & J. Valentine (Eds.), *Project Head Start: A legacy of the war on poverty*. New York: Free Press, 1979.

Ogbu, J. U. *Minority education and caste: The American system in cross-cultural perspective*. New York: Academic Press, 1978.

Ollendick, T., Balla, D., & Zigler, E. Expectancy of success and the probability learning of retarded children. *Journal of Abnormal Psychology*, 1971, 77, 275–281.

O'Malley, J. M. Research perspectives on social competence. *Merrill-Palmer Quarterly*, 1977, 23, 29–44.

Palmer, F. H., & Anderson, L. W. Long-term gains from early intervention: Findings from longitudinal studies. In E. Zigler & J. Valentine (Eds.), *Project Head Start: A legacy of the war on poverty*. New York: Free Press, 1979.

Palmer, F. H., & Semlear, T. Early intervention: The Harlem Study. In R. M. Liebert, R. W. Poulos, & G. Marmor (Eds.), *Developmental psychology*. Englewood Cliffs, N.J.: Prentice-Hall, 1976.

Palmer, F. H., & Siegel, R. J. Minimal intervention at ages two and three and subsequent intellective changes. In M. C. Day & R. K. Parker (Eds.), *The preschool in action: Exploring early childhood programs* (2nd ed.). Boston: Allyn & Bacon, 1977.

Pavenstedt, E. A comparison of the child-rearing environment of upper-lower and very low-lower class families. *American Journal of Orthopsychiatry*, 1965, 35, 89–98.

Pechman, J. A., & Timpane, P. M. (Eds.). *Work incentives and income guarantees: The New Jersey negative income tax experiment*. Washington, D.C.: Brookings, 1975.

Penrose, L. S. *The biology of mental defect*. London: Sidgwick & Jackson, 1963.

Piaget, J. *The moral judgment of the child*. Glencoe, Ill.: Free Press, 1948.

Piaget, J. Piaget's theory. In P. H. Mussen (Ed.), *Carmichael's manual of child psychology* (3rd ed.; Vol. 1). New York: Wiley, 1970.

Pollitt, E., & Thomson, C. Protein-calorie malnutrition and behavior: A view from psychology. In R. J. Wurtman & J. J. Wurtman (Eds.), *Nutrition and the brain* (Vol. 2). New York: Raven, 1977.

Provence, S., Naylor, A., & Patterson, J. *The challenge of daycare*. New Haven: Yale University Press, 1977.

Quay, L. C. Academic skills. In N. R. Ellis (Ed.), *Handbook of mental deficiency*. New York: McGraw-Hill, 1963.

Ramey, C. T., Collier, A. M., Sparling, J. J., Loda, R. A., Campbell, F. A., Ingram, D. L., & Finkelstein, N. W. The Carolina Abecedarian Project: A longitudinal and multidisciplinary approach to the prevention of developmental retardation. In T. Tjossem (Ed.), *Intervention strategies for high-risk infants and young children*. Baltimore: University Park Press, 1976.

Ramey, C. T., & Haskins, R. The causes and treatment of school failure: Insights from the Carolina Abecedarian Project. In M. J. Begab, H. Garber, & H. C. Haywood (Eds.), *Prevention of retarded development in psychosocially disadvantaged children*. Baltimore: University Park Press, 1981.

Rand, Y., Feuerstein, R., Hoffman, M., Hoffman, L., & Miller, M. Cognitive modifiability in retarded adolescents: Effects of instrumental enrichment. *American Journal of Mental Deficiency*, 1979, 83, 539–550.

Rescorla, L. A., Provence, S., & Naylor, A. *The Yale Child Welfare Research Program: Description and results*. Paper presented at the biennial meeting of the Society for Research in Child Development, San Francisco, 1979.

Ricciuti, H. N. Malnutrition, learning and intellectual development: Research and remediation. In *Psychology and the problems of society*. Washington, D.C.: American Psychological Association, 1970.

Ricciuti, H. N. Early intervention studies: Problems of linking research and policy objectives. In M. J. Begab, H. Barber, & H. C. Haywood (Eds.), *Prevention of retarded development in psychosocially disadvantaged children*. Baltimore: University Park Press, 1981.

Rich, R. F., & Caplan, N. S. *Instrumental and conceptual uses of social science knowledge in policy-making at the national level: Means/ends matching versus understanding*. Unpublished manuscript, University of Michigan, 1976.

Riesen, A. H. Plasticity of behavior: Psychological aspects. In H. F. Harlow & C. N. Woolsey (Eds.), *Biological and biochemical bases of behavior*. Madison: University of Wisconsin Press, 1958.

Rist, R. C. Student social class and teacher expectations: The self-fulfilling prophecy in ghetto education. *Harvard Educational Review*, 1970, 40, 411–451.

Robertson, A. B. *Group day care and children's social-motivational development*. Unpublished doctoral dissertation, Yale University, 1978.

Rutter, M., Maughan, B., Martimore, P., & Ouston, J. *Fifteen thousand hours: Secondary schools and their effects on children*. Cambridge, Mass.: Harvard University Press, 1979.

Ryan, S. *A report on longitudinal evaluations of preschool programs* (DHEW Publication No. OHD-74-27). Washington, D.C.: Office of Human Development, 1974.

St. John, N. H. Desegregation and minority group performance. *AERA Review of Educational Research*, 1970, 40, 111–134.

Sameroff, A. J., & Chandler, M. J. Reproductive risk and the continuum of caretaking casualty. In F. D. Horowitz, E. M. Hetherington, S. Scarr-Salapatek, & G. Siegel (Eds.), *Review of child development research* (Vol. 4). Chicago: University of Chicago Press, 1975.

Sarason, S. B. *Psychological problems in mental deficiency*. New York: Harper, 1953.

Scarr, S., & Weinberg, R. IQ test performance of black children adopted by white families. *American Psychologist*, 1976, 31, 726–739.

Schaefer, E. S. Factors that impede the process of socialization. In M. J. Begab & S. A. Richardson (Eds.), *The mentally retarded and society: A social science perspective*. Baltimore: University Park Press, 1976.

Schiff, M., Duyme, M., Dumaret, A., Stewart, J., Tomkiewicz, S., & Feingold, J. Intellectual status of working-class children adopted early into upper-middle-class families. *Science*, 1978, 200, 1503–1504.

Scott, J. P. Critical periods in behavioral development. *Science*, 1962 138, 949–958.

Seitz, V., Abelson, W. D., Levine, E., & Zigler, E. Effects of place of testing on the Peabody Picture Vocabulary Test scores of disadvantaged Head Start and non–Head Start children. *Child Development*, 1975, 46, 481–486.

Seitz, V., Apfel, N. H., & Efron, C. Long-term effects of early intervention: The New Haven Project. In B. Brown (Ed.), *Found: Long-term gains from early intervention* (AAAS 1977 Selected Symposium 8). Boulder, Colo.: Westview Press, 1978.

Seitz, V., Apfel, N. H., & Rosenbaum, L. Projects Head Start and Follow Through: A longitudinal evaluation of adolescents. In M. J. Begab, H. Garber, & H. C. Haywood (Eds.), *Prevention of retarded development in psychosocially disadvantaged children*. Baltimore: University Park Press, 1981.

Simeonsson, R. J. Social competence: Dimensions and directions. In J. Wortis (Ed.), *Annual review of mental retardation and developmental disabilities* (Vol. 10). New York: Brunner/Mazel, 1978.

Skeels, H. M. Adult status of children with contrasting early life experiences: A follow-up study. *Monographs of the Society for Research in Child Development*, 1966, *31*(3, Serial No. 105).

Skodak, M., & Skeels, H. M. A follow-up study of children in adoptive homes. *Journal of Genetic Psychology*, 1945, *66*, 21–58.

Skodak, M., & Skeels, H. M. A final follow-up study of one hundred adopted children. *Journal of Genetic Psychology*, 1949, *75*, 85–125.

Smith, A. *The human pedigree*. New York: Lippincott, 1975.

Smith, M. S., & Bissell, J. S. Report analysis: The impact of Head Start. *Harvard Educational Review*, 1970, *40*, 51–104.

Solkoff, J. Strictly from hunger. *New Republic*, June 11, 1977, pp. 13–15.

Sparling, J. Carolina infant curriculum. In C. Heriza (Ed.), *The comprehensive management of infants at risk for CNS deficits*. Chapel Hill: University of North Carolina School of Medicine, 1975.

Sparling, J., & Lewis, I. *Infant learning games: Resources for parental–child partnership*. Chapel Hill: University of North Carolina, 1978.

Stipek, D. J. *Changes during first grade in children's social-motivational development*. Unpublished doctoral dissertation, Yale University, 1977.

Stodolsky, S., & Lesser, G. Learning patterns in the disadvantaged. *Harvard Educational Review*, 1967, *37*, 546–593.

Struening, E. L., & Guttentag, M. (Eds.). *Handbook of evaluation research* (Vol. 1). Beverly Hills, Calif.: Sage Publications, 1975.

Sundberg, N. D., Snowden, L. R., & Reynolds, W. M. Toward assessment of personal competence and incompetence in life situations. In M. R. Rosenzweig & L. W. Porter (Eds.), *Annual review of psychology* (Vol. 29). Palo Alto, Calif.: Annual Reviews, 1978.

Tanner, J. M. *Fetus into man: Physical growth from conception to maturity*. Cambridge, Mass.: Harvard University Press, 1978.

Terman, L. M., & Merrill, M. A. *Stanford–Binet Intelligence Scale: manual for the third revision, Form L-M*. Boston: Houghton Mifflin, 1973.

Thorndike, R. L. *The concepts of over- and underachievement*. New York: Columbia University, Teachers College, 1963.

Thorndike, R. L. *Reading comprehension education in fifteen countries*. New York: Wiley, 1973.

Tizard, J. The prevalence of mental subnormality. *Bulletin of the World Health Organization*, 1953, *9*, 423–440.

Trickett, P. K., Apfel, N. H., Rosenbaum, L. K., & Zigler, E. *Yale Child Welfare Research Program: An independent follow-up five years later*. Paper presented at the biennial meeting of the Society for Research in Child Development, San Francisco, 1979.

Tulkin, S. R., & Konner, M. J. Alternative conceptions of intellectual functioning. *Human Development*, 1973, *16*, 33–52.

Turnure, J., & Zigler, E. Outer-directedness in the problem solving of normal and retarded children. *Journal of Abnormal and Social Psychology*, 1964, *69*, 427–436.

United States Department of Health, Education, and Welfare. *The maternity and infant care projects: Reducing risks for mothers and babies* (DHEW Publication No. [HSA] 75-5012). Washington, D.C.: U.S. Government Printing Office, 1975.

United States Department of Health, Education, and Welfare. *The rural income maintenance experiment: Summary report*. Washington, D.C.: U.S. Government Printing Office, 1976.

Venezsky, R. L. Nonstandard language and reading. *Elementary English*, 1970, *47*, 334–345.

Watts, H. W., & Rees, A. (Eds.). *Final report of the New Jersey Graduated Work Incentive Experiment* (Vols. 1–3). Madison, Wis.: Institute for Research on Poverty, 1973.

Weaver, S. J., Balla, D., & Zigler, E. Social approach and avoidance tendencies of institutionalized and noninstitutionalized retarded and normal children. *Journal of Experimental Research in Personality*, 1971, *5*, 98–110.

Weaver, T. R. The incidence of maladjustment among mental defectives in military environments. *American Journal of Mental Deficiency*, 1946, *51*, 238–246.

Weber, G. *Inner city children can be taught to read: Four successful schools*. Washington, D.C.: Council for Basic Education, 1973.

Weikart, D., Delona, D., Lawser, S., & Wiegerink, R. *Longitudinal results of the Ypsilanti Perry Preschool Project.* Ypsilanti, Mich.: High/Scope Educational Research Foundation, 1970.

Weiss, C. H. Introduction. In C. H. Weiss (Ed.), *Using social research in public policy making.* Lexington, Mass.: Lexington Books, 1977.

Weiss, C. H. Improving the linkage between social research and public policy. In Study Project on Social Research and Development (Eds.), *Knowledge and policy: The uncertain connection.* Washington, D.C.: National Academy of Sciences, 1978.

Weiss, C. H., & Bucuvalas, M. J. The challenge of social research to decision making. In C. H. Weiss (Ed.), *Using social research in public policy making.* Lexington, Mass.: Lexington Books, 1977.

Weisz, J. R. *A developmental analysis of relations among hypothesis behavior, helplessness and IQ.* Unpublished doctoral dissertation, Yale University, 1975.

Weisz, J. R. Transcontextual validity in developmental research. *Child Development,* 1978, 49, 1–12.

White, B. L. *The first three years of life.* Englewood Cliffs, N.J.: Prentice-Hall, 1975.

White, R. C. Motivation reconsidered: The concept of competence. *Psychological Review,* 1959, 66, 297–333.

White, S. H. The national impact study of Head Start. In J. Hellmuth (Ed.), *Disadvantaged child* (Vol. 3). New York: Brunner/Mazel, 1970.

Whitney, E. A. Mental deficiency – 1955. *American Journal of Mental Deficiency,* 1956, 60, 676–683.

Windle, C. Prognosis of mental subnormals. *American Journal of Mental Deficiency,* 1962, 66, (Monograph Supplement to No. 5).

Winick, M. *Malnutrition and brain development.* New York: Oxford University Press, 1976.

Woolman, M. *Learning for cognition: The micro-social learning system.* Report to the New Jersey State Department of Education, 1971.

Work, H. H. Mental retardation. In J. D. Noshpitz (Ed.), *Basic handbook of child psychiatry.* Vol. 2: *Disturbances in development.* New York: Basic Books, 1979.

Yando, R. M., Seitz, V., & Zigler, E. *Intellectual and personality characteristics of children: Social class and ethnic group differences.* Hillsdale, N.J.: Erlbaum, 1979.

Zigler, E. Social deprivation and rigidity in the performance of feebleminded children. *Journal of Abnormal Psychology,* 1961, 62, 412–421.

Zigler, E. Research on personality structure in the retardate. In N. R. Ellis (Ed.), *International review of research in mental retardation* (Vol. 1). New York: Academic Press, 1966.

Zigler, E. Familial mental retardation: A continuing dilemma. *Science,* 1967, 155, 292–298.

Zigler, E. The environmental mystique: Training the intellect versus development of the child. *Childhood Education,* 1970, 46, 402–412.

Zigler, E. Project Head Start: Success or failure? *Learning,* 1973, 1, 43–47.

Zigler, E. National crisis in mental retardation research. *American Journal of Mental Deficiency,* 1978, 83, 1–8.

Zigler, E., Abelson, W. D., & Seitz, V. Motivational factors in the performance of economically disadvantaged children on the Peabody Picture Vocabulary Test. *Child Development,* 1973, 44, 294–303.

Zigler, E., Abelson, W. D., Trickett, P. K., & Seitz, V. Is an intervention program really necessary to raise disadvantaged children's IQ scores? *Child Development,* in press.

Zigler, E., & Balla, D. Developmental course of responsiveness to social reinforcement in normal children and institutionalized retarded children. *Developmental Psychology,* 1972, 6, 66–73.

Zigler, E., & Balla, D. The impact of institutionalized experience on the behavior and development of retarded persons. *American Journal of Mental Deficiency,* 1977, 82, 1–11. (a)

Zigler, E., & Balla, D. The social policy implications of a research program on the effects of institutionalization on retarded persons. In P. Mittler & J. M. deJong (Eds.), *Research to practice in mental retardation.* Vol. 1: *Care and intervention.* Baltimore: University Park Press, 1977. (b)

Zigler, E., & Balla, D. Personality development in retarded individuals. In N. R. Ellis (Ed.), *Handbook of mental deficiency* (2nd ed.). Hillsdale, N.J.: Erlbaum, 1979.

Zigler, E., Balla, D., & Butterfield, E. C. A longitudinal investigation of the relationship between preinstitutional social deprivation and social motivation in institutionalized retardates. *Journal of Personality and Social Psychology,* 1968, 10, 437–445.

Zigler, E., Balla, D., & Watson, N. Developmental and experimental determinants of self-image disparity in institutionalized and noninstitutionalized retarded and normal children. *Journal of Personality and Social Psychology,* 1972, *23,* 81–87.

Zigler, E., & Butterfield, E. C. Motivational aspects of changes in IQ test performance of culturally deprived nursery school children. *Child Development,* 1968, *39,* 1–14.

Zigler, E., Butterfield, E. C., & Capobianco, F. Institutionalization and the effectiveness of social reinforcement: A five- and eight-year follow-up study. *Developmental Psychology,* 1970, *3,* 255–263.

Zigler, E., Butterfield, E. C., & Goff, G. A. A measure of preinstitutional social deprivation for institutionalized retardates. *American Journal of Mental Deficiency,* 1966, *70,* 873–885.

Zigler, E., & Harter, S. Socialization of the mentally retarded. In D. A. Goslin (Ed.), *Handbook of socialization theory and research.* Chicago: Rand McNally, 1969.

Zigler, E., & Muenchow, S. Mainstreaming: The proof is in the implementation. *American Psychologist,* 1979, *34,* 993–996.

Zigler, E., & Trickett, P. K. IQ, social competence, and evaluation of early childhood intervention programs. *American Psychologist,* 1978, *33,* 789–798.

Zigler, E., & Valentine, J. (Eds.). *Project Head Start: A legacy of the war on poverty.* New York: Free Press, 1979.

Zigler, E., & Williams, J. Institutionalization and the effectiveness of social reinforcement: A three-year follow-up study. *Journal of Abnormal and Social Psychology,* 1963, *66,* 197–205.

11 *Culture and intelligence*

LABORATORY OF COMPARATIVE HUMAN COGNITION

11.1. INTRODUCTION

SOME CROTCHETY DISCLAIMERS AND DOUBTS

A chapter entitled "Culture and intelligence" encountered in a book written largely by experimental psychologists ought to promise the reader a satisfactory answer to a seemingly straightforward question: How do differences in culturally organized experience affect the development of powerful and efficient problem-solving skills (intelligence)? It appears to be a question of the form: How does independent variable C effect dependent variable I? Unfortunately, there is no accepted or acceptable answer to this question. The question itself may be a non-sequitur.

Not the least of our difficulties arises because the phenomena we seek to designate as *culture* and *intelligence* are by no means well specified. Definitions of both terms abound. Depending upon which rather poorly specified definitions of individual investigators one uses, a very wide variety of phenomena can be subsumed under both the independent and the dependent variable sides of the functional equation $I = f(C)$. Furthermore, relationships among the variables on each side of the equation are as poorly understood as the relationships between them.

We begin this chapter with a brief review of the essential procedures developed within academic psychology for making comparative statements about intelligence. Central to these psychological procedures are the requirements (a) to identify the task that individuals are working on; (b) to demonstrate that the task embodies the properties that require intelligent behavior; and (c) to equate prior experience with this and similar tasks.

When considered from the perspective of cultural anthropology, these psychological requirements produce many difficulties. Anthropologically, cultures are widely treated as socially organized designs for living that render the experience of people growing up in different parts of the world systematically different. The anthropologist recognizes that prior experiences with a given intellectual task are very unlikely to be equivalent. These systematic differences in life experience invalidate the third psychological requirement. Anthropologists also emphasize that it is extremely difficult to identify the task from the participant's point of view at any given moment in the course of ongoing activity. Finally, the criteria for defining intelligent behavior are believed to vary from one cultural setting to another, a matter that calls the second requirement into question.

These diametrically opposed assumptions set up by students of intelligence and culture, considered separately, render normal procedures of comparison problematic. Despite these fundamental contradictions, psychologists have made cross-cultural comparisons of intellectual performance for a good many years. Two major approaches to such research will be contrasted in Section 11.3–11.8. The first assumes that both culture and cognition can be treated as relatively uniform phenomena: Uniform characteristics of culturally organized experience give rise to uniform characteristics of cognition. The second approach emphasizes the heterogeneity of both experience and cognition. Context-specific, culturally organized experiences are the bases that generally reveal abilities under certain conditions on certain occasions.

In the course of this discussion, we will show how the tension between the universalistic approach of the psychologist and the culture-bound approach of the anthropologist renders conclusions about cultural differences in cognition in general, and intelligence in particular, extremely tentative. The chapter concludes by outlining a framework for the study of culture and cognition in which intelligence, as a cultural phenomenon, is shown to depend upon cultural practice.

INTELLIGENCE

The nature of intelligence is a long-standing topic within psychology. The chapters in this handbook are representative of opinion on the the subject; many other relevant discussions are cited in their reference lists.

Judging from the current evidence, there is no broad agreement about the nature of intelligence. Part of the problem in arriving at a common conception is that the primary criterion for measuring intelligence has long been success in predicting performance in school (Estes, 1974; Resnick, 1976). The efficiency of intelligence tests for sorting individuals into productive roles in a modern, technological society has been sufficiently impressive to allow psychologists to define, albeit grudgingly, intelligence as what intelligence tests measure (Tyack, 1974). The necessary conditions for comparing the intellectual power of two or more people have not been challenged since the early days of testing: We sample the performance of persons who have been given an equal opportunity to learn to solve a tightly specified problem. Then "A is rated as more intelligent than B because he produces a better product, essay written, answer found, choice made . . . , or produces an equally good product a better way, more quickly, or by inference rather than by rote memory, or by more ingenious use of the material at hand" (Thorndike, 1926, p. 11; quoted in Estes, 1974, p. 740).

Three sources of difficulty arise when psychologists try to penetrate the empirical relationships produced by the testing movement to determine the principles governing behavior in the tasks selected as defining intelligence.

First, and most important, it is virtually impossible to ensure that people are given equal opportunities to learn. Not only does direct practice on tasks such as those sampled on standard IQ tests differ among people and groups that are parts of a large and heterogeneous society, but indirect opportunities to practice such problems vary as well. The inability to specify what constitutes equal opportunity to learn fuels the controversy over racial differences in intelligence and vitiates all attempts at standardized intelligence testing that compare groups from different home and community environments.

The second problem arises because the pragmatic procedures that yield tests and theories of intelligence rely on correlations between the products of two complex arenas of activity: (a) the person's cognitive activity when he or she is confronted with specific intellectual tasks, and (b) the person's activities in academic settings. Although correlations between experimental and school tasks are not trivial, they are by no means overwhelming. Even if they were considerably higher, we would still be left wondering what psychological and social processes gave rise to the performances that we correlated. We cannot improve upon Estes's (1974) characterization of the quandaries produced when analysts rely on correlations with external criteria such as schooling: "Little can be accomplished in this direction with present instruments for measuring intelligence because these operate primarily by sampling performance, and in every type of intellectual task any given level of performance can arise in many different ways" (p. 749).

Considerations such as these have led a number of cognitive psychologists (including many of the contributors to this handbook) to eschew the aim of obtaining a more valid IQ-testing device. Instead they follow the route suggested by Estes, applying the knowledge and techniques of modern experimental studies of intellectual behavior to arrive at a description of behavior based upon an explicit theory of individual–task interactions. The basic processes specified by the theory are then used to localize the sources of performance differences that lead to inferences about differential learning ability.

We believe that recent efforts to provide a principled account of the behaviors that assemble the products of intellectual tasks is one important source of information upon which to develop a theory of culture and intelligence. But current psychological methods will not be able to carry the full burden of theory construction. It is necessary to determine what prior life experiences materially affect component processes in the tasks employed by cognitive psychologists.

A third class of difficulties with present procedures is highlighted when we move to different cultural settings in cultural groups both outside and inside the borders of the United States. It is not clear whether all cultures agree with the U.S. definition of intelligent behavior. Without prejudging this issue, we can note that in many areas of the world there are still no schools, and the tasks that people routinely must accomplish to maintain themselves bear no obvious relation to the tasks that yield our basic definitions of intelligence (see Sharp, Cole, & Lave, 1979; Super & Harkness, 1980).

CULTURE

If the view from cognitive psychology is discouraging, consider the situation from the perspective of cultural anthropology. As documented by Stocking (1968), the modern concept of culture took shape at the end of the 19th century and the beginning of the 20th. Early anthropologists struggled to accumulate as much basic, descriptive information as possible about the great variety of human arrangements for living that were at that very moment being homogenized in the great blender of modern industrial technology. The founders of anthropology hoped that their records of the lifeways of contemporary peoples would make it possible to reconstruct a plausible picture of mankind's history (Tylor, 1874). As ethnographers began to collect and collate more and more information about diverse groups, a basic challenge to the assumptions of a universal design of living began to emerge.

Tylor and other social scientists of the mid-19th century constructed a developmental history of *culture;* societies were said to progress through stages from less to more complex, culminating in modern industrial culture with its artistic and intellectual traditions. Cultural development in this evolutionary model looked promising in the flush of post-Darwinian enthusiasm. But field studies of various indigenous groups failed to yield any clear, encompassing progression of stages. Rather, different human groups seemed to have constructed different, collective "designs for living" in response to unique patterns of ecological-historical experience.

What were the defining characteristics of a culture? That question posed to anthropologists yields no fewer answers than the question What is intelligence? will evoke from psychologists. The starting point is provided by Tylor: "Culture or Civilization, taken in its wide ethnographic sense, is that complex whole which includes knowledge, belief, art, morals, law, custom, and any other capabilities and habits acquired by man as a member of society" (p. 1).

Some 75 years and hundreds of definitions later, Kroeber and Kluckhohn (1952) offered the following definition of culture, which is widely cited in cross-cultural psychology:

Culture consists of patterns, explicit and implicit, of and for behavior acquired and transmitted by symbols, constituting the distinctive achievement of human groups, including their embodiments in artifacts; the essential core of culture consists of traditional (i.e., historically derived and selected) ideas and especially their attached values; culture systems may, on the one hand, be considered as products of action, on the other as conditioning elements of further action. [Quoted in Brislin, Lonner, & Thorndike, 1973, pp. 4–5]

Details of differences in the two definitions notwithstanding, the difficulty from the point of view of a psychologist interested in discovering how culture influences intelligence is that there are so many aspects of human experience common to *all* anthropological definitions of culture. Assuming that we could separate certain aspects of culture to use as antecedents affecting intelligence, which should we choose?

Once we solve this problem, the anthropological concept of culture presents us with some others. For either Tylor or Kroeber and Kluckhohn, the *patterning* or *configuration* of potentially isolable cultural elements is emphasized. Thus, not only does the psychologist have a plethora of independent variables to choose among, and not only are many of those independent variables defined so generally as to defy efforts at quantification, but the real stuff of culture is believed to reside in the interaction among elements; *the independent variables are not independent.*

Three additional aspects of culture must be considered if we are interested in linking culturally organized experience to cognitive activity. First, we cannot assume a one-way causal relation between culture and intelligence. If one is willing to assume that some aspect of experience makes individuals more intelligent, then a culture that provides the needed experience is going to produce more intelligent members. These people in turn ought to be expected to produce more propitious patterns of experience for their fellows and offspring, thereby further enhancing the cultural experience (and hence intelligence) of later generations.

We must also acknowledge the relationships between cultural and biological variation. Although the notion that cultural differences are the direct result of inherited mental differences was discredited by Boas (1911) many years ago, the idea that cultures are evolved patterns of adaptation to specialized environments leaves open the possibility that biological selection has accompanied cultural adaptation, at least in some cases. Certainly, in a formal sense, biological and cultural differences often covary, a fact with which cross-cultural comparative research must contend insofar as it is concerned with specifying causal mechanisms, not just patterns of correlation.

Finally, we must consider the interdependence of culture, ecology, and historical circumstances. Modern anthropology insists that cultures represent designs for living that are adapted to very different physical and historical circumstances. The adaptive problems that people have faced over the millennia reflect certain common elements if we consider the issue at a sufficiently general level (e.g., calorie intake must exceed the amount expended on obtaining food). But adaptations have been extremely diverse in their details. The notion that solutions to similar problems can be arrived at by quite diverse routes is as applicable to cultural groups as to individuals; Boas is in complete agreement with Estes that one cannot, with any confidence, infer problem-solving *process* from problem-solving *products*.

When we combine these anthropological approaches to thinking about culture with psychological approaches to thinking about intelligence, our sense of consternation must deepen. We have no a priori reason to believe that the set of problems we have learned to analyze as cognitive psychologists and the set of problems that underpin our definition of intelligence will be of any relevance whatsoever to people living in very different cultural circumstances. On the face of it, we should expect many activities in other cultures to serve a social role similar to the role played by the puzzles upon which we base our judgments and theories of intelligence. Our current technology for the study of intelligence imposes limits upon its range of applicability similar to its theoretical limitations.

11.2.   EARLY APPROACHES

These dour comments should be sufficient to induce a high degree of skepticism among psychologists who have harbored the hope that existing controversies concerning intelligence could be settled more easily if cross-cultural data were added to the discussion. However, our cautionary remarks should not be taken as a conclusion that nothing can be learned from studies of cognitive activity in other cultures. In fact, the idea that culture affects the nature of adult thinking (and for some people, the *level* of adult thinking, or intelligence) is as old and respectable as psychology and anthropology. Tylor (1874), who gave us the "classic" definition of culture, also provided us with a theory of the relationship between culture and mind; he proposed that thought, known by its products, is indistinguishable from culture, known by its products.

Because Tylor subscribed to a developmental, evolutionary view of culture, a developmental theory of mind followed as a natural consequence. Culture varies in level, and so does thought. Herbert Spencer (1886) provided a psychological theory to justify the intertwining of levels of thought with levels of culture:

During early stages of human progress, the circumstances under which wandering families live, furnish experiences comparatively limited in their numbers and kinds; and consequently there can be no considerable exercise of faculty which takes cognizance of the *general truths* displayed throughout many special truths . . . in a like manner it is clear that only after there have been received many experiences which differ in their kinds but present some relation in common, can the first step be taken towards the conception of a truth higher in generality than these different experiences themselves. . . . general ideas can arise only as fast as social conditions render experiences more multitudinous and varied. [Pp. 521–522]

When the psychological and social aspects of these early anthropological theorists are put together, they provide the three commonly held assumptions that served as the essential rationale for the belief that "primitives think like children":

1. Cultures vary in their level on an evolutionary scale.
2. The level of culture is coextensive with the level of mind.
3. The level of children's thinking is lower than that of adults in any society; adult thinking evolves out of children's thinking.

When these assumptions were combined with the belief that 19th-century European science, arts, and technology represented the most evolved form of culture, a scientific basis was laid for claims about both the material and the mental poverty of nontechnological societies (Gould, 1976, chap. 5).

Though some early anthropologists did not shy away from the conclusion that "primitive culture produces primitive mind" (e.g., Spencer, 1874), the traditional anthropological position concerning cultural variations in thought stringently limits this conclusion. Adopting a position known as the "doctrine of psychic unity," anthropologists since the middle of the 19th century have claimed that the basic processes of human reason (the process of making generalizations in the passage quoted from Spencer) are *universal* in *Homo sapiens*. This was not a conclusion reached on the basis of direct evidence. Rather, anthropologists, as scientists concerned with explaining human nature by unraveling its prehistory, needed the assumption of psychic unity so that they could "reconstruct lost history without scruple, trusting to general knowledge of the principles of human thought and action as a guide to putting the facts in their proper order" (Tylor, quoted in Stocking, 1968, p. 115).

There has always been ambiguity in the doctrine of psychic unity; its conceptual uses within anthropology have changed as the dominant theoretical concerns within anthropology have changed (see Harris, 1968). Yet two ideas conveyed by the concept appear to have remained stable across different overall interpretations. First, as Chamberlain (1901) put it, "Not the mind so much as the schools of the two stages of human evolution differ" (p. 456). That is, the minds represented in Spencer's thought experiment would be made of the same stuff in a "one-event" or a "many-event" culture; just the complexity of what the minds could do would differ. Second, it is not legitimate to explain cultural differences in the products of thought solely by reference to differences in basic mental processes. Rather, cultural variations must be used to explain whatever mental differences seem to be present.

Such were the dominant views in anthropology at the end of the 19th century when Galton (1883) proposed the possibility of intelligence tests as a way to obtain quantitative measures of the mental differences associated with various cultural differences. These conjoint developments are crucial for cross-cultural studies of culture and cognition (Rivers, 1901).

The evolutionary social scheme proposed by Tylor (1874), Morgan (1877), and Spencer (1886), accompanied by a developmental interpretation of mind and the belief that products of mind are direct evidence of its processes, served as a common framework within which to pursue studies of culture and cognition.

Despite the power of such evolutionary theorizing, Boas, once a student of Wilhelm Wundt, challenged the notion of invariant evolutionary sciences.

Boas criticized previous evolutionary anthropological theory for its cultural uniformity assumption. This assumption was essential for comparisons of societies by cultural level. To admit that different aspects of culture could be at different levels would mean that overall comparisons were impossible: Level of technology and level of rhetorical skill (for example) could not be used interchangeably to measure the level of culture and thought.

In addition to uniformity of cultural features within a group, evolutionary anthropological theorists assumed that there would be similarity of cultural features among closely neighboring groups. After all, neighbors are likely to inhabit the same general ecology and to share a good deal of history. So it was reasonable to expect both that neighboring societies would be at roughly the same evolutionary stages and that consistent evidence could be found of evolutionary stages in all areas of cultural life – "sequences of art forms, of marriage forms, of stages in the development of myth, religion and so forth" (Stocking, 1968; p. 211).

It was these expectations that Boas set out to evaluate in his early trips to the American Northwest, where he sought to determine, through an analysis of language and myth, as well as material culture and social organization, the reasons why groups in a single area participated in a common culture.

But the pattern of language, custom, and myth that he encountered shattered his initial expectations. (See Stocking, 1968, for an excellent discussion of Boas's work.) Instead of uniformity of cultural features, he found diversity that defied either a simple diffusionist or an independent-invention explanation: Tribes with the same basic languages were found to adhere to very different myths and beliefs, and tribes with very different languages were found to have almost identical myths and beliefs. Nor was it possible to assign cultural levels to individual cultures on the assumption that the course of their development and their current form could be deduced from a common set of diachronic process rules. Boas's study of Kwakiutl art emphasized the abstract intellectual work involved in the representation of natural forms. His work on social organization revealed a complexity that badly damaged evolutionary theories of kinship and marriage forms. For example, kinship regulations among the Kwakiutl appeared to result from a mixture of "maternal laws" by a group that was expected to be at a "paternal" stage according to other accepted criteria. This conclusion directly contradicted the traditional evolutionary sequence from maternal to paternal forms of kinship regulation.

Moreover, the assumption that different cultural elements would cohere in a uniform manner proved to be incorrect, so that even if a particular cultural product could be said to have been produced by the same historical-cultural process in two cultures, it was unsafe to assume that the same laws applied to other domains within those cultures. Each aspect of culture had to be examined in its own right and its relations to other aspects within the same society examined to discover the pattern of adaptation that organized the parts; uniform complexity as a principle of cultural organization was unacceptable. In short, cultural features did *not* cohere with respect to any known rules that seemed to apply to all cultures in all places. Boas was forced to conclude that each culture represents a combination of locally developed and borrowed features, the configuration of which is an adaptation to the special constraints operating on the people in question.

Boas's anthropological attack on the evidence for a universal, evolutionary sequence of culture had an inevitable effect on the accompanying theory of mind. A close association between culture and cognition is maintained in this revised conception. But if cultures are not internally uniform with respect to levels of culture, then minds will not be uniform with respect to intellectual accomplishments. It will always be possible to pick some aspect of culture or mind and to rank cultures using some chosen criterion. But the ranking in one domain will not apply uniformly across cultures; which culture looks superior will depend upon the domain of activity chosen for comparisons. This conclusion holds for intellectual as well as other kinds of activity: A member of a nonliterate, low-technology culture, who fails miserably at IQ-like tests, may still demonstrate conceptual and rhetorical subtlety of the highest intellectual order (Bellman, 1978; Radin, 1957).

The evolutionary and culture-specific approaches to understanding the relationships between people in terms of cultural and intellectual achievement provide an important framework within which to understand contemporary psychological studies of culture and cognition. At one pole, we see evolutionary cultural theorists who rank individual intellectual achievements as cultural products. At the other pole, we see great skepticism about the evolutionary sequences and a reluctance to extract elements of culture (or cognition) that could serve the purposes of comparative ranking. Instead, behavior at both cultural and cognitive levels is interpreted in terms of specific configurations of adaptation.

Despite sporadic interest in questions of culture and cognition during the first several decades of the 20th century (see Berry & Dasen, 1974; and Klineberg, 1980, for summaries), no really comprehensive attack on this topic occurred until the 1930s, when several scholars undertook systematic accounts of the relationship between culture and *personality* (see Bock, 1980, especially chaps. 3–6). Culture and personality theorists, despite many differences, agree that just as historical forces mold the configuration of social institutions, beliefs, and technology that characterizes a culture, so cultures mold children socialized into them to form those psychological characteristics that can function most effectively under the given cultural circumstances.

The meaning of the term *personality* has been quite amorphous in the culture and personality tradition, as it is in psychology today. A major concern among early researchers was to prove (or disprove) the universality of psychological phenomena made famous by Freud, as exemplified by Malinowski's (1927) claim that the Oedipus complex was absent among Trobriand Islanders or by Mead's (1928) work on adolescent sexuality and social adjustment in Samoa. "Cognitive orientations" and other phenomena considered more nearly intellectual were sometimes acknowledged to be a part of personality. But data provided by informants' autobiographies, Rorschach tests, and Thematic Apperception Tests (TATs) were the primary source of evidence concerning personality, yielding hypotheses about the cultural sources of aggression, nurturance, anxiety, and other such "clinically" oriented concepts.

This research, carried out within a largely relativist framework on the anthropological side (derived from Boas), rarely concerned itself with questions that might seem relevant to issues of intelligence. To use Bateson's fashionable phrase, they were concerned more with the ethos than with the eidos of culture and mind. The major exception to this generalization concerned IQ testing. Here culture and personality theorists, extending Boas's basic position, argued forcefully against racial theories of intelligence based on cross-cultural applications of standardized tests (see Mead, 1928, p. 289, for early discussion).

11.3.   THE ECO-CULTURAL FRAMEWORK

Despite its concentration on personality constructs, early anthropological work provided the study of culture and cognition with a general framework that has influenced the major culture–cognition theories of the 1970s and 1980s. Operating in this framework, anthropologists and psychologists interested in how culture shapes mind concentrated their attention on an analysis of the sources of culturally organized adult personalities. The general framework is presented in Figure 11.1, which is representative of block diagrams that can be found in a number of important publications bearing on the psychological consequences of cultural experience (e.g., Berry, 1976; Serpell, 1976; J. Whiting, 1969).

There are a number of common elements in all versions of this framework. They include the following assumptions: (a) The kinds of cultural activities that can be engaged in are constrained by physical ecology; (b) cultures elaborate different kinds of social organization to deal with the basic life predicaments that their members have encountered; (c) cultures transmit their acquired patterns of adaptation to their children in ways that are shaped by the ecology and necessary maintenance activities of adults; and (d) all of these influences, separately and in concert, affect the development of cognitive skills.

It is also commonly agreed that this kind of diagram is a serious oversimplification; a great number of elements may be needed in the basic model, and feedback between elements of the model is an acknowledged necessity. Berry (1976) underscores the dilemma that the full eco-cultural model shown in Figure 11.1 presents to the analyst. That dilemma led Frijda and Jahoda (1966) to lament that culture and behavior, as a system of interlocking variables, "defies causal analysis by methods at present at our disposal" (p. 114).

Dilemmas or no, the idea of an embedded set of eco-cultural constraints is the implicit or explicit framework for most cross-cultural work on cognition. Though it does not specify how those constraints shape culture or mind in any detail, it provides the source of the independent variables that distinguish between cultures and serve as the predictors in the equation $I = f(C)$.

RESEARCH WITHIN THE ECO-CULTURAL FRAMEWORK

A clear example of the style and logic of cross-cultural work among anthropologists is provided by Munroe and Munroe (1977). This study, which is one of a larger set of similar studies conducted by the Munroes and their colleagues, purports to show "how variable land holdings affect the proportion of time a woman spends in subsistence activities, and how this in turn influences her socialization [practices] and ultimately shapes the cognitive functioning of her children" (p. 309).

These propositions were tested in the following way. The size of the family farming plot was measured on the ground or from aerial photographs. Direct observation yielded a measure of women's involvement in subsistence activities; a structured interview modeled on something like a projective test with fixed alter-

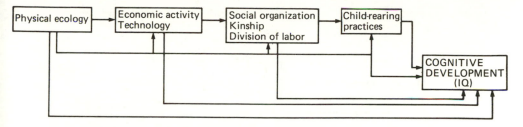

Figure 11.1. The normative eco-cultural theory of culture and cognitive development.

natives yielded the socialization practices measure; and performance on a Piagetian conservation-of-mass problem was the measure of cognitive development. Drawing on B. B. Whiting and J. W. M. Whiting (1975) the Munroes hypothesized that greater involvement in subsistence activities would result in stricter socialization practices and that strict socialization practices would be associated with "either an inhibition of cognitive performance or a deficit in cognitive capacity" (Munroe & Munroe, 1977, p. 311).

Sixteen children were administered the Piagetian task, and their performance was correlated with the amount of land their mothers had to work, their mothers' involvement in farming, and their mothers' repsonses to the test of compliance pressures used in socialization practices. All variables worked in the predicted direction and to roughly the same degree, yielding a significant relation between conservation performance (the index of cognitive development) and compliance pressure as the socialization variable at the end of the hypothesized causal chain.

The Munroes are not psychologists, and their study does not claim to test a psychological theory; rather, it borrows from an existing theory (Piaget's in this case) to make its general point about culture–cognition relationships. Nonetheless, it is a useful case with which to highlight psychological assumptions and methodological issues common to a good deal of psychological research within the eco-cultural framework.

A major psychological assumption embodied in the Munroes' study is the idea that performance on a conservation task is a useful index of the level of a person's cognitive development much as the size of the family farm plot is an index of economic activity; larger farms require that more (or more sophisticated) work be done, better test performance means that more (or more sophisticated) mental work was carried out.

The implicit theory of the processes that mediate such effects can be illustrated by reference to Figure 11.2, which represents what we will call a central processor notion of cognition. Its basic thrust is to assume that experience operates on the current state of some central cognitive structures (perhaps characterized by stagelike features, perhaps characterized only by level). Each learning experience $(E_1, E_2, E_3, \ldots E_n)$ contributes some increment in power (level, amount) to the central processing machinery that is then deployed to deal with individual performance tasks $T_1, T_2, T_3, \ldots T_n)$. This kind of formulation provides a scale that can be used to compare people across cultures because it provides a characterization of the level of mental functioning in general.

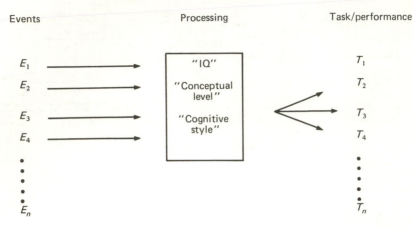

Figure 11.2.　The general processor model.

It is not logically necessary to combine an eco-cultural framework with the notion that eco-cultural pressures operate on a central processing capacity. However, this combination is the one most often used in cross-cultural cognitive research. We will presently describe the application of the eco-cultural framework and the central processor assumption in two major psychological theories of culture and cognition. First, however, we need to discuss three methodological problems that arise in pursuing this analytic path.

Multicolinearity.　When introducing the eco-cultural framework, we pointed out that it posed a severe analytic difficulty: The presumed causal factors are theoretically interrelated and are suspected to have similar effects on behavior. This problem exists independently of one's choice of psychological theory. It is very widely acknowledged by those who use the eco-cultural framework, but the acknowledgement fails to deter the use of data-analytic techniques and interpretations based on the assumption that the problem does not exist.

We can consider the multicolinearity problem by examining the claims of Munroe and Munroe (1977). In the introduction to their study, these authors caution that its analytic power and generalizability may be limited: "The sample size is small, the variables are tapped by means of a single measure, and the findings perhaps can not be generalized beyond the configuration of factors that together comprise a unique sociocultural system" (p. 309). These cautions are less evident in the paper's abstract, where we learn that "ecological variables begin a chain of relationships that carries into subsistence and socialization and ends with effects on cognition" (p. 309).

The Munroes' study exhibits the attractiveness as well as the shortcomings of a good deal of the research within the eco-cultural, central processor tradition. The hypothesized range of variables is neatly laid out; each step in the causal chain is sampled by a quantifiable index; and an extensive network of prior research establishes the plausibility of relations among the most proximal independent variable and behavior. On the other hand, there really *is* a problem of nonindependent antecedent variables.

The Munroes correlate three indexes of eco-cultural variables with cognitive performance: farm plot size, involvement in subsistence activities, and pressure on children to be compliant. These variables intercorrelate at a level as great as their correlation with the dependent variable. When all three factors were entered into a single regression equation, none were significant and only the compliance pressure measure produced a significant correlation with the dependent variable in isolation.[1] Clearly, there is no statistical evidence to support the authors' claims concerning the causal sequence of eco-cultural variables.

A more sophisticated approach to this same set of problems is addressed in Berry's (1976) major study of his eco-cultural model. In some of his early studies, Berry treated indexes of each stage of the eco-cultural system as if they yielded independent confirmation of his hypotheses. In the more recent work, however, Berry reduces the set of independent variables to two, each representing a different cluster of variables. He aggregates the elements of the full model into a single "ecocultural" index, whereas factors such as education and urbanization are converted into an "acculturation" index. This approach has the virtue of removing the mirage that independent contributions of different sources of behavioral variation are being assessed when they are not. However, it represents a retreat from one of the major goals of cross-cultural research, because it reduces a great variety of cultural configurations to a single scale. For example, we can no longer accept as a goal, let alone a specific claim, the ability to specify how the visual ecology of the Eskimo per se affects the development of Eskimo visual skills. In like manner, although Dasen can entitle a paper, "The Influence of Ecology, Culture and European Contact on Cognitive Development in Australian Aborigines" (1974), he must conclude that "the present study does not enable us to assess the relative importance of any of these factors" (p. 407).

The problem of behavioral generality. The rightmost box in Figure 11.1, cognitive development, is not without its own difficulties as an analytic category.

Here we encounter doubts about the extent to which a particular cognitive achievement (conservation performance, for example) can legitimately stand as a proxy for cognitive development in general. The generality assumption really represents an ideal, which is only approximated in real psychological functioning. The important issue for research in the eco-cultural tradition is to establish generality with a sufficient degree of plausibility to permit nontrivial tests of the particular relationships at issue.

In a recent series of articles, Shweder (1979a, 1979b, 1980) reviews the evidence concerning the intersituational generality of culture–personality relations in a manner that addresses culture–cognition research in equal measure:

Any attempt to describe either personality or culture must address two basic questions: (1) How widely do the thoughts, emotions, and actions of a person or a people generalize across diverse stimuli, contexts, or domains? (2) To what extent can the thinking, feelings, and doings of a person or a people be sorted into a limited number of descriptive categories? The two questions are interrelated. If behavior is widely generalized it can be described with fewer categories, and vice versa. [Shweder, 1979a, p. 258]

As Shweder points out, all global trait theories claim to be able to characterize individual behavior using a small number of categories (e.g., field-dependent vs.

field-independent, concrete-operational vs. formal-operational). Yet the evidence in culture and personality research fails to support such claims of intersituational consistency for that psychological domain:

The more assertive child at the breakfast table is not the more assertive child in the playroom. The child who seeks help more than others is not the one who is more inclined to seek physical nearness. The man who is more likely to express his emotions to his wife is not the one who is more likely to express his emotions to his friends. . . . Individual differences in the one context do not predict individual differences in the other. Different situations, stimuli or domains seem to affect different people differently. [Shweder, 1979a, p. 259]

The issue of intersituational generality can be seen to be central to cognitive psychology as well, for Shweder follows other culture–personality theorists in treating cognition as a subcategory of personality. To be sure, the contents of the behaviors being compared are different (Block sorting, water pouring, and word-list recall instead of "offers help" or "makes suggestion"). But the underlying logic of establishing the general significance of specific culture–cognition relations remains unchanged. In the research that we review herein, issues of generality will come up in several guises.

First, we must determine if the research even addresses the issue. A good many studies (of which the 1977 Munroe & Munroe study is but one example) simply *assume* generality, rendering it a moot issue. Studies that employ multiple tasks with the same population of subjects embody a minimum requirement for such research.

Second, we must determine if the range of tasks used to sample a hypothetical domain of intellectual activity (perceptual functioning, cognition, etc.) actually covers the domain in a representative manner.

Third (and crucial to cross-cultural research), we must be certain that the *tasks used to sample the domain in question do so for the culture in question*. The issue was put squarely by Goodenough many years ago:

If we are to look upon intelligence tests as samples of the intellectual requirements of a given culture-group, what basis is there left for applying such a sample of tasks to individuals from another group whose cultural patterns differ widely from those of the original group for whom the test was designed? Very little, I think. [Goodenough, 1936, p. 8]

Without adequate sampling, then, it is clear that not only will we be unable to gain an accurate picture of what skills people do possess, but we will also be unable to make valid inferences to any basic cognitive competence or capacity. [Quoted in Berry & Dasen, 1974, p. 229]

Or, as Wober (1969) remarked, we must ask not only "How well *they* do *our* tricks but How well can *they* do *their tricks*?" (p. 488).

Ideally, then, one should begin cross-cultural cognitive research with a study of those situations arising in different cultures in which the ability in question is manifested. Or, if one is interested only in behaviors that occur in a restricted set of situations, this set should be specified as fully as possible.

The problem of theoretical specificity. We need to discuss one further difficulty common to all cross-cultural cognitive research prior to considering the main lines of evidence.

Contrast the following two characterizations of the processes involved in solving the Piagetian three-mountain problem, the first offered by Dasen, Berry, &

Witkin (1979) in the context of psychological differentiation theory, the second from Kirk's (1977) analysis of the three-mountain problem:

> . . . cognitive restructuring tasks – that is, tasks which require the person to act on percepts or symbolic representations rather than to adhere to their dominant properties as given. A well-known example of a restructuring task is provided by the Embedded Figures Test. . . . Other examples of cognitive restructuring tasks [include] the Piagetian conservation, 3-mountain and water-level problems. [Dasen, Berry, & Witkin, 1979, p. 72]

> There are probably several skills involved in successful response to this task. The first is the "mental shuffling" [Goodnow, 1969], or mental reversal of the child's image. . . . A second is the projection of the child's vision into the doll; that is understanding that he is supposed to try to imagine seeing what the doll sees. . . . A third is perceptual: the decoding of two-dimensional (the color photographs) into three dimensional images. [Kirk, 1977, pp. 282–283]

The first characterization is quite general, befitting the authors' claim that such processes characterize the individual's style of interacting with the world; the three-mountain problem requires people to act on percepts, not on dominant properties as given.

Kirk is more specific. She suggests three component skills needed to solve the problem. Though it may well be that these three skills all fit the definition of cognitive restructuring proposed by Dasen and his associates, we really cannot be sure because no characterization of the cognitive restructuring required by the three-mountain problem is provided.

When we consider carefully the activities required to perform any of the cognitive tasks that are the contexts from which the dependent variables in cross-cultural research arise, we quickly realize, along with Kirk, that a great many skills must be brought into play in a well-integrated fashion. It is widely agreed that no tests of cognitive activity yield pure measures of any of the processes that psychologists designate as *the* process under consideration. Rather, each test must be considered as a system of activity in which elementary processes combine to produce the behavior that we use as a criterion (Cole & Scribner, 1974; Luria, 1932, 1979). Estes (1979) puts the matter very clearly in his discussion of the relation between intelligence and learning:

> The behavior we tap when we give tests or scales of intelligence . . . must *always* be assumed to depend on all [the factors in the theory]. Thus to measure any one component it is necessary either to hold all of the others constant, which may often be impossible of realization, or to understand the interactions well enough to partial out the effects of components other than the one that is being measured. [P. 14]

The interaction of system components operating within any task environment is the object of study of cognitive scientists. As any review of the literature on this subject (e.g., Estes, 1975–1979, Vols. 1–6) quickly reveals, there are many competing theories of the way in which children assemble components for the kinds of tasks used by the major investigators working within the eco-cultural framework. (Cf., e.g., Dasen et al., 1979; Kirk, 1977; and Pascual-Leone, n.d.; with Klahr, 1976; and Resnick & Glaser, 1976.) This situation has at least two implications for cross-cultural cognitive studies.

First, test scores *cannot* confidently be ascribed to any particular underlying process; there are likely to be plausible alternative process explanations that can do the job. This statement is a trivial truism in domestic research, the aim of which is to build workable models of task-specific behavior. But it is damaging to the kind of cross-cultural work we have been describing, because what the cognitive psychologist treats as a model system *to be explained,* the cross-cultural psychologist uses as a *test* of a specific, hypothetical process. The cross-cultural researcher's independent variable is dictated by a hypothesis about the behaviors required to generate the dependent variable. Insofar as the analyst's hypotheses about the nature of the dependent variable are inaccurate, the entire enterprise is vitiated. In effect, the hypothesis is not being tested.

Consider another aspect of Kirk's research. In addition to posing the three-mountain problem, she asked mothers to direct their children in constructing a model toy, and she gave the children a conservation task. One of her findings was that the age at which children achieve conservation of quantity is predicted by the degree to which their mothers emphasize relationships among elements when they teach the construction task. One can make the case (as Kirk does) that "precision in relational thinking" is an important factor in cognitive growth within a Piagetian framework.[2] Problems arise because this aspect of mothers' teaching style is *not* related to performance on the three-mountain problem, even though that task is also said to depend critically upon relational thinking. A new factor (exposure to photographs) can be offered to explain the failure of prediction. But such explanations are not confirmations of theory. When the investigator has to resort to them, they raise questions about the positive results as well, because the underlying theory is supposed to account for behavior changes in *both* sets of problems by the same mechanisms. Appeals to other factors simply threaten the confidence with which we can ascribe the behavior differences in the experiment to the proposed underlying process of "precision in relational thinking." Other, facilitating factors are as likely to have occurred here as other, debilitating factors are to have occurred with the mountains problem.

The second problem caused by lack of specificity when describing behavior in testlike situations is that it is likely to reduce the magnitude of effect that could possibly be achieved. Again, Estes (1979) makes a crucial point:

Each laboratory test used in an attempt to get at some constituent of learning ability calls on some pattern of cognitive operations to carry out a given task and has its unique requirements with regard to products of previous learning, both in kind and in degree, that are prerequisite to the performance called for. Thus the low correlations commonly observed in laboratory tasks used to measure learning abilities may simply reflect variation in contexts rather than independence of the abilities. [P. 15]

Translated into the independent-variable–dependent-variable framework that characterizes most cross-cultural research, this dismal conclusion means that even when a theory is correct, we may expect to find only modest correlations among theoretically central variables.

Recognition of this difficulty among cognitive psychologists interested in establishing intertask consistency has led many researchers, such as Hunt and his colleagues (see Hunt, 1976), to eschew comparisons based upon raw test scores and to depend instead upon parameters of the data derived from explicit, mathematically formulated models (see Cooper and Regan, Chapter 3). In the same spirit, Pascual-Leone (n.d.) has used the embedded-figures test as a "control" to assess the disembedding aspect of Piagetian problems, a line of work currently being pursued by Case (1978). To date, there has been little cross-cultural research building on a strong model of behavior in a well-specified cognitive task.

GOING AHEAD ANYWAY

It should be obvious that even under the best of circumstances, cross-cultural cognitive research is a risky enterprise. This is true even before we consider obvious difficulties that arise from attempting to communicate with people whose life experiences do not include exposure to electronic media, two-dimensional representations of objects such as photographs, writing, or the kinds of dialogue upon which most cross-cultural cognitive research is based.

Rather than continue this litany of difficulties, we will turn to the major lines of cross-cultural research that bear on the question of culture and intelligence. Because the more general topic of culture and cognitive development has been extensively reviewed in several publications (e.g., Berry & Dasen, 1974; LCHC, 1979, 1982; Scribner & Cole, 1973; Serpell, 1976), we will be selective in our review, choosing studies that illustrate the central logic of different approaches and lines of evidence that have been underrepresented in previous reviews. Issues of method will be dealt with in the context of specific lines of theorizing. As we shall see, issues of method cannot be treated completely independently of the-oretical aims.

We begin our review with the two major approaches based upon the central processor assumptions described earlier. After summarizing their achievements and difficulties, we will consider an alternative approach that begins from quite different assumptions.

11.4.   COGNITIVE STYLES

Perhaps the largest program of research in cross-cultural cognitive psychology has been pursued by John Berry and the late Herman Witkin within a framework that combines the notion of culture as an interlocking configuration of activities with the concept of psychological differentiation. Their specific theoretical claims have undergone considerable change in recent years (contrast Witkin, 1967, with Dasen, Berry, & Witkin, 1979). But the underlying framework for relating adap-tive behavior to prior experience has remained largely intact. Moreover, charting the changes in theory and research strategy helps to highlight special points of difficulty in the enterprise.

In early research, Berry argued that ecological demands, when combined with cultural adaptions to those demands (e.g., linguistic categories, arts, and crafts), produce identifiable patterns of perceptual skill. For example, Berry (1974) con-ducted an extensive study of 10 subsistence-level groups to test the hypothesis that people whose culture is an adaptation to circumstances that make hunting an adaptive activity should

possess good visual discrimination and spatial skills, and their cultures are expected to be supportive of the development of these skills through the presence of a high number of "geometric spatial" concepts, a highly developed and generally shared arts and crafts produc-tion, and socialization practices whose content emphasizes independence, and self-reliance, and whose techniques are supportive and encouraging of separate development. [P. 133]

To test this hypothesis, Berry ranked his cultural groups according to the im-portance of hunting to their existence and compared these eco-cultural rankings with the average test scores for discrimination and perceptual skills (as man-ifested in such tasks as the Kohs blocks test, Raven's matrices, and the embed-ded-figures test). As predicted, the more central the role of hunting to a culture, the better the psychological test scores, a finding that led Berry to conclude: "It is apparent from the data that the visual skills are developed to a degree predictable from an analysis of the ecological demands facing the group and the cultural aids developed by them" (Berry, 1971, reprinted in Berry & Dasen, 1974, p. 140).

Even in his early work, Berry was aware of Witkin's work relating socialization to perceptual behavior in terms of a "style" of responding that could be characterized as field-dependent (where there is difficulty in overcoming the influence of the surrounding field, or in separating items from context). Socialization factors (which were central to Witkin's work: See, e.g., Witkin, Dyk, Faterson, Goodenough, & Karp, 1962) were included in Berry's early model, but primarily as they affected *perceptual* functioning. In later work, Berry began to collaborate with Witkin in a series of studies and theoretical writings that broadened his early efforts (see Berry, 1966; Dawson, 1967) into a theory of culture and cognitive style in which it was hypothesized that, through the combination of techniques of socialization with ecological and other cultural factors, specific skills are welded into "characteristic, self-consistent modes of functioning found pervasively throughout an individual's cognition, that is perceptual and intellectual activities" (Witkin, 1966, reprinted in Berry & Dasen, 1974).

Berry (1976) used two different techniques to obtain indicators of the restrictiveness of socialization. First, he used a scale of "compliance–assertion" that had been developed by Barry, Bacon, and Child (1957) to relate child-training techniques to economy and sex differences in socialization (see also Barry, Child, & Bacon, 1959). Barry and associates had constructed their scale out of ratings in six categories of interaction involving child rearing: Obedience training, responsibility training, nurturance, achievement, self-reliance, and general independence training. Using the Human Relations Area files, they had obtained significant relations between economic activities and socialization practices: Compliance increases as food accumulation increases.

To these ratings on societies, Berry added a question about how his subjects rated their own socialization: Subjects were asked how strict their upbringing was. These two measures of restrictive socialization practices, which were highly correlated, were combined into a standardized socialization score.

To complete the framework for evaluating the overall theory, Berry needed indexes of ecological factors, acculturation factors, and social stratification (differentiation). For ecological indexes, he used Murdock's classification of subsistence societies in terms of exploitative pattern (animal husbandry, agriculture, etc.), settlement pattern, and size of communities. Acculturation factors included levels of wage labor and education. To these he added an index of social differentiation made up of rankings by political stratification and family organization.

With the exception of education and socialization self-ratings, indicators relevant to the eco-cultural part of the theory were gathered for 18 subsistence cultural groups ranging from West Africa to northern Canada to Australia and three industrialized groups. Data from the Human Area Files were used to code the information about ecological, acculturative, and cultural elements that had been related theoretically to sociocultural differentiation. Tests of cognitive style and some control tests were administered to samples within each cultural group. Then the relationships among variables were calculated, using correlational analysis of variance and multiple regression techniques. The relationships that Berry reported led him to summarize the results as follows:

This pattern of support constitutes a powerful indicator that there is systematic covariation between the set of independent variables and the differentiated and acculturative stress behaviors. Cultural groups [and individuals] which are hunting and gathering in subsistence pattern, nomadic in settlement pattern, and loose in sociopolitical stratification emerge as clearly different in cognitive style from those which are agricultural, sedentary, and tight. And within this range of ecological and cultural adaptations, those which occupy intermediate positions eco-culturally also exhibit intermediate behavioral adaptations. . . .

. . . Taken at the level of a general overview, it is difficult to avoid the conclusion that the hypothesized relationships have been confirmed. [P. 200]

These generalizations have been bolstered by similar studies conducted in many parts of the world on many different populations (see Werner, 1979, for a recent review), so that the Berry–Witkin approach to culture and cognitive development is one of the most extensively tested and persuasive theories available at the present time. Located within a long tradition of eco-cultural research on the "fit" between configurations of culture and configurations of mind, this approach has the added attractive feature of uniting cognitive and personality research into a single enterprise.

DIFFICULTIES WITH THE COGNITIVE-STYLE APPROACH

Despite these attractive features, there are a number of reasons to question whether the theoretical relationships are either as strong or as broad as they appear to be.

One of the major questions raised in recent discussions of the psychological-differentiation–cognitive-styles approach is the issue of domain consistency. The use of the term *style* is motivated by the claim that differentiation manifests itself in all areas of psychological functioning. Key behavioral indicators of field independence should cluster within domains (perceptual, cognitive, social, affective) and correlate highly across domains.

As other writers have noted (e.g., Jahoda, 1980; Werner, 1979), the evidence of domain consistency is not at all strong when one moves from the perceptual/cognitive tasks to the social/affective indicators. Although domain consistency is claimed for intracultural data from the United States, the failure to obtain expected correlations in the cross-cultural arena is considered a problem, not only by others but by the participants in the psychocultural-differentiation research perspective (e.g., Dasen, Berry, & Witkin, 1979; Witkin & Berry, 1975, pp. 29–30). There is still the apparent consistency across perceptual and cognitive domains to be considered, however.

Berry's own massive review suggests that a narrower interpretation of his results than implied by the notion of cognitive style ought to be considered. We have already described the tasks used to index differentiation in the cognitive and perceptual domains. Here it seems appropriate to question the assignment of task to domain. Berry's own comments on this problem are instructive: "In cognition (where perception is also inevitably implicated) differentiation involves the ability to break up or analyze a problem as a step towards its solution, in addition, of course, to many other components (such as background knowledge, general competence, etc.)" (Berry, 1976, p. 28). Goodenough and Karp (1961) are cited as being of the opinion that standard psychometric tests such as block designs, picture completions, mazes, and puzzles appear to involve a capacity to "overcome embeddedness." With this justification, supplemented by references to other tasks such as conservation and concept attainment, the separateness of perceptual and cognitive domains is established.

As Jahoda (1980) comments, the lack of process specification in the psychological-differentiation approach can cause analytic difficulties in attempts to evaluate the theory. Nowhere is this truer than in trying to decide if the tasks used to represent cognitive and perceptual domains are sufficiently distinct to warrant the use of the term *cognitive style* when intertask correlations are observed. This issue takes on an added significance in evaluating generalizations from the data because Kohs blocks and Raven's matrices are widely accepted in American psychological research as indicators of intelligence.[3] The Morrisby shapes are out of the same mold. Berry would not accept this characterization, but in the absence of a process theory of performance on these tasks, it poses a problem for claiming *differentiation* as the process variable implicated in their performance. A "perceptual" task such as the embedded-figures test (EFT) appears to be no less cognitive than the "cognitive tasks."

Our own view is that evidence of domain consistency is less convincing than current discussions suggest, even for the perceptual and cognitive domains. Serpell (1976) reviewed several studies, proposing that what Witkin and Berry label as cognitive style is best thought of as increased skill in dealing with pictorial stimuli. For example, Okonji (1969) found the expected correlation between EFT and Raven's matrices, but these two tests did not correlate with the rod-and-frame test. Okonji also failed to find the expected correlation among EFT, rod-and-frame test (RFT), and socialization factors (see also Siann, 1972). In Berry's (1976) study, the rod-and-frame test correlated least with the other measures of field dependence and not at all with measures of socialization or education.

These issues of domain independence and the strength of existing evidence for the theory force themselves on us in two ways. First, they are important to evaluating claims that differentiation (disembedding) is the process implicated in the pattern of performance. Berry (1976) quite properly included in his battery a test of perceptual discrimination as a process "prior to disembedding (and separate from it . . .)" (p. 146). Geometric shapes with gaps in them were presented tachistoscopically, and a discrimination score was assigned on the size of a gap necessary to produce recognition. Subjects responded by drawing the figure they saw.[4]

The logic of Berry's analysis leads us to expect that performance on the discrimination task will not correlate highly with performance on the disembedding tasks, and will not correlate well with the predicted antecedents of disembedding. Only the first of these expectations is supported by the data: Discrimination performance is not as highly correlated with the disembedding tasks as the disembedding tasks are with each other, although the correlation is substantial. But discrimination *is* highly predicted by major antecedents. In some cases it is predicted as well as the disembedding task. In light of the truncated range of these scores, owing to deleted subjects, the success of the independent variables in predicting discrimination performance is a problem of the sort that motivates perceptual-skills interpretation. According to Berry's statements about the priority of discrimination in the perceptual–analytic process, it would have been interesting to see tests of the effect of eco-cultural antecedents with discrimination performance partialed out. No such analysis is offered.

A second concern about the extent to which the implicated differentiation is the major process variable controlling performance is the way in which performances generate the classification of subjects in terms of cognitive style.

For a task like the rod-and-frame test, the analogy relating performance to process is relatively clear: Field independence is indicated when the subject ignores the wooden frame and sets the rod upright with respect to the ground. Field-dependent subjects "depend" on the wooden frame. There are no right or wrong answers, simply different sources of information used to deal with an ambiguous situation.[5]

But for the other tasks used by Berry, there are clear right and wrong answers. There seems to be no alternative to labeling the performance of someone who cannot identify any of the hidden figures in the EFT as "poor." Certainly, when used as psychometric tests, performances like those of many of Berry's groups are so labeled, and the educational researchers focus on remediation through "direct [and] vicarious experiences encouraging conceptual development" (MacArthur, 1973, p. 24).

This close identification between performances on the various indicators of perceptual/cognitive ability is echoed in a recent, comprehensive study of culture and child development: "Studies in both the Western and developing world have shown that children progress from relative field dependence, in which their perception is dominated by the organization of the surrounding field, to relative field independence" (Werner, 1979, p. 187).

One might be tempted to conclude from these and similar remarks in the literature that *field-dependent* and *less-developed* are in some way synonymous, at least within the confines of differentiation theory (Scribner & Cole, 1978). Less-differentiated people, like young children, perform poorly on a variety of perceptual/cognitive tasks.

It is this web of factors vitiating claims of interdomain consistency and this pattern of mixing tasks interpreted as having right and wrong answers with tasks having different kinds of answers that lead us to prefer the idea that Berry and his colleagues have been dealing with a less pervasive set of individual accomplishments than their theory commits them to. By using behavioral indicators that have clear implications of higher and lower levels of performance, they leave open an interpretation that links field dependence (the style that generates low performance) to lower stages of development.

Dasen, Witkin, and Berry (1979) strenuously object to this interpretation of their work. Their basic strategy for divorcing differentiation theory from implications of higher and lower levels of development is to invoke the distinction between general and specific evolution, and to choose the specific-evolution option according to which adaptive improvement is judged by the adaptive problem. Applied to cross-cultural research on cognitive differentiation, this strategy has led differentiation theorists to suggest that the field-dependent and field-independent styles are adaptive to different environments:

Relatively field-independent people are better at cognitive restructuring tasks – that is, tasks which require the person to act on percepts or symbolic representations rather than to adhere to their dominant properties as given. . . .

. . . relatively field-dependent people are more sensitive . . . to social cues provided by others; they choose to be among others which gives them more experience with people; they have characteristics which are likely to be helpful in relating to other people such as having an interest in others, wanting to help others, and having concern for others. [Dasen, Witkin, & Berry, 1979, pp. 71, 72]

This domain-specificity of the adaptiveness of the two styles is the framework for the specific-evolution formulation that allows Berry and his co-workers to characterize the theory as "bipolar" and "value-free."

Although the claim is not made explicit, it appears that this most recent statement of the theory conceives of societies as either people-oriented or object- and symbol-oriented in varying and complementary degrees. "The proposal is that the field-dependent and field-independent cognitive styles, which are process variables, influence the development of patterns of abilities – in this instance, cognitive restructuring skills and interpersonal competencies, combined in an inverse relationship" (Dasen, Berry, & Witkin, 1979, p. 72).

This is an interesting suggestion, but its empirical basis has to be considered very shaky at best because it rests heavily on claims about domain-specific patterns of reciprocally adaptive behavior that no one claims in any cross-cultural developmental work. What one seeks are a series of "bipolar" tasks (such as the RFT) that sample each of the domains in question. Then it needs to be shown that subjects who do well in one domain do poorly in the other *while maintaining the same cognitive style*.

A thought experiment can illustrate how difficult empirical tests may be. Eskimos are often characterized as field-independent. Their talents, therefore, would seem to lie in the cognitive-restructuring domain. But do we want to claim of Eskimos that they have less "experience with people," less "interest in others," and less "concern for others" than the Temne? Do they have less ability to deal with people than with objects? And if we want to make such claims, how should we establish their validity?

Existing guesses about the real-world analogies for Berry's perceptual tasks also indicate sources of uncertainty in the presumed validity of the perceptual tasks. Berry (1976) offers his gap-detecting discrimination task as an experimental analogy to the task facing a hunter: "For Discrimination disembedding is not involved; rather the task is to detect an element from a fairly simple gestalt" (p. 147). But Wagner (1978), noting the precocity of 7- to 8-year-old Berber sheepherders on the EFT, surmises, "One might hypothesize that these boys, who are Berbers and who were raised as shepherds before they went to school, had developed certain perceptual skills (such as location of sheep in a variegated terrain)" (p. 150).

Yet another concern is the relationship between psychological-differentiation theory as a theory of individual differences related to experiences within cultures and the data offered in the cross-cultural literature. Berry (1976) offers analyses at both individual and cultural sample levels of analysis – or so it appears. However, when one considers the nature of the independent variables, it is quickly apparent that with two exceptions, *the same independent-variable codes must apply to all subjects within a cultural group*. The exceptions are years of education and self-rated strictness of child rearing.

Cognizant of this problem, but limited in his ability to carry out within-cultures analyses, owing to limited variation in the eco-cultural index within the cultures, Berry (1976) presents within-cultures analyses for each group he studies relating complaint socialization self-ratings and education to cognitive performance (pp. 155–157). Though substantial correlations between cognitive performance and education are obtained, correlations with the socialization index are variable and quite low on the average, in sharp contrast to the general picture given by the between-cultures analyses.

Concern that failure to provide within-cultures evidence may give a false picture of the factors at work is heightened by reports such as that from Irwin, Engle, Klein, and Yarbrough (1976), who studied the relationship between EFT performance and mother's traditionalism. Similarity of items on their traditionalism scale and Witkin's characterization of the antecedents of field dependence had led them to hypothesize a positive relationship between traditionalism of mothers and field dependence of children. No such relationship was found. However, ratings of sources of intellectual stimulation did predict EFT performance. The authors argue that previous research linking field dependence to traditionalism was confounded by variables such as availability of intellectual stimulation.

IMPLICATIONS FOR INTELLIGENCE

Couched as it is in culture-specific terms, the psychological-differentiation approach rejects the idea that cross-cultural comparisons of intelligence are possible. In his earliest research, Berry had shown large differences in performance between neighboring African tribes and between acculturated (e.g., urban-educated) and traditional members of the same tribe. He had also demonstrated excellent performance in Eskimos when compared with Scots. These findings led him to conclude that tests of cognitive ability must be culture-dependent, because "peoples with differing cultures and ecologies tend to develop and maintain different sets of skills," so that the concept of intelligence (or its equivalent) would differ from one society to the next. "It follows from this that the search for a 'culture-free' test is futile insofar as it is hoped to find a *universally* valid test; although some tests might be used with fairness in a limited number of societies, this still leaves us with the problem of comparing the results between these various 'test-fair' units." (Berry, 1966, p. 229).

In a later discussion devoted explicitly to the problem of intelligence, Berry (1971) adopted what he called a radical cultural relativist position. In addition to reaffirming the cultural specificity of the abilities that people will develop, Berry acknowledged the central importance of sampling those areas of activity that are crucial to the people in question: "Without adequate sampling . . . it is clear that not only will we be unable to gain an accurate picture of what skills people do possess, but we will also be unable to make valid inferences to any basic cognitive competence or capacity" (Berry, 1971, reprinted in Berry & Dasen, 1974, p. 229).

11.5. COGNITIVE UNIVERSALS: PIAGET

The second major research program concerned with the cultural antecedents of cognitive development has tested hypotheses derived from the theory of Jean Piaget. Like the research on cognitive styles, Piagetian-inspired research has been the subject of extensive discussion and review (e.g., Dasen, 1972, 1977; Glick, 1975; Greenfield, 1976; Jahoda, 1980; LCHC, 1979; Price-Williams, 1981). Consequently, our discussion will be highly selective, focusing on central areas of accomplishment and uncertainty.

The cognitive processes that Piaget's theory is intended to explain are the acquisitions of very general schemata that are related to each other in a logical, hierarchially organized sequence.

The basic assumption underlying the bulk of Piaget's work prior to the 1960s was that the basic cognitive achievements observed in Genevan children would be universal. (For a brief but comprehensive review by the man himself, see Piaget, 1970.) The basis for this assumption was Piaget's belief that the possible basic forms of interaction between the growing child and his or her environment are defining characteristics of *Homo sapiens*.

However, from very early in his career, Piaget manifested a keen interest in the work of the French sociological school, and particularly the speculation about cultural differences in mind proposed by Lucien Levy-Bruhl (Piaget, 1955, p. 21). But early remarks about the minds of primitives and children have amounted to no more than speculation on Piaget's part. Almost no appropriate data were at hand to provide concrete tests of such ideas.

An interesting exception to this generalization was provided by Margaret Mead during her early field work in Samoa. Mead disagreed with remarks supportive of Levy-Bruhl that she encountered in Piaget's first book on cognitive development (1926). ("In Piaget I found the assumption that the 'savage' and the 'child' think alike"; Mead, 1978, p. 96.) The particular aspect of Piaget's ideas studied by Mead was animism, the attribution of the properties of animate creatures to inanimate objects. She observed children at play as well as engaged in tasks that she designed to elicit animistic responses. Her conclusions are a straightforward assertion of cultural determination in this cognitive domain: "[My results are] a direct contradiction of findings in our own society, in which the child has been found to be more animistic . . . than are his elders. When such a reversal is found in two contrasting societies, the explanation must obviously be sought in terms of the culture; a purely psychological explanation in inadequate" (Mead, 1980, p. 115).

Piaget did not systematically take up the issue of cultural variations in cognitive development until the mid-1960s. Processes of cognitive development are treated in his writings as roughly equivalent to processes of intelligence. "Intelligence itself does not consist of an isolated and sharply differentiated class of cognitive processes. It is not, properly speaking, one form of structuring among others; it is the form of equilibration towards which all structures arising out of perception, habit and elementary sensori-motor mechanisms tend" (Piaget, 1963, p. 6).[6]

FOUR FACTORS CONTRIBUTING TO DEVELOPMENT

Responding to the growing number of researchers exporting his tasks to non-Western cultures, Piaget (1966) attempted to clarify the possible contributions of cross-cultural research to his theory. He did so by means of four theoretically distinct factors that would be expected to contribute to the process of development.

It has proved difficult to interpret Piaget's four factors according to cultural variations in experience, particularly his notion of equilibration. On the basis of Piaget's 1966 article, Dasen (1972) and others interpreted equilibration vaguely as "factors, which arise as the young organism interacts with its physical environment" (LCHC, 1978, p. 148). A more thorough examination of Piaget's writing indicates that this interpretation is too narrow, although it describes the vast majority of Piagetian research.

Piaget's four factors are:

1. *Biological factors.* Piaget (1963) draws heavily upon biology and particularly biological evolution for his explanation of ontological development. But, as indicated in the passage already quoted, he is careful to distinguish the process of cognitive development from the maturational process of physical development. If biological factors dominate cognitive development, Piaget would expect little or no effect of the cultural environment either on the developmental sequence that unfolds or on the rate at which the unfolding occurs.

2. *Equilibration factors.* These factors are at the heart of Piaget's theory of development (Piaget, 1970, 1977). What children come to know about the logic of their world is not based solely on relations that are preexisting in the environment nor on the teachings of their caretakers; rather, children must act on and interact with their environment. What they come to know is the form of this interaction. Piaget does not deny that children are taught much of what they know or that explicit teaching is not dominated by equilibration factors. But he does claim that the acquisition of fundamental logical knowledge structures is dominated by this process of equilibration.

The process of equilibration is best considered to be both universal *and* sensitive to the environments created by specific cultures. Cultures may differ in the extent to which their particular practices provide opportunities for experiences or "operational exercises" of the required kind. To the extent that such variations exist, Piaget predicts that different cultures will retard or accelerate the equilibration process but that the sequence of knowledge structures will be universal.

3. *Social factors of interpersonal coordination.* Piaget distinguishes between the effect of the teachings of a particular culture (Factor 4) and the effects on development of the features that all societies have in common. In all cultures there is a socialization process involving social exchanges among children and between children and adults.

Both theoretically and practically, this factor enters into exceedingly complex relations with Factors 2 and 4. To understand the difficulty of distinguishing this social factor from equilibration, we must consider more carefully Piaget's conception of the relationship between the individual and society.

Piaget (1967) describes children engaged in an activity in which they are free to work together or alone:

Among the younger children, there is no distinct dividing line between individual activity and collaboration. The young children talk, but one does not know whether they listen. Several of them may be at work on the same project, but one does not know if they are really helping one another. Among the older children, there is progress in two directions: individual concentration when the subject is working by himself and effective collaboration in the group. [P. 39]

In contrasting younger and older children in this passage, Piaget shows that he considers "egocentricity" or the lack of it to be a feature of both the children's intellectual structures and the social organization of the work group. The same process of equilibration operates both to coordinate the schemata of the individual and to coordinate collective action. This process operates whether the collective actions include those among peers or those between children and cooperative (rather than coercive) adults. If we ask whether the intellectual operations are the cause or effect of cooperation, Piaget answers that it is like the question whether the chicken appears before the egg: "Logic constitutes the system of relationships which permit the coordination of points of view corresponding to different individuals, as well as those which correspond to the successive percepts or intuitions of the same individual" (p. 41). A new structure of knowledge (logic) cannot arise simply from the internalization of cooperative action, because the internal coordination is necessary for cooperation to take place. And it must take place to be available in the child's environment to be internalized.

Then how can "interpersonal coordination" be considered a factor having an independent effect? The distinction can be made, if at all, by shifting our focus from a structural description of the equilibrium of internal and external structures, and instead considering the process by which an individual might achieve that coordination. Piaget (1967) has suggested, and current Genevan research (Doise, Mugny, & Perret-Clermont, 1975) is exploring the hypothesis of a unique role for the fact that "in any environment individuals ask questions, exchange information, work together, argue, object, etc." (Piaget, 1966, p. 302). Essentially, the idea is that two children working together may each notice different aspects of the same situation and need to coordinate these perceptions, whereas a child working alone would notice only one aspect, which would not need to be coordinated.

Although the general structure of interpersonal coordination is independent of content and universal, cultures may vary in the number or nature of opportunities they provide for such interpersonal experiences.

4. *Factors of educational and cultural transmission.* The final factor includes all the specific features that make the social environment of one culture different from that of another. The child learns specific skills and beliefs through both formal and informal education. This is not to say that learning particular cultural practices does not also include a certain amount of more general experience. In fact, a particular craft, pottery, for example, may provide more operational exercises of some kinds than other practices, such as map making. If some societies provide more overall experience relevant to discovering the nature of the environment than others, true developmental differences would exist between those cultures in either the rate or the asymptote of development.

It is Piaget's characterization of the four factors and their contribution to development that causes us to include him within the eco-cultural framework. Although he did not, himself formulate the problem in this way, Dasen (1974, 1977), a major interpreter, has formally acknowledged this framework as appropriate to applying Piagetian theory cross-culturally.

It should also be clear from the previous discussion that the final three factors all operate singly and in common to increase the level of a child's thinking through a series of stages and substages. More operational exercise is possible in all three realms; a little more operational exercise leads to a little more development. The problem, then, is to identify dimensions of cultural difference that are theoretically significant, in order to predict the course of cognitive development in different cultures.

OVERALL STAGES

Piaget describes four major stages of development, which form an invariant sequence. Many tests of Piaget's developmental theory cross-culturally are formulated as attempts to confirm the presence of one or more of these four stages.

Typically, several age groups are sampled and the ages at which given percentages of the various groups "pass" the test are compared to each other and to the studies conducted in Geneva (or in other cultures of interest). "Passing" may consist only of giving the answer to the problem that is associated with the stage in question, but it may also include giving an appropriate justification for the answer. Correct performance on these tasks is used as an index of the presence of the mental operations that are assumed to be necessary for that task.

Obviously, researchers working in the field cannot try out all the tasks that have been used to create modern Piagetian theory. For the most part, the cross-cultural research has focused on the concrete-operational stage, which among Swiss children studied by Piaget and his colleagues begins at about 7 years. It is supplanted by the formal-operational stage at around 12 years.

Concrete operations. Attainment of concrete operations is the aspect of Piaget's developmental theory that is most frequently studied cross-culturally. There are perhaps two reasons why this is so. The first involves the nature of the tasks: Concrete-operational tasks require the manipulation of physical materials that can be easily transported to exotic cultures or constructed on the spot. A second reason has to do with the activities that constitute the tasks: They can be scored "right" or "wrong." Western psychologists who work in a tradition of quantitative assessment of psychological processes find it easy to standardize the application. Although, in fact, the "clinical" aspect of the concrete-operational tasks is fundamental to interpreting responses, the complex interaction required by Piaget tends to drop out of many cross-cultural analyses (cf. Kamara, 1971; Nyiti, 1973).

Population samples from other cultures have been found to achieve concrete operations sooner than, at the same time as, or later than European and American samples. In some studies a significant proportion of adults has failed to achieve concrete operations. A variety of explanations, which we will discuss shortly, have been offered to account for these results.

Formal operations. Piaget (1972) characterizes the thinking process of young children as "concrete"-operational because it relies on the actual manipulation of objects and events in the immediately present context. Formal operations are not tied to reality in the same way. They enable the adolescent to reason in terms of verbally stated hypotheses.

A second difference between concrete operations and formal operations results from the development of a new organization of cognitive structures. Whereas the concrete-operational child reasons from one element to the next, with no overall structure for representing relationships, formal-operational adolescents are able to consider systematically the complete set of possibilities.

Genevan adolescents were found to reach the 75% success criterion for each of the substages between 11 and 15 years of age. That is a rare, high level of success.

Although Inhelder and Piaget (1958) used 15 different formal tasks, attempts to assess the presence or absence of formal operations typically use a single task and draw inferences about the whole mental organization of the mind on the basis of this single task. Neimark's (1975) review of these studies reports a consensus that the level of performance is lower in other cultures than the level reported for comparable ages in Geneva. The older cross-cultural research generally failed to find evidence of formal-operational thought among nonschooled, non-Western populations. Recently there has been some evidence for the existence of formal-operational thought in non-Western, schooled populations. Za'rour and Khuri (1977) found evidence of a shift from concrete performance to formal-operational performance on time–distance problems in Jordanian children at about 13 years of age. Saxe (1979) also documented the presence of formal operations in a population of schooled children from Papua, New Guinea. His work represents a break from other studies of formal operations in exotic cultures because he utilized an *indigenous* knowledge system, the birth-order system. Saxe explored the development of the ability to coordinate two reference systems and to generate the possible or hypothetical combinations of birth orders in a family (combinatory logic). He found evidence of a shift from concrete to formal understandings between the ages of 13 and 19.

Jahoda (1980) presents an especially helpful discussion of the implications of the formal-operations cross-cultural research. Citing evidence from the informal reports of explorers and the more formal reports of anthropologists, Jahoda illustrates behaviors that apparently require formal-operational thinking among people who have not manifested such thinking in experimental settings. Jahoda's central conclusion is that Piaget's reliance on actions in the physical world is a "bias that may be unjustified, resulting in a misclassification of subjects in traditional societies whose logic gets the main chance to manifest itself in verbal behavior in the social domain" (p. 119).

Jahoda's suggestion and the possibility of domain-specific stage acquisition are two major directions that research on culture and cognitive development have been taking. These themes will recur frequently in the remaining discussion.

WITHIN-STAGES VARIABILITY

In addition to variability in the age at which children from different cultural groups attain one or another of the global Piagetian stages, there is variability to be accounted for in the manifestation of stage-appropriate behavior *within* stages. Within a Piagetian framework, this kind of variability has traditionally been referred to as *horizontal decalage*. Among Genevan children, for example, there is an ordering of the acquisition of conservation that begins with conservation of quantity, then moves to conservation of weight, then to volume.

Strictly speaking, studies of horizontal decalage are not motivated by Piaget's theory, because he does not predict within-stages sequences of concept acquisition. They have been of interest to Piagetians partially because they are not properly incorporated into the theory and because obvious lines of accommodation of facts to theory suggest ways in which experience might influence development.

The cross-cultural evidence with respect to invariance of within-stages concept acquisitions is ambiguous. Early studies found the order of conservation of quantity, weight, and volume to be consistent with Piaget's description among Iranians (Mosheni, 1966), Sicilians (Peluffo, 1967), and Chinese (Goodnow, 1962). Dasen (1970, 1972), Boonsong (1968), and Prince (1968, 1969) found these concepts all developing at the same time, and Bovet (1974) and Otaala (1971) found different sequences of within-stages operational development in their samples. Dempsey (1971), using different cultural groups in the United States, found differing decalage among them on time-conservation tasks. Kelly (1977) found effects of schooling on decalage among conservation tasks with New Guinea children.[7]

Piagetian treatments of variability. Evaluating the mounting evidence of both variability in the age at which various "universal" cognitive operations were achieved and within-stages variability connected with the specific materials being manipulated, Piaget (1972) offered three global courses that an explanation of performance variability might take.

First, "different speeds [might] be due to the quality and frequency of intellectual stimulation received from adults or obtained from the possibilities available to children in their environment" (Piaget, 1972, p. 7). Second, formal operations might be not the expression of a universal stage, but a form of cognitive specialization (in the manner of an aptitude) that permits certain individuals to penetrate particular domains of experience more deeply than others. The third possibility, which Piaget favored, was that all individuals reach a universal stage of formal operations, but that formal operations are acquired first (and perhaps only) in fields of adult specialization or in connection with special aptitudes.

None of these possibilities was pursued by Piaget himself, and it is not entirely clear how "aptitude" as a theoretical entity should enter Piagetian theory. However, a number of investigators have been attempting to reconcile Piagetian theory with the evidence that differences in cultural experience underlie developmental delays in performance on Piagetian tasks. In some cases this reconciliation seeks to explain away the performance differences as the result of experimental artifact; in others the theory is modified to accommodate the data.

The most traditional approach to this set of problems is to claim that reported cultural differences in cognitive achievement are the result of methodological artifacts: *Real* cognitive development is universal; psychologists simply get a mistaken impression of their subjects' competence because of the specific assessment activities that they depend upon.

This conclusion was suggested by Kamara and Easley (1977) and Nyiti (1976). Their investigations used as the experimenter a native speaker who was also a psychologist trained in clinical interviewing. The developmental curves of these results approximate European norms. Unhappily for the theory, these studies did not manipulate the factors of language and cultural membership of the experimenter. There has been enough variability in previous between-studies comparisons to make it unlikely that these factors alone are sufficient to account for many of the cultural differences that have been reported (e.g., in Dasen, 1977).

However, there is no doubt that features of the interactions involved in assessing Piagetian development can materially affect the results. For example, Irvine (1978) sought to reevaluate the difficulties reported for Greenfield's Wolof (Senegalese) subjects who were asked to deal with a conservation-of-liquids problem. As a part of her assessment, Irvine asked subjects to play the role of an informant whose job it was to clarify *for the experimenter* the Wolof terms for resemblance and equivalence. When confronted with the typical Piagetian conflict situation, Irvine's "linguistic informants" gave the "wrong" response: The beaker with water higher on its sides was said to contain more liquid. However, in their role as linguistic informants, these same subjects went on to explain that while the level of the water was "more" the quantity was the same. In her 1966 study, Greenfield herself had noted that conservation was achieved if the children poured the liquids themselves, a finding which suggested that the European-based procedure was eliciting an irrelevant interpretation of the task.[8]

A closely related interpretation of culturally linked performance differences on

Piagetian tasks invokes the distinction between cognitive competence and cognitive performance. Dasen (1977) introduced this distinction into the cross-cultural Piagetian literature, drawing upon a formulation offered earlier by Flavell and Wohlwill (1969). Flavell and Wohlwill had suggested that the correct response to a Piagetian task should be considered a joint product of the probability that the child has acquired the operational structure and the probability that the relevant task-specific knowledge is applied. To this, Dasen added a third factor identified with cultural factors affecting the probability that the proper knowledge would be brought to bear in "a given cultural milieu."

A major strategy offered by Dasen and his colleagues to address the competence–performance distinction is the conducting of training studies, the procedures of which embody a Piagetian theory of the interactions necessary to produce development. For example, Dasen, Lavallee, and Reschitzki (1979) conducted a training study with a large number of Baoule (Ivory Coast) children, to determine both changes in level of responding to the training task and transfer of training to a variety of other problems requiring the same operations. The central goal in this research was to determine if training occurred rapidly and to the hypothetically maximum level. Very rapid and marked effects of training were taken as evidence that the underlying competence existed, but its expression was inhibited. Training in this case was believed to act on the relevant performance factors. Slow learning was interpreted as evidence that the essential competence was initially absent, but was instilled by the training. In this study, Dasen and his associates obtained evidence for learning during the training sessions; the level of performance improved between pre- and posttests. But change was slow enough to fit best the notion that training actually changed the basic competence of the subjects, instead of "triggering" an already existing competence. This newly acquired competence transferred to the other appropriate operational tasks. In other studies, change was rapid enough to implicate performance factors; in still other cases, training was not completely successful (see Dasen, Ngini, & Lavallee, 1979).

Dasen (1974, 1977) has sought to provide the most systematic account of performance variability within the overall eco-cultural framework summarized in Figure 11.1. Acknowledging the need for methodological rigor in the conduct of studies, Dasen has continued to assume that there are real developmental differences associated with special cultural experience. However, in order to make theory and data fit, he has to follow that line of Piaget's speculations which relaxed assumptions about the uniformity of developmental levels. (See Dasen, Berry, & Witkin, 1979, for the most extreme statement of this viewpoint.) Working with two groups of Australian aborigines who differed in the degree of contact they maintained with Euro-Australian culture, Dasen (1974) contrasted performance for two classes of concrete-operational tasks. He presented three tasks designed to sample spatial thinking, on the grounds that traditional aborigine culture depends heavily for its survival on the ability to orient in space using cues deemed subtle and obscure to strangers. These spatial tasks were contrasted with standard conservation-of-number, -quantity, -volume, and -length and seriation tasks, in which, according to the theory, "logico-mathematical" concepts dominate. Dasen cites reports that aborigine numerical concepts are few and seldom used to motivate the hypothesis that tasks embodying such concepts will be learned more slowly by aborigines than spatial tasks, for which the aborigines have dense practice and cultural aids. On the basis of prior evidence, Dasen predicts the opposite relation among tasks for the European population tested.

The results of this study confirmed differences in both the age of acquisition of general stages and differences between cognitive domains in the direction Dasen predicted. European contact increased performance of the aborigine populations for the logico-mathematical tasks, and the aborigines found those problems relatively more difficult than the spatial tasks. Linking within-stages performance variations to environmental variations is an important extension of Piagetian research. In recent years, Dasen has systematically explored a variety of strategies for bringing the European-based theory into line with cross-cultural research while maintaining its basic thrust (see Dasen, 1980, for a recent overview).

IMPLICATIONS FOR UNDERSTANDING CULTURE AND INTELLIGENCE

The implications of cross-cultural Piagetian work for theories of culture and intelligence are difficult to spell out, because one's interpretation of culture–intelligence relations will depend heavily on decisions about what general interpretation one gives to the cross-cultural evidence, and that will depend upon what set of assertions is adopted as *the* theory (and also upon relevant evidence).

From "classical" Piagetian writings (such as *The Psychology of Intelligence,* 1973), it is clear that Piaget defines intelligence in terms of his overall theory of development, for which he contends that he has established an identifiable hierarchy of logically embedded relations, from sensorimotor to logicomathematical. The processes of reciprocal transformation between organism and environment *are* intelligence for Piaget. Within this framework, comparisons of intelligence are straightforward; it is the rules for assessing the applicability of the framework that are in dispute. People who advance further in the hierarchy of developmental levels (in effect, people who penetrate deeper into that theory of the world embodied in European physical science) are more intelligent than people who operate on the world in accordance with a lower level of operations.

The first issue, of course, is to determine if there are nonartifactual cultural differences in rate of cognitive development. With the exception of those who maintain that all such variability is artifactual (e.g., Kamara & Easley, 1977), the general consensus seems to be that cultural differences in development (as defined by Piaget) are real. Feldman and Stone (1978), for example, offer a series of experiments using a colored-blocks test (CBT) "designed to tap the central cognitive abilities associated with each of the major periods of intellectual development. . . . The CBT is a single test battery appropriate for a wide range of ages. It makes use of substantially identical materials and the same test format" (p. 5). Adding the claim that these test materials and formats are familiar across cultures is all one needs to arrive at the Piagetian equivalent of a culture-free intelligence test. Feldman and Stone do not make this strong argument, and they note especially the reticence of the Hawaiian children they studied. However, they do claim to have a useful cross-cultural testing device; so their work stands as a reasonable example of studies within the classical Piagetian tradition. They also observed differences between the populations contrasted (urban Chicago, rural Hawaii); even from a classical position, cross-cultural differences in development (or intelligence) must be accounted for.

In making such comparisons, it must be assumed that for cultures that fall within the classical framework, the explanation of such differences is provided in a general way by Piaget: It must be assumed that cultures that provide for more operational exercise will produce more intelligent members, because such people will progress further in the hierarchy of stages.

The relative simplicity of this viewpoint may be its strongest feature. It permits one to abstract highly specialized interactional patterns from the endless particulars of everyday life (such as a conservation problem) that can be used across cultures in a uniform manner (on the assumption that such interactions are universal in the species). Each such task embodying a universal cognitive operation is representative of the particulars; so one can assume that pervasive stages are being tapped. Finally, one knows where to intervene if cultural differences in intelligence (development) are observed: Look to the amount of relevant operational exercise, and increase it if the culture does not do so spontaneously.

There are, of course, many objections to this course of action, as we have shown in our prior discussions. It is probably worth reporting, however, that even operating as if standard, competently executed Piagetian tests measured intelligence, there is evidence that this intelligence is *not* what intelligence tests measure, and it is not predictive of performance in the schools of Third World peoples. For example, Heron (1971) failed to find a correlation between Piagetian logico-mathematical performance and school performance for subjects that hypothetically required the same kinds of knowledge. This finding would not particularly bother Piaget, who evidences no great love for the manner in which problem-solving activities are organized in schools (Piaget, 1935/1970). But it does pose a problem for those who wish to construct a universally valid theory of intelligence for which there is a universally valid set of tests. Advance in school presumes mastery of precisely that domain of knowledge (Euro-American science) which is the source of hierarchy in Piaget's theory. Perhaps because there are so many problems associated with it, on both empirical and theoretical grounds, the classical formulation of Piagetian theory is probably not a useful one to employ as the standard against which to judge this approach to culture and cognition. However, alternatives are not without their difficulties.

If one acknowledges some kind of competence–performance distinction in cross-cultural Piagetian problem-solving studies, the general logic applied to the classical theory remains. It becomes the investigator's duty "simply" to make clear whether his or her dependent variables reflect competence, which, being universal and accessible to measurement, becomes the standard for comparison. The quotation marks around *simply* in the previous sentence indicate, of course, that it is time-consuming to make the additional observations necessary to sustain a competence–performance distinction, so that the investigator needs to construct a new kind of testing procedure within which the distinction attains consistent meaning. Considering the complexities of the training procedures used by Dasen to warrant competence–performance distinctions, this line of work faces formidable obstacles. (We might note, parenthetically, that Dasen's procedural approach to assessing levels of cognitive development bears a strong family relation to Vygotsky's early notations of ways to measure intelligence, e.g., Vygotsky, 1934/1978.)

A quite different set of difficulties for comparative judgments of intelligence arises if one takes as the working model the most recent writings by Piaget on the domain-specificity of cognitive achievements (e.g., Piaget, 1972; Dasen's relativist interpretation of Piagetian cognitive development, Dasen, 1977; Dasen, Berry, & Witkin, 1979). Because this line of reasoning has not been well developed within Piagetian theory and because it will form the basis for an alternative framework for understanding culture, intelligence, and development, we will postpone further discussion of modified Piagetian theory until the remaining alternative framework has been explored.

11.6. REEXAMINING BASIC ASSUMPTIONS

As outlined in previous sections, the dominant theories relating culture to cognitive development have sought to account for broad regularities in psychological functioning. For Piaget, these regularities find expression in stages of development that characterize qualitatively distinct modes of interaction between person and environment. For psychological-differentiation theorists, a limited number of global styles are hypothesized to control the quantity and quality of problem solving in different behavioral domains.

This central processor approach was diagrammed schematically in Figure 11.2. In applications of this approach, we saw how a variety of ecological conditions and child-rearing experiences may serve to foster field-independence or field-dependence (as in Witkin & Berry, 1975) or level of cognitive development (Piagetian tradition) or the sophistication of schemata (Kagan, Kearsley, & Zelazo, 1978). This kind of formulation provides a scale on which to rank individuals and cultures because it provides a *general* characterization of mental functioning, consistent with the properties of the central processing mechanism that experiences of the right kind promote.

The great strength of the central processor approach is that it brings order out of a welter of details. It is by no means obvious that the sequences of behaviors describing the problem solving of children in the Arctic Circle, Chicago and Hawaii should be the same (Feldman & Stone, 1978). It cannot be considered self-evident that men from the Mende tribe of Sierra Leone would be more proficient in picking geometric figures from an embedded-figures test or in matching Kohs blocks than their neighbors, the Temne (Berry, 1966, p. 229). Nor would we necessarily expect people who are good at picking out embedded figures to be relatively insensitive to their position in space when judging lines as upright. When such behavioral patterns are found in a far-off human group, and when it is further shown (as theoretically predicted) that the behavior patterns in question are related to child-rearing or economic practices, the theories are scientifically useful tools for understanding the conditions that promote global configurations of intellectual functioning.

As theories designed to explain uniformities across broad ranges of behavioral functioning, these approaches face a common problem; they find it difficult to account for variability within the stages or styles whose uniformity is a basic assumption. In each case, behavioral variability is accounted for by secondary mechanisms, either in the form of quasi-theoretical principles, such as horizontal decalage, or as methodological problems, such as the influence of stimulus familiarity on thinking *within* cognitive domains.

We have reviewed briefly efforts within a Piagetian framework to deal with such unwanted behavioral variability, for example, Dasen's invocation of a competence–performance distinction and his use of training studies as a means of

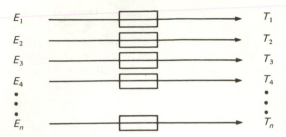

Figure 11.3.   The specific learning model.

reconciling a universalistic theory with variable data. Witkin, too, recognized the problem when he emphasized that factors controlling cognitive style are only part of what must be accounted for in obtaining evidence of interdomain consistency.[9]

Rather than pursue this discussion as a critique of existing theories, we propose in the remainder of this chapter to explore an alternative formulation of the same problems, a formulation that retains the basic eco-cultural framework, but rejects the central processor assumption as the organizing metaphor for culture's effect on cognition. Instead, we will advocate turning the Piagetian approach on its head; we will assume that learning is *context-specific,* so that context-specific intellectual achievements are the *primary* basis for cognitive development. We will not deny intercontextual generality of behavior, which must be accounted for. Rather, intercontextual generality will be treated as a secondary phenomenon, in which the cultural organization of experience plays a major role.

The idea that a theory of cognitive development powerful enough to handle major Piagetian phenomena could be built in such a "bottom-up" fashion is not original with us. It is to be found in early Soviet challenges to Piaget (see Zaporozhets, 1939/1980, for an early statement) and in contemporary research in cognitive development, which we review presently in an abbreviated manner. We came to these ideas through our own attempts to deal with behavioral variability in cross-cultural research (e.g., Cole, Gay, Glick, & Sharp, 1971).

The basic thrust of this approach is diagrammed in Figure 11.3, which is designed to contrast with Figure 11.2. Like central processor approaches, the framework schematized in Figure 11.3 also seeks to link experiences (E_n) to task performance (T_n). But in this case, there is no "central processor" or general ability intervening between the experiences we have called events and tasks. This does not imply that there is no organism mediating between events at one time (E_n) and events at another (T_n). Rather, the general framework assumes that learning is *predominantly* event- or context-specific. The extent to which learning in one context controls performance in another will depend upon (a) what the person learns on the basis of experience in the first context, (b) the similarity between the two events, and (c) the activity of other people in the second context. Generalized response tendencies derive from common features shared by the current task (T_n) and prior contexts (E_n). Without subscribing to an associationist theory of learning, we are adopting a position championed 75 years ago by Thorndike when he insisted that the extent to which learning in one setting transfers to learning and performance in others depends upon the similarity between settings. Like

Thorndike (1931), we find little virtue in believing that transfer can be provided by "mental exercise." The central processor approach treats transfer very much in this latter tradition. We will term our alternative approach a *cultural practice* framework, for reasons that will become apparent presently.

11.7. CONTEXT-SPECIFIC APPROACHES

In case it is necessary, let us hasten to acknowledge that, as sketched in Figure 11.3, our framework is absurdly underspecified. We present no characterization of the tasks, no characterization of how to identify what is learned, no theory of similarity between learning contexts and performance contexts (E_n and T_n), and no way to account for the obvious generalized competencies that are the bread and butter of cross-cultural cognitive research. This skeleton of a framework is no competitor for the masses of data and associated theory represented by the approaches we have just reviewed.

In the material that follows, we will attempt to fill in enough raw material to make a cultural practice approach seem plausible as an alternative to existing theory. We will begin by presenting examples of concrete research that challenge the central processor model already discussed and that provide a starting point for the formation of a cultural practice approach. With these data as background, we will then return to our theoretical framework in an attempt to show what it needs to accomplish in order to become a real alternative to existing theories.

11.8. CONTEXT SPECIFICITY AND CULTURAL DIFFERENCES

INFANCY

All of the measurement problems and assumptions about the generalized nature of developmental patterns can be seen in the earliest assessments of infants, particularly in comparisons between infants in different cultural settings. A number of different assessment techniques (Bayley's motor and mental development scales, 1965; the Neonatal Behavior Assessment Scale developed by Brazelton (1973); Gesell Scales, by Gesell & Amatruda, 1947) sample the behavior of the infant to arrive at a general measure of both mental and motor development (Bayley, 1965; Gesell & Amatruda, 1947). One infant is said to be more mature or advanced than another if he or she receives higher scores on these scales. In cross-cultural comparisons, one group of infants is said to be more mature or advanced if its mean scores on these scales are higher. Such evaluations have led some researchers to claim an early, general precocity in the mental and motor development of infants from sub-Saharan Africa (Geber, 1956, 1958, 1961, 1974; Geber & Dean, 1957, 1958; for a review, see Dasen, 1972; Super, 1981; Wober, 1975). Though it is claimed that infants in Africa have a head start in development during their first year, they are also found to drop below Western standards in their second or third year.

Super reviews the cross-cultural comparisons of infant development based on infant-development scales. Contrary to the accepted wisdom, he finds no reliable corroboration of claims for neurological precocity in African newborns (Super, 1981), and he objects to the use of such general terms as *maturity* or *precocity* to characterize differences in developmental patterns. Although infants from different racial groups have different characteristics at birth, and differences in patterns of development, there is no evidence to justify claims of different levels of general maturity in either mental or motor development for different cultural groups.

Super entreats the reader to consider carefully the relationship between the specific items used on scales of development and the cultural system in which they are embedded. For example, in one review of the "infant-scale" literature, Super (1976) finds reliable evidence that sub-Saharan African infants sit and walk earlier than do their U.S. and European counterparts (despite many uncertainties in the individual studies). To support his claim that these differences are specific ones, Super investigates the functional tie between these behavior patterns and their cultural organization. Using spot observations[10] of East African mothers and infants, as well as interviews with the mothers, Super reports a self-conscious effort to teach babies to sit and walk. Within Kipsigi (Kenyan) and other African cultures, there are standard procedures for this instruction and particular words in the language for characterizing this process. Super observed mothers teaching their babies to sit. The babies are placed in a hole in the ground with blankets rolled up to provide support. Infants are left in this "sitting" position long before they are able to sit on their own. When asked what they were doing on such occasions, the mothers explained that they were teaching their children to sit, confirming the deliberate nature of the event. Spot observations showed that the Kenyan infants are in a sitting position two-thirds again as often as infants of comparable age in Cambridge, Massachusetts.

As early as the infant's second month of life, Kpsigi mothers attempt to teach walking skills by holding the infant's arms and encouraging him or her to jump. This particular behavioral practice is very similar to the test item found on the Bayley motor scales that is used to indicate readiness to walk.

In summarizing his findings, as well as the research of others, Super concludes that African infants are only more advanced in those behaviors that are (a) specifically taught or (b) encouraged through the provision of opportunities for practice or (c) both. The early advancement of particular motor milestones does *not* mean that other behaviors are also advanced. For example, the group of infants who were found to sit and walk early were found to crawl several weeks *later* than the norms established by U.S. infants. This behavioral outcome is connected with the fact that Kpsigi infants spent only a third as much time on the ground as infants in Cambridge did.

The attitudes of the parents, the relative importance of a particular behavior, and the amount of time that infants were left in a position that afforded opportunities for practice were the reliable predictors of the onset of particular motor milestones, a finding which supports the idea that variation in infant behavior is a reflection of variation in the caretaking environment. It may appear to be general if scores from many subtests are aggregated, but such a procedure serves only to mask the important functional antecedents of specific acquisitions.

Super and Harkness (1980) have continued this analysis of the relationship between the infant's behavior and the immediate social environment. They term the behavior-support system the infant's *niche*. This niche is structured by (a) biological needs, (b) social and physical constraints operating on the infant, and

(c) the cultural needs or constraints operating on the social group of which the infant is a member. Economic activities, social and family structure, the physical ecology, and the values of the caretakers (coded in their language and belief systems) all structure the environment. Cultural differences in the structuring of practice are responsible for cultural differences in patterns of development. Such differences in cultural practice may totally change the significance of "developmental indicators."

To demonstrate this point, Super and Harkness provide a detailed comparison of the sleep–awake cycles in infants in rural Kenya and the urban United States. The length of the infant's longest sleep period (occurring most often during the night hours) is an accepted behavioral index of the neurological maturity of the brain. By the third or fourth month, American infants who are developing normally are expected to have maximum sleep periods that last on the average 8 hours. Another assumption about the normal pattern of infant development is that, as the infant becomes more mature, fewer hours of sleep will be necessary. These developments in the infant's sleep–awake cycle have been assumed to be regulated by universal biological needs and not by cultural factors.

Sleep patterns for Kenyan and American babies are relatively similar during the first few months, but then consistent differences develop. By the fourth month, the Kokwet babies are awake, on the average, 2 hours more than the U.S. babies in any 24-hour period. Another change is that, between the third and fourth months of life, U.S. babies begin to concentrate their sleeping into fewer and longer bouts, so that the longest single period of sleep lasts on the average 8 hours and roughly coincides with the sleeping patterns of adults. This is not the case with the Kokwet sample. They continue to have maximum sleep periods of about 4 hours throughout their first year of life. These differences in sleep–awake patterns are paralleled with differences in adult structuring of the infants' experience. The caretaking patterns in Kenya are much different from those Americans consider normal. Babies are frequently carried in slings by the mother or some other family member. The productivity of the mother is independent of the sleep–awake cycle of the baby so long as the baby does not become too active, in which case carrying it in the sling is impossible. Babies sleep in skin-to-skin contact with their mothers, who sleep, except for the infant, alone. The mother's sleep pattern is only minimally disturbed by a baby who is awake or nursing.

The difference in environmental situations of these two cultural groups controls the amount of flexibility in the development of behaviors that are assumed to be determined by biological needs. This is not to claim that the child is completely malleable. Super and Harkness point out that the rate of sudden infant death syndrome increases dramatically during the third month in the United States, and this increase coincides with the change in sleep patterns from 4 to 8 hours. They do not claim that crib death is caused by these caretaking patterns, only that the change may well tax the limits of the infant's flexibility.

Cross-cultural assessments of infant mental development are similarly function-specific. In reviewing the studies of cultural variations in the assessment of infant mental development, Super (1981) concludes that, except for conditions of minimal stimulation and/or malnutrition, there is *no* cultural group that shows more rapid general cognitive development than another. The literature does, however, provide a number of examples of environmental influences on particular items.

In a longitudinal research project, in which the Kilbrides demonstrate an empirical correspondence between patterns of specific item precocity in Uganda infants and the culture's child-care practices (Kilbride & Kilbride, 1975), frequency of being in the supine position was related to early grasping and manipulative behaviors; frequency of being carried at shoulder level was correlated with performance on a task of visual skills; and cultural emphasis on early smiling and social behaviors was related to early smiling (see also Grantham-McGregor & Hawke, 1971; Leiderman, Tulkin, & Rosenfeld, 1977).

Although we realize that assessments of motor or mental development in infancy have not been found to correlate with scores on later intelligence scales, these examples have been provided to indicate the problems that are identical with attempts to measure mental abilities at a later age. If specific behavioral accomplishments are isolated and this performance is used to make general claims about the overall state of development, then individuals who have had the most opportunity to practice those skills and whose environment is organized so that those skills are highly prized accomplishments will be evaluated as more intelligent or more advanced than those for whom this is not the case.

Some authors seek general developmental influences linked to overall *levels* of stimulation provided by a culture (e.g., Kagan, Kearsley, & Zelazo, 1978). In our view, this position allows too much latitude for the theorist and too little specification (other than experimentally induced levels of discrepancy) of how culture causes behavioral change. We will discuss the generality issue again in Section 11.9. For the moment, we wish to take the following lesson from the cross-cultural infant-development literature: Unless one can be assured that a particular behavioral skill has the same functional value within the cultural experiences of the individuals tested and that the individuals have had roughly the same opportunity to practice that skill, no inference about their general mental abilities is warranted. Regularities among behavioral patterns are viewed as reflections of regularities in cultural patterns. There are two points to these examples: (a) the importance of examining the relationship between specific skills and environmental pressures, and (b) the problem of generalizing from differences in sampled behaviors to differences in underlying general capacities.

PERCEPTUAL SKILLS

Past infancy, there are a number of studies that relate specific cognitive change to specific experience, where common wisdom has supposed differences to reflect an underlying general mental ability. One such example is provided by Serpell (1979). Just as the early literature suggested a general motor precocity in African infants, a sizable body of literature suggested that African tribal children perform less well than European or American subjects of similar age when asked to represent an object or pattern using either pen and paper or block designs. Performance on these tasks is often interpreted as indexing the presence or absence of general cognitive abilities (differences in "practical intelligence" [Vernon, 1969]; "cognitive style" [Witkin & Berry, 1975]; "attitudes toward perception" [McFie, 1961]; "Sensotypes" [Wober, 1966]; "imagined transformations" [Goodnow, 1969]; and "response organizations" [Serpell, 1969]).

These *general characterizations of mental ability* are then commonly related to *general environmental contingencies*. Vernon (1969) suggests that retarded practical intelligence is the result of inadequate psychomotor experience and the absence of constructive play or cultural pressures to practical achievements. As we have already mentioned, Witkin and Berry (1975) attribute the field-dependent cognitive style to a complex of environmental relationships, particularly to using strict socialization practices to enforce this conformance and also by tight social organization. McFie (1961) suggests that lack of toys and construction games that encourage accurate standards of orientation and imitation are the cause of these perceptual differences. These studies serve as examples of the way in which central processor approaches use performance on a particular test or set of tests to serve as an index of an intellectual ability – in this case, perception – and then relate this capacity to general aspects of the ecological-social conditions.

Suspicious of such inferences, Serpell (1979) designed a study to distinguish between generalized interpretations and more specific accounts. He selected four perceptual tasks that, according to a general process interpretation, should result in lower performance scores for Zambian than for English children. One required the child to copy the positions of the experimenter's hands (mimicry), the second required the child to copy two-dimensional figures with pen and paper (drawing), the third required him or her to construct two-dimensional wire objects with strips of wire (molding), and the fourth involved making copies of three-dimensional objects from clay (modeling). Serpell chose precisely these four tasks because he knew something about the prior experiences of each of the cultural groups on the specific tasks; he based his predictions concerning patterns of cultural differences on a function-specific culture–cognition hypothesis.

Because skill learning in any culture requires children to attend to and imitate the hand positions of the more competent members, both groups of children should do equally well on the mimicry. Children in both cultures also had experience modeling with clay (or plasticine); so no differences were expected. Two-dimensional representation with pen and paper is an activity that English children have encountered frequently in their school experience, whereas Zambian children have had more practice molding wire into two-dimensional objects. Therefore, Serpell predicted that the English children would score high on the pen-and-paper task, but not as high on the wire-shaping task. For the Zambian children, he made the opposite prediction.

Serpell also wanted to investigate a claim by Wober that African subjects process information from different senses in ways that are different from Europeans'. For both groups of children, he established a "visual" condition and a blindfolded or "haptic" condition. According to Wober, the Africans should do better in the haptic condition, whereas Europeans should do better in the visual condition. The major comparisons were drawn between 8-year-olds in the second grade in Zambian and English primary schools.

The findings confirm the specific experience hypothesis and present evidence that is difficult to interpret from a general, perceptual-deficit approach. The English children did better than the Zambian children in the drawing task and the Zambian children did better in the wire-molding task, as was predicted on the basis of Serpell's analysis of their prior experiences. There were no significant differences between the groups on the clay-modeling or hand-mimicry tasks. The modality of the task, visual or haptic, did not result in any differences between the cultural groups. Each group performed better in the visual condition, contrary to a sensotype interpretation.

LEARNING AND PROBLEM SOLVING

A great variety of problem-solving and learning tasks derived from American and European studies of cognition and cognitive development have been used in cross-cultural research. Where such studies have been restricted to new replications of procedures used in the source culture, the results are virtually uninterpretable in terms of causal, cultural factors (particularly when a single "test instrument" is used) (for excellent discussions, see Campbell, 1964; Price-Williams, 1975; Shweder, 1979a, 1979b). However, where the researcher uses multiple conditions of problem presentation, especially when those conditions are chosen because of a specific, prior hypothesis about cultural influences, the issue of context-specificity or generality of performance can often be evaluated.

In this section, we will review a selected cross-section of research that permits some evaluation of the specificity or generality of cognitive differences associated with cultural differences.

IQ-test studies. As in the infant literature, tests of mental ability designed to tap universal cognitive skills have been prominent in cross-cultural problem-solving work. An early, but seldom discussed, study by Nissen, Machover, and Kinder (1935) is interesting as an example of the early use of an IQ test that was related to cultural differences by claims that clusters of subtests related *differentially* to performance. Although overall performance was sufficiently low to warrant the conclusion (based on American norms) that the investigators' West African subjects were incapable of "managing their affairs with ordinary prudence" (p. 346), the unevenness of performance on different subtests (to say nothing of observations from common interactions) led Nissen and his associates to conclude that "as the content and activities involved in each [subtest] correspond more to specialized experience in a civilized environment, they provide greater difficulties for our culturally primitive subjects. Conversely, as the content and activities involved in each correspond more to the common matrix of universal experience they provide less difficulty for our subjects" (p. 338).

Naturally, because none of the subtests were designed on the basis of West African experiences, there were no data to demonstrate a reversal of difficulty in which the "primitive" subjects might outperform their "civilized" brethren.

In a recent review of 91 cross-cultural studies using factor analysis to uncover general clusters of ability, Irvine (1978) found "six comprehensive broad-spectrum groupings . . . : *reasoning, verbal abilities and skills, spatial/perceptual processes, numerical observations, memory functions, and physical/temperamental quickness*" (p. 315).

Irvine, one of the most sophisticated and thorough cross-cultural psychologists using IQ tests as a technique for linking culture and cognition, is quite measured in his claims for utility:

Cross-cultural factor analyses show that psychologists can measure consistently individual differences in cognition along several broad dimensions. The analyses also show that the definition of these dimensions is by no means complete and that reasons for the correlation or lack of it among factors are difficult to come by. The problems that faced early theorists have not been solved by a lateral arabesque through other cultures. They have simply appeared once again. [P. 326]

He urges expansion of tests' theoretical utility by combining (a) IQ tests; (b) experimental cognitive methodology in the manner reviewed by Estes and others in this handbook; and (c) systematic investigation of cultural independent variables.

As might be anticipated from our earlier discussion, we find continual reliance on IQ methodology, even when elaborated in an experimental direction, extremely limited. A key difference between our view and Irvine's can be seen in his use of the term *broad dimensions* of cognition as a marker of the generality of test results. These dimensions reflect patterns of correlation among cognitive tasks, all of which share the characteristics of Binet's early sampling procedures. The "dimensions" referred to are cognitive process names. No evidence of the breadth of contexts represented by the behavior samples used in tests to represent broad dimensions of mind are offered, nor is a *cultural* theory of intelligence.

A persistent question in this cross-cultural research is the extent to which there are universal conceptions of what intelligence is, regardless of the specific cultural content of activity. In effect, such research seeks to establish common dimensions for both a French and a Western African Binet (in terms of our early examples). When specific efforts have been made to determine if the dimensions of mind arrived at from IQ tests match the conception of IQ arrived at by traditional, nonliterate peoples, the results have been ambiguous.

An early study by Klein, Freeman, and Millet (1973) provided evidence that traditional people judge intelligence much as do test constructors and the American person-on-the-street. They had formed the impression that adult members of the isolated Guatemalan village where they were working made judgments about children's abilities that bore some relation to North American notions of intelligence. In interviews with several adults, they found that the Spanish term *listura* seemed to be an appropriate gloss of *intelligent,* so they asked a number of villagers to rank 7-year-old boys of their acquaintance in terms of *listura*. The average *listura* ratings were correlated with performance on a number of psychological tests designed to measure intelligence in North American populations. Correlations varied from test to test, from a low of .11 to a high of .75 (which was statistically significant), leading the authors to conclude that they had preliminary evidence for "uniform" characteristics of cognitive competence across cultures.

Nerlove, Roberts, Klein, Yarbrough, and Habicht (1974) extended this line of work by seeking "natural indicators" of intelligent behavior leading to judgments of *listura* that would correspond to the "formal" indicators derived from psychological tests. Using the method of spot observations, in which children are observed at selected intervals of the day, they divided all work and play activities into those involving "self-managed sequences" – those which, they believed, require the children to engage in behaviors also required by tests of analytic ability. They obtained significant correlations between ratings of self-managed behavior and test performance, which led them to conclude that such indicators could form the basis for tests of intelligence valid across cultures.

In a quite different part of the world, Dube (1977) studied Botswanian categories related to our conceptions of intelligent behavior. He related Botswanian conceptions to recall ability on specially constructed story materials.

Dube succeeded in showing that ratings of intelligence in a traditional culture related to recall of stories: The higher the rated intelligence, the better the recall. Two other of Dube's results are of interest. First, the same relationship was found between rated intelligence and memory performance in nonliterate groups (where the criterion was grades in school). Second, the African subjects outperformed American subjects on this task (see also Ross & Millsom, 1968).

Both Dube and Nerlove and his associates explain these results by assuming that adults have had many opportunities to judge children's performance across a wide variety of tasks, so that natural indicators, whether arrived at formally or informally, yield a measure of competence that is not bound to any particular task.

Before discussing the possible implications of such findings, we need to consider the strength of the evidence that this research provides. As Serpell (1977) points out, there are ambiguities that need to be dealt with. Correlational studies such as that conducted by Klein and his co-workers (1973), in which the investigators first attempt to find the local equivalent of *intelligence,* are especially troublesome when correlations between ratings are variable (as they are); how are we to explain such variability when the dependent variables are presumably interchangeable indexes of a single, unitary ability? And even where correlations are substantial, we cannot be certain of their meaning, because the bilingual informants who assist in choosing the appropriate local gloss may be doing no more than choosing the word that singles out behaviors appropriate to Western tests.

Dube's results appear to demonstrate that a characteristic of people identified as intelligent, which is said to accord well with North American folk theories about intelligence, is memory for stories. A key part of his logic is the demonstration that memory ability is not a part of the definition of intelligence, or he would merely be showing that people who are judged to remember well remember stories well. Although it appears that he has accomplished this aim in that part of his study in which elders described the criteria for characterizing a person as intelligent, Dube himself is not certain that he has really made the proper separation. When school grades are used as a definition, there are obvious doubts about the separability of "intelligence in general" and "ability to remember things" in particular. But these doubts extend back to the traditional, nonliterate subjects:

Wisdom seems to be an important defining characteristic of the non-literate Botswan's view of "intelligence." Memory, however, does not seem to be, even though it is mentioned in all those words which seem to define "intelligence" among these people. One possible reason for this poor showing by "memory" is probably that "memory" might be [so] taken for granted by these people as a defining concept of "intelligence" that they probably did not see the need to mention it often. [Dube, 1977, p. 45]

In short, Dube's subjects may well have been identifying children on the basis of presumed memory abilities, and may have discovered that they remember better when asked to do so.

In addition to doubts about the basis for successful demonstrations of a link between primitive conceptions of intellectual acumen and American-based intellectual tasks, there are some important unsuccessful attempts to demonstrate such relations. Serpell (1977) reports a study in which he asked village elders to select children whom they would be likely to assign responsibilities for a wide variety of common chores and special, but accepted, tasks that arise in daily village life. These same adults were also asked to make direct judgments across the two tasks; children assigned more responsibility were judged more intelligent.

But different informants did not agree with each other about who should be assigned responsibility for which task; so no unified notion of intelligence emerged. One important cause for the discrepancy was that in this Zambian group, there was a strong emphasis on cooperation in the basic concept of intelligence, a finding which indicates that positive correlations obtained with standard test scores, even if obtainable, would have to be treated with extreme caution.

A different difficulty arose in Rogoff's (1977) work in Guatemala, where she attempted to follow the strategy of Nerlove and his associates (1974), using spot observations to measure differences in experience and culturally defined competence as predictors of visual and verbal memory ability. Not only did her spot observations fail to be correlated with performance, but she was unable to obtain such correlations when she attempted to combine individual categories into a category of "self-managed sequences." Whether her failure arose from an inability to replicate the creation of appropriate categories, or whether her dependent variables (recall tasks involving model recreations of familiar scenes) were not reasonable samples of intellectual behavior, is uncertain. What is certain is that this line of work remains fraught with ambiguity and uncertainty.

Despite ambiguities, we can discern the common logic underlying such attempts. Those who would come up with a culture-free set of natural indicators of intelligence are, in effect, following Piaget's lead in assuming that there is a common core of problem-solving situations that are a part of the complex interactions making up the cultural experience of any member of *Homo sapiens*. Insofar as these tasks are known to us and we depend upon others to help us fulfill them, we can build up an overall impression indicating who picks up new tasks quickly and effectively. We might expect, on this basis, that there would be quite good agreement across cultures concerning at least some aspects of human intellectual functioning, and there is evidence, shaky, but present nonetheless, to indicate that some degree of agreement on common criteria of intellectual competence does exist across cultures. However, as in the case of Piagetian theory, the amount of variability in ideas of intelligence associated with cultural variations in social organization and technological demands is very great indeed, and needs to be accounted for.

Other problem-solving studies. Here we will review selected cross-cultural studies of learning and problem solving that yield some idea of the variability that can be observed within the confines of relatively circumscribed experimental tasks. Instead of guessing at natural equivalents to the demands of intelligence tests and relying on correlational procedures, these studies attempt to vary the specific conditions that instantiate a particular set of task demands, seeking variations in performance that can be linked to variations in prior cultural experience.

Irwin and his colleagues (Irwin & McLaughlin, 1970; Irwin, Schafer, & Feiden, 1974) were skeptical of claims based on poor performance in sorting geometric shapes that unschooled Liberians (Mano) generally lack the ability to classify. Gay and Cole (1967) had attempted to create stimuli more culturally appropriate for people in a neighboring tribal group (the Vai) by using stylized drawings of culturally appropriate scenes. But their attempt at embodying a classification task with Vai content was unsuccessful. Examination of the cultural practices established that sorting rice is a center of Mano economic activity. Rice variations were talked about in everyday speech, and these distinctions could be used as the logical equivalent to the classification of geometric shapes. Two sets of tasks, one using bowls of rice and the other using geometric blocks, were presented to schooled and unschooled Liberians and to U.S. schooled subjects. Subjects had to categorize and, if possible, reclassify each set along three dimensions. Uneducated Liberian subjects, as past research indicated, had greater difficulty sorting geometric shapes than did Americans. The American subjects performed very well with these stimuli. But when the material to be sorted was changed to rice, the results were reversed. The African subjects were able to sort the rice, sifting dimensions and accounting for their sorts as skillfully as did the U.S. sample when the task involved geometric shapes. When U.S. children were faced with sorting bowls of rice, they demonstrated the same hesitation and bewilderment as the Africans displayed when faced with geometric shapes. Similar results have been obtained by Price-Williams (1962).

Other evidence of content specificity in classification, this time embodied in a communicative task, comes from the work of Lantz (1979). Lantz sought to evaluate the suggestion of Bruner, Olver, and Greenfield (1966) that rural unschooled children lack symbolic representational skills because their linguistic ability is tied to the immediate context of the referent. Formal education, they said, facilitates the development of language into a fully symbolic tool that can be used for communicating about things in their absence and for mediating other cognitive processes, such as classification and memory.

Lantz designed a study that would distinguish between the *absence* of symbolic representational skills and the *variable manifestations* of these skills. She selected a coding task to measure communicative accuracy as well as classificatory skills and memory. Children were shown an array of objects and asked to describe each item so that it could be distinguished from the others. They were told sometimes that they were describing stimuli for themselves (Condition 1) and sometimes that they were providing descriptions for another child to use at a later time (Condition 2). The subjects in this study were rural, unschooled and schooled Indian children and U.S. schoolchildren at three ages. Two stimulus arrays were used: a color array and a grain and seed array.

Lantz reasoned that although the Indian children have a complex color terminology, colors in their culture are more often substituted for one another with no functional consequence than is the case in the United States. Grains, on the other hand, are an extremely important part of the village life. Communication about them is significant in many contexts. Just the opposite relation between task content and culture is true for Americans.

As predicted from a context-specific perspective, the unschooled rural children coded and decoded the grain and seed array with no difficulty, performing at a higher level than either of the two schooled groups at all ages. The schooled rural children also scored significantly higher than the U.S. schooled children. This finding clearly shows that children from a nontechnical society without the benefit of formal schooling are able to separate language symbols from the physical referent and to use those symbols for communicating accurately in an artificial situation.

A very different pattern emerges for the results from the color array. The U.S. children scored significantly higher than both Indian groups. The unschooled Indian children did very poorly on this task. They were unable to decode even their own labels, let alone those produced by other children. The schooled Indian children did show higher performance on their own labels, a finding which indicates that some useful information could be coded, but their performance was poor relative to the U.S. sample.

This study shows that both groups were affected by the content of the stimulus materials. Communicative accuracy was closely related to the functional importance placed on making fine distinctions between the particular items used in one's prior cultural experiences. Here we also see that increased levels of schooling improve performance in a manner that appears task-specific, not generalized, contrary to explanations of a central processor variety (cf. Scribner & Cole, 1973).

There is also evidence to suggest that supposed *general* cultural differences in memory are far more specific than heretofore suspected. In considering this issue, it is important to keep in mind that almost all memory tasks that have been used are highly similar to the kinds of tasks that are required of children in school. When variations on the traditional memory tasks have been used, the differences are not as clear. Studies of the use of memory skills within various cultural settings indicate that traditional people often have excellent memories for spatial and visual information (Kearins, 1980; Kleinfeld, 1971; Meacham, 1975) and that some members within the traditional culture have excellent memories for narratives (Dube, 1977).

A series of studies by Cole and his associates (summarized in Cole & Scribner, 1974) demonstrates that matching the instantiation of standard cognitive tasks to locally organized activities cannot be restricted to the content of the objects or words to be manipulated. Many theoretically distinct features of memory tasks are important to performance and can serve as the focus of performance differences in cross-cultural comparisons. The crucial factor in this research was the extent to which the coherence or structure of the to-be-recalled materials was made manifest. It appears that the impact of schooling on a wide range of developmentally sensitive memory tasks occurs because schooling provides a great deal of practice in imposing structure on initially meaningless strings of words or objects. A crucial issue highlighted by this work is the need to understand how our theoretically motivated task fits into the overall structure of people's activities. Without such an ability to "locate" tasks in relation to culturally organized experience, we are greatly weakened in our ability to link cognitive performance and prior cultural practice.

In a test of culture-specific learning that hypothesized *nonliterate superiority,* Kearins (1980) designed a series of experiments specifically motivated by her educated guesses concerning special kinds of cultural practice.

The aboriginal inhabitants of the western desert region of Australia, like those of many other nonindustrial societies, have been shown to perform poorly on a number of standard psychology tests (Dasen, 1972; de Lemos, 1969; McElwain & Kearney, 1973). These measures of intellectual ability contrast with a long history of successful adaptation in a desert region that recent European settlers find uninhabitable. The reports of aborigine skill in "navigating" terrain perceived as featureless wastelands by Europeans are legion (e.g., Lewis, 1976). Kearins reasoned that requirements of survival in such an environment might result in the development of perceptual skills, particularly the ability to attend to small changes in spatial relationships.

In a series of experiments, she compared spatial memory strategies and skills of aboriginal Australian children with those of white Australian children. The children were shown a number of items arranged in matrices of different sizes. They were shown the display for 30 sec and then after a few seconds were asked to replace the items in the order in which they had been seen. She controlled for object familiarity by using two different types of materials: "natural" objects (a stone, leaves, a stick, etc.) and "artifactual" objects (a bottle, a knife, a matchbook). To test for differences in the use of verbal and visual strategies, in some displays Kearins combined objects that came from the same lexical category (i.e., rocks), but were varied in size and shape; other displays were made up of objects each from a different lexical category.

The aboriginal children were consistently better able to reproduce the display, regardless of the size of the matrix, the type of materials used, or the degree of similarity among the objects. In addition to better overall scores, significantly more aboriginal children had perfect scores on one or more of the displays. The white Australian children's best performance was on the artifactual display in which the objects all came from different lexical categories, but even on this task their score was significantly lower than that of the aboriginal group.

There were clear behavioral differences in the way each group approached and worked on the problem. Aboriginal children viewed the display in silence and, after stabilizing their position, sat motionless during the 30-sec observation period. When replacing the items, they tended to work at a constant rate, usually holding an item above a location before placing it and rarely moving objects after they had been placed. When asked how they remembered the display, their most frequent response was that they remembered the "look" of it.

The white Australian children were more likely to move around the display and pick up and point to objects, and they could be heard whispering, muttering, or naming objects. They moved about restlessly while waiting to replace the items and then generally replaced four or five immediately, and then the rest at a much slower rate. These children were also more likely to move objects around after they had been placed. Their accounts of their remembering suggest the use of verbal strategies: "'I tried to learn around the outside by saying the colors of the bottles,'" or "'I remembered what was in it, the shape, the color. . . . I described them to myself'" (Kearins, 1980).

Conservation tasks, developed by Piaget, have also been used cross-culturally to determine relations between task-specific performance and special cultural practice (Price-Williams, Gordon, & Ramirez, 1969).

Price-Williams and his colleagues compared the pottery-making experience of children in two Mexican villages, where some children worked in pottery and some did not. They found earlier development of conservation of quantity in those children who worked often with clay. They explain the early development of conservation in these children by noting that the children have learning experiences that are very similar to the conservation tasks. Making pottery in both villages involves fitting balls of clay into molds. The shape of the clay is transformed while the weight and the amount of clay remains constant. When errors are made, the clay is removed from the mold and once again returned to the shape of the ball. Thus transformation in form and reversibility activity necessary for conservation learning are practiced daily.

Children from one of the villages showed no *general* advance in conservation ability; they improved only on quantity. Children of the other village were advanced in other conservation tasks as well (numbers, area, etc.). In this latter case the investigators found that the childrens' pottery experience was unusual in that they were actively involved not only in manufacture but also in the commercial aspects of selling their pots, which provided additional kinds of practice relevant to the other conservation tasks.

The need to examine carefully the specific experiences of children and their relationship to skilled performances is emphasized by the contrast between the findings of Price-Williams and his co-workers and those of Steinberg and Dunn (1976). Steinberg and Dunn gave conservation tasks to children who were the sons of potters in another Mexican village and found no relationship between early conservation of quantity and experience of working with clay. This finding is understood when the villages' methods of building pots are compared. In the village studied by Steinberg and Dunn, the clay is rolled out into coils, and pots are built by adding layers of coils. This experience with clay does not provide the practice in the conservation skills that Price-Williams and his associates found in their research. It is only when the experience that occurs in one's everyday life is highly similar to the task requirements that a high degree of transfer is observed.

TOWARD A CHANGE IN PERSPECTIVE: FAMILIARITY RECONSIDERED

It would be possible to add to the list of examples of cultural influences on problem solving (see reviews by Cole & Means, 1981; Glick, 1975; LCHC, 1979a, 1979b, 1982). However, the examples presented thus far are sufficient to explain why one might conclude that "cultural differences in cognition reside more in the situations to which particular cognitive processes are applied than in the existence of a process in one cultural group, and its absence in another" (Cole et al., 1971, p. 233). Moreover, it appears that a simple rule applied to situations: The more familiar and culturally relevant the situation being observed, the more likely people are to perform competently.

The concept of stimulus familiarity is at the heart of methodological disputes in cross-cultural research, because familiarity is widely acknowledged to be a central requirement for establishing *stimulus equivalence*. It is also agreed that "a naive descriptive equivalence" of tasks is often not sufficient to ensure that a psychological task is the same for two different cultural groups (Glick, 1975; Greenfield, 1974; Price-Williams, 1975). Rather, what one seeks is *functional equivalence*. But, as Berry (1969) puts it, "These functional equivalents must pre-exist as naturally occurring phenomena; they are discovered and cannot be created or manipulated by the cross-cultural psychologist" (p. 122).

Putting all of these facts together, we can see the special risks of cross-cultural cognitive inferences: Our theories acknowledge the importance of knowledge base, and our methods assume the need to equate knowledge base to abstract "process" from the system of interactions we observe, but we engaged in the process in the first place because we wanted to study people who differed systematically in their knowledge and experience of the world. It is also agreed that *differences in knowledge can masquerade as differences in process*. Here, by yet another route, we come to the conundrum blocking cross-cultural comparisons in general, and comparisons based on the idea of unitary, underlying response proclivities in particular.

It is not clear that there is any single solution to this problem. Rather, the kind of solution that is sought will depend upon the kind of theory one is building. From a central processor point of view, familiarity has been handled by secondary mechanisms like decalage within the Piagetian framework. As Dasen (1977) has remarked, decalage is not systematically accounted for within Piaget's theory.

Dasen's entire research program can be viewed as an attempt to bring systematic cultural variability into a theory that has been built upon the notion of universal structures of mind corresponding to universal structures of interaction, for example, as an attempt to make differences in familiarity an important part of the theory.

Familiarity with what?   So far we have discussed familiarity as if its referents were easily understood but, in fact, we have used the term to indicate quite different kinds of familiarity: familiarity with the stimuli being used, with the operations to be performed, and with "the task." Glick (1975), Greenfield (1974), and Price-Williams (1975) offer structured schemes for ordering familiarity effects as they enter cognitive research. These are nicely summarized by Price-Williams (1975) in his idea of a "graduated steps" design in cross-cultural research. At one end of the set of steps is the naturally occurring situation embodying a particular cognitive demand. At the other is the standard cognitive experimental task embodying the same demand. The goal is to construct contexts of observation that vary in graduated steps of increasing distance from the naturally occurring situations.

Price-Williams constructs his steps within a three-part concept of the standard experiment consisting of the task, the materials, and the context. In the natural situation, all three elements are familiar. By mixing familiar elements for each component of the performance situation, it should be possible to map the traditional domains of thought, and also to "find out within any culture the extent to which its population thinks outside of its accustomed experience" (p. 49). This last claim is important to the study of culture and intelligence because it implies Price-Williams's belief that some cultures may give systematic practice in "thinking outside one's common experience." Such speculations, if they can be sustained by empirical evidence, would be one basis for claims that some cultures produce more powerful and more general modes of thought.[11]

The research strategy described by Glick, Greenfield, and Price-Williams has rarely been carried out. From those studies that have been conducted, however, it is clear that our understanding of the enterprise will have to be more complicated than the three-part category system used by Price-Williams. The basic issue is the difficulty of specifying "task" and "context." For example, Greenfield (1974) conducted a study that varied different kinds of familiarity in object sorting, but found no familiarity-linked improvements in performance. In fact, some of her younger subjects seemed to be more rigid categorizers when using familiar materials. We can explain such results by saying that only the materials were varied in familiarity; but how are we to interpret plausible experimental manipulations within the task–materials–context framework? If we change the instructions, do we change the task or the context? If we are working in a culture where adults do not ask children known-answer questions, or where one-to-one dialogue with a strange adult is unknown, or where sleight of hand is a culturally valued practice, how are we to make the task familiar when it is, *because of differences in culturally organized contexts for thinking,* an unfamiliar form of interaction?

These logical difficulties are sufficiently clear to provoke Jean Lave (1980) into suggesting the total inappropriateness of standard psychological techniques for assessing cognition across cultures or across contexts within cultures. Her view will not be welcomed by psychologists interested in cross-cultural comparisons with standardized instruments. But it does focus attention on the severe limits to "equating for familiarity" that experimentally derived observational technology permits.

An extremely interesting common thread runs through all of the discussions that have stressed functional stimulus equivalence. All discussions point to the need to take very seriously the everyday activities of people as the starting point for comparative analysis. Even more specifically, researchers who have tried to make cross-cultural studies of culture's impact on thinking have turned to areas of activity that are believed to require skill and training *by people in the cultures to be compared* as basic contexts of observation.

Price-Williams (1975) suggests that the steps between artificial experiment and natural activity can best be filled in by studying

the skills of a culture. Perhaps we ought to focus upon *homo faber* as our target. Traditionally in psychology, skills and crafts are more often inspected from the vantage point of aptitudes and manual dexterity than from perception of information processing generally. . . . We need to take such a craft as this . . . and interfere just slightly in the sequence of operations. [P. 47]

Glick (1975) expands upon this theme:

Everyday activities, such as speaking, doing ordinary tasks, and, in general, being a competent human being – whether in hunting, gathering, working a computer, or telling and understanding a myth – are regarded as important data inputs about the human cognizer's abilities. The cognitive structural description of these activities becomes then a "theory" of cognitive abilities that might be manifested in specifically designed experiments. [P. 648]

The list of research efforts that attempt to implement such a research strategy is small but growing (see Hutchins, 1980; Lave, n.d.). We will describe one such project, in which the issues of familiarity and breadth of transfer are addressed in ways that provide a good basis for reformulation of the problem of culture and thought.

The cognitive consequences of literacy. Early research on the consequences of literacy based on historical and ethnographic data suggested very general cognitive consequences of learning to read and write: changes in the nature of deliberate remembering (Havelock, 1978), logical reasoning (Goody & Watt, 1963/1968), and uses of language in a variety of settings (Olson, 1977). (See also McLuhan, 1962; Vygotsky, 1962.)

Some experimental work aimed at testing these ideas was carried out in the 1960s and early 1970s. But this research all rested on comparisons involving *schooling* (e.g., Greenfield, 1966/1969). Though reading and writing are clearly central to schooling as we know it, there are many reasons for thinking that practice at learning and reproducing large amounts of novel information organized around modern scientific and social concepts, not the ability to read or write per se, is the basis for widely reported differences between schooled and unschooled populations on relevant cognitive tasks.

Scribner and Cole (1981) carried out research in a culture that provided an unusual opportunity to disentangle literacy from schooling. For the past 100–150 years, the Vai people of Liberia have been employing a syllabic script of their own invention. The Vai syllabary is known and used by approximately 20% of Vai men, primarily for letter writing and record keeping. Unlike literacy acquired in school,

Vai literacy does not prepare the learner for a variety of new kinds of economic and social activity. Learning is almost always a personal affair carried out in the context of daily activities (most often, when a friend or relative agrees to teach the learner how to read and write letters). The Vai are primarily upland rice farmers, small business entrepreneurs, and craftsmen. Their literate skills play a useful role in those traditional occupations, but a more restricted role than we usually associate with school-based literacy practices. There is no tradition of text production for mass distribution; no traditional occupations depend upon being literate. Nonliterates can engage in the same basic economic activities as literates. The contrast between Vai literacy and literacy acquired in school (some Vai have attended American-style schools) provided Scribner and Cole with one line of evidence on the consequences of literacy, independent of schooling.

Because the Vai have been influenced by Islam for about as long as the existence of the Vai script, a third kind of literacy also flourishes in Vai country, literacy in Arabic. Actually, Arabic literacy consists of two distinct kinds of literate skills. Most Vai who read Arabic do not understand the words they read. Rather, they have learned to decode the characters of the alphabet in order to help them recite the Koran at religious services. However, some Vai have mastered sufficient Arabic to keep records, and in some cases to write letters or read books such as commentaries on the Koran. We will distinguish these groups by referring to those who have used Arabic only to recite the Koran as Koranic literates, reserving the term *Arabic literate* for those who can write and read Arabic more generally.

Using these four groups (English, Vai, Arabic, and Koranic literates) to contrast with nonliteracy and one another, Scribner and Cole conducted several series of studies to determine the nature and generality of cognitive skills generated by each kind of literate practice.

In their initial investigations, they selected a variety of classification, memory, and logical reasoning tasks that had produced improved performance for *schooled* literates in previous research (Rogoff, 1980; Sharp et al., 1979). The results of this phase of the work were as clear as negative results can be. English schooling produced changes in many, but not all, of the tasks; the other literacies produced almost none. The most consistent effect of schooling was to improve individual's abilities to explain the basis of performance on cognitive tasks.

Finding no measurable consequences of Vai literacy, Scribner and Cole then narrowed their focus. Noting that a core of all speculations about literacy's impact is the notion that practice in reading and writing should change a person's knowledge of the properties of spoken language, they designed a new series of tests to demonstrate *metalinguistic* consequences of becoming literate. Very little evidence for effects of any of the literacies encountered in Vai country were found in this phase of the work. The strongest result to emerge was increased skill among schooled and Vai literates when they were asked to explain the basis for judgments of grammaticality.

The combined results of these two lines of study discouraged the notion that literacy per se produces the general cognitive changes previously associated with schooling. Indeed, although schooling produced changes in performance on many tasks, its effects were by no means uniform.

At this point, Scribner and Cole began designing studies that were intended to test very specific hypotheses about cognitive effects growing directly out of analyses of literate practices. From analysis of a large corpus of letters, they hypothesized that Vai literates ought to be able to communicate quite effectively with someone in a remote place, because writing letters requires practice in formulating descriptions for someone who does not share one's knowledge of the events to be described. Vai literates ought to produce fuller, less egocentric, descriptions. Utilizing an analysis of the reading and writing process used by Vai literates, Scribner constructed rebuslike tasks, which required people to code and decode simple graphic symbols that could form propositions. To differentiate among the various literate groups (all of which engage in such activities in order to read or write), they constructed one task based on syllables (the units of analysis central to Vai script, but only implicit in Arabic or English) and another based on words as the basic units.

The outcome of these studies designed to model various literate practices observed in Vai country yielded clear-cut evidence of *function-specific* cognitive change, where functions were implemented within different, but overlapping, configurations of cultural practice. As hypothesized, the two literacies used widely for letter writing, Vai and English, both improved performance on the communication task. All the literacies in which understanding the text was important improved performance on the rebus tasks. However, only Vai literacy produced improved performance when the basic graphic units referred to *syllables*.[12]

Completing the case for function-specific consequences of literacy were results from the only experiment designed to test a hypothesis favoring Koranic literacy. Using a memory procedure proposed by Mandler and Dean (1969), in which lists of words are built up by starting with a list length of one item and adding one item per trial (called the incremental recall task), Scribner and Cole (1981) found that practice reciting the Koran (associated with both Koranic and Arabic literacy) was the only literacy factor that improved serial recall performance.

The pattern of results obtained from this series of studies is shown in Figure 11.4. Figure 11.4 clearly displays the fact that schooling has more effects than any of the other literacies. When tasks call for explanation of the basis for performing a task, schooling is the *only* literacy contributor, with two significant exceptions: Vai literacy enhances the descriptive power of communications at a distance and the ability to justify grammatical judgments. Scribner and Cole attribute this latter result not to Vai reading or writing in general, but rather to the specific practice in arguing the merits of various propositional forms that is common among Vai literates.

Following Scribner and Cole, we wish to interpret these results within a context-specific theory that specifies the within-context structures of activity. In those cases in which an outcome does appear to be directly related to reading and writing, analysis of the social organization and purposes of writing points at literacy-related *practice* as the crucial experience. Thus the increased ability to explain the basis for one's cognitive performance is attributed to modes of classroom discourse in the case of the schooled students for whom questions and requests such as "How did you know that?" "What makes you say that?" "Go to the board and show us how you do that" are a routine accompaniment to becoming literate. The improved ability of the Vai literates on the communication task has a straightforward interpretation based on the structure of Vai literacy practices. The ability of Vai literates to explain the basis of grammatical judgments (but not other cognitive judgments) is again attributed to their custom of discussing the proper-

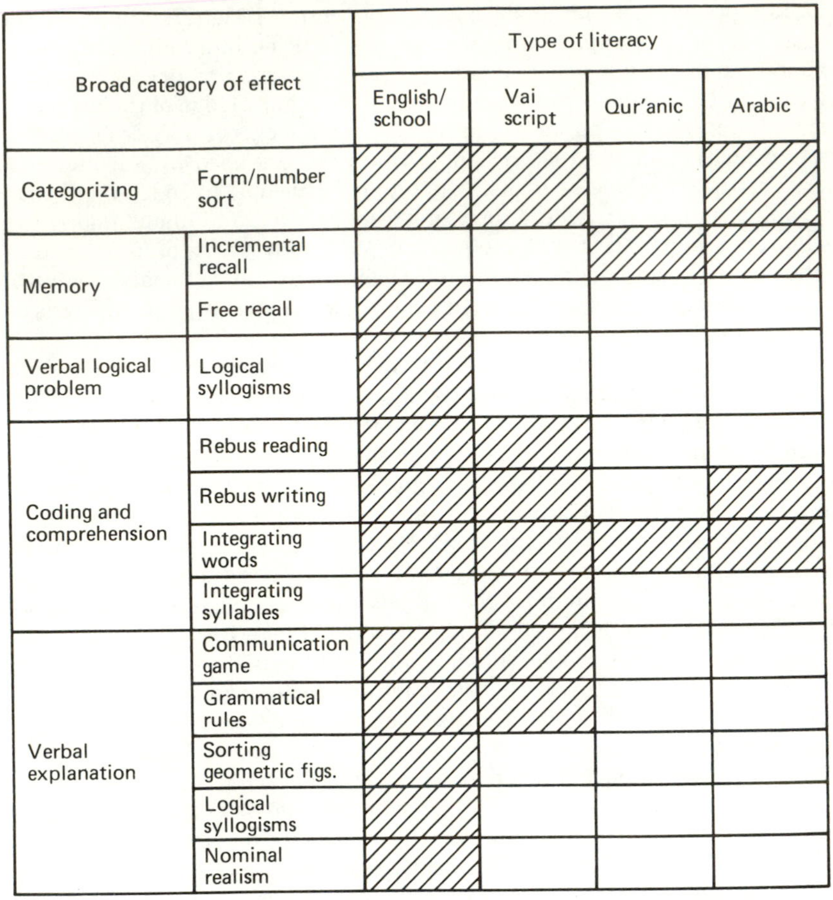

Broad category of effect		Type of literacy			
		English/ school	Vai script	Qur'anic	Arabic
Categorizing	Form/number sort	▨	▨		▨
Memory	Incremental recall			▨	▨
	Free recall	▨			
Verbal logical problem	Logical syllogisms	▨			
Coding and comprehension	Rebus reading	▨	▨		
	Rebus writing	▨	▨		▨
	Integrating words	▨	▨	▨	▨
	Integrating syllables		▨		
Verbal explanation	Communication game	▨	▨		
	Grammatical rules	▨	▨		
	Sorting geometric figs.	▨			
	Logical syllogisms	▨			
	Nominal realism	▨			

Figure 11.4.   Schematic representation of effects associated with each literacy practice in Vai country.

ties of correct Vai speech, a custom occasioned by letters containing unusual constructions. Finally, the evidence that English schooling and Koranic and Arabic literacy improve performance on memory tasks, although weak and spotty, is consistent with the fact that these three literacies, but not Vai, require practice in remembering large amounts of novel material, material that is often devoid of specific meaning to the rememberer.

11.9.   REORIENTING THE DISCUSSION

The research reviewed in the preceding section provides the basis for a reformulation of the relationship between cultural experience and cognitive development, as schematically represented in Figure 11.4. A theory about the way in which culture influences cognitive development must account for the patterning of performance across a wide variety of cultural contexts. We assume that a requirement of such a theory must be the ability to account for the cultural practices that promote this rapid and extensive learning.

The central processor theories begin with theoretical assumptions about universal configurations of constraints on domains. For Piaget, this domain is the set of abstract schemata that underlie universal patterns of human interaction with the world. For the cognitive-style theorist, this domain is the set of constraints created by culture-wide, culture-specific adaptations to members' common experience of the physical world and their historically accumulated patterns of response to these constraints. The psychological processes that are the "inside" consequence of the "outside" constraints operate in a "top-down" manner to control the way in which the world is interpreted and acted upon. From the point of view of these central processor approaches, differences in familiarity are noise in the system of observation. The theory specifies the most general aspects of hypothetical patterns of interaction between individual and environment. However, few interpretive rules leading from an abstract central processing mechanism to the everyday scenes that embody these principles are provided. As a consequence, systematic response variability and familiarity effects sometimes are a real difficulty for central processor theories.

From the context-specific approach diagrammed in Figure 11.4, the primary unit of analysis is neither universal operations nor culture-wide patterns of styles (or their external counterparts, culture-wide constraints). Rather, the basic unit of analysis is the set of structured activities of people that we have variously referred to as contexts or events. Beginning with contexts as basic units of analysis, the challenge for a context theory is to show how behavior is brought under the control of patterns of events embodying the stages, or patterns, of cognitive behavior that have been identified by other theorists. That is, one must demonstrate how one moves from specific contexts to general knowledge. In proposing a theory to account for this basic issue in culture and cognition, we will argue that a great deal of the "top-down" processing that is treated as a psychological process by central processor theorists is usefully thought of as an interpersonal, cultural process in a context-specific approach to culture and cognition. In this section we will first specify more clearly how the term *context* should be used in culture–cognition research. We will show that there are parallel concepts in both psychology and anthropology that point to contexts as the basic units of analysis for *both* sciences. Using our psychocultural notion of context, we will sketch the way in which this approach interprets cultural differences in the organization of cognitive skills. We will close by discussing the implication of this and alternative theories for the concept of intelligence and its cultural determinants.

THE NOTION OF CONTEXT

As we have been emphasizing, participation in interaction takes place in cultural contexts. Contexts are not to be equated with the physical surroundings of settings, like classrooms, churches, kitchens. As McDermott and Roth (1978) have put it, contexts are constituted by what people are doing, as well as by when and where they are doing it. That is, people in interaction serve as contexts for one another. Ultimately, social contexts consist of mutually ratified and constructed environments.

S. F. Nadel (1951), while discussing social anthropology as a science, recommends units embodying our notion of "contexts" as basic units of anthropological theorizing. The difficulty of defining basic units of analysis for anthropological observation and description, Nadel tells us, "is resolved if the units we seek to isolate satisfy the condition of the whole, this is, if each bears the characteristics pertaining to that total entity, culture or society" (p. 75). To this statement we must add that the unit must also bear the characteristics pertaining to individuals. This additional requirement, as we shall see, can prove no burden for Nadel, because his basic unit includes the person.

Society and culture are broken down, not to, say, individuals, nor to the "works of man" (Kroeber), but to *man-acting*. In this sense no legitimate isolate can be discovered [other] than that of a standardized pattern of behavior *rendered unitary and relatively self-contained by its task-like* nature and its direction upon a single aim. [P. 75, emphases added]

This principle of "methodological individualism" (Nagel, 1961) is also well developed in phenomenologically influenced sociology. Compare the following statement by Alfred Schutz (1964) with that of Nadel:

Whenever the problem under inquiry makes it necessary, the social scientist must have the possibility of shifting the level of his research to that of individual human activity.

We want . . . to understand social phenomena, and we cannot understand them apart from their placement within the scheme of human motives, human means and ends, human planning – in short – within the categories of human action. [P. 15]

"Action," then, refers to behavior assembled by people in concert with one another. It is for this reason that we have adopted cultural contexts, that is, interactionally assembled situations, not individual persons and not abstract cultural entities, as the unit of analysis for the study of culture and cognition. A very similar idea is proposed by Fortes (1970) in his discussion of traditional forms of education. For Fortes, the "man-acting" unit is called a "social space" and is discussed in connection with the growing child's interactions with its environment. Fortes characterized the social space as "the part of the society and habitat that the child is in effective contact with" (p. 27) and emphasized the crucial role of adults in controlling access to, and behavior in, the important contexts of adult life.

These anthropological and sociological characterizations of a basic unit in terms of person-acting units have important parallels in psychology that are an intellectual resource for a context-specific approach to culture and development.

First, there is the very important work of Barker and his colleagues (Barker, 1968) in which the basic unit of analysis is the behavior setting. In Barker's concept of a behavior setting, the term *behavior* refers to patterns of behavior–environment interactions; further, the settings are nonrandomly "fitted" to the behaviors that are appropriate in that setting. Barker referred to this fit as "synomorphism": The environment and behavior are adapted to each other. This is analogous to what Fortes called a social space.

Neither Fortes's nor Barker's idea of a basic unit of analysis has been taken up by people studying culture and cognition, for reasons that go beyond the limits of this discussion. However, there are two traditions in psychology that have brought versions of this concept to the very core of cognitive psychology. The first tradition is represented by schema theory as embodied in the writings of J. Mandler (in press) and Rumelhart and Norman (1980). (For alternative formulations see Minsky, 1975; Schank & Abelson, 1975.) The second comes from the Soviet work of Vygotsky and his students.

Consider the very recent characterization of schemata by Rumelhart and Norman (1980). Condensing their discussion slightly, we can say that schema theory attempts to account for the representation and application of human knowledge. According to this and all other schema theories, knowledge is represented as schemata. Schemata consist of subschemata. Different theories pursue the microstructure of schemata to different degrees. We will be concerned here only with schemata and subschemata that can be related in some way to cultural variations in experience. When we look to the hypothetical content of schemata, the relationship to anthropological units such as person-acting becomes immediately apparent. Rumelhart (1980) tell us that there are schemata representing "our knowledge about all concepts: those underlying objects, situations, events, sequences of events, actions and sequences of actions. A schema contains, as part of its specification, the network of inter-relations that is believed normally to hold among constituents of the concept in question" (p. 34).

Moreover, a schema theory is based upon a prototype theory of concepts (see Smith & Medin, 1981). That is, because schemata are closely identified with the meanings of concepts, meanings are assumed to represent the typical or normal situations and events that are instances of the schemata. The context-specificity of schema theory is nicely captured by Rumelhart's (1980) statement that "schemata play a central role in all of our reasoning processes. Most of the reasoning we do apparently *does not* involve the application of general purpose reasoning skills. Rather, it seems that most of our reasoning ability is tied to particular bodies of knowledge" (p. 55).

We see in these ideas about schemata the cognitive psychological, "internal" version of the "outside" context of person-acting. Concerned as we are with specifying how the outside influences the inside and vice versa, we cannot proceed leaving these two systems as independent entities. Somehow, we must deal with the problem of inside and outside together, as mutually influencing systems. This task has not been attempted by modern American cognitive psychology, but it was a concern of Piaget's, and it has been the subject of systematic investigation by Vygotsky and his students in the Soviet Union for half a century (see Luria, 1932, 1976; Vygotsky, 1934/1978; 1962). From a contemporary Vygotskian perspective, the basic unit of analysis is called *activity*. Like the idea of a social space or a behavior setting, the idea of activity emphasizes the interactions between social unit and individuals, in the process of which they take on their defining characteristics. As Leontiev put it,

In activity the object is transformed into its subjective form or image. At the same time, activity is converted into its objective results. . . . activity emerges as a process of reciprocal transformations between the subject and object poles. . . . In society humans do not simply find external conditions to which they must adapt their activity. Rather, these (external) social conditions carry within them the motives and goals of their activity, its means and modes. In a word, society produces the activity of the individuals that it forms. [Quoted in Wertsch, 1981]

In this statement we see the major elements of the anthropological concept of contexts as person-acting units that interact to define each other, a psychological, schema-based unit as the "subjective form or image" and *an explicit statement of the idea that interactions between external and internal "poles" create "mind" at one end and "society" at the other*. It is these properties that are assumed in the bare-bones outline of a context-specific approach to culture–cognition relations that is given schematically in Figure 11.4.

When applied to the problem of accounting for cultural differences in thinking, we find it useful, following Scribner (1977), to characterize contexts in terms of the cultural practices that they embody. Following Scribner and Cole (1981), we characterize a cultural practice as

a recurrent, goal-directed sequence of activities using a particular technology and particular systems of knowledge. We use the term *skills* to refer to the coordinated sets of actions involved in applying this knowledge in particular settings. A practice, then, consists of three components: technology, knowledge, and skills. We can apply this concept to spheres of activity that are predominately conceptual (e.g., the practice of law) as well as to those that are predominately sensori-motor (e.g., the practice of weaving). All practices involve interrelated tasks that share common tools, knowledge base and skills. But we may construe them more or less broadly to refer to entire domains of activity around a common object (e.g., law) or to more specific endeavors within such domains (e.g., cross-examination or legal research). Whether defined in broad or narrow terms, practice always refers to socially developed and patterned ways of using technology and knowledge to accomplish tasks. Conversely, tasks that individuals engage in constitute a social practice when they are directed to socially recognized goals and make use of a shared technology and knowledge system. [P. 236]

A full description of a context-specific theory is beyond the scope of this chapter (see LCHC, 1982, for additional specification), but further treatment of two closely related issues must be provided if the implications of this alternative are to be made explicit. Central is the question how context-specific achievements can produce seemingly context-free abilities; how we can get from the specific to the general. We will address this specific-to-general problem in two ways. First, we will show how contemporary developmental theories of cognition built on experimental model systems have formulated congitive development in specific-to-general terms. Second, we will show how contemporary developments in ethnography and interactional cognitive analysis point to the interpersonal sources of cognitive change. These two lines of work will provide the basis for several conclusions regarding culture–cognition relations, including a resolution of the dilemmas regarding inferences about culture and cognition with which we began this long discussion.

FROM THE CONTEXT-SPECIFIC TO THE CONTEXT-FREE IN COGNITIVE
DEVELOPMENT

The beginning of a viable alternative to central processor theories (including Piagetian theory) is to be found in an ever-increasing number of developmental studies that emphasize the accumulation of context-specific knowledge as a major force in development. Significantly for our argument, these formulations bear a very close relation to the conclusion of Cole and his colleagues (1971) that cultural differences in cognition arise more from differences in contexts than from differences in basic psychological processes. For example, Siegler and Richards (Chapter 14) conclude, on the basis of their studies of the development of problem solving, that "intellectual development on the task seems to involve improvement in the range of conditions under which appropriate representations are formed more than improvements in the inference process itself" (Siegler and Richards, Chapter 14). They then provide the central reformulation:

Developmental psychologists until recently devoted almost no attention to changes in children's knowledge of specific content. . . . Recently, however, several researchers have hypothesized that knowledge of specific content domains is a crucial dimension of development in its own right, and that *changes in such knowledge may underlie other changes* previously attributed to the growth of capacities and strategies. [Siegler, in press, emphasis added][13]

Consider children's understanding of time, embodied in a task in which two trains move down a track at different speeds to different locations. The trains can start from different places, end up in different places, and go at different speeds. By controlling these variables carefully, it is possible to determine the basis for judgments such as which train moved fastest, which train went furthest, and which train took the most time from start to finish. Concentrating on the time question, Siegler and Richards found that 5-year-olds respond to questions about time by noting where the train stopped: The one that had reached the most extreme point on the tracks was judged as having taken the most time, no matter where it started from. Older children, however, associated *time* with the *total distance* traveled, no matter how fast the train was going.

Of course, each of these explanations can be consistent with what we consider a correct theory of elapsed time. All other things being equal, the train that went the farthest (or the train that traveled the greatest distance) is the one that took the most time. Of course, in the real world, trains do not always travel at the same speed, nor do they always start in the same place, so these generalizations as a basis for judgments of elapsed time will sometimes err. The crucial questions are: *Under what circumstances will a generalized rule or theory err?* Under what circumstances will the limited generalizations that children achieve give way to more powerful generalizations? Siegler and Richards answer these questions by showing that generalizations of increased power will not come about through repeated exposure to moving trains *unless the information carried in that exposure makes clear to the children* the error in their generalization and provides information that can be the basis of a more powerful (general) rule.

The experiences that will lead to such change are different, depending upon the rule one begins with. For the 5-year-olds whose rule is based on the end point the trains reach, exposure to problems that vary the end point while holding time constant are needed. For the slightly older children whose rule is total distance, the training must consist of problems that discriminate time and distance in a different way.

Because Siegler and Richards had a strong theory of relevant events based on their knowledge of our culture's theories of the task they present, and because they took trouble to ensure that children were, in fact, doing their task, they could classify subjects according to the rule they used. Because they had several different rules to work with, and because they knew that the rules followed each other in typical developmental sequences (sequences that map directly onto Siegler and Richards's theory of the relationship between events in the world of moving trains), they could arrange carefully constructed experiments between the child's current state of knowledge and the learning environment. In other words, they could provide specific kinds of feedback. They could also show that if a child got *too much new information,* no learning would occur. Here is how they express it:

When 5-year-olds were presented problems that did not discriminate their existing rule from the time rule . . . they continued to rely on end points. When they were presented problems that disconfirmed their existing rule but not the rule that they would be expected to adopt next . . . they began to rely on the new rule. However, when presented with problems that disconfirmed both their existing rule and the rule that they would not typically acquire next, . . . they simply became confused, not relying on any apparent cue. [Siegler & Richards, Chapter 14]

Siegler and Richards's study represents a microcosm of the general pattern of development. Individual experiences are compatible with many explanations of variability in the world. But the number of explanations that fit several experiences *simultaneously* will be much smaller. Development is the acquisition of more and more general rules (or explanations, or habits) that apply to a progressively larger set of specific domains of experience. Development in this view is virtually *never* general. That is, explanations are not likely to be totally general. As Siegler and Richards point out with respect to time, even physicists and philosophers have context-bound theories; it is just that their contexts are less restricted than ours.

Roughly speaking, the theory of development suggested by the work of Siegler and Richards (and many others – e.g., Feldman, 1980; Fischer, 1980; Zaporozhets, 1980) yields the following account of how thinking goes from the specific to the general: Viewed at any given time period, the child's mental processes can draw upon a large repertoire of remembered interactions with the social and nonsocial environment. Elements of that historically accumulated experience are represented by "events" in Figure 11.3. The various events that the child has experienced form the basis for a large set of rather specific adaptations (where "adaptation" can be conceived of as the content of knowledge that answers the ethnographer's question. What's going on here?). By the time a child has reached the age at which typical cognitive research is carried out (2–3 years of age, say), he or she has learned a good deal about the properties of objects and events in the world. But this information is limited because the variety of events that the child has encountered and formed theories about is limited in both scope and quantity.

In any specific problem domain (say, for example, judging elapsed time), the child's experience is certain to be limited with respect to the variety of parametric variations that he or she has experienced. Not enough information has been assimilated to allow for very many (lateral) or very inclusive (vertical) generalizations about the properties of the objects and events that determine the aspects of what the child has encountered (e.g., rarely is common experience organized so that judgments about elapsed time err in a detectable way under the special conditions that will permit formulation of a next-higher level of correct generalization). Basing judgments on a limited number of configurations of objects and events, children are very often correct, only sometimes in error. Changes of the sort associated with major reorganization of generalizations can occur only when there are errors (an assumption strongly supported by more than a decade of research in problem solving [but cf. Levine, 1966]). The engine of change is experience of a very special kind – experience tailored to the child's current level of understanding, experience that provokes contradictions of just the right kind. These contradictions are invitations to form a next-higher-order generalization. These "invitations," of course, may be refused.[14]

From this point of view, the concept of stage is secondary. Depending upon how long it takes for the world to provide the child with appropriately informative experiences, the child will respond to problems in a given domain in a characteristic way, that is, using a current generalization.[15] The rule describing that generalization is equivalent to a stage, but it is posited to exist and operate only within the specific content domain. Development proceeds both laterally, at a given level of generalization, and vertically, to generalizations that subsume current examples and work for a broader range as well (as in Gagné, 1968). Thus the child will make time judgments of many objects in many events on the basis of a given rule, so long as no contradictions arise (lateral development). He or she will also, on occasion, learn new generalizations that can cover a wider range of enabling circumstances (vertical development). But this development will be *domain-specific*. The content and range of conditions of the domain will govern how general a psychological process appears. So long as our psychological test samples within domains, the child will appear to be at a given, general level. But move outside that domain (laterally or vertically) and the limits of the stage will quickly manifest themselves. This is as true for adults as for children: Everyone's knowledge is domain-specific. The issue is to specify the domains and the prior conditions that determine their limits.

Experiments and contexts: introducing interaction. We now have several elements necessary for filling out a context-specific approach to culture and cognitive development. We have identified an "outside" unit of analysis variously identified as a context or event by anthropologists and a corresponding "inside" unit called a schema by contemporary cognitive psychologists. In the carefully designed experiments of developmental cognitive psychologists, we have obtained a model of the structuring of events that produces cognitive development as increase in range of contexts.

Viewed in this way, experiments of the sort constructed by Siegler and Richards represent one kind of person-acting unit, one kind of context. It is a context designed to highlight the child's independent discovery of generalizations that embody adult theories of how things work. So little significance is attributed to the adult in this kind of arrangement that adult behaviors go undescribed, except insofar as the procedures and instructions are provided in the description of the experiment. In effect, the interactions that construct an experiment on learning to understand the concept of time are made transparent by the strong constraints of the experimental procedures that highlight the child's behaviors. These restrictions on the nature of the model system represented by standard cognitive experiments are very important to keep in mind when attempting to use the system as a basis for constructing a theory of culture and cognitive development, because we have emphasized the *interactive nature of the events that are our basic units of analysis*. It becomes very important, from this point of view, to look at the interactions that take place in naturally occurring contexts where adults arrange for children to learn things in order to discover how the interactions in these settings differ from those that we have studied in the laboratory. This requirement is motivated by more than a desire for methodological rigor. It is urged upon us by the data. For example, Fortes, in his work on traditional education (1970), makes it clear that crucial events in the child's "social space" cannot be treated as static elements of the environment: "The individual creates his social space and is in turn formed by it. On the one hand, his range of experiences and behavior [is] controlled by his social space, and on the other, everything he learns causes it to expand and become more differentiated" (p. 27).

In seeking a theoretical formulation that will encompass all the elements of a theory of culture and cognition that we have discussed so far, we have found the ideas of L. S. Vygotsky and his students particularly useful. Especially pertinent to this discussion is Vygotsky's idea of a "zone of proximal development," which, combined with his general views on the central role of interaction in development, provides a very useful framework.

Interactional mechanisms of cognitive change. For Vygotsky and his students, it was a fundamental tenet that adult human cognitive functioning emerges from culturally organized forms of social interaction. Variously called a "cultural" or "sociohistorical" school of psychology, Vygotsky's approach includes several proposals about the ways in which culturally organized social interactional patterns shape the psychological development of the child. Thus, Vygotsky (1981) wrote: "To paraphrase a well-known position of Marx, we could say that humans' psychological nature represents the aggregate of internalized social relations which have become functions for the individual and the structure of individual behavior" (p. 164).

Vygotsky and his colleagues also specified some of the processes that make possible the transition from social to individual functioning. The basic points in this argument can be found in Vygotsky's "general law of cultural development," in the formulation of which he wrote:

Any function in children's cultural development appears twice, or on two planes. First it appears on the social plane and then on the psychological plane. First it appears between people as an interpsychological category and then within the individual child as an intrapsychological category. This is equally true with regard to voluntary attention, logical memory, the formation of concepts and the development of volition. [Vygotsky, 1934/1978, p. 57]

Like Carey, Fisher, and Siegler, proponents of the sociohistorical school view development as the acquisition of ever-wider ranges of contexts to which a constant set of basic cognitive capacities and more powerful (general) rules for interpreting the phenomena of the environment are applied (see *Soviet Psychology*, Winter 1979–1980).

Unlike Siegler and most American researchers, however, the Soviet sociohistorical theorists add to their analyses of the physical situation facing the child and the child's current stage of knowledge an analysis of the way in which adults structure learning environments. They ask the following crucial questions: What factors shape the child's interpretation of experiences, and what factors determine whether a child will encounter experiences of the kind that are necessary to produce change from one stage of generalization to the next (understanding *stage* always to mean "stage within context")? In the American experimental work previously reviewed, these questions do not arise because the experiments are designed to display what experiences lead to change, not how those experiences come into play or what the child's role is in bringing about the necessary experiences. The experimenter makes certain that the experiences occur because of his or her interest in specifying their logical connection to existing states of knowledge. Learning "just happens" if the right circumstances occur. The circumstances are not an object of inquiry.

It is precisely in addressing the circumstances that control the timely occurrence of needed experience that insights of the sociohistorical school become crucial. The environments a child encounters are not a sequence of random events. Eco-cultural psychologists and anthropologists postulate that the environments that make up our lives are highly constrained by ecological and adapted sociocultural circumstances (Berry, 1976; B. Whiting, 1980). As generations of anthropologists have documented, those adaptations take a variety of forms that rival the wonders of all natural phenomena (Mead, 1958). As ecological psychologists have shown, the environments in which cognition occurs (which is to say, all human environments) are highly organized (Barker, 1968). Micro-ethnographers have shown that this organization extends down to the organization of minute aspects of our interactions with each other (McDermott & Roth, 1978) – and, we would claim, to the interactions we engage in "between our ears."

Thus, to the sequence of learning steps that characterizes the order of acquiring generalizations about the world, the sociohistorical psychologist adds the study of how the culture organizes for the next step of development to occur. How might this happen? From a sociohistorical perspective such as that adopted by Vygotsky and his followers, culture influences the organization of children's environments in four ways.

First, it arranges for the raw *occurrence* or *nonoccurrence* of specific basic problem-solving environments. Infants are taught to crawl or climb, sleep briefly or sleep for long periods. Preschoolers learn to model with wire or to draw, that is, to model with pen and paper. Students chant the Koran or read the Bible.

Second, the *frequency* of the same kinds of events is culturally organized in these learning environments. Does one read daily in class or weekly in church? When is it necessary to sort grains? How many times a day does one engage in pottery making and with how many products? Does one sell pottery as well as make it? Culture exerts an overwhelming power in answering such questions.

Third, culture shapes the *patterning* or co-occurrence of events. One measures rice when selling and buying by using related-quantity tins but measures cloth and tables with unrelated quantities. One culture provides for recalls of spatial arrays with rehearsal strategies, and another does without them.

Fourth, culture *regulates the level of difficulty* of the task. This regulation increases the likelihood both that potentially crucial learning events will occur and that costly failure will be averted (Lave, n.d.). Teaching children to sit by propping them up in a hole with a blanket might be a starter task for walking, just as sewing the buttons on a shirt for the master tailor is a starter task for tailoring.

This regulative function of the culture was studied by Vygotsky under the rubric "the zone of proximal development," which he defined as "the distance between the actual developmental level as determined by independent problem solving and the level of potential development as determined through problem solving under adult guidance or in collaboration with more capable peers" (Vygotsky, 1934/1978, p. 86).[16]

Problem solving and social regulation within the zone of proximal development are not restricted to contexts formally established for instruction. It can be seen in cases like the tailoring apprentice system (Lave, n.d.), which is intimately related to the actual day-to-day problems of the "tutor."

The basic idea expressed in all of this work is an elaboration of the educational homily: *Teach children by starting with what they know* and by moving them from that starting point nearer to the end point defined by the teacher. Psychological research on this problem using the concept of a zone of proximal development adds three points to the educational homily:

1. a theory of the structure of the task that yields information about the proper distance between teacher and students;
2. a theory of the role of the adult in this process; and
3. a description of the system of interactions between adult and child during which the child comes to take responsibility for doing more and more of the task.

An example of a *part of the structure* of one kind of zone of proximal development is given in Siegler and Richards's experiments, described previously. The various generalizations that a child must form in order to arrive at what we call adult concepts are specified in terms of the logically available kinds of information. A definition of what constitutes too much or the wrong kind of information is also given by the task analysis. The role of the adult is restricted to arranging environmental events so that these match, or exceed by specified amounts, the knowledge base with which the child enters the experiment.

What is not obvious in such experiments is the role played by the social environment; yet it is there in the form of experimental procedures, which select each step in the series of problems that the child will next confront. The experimenter is, of course, doing a great deal more. This extra work is seldom the object of analysis, but it is crucial to understanding how development occurs. The experimenter guides the child's attention to the relevant features of the problem in the way in which he or she has arranged the physical arrays and in the language used both as "instructions" and as social reinforcements necessary to maintain the sensibilities of the social situation during the course of the experiment itself.[17]

Some experimenters have succeeded in making visible for analysis a fuller picture of the way in which adults organize the learning environments of children, using the idea of zones of proximal development. For example, Wertsch and his associates (Wertsch, 1981) have conducted a series of studies on the way in which mothers teach their young children an elementary task such as assembling a relatively simple jigsaw puzzle. The puzzle pieces were cutout parts of a truck picture, which the 2- to 3-year-old children were supposed to put together. Each child was helped by his or her mother through several assemblies of the same puzzle.

The course of the interaction as the child assembled the puzzle, with the mother assisting, usually went something like this. On the first try at the puzzle, the child might pick up pieces and play with them aimlessly. The mother would direct the child's attention to the puzzle and the pieces lying around. She would help the child choose a piece to try in the puzzle, and perhaps guide its placement. Her movements and intonation all helped to focus the child's attention on relevant aspects of the puzzle (as defined by the psychologists and adult) and to keep the child going from one piece to another or constructing alternate tasks. Over the course of a single assembly, the mother contributed less and less to the problem-solving activity. The child began to anticipate what it was necessary to do next. When the child erred and was confused, the mother was there to help, but otherwise, the child was on his or her own. Repeated trials reproduced this pattern, except that the child did more of the work earlier as his or her experience with the puzzle increased.

In this example, the content of the zone of proximal development can be seen to change as the child's experience with the problem increased. Initially, orientation to the task, selection, comparison, and even motor components of the problem were in large measure carried out by the mother, who elicited required motor and verbal compliance from the child. The mother was doing more than the child could do, but not so much more that the child could not participate. As the child came to take over more of the task, the mother shifted the nature of the work she did (e.g., offering praise or pointing to potential trouble a few steps ahead).

One important characteristic of teaching situations such as those described by Wertsch is that the children must be allowed to participate in an activity in which the crucial learning events are relatively dense long before they can deal with such an activity on their own. Not only are they thus exposed to developmentally relevant events, but this exposure is modulated to provide each child with what he or she needs to learn more about the principles guiding those events.

The interactive nature of the learning process is highlighted by two facts, so mundane that they invite inattention. First, one never sees the mother sitting next to the child, blithely putting the puzzle together. The child *is always* a participant, and that participation is made possible by the adult. The *nature* of the participation is interactively negotiated by child and adult. Secondly, the puzzle is always assembled. This puzzle problem is well within the independent problem-solving capacity of one of the participants, so of course it gets done. Putting these two facts together, we can see the basis for a claim that development always occurs in a zone of proximal development. Additionally, that zone is dynamically achieved by the *child and others in a social environment*. At the outset, for any problem, the social environment may seem to be doing more than its share of the work, but progressively, the achievements of the child and mother in interaction with each other (with the mother carrying a heavy cognitive load) are transformed into achievements of the child, with the mother a distant prop.

This kind of progression, played out in many different content domains, is what led Vygotsky to assert that higher psychological functions begin as *interpsychic functions shared between individuals*. Only extensive practice permits a person to carry out the same functions intrapsychically. Moreover, as already indicated, Vygotsky hypothesized that the initial structure of the internal process would be patterned after the external, interactional, one (Vygotsky, 1934/1978; Wertsch, 1980).

The central insight embodied in these ideas about the immediate contexts where development occurs is that crucial events causing change from one level to another heavily involve people (generally older people in the case of young children) who provide an environment that makes likely the necessary learning. In a very important sense, the changes referred to as "cognitive development" are modeled for the child with the child in the role of "apprentice-participant." Next stages in development are provided by socially organized systems of activity in which the child plays a gradually changing role. In some cases the child will quite literally be *told* the necessary information ("You better watch where the trains are coming from, silly!"); in others, adults make only the important factors salient ("Which piece will fit into the corner?"); and in still others they may do no more than make it possible for the child to be present while potential learning events are in progress ("Come sit on my lap while I help your sister figure out this puzzle"). But almost always, directly or indirectly, the social environment is providing important information to sustain and increase the efficiency and the activity in which the subject is engaged. The child's role in this process is no less active and crucial than the adult's; their joint contribution to the ongoing system of interactions is necessary to maintain the context and to provide the opportunity for learning to occur.

Zone of proximal development considered cross-culturally. Sociohistorical psychologists have never exploited the potential of the concept of a zone of proximal development in cross-cultural work. Only one cross-cultural expedition was undertaken at the time these ideas were being developed (Luria, 1931), and few have been entered upon since that time (Tulviste, 1979). Almost all of the scanty Soviet work was concentrated on demonstrating qualitative shifts in the functional systems that dominate for preliterate and industrialized man. No research went into an exploration of how these different kinds of functional systems came into being and how they operate to reproduce themselves across generations.[18]

In view of the fact that the sociocultural theory posits the zone of proximal development as the focus of learning and of the use of higher psychological functions, it may appear surprising that no work was put into comparative studies of concept acquisition. The limited attention given to the problem of culture and cognition in Soviet research is an explanation for this neglect. But the failure runs deeper. A commitment to the sociohistorical approach applied cross-culturally is a commitment to looking at how cultures organize learning environments for their members, especially their young. Following his theory, Luria went to Uzbekistan to discover the cognitive consequences of the dramatic shift from traditional pastoralism to literate, technological activities. He did not begin his research with a study of indigenous reasoning. Instead, he conducted experiments with Uzbekis modeled on practices developed in Russian clinics and laboratories. It is in interaction *between Uzbekis,* not in interactions between Uzbekis and Russians, that Luria's theory sought the operation and acquisition of Uzbeki concepts and problem-solving modes. Consequently, there is an important sense in which Luria failed to carry out the sociohistorical research program. Very little subsequent cross-cultural work has been undertaken by Soviet psychologists; however, a great deal of work has been done that illustrates hypothetical pieces of the enculturation process.

The zone of proximal development in socialization. Cultural anthropologists have described the patterns of family interactions that are sometimes labeled socialization, sometimes education "in the broad sense" (Mead, 1958; Raum, 1940; see Mead, 1958, for a review). Overwhelmingly, in pretechnological societies, whether of hunter-gatherers (Lee & DeVore, 1976) or of agriculturalists or pastoralists (Fortes, 1970; B. Whiting & Whiting, 1975), children are described as participants in a wide variety of social activities that we consider adult. Their role as participants varies as they grow older, but not the fact of their participation. The more detailed ethnographies of the socialization process show that children are routinely assigned tasks commensurate with their current abilities as elements in a larger task guided by their older siblings or adults. Just as Siegler and Richards can point to stages of understanding that correspond to logically connected aspects of the environment, anthropologists have pointed out that the sequences of child acquisitions in naturally organized learning environments have a strong element of necessity imposed by environmental constraints. The idea that one must be able to walk before one can run exemplifies this central fact about psychological development's dependence upon the constraints imposed by biological and environmental structure.

Very often, learning is so embedded in group activity that it is hard to see how individual accomplishments occur.[19] However, where there is specialization of activity, there are more visible environments in which to watch the cultural shaping of learning. This specialization may apply to different groups of people, or to the same people in different contexts.

One example of a specialized skill that is open to all adults and that is learned in specific contexts is given in the work of A. Kulah (1973). In preparatory work, Kulah, who was interested in the way that young Kpelle children come to learn the meaning of proverbs, made a study in their use in the formal and informal rhetorical discussions of Kpelle elders. His investigation showed that, in a very important sense, proverb content and interpretation are not taught; they are "arranged for." The arranging starts long before any child is expected to know or use proverbs. All Kpelle children engage in a variety of verbal games, including riddling and storytelling. One genre of this game requires teams of children to pose riddles to each other. The riddles consist of two parts roughly akin to a question and an answer. Both questions and answers are part of the traditional lore of the group, and they must be learned as pairs. The children line up in two rows and sequentially challenge each other with riddles. The team that answers the most riddles correctly is the winner.

The teams of children are age-graded. Children of a wide span of ages (say, from 5 to 12) may play, with the oldest on each team taking the first turn, then the next oldest, down to the youngest. In this way, even the youngest member of a team is important, and even the youngest is around to learn many new riddles.

This activity is related to adult proverb use in the following way. The question and answer halves of the riddles that the children learn are key phrases that will appear in adult proverbs. It is as if the riddle learning serves to teach children the "alphabet" along the way to learning to "read words." For example, a question might be something like "rolling stone" and the answer, "no moss."

Kulah's research shows that the potential meaning in combining "rolling stone" and "no moss" is not well understood by young children, even if they know many riddle question–answer pairs. When asked to group different riddles by the common meaning that the adult interpretation specifies, young children do not respond as if one riddle is related in any way to another. But as the children grow older, they approximate adult groupings of riddles according to their "message." By the time they are old enough to participate in the adult discussions in which these proverbs are a rhetorical resource, they show the adult pattern of proverb interpretation. They are ready to learn how to use their now-organized alphabet in a new context, as a component in new, adult, tasks.

The zone of proximal development in economic activities.   Contexts in which people can engage in specialized economic activities are a rich source of examples of the cultural organization of zones of proximal development that draw on different mixes of cognitive skills.

Lave (n.d.) has provided the most detailed account of traditional apprenticeship learning. Her description is sufficiently detailed to suggest important principles that must be considered when dealing with nonschool learning tasks as zones of proximal development.

Lave's subjects are tailors and their apprentices in a small tailors' district in Monrovia, Liberia. The tailors' stock in trade is trousers, with a few fancy suits and some simple hats and drawers as the upper and lower bounds of the tailoring skills. Apprentices are young boys, who spend from one to several years learning the trade.

According to Lave, tailoring is learned in five broad stages. The first involves basic skill learning and the second through the fifth, sewing and cutting first of drawers or hats, then of pants, then of gowns, and finally of suits. Within stages, practice is organized as a part of the general business of the shop. The boys learn from the ground up. At first they are the "gofers," a help and a burden. Apprenticeship can be said to be complete when they are only a help, and no longer a burden.

Their early learning contains little explicit instruction, but a good deal of "arranging for." The novice is given tasks that really need doing (holding cloth for the master, pressing pants, sewing on buttons). He is also given scrap material to practice on.

The arrangement of this early skill learning has both pedagogical and business aims. Lave summarized the dynamics as follows:

> The apprentice should learn quickly, but should be able as soon as possible to help the master with the work. The work that can be done with the lowest error cost and least dependence on coordination with the master's work is finishing. The master oversees the apprentice closely until he learns the skills which make him useful. After that it is the apprentice's responsibility to learn at his own pace. [Chap. 5, p. 12]

Once the apprentice has mastered the finishing skills to his master's satisfaction, he is given some very simple garments to make. He is also asked to help the master with more substantial parts of the mature practice of tailoring. Here the stage is subdivided: Sewing and cutting are learned and taught separately. Sewing is learned earlier (although it comes later in the actual sequence of making a garment), because the economic cost of an error is smaller.

At the point where the apprentice begins to deal with trousers, he is expected to know the overall structure of each of the sewing tasks. The tailors say that the way to learn is to watch until you know how to make all of a garment. Once you grasp the overall process, your practice can be effective. Lave presents interesting evidence to show that children understand the overall structure of the garment and steps needed to make it well before they can execute the corresponding actions with sufficient skill.

Although the apprenticeship process involves a good deal of verbal interchange, the only periods during which there is intense teaching interaction occur when the master seems consciously to be teaching in the period between the first execution and the first good approximation of some task. Lave was able to observe brief, intensive sessions of this sort, which she noted for the fine-grained coordination between the apprentice and his master. She also found evidence of an increase even within a single session. Her description of these incidents is very similar to that reported by Wertsch in his mother–child interaction work.

Lave also provides evidence of a kind of learning that is *not* described in the mother–child research, and does not fit neatly within the kind of experimental model favored by developmental psychologists. She observed the many occasions between organized teaching sessions when the apprentices practice on their own tasks within a given stage. The consequences of errors (mismatched seams, buttons falling off trousers) are obvious, as is the necessary action to take to remedy the mistake. Masters systematically work to get their apprentices to notice and remedy their own errors.

The similarity between Lave's description of stages of tailoring and cognitive-psychological models of concept acquisition are striking; in each case practice is organized into a hierarchy of skills, and practice is regulated in difficulty to fit the level of the learner. There are also important differences. We have already mentioned the division of learning stages into periods of "stage" acquisition and periods of skill solidification within stages. We think it significant that the masters formulate the need to understand the overall structure and sequencing of garment construction for each thing the person makes. This overall concept guides specific practice in a top-down manner.

It is also important that one account for the mix of goals in the setting. Lave suggests that, from a strictly pedagogical point of view, practice could be more efficiently organized. But the real-world economic circumstances that constrain master and apprentice alike modify the preferred order of learning, and the participants must adapt. (At one point, after an intense lesson on sewing a hat, the master picks up the garment and completes it, an unthinkable conclusion to most teaching scenes we are likely to think of.)

In this description (see also Childs & Greenfield, 1981; Karmiloff-Smith, 1979), we have an excellent sample of the way in which important cultural practices can be discovered and analyzed. This analysis can then serve as the basis for a study of the context-specificity or generality of the skills learned as a part of tailoring. Lave has also carried out this additional step, demonstrating limited transfer of tailoring skills outside everyday tailoring activities (Lave, 1977).

Additional requirements. We now have some idea of what we mean by contexts embodying cultural practices and the way in which learning is organized within contexts so that successively higher levels of development will be achieved.

A full theory would need to add ways of specifying relationships between contexts so that actions and operations learned in one would be relevant to performance in others. The similarity of actions and operations would be a primary source of transfer, for example, *the generality,* of behaviors that are learned in a context-specific way.

We would also need to consider within-context, interactional mechanisms that render relevant information from other contexts available for thinking. As we have suggested elsewhere (LCHC, 1982), transfer (and hence the generality of behavior) is very often organized by the environment as a process of information exchange *between* people.

IMPLICATIONS FOR THE STUDY OF CULTURE AND INTELLIGENCE

Summary of assumptions concerning development. The general approach to cognitive development sketched in the previous section has several implications for theories about how culture could differentially promote increased ability to deal with intellectual problems. Specific implications of our approach to cognitive development are the following:

1. Learning is context-specific. This implies (a) differences in development depending upon the degree of practice in the domain of activity in question and (b) difficulty in explaining transfer between domains.
2. Development consists of extending the domains to which particular procedures are applied through lateral transfer of a given kind of generalization or replacement of domain-specific formulations by more broadly applicable formulations at the same level of analysis. The evolution of qualitatively new procedures may or may not underlie specific achievements that we wish to refer to as development.

3.   Within-context change often occurs through individual-environment interactions in which adults and more knowledgeable others represent top-down processing agents guiding developmental change.

Summary of assumptions concerning cultural differences. In our review of cross-cultural research on cognitive development, we specified three basic units of analysis that theorists have identified:

1.   units involving species-wide forms of individual–environment interaction governed by universal (for *Homo sapiens*) constraints on behavior;
2.   units organized around culture-wide constraints that arise from adaptations to ecological demands accrued over the long course of a particular group's history of interactions with that environment and other cultures; and
3.   units organized at the level of within-culture person-acting activities embodied in the variety of everyday activities that different people of different ages within different cultures must master.

It should be clear that these three approaches are not mutually exclusive. A plausible case can be made for the importance of all three kinds (levels?) of constraint and their associated internal processing mechanisms. Instead of choosing one kind of unit to the exclusion of others, we need a framework that can encompass them all in a principled manner. This framework must also guide our theories of what constraints are operating in what ways in the scenes that are the basis for our observations of both culture and cognition.

Our strategy for creating such a framework is to begin with a basic unit of analysis in which independent and dependent variables come together so that the mechanisms of mutual causation can be analyzed. The idea of an activity proposed by the Soviet sociohistorical school is attractive for this general methodological reason: It corresponds on the one hand to the anthropological unit of analysis variously called an event or context and on the other to the psychological unit called a schema. Activities provide a unit within which it can plausibly be argued that culture and cognition are created as phenomena for analysis.

An emphasis on culturally organized, standard patterns of interaction that we term cultural practice is a solid basis for such theorizing on more narrow methodological grounds as well. Though Piagetian ideas concerning universal patterns of interaction and cognitive-style ideas concerning culture-wide patterns of interaction are plausible, it is generally accepted that we can come to know such patterns only as they are embodied in the concrete experience of people; the psychological constructs used by such theorists are necessarily abstractions from behavior in a variety of person-acting contexts that instantiate the abstractions.

Although there is a certain attractiveness in assuming that one's specification of the abstract relations underlying a particular form of interaction will necessarily control behavior, the fact of the matter is that in every concrete instance of person-acting, a great variety of constraints are operating simultaneously. A conservation experiment, for example, is not a transparent window on "reversibility" or "mental compensation." Nor is an embedded-figures test a perfect embodiment of field forces in which psychological differentiation can be unambiguously assessed. Rather, each session of a conservation experiment is a set of interactionally constructed exchanges in which Piagetian schemata, Witkinian social conformity pressures, and a variety of culture-specific rules for adult-child interaction concerning objects in the world and social relations are all operative *simultaneously*.

Operating within a single, familiar culture, students of cognitive development can rely (not without some risks) on their ability to construct contexts in which the abstract relations upon which their theories are based will be properly highlighted. Piagetian interviews and embedded-figures tests are two such contexts.

When we enter a different culture, the assumption that the abstract schemata are embodied in the procedures enacted by the participants loses its hold. In effect, what was previously assumed now has to be demonstrated anew. The logical need for establishing the control of theoretically important abstract relations when conducting research in alien cultures, with their own historically unique patterns of interaction, is the root of arguments over the meaning of experimentation and the problem of stimulus equivalence.

Here we want to raise another implication of our context-specific, cultural practice approach. Insofar as patterns of person–environment interaction are embodied in cultural practices, and cultural practices vary from one culture to another, it must be considered an empirical question whether some cultures will provide practice in patterns of interaction that have no equivalent form, even at an abstract level, in other cultures. (We have seen that Piaget came to doubt the universality of formal operations, recognizing that circumstances might limit people's exposure to environments that required the assembly and use of such schemata.)

In traditional developmental theories, the possibility of real discontinuity in the cognitive repertoire of different cultural groups has always been viewed with skepticism, because such theories assumed a hierarchy of processes with uniform levels of processing across all domains of experience.

From a context-specific perspective, the possibility that certain forms of interaction (and their internal equivalents) will have no equivalents in other cultures is an interesting one. However, drawing such a conclusion could never be warranted on the basis of experiments that take one culture's practices as *the* contexts in which the schemata are to be found. Rather, this mode of studying cognition and development requires that analysis begin with mature adult practices, including interpersonal interactions involving regulation of social and economic resources, as the domains in which to seek the operation of abstract schemata. Schools are important contexts of this kind in our culture.

We expect that, as a rule, cultures will vary greatly in the kinds of "operative exercise" that they afford members, with particular operations governing practice in different domains.

A crucial requirement in future work on culture and cognition will be the study of cognition in those settings crucial to the use of mind in different cultures. Our current preoccupation with the manipulation of objects and disembodied information can tell us a great deal about our own cultural practices in the service of modern technology. But it is a limited tool for understanding cultural influences on the development of mind.

Application to the notion of intelligence. The units of analysis upon which a theory of culture and cognition must be based are clearly too global to be of direct use to those seeking to explain differences in cognitive achievement for people growing up in what is assumed to be equivalent environments, for example, environments assumed to fulfill the psychological specification of the conditions needed to establish a difference in intelligence. From a schema-theoretic point of view, Spearman's very early notion that intelligence is the ability to "apprehend analogies" is certainly congenial, because analogizing is the basic mechanism posited by such theories to account for learning (e.g., Rumelhart & Norman,

1980). In relating schema acquisition to cultural experience, however, we have been led to examine the differences in the context made available to individuals by their culture. Postulating a universal analogizing mechanism in which differences in some (unspecified) component process(es) are used to account for individual variation is of no help. In short, a cultural theory of intelligence must rest upon cultural differences in the events out of which people can create schemata.

A clear implication of this line of reasoning is that *intelligence* will be different across cultures (and across contexts within cultures) insofar as there are differences in the kinds of problems that different cultural milieus pose their initiates. *In this sense*, we must adopt the position of cultural relativists, such as Berry (1971) and Boas (1911), that no universal notion of a single, general ability, called intelligence, can be abstracted from the behavior of people whose experiences in the world have systematically been different from birth in response to different life predicaments handed down to them in their ecocultural niche. In this sense, all cultures have to be considered equally effective in producing ways of dealing with the problems of survival of our species under unique patterns of constraint. Unless and until it is demonstrated that there is a common mechanism underlying all schema formation, so that it is possible to claim that some kinds of experience positively influence that single process of formation differentially, no other position is feasible.

However, this radical relativist conclusion does not represent the full position of a context-specific culture–cognition theory of the type we have outlined in this chapter, because it fails to consider the fact that cultures interact. Though it is a logical requirement to adopt radical relativism in the ideal case, we are led to a somewhat different position with respect to the treatment of domain-specific achievements considered cross-culturally in the nonideal case of the contemporary world. Throughout human history, cultural groups in contact have also been in competition for resources. That competition has sometimes been in the form of friendly cooperation, but more often the ability of one group to dominate the other politically (and hence economically) has been crucial to the nature of culturally organized experience in both the dominated and the dominating group. Key resources in such struggles have been culturally elaborated tools (ranging from the bow and arrow to the neutron bomb, from the rudiments of an alphabet to modern computers) for operating on the environment (where *environment* now stands for other peoples as well as one's own people and physical setting). It has been very tempting over the past 400 years to take the level of those technologies associated with "the modern world" as an index of the extent to which the peoples in the groups producing those technologies have developed further than others in the *common* problem of adapting to the planet earth.

This line of reasoning can be recognized as but a subset of the general proposition that if one wishes to abstract a particular kind of activity from its cultural context and assert (a) that it is a universal kind of achievement that differing peoples have mastered to greater or lesser degree, and (b) that one has a true theory of developmental stages in that domain, then it is possible to do a kind of *conditional comparison* in which we can see how different cultures have organized experience to deal with that domain of activity. When this conditionality is forgotten, the door is left open to severe abuses of the scientific method in favor of ethnocentric claims about the true nature of reality.

NOTES

The following members of the Laboratory of Comparative Human Cognition collaborated on this work: Alonzo Anderson, Denise Borders-Simmons, Michael Cole, Esteban Diaz, Peg Griffin, Laura Martin, Bud Mehan, Luis Moll, Jacquelyn Mitchell, Denis Newman, Mitch Rabinowitz, Margaret Riel, Warren Simmons, and Stephanie Stolarz. Substantial assistance in revising and clarifying the ideas expressed was provided by Jean Lave and James Wertsch. Support for this work was provided by Carnegie Corporation DC15 Dept. 06/84; Ford Foundation 780-0639; and National Institute of Mental Health MH 15972-01.

1 Our thanks to Charles Lave for making these calculations.

2 Kirk's failure to measure such precision in the child in any way other than the age at which conservation is achieved makes this explanation less than totally satisfactory.

3 In fact, they have been called culture-free tests of intelligence by Jensen (1980).

4 Not all subjects could draw, and so this task was deleted for some unspecified number of subjects.

5 In earlier versions of this task, in which both person and wooden frame could be tilted, the alternative criteria for judging made the analogy even clearer.

6 It is significant that Piaget took as evidence for this view research that had demonstrated time lags of several years in a group of Third World children whose primary school program is identical to that used in France.

7 Dasen mentions an important difficulty with the studies of decalage: The effects of cultural variables are not discernible in group statistics that present population frequencies of responses at different ages. Individual longitudinal studies would serve to uncover differences in hierarchical development, but such studies are absent from the cross-cultural literature.

8 Glick (1975) offers a useful discussion of the ways in which language factors may enter into Piagetian assessment.

9 As related by Jahoda (1980), Witkin believed that differences between field-independent and field-dependent people could be demonstrated only if the conditions facing the individual had the right degree of structuring. For example, whereas field-dependent people would be expected to make use of external social referents, this expectation would hold only if the circumstances were ill structured and ambiguous. In short, the general process is one whose expression is context-dependent in ways that need to be specified in the theory.

10 The spot-observation technique involves timed samples of behavior of target subjects (see B. Whiting & Whiting, 1975, for a review).

11 It might also be concluded that this last line of speculation is a non sequitur. Once experience is organized to permit practice in thinking outside one's experience, thinking-outside-one's-experience becomes a part of one's experience. This important point underlies doubts about evidence concerning the cognitive efficacy of schooling, and brings us back to the difficulty of specifying familiarity (see Sharp et al., 1979).

12 The only task from the initial series of studies suggesting that literacy would substitute for schooling required subjects to categorize geometric figures on the basis of form and number, a change in salience of those attributes of graphic symbols common to all three writing systems.

13 A great deal of such research has appeared in recent years. Fischer (1980) for example, provides many examples of domain-specific development, in which increasingly complex skills are acquired within "skill domains," and of the ways in which populations of skills change over development. Other examples are provided by Feldman (1980) and Chi (1978).

14 Research by Karmiloff-Smith (1979) suggests that increasingly sophisticated performance within a single "stage" can be engendered by repeated practice in which the child comes to integrate activity. The notion of error in our formulation must be expanded to account for impediments resulting from poorly integrated knowledge components, as well as components that produce obvious contradictions.

15 Insofar as it takes time to undergo the needed experiences, children growing up in similar circumstances are likely to reach the same stages at about the same ages.

16 This concept has been the basis for a wide range of developmental research projects. Studies of play by El'konin and his associates have built upon the idea that fantasy situations provide interactional props allowing more complex intellectual accomplishments (El'konin, 1971). This idea was carried into studies of memory, where the role of event

knowledge and the social structure in remembering and motor-control performance were the objects of attention (Istomina, 1975; Manuilenko, 1975). It has also been applied to design of an elementary-school curriculum in language arts (Cazden, 1979; Markova, 1978–1979), and used in training the mentally retarded (Brown & Ferrara, 1982).

17 Although the role of rapport in eliciting the child's best effort is widely recognized (see, e.g., Jensen, 1969), there are few theoretical accounts of this phenomenon that include the adult's social behaviors (other than those embodied in the instructions) as a resource for the child's problem solving (see, however, Mehan, 1979). From our point of view, *rapport* describes ways in which adults create a more effective zone of proximal development supporting children's overall problem-solving performance. It functions like play in this respect (Saltz & Johnson, 1974; Vygotsky, 1934/1978, chap. 6).

18 The concept did organize the clinical interview strategy applied by Luria (1976). However, his research gathered talk about concepts and objects and involved almost no direct observation of indigenous activities involving those concepts.

19 In fact, the notion of "individual" accomplishment is an abstraction, the problematic status of which is a serious bone of contention dividing social scientists; see Mehan & Wood (1975).

REFERENCES

Barker, R. G. *Ecological psychology: Concepts and methods for studying the environment of human behavior.* Stanford: Stanford University Press, 1968.
Barry, H. Bacon, M., & Child, I. A class-cultural survey of sex differences and socialization. *Journal of Abnormal Social Psychology,* 1957, 55, 327–332.
Barry, H., Child, I., & Bacon, M. Relation of child training to subsistence economy. *American Anthropologist,* 1959, 61, 51–63.
Bayley, N. Comparisons of mental and motor test scores for ages 1–15 months by sex, birth order, race, geographic location, and education of parents. *Child Development,* 1965, 36, 379–411.
Bellman, B. L. Ethnohermeneutics: On the interpretation of subjective meaning. In W. McCormack & W. Wurm (Eds.), *Language and Mind.* The Hague: Mouton, 1978.
Berry, J. W. Temne and Eskimo perceptual skills. *International Journal of Psychology,* 1966, 1, 207–229.
Berry, J. W. Radical cultural relativism and the concept of intelligence. In J. W. Berry & P. R. Dasen (Eds.), *Culture and cognition: Readings in cross-cultural psychology.* London: Methuen, 1974.
Berry, J. W. On cross-cultural comparability. *International Journal of Psychology,* 1969, 4, 119–128.
Berry, J. W. *Human ecology and cognitive style.* New York: Sage-Halsted, 1976.
Berry, J. W., & Dasen, P. R. (Eds.). *Culture and cognition: Readings in cross-cultural psychology.* London: Methuen, 1974.
Boas, F. *The mind of primitive man.* New York: Macmillan, 1911.
Bock, P. K. *Continuities in psychological anthropology.* San Francisco: W. H. Freeman, 1980.
Boonsong, S. *The development of conservation of mass, weight and volume in Thai children.* Unpublished master's thesis, Bangkok College of Education, 1968.
Bovet, M. C. Cognitive processes among illiterate children and adults. In J. W. Berry, & P. R. Dasen (Eds.), *Culture and cognition: Readings in cross-cultural psychology,* London: Methuen, 1974.
Bovet, M. C., Dasen, P. R., & Inhelder, B. Etapes de l'intelligence sensori-motrice chez l'enfant Baoule. *Archives de Psychologie,* 1974, 41, 363–386.
Brazelton, T. B. *Neonatal behavioral assessment scales.* London: Spastics International Medical Publications, 1973.
Brislin, R. W., Lonner, W. J., & Thorndike, R. M. *Cross-cultural research methods.* New York: Wiley, 1973.
Brown, A. L., & Ferrara, R. A. Diagnosing zones of proximal development: An alternative to standardized testing? In J. Wertsch (Ed.), *Culture, communication and cognition: Vygotskian perspectives.* Cambridge: Cambridge University Press, 1982.
Brown, A., & French, L. A. Commentary in D. Sharp, M. Cole, & C. Lave, Education and

cognitive development: The evidence from experimental research. *Monographs of the Society for Research in Child Development,* 1979, 44(1–2, Serial No. 178).

Bruner, J., Olver, R., & Greenfield, P. *Studies in cognitive growth.* New York: Wiley, 1966.

Campbell, D. T. Distinguishing differences of perception from failures of communication in cross-cultural studies. In F. S. C. Northrop & N. H. Livingston (Eds.), *Cross-cultural understanding: Epistemology in anthropology.* New York: Harper & Row, 1964.

Case, R. Intellectual development from birth to adulthood: A neopiagetian interpretation. In R. Siegler, *Children's thinking: What develops?* Hillsdale, N.J.: Erlbaum, 1978.

Cazden, C. Language in education: Variation in the teacher-talk register. *30th Annual Georgetown University Round Table on Languages and Linguistics,* 1979.

Chamberlain, A. F. *The child: A study in the evolution of man.* London: Walter Scott, 1901.

Chi, M. T. H. Knowledge structure and memory development. In R. Siegler (Ed.), *Carnegie Symposium on Cognition.* Hillsdale, N.J.: Erlbaum, 1978.

Childs, C. P., & Greenfield, P. M. Informal modes of learning and teaching: The case of Zinacanto weaving. In N. Warren (Ed.), *Advances in cross-cultural psychology* (Vol. 2). London: Academic Press, 1981.

Cole, M., Gay, J., Glick, J. A., & Sharp, D. W. *The cultural context of learning and thinking.* New York: Basic Books, 1971.

Cole, M., & Means, B. *Comparative studies of how people think.* Cambridge, Mass.: Harvard University Press, 1981.

Cole, M., & Scribner, S. *Culture and thought: A psychological introduction.* New York: Wiley, 1974.

Dasen, P. R. *Cognitive development in aborigines of Central Australia: Concrete operations and perceptual activities.* Unpublished doctoral dissertation, Australian National University, 1970.

Dasen, P. R. Cross-cultural Piagetian research: A summary. *Journal of Cross-cultural Psychology,* 1972, 3(1), 29–39.

Dasen, P. R. The influence of ecology, culture and European contact on cognitive development in Australian aborigines. In J. W. Berry & P. R. Dasen (Eds.), *Culture and cognition.* London: Methuen, 1974.

Dasen, P. R. Are cognitive processes universal? A contribution to cross-cultural Piagetian psychology. In N. Warren (Ed.), *Studies in cross-cultural psychology* (Vol. 1). London: Academic Press, 1977.

Dasen, P. R. Psychological differentiation and operational development: A cross-cultural link. *Quarterly Newsletter of the Laboratory of Comparative Human Cognition,* 1980, 2(4).

Dasen, P. R., Berry, J. W., & Witkin, H. A. The use of developmental theories cross-culturally. In L. Eckensberger, Y. Poortinga, & W. Lonner (Eds.), *Cross-cultural contributions to psychology.* Amsterdam: Swets & Zeitlinger, 1979.

Dasen, P. R., Lavallee, M., & Reschitzki, J. Training conservation of quantity (liquids) in West African (Baoulé) children. *International Journal of Psychology,* 1979, 14(1), 57–68.

Dasen, P. R., Ngini, L., & Lavallee, M. Cross-cultural training studies of concrete operations. In L. H. Eckensberger, W. J. Lonner & Y. H. Poortinga (Eds.), *Cross-cultural contributions to psychology.* Amsterdam: Swets & Zeitlinger, 1979.

Dawson, J. L. M. Cultural and physiological influences upon spatial-perceptual processes in West Africa: Part I. *International Journal of Psychology,* 1967, 2(2), 115–128.

deLemos, M. M. The development of conservation in aboriginal children. *International Journal of Psychology,* 1969, 4, 225–269.

Dempsey, A. D. Time conservation across cultures. *International Journal of Psychology,* 1971, 6, 115–120.

Doise, W., Mugny, G., & Perret-Clermont, A. Social interaction and the development of cognitive operations. *European Journal of Social Psychology,* 1975, 5, 367–383.

Dube, E. F. *A cross-cultural study of the relationship between "intelligence" level and story recall.* Unpublished doctoral dissertation, Cornell University, 1977.

El'konin, D. Symbolics and its functions in the play of children. In R. E. Herron, & B. Sutton-Smith (Eds.), *Child's play.* New York: Wiley, 1971.

Estes, W. K. Learning theory and intelligence. *American Psychologist,* 1974, 29(10).

Estes, W. K. (Ed.). *Handbook of learning and cognitive processes* (Vols. 1–6). Hillsdale, N.J.: Erlbaum, 1975–1979.

Estes, W. K. *Intelligence and learning.* Unpublished manuscript, Harvard University, 1979.

Feldman, D. H. *Beyond universals in cognitive development*. Norwood, N.J.: Ablex, 1980.

Feldman, C. F., & Stone, A. Colored blocks test: Culture-general measure of cognitive development. *Journal of Cross-cultural Psychology*, 1978, *9*(1), 3–23.

Fischer, K. W. A theory of cognitive development. *Psychological Review*, 1980, 87(6), 477–531.

Flavell, J. H., & Wohlwill, J. F. Formal and functional aspects of cognitive development. In D. Elkind & J. H. Flavell (Eds.), *Studies in cognitive development*. New York: Oxford University Press, 1969.

Fortes, M. Social and psychological aspects of education in Taleland. In J. Middleton (Ed.), *From child to adult: Studies in the anthropology of education*. New York: Natural History Press, 1970.

Frijda, N., & Jahoda, G. On the scope and methods of cross-cultural research. *International Journal of Psychology*, 1966, *1*, 109–127.

Gagné, R. M. Learning hierarchies. *Educational Psychologist*, 1968, 6, 1–9.

Galton, F. *Inquiries into human faculty and its development*. London: Macmillan, 1883.

Gay, J., & Cole, M. *The new mathematics and an old culture*. New York: Holt, Rinehart & Winston, 1967.

Gerber, M. Développement psychomoteur de l'enfant africain. *Courrier*, 1956, 6, 17–29.

Geber, M. L'enfant africain occidentalise et de niveau social supérieur en Ouganga. *Courrier*, 1958, 8, 517–523.

Geber, M. Développement psychomoteur des petits Baganda de la naissance a six ans. *Journal Suisse de Psychologie*, 1961, 20, 345–357.

Geber, M. La recherche sur le développement psychomoteur et mental a Kampala. *Compte-rendu de la XII Réunion des Equipes Chargées des Etudes sur la Croissance et de développement de l'enfant normal*. Paris: Centre Internationale de l'Enfance, 1974.

Geber, M., & Dean, R. F. A. Gesell tests on African children. *Pediatrics*, 1957, 20, 1055–1065.

Geber, M., & Dean, R. F. A. Psychomotor development in African children: The effects of proved tests. *Bulletin of the World Health Organization*, 1958, *18*, 471–476.

Gesell, A., & Amatruda, C. S. *Developmental diagnosis* (2nd ed.). New York: Hoeber, 1947.

Glick, J. Cognitive development in cross-cultural perspective. In T. D. Horowitz (ed.), *Review of child development research*. Chicago: University of Chicago Press, 1975.

Goodenough, F. The measurement of mental functions in primitive groups. *American Anthropologist*, 1936, *38*, 1–11.

Goodenough, D. R., & Karp, S. A. Field dependence and intellectual functioning. *Journal of Abnormal and Social Psychology*, 1961, 63, 241–246.

Goodnow, J. J. A test of milieu differences with some of Piaget's tasks. *Psychological Monographs*, 1962, 76(36, Whole No. 555).

Goodnow, J. Rules and repertoires, rituals and tricks of the trade: Social and informational aspects to cognitive and representational development. In S. Farnham-Diggory (Ed.), *Information processing in children*. New York: Academic Press, 1969.

Goody, J., & Watt, I. The consequences of literacy. In J. Goody (Ed.), *Literacy in traditional societies*. Cambridge: Cambridge University Press, 1968. (Originally published in *Comparative Studies in Society and History*, 1963, 5, 27–68.)

Gould, S. J. *Ontogeny and phylogeny*. Cambridge, Mass.: Harvard University Press, 1976.

Grantham-McGregor, S. M., & Hawke, W. A. Developmental assessment of Jamaican infants. *Developmental Medicine and Child Neurology*, 1971, *13*, 582–589.

Greenfield, P. M. On culture and conservation. In J. S. Bruner, R. P. Oliver, & P. M. Greenfield (Eds.), *Studies in cognitive growth*. New York: Wiley, 1966.

Greenfield, P. M. Comparing dimensional categorization in natural and artificial contexts: A developmental study among the Zinacantecos of Mexico. *Journal of Social Psychology*, 1974, *93*, 157–171.

Greenfield, P. M. Cross-cultural research and Piagetian theory: Paradox and progress. In K. F. Riegel, & J. A. Meacham (Eds.), *The developing individual in a changing world*. Vol. 1: *Historical and cultural issues*. Chicago: Aldine, 1976.

Harris, M. *The rise of anthropological theory*. New York: Crowell, 1968.

Havelock, E. A. *The Greek concept of justice: From its shadow in Homer to its substance in Plato*. Cambridge, Mass.: Harvard University Press, 1978.

Heron, A. Concrete operations, "g" and achievement in Zambian children: A non-verbal approach. *Journal of Cross-cultural Psychology*, 1971, 2, 325–336.

Hunt, E. Varieties of cognitive power. In L. B. Resnick (Ed.), *The nature of intelligence.* Hillsdale, N.J.: Erlbaum, 1976.

Hutchins, E. *Culture and inference.* Cambridge, Mass.: Harvard University Press, 1980.

Inhelder, B., & Piaget, J. *The growth of logical thinking from childhood to adolescence.* New York: Basic Books, 1958.

Irvine, J. Wolof "Magical Thinking: Culture and conservation revisited." *Journal of Cross-cultural Psychology,* 1978, *9,* 300–310.

Irwin, M., Engle, P. L., Klein, R. E., & Yarbrough, C. Traditionalism and field dependence. *Journal of Cross-cultural Psychology,* 1976, *7*(4), 463–471.

Irwin, M. H., & McLaughlin, D. H. Ability and preference in category sorting by Mano school children and adults. *Journal of Social Psychology,* 1970, *82,* 15–24.

Irwin, M. H., Schafer, G. N., & Feiden, C. P. Emic and unfamiliar category sorting of Mano farmers and U.S. undergraduates. *Journal of Cross-cultural Psychology,* 1974, *5,* 407–423.

Istomina, Z. M. The development of voluntary memory in preschool-age children. *Soviet Psychology,* 1975, *13*(4), 5–64.

Jahoda, G. Theoretical and systematic approaches in cross-cultural psychology. In H. C. Triandis & W. W. Lambert (Eds.), *Handbook of cross-cultural psychology* (Vol. 1). Boston: Allyn & Bacon, 1980.

Jensen, A. R. How much can we boost IQ and scholastic achievement? *Harvard Educational Review,* 1969, *39,* 1–123.

Jensen, A. R. *Bias in mental testing.* New York: Free Press, 1980.

Kagan, J., Kearsley, R., & Zelazo, P. *Infancy.* Cambridge, Mass.: Harvard University Press, 1978.

Kamara, A. I. *Cognitive development among school-age Themne children of Sierra Leone.* Unpublished doctoral dissertation, University of Illinois, 1971.

Kamara, A. I., & Easley, J. A., Jr. Is the rate of cognitive development uniform across cultures? – A methodological critique with new evidence from Themne children. In P. R. Dasen (Ed.), *Piagetian psychology.* New York: Gardner, 1977.

Karmiloff-Smith, A. Micro- and macrodevelopmental changes in language acquisition and other representational systems. *Cognitive Science,* 1979, *3,* 91–118.

Kearins, J. M. Visual spatial memory in Australian aboriginal children of desert regions. *Cognitive Psychology,* 1981, *3*(4), 434–460.

Kelly, M. Papua New Guinea and Piaget – An eight-year study. In P. R. Dasen (Ed.), *Piagetian psychology: Cross-cultural contributions.* New York: Gardner Press, 1977.

Kilbride, J. E., & Kilbride, P. L. Sitting and smiling behavior of Baganda infants: The influence of culturally constituted experiences. *Journal of Cross-cultural Psychology,* 1975, *6,* 88–106.

Kirk, L. Maternal and subcultural correlates of cognitive growth rate: The Ga pattern. In P. R. Dasen (Ed.), *Piagetian psychology: Cross-cultural contributions.* New York: Gardner Press, 1977.

Klahr, D. Steps toward the simulation of intellectual development. In L. Resnick (Ed.), *The nature of intelligence.* Hillsdale, N.J.: Erlbaum, 1976.

Klein, R., Freeman, H. E., & Millet, R. Psychological test performance and indigenous conceptions of intelligence. *Journal of Psychology,* 1973, *84,* 219–222.

Kleinfeld, J. Visual memory in village Eskimo and urban Caucasian children. *Artic,* 1971, *24,* 132–137.

Klineberg, O. Historical perspectives: Cross-cultural psychology before 1960. In H. C. Triandis & W. W. Lambert (Eds.), *Handbook of cross-cultural psychology* (Vol. 1). Boston: Allyn & Bacon, 1980.

Kroeber, A., & Kluckhohn, C. Culture: A critical review of concepts and definitions. *Papers of the Peabody Museum of American Archaeology and Ethnology, Harvard University,* 1952, 47.

Kulah, A. A. *The organization and learning of proverbs among the Kpelle of Liberia.* Unpublished doctoral dissertation, University of California, Irvine, 1973.

Laboratory of Comparative Human Cognition. Cognition as a residual category in anthropology. *Annual Review of Anthropology,* 1978, *7,* 51–69.

Laboratory of Comparative Human Cognition. What's cultural about cross-cultural cognitive psychology? *Annual Review of Psychology,* 1979, *30,* 145–172. (a)

Laboratory of Comparative Human Cognition. Cross-cultural psychology's challenges to our ideas of children and development. *American Psychologist*, 1979, *34*(10), 827–833. (b)

Laboratory of Comparative Human Cognition. Culture and cognitive development. In W. Kessen (Ed.), *Mussen handbook of child development* (Vol. 1). New York: Wiley, 1982.

Lantz, D. A cross-cultural comparison of communication abilities: Some effects of age, schooling and culture. *International Journal of Psychology*, 1979, *14*, 171–183.

Lave, J. Tailor-made experiments and evaluating the intellectual consequences of apprenticeship training. *Quarterly Newsletter of the Institute for Comparative Human Development*, 1977, *1*(2), 1–3.

Lave, J. What's special about experiments as contexts for thinking? *Quarterly Newsletter of the Laboratory of Comparative Human Cognition*, 1980, 2(4), 86–91.

Lave, J. *Apprenticeship and a cultural theory of learning*. Unpublished manuscript, University of California, Irvine, n.d.

Lee, R. B., & DeVore, I. (Eds.). *Kalahari hunter-gatherers*. Cambridge, Mass.: Harvard University Press, 1976.

Leiderman, P. H., Tulkin, S. R., & Rosenfeld, A. (Eds.). *Culture and infancy: Variations in the human experience*. New York: Academic Press, 1977.

Leontiev, A. N. The problem of activity in psychology. In J. V. Wertsch (Ed.), *The concept of activity in Soviet psychology*. White Plains, N.Y.: Sharpe, in press.

Levine, M. Hypothesis behavior by humans during discrimination learning. *Journal of Experimental Psychology*, 1966, *71*, 331–338.

Lewis, D. Observations on route finding and spatial orientation among the aboriginal peoples of the Western Desert region of Central Australia. *Oceania*, 1976, *46*(4), 249–282.

Luria, A. R. Psychological expedition to central Asia. *Science*, 1931, *74*(1920), 383–384.

Luria, A. R. *The nature of human conflicts*. New York: Liveright, 1932.

Luria, A. R. *Cognitive development*. Cambridge, Mass.: Harvard University Press, 1976.

Luria, A. R. The development of writing in the child. In M. Cole (Ed.), *The selected writings of A. R. Luria*. White Plains, N.Y.: Sharpe, 1978.

Luria, A. R. *The making of mind: A personal account of Societ psychology* (M. Cole & S. Cole, Eds.). Cambridge, Mass.: Harvard University Press, 1979.

MacArthur, R. S. Some ability patterns: Central Eskimos and Ngenga Africans. *International Journal of Psychology*, 1973, *8*, 239–247.

Malinowski, B. *The father in primitive psychology*. New York: Norton, 1927.

Mandler, G., & Dean, P. J. Seriation: The development of serial order in free recall. *Journal of Experimental Psychology*, 1969, *81*, 207–215.

Mandler, J. Structural invariance in development. In L. S. Liben (Ed.), *Piaget and the foundation of knowledge*. Hillsdale, N.J.: Erlbaum, in press.

Manuilenko, Z. V. The development of voluntary behavior in preschool-age children. *Soviet Psychology*, 1975, *13*, 65–116.

Markova, A. K. *The teaching and mastery of language*. White Plains, N.Y.: M. E. Sharpe, 1979.

McDermott, R. P., & Roth, D. R. The social organization of behavior: Interactional approaches. *Annual Review of Anthropology*, 1978, 7, 321–345.

McElwain, D. W., & Kearney, G. E. Intellectual development. In G. E. Kearney, P. R. deLacey, & G. R. Davidson (Eds.), *The psychology of aboriginal Australians*. Sydney: Wiley, 1973.

McFie, J. The effect of education on African performance on a group of intellectual tests. *British Journal of Educational Psychology*, 1961, *31*, 232–240.

McLuhan, M. *The Gutenberg galaxy*. Toronto: University of Toronto Press, 1962.

Meacham, J. A. Patterns of memory abilities in two cultures. *Developmental Psychology*, 1975, *11*, 50–53.

Mead, M. *Coming of age in Samoa*. New York: Morrow, 1928.

Mead, M. *Continuities and discontinuities in cultural evolution*. New Haven: Yale University Press, 1958.

Mead, M. The evocation of psychologically relevant responses in ethnological field work. In G. D. Spindler (Ed.), *The making of psychological anthropology*. Berkeley and Los Angeles: University of California Press, 1978.

Mead, M. Samoan children at work and play. *Natural History*, 1980, 89(4), 103–105.

Mehan, H. *Learning lessons*. Cambridge, Mass.: Harvard University Press, 1979.

Mehan, H., & Wood, H. *The reality of ethnomethodology*. New York: Wiley, 1975.

Minsky, M. A framework for representing knowledge. In P. H. Winston (Ed.), *The psychology of computer vision*. New York: McGraw-Hill, 1975.

Morgan, L. H. *Ancient society*. New York: Holt, 1877.

Mosheni, N. *La comparaison des réactions aux épreuves d'intelligence en Iran et en Europe*. Unpublished thesis, University of Paris, 1966.

Munroe, R. H., & Munroe, R. L. Land, labor, and the child's cognitive performance among the Logoli. *American Ethnologist*, 1977, 4(2).

Nadel, S. F. *Foundations of social anthropology*. London: Cohen & West, 1951.

Nagel, E. *The structure of science*. New York: Harcourt, Brace & World, 1961.

Neimark, E. D. Intellectual development during adolescence. In F. D. Horowitz (Ed.), *Review of child development research* (Vol. 4). Chicago: University of Chicago Press, 1975.

Nerlove, S. B., Roberts, J. M., Klein, R., Yarbrough, C., & Habicht, J. P. Natural indicators of cognitive development: An observational study of rural Guatemalan children. *Ethos*, 1974, 2(3), 265–295.

Nissen, H. W., Machover, S., & Kinder, E. T. A study of performance tests given to a group of native African Negro children. *British Journal of Psychology*, 1935, 25, 308–355.

Nyiti, R. *A study of conservation among Meru children of Tanzania*. Unpublished doctoral dissertation, University of Illinois, 1973.

Nyiti, R. M. The development of conservation in the Meru children of Tanzania. *Child Development*, 1976, 47, 1122–1129.

Okonji, M. O. The differential effects of rural and urban upbringing on the development of cognitive styles. *International Journal of Psychology*, 1969, 4, 293–305.

Olson, D. R. From utterance to text: The bias of language in speech and writing. *Harvard Educational Review*, 1977, 47, 257–281.

Otaala, B. *The development of operational thinking in primary school children: An examination of some aspects of Piaget's theory among the Itseo children of Uganda*. Unpublished doctoral dissertation, Teachers College, Columbia University, 1971.

Pascual-Leone, J. *Piaget's period of concrete operations and Witkin's field dependence: A study on college students and children*. Unpublished manuscript, University of British Columbia, n.d.

Peluffo, N. Culture and cognitive problems. *International Journal of Psychology*, 1967, 2(3), 187–198.

Piaget, J. *The language and thought of the child*. New York: Meridian, 1926.

Piaget, J. *Science of education and the psychology of the child*. New York: Grossman, 1970. (Originally published, 1953.)

Piaget, J. *The language and thought of the child*. New York: World, 1955.

Piaget, J. *The origins of intelligence in children*. New York: Norton, 1963.

Piaget, J. Need and significance of cross-cultural studies in genetic psychology. *International Journal of Psychology*, 1966, 1, 3–13.

Piaget, J. *Six psychological studies*. New York: Vintage, 1967.

Piaget, J. Piaget's theory. In P. H. Mussen (Ed.), *Carmichael's manual of child psychology* (3rd ed.). New York: Wiley, 1970.

Piaget, J. Intellectual evolution from adolescence to adulthood. *Human Development*, 1972, 15, 1–12.

Piaget, J. *The psychology of intelligence*. Totowa, N.J.: Littlefield & Adams, 1973.

Piaget, J. *The development of thought: Equilibration of cognitive structures*. New York: Viking, 1977.

Price-Williams, D. R. Abstract and concrete modes of classification in a primitive society. *British Journal of Educational Psychology*, 1962, 32, 50–61.

Price-Williams, D. R. (Ed.). *Explorations in cross-cultural psychology*. San Francisco: Chandler & Sharp, 1975.

Price-Williams, D. Concrete and formal operations. In R. H. Munroe, R. L. Munroe, & B. Whiting (Eds.), *Handbook of cross-cultural human development*. New York: Garland STPM Press, 1981.

Price-Williams, D., Gordon, W., & Ramirez, M. Skill and conservation: A study of pottery-making children. *Developmental Psychology*, 1969, 1, 769.

Prince, J. R. The effect of Western education on science conceptualization in New Guinea. *British Journal of Educational Psychology*, 1968, 38, 64–74.

Prince, J. R. *Science concepts in a Pacific culture*. Sydney: Angus & Robertson, 1969.

Radin, P. *Primitive man as philosopher*. New York: Dover, 1957.

Raum, O. F. *Chaga childhood*. London: Oxford University Press, 1940.

Resnick, L. (Ed.). *The nature of intelligence*. Hillsdale, N. J.: Erlbaum, 1976.

Resnick, L. B., & Glaser, R. Problem solving and intelligence. In L. Resnick (Ed.), *The nature of intelligence*. Hillsdale, N.J.: Erlbaum, 1976.

Rivers, W. H. R. Vision. In A. C. Haddon (Ed.), *Reports of the Cambridge Anthropological Expedition to the Torres Straits* (Vol. 2). Cambridge: Cambridge University Press, 1901.

Rogoff, B. *Mother's teaching style and child memory: A Highland Guatemala study*. Paper presented to the meeting of the Society for Research in Child Development, New Orleans, 1977.

Rogoff, B. Schooling and the development of cognitive skills. In H. C. Triandis & A. Heron (Eds.), *Handbook of cross-cultural psychology* (Vol. 4). Boston: Allyn & Bacon, 1980.

Ross, M. B., and Millsom, C. Repeated memory of oral prose in Ghana and New York. *International Journal of Psychology*, 1968, 5(3), 172–181.

Rumelhart, D. E. Schemata: The building blocks of cognition. In R. Spiro, B. Bruce, & W. Brewer (Eds.), *Theoretical issues in reading comprehension*. Hillsdale, N.J.: Erlbaum, 1980.

Rumelhart, D. E., & Norman, D. A. Analogical processes in learning. In J. R. Anderson (Ed.), *Cognitive skills and their acquisition*. Hillsdale, N.J.: Erlbaum, 1981.

Saltz, E., & Johnson, J. Training for thematic-fantasy play in culturally disadvantaged children: Preliminary results. *Journal of Educational Psychology*, 1974, 66(4), 623–630.

Saxe, G. B. A comparative analysis of the acquisition of numeration: Studies from Papua New Guinea. *Quarterly Newsletter of the Laboratory of Comparative Human Cognition*, 1979, 1(3), 37–43.

Schank, R. C., & Abelson, R. P. Scripts, plans, and knowledge. *Advance Papers of the Fourth International Joint Conference on Artificial Intelligence*, Tbilisi, Georgia, USSR, 1975, pp. 151–157.

Schutz, A. *Collected papers* (Vol. 2). The Hague: Mouton, 1964.

Scribner, S. Modes of thinking and ways of speaking: Culture and logic reconsidered. In P. N. Johnson-Laird & P. C. Wason (Eds.), *Thinking: Readings in cognitive science*. Cambridge: Cambridge University Press, 1977.

Scribner, S., & Cole, M. Cognitive consequences of formal and informal education. *Science*, 1973, 182, 553–559.

Scribner, S., & Cole, M. Literacy without schooling: Testing for intellectual effects. *Harvard Educational Review*, 1978, 48(4), 448–461.

Scribner, S., & Cole, M. *The psychology of literacy*. Cambridge, Mass.: Harvard University Press, 1981.

Serpell, R. The influence of language, education and culture on attentional preference between colour and form. *International Journal of Psychology*, 1969, 4, 183–194.

Serpell, R. *Culture's influence on behaviour*. London: Methuen, 1976.

Serpell, R. Strategies for investigating intelligence in its cultural context. *Quarterly Newsletter of the Laboratory of Comparative Human Cognition*, 1977, 1(3), 11–15.

Serpell, R. How specific are perceptual skills? A cross-cultural study of pattern reproduction. *British Journal of Psychology*, 1979, 70, 365–380.

Sharp, D. W., Cole, M., & Lave, C. Education and cognitive development: The evidence from experimental research. *Monographs of the Society for Research in Child Development*, 1979, 44(1–2, Serial No. 178).

Shweder, R. A. Rethinking culture and personality theory: Part I. A critical examination of two classical postulates. *Ethos*, 1979, 7, 255–278.(a)

Shweder, R. A. Rethinking culture and personality theory: Part II. A critical examination of two classical postulates. *Ethos*, 1979, 7, 279–311. (b)

Shweder, R. A. Rethinking culture and personality theory: Part III. From genesis and typology to hermeneutics and dynamics. *Ethos*, 1980, 8, 60–94.

Siann, G. Measuring field dependence in Zambia. *International Journal of Psychology*, 1972, 7, 87–96.

Siegler, R. S. Information processing approaches to development. In P. H. Mussen (Ed.) *Handbook of child psychology* (History, theories, and methods volume (W. Kessen (Ed.)). New York: Wiley, in press.

Smith, E., & Medin, D. *Categories and concepts*. Cambridge, Mass.: Harvard University Press, 1981.

Spencer, H. *The principles of psychology* (Vol. 5). New York: D. Appleton, 1886.

Steinberg, B. M., & Dunn, L. A. Conservation competence and performance in Chiapas. *Human Development*, 1976, 19, 14–25.

Stocking, G. *Race, culture and evolution.* New York: Free Press, 1968.

Super, C. M. Environmental effects on motor development: The case of African infant precocity. *Developmental Medicine and Child Neurology,* 1976, *18*(5), 561–567.

Super, C. Behavioral development in infancy. In R. H. Munroe, R. L. Munroe, & B. Whiting (Eds.), *Handbook of cross-cultural human development.* New York: Garland STPM Press, 1981.

Super, C. M., & Harkness, S. The infant's niche in rural Kenya and metropolitan America. In L. L. Adler (Ed.), *Issues in cross-cultural research.* New York: Academic Press, 1980.

Thorndike, E. L. *Measurement of intelligence.* New York: Teachers College, Columbia University, 1926.

Thorndike, E. L. *Human learning.* New York: Century, 1931.

Tulviste, P. On the origins of theoretic syllogistic reasoning in culture and the child (Annotated bibliography). *Quarterly Newsletter of the Laboratory of Comparative Human Cognition,* 1979, *1*(4), 73–80.

Tyack, D. B. *The one best system: A history of American urban education.* Cambridge, Mass.: Harvard University Press, 1974.

Tylor, E. B. *Primitive culture.* London: John Murray, 1874.

University of Liberia. *The standard Vai script.* African Studies Program, August 1962.

Vernon, P. E. *Intelligence and cultural environment.* London: Methuen, 1969.

Vygotsky, L. S. *Mind in society: The development of higher psychological processes.* Cambridge, Mass.: Harvard University Press, 1978.

Vygotsky, L. S. *Thought and language.* Cambridge, Mass.: MIT Press, 1962.

Vygotsky, L. S. The genesis of higher mental functions. In J. V. Wertsch (Ed.), *The concept of activity in Soviet psychology.* White Plains, N.Y.: Sharpe, 1981.

Wagner, D. A. The effects of formal schooling on cognitive style. *Journal of Social Psychology,* 1978, *106,* 145–151.

Werner, E. E. *Cross-cultural child development.* Monterey, Calif.: Brooks/Cole, 1979.

Wertsch, J. *From social interaction to higher psychological processes: A clarification and application of Vygotsky's theory.* Paper presented at the Working Conference on the Social Foundations of Language and Thought, Center for Psychosocial Studies, Chicago, Ill., September 8–10, 1978. Revised as from social interaction to higher psychological processes: A clarification and application of Vygotsky's theory. *Human Development,* 1979, *22*(1), 1–22.

Wertsch, J. V. (Ed.). *The concept of activity in Soviet psychology.* White Plains, N.Y.: Sharpe, 1981.

Whiting, B. B. Culture and social behavior: A model for the development of social behavior. *Ethos,* 1980, *8,* 95–116.

Whiting, B. B., & Whiting, J. W. M. *Children of six cultures: A psychocultural analysis.* Cambridge, Mass.: Harvard University Press, 1975.

Whiting, J. W. M. Methods and problems in cross-cultural research. In G. Lindzey & E. Aronson (Eds.), *The handbook of social psychology* (Vol. 2). Reading, Mass.: Addison-Wesley, 1969.

Witkin, H. A. Cognitive styles across cultures: A cognitive style approach to cross-cultural research. *International Journal of Psychology,* 1967, *2*(4), 233–250.

Witkin, H. A., & Berry, J. W. Psychological differentiation in cross-cultural perspective. *Journal of Cross-cultural Psychology,* 1975, *6,* 4–87.

Witkin, H. A., Dyk, R. B., Faterson, H. F., Goodenough, D. R., & Karp, S. A. *Psychological differentiation.* New York: Wiley, 1962.

Wober, M. Sensotypes. *Journal of Social Psychology,* 1966, *70,* 181–189.

Wober, M. Distinguishing centri-cultural from cross-cultural tests and research. *Perceptual and Motor Skills,* 1969, *28,* 488.

Wober, M. *Psychology in Africa.* London: International African Institute, 1975.

Zaporozhets, A. V. Thought and activity in children. *Soviet Psychology,* 1980, *18*(2), 9–23. (Originally published, 1939.)

Za'rour, G. I., & Khuri, G. A. The development of the concept of speed by Jordanian school children in Amman. In P. R. Dasen (Ed.), *Piagetian psychology: Cross-cultural contributions.* New York: Gardner Press, 1977.

PART IV

The phylogeny and ontogeny of intelligence

12 *The evolution of biological intelligence*

HARRY J. JERISON

> I have endeavoured to show that no absolute structural line of demarca-
> tion, wider than that between the animals which immediately succeed us
> in the scale, can be drawn between the animal world and ourselves; and I
> may add the expression of my belief that the attempt to draw a psychical
> distinction is equally futile, and that even the highest faculties of feeling
> and intellect begin to germinate in lower forms of life.
>
> *T. H. Huxley*

Thomas Henry Huxley (1825–1895) presented the first challenge by an evolutionist
to conventional mid-19th-century wisdom about the uniqueness of the human mind.
His statement, given in the epigraph to this chapter, was in one of "Six Lectures to
Workingmen" presented in 1860 and is from the second chapter of *Man's Place in
Nature* (Huxley, 1863/1899). Evolutionary theory no longer insists on continuity in
the "scale" of nature (Gould, 1980; Stanley, 1979); uniqueness, continuity, and
progress are now treated in more technical ways in the analysis of adaptation of
structure and function (including behavior) in animal species. But for biological
intelligence, Huxley's statement strikes exactly the right note, emphasizing its origins in "lower forms of life" and suggesting that there is a scientific issue in tracing
the progressive evolution of intelligence as a biological character. This chapter reviews the present understanding of that evolution, with emphasis on the structural
evolution of the brain.

The working definition of intelligence here is broad enough to cover a variety of
animal intelligences. It ties behavior to neural structure and enables us to analyze
the fossil evidence of the brain as evidence on the evolution of intelligence:

*Intelligence is the behavioral consequence of the total neural information-processing capacity
in representative adults of a species, adjusted for the capacity to control routine bodily
functions.*

Total neural information-processing capacity is estimated from brain size, and the
adjustment for bodily functions is made on the basis of brain–body allometry, as
discussed later in this chapter.

This definition applies to differences among species and is only indirectly related
to individual differences within a species. Although an animal may use its processing capacity in species-typical ways, the various unique behavioral adaptations of
different species may be compared with one another according to the processing
capacity that they encumber, and so may contribute to a measure of between-species
intelligence. For a comparative and evolutionary perspective, it is helpful to think of
intelligences in the plural, and to keep in mind that a specific grade of capacity may
refer to rather different sets of behavioral adaptations. Human intelligence can be

related to this framework in that cognitive processing capacity is correlated with psychometric intelligence (Carroll, 1980; Carroll & Maxwell, 1979; Hunt, 1978; Hunt, Lunneborg, & Lewis, 1975; Jensen, 1979), although this is an intraspecific correlation. Interspecifically, "man's place in nature" is established by the very large human brain and extraordinary grade of encephalization and by species-typical human adaptations.

The connection between a neural measure of intelligence and behavioral approaches was suggested in the following observation by Karl Lashley (1890–1958) in his presidential address to the American Society of Naturalists:

The only neurological character for which a correlation with behavioral capacity in different animals is supported by significant evidence is the total mass of tissue, or rather, the index of cephalization, measured by the ratio of brain to [the 2/3-power of] body weight, which seems to represent the amount of brain tissue in excess of that required for transmitting impulses to and from the integrative centers. [Lashley, 1949, p. 33]

Lashley's "correlation" becomes our definition by reversing the direction of the implicit causal arrow to place the nervous system at the center of the concept.

The history of the ideas that shaped our understanding of biological intelligence is the topic of the next section of this chapter. This is followed by a section on modern evolutionary theory relevant to that understanding. Intelligence as a behavioral trait has been the subject of an enormous psychological and ethological literature, which is covered very selectively in the third section of the chapter. The evolution of intelligence is (for us) also the evolution of information-processing capacity, which is the history of encephalization. That history of the evolving brain, based on direct fossil evidence, is the topic of the fourth and final section.

Various specific behavioral adaptations in various animal species will be analyzed with concern for human intelligence as a biological adaptation. Human intelligence is biologically unique because of the role of language as a species-typical human cognitive adaptation. Other intelligences should also be presumed unique, but in different ways, of course.

12.1.   HISTORY AND PHILOSOPHY

Huxley's idea of continuity of variation of intelligence in the animal kingdom, quoted in the epigraph, was an extension of the great thesis of Charles Darwin (1809–1882) that species originated by "natural selection" from the normal variations within earlier species (Darwin, 1859/1872/1936). As an idea, mental continuity among animal species was a materialist challenge to two rather distinct alternatives: the rationalist, dualist view in the tradition of Aristotle (384 B.C.–322 B.C.) and René Descartes (1596–1650), and the mystical view of revealed religion. The history of our topic is to a significant extent a history of the philosophy of mind. In reading this section, it may be helpful to refer to Bertrand Russell (1945) as a guide to the philosophical language and for a broader view of the ideas.

Within nonmystical styles of thinking, differences among animal species can be described as easily in a nonevolutionary as in an evolutionary framework. The classic *scala naturae* of Linnaeus (1707–1778), in which each animal species is at its God-created discrete grade in the great "chain of being," is readily reinterpreted in modern terms. In evolutionary translation, the discrete grades are on an anagenetic evolutionary scale, which represents the progressive evolution of an adaptation (J.

Huxley, 1958; Gould, 1976; cf. Hodos & Campbell, 1969). Discontinuity is, thus, consistent with materialistic evolutionary analysis, with nonevolutionary Cartesian rationalism, and with a philosophical idealism that is comfortable with theories of animal "types." Continuity, on the other hand, is inconsistent with nonevolutionary analysis, depending as it does on the role of variation, which makes typologies untenable and change almost inevitable. Continuity of mind has additional philosophical implications if mind and body (or brain) are seen as comparable products of organic evolution. Evolutionists were likely to be philosophical monists (Morgan, 1894), and not dualists or mystics (Rieber, 1980).

The truly radical break in Huxley's assertion is with religious mysticism, a muddy dualism that allows mind to be viewed as entirely independent of body and can take seriously ideas like reincarnation and metempsychosis (transference of souls among bodies, migration of souls). The attraction of this kind of mythology is so great that it continues to support major popular industries based on fakery and delusions.

The advance to rationality has been slow. Giordano Bruno (1548–1600) recognized the inherent difficulties with mysticism, but consider what Bruno was able to make of them: "Is then the body not the habitation of the soul? No, for the soul is in the body not as location but as intrinsic form, extrinsic formative influence. . . . The body is in the soul, soul in mind. Mind either is God or is in God, as said Plotinus" (quoted in Singer, 1950, p. 127). Could a model of the evolution of intelligence as a topic in organic evolution ever be developed from such meanderings? Like Bruno, we probably have to answer no.

Some of these historical questions have been discussed more extensively by the great comparative psychologist Theodore C. Schneirla (1958). Although most neurobiologists now accept a mind–brain equivalence at least as a working hypothesis, there are convinced dualists among outstanding neurobiologists of our time. By tying mind (= self-consciousness, thoughts, feelings, memories, dreams, imaginings, intentions, the "will," and perception) to the world of the brain, they have accommodated dualism to the scientific problems of evolutionary analysis (Eccles, 1979; Popper & Eccles, 1977). The murkiness is not dissolved; the knot between mind and brain is not unraveled. But a connection is asserted that would have mind somehow connected to a functioning brain. It would be impossible to imagine a manlike mind associated with an ant's brain (cf. Schneirla, 1958) in the neurologically sophisticated modern dualism of Sir John Eccles.

The history of these ideas is a story of efforts to replace mysticism with science. To the extent that this has been accomplished, it has been done by tying mind to brain and associating mental phenomena with the work of the brain. There have been intriguing accounts of the evolution of consciousness developed in such a framework (e.g., Jaynes, 1977 – a book that includes perhaps the best and certainly the most readable review of the concept of consciousness that is available). On issues of this kind, I have taken the position that consciousness is part of the work of the brain, which includes constructing the real world of everyday experience (Jerison, 1973, 1976a). The construction is an aspect of the brain's hierarchical organization and is a way to handle the otherwise overwhelming load of neural information that is processed. Our experienced real world, according to this view, is a possible world that is constructed in a way that makes the neural information reasonably self-consistent. Animals with different kinds of neural information, for example, ones lacking color vision or having limbs that functioned as wings or flippers, would construct at least slightly different realities. The position is a familiar one to comparative psychologists (Craik, 1943/1967; Morgan, 1890/1891, pp. 312, 338) and has been charmingly illustrated by von Uexküll (1934/1957), who evoked some of these worlds by reconstructing the experiences of various animal species.

It should be emphasized that there remains a gap in our understanding between objective descriptions of the brain's work and subjective experience. The gap has not been completely bridged, but many of the events in experience are now known to be tightly tied to activity in the brain. The bridge is under construction.

BRAIN AND INTELLIGENCE

When the spleen or the pineal body was suggested as the seat of intelligence or mind, there were logical reasons for the bizarre localization. Modern philosophers are not above comparable logical games that avoid known facts (see Malcolm, 1971; Ryle, 1949), but the brain as a whole has been assigned a more or less correct place in the picture since the middle of the 18th century. A correct assignment is really not obvious. The only intuitive evidence in its favor comes from the relationship between blows to the head and alterations (and loss) of consciousness.

The modern understanding was developed in the 19th century (Young, 1970), beginning with Franz Joseph Gall (1758–1828), who is better known as the originator of the pseudoscience of phrenology. Gall was the greatest neuroanatomist of his time. Lacking stain technology, he nevertheless successfully traced many of the major neural pathways in the brain, and correctly presented the doctrine of localization of functions in the cerebral cortex. (The functions – philoprogenetiveness, friendship, etc. – were not the ones eventually localized, but that was just bad psychology. Better functions and better names were soon discovered: vision, hearing, somaesthesis, etc.; see Jerison, 1977b, Young, 1970).

There followed a strange paradoxical twist in the argument. Gall's scientific reputation was destroyed by his connection with phrenology, and the attack came from Pierre Jean Marie Flourens (1794–1867), who opposed localization and supported a kind of mass-action theory for the cerebral cortex, the idea that the cortex worked as a whole. Gall's scientific doctrine on localization was supported by some leading neurologists, however, and was eventually vindicated by the demonstration of Pierre Paul Broca (1824–1880) that the third left frontal convolution of the cerebral cortex was a "speech and language area" related to aphasia (Broca, 1861). Localization of motor functions at the cortical level was demonstrated shortly afterward by studies involving experimental surgery in animals (Ferrier, 1876, and others; see Young, 1970).

The paradox was that, despite the eventual victory for Gall's doctrine of localization, another facet of Gall's influence had led to the view that total brain size should be correlated with intelligence, an idea that implied Flourens's mass action, and thousands of human skulls were examined and measured during the 19th and early 20th centuries for information on cranial capacity. (The mammalian brain pretty much fills the cranial cavity and has a specific gravity of very nearly 1; cranial capacity is, therefore, more or less equal to brain weight – numerically equal if the measures are in cubic centimeters and grams.) This "craniology" was systematized by Broca and others as a branch of anthropology, a branch that has still not been properly evaluated. Its 19th-century biases on race differences have been exposed (Gould, 1978), but the possible correlations between brain size and intelligence within a population have not been determined. On theoretical grounds, the correlation should be low but not zero, as we shall see in the analysis of heritability and of within-species variations in encephalization.

After Broca, the mainstream of brain research moved away from gross measures and, increasingly, toward microscopic analysis. Theodor Schwann (1810–1882) had enunciated the cell doctrine, and the discovery of stain technology made it possible to see individual neurons under the microscope. This view of individual neurons led to the discovery of synaptic transmission and the modern analysis of the activity of single nerve cells in the nervous system. The fundamental task appeared to be to reduce, as much as possible, the understanding of the brain to an understanding of its elementary units and their integrative action (Sherrington, 1906). Yet theoretical understanding clearly had to be in terms of larger assemblies of cells (cf. Bindra, 1976; Hebb, 1949; Konorski, 1967). It has been only within the past decade that part of the mainstream of neurology has discovered a method of experimental analysis of cell assemblies ("modules") that may be appropriate for making the connection between intelligence and the brain (Eccles, 1979; Mountcastle, 1978; Szentágothai, 1978).

We should appreciate that, before the discovery of stain technology, the brain had to be studied primarily by gross dissection. Grossly, the brain looks like a large gland, with functions only suggested by the stalks that connect it to eye (optic nerve), ear (auditory and vestibular nerve), and body (other cranial nerves, medulla, and spinal cord). That the brain is at the confluence of tracts connecting it to sensory organs and the body did, of course, suggest that it had something to do with sensation and movement, but the something had to be guessed. That the something might be called "mind," or an equally nebulous thing, was almost pure speculation.

BRAIN–BODY RELATIONS

One reason for the correct assignment of mental functions to the brain before the discovery of the most elementary microscopic and physiological justifications was the observation that the brain differed in gross ways in different animal species. The first such observation may have been Aristotle's, when he wrote: "Of all the animals, man has the largest brain in proportion to his size" (Aristotle, ca. 335 B.C./1952; see Jerison, 1977a). In the middle of the 18th century, Albrecht Von Haller (1708–1777) included systematic observations of relative brain size in his textbook of physiology (von Haller, 1762), the major medical text of that period. The observations were presented quantitatively as ratios of brain weight to body weight and were related to the "organic efficiency" (running speed, etc.) of various species. Recall that Descartes and Aristotle were then the authorities on mind and body, and had argued strongly that animal nature was fundamentally different from human nature. Animal nature for them provided reflex control and was reflected in motor efficiency; human nature was based on rational intelligence. Von Haller's "organic efficiency" is transformed into "intelligence in lower forms" when Thomas Huxley replaces Aristotle, and listing brain–body ratios is a comparative approach to intelligence.

Lists of brain–body ratios became common in the century after von Haller, culminating in the work of François Leuret (1797–1851) and Louis Pierre Gratiolet (1815–1865). It was notably difficult to make sense of these ratios, a problem that did not deter the authors from reporting them. For example, Leuret and Gratiolet (1857) reported that the mean ratio "among the mammals is 1/186; the range is 1/22 to 1/860" (Vol. 1, p. 453). This is the report. There was no interpretation, because the ratio was uninterpretable. The authors reported comparable means and more or less comparable ranges in birds. Leuret and Gratiolet's text was, as its title indicates, a comparative anatomy of the nervous system in its relation to intelligence. As committed positivists and materialists, these investigators trusted that knowledge and understanding would follow inevitably if only the data were presented clearly. Their Baconian faith in induction may not have been justified, but they presented some of their "data" as beautiful illustrations of brains, which are still used in modern texts. They had less useful observations on intelligence: "Carnivores are generally more industrious and more intelligent than herbivores. . . . Training does not develop in any animal as much intelligence as or better sentiments than in the dog. . . . In intelligence, bears, martens and civets are inferior to dogs, but superior to cats" (Vol. 1, p. 541). This was the level of description, and it was based entirely on anecdotes and casual observations. It was also wrong.

Despite obvious inadequacies, the scientific condition of our topic prior to Darwin's *Origin* was healthy in some ways. Leuret and Gratiolet (and others) were obviously prepared to see a connection between animal and human intelligence that anticipated Huxley. They had also begun taking measurements that were eventually to lead to the modern view of encephalization.

Paul Broca, the discoverer of Broca's language area in the brain and the founder of physical anthropology in France, played an inadequately appreciated role in this development. Broca was a modern in many respects, one of the founders of anthropology, a prodigious worker, a great collector of skulls and measurer of cranial capacities (Schiller, 1979). He organized clubs, societies, and institutes, and created scientific journals. For his time, he was an extraordinary scientific entrepreneur. Broca was also an extraordinary scientist. He wrote major monographs on the comparative anatomy of primates; he named and described the limbic system (the "great limbic lobe") of the brain, and he wrote extensively on evolution and intelligence. Craniology, the measurement of skulls and brain size, was a persistent theme throughout his life, and it is a bit surprising that this creative scientist never published a theoretical contribution on brain size and intelligence. There is evidence that he may have achieved some closure on this issue, perhaps with the help of his senior student, Léonce-Pierre Manouvrier (1850–1927).

Broca died suddenly on July 7, 1880, at the age of 56. On December 31, 1880, Manouvrier deposited a major document on the interpretation of brain size with the Société d'Anthropologie in Paris, a society that Broca had founded 20 years earlier. This was part of Manouvrier's doctoral research and was published a few years later (1883). It probably represents Broca's final view as well as Manouvrier's carefully developed conclusion. My approach to the evolution of intelligence in this chapter can be traced to that document, prepared a century ago, in Manouvrier's suggestion of the analytic goal: "to divide *abstractly* the weight of the brain into two quantities . . . analyzing the influence on the development of the brain of each of these two great orders of cerebral function: psychic functions and motor functions, intimately associated one with the other. The correlates of each of these two quantities may be expressed numerically" (p. 144). Manouvrier recognized that he did not have the mathematical training to make that abstract division, but he predicted that this approach would lead to "a theory that is unequivocally positivistic [operational] and founded entirely on universally accepted anatomical and physiological principles." The issue is not especially difficult from the perspective of another century of research; a possible theory (Jerison, 1977a) is summarized later in this chapter.

The main conceptual path had now been set, although it was abandoned by the mainstream of anatomical and physiological research on the brain, which, as noted earlier, became increasingly microscopic. There remained one tradition in brain research, often associated with anthropometry and biometrics, rather than biomedical and psychological analysis, which built on Manouvrier's proposal.

BIOMETRICS, ALLOMETRY, AND ENCEPHALIZATION

Insight came slowly. The program suggested by Manouvrier required no fundamentally new mathematics, and Broca's premedical background, which was in mathematics and engineering, would have equipped him adequately for the job had it not been for his early death. To appreciate what had to be done, let us look more closely at Manouvrier's proposal and at the data that were available.

Manouvrier wanted to separate "psychical" from motor ("somatic") quantities. He did not realize, apparently, that factoring out a "somatic" component in brain size was the real purpose of using a brain:body weight ratio, because the rationale for using body weight as a divisor must be to fraction out the part of brain weight that controls the body. The ratio should then enable one to compare species that differ in body size with respect to "intelligence" – the psychical factor. If a brain:body *weight* ratio did not work (as it manifestly did not), perhaps the body factor could enter the equation in a different way. There are many different ways to measure size. For example, body size can be the area of the body's surface, which is proportional to the 2/3 power of body weight. Interestingly, a brain-weight:body-surface ratio agrees rather well with our intuitions about animal intelligence (Jerison, 1973; von Bonin, 1937). This ratio is the "cephalization index" mentioned by Lashley (1949) in the address to the American Society of Naturalists quoted earlier.

It should not have been too difficult a step for mathematically inclined biologists. A formally comparable problem had arisen in the analysis of brain size in then-well-known work by Baillarger (1853), who showed that the ratio of cortical surface to brain weight had to become smaller in humans than in sheep and smaller in sheep than in rabbits. Baillarger pointed out that surface of a solid body such as the brain increases as the square of length, whereas weight (= volume) increases as the cube; hence the surface:volume ratio in larger brains had to decrease. Dareste (1862), in a paper sponsored by Broca, appreciated this conclusion and its implication that the brain's convolutedness was related to total brain size (between species) rather than to intelligence. The idea that brain size was generally proportional to body surface and not to body weight or volume had also been proposed in just these terms by Alexandre Brandt, Jr. (1867), in a paper that was actually discussed at length by Manouvrier (1883, pp. 301–303). Yet the idea that size had to be given an appropriate dimension, that it was important to know whether it was surface or volume, did not penetrate.

Part of the problem was certainly that neither Manouvrier nor his contemporaries knew how to think about partitioning, or how to partition a variable quantity like the brain in an abstract way. This is not surprising. People still have this problem, and people still report simple brain:body-weight ratios, usually unaware that they imply a false linear model for the partitioning.

A formal approach to partitioning a variable trait was discovered shortly after Manouvrier's publication. Francis Galton (1822–1911) and Karl Pearson (1857–1936), the founders of biometrics, created the methods in order to analyze the heredity of certain traits. They constructed a scatter diagram of points in which the x coordinate of each point was the parental value of the trait and the y coordinate was the offspring's value. This procedure came to be called "regression analysis" (Galton, 1885; Pearson, 1896, 1900), because the cloud of points that was generated always had a slope less than 1.0: Offspring "regress" toward the mean of the parental generation. Pearson developed rational methods for fitting a line through the cloud of points and analyzed the variability ("variance") of the system into a component attributable to the slope of the line and another component described as residual, that is, deviations from the regression line. For Pearson and his colleagues in biometrics, the residual was a random or error effect; it was based on the theory of errors used for curve fitting by least squares. Manouvrier's problem was not attacked with this method until von Bonin's (1937) work much later. Use of this method led to the present understanding that Manouvrier's two factors are essentially a regression (somatic) factor and a residual (psychic-encephalization) factor (see Jerison, 1977a).

Manouvrier's program did not have to wait for the resolution of these statistical problems. Its development began with the appreciation that dimensional issues and the principle of "similitude" were involved. As mentioned earlier, Baillarger (1853) had used this principle in his analysis of surface–volume relations in the brain, and Brandt (1867) had used the idea that brain size should be proportional to body surface in comparing brain size in different species. The principle was well known: Galileo explained it and used it in classic analyses of the limits on the maximum size of organisms (see Bridgman, 1931; D. Thompson, 1942). Following Brandt, Snell (1891) worked out the mathematics of Manouvrier's problem and showed that the expected size of the brain in animals of different body size should follow the equation

$$E = kP^\alpha \tag{1}$$

in which E is brain weight, P is body weight, and k is an empirical constant. Snell noted that if brain size is proportional to body surface, the exponent α is 2/3. Equation 1 could then be rewritten in its logarithmic form as a computational formula:

$$\log E = 2/3 \log P + \log k \tag{2}$$

Snell was able to show that k computed for several animal species provided a reasonable measure of relative brain size, or encephalization.

Snell's work was immediately followed up by Eugene Dubois (1858–1940), the outstanding early figure in developing a quantitative analysis of encephalization. A Dutch physician working in Java, Dubois was fascinated by the theory of evolution and inspired by the prospect of finding a "missing link" for human evolution from an apelike creature. He was also convinced that human origins were in Asia and perhaps on his island, Java. Within a few years after his arrival he discovered the bones of a proper specimen, a fossil hominid skullcap (calvaria) and a nearby straight fossil femur. He named his find "*Pithecanthropus erectus*," the erect ape-man. The creature was apelike, he reasoned, because of extraordinarily heavy browridges and small cranial capacity. The latter he estimated to have been 855 cc (Dubois, 1898), which was much less than that of other fossil hominids known at the time, such as the Neandertals. The femur was straight; hence the creature must have walked like a man. We now know that the femur was from a later human fossil, and the cranial capacity has been reestimated as about 900 cc (Kennedy, 1980; Tobias, 1971). But this newer knowledge (and our present classification of pithecanthropus as *Homo erectus*) would not have resolved Dubois's basic problem in analyzing his find: What was the significance of the cranial capacity, and how could he measure the significance?

Dubois used Snell's approach to analyze the significance of cranial capacity, but he rejected the arbitrary surface–volume association, by deciding that α in Equation 1 should be determined empirically. He could make this determination by taking pairs of species that differed in brain and body size and were equal in the psychic component, in intelligence, and solving for α in Equation 1 as a pair of simultaneous equations. There was, of course, a problem in deciding when species were equal in intelligence, a point mentioned by at least some of Dareste's critics (see Dareste, 1862). But Dubois did not sense the difficulty. His instinct was right, though his science was weak. He relied on common sense. His pairs were house cat and puma, jackal and wolf, and the like. With this kind of curve fitting he found that the exponent in Equation 1, the slope of Equation 2, was about .56. He then calculated many coefficients k (see e.g., Dubois, 1897, 1930), which are measures of the residual if Equation 2 is treated as a regression equation. These coefficients have continued to appear in the later literature when questions of animal intelligence and its morphological basis have arisen (e.g., Lenneberg, 1967). By the turn of the century, Lapique (1866–1952) extended Dubois's method to show that within a species – among breeds of dogs – the slope was about .25 (Lapique, 1898, 1907).

We enter modern times with von Bonin's (1937) work, which was also empirical. It differed from Dubois's work, however, in not attempting a definition of intelligence prior to measurement. Von Bonin graphed a large number of brain and body weights and determined the slope of the regression line using Pearson's method of correlational analysis ("least squares"). It was approximately 2/3, and supported the a priori analysis of Brandt and Snell, rather than Dubois's empiricism. The entire issue is reviewed at length in Jerison (1973).

The regression factor has since been named more appropriately by Julian Huxley (Thomas Huxley's grandson) as an "allometric" factor, reflecting the relative sizes of organs of the body (Huxley, 1932); it should be determined as a "principal axis" rather than "statistical regression" in formal statistics. I have updated the analysis of the residual factor, and called it an "encephalization" factor for the brain, relating it once again to surface–volume issues, but the surface is now a surface of a map in the brain. The 2/3 exponent can be derived from neurology and dimensional aspects of brain maps, and departures from it such as that found by Lapique are explained on the basis of the organization of living brains (Jerison, 1977a).

FOSSIL BRAINS

An unusual but important contribution of 19th-century science to the analysis of the evolution of intelligence was the discovery and analysis of fossil brains. These are not really brains; they are endocasts: casts for which the endocranial cavity of the skull is the mold. In all species of birds and mammals, such casts provide enough information about the brain for a good estimation of brain size. In almost all species, the endocast looks remarkably like a brain, including a detailed reproduction of the external gyri and sulci and blood vessels. The pattern is less adequately reproduced in some large-brained species – humans, great apes, whales, and elephants – but it is still possible to estimate brain size, and many significant details of the brain can be reconstructed (Jerison, 1973, 1976a; Radinsky, 1974; Tobias, 1971).

The first demonstration of fossil endocasts was by the French naturalist, Baron Cuvier, in 1803, and there were occasional reports of these fossils during the half-century that followed (see Edinger, 1975, for a bibliography; Jerison, 1973, for more detailed history). These fossils were known to early evolutionists, although their significance was not fully appreciated. Discovered in 1856, Neandertal man yielded an endocast described by Schaaffhausen (1863), and skeletal information as well as information about its brain was included in later editions of T. H. Huxley (1863). Huxley described its skull as the most apelike ("pithecoid") of human skulls that he had seen, but clearly within the range of variation of living human skulls. We now see the Neandertals as a subspecies of *Homo sapiens* (Kennedy, 1980), and at least one Neandertal endocast has been analyzed for information about the evolution of asymmetric lateralization (LeMay, 1975). The story of the endocast of *Homo erectus*, discovered at the end of the century (Dubois, 1898), was told earlier.

After Darwin, endocasts took on new importance. There is one major generalization that can be made on the basis of fossil evidence of the brain: "The further back that mammals went into geological time, the more was the volume of their brain reduced in relation to the volume of their head and to the overall dimensions of their body" (Lartet, 1868, p. 1120). This generalization, stated positively, is that encephalization occurred. It was extended by O. C. Marsh (1831–1899), a professor of paleontology at Yale and one of the leading figures in American science during the latter half of the 19th century. Marsh collected many fossil specimens, prepared many fossil endocasts, and published many, many reports on all of these (e.g., Marsh, 1874, 1886). He was joined in this effort by both rivals and associates, although he seemed to have a talent for disaffecting his colleagues. Perhaps for this reason, his "laws" of brain evolution, which related the fossil evidence to the adaptive value of brain size, were rejected by many paleontologists (see Edinger, 1962). The mythology of unusually small-brained dinosaurs and of universal evolution toward higher levels of organization and intelligence is traceable partly to Marsh's work, but that work is also the source of many presently accepted generalizations about the pattern of evolution of intelligence in the vertebrates (Jerison, 1973, pp. 14–15).

The evidence of fossil endocasts is the most direct evidence on the evolution of the brain and encephalization. To the extent that encephalization can be related to intelligence, these fossil brains provide unusual data on fossil intelligence, unique "psychological" data.

INTELLIGENCE, BEHAVIOR, AND SOCIETY

The connection between brain and mind (or intelligence) was the basis for the morphological approach, which has just been discussed in so much detail. The analysis of brain size provided the first scientific approach to biological intelligence. A connection between brain and intelligence was accepted, and the idea that the mass of tissue in the brain was important was also accepted, but ideas on the meaning of intelligence were primitive. The word was used, but until early in this century there was surprisingly little interest or concern with its precise meaning. Intuitive understanding of the nature of intelligence may have been so compelling that its inadequacy as a scientific concept was missed.

The idea of mind or intelligence is both ancient and primitive. To state that "the serpent was more subtle than all of the beasts of the field" (Genesis 3:1) was to accept the possibility of an animal intelligence that was smart enough and *human* enough to compete successfully with Eve's. Wheeler (see Schneirla, 1958) presented observations by Roman naturalists of the behavior of ants, one aspect of which the Romans interpreted as a funeral complete with eulogy and cemetery. Legends of sly foxes, noble lions, and the varieties of mind in animals, trees, and even stones are familiar elements in the ethnologist's work. They are more than metaphorical. They are expressions of concerns with the possible, like tales of transmigration of souls that are titillations of modern "science" fiction. The dualism implicit in such stories, like that implicit in work on extrasensory "perception" (Thouless, 1963), continues to be a main current in contemporary thought.

It is impossible to discuss intelligence sensibly, at least in a comparative and evolutionary framework and perhaps in all frameworks, without awareness of the deep influence of both philosophy and society on one's ideas. The animism of the ancients and the mysticism of the moderns were possible only because of fundamental features in their view of the nature of reality. Consider the problem of solipsism, of assuming that there exists no reality beyond one's self. Descartes resolved this problem by first asserting his own reality: "I think, therefore, I am." The rest more or less followed. But it took the analytic philosophy of Bertrand Russell (1912/1959, 1956), applied in a surprisingly commonsense way, to put that problem in a proper context – and to lay it to rest. The resolution: Solipsism cannot be categorically refuted; it is merely much simpler to assume that there is a reality beyond one's own mind, because of the elaborate and often counterintuitive nature of events in the perceived world. The alternative is a God-like infallible intelligence, somehow buried within one's self, which plays capricious games with reality. Because one is unaware, or at best less directly aware, of that God-like intelligence than one is of "external reality," it is simpler to assume the reality of "reality" than that of the intelligence. QED.

For philosophers, animism represents the most extreme dualism, in which there is a capricious association between mind and body. Solipsism represents an equally capricious monism, based on the recognition that the knowledge of reality depends on perception and conscious experience. I have the impression that the discovery of solipsism is an almost universal event among philosophically inclined adolescents. It is clearly also evidence of developing insight into the nature of mind, and an advance over a naive realism that does not question the nature of the universe or of the knower (experiencer) of the universe.

There were several strands in the development of a scientific understanding of intelligence during the 19th and early 20th centuries. The first, a morphological understanding based on assumptions about the connection between brain and mind, is the basis for a direct evolutionary and quantitative analysis that can transcend species-typical adaptations. The second is philosophical, requiring careful reflection on one's own experience in the context of the science of one's time. We have seen from Bruno's effort at stating the mind–body problem, as quoted earlier, that this approach is difficult. Psychologists, as working scientists, tend to ignore formal philosophy. Yet this philosophical strand is fundamental to all the others. It is this strand that enables us to frame questions and reach decisions on what issues are important. There is, finally, the recognized scientific program of observing and recording (measuring) intelligence, however that is defined, and placing it in our understanding of nature. These paths to understanding have interacted with one another within a historical intellectual and social (including economic) milieu that must also be taken into account in evaluating the ideas, philosophies, models of reality, or scientific paradigms – whatever words we use to designate the framework that makes a science possible.

I have written enough about morphology in this historical section. There will be more later in the chapter. On philosophical questions, dualism and monism were discussed earlier as resolutions of the mind–body problem (Rieber, 1980). There are other classic philosophical categories that are important. Darwinists were usually "materialists" rather than "idealists," for example. They accepted the stuff of nature as real and independent of experience. It was this sort of thing that led William James (1890) to write about evolution as implying the existence of a "mind-stuff" (Vol. 1, p. 146).

Despite their ethereal quality, philosophical "quibbles" have led to important divergences. Recent work in the philosophy and sociology of science has led to the recognition that accepted paradigms can act to screen ideas (Kuhn, 1970). Scientists have been all too fallible when driven by strongly held convictions, a situation that can lead to public skepticism about scientific truth. We are amused to discover that Isaac Newton fudged his data to show that he had discovered God's clockwork, which ran His physical universe (Westfall, 1973). We are not surprised, though less amused, to read of Darwin and his contemporaries as fashioning biological theories consistent with the cutthroat economic world within which they lived and worked (Buss, 1979; Gould, 1978). And we are shocked to discover outright fraud in science designed to further an evolutionary doctrine about human origins (Weiner, 1955). When the fraud, or the "cooking" of data, is discovered with respect to the interpretation of data on human intelligence, as discussed in critiques of the work of Cyril Burt (Cronbach, 1979; Hearnshaw, 1979), the interaction between science and culture strikes home. Inevitably, this kind of criticism is applied to the analysis of animal intelligence (Garcia, 1975).

The recognition of the importance of the cultural broth within which science grows began with Karl Marx (1818–1883) and Friedrich Engels (1820–1895). Engels, especially, was concerned with extending the philosophy of dialectical materialism to natural phenomena (Engels, 1940), although he was a philosophical conservative in his understanding of the role of the dialectic (cf. Russell, 1934). Engels reads as if he were an unconscious dualist, trying to have nature represented by its thesis, antithesis, and eventual Hegelian synthesis, while maintaining a distinction between nature's problems and those of its human observers. His naive "Marxism" has bred occasionally odd science (Kochetkova, 1973/1978). Marx was more consistent. Among the conflicts that he saw as resolvable (at least as I understand him) was one between nature and the observer – its human observer. As he saw it, the reality of nature was a synthesis of events generated by the observed and the observer, a conclusion which implied that the observer was a part of nature whose observations determined the reality, the truth, about nature.

Many bits of modern Marxist doctrine fall into place when this really deep philosophical (metaphysical, as it were, despite the antipathy toward metaphysics shared by Marx, Engels, and most modern scientists) point is made. On this issue Marx was concerned with classic epistemological and metaphysical problems: how we *know* reality and the nature of *reality*. Engels missed the problem of how *we* know and so missed the meat of the matter. The important point made by Marx, and accepted by many non-Marxist philosophers, is that the knowable truths about nature (including intelligence) must be known as an interaction between the knower and the data.

John Dewey (see Russell, 1945) made almost exactly the same point a bit later, and the revolution in physics that we associate with Einstein and Heisenberg gives physical meaning to many counterintuitive interactions between the measuring instrument and the measured object (Bridgman, 1959).

For the analysis of intelligence and its evolution, this kind of interaction is especially critical, because that analysis is performed by an intelligence, that of a human analyst or observer. We are in the role of an electron, or other particle, trying to create particle physics from the particle's perspective. Concern with this kind of philosophizing is neither trivial nor "precious" when the topic is the evolution of intelligence.

INTELLIGENCE AS A SCIENTIFIC ISSUE

Divorced from philosophy, biological intelligence had first to be identified, to be defined. There is little history of the scientific definition. We are still working on it, and that is why this chapter had to begin with a definition. The definition offered in this section of the handbook can resolve this problem, of course, and if it does, the rest of this section can be read as the historical background for the achievement of a consensus. (Halstead, 1947, wrote a book on "biological intelligence," which dealt with the physiological correlates of human performance on intelligence tests, not with intelligence as a trait with an evolutionary dimension.)

It is astonishing to a modern reader to browse through works on intelligence by any of the authors whose expertise was recognized in the 19th century. None of them saw an issue in specifying the trait behaviorally. Always astute, always erudite, and always literate, Darwin relied entirely on anecdotes – careful observation, carefully reported in many instances, and methodologically not far from modern ethological work. But the analysis was arid because it had no support from the kind of solid science that we have since learned to enjoy. It had no experimental foundation.

All 19th-century evolutionists were concerned with analyzing animal intelligence. Darwin (1871/1936) himself accepted the challenge, beginning with a passage almost identical with Huxley's and then developing the position. He is worth quoting at length:

My object in this chapter is to shew that there is no fundamental difference between man and the higher mammals in their mental faculties. . . . [T]he first dawnings of intelligence, according to Mr. Herbert Spencer (*The Principles of Psychology*, 2nd edit., 1870, pp. 418–443), have been developed through the multiplication and co-ordination of reflex actions. . . . All animals feel *Wonder,* and many exhibit *Curiosity.* . . . Brehm gives a curious account of the instinctive dread, which his monkeys exhibited, for snakes. . . . I was so surprised at this account, that I took a stuffed and coiled-up snake into the monkey-house at the Zoological Gardens, and the excitement thus caused was one of the most curious spectacles which I ever beheld. Three species of Cercopithecus were the most alarmed; they dashed about their cages, and uttered sharp cries of danger, which were understood by the other monkeys. [P. 450]

The example of Brehm's monkeys anticipates Klüver (1933) and Seyfarth, Cheney, and Marler (1980), who showed how to experiment on this "instinct." Darwin continues in this vein, with examples of *Imitation, Attention, Memory, Imagination, Reason,* and toolmaking. He stops short of attributing *Abstraction, General Conceptions, Self-Consciousness,* and *Mental Individuality* (his emphases throughout) to animals, but only because of "the impossibility of judging what passes through the mind of an animal" (p. 460). These categories appeared to define intelligence for

Darwin, and they would satisfy most of us as intuitively appropriate. They are not easy categories to use for objective analyses, however, a difficulty that was recognized at the time as clearly as it is recognized today.

There was then no experimental psychology or ethology, although the earliest formal experiments on animal intelligence date from that period. In about 1882, Sir John Lubbock taught his dog Van to ask for food or tea by bringing a card on which the correct word was printed (Lubbock, 1888). He controlled for effects of odor by using a fresh card for each trial, and he recorded and reported his dog's performance. The important point was that controls were attempted, and the report included actual data on successes and failures (the latter rather inadequately). This quantification would eventually lead to science. Lubbock's work with Van was cited by Lloyd Morgan (1894, 1896), but without clear recognition that such experimental work had to be performed and reported to clarify the mental concepts that concerned evolutionists. There was, in fact, no real advance in the behavioral understanding of intelligence until the challenge of behaviorism (Watson, 1913), based on the iconoclastic experimentalism of E. L. Thorndike (1898) and his successors at the beginning of the 20th century: Pavlov (1903/1928), Watson (1903), and Yerkes (1907). It was then that the need for objective definitions of the psychological concepts became clear.

The most nearly standard work until then was Romanes's (1883), which was comparable to Darwin's in method – an expanded set of tales. Morgan (1890/1891, 1894, 1896) was heralded by the 20th-century iconoclasts as supporting the experimental method. Though he contributed little beyond support to that method, he did contribute his "canon": *In no case may we interpret an action as the outcome of the exercise of a higher psychical faculty, if it can be interpreted as the outcome of the exercise of one which stands lower in the psychological scale*" (Morgan, 1894, p. 53). This canon was widely accepted and cited by students of animal behavior as a principle of parsimony, and it had the helpful effect of reducing reliance on anecdote, though it also encouraged a simpleminded reductionism. In any event, these were the drives toward a science of animal behavior that heralded the advances of the 20th century.

For intelligence as a concept, the variety of traits mentioned by Darwin was reduced by Romanes to the idea that profiting from experience, that is, learning, was the central feature of intelligence, a view shared by most later comparative psychologists, as well as by their contemporaries – rivals or associates – the ethologists, whose roots were in zoology rather than in psychology and physiology. It is a view that is rejected in this chapter.

CONCLUDING REMARKS

The reason for devoting so long a section to historical and philosophical issues is that these remain insufficiently resolved. Too many students are ignorant about history and scornful (as well as ignorant) about philosophy.

These issues are at the core of the present "IQ controversy" on the role of genetic and environmental contributions to human intelligence, the definition of human as well as animal intelligence, the role of culture in intelligence, and the concept of intelligence as a dimension (or dimensions) of mind. If we are to analyze intelligence as a trait that evolved, we need closure on its nature as a trait. To know its history as a concept may help provide that closure. Modern views and modern data are presented in a later section, but we need to take space now for a more or less didactic section on evolutionary theory.

12.2.   ON EVOLUTIONARY THEORY

The evolution of neural processing capacity and intelligence in the history of animal life is a topic in macroevolution – above the species level (Rensch, 1959; Simpson, 1953; Stanley, 1979). Processing capacity is measurable in any species with a nervous system, and the data of such measurements are orderly and easily interpreted as evolutionary (Jerison, 1973). Present behavioral diversity among species can also be interpreted as evolutionary. To point out the limits of the interpretations, I review selected topics in evolutionary theory in this section.

Public challenges by "creationists" during the past decade may have left non-specialists uncertain about the scientific status of evolution. Among biologists familiar with the evidence, there is no debate about the basic facts, which lead to the conclusion that presently living species evolved from earlier forms. The evidence is overwhelming. The fossil evidence has been described in countless publications, and I will review that evidence for the brain in a later section. There is equally compelling evidence of evolution in the recent history and present diversity of living things at the species, organismic, and molecular levels. There is debate about the theory, however, and there appears to be a new synthesis arising from that debate (Gould, 1980). But the fundamentals are still fundamental: a hereditary material (genes and chromosomes), a mechanism of change of the material (mutation and recombination), an internal and external environment within which growth and development take place, and natural selection.

The debate is primarily about microevolution in populations of organisms as an explanation or model of macroevolution of species or higher taxonomic categories (genera, families, orders, classes, and phyla). One of the more important conclusions is that macroevolution may emphasize other kinds of genetic change than those emphasized by microevolution, and because we are considering the macroevolution of intelligence in this chapter, we should understand the emerging perspective.

At the molecular level, evolution is reflected in biochemical differences among organisms in the genetic material. There is enormous variation within species in structural genes, often greater within populations than between populations (Lewontin, 1974). Important morphological (phenotypic) differences are sometimes poorly correlated with measurable genetic differences at the molecular level. The outstanding example from a human perspective is the near identity of man and chimpanzee with respect to genetic structure determined in this way (King & Wilson, 1975), despite obviously major phenotypic differences.

Evolutionary analysis at the molecular level can also be significantly non-Darwinian. That is, some evolutionary changes can be explained by "genetic drift," or the "neutralist" view, without recourse to Darwin's central concept of natural selection. The analysis is formalistic, and natural selection is usually represented by one or two terms in a complex mathematical expression. The non-Darwinian feature is simply that the "selection-pressure" term can have a value of zero or nearly zero, and the expression still explains the measured variability of evolving populations (see Dobzhansky, 1970, chap. 8; Lande, 1976; Lewontin, 1974).

Recent analysis of macroevolution emphasizes the likelihood that its genetic basis is probably more in mutations of regulatory genes than in those of structural genes

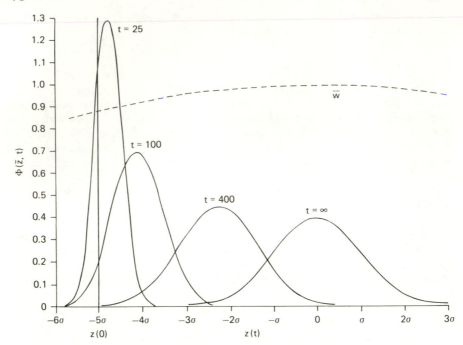

Figure 12.1.   Lande's model for the course of evolution of a phenotypic trait over the course of t generations. The initial value of the trait at $t = 0$ is set at 5 standard deviations below its optimum value (arbitrarily set at o on the x axis). The optimum value of the trait is the mean value of the adaptive zone of shape $\overline{W}$ (dashed line). The set of normal curves are the distributions of the trait at the indicated values of t. Other assumptions: Population size $N = 50$; heritability $h^2 = .2$. (From "Natural Selection and Random Genetic Drift in Phenotypic Evolution" by R. Lande, *Evolution*, 1976, *30*, 314–334. Copyright © 1976 by the Society for the Study of Evolution and the University of Chicago Press. All rights reserved. Reprinted by permission.)

and in recombination of genetic material at the level of the chromosome (Valentine & Campbell, 1975). Selection pressures that actually arose in history were strong, according to the new view, and produced effects in relatively short periods of time (relatively few generations, thousands rather than millions of years, or a few million years rather than tens of millions). Periods of rapid change were followed by long periods of genetic equilibria in stable environments. According to the new view, evolution was a series of "punctuated equilibria," the phrase that describes the model. This view is as consistent with the fossil evidence as a model that assumes that large changes are simply the cumulative effects of the small changes of micro-evolution (Eldredge & Cracraft, 1980; Gould, 1980; Stanley, 1979; cf. Lande, 1976, 1980a, 1980b).

The kind of continuity assumed by Darwin and Thomas Huxley, in which variations among species were seen as outgrowths of individual differences within species, can be replaced by a discontinuity, at least in the sense that between-species variations may be decoupled from within-species variations (see Lande, 1979, on decoupling). But natural selection retains its central role; it is Darwin's "demon," and it picks the animals from one generation that will be parents of the next generation. Accounts of how this may occur for behavioral phenotypes, and some of the unusual implications for "kin selection" and "altruism," are now the familiar material of sociobiology (Dawkins, 1976; Wilson, 1975, 1978). In macroevolution there is species selection, as it were, as the effect of natural selection (Stanley, 1979; cf. Lande, 1980a, 1980b).

There are several ways in which to explain the evolutionary process. The first formal theories grew out of the rapprochement between Mendelian genetics and Darwinian selectionism and were essentially descriptions of the rate of change of the genetic pool. These were developed about 50 years ago, more or less independently, by R. A. Fisher, J. B. S. Haldane, and Sewall Wright (see Johnson, 1976). Russell Lande (1976) developed an elegant extension of genotypic theories to phenotypic evolution, and Figure 12.1 is an example of this kind of theorizing.

The series of normal curves represents the distribution of a trait (e.g., body size) in a population or set of populations after t generations. Above these normal curves there is a dashed curve labeled $\bar{W}$, which is a segment of another normal curve that characterizes an environment, an adaptive zone within which the evolution takes place. The zero on the abscissa is an arbitrarily chosen "optimum" numerical value of the trait for the adaptive zone, that is, the average value of a perfectly adapted phenotype for that adaptive zone. I have presented Figure 12.1 as an example of how both the rate of evolution and the diversity of a particular trait under natural selection are described by modern theory. It requires relatively simple assumptions about the variability of the trait, about its heritability, h^2, and about the nature of the environment in which organisms are evolving. Notice how the evolution and distribution of the trait depend on both its heritability and the environment, with the latter specified by the curve $\bar{W}$. A precisely defined environment – the function $\bar{W}$ – is part of the requirement of a theory of the evolution of the genetic material and its phenotypic expression.

ANAGENETICS (PROGRESS) AND CLADISTICS (SPECIATION)

Figure 12.1 shows how progress, or *anagenesis,* would occur in a trait under natural selection with the passage of time, according to present models of evolution. The 400th generation ($t = 400$) is more advanced than the 100th generation, though there is some overlap between the distributions. We might imagine another set of populations evolving in a different environment that is characterized by an optimal phenotypic value: $\bar{z}(\infty) = -4\sigma$. After 400 generations this set of populations would approach stability at the $t = 100$ curve of Figure 12.1. The two sets of populations would then be statistically distinguishable; the classic evolutionary model would assert that subspecies and species always become differentiated in this way. Lande (1980a) has shown that the classic model works for macroevolution.

The next example, taken from my work on the evolution of encephalization in mammals during the past 60 million years (Figure 12.2), is an example of macroevolutionary anagenetic analysis. Figure 12.2 shows how the distribution of relative brain size among genera of living and fossil carnivores and ungulates has progressed (for more on the data, see Jerison, 1979a; Radinsky, 1978). The curves are remarkably similar to those in Figure 12.1 in appearance, but are quite different in significance. The curves in Figure 12.1 are theoretical curves, based on a mathematical model that relates phenotypic distributions to genotypic distributions and shows how these would change in a particular environment. The curves in Figure

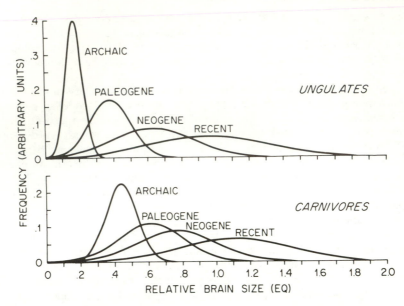

Figure 12.2.   Changing distributions of relative brain size. (From *Evolution of the Brain and Intelligence* by H. J. Jerison [New York: Academic Press, 1973]. Copyright © 1973 by Academic Press. Reprinted by permission.)

12.2, on the other hand, are normal curves fitted to empirical data. Each one represents a population of genera of radically different genetic structure. The "Recent Ungulates" for example, include zebra, rhino, tapir, deer, camel, giraffe, and so on.

One interpretation of Figure 12.2 is as curves characterizing the change in the adaptive zone. The "Recent Ungulates" curve would characterize the demands of present ungulate environmental niches with respect to neural information-processing capacity. There are many such niches, some with heavier demands and others with lighter demands; the present diversity of species in encephalization may be thought of as corresponding to the diversity of the niches, which combine to define the ungulate adaptive zone. Curve $\bar{W}$ in Figure 12.1, which characterizes the adaptive zone, is therefore closer conceptually than the other curves in Figure 12.1 to each curve in Figure 12.2. Figure 12.2 is a characterization of changing environmental demands, as well as the distributions of a particular morphological trait (relative brain size) in those changing environments. Figure 12.1 shows one environment, $\bar{W}$, and the anagenetic evolution in that environment.

The process of splitting of groups, whatever its mechanism, is called *cladogenesis*, and the study of its effects is called *cladistics*. It is the usual view of what evolution is about: tracing family trees and determining ancestor–descendant relations among species. A *clade* is a cluster of related species, that is, species derived from a common ancestor. Anagenetic advances are represented by the presence of different *grades* with respect to an adaptation. If we think of progress and phyletic relationship, of grades and clades, Figure 12.2 is entirely about grades, about anagenesis, or progress, and it is above the species level.

Macroevolutionary analysis is not restricted to nor is it primarily about anagenetic matters. Cladograms, or phylogenetic trees, have been constructed for "speciation"

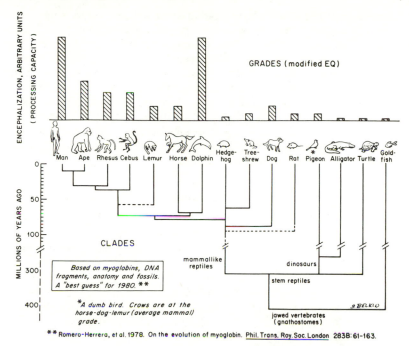

Figure 12.3. Cladistic (*bottom*) and anagenetic (*top*) analyses of vertebrate evolution.

at the level of families, orders, and even classes of vertebrates. One such tree, based on biochemical, morphological, and paleontological information, is presented in the lower part of Figure 12.3. Such analyses are obviously important for suggesting degrees of relationship among species. The time dimension is supplied by paleontological data and assumptions about mutation rates. In other respects, the network was developed to meet criteria of parsimony in describing relationships.

A purely anagenetic analysis of the species that produced the cladogram of Figure 12.3 is presented in the upper half of this illustration. Here the species are rated with respect to encephalization. Figure 12.3 was prepared to contrast anagenetic and cladistic analyses and to emphasize their complementary nature. It also illustrates some of the pitfalls in the analysis of the evolution of processing capacity and intelligence. As an anagenetic trait, this capacity has evolved to comparable grades in species with radically different adaptations. Man and dolphin (*Tursiops*, the bottlenose dolphin) are at comparable grades; great apes and the harbor porpoise, *Phocaena* (not shown in Figure 12.3), are comparable, but are at a lower grade; horses and dogs are at comparable grades and (from more extensive analyses) are known to represent an average mammalian grade – at which they are joined by lemurs (which are primates) and crows! One of the problems in the analysis of the evolution of intelligence is to make sense of these anagenetic data in a context compatible with the cladistic information.

Although evolution can be measured by specific traits (Figure 12.3, top), the evolutionary process refers to whole organisms (Figure 12.3, bottom). The course of evolution is displayed as the adaptive radiation of species, a branching tree showing new and different species, genera, and so on with the passage of time. This cladistic perspective has been emphasized by ethologists, and is reflected in their program of developing as complete an ethogram for each species as possible, in addition to attempting to analyze individual traits in between-species comparisons. It should be a sobering view for those comparative psychologists who have sought to evaluate intelligence (learning ability, or behavioral capacity) as an anagenetic trait in different species (e.g., Bitterman, 1975; Parker & Gibson, 1979). The problem, of course, is in the species-typical traits of each species, which may assist or interfere with performance on the tasks used for the evaluation (see pp. 753–754; Hinde & Stevenson-Hinde, 1973; Seligman & Hager, 1972).

PROCESSING CAPACITY WITHIN AND BETWEEN SPECIES

Neural information-processing capacity is related to gross brain size in an interesting way, which illustrates the distinction between analysis at the within-species level and at higher levels. The analysis is fundamental background for the use of encephalization as a measure of adjusted processing capacity (biological intelligence).

The unit of information processing in the mammalian cerebral cortex appears to be a module (column, or barrel) of neocortical tissue about 0.5 mm in diameter and extending the full depth of the cortex, about 0.5–4.0 mm, depending on the species (Eccles, 1979; Mountcastle, 1978; Szentágothai, 1978). Modules may be surprisingly uniform in structure between species, and may contain about 2,000 neurons. Because the number of modules is proportional to the surface area of the cortex, that area estimates processing capacity, at least as a first approximation.

There is an extremely orderly relation between cortical surface and gross brain size in mammals, which is shown in Figure 12.4. The data are on 48 species, including monotremes, marsupials, and "primitive" as well as "advanced" placentals (e.g., insectivores, rodents, ungulates, carnivores, cetaceans, elephants, and primates, including *Homo sapiens*). Figure 12.4 shows that the between-species diversity in processing capacity (cortical surface area) in the mammals is "explained" by brain size. Gross size, surface area, and many of the details of its final structure are determined by constraints on growth of the brain, by the environment in which growth occurs (extracellular space, other cells growing, etc.), and by the interactions of each growing neuron with that environment. Such constraints reflect the role of regulatory genes designed to control growth in normal environments.

In a sense, Figure 12.4 is a map of the effect of such constraints. The correlation ($r = .995$) is so strong that it amounts to a functional rather than a merely statistical relation. A mammal with "design characteristics" for a certain amount of processing capacity, y, in its brain, *must* develop a brain of x size with which there *must* be associated a surface z to contain the neural processing machinery. These constraints are at the interspecific level. We can write them as equations: $y = kz$ and $z = 3.9x^{.91}$, where z and x are in cm² and cm³, respectively. It is easy, and really right, to think in this mechanistic way at this level of analysis.

When we examine the same sort of thing within a species, the system falls apart. The intraspecific "function" that relates cortical surface to brain size (Figure 12.5) within the human species is no function at all. At best it is a statistical map, suggesting some slight association between the two dimensions of analysis, and even that

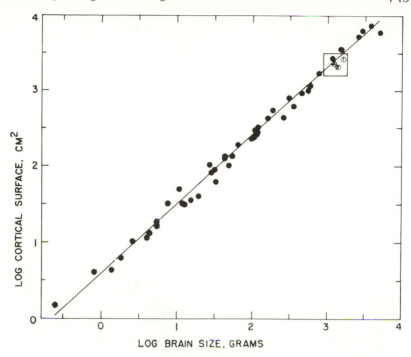

Figure 12.4. Cortical surface and brain size in 48 species of mammals. The small square contains three human data points (open circles) and one *Tursiops* data point (filled circle). (Data from "Neue Forschungsergebnisse der Grosshirnrin-denanatomie mit besonderer Berucksichtung anthropologischer Fragen" by K. Brodmann, *Verhandlungen des 85ste Versammlung Deutscher Naturforscher und Aerzte in Wien*, 1913, 200–240 and "Cerebro-cortical Surface Areas, Volumes, Lengths of Gyri and Their Interdependence in Mammals, Including Man," by H. Elias and D. Schwartz, *Zeitschrift für Säugetierkunde,* 1971, 36, 147–163. Figure from "Allometry, Brain Size, Cortical Surface, and Convolutedness" by H. J. Jerison, in E. Armstrong and D. Falk [Eds.], *Primate Brain Evolution: Methods and Concepts* [New York: Plenum, in press]. Copyright © 1982 by Plenum Press. Reprinted by permission.)

slight association may be an artifact owing to a few outliers – atypical brains. In any case, the intraspecific picture shows none of the orderliness of the interspecific picture. Individual variation, the source of microevolution, seems to be decoupled from interspecific variation, which represents the effect of macroevolution.

Before we accept the story suggested by Figures 12.4 and 12.5, there is a methodological artifact to be appreciated. The intraspecific data of Figure 12.5 would be contained in the small square in Figure 12.4 that contains three human data points (open circles) and a data point for *Tursiops* (D in Figure 12.5; filled circle in the small square in Figure 12.4). Some of the strong associations between cortical surface and brain size in the mammals evident in Figure 12.4 are clearly related to the enormous range of brain sizes being examined. Restricting the range in a bivariate system of data always reduces the correlation. The low surface–volume correlation in humans is at least partly an effect of the restricted range of measures.

According to modern evolutionary and genetic theory, as emphasized earlier, be-

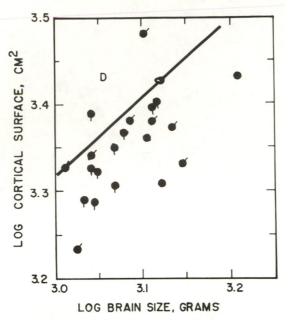

Figure 12.5. Cortical surface and brain size in 20 human brains. Diagonal marks are males; vertical marks, females. *D* is a data point for the bottlenose dolphin, *Tursiops.* (Data from "Cerebro-cortical Surface Areas, Volumes, Lengths of Gyri and Their Interdependence in Mammals, Including Man," by H. Elias and D. Schwartz, *Zeitschrift für Säugetierkunde,* 1971, *36,* 147–163.)

tween-species and within-species comparisons may involve significantly different and almost independent dimensions. There are paradoxical effects that would be expected in that case, especially for the heritability of human intelligence; they are discussed in the next paragraphs.

HERITABILITY, EVOLUTION, AND THE ENVIRONMENT

Heritability, h^2 in the narrow sense, is the fraction of phenotypic variance attributable to additive genetic variance. In his "fundamental theorem of natural selection," R. A. Fisher (1930/1958) showed that evolutionary change in relative fitness per generation is equal to this additive genetic variance. As McClearn and DeFries (1973) have pointed out, this implies that, "for a species well adapted to its particular ecological niche, fitness must be relatively constant from generation to generation; thus, additive genetic variance for characters that are major components of fitness must be near zero for such populations" (p. 218). To the extent that within-species variation in processing capacity is related to human psychometric intelligence (cf. Hunt, 1978), and to the extent that this has been an important trait in human evolution, we should anticipate that its heritability would be low. The presently accepted heritability for psychometric intelligence (DeFries, Vandenberg & McClearn, 1976; Rose, Harris, Christian, & Nance, 1979) of about .50 is, thus, unusual in evolutionary perspective (Whitney, 1976), and implies that psychometric intelligence has only recently become an important adaptive trait, that its heritability is unusually complex, or that it does not contribute significantly to genetic fitness (cf. Falconer, 1960, p. 167).

If the between-species correlation of brain size and processing capacity shown in Figure 12.4 is derived from the within-species correlation of Figure 12.5, the latter correlation should also be low but not zero. The same should be true of the correlation between brain size and intelligence within human populations: It should be low but positive. Van Valen (1974b) analyzed this heritability as a theoretical problem, suggesting a value for the correlation of .30. A more likely value, however, given the limited good evidence (Robinow, 1968; see Jerison, 1979b), is of the order of .01, certainly no more than .05. Demonstrating such low correlations as real, rather than sampling artifacts, is a formidable biometric problem. Almost 40,000 measurements would be needed to show that a measured correlation $r = .01$ was "significantly" different from zero ($p < .05$), and over 1,500 measurements would be needed to demonstrate this for $r = .05$.

Recent views of macroevolution discussed earlier (e.g., Stanley, 1979) treat it as decoupled from microevolution with respect to genetic mechanisms. If Figure 12.4 reflects the action of regulatory genes and Figure 12.5 is simply the result of random variation about the human grade of surface–volume association, there may be no connection at all between the systems.

Another example, from the relationship between encephalization and intelligence, illustrates the decoupling. Because of their similarity in body size, the difference in encephalization between human and chimpanzee is proportional to the absolute difference in their brain sizes. Typical adult chimpanzee brains weigh about 400 g, and the human brain weighs about 1,400 g. There have been, however, microcephalic human brains that weighed about 300 g, in people who functioned not as chimpanzees but as severely retarded humans, with some speech and reasonable sensory and motor abilities (Jensen-Jazbutis, 1970). Although there are problems in placing such pathological brains within an appropriately defined population of human brains, there is no question that it is within a human, not a chimpanzee, population that such brains have to be placed. The mechanisms that produce human microcephaly are not related to the mechanisms that produce normal chimpanzee brains. In short, an interspecific comparison of human and chimpanzee has to be with respect to a species value, not to values of aberrant individuals of a species.

Yet another problem arises in comparisons among closely related species or among well-differentiated populations within a species. The latter are especially difficult and include the analysis of sex differences and race differences, thorny questions with implications beyond the purely scientific issues. There are real differences between the sexes with respect to the brain that probably involve processing capacity, but not necessarily intelligence as defined here. They are poorly understood but will be discussed in Section 12.4. Although there appear to be race differences in brain size within the human species, they are smaller than the sex differences and are even less well understood. These differences, too, will be discussed briefly in Section 12.4. These population differences are worth studying on scientific grounds because of the insights that may result about the nature of human intelligence. But they may be impossible to study because of confounding interactions between observer and observed, discussed in Section 12.1, as well as because of problems that incompletely understood studies can raise for public policy. Such studies can be and have been done in nonhuman species, where the effects of experimental and interpretive errors are less devastating. There are now studies by

Riddell and his associates (Riddell, 1979) showing some relationship between encephalization and learning ability, but there appears to be no relationship within species in well-controlled studies of the behavior of strains of mice bred for small and large brains (Hahn, Jensen, & Dudek, 1979).

We cannot escape at least a few words on the old theme of nature and nurture, heredity and environment. The hereditary materials provide information – blueprints – for bodily structures, but the structures are built in an environment, and the whole organism is always a result of an intricate gene–environment interaction. Adapted organisms, especially mammals, are adapted to their environments as a result of experience as well as of growth; so the interaction between organism and environment can involve many capricious environmental elements. The growth of the brain, like the development of intelligence, is determined by the interaction of a genetic program with the environment in which growth occurs. The environment is deeply involved, and has major effects on the anatomy as well as the physiology of the brain (Buell & Coleman, 1979; Greenough & Juraska, 1979; Rosenzweig, 1979).

When heritability is distinguished from "environmentality," the distinction is statistical. It is an analysis of components of variance that contribute to the overall measured variance of traits. Such an analysis can be performed for brain size, intelligence, or any other measured trait (DeFries, 1973; Whitney, 1976). The high heritability of psychometric intelligence might be interpreted as distinguishing it from what has been termed here *biological intelligence*. The latter, as is emphasized later in this chapter, is properly associated with imagery and cognition as species-typical phenomena and the correlated consciousness, or awareness. It is a reasonable conjecture that biological intelligence, despite the extent to which it is controlled by hereditary mechanisms, would display low heritability within each species, because the additive genetic variance would have been "depleted" in its long evolution (Falconer, 1960).

THE RED QUEEN AND THE COURSE OF EVOLUTION

According to Van Valen (1973, 1974a), nature is like Alice's Red Queen: Species evolve to higher and higher grades not so much to win a competition as to keep pace with their competitors. Like the Red Queen, they may have to run, that is, evolve, as fast as they can merely to stay in place. Maynard Smith (1978a), Lewontin (1978), and others have found this an attractive evolutionary hypothesis for macroevolution. It is supported by paleontological data on extinction rates (Stanley, 1979; Van Valen, 1979), and it fits in well with the data on the evolution of relative brain size, as illustrated in Figure 12.2. The central feature of the hypothesis is the assumption that any gain in adaptation in one species is offset by an equal loss in other species – that evolution is a zero-sum game (Maynard Smith, 1978b). The view emphasizes interaction among species and the fact that other species and other individual animals constitute a major aspect of the environment.

The Red Queen hypothesis implies that there will be coordinated change in many species during the course of evolution in any phenotypic trait that is measurable on the same scale in different species. Information-processing capacity is such a trait, and we should expect exactly the sort of curves shown in Figure 12.2. Each curve represents about 20 million years of evolution, and each distribution represents the coevolution of species with respect to relative brain size as sampled in successive 20-million-year slices. To be proper carnivores or ungulates, for example, species generally have larger brains today than, say, 60 million years ago, when other species were generally from small-brained "archaic" orders. The part of the environment that is defined by "other species" has become more demanding, and all surviving species must measure up to the demands.

There are interesting implications here for intelligence as a macroevolutionary trait. The idea that living species should be placed on a smart–stupid scale makes less sense than early evolutionists suggested. At any slice in time, according to the Red Queen hypothesis, there should be a balance of intelligence – a kind of equilibrium with respect to the distribution of processing capacity. Depending on its niche, each species would have evolved brain and behavior characterizable in relation to processing capacity and designed to control the repertoire of behaviors spelled out in the ethogram of the species. In successive geological strata there were, on the average, increments in processing capacity in species within comparable niches; that is the evidence of Figure 12.2. But the interpretation is that a balance of species, an equilibrium, was maintained.

We are not surprised to find reversals as well, such as the one that occurred within an adaptive zone for rodentlike animals. Such niches were apparently occupied, successively, by multituberculates (an archaic order of mammals dominant in this adaptive zone between about 70 and 150 million years ago), by condylarths (a later archaic order), by primates (plesiadapids: a family of primates that probably fathered the earliest prosimians), and finally by true rodents about 35 million years ago (Gingerich, 1976). It takes more than brains to make a living in some niches, and this particular macroevolutionary sequence is one that has small-brained rodents replacing large-brained primates in the course of evolutionary history.

This section was planned as a kind of primer on evolution to inform psychologists about recent approaches. It cannot be emphasized too strongly that the basic facts and many of the principles of evolution continue to provide a fundamental structure for biology. It would be appropriate to conclude a primer with a review of facts – of what happened, when it happened, and what life was like at various times in the past. There is simply not enough space for such a review; the reader must find appropriate references elsewhere. The September 1978 issue of *Scientific American* was devoted entirely to evolution and is an excellent and up-to-date introduction, parts of which have been cited here (Lewontin, 1978; Maynard Smith, 1978b). Other publications cited here, for example, Simpson (1953) and Stanley (1979), can also be used as general references.

It is important to try to keep some key dates and trends in mind: Vertebrate life has spanned some 500 million years of geological time. The reptiles appeared over 300 million years ago, the mammals about 200 million years ago, birds at least 150 million years ago, and primates about 75 million years ago. The major modern orders of mammals were all present about 40 million years ago, "higher" primates about 30 million years ago, hominids about 10 million years ago, some species of *Homo* at least 2 million years ago, and *Homo sapiens* about 250,000 years ago. The appearance and disappearance of species is the fundamental information for the Red Queen hypothesis and is also fundamental to the reconstruction of the evolution of specific adaptations. It was the basis for my effort at reconstructing the evolution of intelligence (Jerison, 1973), which is summarized and updated in this chapter.

Evolution as the history of life is, in cladistic perspective, a reconstruction of family trees. In anagenetic perspective, it is a story of changing patterns of structural and functional adaptations. The evolution of intelligence may be traceable within family trees, perhaps within the higher primates or the hominoids. This is the cladistic perspective. Anagenetically, it is traceable as changing distributions of processing capacities among evolving species. The main objective of this section has been to explain these perspectives, both of which are necessary for a proper analysis, while giving some flavor of recent advances in evolutionary theory.

12.3.   ON INTELLIGENT BEHAVIOR

Because of its great complexity, the strictly behavioral dimension is less well understood in evolutionary perspective than other dimensions of intelligence considered here. When he reviewed the subject for Stevens's *Handbook* three decades ago, Henry Nissen (1951) summed it up with Figure 12.6, a programmatic conjecture based on a few data. If the "data" generating the psychometric functions in Nissen's graph are species points, then the graph can be thought of as a kind of mathematical integral of Figure 12.2. (Nissen extends it to the entire animal kingdom.) Figure 12.6 still represents the best that can be done in describing the likely progress and discontinuities among phyletic groups (see Hodos & Campbell, 1969). The anagenetic trend can be imagined by connecting the midpoints of the psychometric functions.

When actual data are used, it is more difficult to illustrate progress among species. The nearest thing to such evidence is in research on learning sets, which has been summarized by Passingham (1981) and is presented here in Figure 12.7. The advance from the conceptually clear but data-poor picture offered by Nissen to the less grand, factual picture offered by Passingham is a central theme of this section. These are ways to analyze an anagenetic trait, the sort of thing one likes to see in handbooks.

The behavioral literature comes from at least three disciplines – psychology, zoology, and anthropology – and there are also contributions from linguistics. One purpose of this chapter is to integrate this inevitably diverse knowledge. A list, such as the following one, of important reviews of literature can accomplish part of the integration. In psychology the great emphasis has been on laboratory studies of learning, the results of which have been reviewed from a variety of perspectives by Bitterman (1975), Brookshire (1976), Herman (1980), Mackintosh (1974), Passingham (1981), Riddell (1979), and Warren (1977). Ethologists, as zoologists concerned with behavior, have tended to emphasize species-typical behaviors and cladistic rather than anagenetic dimensions. Hinde's (1969) textbook represented a major ethological and psychological synthesis, and there are now several collections of articles concerned with such a synthesis (Bateson & Hinde, 1976; Hinde & Stevenson-Hinde, 1973; Seligman & Hager, 1972). Contributions from anthropology and archaeology (Isaac, 1976; Marshack, 1976; Washburn & Harding, 1970) are increasingly recognized as relevant to the other areas, and were especially emphasized within a more general review by Parker and Gibson (1979). The most recent development, covering all the disciplines, has been the discovery of "language" in apes, an issue in cognitive science as much as in the analysis of communication (Gardner & Gardner, 1971; Hill, 1978; O'Sullivan, Fouts, Hannum, & Schneider, in press; Premack, 1976; Savage-Rumbaugh, Rumbaugh, and Boysen, 1980; Seidenberg & Petitto, 1979; Terrace, Petitto, Sanders, & Bever, 1979).

There are several other kinds of integrative contributions that should be added to the "library" of readings just listed. E. O. Wilson's (1975) landmark publication

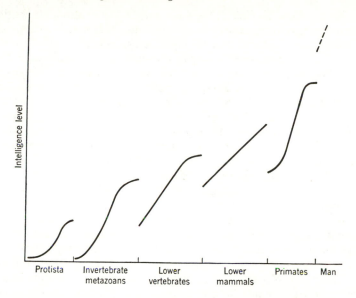

Figure 12.6. Henry Nissen's estimate of comparative intelligence in animals. (From "Phylogenetic Comparison" by H. W. Nissen, in S. S. Stevens [Ed.], *Handbook of Experimental Psychology* [New York: Wiley, 1951]. Reprinted by permission.)

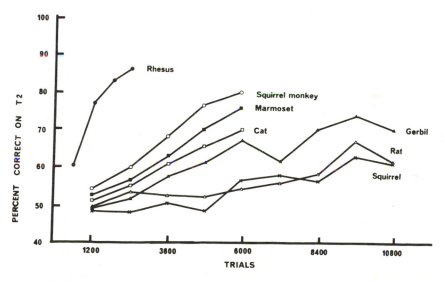

Figure 12.7. Performance by various species on Trial 2 (T2) of 6-trial exposures to each of many learning-sets problems as a function of total number of trials. (From "Primate Specialization in Brain and Intelligence" by R. E. Passingham, *Symposia of the Zoological Society, London*, 1981, *46*, 361–388. Reprinted by permission.)

introducing "sociobiology" as a discipline has a special place. Although not directly concerned with intelligence as a trait or system of traits, sociobiology presents a style of biological analysis of adaptation that can easily be applied to our topic. There have been several thoughtful, philosophical works by eminent biologists, some of which have been cited before, which deserve special mention and attention: Eccles (1979), Griffin (1976), Lorenz (1965), and Thorpe (1974). Several recent symposia (Dimond & Blizard, 1977; Harnad, Steklis, & Lancaster, 1976) have included important papers close to this topic. Finally, there are the results of the recent revival of interest in the evolution of cognitive processes that are not measured with learning tasks (Gallup, 1977, 1979; Humphrey, 1978; Jerison, 1973; Mason, 1976). A number of the other authors cited earlier, especially Griffin, Herman, Premack, and Warren, and students of ape "language," have discussed such cognitive dimensions.

My intention in presenting this lengthy reading list was to balance a necessarily personal brief summary and evaluation of data. I would start with Warren (1977) and Passingham (1981) to enter this literature, and then Bitterman (1975) for an exposition of one research program as well as a good evaluation of methodological problems. The major defect in this literature arises from overemphasis on learning, as studied in psychological laboratories, and a misunderstanding of the contribution of ethology. Parker and Gibson's (1979) review, in which cognitive dimensions are considered, is a helpful antidote to the too-close tie to learning. For a subject as intrinsically interesting as the source of mind, the scientific literature is disappointingly dull. The richness that we know intuitively has simply been lost in the effort to treat intelligence scientifically. In my own monograph (Jerison, 1973), I have often relied on anecdote and the evocation of experiences that readers are likely to have shared, as a way of maintaining a connection with our intuitions about intelligence. In the pages that follow, I evaluate the more recent scientific evidence and try to suggest ways to improve it.

COMPARATIVE PSYCHOLOGY VERSUS ETHOLOGY

There are differences between the psychological and zoological approaches, which are sometimes glossed over or dismissed apologetically. But these are fundamental; they parallel the distinction between anagenetic and cladistic analyses, and they distinguish comparative psychology from ethology. Psychologists have been concerned traditionally with manifestations of the human mind: observable behaviors that can be analyzed and described by essentially mathematical functions, rationalizable curves on graphs. The species has usually been unimportant in stating such functions (Skinner, 1957). Animal psychology was developed as a kind of physiology of mind to provide animal models in which the functions could be studied. The albino rat was chosen for convenience, and it was replaced by the pigeon in some laboratories for the same reason. As biologists, comparative psychologists followed the physiological rather than zoological tradition. It was only a casual acknowledgment of systematic zoology that led to the introduction of monkeys as "closer to man" into the psychological laboratory, but in every instance experiments that might be relevant to intelligence were experiments on "functions" that could be defined in human terms.

Without defending the willful ignorance and arrogance of this scientific pose, I suggest that it is possible to recognize some validity in it for the study of intelligence.

We have learned from ethology the tight coupling of animal behavior to the demands of adaptation, and the ethological program has successfully shown how even small elements of an "ethogram" fit into the requirements of an environmental niche. As Maynard Smith (1978b) put it, ethologists "have shown that the animal brain possesses certain specific competences, that animals have an innate capacity for performing complex acts in response to simple stimuli" (p. 178).

To the extent that animal brains are organized in terms of specific competences, the analysis of intelligence as a general competence is clearly a different dimension of analysis. The specific competences, "fixed action patterns" in response to "sign stimuli," are specific to a species and could be used as part of a taxonomic key to classify species. This is the evolutionary program of ethology, to generate clado-grams (at the level of species and subspecies) of the kind shown in the lower half of Figure 12.3, but based on behavioral data. The analysis of animal intelligence, as a general competence, would yield an anagenetic picture of the type indicated in the upper half of Figure 12.3, and the anagenetic measure could be functional and entirely independent of species. This has been the evolutionary program of comparative psychology.

Functions relevant to intelligent behavior have usually been associated in some way with learning and learning ability. Bitterman (1975) has pointed out that such functions appear to be the same in many vertebrate species, at least as studied by Thorndike and his successors. Skinner (1957) demonstrated impressively that the effects of various schedules of reinforcement on operant conditioning are essentially the same in pigeons, rats, monkeys, and humans. Animals working in Skinnerian paradigms are no longer learning when tested, of course. They learned during the period of "shaping" of the response (Bailey & Bailey, 1980), and the similar performance curves that are obtained in different species are evidence of another kind of uniformity, an optimization by the animal – a balancing of the cost of responding against the benefit of reinforcement in an animal that has learned about responses and reinforcements. The control of behavior under these circumstances could in principle involve some systematic differences among species. That it does not is an empirical fact. If differences among species in processing capacity are reflected in the costs–benefit analysis, these differences have not yet been measured and reported. More subtle and perhaps more difficult learning tasks have been developed that do show differences among species.

LABORATORY STUDIES OF ANIMAL LEARNING

The most straightforward demonstration of species differences in learning capacity has been with learning sets, in which an animal "learns to learn." Adapted by Harlow (1949) from Klüver's (1933) work on "equivalent stimuli," the procedure is based on learning a response strategy, or set of rules, to handle sequences of problems based on a common principle. For example, the problems might all involve choosing a "correct" box when a baited and an unbaited box are marked to be discriminably different. When an animal learns to look for and use the right kind of discriminable features to guide its choice, it needs only one trial on the task to get all the information necessary for correct responses. Performance on the second trial (T2) of a set of trials can then be perfect if the animal adopts a "win–stay, lose–shift" strategy in response to the markings. Passingham's summary of performance of animals of different species in Figure 12.7 is on this sort of task and is based on training procedures in which all problems were presented for six and only six trials with data in terms of success on T2.

The differences among species suggested in Figure 12.7 are consistent with our intuitions and with data on encephalization (Riddell, 1979). Passingham chose the data in this illustration to meet Warren's (1974) criticisms of the learning-set paradigm as providing a measure of animal intelligence, primarily by controlling the number of trials per problem. Other data, less adequately controlled in this respect (see Passingham, 1981), suggest how the picture would probably be filled out. Cebus and spider monkeys perform better than squirrel monkeys, chimpanzees better than rhesus monkeys, minks and ferrets better than cats and skunks. Birds can also do this sort of thing: pigeons, myna birds, and blue jays have been studied and do at least as well as cats.

Learning sets involve a cognitive dimension. The animal has to learn the principle of its task. The behaviorist tradition, emphasizing associative learning, fostered an enormous literature on presumably simpler problems faced by rats in mazes, runways, and various puzzle boxes, such as Skinner boxes. As noted earlier, this performance is remarkably similar among most vertebrate species that have been studied within the constraints of the procedure. Capitalizing on this finding. Bitterman (1975) considered the questions that had arisen in exceptional cases, when rats had performed in ways that were difficult for stimulus-response (S-R) association theory to handle. Was it possible that species from "lower" classes of vertebrates (fish, reptiles, birds) would perform in ways consistent with S-R theory in comparable tasks? The idea was that associative learning was simpler than ideational learning involving expectations and other cognitive mysteries. In cases in which rats seemed to use higher (cognitive) processes, lower vertebrate species might be limited to lower processes, and their performance would be consistent with S-R theory. (Birds are "higher" vertebrates in encephalization, and Passingham, 1981, emphasizes their "higher" behavioral grade. Their status was not clear when Bitterman undertook his research program.)

At least seven learning paradigms of the type studied in rats turned out to work in more or less this way, to differentiate species of vertebrates. These will not be considered in detail here (see Warren, 1977, for a succinct account and Bitterman, 1975, for more detail and an extensive bibliography). There are no clear formal statements that can enable us to differentiate the "higher" from the "lower" capacities that turn up in this work. Working at "higher" capacity seems to mean behaving sensibly in a way in which we as humans can imagine ourselves behaving in these environments. One example is in studies of contrast effects. The classic effect, described by Tolman (1932) and based on Elliott's (1928) work, was that rats trained in mazes with mash as reward began to make more errors when the reward was changed to sunflower seed. Their performance became poorer than that of other rats trained on sunflower seeds throughout. The behavior is like human disappointment when an expectation about what will be in the goal box is not met. This kind of contrast effect has not been found in goldfish or turtles (Bitterman, 1975). Such contrast effects in rats were among the early embarrassments to S-R learning theory (Mackintosh, 1974). The behavior in goldfish, as Bitterman put it, shows that "goldfish do have some respect for the S-R reinforcement principle" (p. 701). They do not behave as if they were disappointed; they are proper automatons, as it were.

Other categories of performance studied by Bitterman – the partial reinforcement effect, probability (versus minimax) matching, the overtraining reversal effect, over-shadowing, inter- and intradimensional transfer – all have been used to discriminate among vertebrate classes as represented by goldfish, painted turtle, pigeon, and rat. The common feature is the extent to which S-R theory is embarrassed by the performance of rats (or other "higher" species) and not embarrassed by that of a lower species. The results show without much question that the distinctions among species should be made, and the interpretation is that rats have more performance strategies (the S-R "strategy" as well as various cognitive strategies) available to them than have representatives of the lower classes.

This kind of straightforward empiricism in the analysis of grades of intelligence in different species can work in a variety of frameworks. Bitterman used S-R theory as a cutting edge to separate stupid from smart species: To the extent that S-R rather than cognitive theory worked for them, the species were stupid.

Other criteria can be derived from brain–behavior data, as Masterton and Skeen (1972) have shown. The prefrontal neocortex of the mammalian brain is implicated in a number of behaviors studied in monkeys, such as the delayed-alternation response, one of the tricks of the animal laboratory. There is a well-validated literature demonstrating that after ablation of prefrontal brain, cats and monkeys have shorter maximum latencies for delayed-reaction tests. Masterton and Skeen did an evolutionary rather than surgical experiment of this type, comparing performance of hedgehogs, tree shrews, and bush babies, species of mammals that differ dramatically in both absolute and relative amounts of prefrontal cortex. The results confirmed expectations: Whether the amount of prefrontal cortex in an animal is determined by surgery or by evolution, it is correlated with performance on delayed-alternation tasks.

I have not spelled out the details of the tasks. They are described by Masterton and Skeen (1972), and details of procedure are too important to risk the misunderstandings that can follow a brief summary. The procedures were developed from Hunter's (1913) original work, designed to study covert (mental) processes by delaying some of the information required to make an "association"; if the association was successfully made, as shown by a correct response despite the delay, it was assumed that mental work must have been going on, and that memory and ideation were probably involved.

CRITICISMS OF LEARNING MODELS: PREPAREDNESS

Research of the kind just cited involves few theoretical assumptions. Success on a task implies "smart" and failure implies "stupid," and when species regularly succeed or fail, they are placed on an intelligence scale relative to one another. This "IQ" approach can be criticized for many reasons (Warren, 1977), most cogently on the ground that specialized evolutionary adaptations of a species may interact with the task in ways that result in advantages or disadvantages. Rats as animals that normally live in burrows may be especially adapted to learn mazes, but they may do poorly in learning sets because their natural strategy is "win–shift" (Olton, 1979). In general, species are "prepared" (Seligman, 1970) by their adaptations to learn some tasks and fail in others, independently of our intuitions about intelligence.

The most obvious preparedness is with respect to sensory information to be handled in discrimination tasks. Primates are adapted for handling visual information, and human experimenters may erroneously assume that other species see more or less what we see when presented with visual stimuli. When dolphins (*Tursiops*) have been studied for their ability at discrimination learning, some of the tasks involved visual discriminations of the kind used in rats and monkeys: triangle versus square, vertical versus horizontal stripes, and so on. This large-brained cetacean at first seemed curiously inept when such visual discriminations were used to test its ability at complex tasks. We know that these are smart animals not only because of their enormous brains (see Figure 12.3), but also because they handle auditory tasks quite well. The paradoxical effect was eventually resolved: Dolphins improved considerably in visual work when the displays were made less static – jiggled a bit rather than kept fixed. They are not "prepared" to respond to static visual displays. The story is reviewed by Herman (1980). In general, the perceptual world, the *Umwelt* (von Uexküll, 1934/1957), of a species has to be understood and taken into account when species are compared.

Seligman's (1970) idea of preparedness was introduced with an order of effects somewhat different from the straightforwardly perceptual. The questions were about the generality of "laws" of learning for any stimulus, any response, and any species. Seligman cited the difficulty in using movements of the scratch reflex as an operant for other behaviors in cats as an example of preparedness (or its opposite). In Rozin's (1976) terms, the scratch reflex is not a response "accessible" to other behavioral systems. Learning when stimuli are gustatory and the reinforcement is illness seems to have radically different "laws" from that when stimuli and reinforcement are "exteroceptive" (Garcia, 1975; Garcia, Hankins, & Rusiniak, 1974). It is almost certain, in short, that the laws differ for different dimensions of stimulus, response, and reinforcement; a general S-R theory, in which anything can be an S or an R, must be impossible.

Warren (1977) made the same point in the analysis of species differences in forming learning sets and other discriminations; rats do much better if the stimulus dimension is olfactory rather than visual, and we have already noted the auditory "preparedness" of dolphins. Warren's concluding remarks contrasted within-species with between-species results and presented a behavioral definition. He emphasized the absence of reliable within-species differences. Between species, he concluded:

There are no significant differences among vertebrate species in simple associative learning. . . . The concept of intelligence is helpful in describing the set of qualitative differences observed between species of vertebrates in characteristics like: breadth of spatial capacity for processing sensory information, rule learning, language-like behavior and self-recognition. The evolution of intelligence consists of the development of new and more sophisticated skills for learning and solving problems in the more progressive levels. [P. 54]

Phrased another way, the definition equates animal intelligence with the number of alternate strategies available to members of a species in coping with environmental problems. Warren (personal communication) sees this as a behavioral definition consistent with the definition in terms of processing capacity used in the present chapter.

COGNITION

Learning has been an unfortunate psychological anchor for intelligence. It is too dry a topic, at least as developed by academic psychologists, who have been committed to a behaviorism and reductionism that inevitably miss the essence of intelligence.

Where intelligent behavior is flexible and at least somewhat unpredictable, "learned behavior" in the laboratory is the reverse, successfully studied when it is most predictable and governed by rules that are deterministic in their force, even when described as probabilistic in statistical theories of learning. The probabilities in learning theory are of responses that, in their simplicity, are not easy to define biologically. An animal in a puzzle box moves a lever which closes a switch which operates a relay which moves a chain to which a pen is attached, and a "cumulative record" of performance is written by the animal. The result can make science fun to do, and it has enabled us to write many important rules about performance in its relation to schedules of reinforcement. But the rules are not about intelligent performance, except incidentally. The rules are about probabilities that arbitrary responses will occur, and not about response strategies.

The unit of intelligent behavior is not a single response but a system of responses in an environmental (stimulus) context. The system is a strategy, as it were, for coping with an environment. Learning sets involve intelligence because they are based on the subject's having learned a strategy, a set of rules about how to cope with a variety of settings, rather than rigid behaviors for unique settings. The response of moving a hand toward a lever or a baited box is trivial in itself, but intelligent or stupid when based on (and a measure of) an animal's choice in the face of uncertainty. Yet the single response, the movement of a pen on a recorder, charms and soothes the scientific spirit. Behaviorism, psychology's operationalism, won the battles of the first half of the 20th century; operationalism is the essence of modern science, an ideal philosophy for scientists, and no one willingly rejects it.

The real problem is to operationalize the "higher" functions of intelligence. Learning situations such as the learning-sets task, reversal learning, the various contrasts experiments, overshadowing, and so on, as described or mentioned earlier, operationalize the analysis of cognitive processes. It is unfortunate that the metaphor has to be mechanistic – that we must imagine a machine that follows appropriate rules, and thus mimics the intelligent behavior of a living animal.

Emphasis on cognition per se, redeveloped by scientific psychologists, has been accompanied by several new analyses of animal behavior that are related to intelligence. The most spectacular grew out of a problem on the uniqueness of language as a species-typical human character. In an effort to test the limits of the assertion of uniqueness, the Gardners (1971) and Premack (1976) undertook to train chimpanzees to communicate with human experimenters, using artificial systems of signs that met linguists' criteria for language. During the decade that followed, it became clear that such studies were direct approaches to mind in apes – that procedures developed from studies of "language" in chimpanzees could be used to prepare queries referring to cognitive processes in the animals, like items on a human intelligence test (Premack, Woodruff, & Kennel, 1978).

APE LANGUAGE AND INTELLIGENCE

The emerging consensus about studies of language in chimpanzees and other great apes is that the performance of the animals demonstrates much greater cognitive capacities than had been recognized by psychologists in the past, but that the actual performance cannot be correctly described as language in a strictly human sense (Savage-Rumbaugh et al., 1980). Fouts and his associates (O'Sullivan et al., in press) argue an even stronger view favoring "continuity" for language. The issue is by no means settled, and the history of comparative psychology suggests that judgment should generally be deferred when the issue is about upper limits of a precisely defined ability in a species. Linguists have sometimes attempted the analysis of language as a human ability by listing "design features" of language as communication (Hockett, 1960), to suggest the kind of machine involved in the production of language; but there is no uniquely human machine that differs fundamentally from animal machines. The approach is wrong for an evolutionary analysis, limited as it is by mechanistic reductionism. Working scientists studying animal "intelligence" have long recognized that the apparent limits on the ability of any given species are often limitations of the imagination of the experimenter in devising a procedure in which the ability can be manifested. The successful teaching of "language" to apes is an outstanding example, regardless of our eventual conclusions about the nature of the language.

The general impression of levels of intelligence in living primates is summed up by Mason (1976), who wrote: "I am persuaded that apes and man have entered a cognitive domain that sets them apart from all other primates" (p. 293). Woodruff, Premack, and Kennel (1978) point in the same direction in demonstrations that Piagetian "conservation" principles were followed by their chimpanzee. Parker and Gibson (1979) reviewed an extensive literature to support the contention that great apes were at more advanced Piagetian stages than were monkeys – at the beginnings of "preoperational intelligence" rather than merely at "sensorimotor intelligence," the level at which they place monkeys. (Parker & Gibson have attempted a detailed application of Piaget's methods to rate various species of primates with respect to intelligence, an interesting effort that is probably limited by anthropocentrism – see the commentary following their article; Jerison, 1982b; and other later commentary on the same article.) In any event, the consensus is with Mason (1976) that the essential differences are in the way reality is represented in the animal's mind, and that the reality, the *Umwelt*, of apes is similar to that of humans in synthesizing "heterogeneous attributes as different properties of the same 'object'" (p. 284). The greater gap may be between great apes and "lower" primates. Premack's (1978) analysis of the ape's "theory of mind" develops a similar position on the ape's world.

SMART CETACEANS

The major incompletely resolved problems are on operationalizing intelligence behaviorally, on prescribing behavioral methods to measure intelligence in animals. Many of the measures have to be derived from learning theory, as discussed by Bitterman (1975), Passingham (1981), Warren (1977), and others. Observational methods discussed by Parker and Gibson (1979), especially as developed by students of ape languages into quasi-experimental or fully experimental methods, broaden the scope of the defining properties. Herman (1980) has published an outstanding review of operationally defined cognitive processes in bottlenosed dolphins, which can be a model for such reviews for other species.

Herman discusses cognition in dolphins in terms of memory, of conceptual processes, and of language. The studies of memory include matching-to-sample, delayed matching, delayed discrimination, and so forth. In general, his bottlenose dolphins performed extremely well, at levels comparable to those of chimpanzees or humans on such tests, when auditory stimuli were used. The dolphins performed poorly when visual stimuli were used, but, as mentioned earlier, they approached the high-primate level when dynamic displays replaced static displays. Conceptual processes for Herman (1980) "involve the manipulation of information" (p. 390) (transforming, organizing, operating on according to rules, etc.). The learning sets and reversal learning problems are in this category. As in the case of memory, these "conceptual processes" show "substantial differences between the auditory and visual information-processing capabilities of the dolphin" (p. 407). Herman reports instances of true motor and vocal mimicry and observational learning in dolphins. These include the learning of elaborate behaviors that could be used for public performances, behaviors that normally take months to develop in an isolated naive dolphin.

The most dramatic examples of observational learning are from work on "language" in dolphins, in which the procedure is formally like Premack's with chimpanzees. For instance,

Maui [a dolphin] was trained to emit an echolocation sound on hearing a three-word command preceded by a sound for his name. Later, without training, Puka [another dolphin housed with Maui] was given the same three-word command, preceded by her name, and responded with her echolocation signal. In another test, Maui was trained to raise his flukes clear of the water on a three-word command preceded by his name. Subsequently, when the command was given to Puka, she slapped her flukes on the water. [Herman, 1980, p. 407, reporting work by D. W. Batteau & P. R. Markey of about a decade ago. Unpublished results from Herman's group in 1980–1981 are better documented and even more spectacular.]

These examples are important illustrations of cognitive capacities. Herman is conservative in assessing these capacities in dolphins, concluding only that, "though their evolutionary lines have been divergent for tens of millions of years, there seem to be many areas of cognitive convergence between some of the delphinids and some of the advanced simian primates. In many ways the two groups are cognitive cousins, though at opposite poles in sensory specialization" (p. 421). He continues in this vein, summarizing the points of comparison and implying equality of dolphin and chimpanzee. In view of the difficulty of establishing communication with dolphins and the ease of doing so with chimpanzees, Herman's successes warrant a less conservative interpretation than he offers. The chimpanzee grade that he suggests is clearly a minimum; the evidence is not inconsistent with much more radical suggestions.

The best known of the radical suggestions about cetacean intelligence are certainly Lilly's (1975, 1978). Arguing essentially from information on absolute brain size, Lilly ties brain size to language systems and to an idea of a kind of cerebral Rubicon for language that is reminiscent of Sir Arthur Keith's long-discredited ideas (see Lenneberg, 1967, but also Jerison, 1976b). Lilly's picture of a possible cetacean natural language is anthropomorphic but not naively so. His view is that dolphins (*Tursiops*) are so smart that they can descend to a human level and communicate vocally with appropriately sensitive human scientists with whom they establish close social relations. (The strong human–dolphin social bond is crucial for his argument, and it is generally agreed that this is a major feature of work with dolphins.) Despite severe criticisms of Lilly's views (Herman & Tavolga, 1980), there is no present evidence that would force rejection of their conclusions, and there is now evidence (Richards, Wolz, & Herman, 1981) of unusual capacities for vocal mimicry in dolphins that could justify Lilly's proposals on developing a working communication system between man and dolphin. Because of its basis in an auditory–vocal mode, it might be even more effective than the system established by "language" tutoring of chimpanzees.

Analyzing cognitive capacities in animals requires imagination as well as restraint, a willingness to entertain unusual suggestions, such as some of Lilly's, at least as working hypotheses, while keeping in mind Lloyd Morgan's canon and the importance of laboratory studies to control for experimenter error, including the "Clever Hans" phenomenon (see Lilly, 1975, pp. 383, 402). "Clever Hans" was a horse presented at the turn of the century as being able to do arithmetic, giving answers in hoofbeats. Hans was indeed clever, as it turned out, responding to cues from his trainer of which the trainer himself was unaware: a slight nod of the head or other gesture that was the cue for stopping the hoofbeats. The horse was a clever observer but not a mathematician.

COGNITION: FIELD OBSERVATIONS

Some of the most important evidence about cognitive capacities comes from field observations, in which controls for experimenter errors are impossible. Tool use by chimpanzees, for example, has been described by Goodall (Van Lawick-Goodall, 1970) and Telecki (1974) and reviewed by Parker and Gibson (1979). These field observations contribute significantly to our understanding of the grade of intelligence of chimpanzees. The descriptions make clear that the tool use is culturally determined. Parents teach offspring; specific tools differ in size and shape, and seem to be fashioned for particular jobs (in the case of reeds used to pick termites); and Teleki's descriptions of his own strenuous efforts to learn to do as well as the chimpanzees at termiting attest to the level of skill attained by the apes that taught him.

The evidence from tool use for intelligence is not in the use per se. Many vertebrates and invertebrates construct and use tools; the spider's web is a familiar example. At least one orangutan has been trained to use and make stone tools (Wright, 1978). The evidence for intelligence is in the cognitive capacities involved in the use of tools, and these capacities may be difficult to demonstrate. Part of the demonstration can be to show that there are cultural effects in natural populations, such as those noted in chimpanzees. The evolution of human intelligence has also been recorded in the fossil record of stone tools, and may be measurable by an analysis of the skills required to shape the tools (Isaac, 1976).

Field observations have established the importance of learning in natural animal communities. The outstanding example is, perhaps, the diffusion of the habit of washing potatoes in a troop of Japanese macaques (Itani & Nishimura, 1973; Kawai, 1965). Observers of the natural behavior of wolves have been impressed by their ability to navigate enormous ranges, which clearly involves learning a cognitive map (Peters & Mech, 1975). That map is established on the basis of olfactory as well as visual cues, depending heavily on urine marks, and is one of many examples of labile olfactory communication systems in mammals (Eisenberg & Kleiman, 1972).

There may be some tendency to think about the cognitive dimension anthropomorphically, emphasizing human categories. Lilly's suggestions about delphinid intelligence are presented as if *Tursiops* had a modified human language. Perhaps a didactic device, reflecting the general audience for which Lilly has often written, this anthropomorphic suggestion also shows how difficult it is to imagine a truly exotic intelligence. (Lilly goes to some length to raise exactly this kind of point, citing the Clever Hans problem, for example.) Anthropomorphizing enters into many analyses, however. The idea of a cognitive map is easy to work with, because it makes intuitive sense and is also supported by a major literature (Olton, 1979; Tolman, 1948). But classic statements about tool use have been naive, as if this were a magical adaptation that distinguished man from apes and other creatures. Man was *Homo faber,* uniquely the toolmaker, for some authors, and it required a special analysis of the prevalence of tool using in animals to put the issue in perspective (e.g., Hall, 1963).

Anthropomorphizing about cognition has us imagining an animal "cognizing" by "reasoning," that is, performing a kind of logical operation on the information available to it – thinking like a person who is solving a problem. This might not be a bad model if we demystify human problem solving and think of it as something that a machine, a computer, might do in a human way, given an appropriate program. The mystical side of the analysis occurs when we try to imagine experience in another species, an individual animal's consciousness or awareness. This does not have to be mystical. Consciousness is as important a problem as any in the analysis of intelligence. It surely represents an adaptation related to information processing of a high order, and it can be analyzed in a reasonably objective way.

CONSCIOUSNESS AND HIERARCHICAL ORGANIZATION

It would be fair to assert that the idea of consciousness, or awareness (the words are used as synonyms), and the extent to which various species of animals are conscious in the same general ways are at the core of most approaches to the evolution of mind and intelligence. Difficulties in operationalizing consciousness have kept it from the center of scientific analysis, but many students of evolution of brain and mind have written thoughtfully and cogently on it. Mason (1976) and Jaynes (1977) are among the more imaginative recent reviewers, and Griffin (1976) has presented a scholarly and detailed analysis that is likely to reestablish the legitimacy of consciousness as a topic in biology. The difficulties are primarily in deciding exactly what we mean by consciousness, beyond our intuitive understanding. In the following paragraphs, I present a view of the nature of consciousness developed in Jerison (1973), which is reasonably consistent with the present consensus, to the extent that a consensus has been achieved.

Although most authors mean self-awareness when they write of consciousness, it may be wisest to keep *self* out of the definition at the start. I believe that the place of *self* is less fundamental than the problem of simple awareness, which is the problem of how we know and represent reality. (See Humphrey, 1978, for another view.) Early in this chapter, I presented the view that awareness is an almost arbitrary construction of the brain; its role in the work of the brain is as a model, in Kenneth Craik's (1943/1967) sense, constructed at a particular hierarchical level of the brain's work to "explain" the otherwise overwhelming amount of information in ongoing neural activity. The model cannot really be arbitrary, of course. Physical environmental information is a rigid constraint on the activity of sensory (and motor) surfaces, and these are the sources of information processed by the nervous system. The nature and organization of the neural material are further constraints on the model. The model is a possible world, which is a reality made by a brain. To the extent that brains are similar, the models should be similar, and to the extent that they differ, the models should differ. For each of us the model *is* reality, the real world of everyday experience, although there has long been a philosophical appreciation that there is a problem in validating our knowledge of reality, a recognition of its constructed nature.

Consciousness is thus a description of one level of activity of a very large hierarchically organized information-processing system. The lowest level of organization is the single nerve cell. Intermediate hierarchical levels mentioned earlier include cell assemblies, or modules, of neuronal material. But there are too many even of these (they number in the millions) for efficient processing to take place, and they have to be organized into fewer chunks (Simon, 1974). The reality of which we are aware is at a higher hierarchical grade, a set of chunks assembled into an "image" of reality. It is (for us) a visual three-dimensional "representation" (Mason, 1976) of an active world, enhanced by sounds and odors, verified by touch, illuminated by our emotions, which accompany the view and attract us to some parts, repel us from others, and leave us passive, neutral, with respect to still others. For us (perhaps as a species-typical adaptation), it is also meaningful in that we see it not only as sights and sounds but as verbally describable. The raw information changes from instant to instant and is incorporated into this hierarchical structure as sensible change over time with respect to the things in our space and, occasionally, with respect to the space itself.

It takes an almost poetic language to present this kind of idea, to evoke an appropriate image. The idea is important for a comparative analysis because it suggests how the *Umwelten* of various species, which are models of reality of the species, are related to one another. The kinds of intermediate-level analyses that take place in the hierarchies of a group of species produce each *Umwelt* in contrast with other *Umwelten*. When we discover that there are bat worlds built with living sonar systems, for example, in which sound emission and echolocation are so significant that enormous amounts of neural tissue are co-opted (Suga & Jen, 1976), we appreciate that these animals live in a special world that we humans might describe as full of ultrasonic squeaks and echoes. For insect-feeding bats, "squeaks" and "echoes" must surely be transformed into something equivalent to "prey insects" at some specified "distance" within a specified "space" and moving at a "speed" that must define "time" as well (cf. Griffin, 1976).

The quotation marks are to suggest a translation from the bat's *Umwelt* to that of man. The translation may be more vivid if we impose an additional stage in information-processing for a human observer: a television camera recording a scene and a man watching a television screen on which the scene is projected. An intelligent bat watching the man watching the screen would record a remarkable skill: Information from a changing pattern of illuminated dots on the screen is clearly being converted into some image of reality, a "real world" almost unimaginable to the intelligent bat. The idea of awareness or consciousness becomes necessary when sequences of dots or other fairly elementary events (edges, lines, surfaces) are organized to become "objects" in "space" and "time." To the extent that "squeaks" and their "echoes" become "insects in flight" or "edibles in motion" for bats, these small mammals are aware, or conscious, in our terms (Griffin, 1976).

The problem is deeper, but it is too difficult to develop much further here. Is the equivalence of "insects" with "edibles" for bats comparable to its equivalence for humans? This is the sort of issue that Klüver (1933) faced and resolved operationally with his "method of equivalent stimuli." Klüver did not question the existence of more or less equivalent codes in monkey (the cebus was his favorite) and man that transformed a pattern of neural activity into an image of some kind in conscious awareness. His question was, Given the transformation into an image, into consciousness, was the structure of the image the same in man and monkey? The issue is the same as that raised by Posner (1978), in which the cognitive equivalence of *A* and *a* for English language readers is recognized. Earlier in this section, Herman's (1980) work on visual discrimination of static and dynamic shapes by dolphins was described. To me this suggests that dolphins do not know (see) these shapes the way we do. When the shapes do not move, they may not enter the dolphin's real world, and it is only when they move at least a bit that they are used as information for further analysis. Static and dynamic visual displays that are "equivalent stimuli" for human observers are probably not equivalent for dolphins.

In these several examples, one should get a sense of the problem of defining consciousness, or awareness. It is the problem of defining a mental image as opposed to some simpler central state or pattern of neural activity. To assume that members of other species do not have images is so strange that it is something of an effort to describe their worlds without using words that evoke elaborate ("insect") as opposed to simple ("squeak" and "echo") central states; the ideas "elaborate" and "simple" can easily lead to further regressive semantic games, and a "central state" must be an image of sorts with a new name.

We have a clue to the operational behavioral analysis of this kind of consciousness in some of the preceding discussion. It is not so much a matter of determining the pattern of equivalences among the stimuli in various animal worlds as it is a matching of animal and human performance. Morgan's canon, the principle of parsimony, would direct us to as simple an interpretation of such equivalences as possible, but simplicity should not falsely be equated with operations at lower hierarchical levels of the brain's work. The behavioral definition of consciousness is properly based on the idea that hierarchical organization is simple organization for the work of elaborate systems such as brains.

It is simpler to assume that a brain is hierarchically organized than that it is organized with a minimum of hierarchy. The most efficient system is hierarchical. It is difficult to imagine a computer program of more than a few hundred steps that works efficiently without subroutines, and this is the general model for any hierarchical system. In the computer, it is subroutines nested within subroutines; in the brain, it is chunks within chunks, sets of metaphors, as Jaynes (1977) might describe the system. When a reasonably elaborate behavioral experiment with humans is known to involve conscious awareness, animals performing in a comparable way in a comparable experiment should, on the assumption of parsimony, be granted conscious awareness as part of the strategy for coping with the experimental procedure.

BEHAVIORAL ANALYSIS OF CONSCIOUSNESS

The evidence on animal awareness is based on more than inference from human experience. The direction of inference in certain crucial experiments has been from judgments about unusual kinds of awareness in the animals being tested, which led to new observations and eventual confirmation of comparably unusual awareness in human subjects. One series of experiments was on visually guided behavior in monkeys following complete bilateral ablation of primary visual cortex. A second series of experiments was on unusual learning in cats and monkeys following complete transection of the corpus callosum and other commissural systems, the original "split brain" preparations. Both groups of experiments and their application to ideas about human consciousness are reviewed.

After ablation of the visual cortex, some rhesus monkeys recovered visual function, but their behavior suggested that they experienced a kind of surprise about visual events – that they were not fully aware of what they were seeing (Humphrey, 1974). Tests with human neurological patients suffering from comparable lesions explained the surprise. Such patients are usually completely blind as far as they or anyone else is concerned – at least that has been the general consensus. Partial lesions are correlated with complete blindness for part of the visual field, and the blind area is mapped as a kind of enlarged "blind spot." Clinical neuropsychologists routinely map the lesion by recording where in the visual field objects are reported as seen and not seen by patients. Because of the orderly projection of the retina onto the primary visual cortex, there is a good correspondence between the lesion in the brain and the blind area of the visual field.

Humphrey's observations in monkeys suggested that human patients might be able to use visual information presented to the blind area to guide their behavior, and this was found to be the case. Patients found the test peculiar, because they were asked to point to things they could not see, yet their pointing was perfect (Weiskrantz, 1977), a behavior that has been felicitously called "blindsight." It is vision of a sort, without awareness, and it was discovered by using inferences about an aberration of awareness in monkeys.

In the 1950s, animal studies showed that cats and monkeys in which the commissures were cut could be trained to develop incompatible competing habits if the information for each habit was presented to a different half of the brain (Myers, 1956; Sperry, Stamm, & Miner, 1956; see Sperry, 1974). The results suggested an unsuspected independence of the two halves of the brain. When the same surgical procedure was developed by Bogen, Sperry, and their associates to control human epilepsy, it was discovered that, beyond their functional differences with respect to language, the hemispheres of the human brain seemed to maintain separate consciousness after sectioning of the commissures. The dominant hemisphere, the language hemisphere, seems to be the seat of what we think of as the self-conscious ego (Dimond, 1979; Eccles, 1979). Once again, an inference about awareness in animals led to discoveries about human awareness.

Self-awareness in animals has to be studied with procedures modeled on human experience, and in recent years an appropriate approach has been discovered. In a series of studies of consciousness and self-recognition in various species of animals, including monkeys and chimpanzees, Gallup (1979) has reported that only the great apes responded to their reflections in mirrors as reflections of themselves rather than of another individual. When their faces were painted, their responses were typically to touch their own faces rather than reach to the mirror to explore a "compatriot" there. This response pattern implies a concept of self as a distinctive kind of object with properties different from those of other objects. It was this kind of evidence, in addition to the results of studies of "language," that led Mason (1976) to the view that the *Umwelt* of great apes, their representation of reality, is significantly closer to the human condition than is that of any other primate.

Humphrey (1976, 1978) has argued that intelligence should be widely distributed among animal species because it should contribute directly to fitness, and that consciousness, including self-consciousness, should be an attribute of such intelligence. His argument for self-consciousness as a contributor is ingenious, involving the problem of anticipating the actions of other animals on the basis of projecting oneself into the other animal's situation. There is little question that consciousness as intelligence, and intelligence as a broad capacity to adopt many behavioral strategies in the face of environmental challenges, might be justified as an evolutionary investment by many lineages of organisms. It should be appreciated, however, that in the broad range of living creatures and their behavioral adaptations, the most frequent adaptations are relatively automatic and deserve the old ethological descriptions as "fixed action patterns." Intelligence – a major increment in neural processing capacity – is an expensive way to cope with the challenge of the environment. It is cheaper to evolve specialized, perhaps unconscious, behaviors (and neural control systems) for specialized environments, and that has been the universal invertebrate and typical vertebrate mode.

Operationalizing animal awareness evidently requires (is based on) analogies from patterns of behavior in animals to the corresponding patterns in humans in which awareness has a role. We assume that Humphrey's monkeys, like Weiskrantz's patients, *experienced* a "blindsight" of some kind in their visually guided behavior after lesions of the primary visual cortex. We assume that the learning with the left hemisphere by Sperry's and Myers's callosal cats and monkeys was organized by experience that was independent from that learned by the right hemisphere. (The functional differentiation of the two hemispheres in cats and in monkeys is not nearly as dramatic as in humans. In cats and monkeys the two hemispheres more nearly duplicate one another and are equipotential [Casseday & Diamond, 1977; Hamilton, 1977].) But the nature of the cat's and monkey's awareness is surely an elaborate image of a world, a reality comparable in many ways to human realities.

Operationalizing is direct in Gallup's experiments with mirrors. The development of superior methods of communicating with other species, ape languages and their extensions for dolphins, may make it possible to ask equally direct questions about an animal's experience or to inquire indirectly about its mental images. The procedures could be similar to those used to study mental imagery in humans (Kosslyn, 1980), though one should expect difficulties analogous to those that might occur if the human subjects were severely retarded.

SELF-CONSCIOUSNESS AND LANGUAGE

Self-consciousness is the awareness of self as a unique object in space and time, and the awareness of being aware, of attending to one's own thoughts. There are no operational approaches to all of this, though Gallup's (1979) procedures make it clear that chimpanzees, like humans, see their images in mirrors as images of themselves. To a monkey, on the other hand, its reflection in a mirror is another monkey. Attending to one's thoughts and the concept of self for humans are probably associated with the evolution of human language, and I would argue that the human self differs from the chimpanzee's as much as or more than the chimpanzee's differs from the monkey's. The difference is due to language, human language.

I have argued (Jerison, 1973, 1976a, 1976b) that human language evolved in response to an environmental demand for additional cognitive capacity in early hominids, not specifically for a new and better communicational skill. The distinction is important for an evolutionary perspective, because, typically, communication is rigid in mammals, based on a limited number of signs, and the behaviors tend to be genetically fixed. Cognition (literally, "knowing"), on the other hand, is what has been referred to earlier as the construction of a real world of experience. It is based on the processing of sensory information (including information from feedback from motor systems and motor activity), and it is clearly related rather directly to the intelligence and consciousness that is our subject here. Communication is less clearly related. Typical communication is with fixed action patterns, the most efficient way to communicate reliably and unequivocally; the typical messages are approach, withdraw, watch out, or run (alarms).

According to my argument, human language began as a relatively simple adaptation in small-brained early hominids in which auditory–vocal marks were used as the functional equivalents of olfactory–scent marks in the cognitive worlds of social carnivores, such as wolves (cf. Peters & Mech, 1975). The argument is speculative, based on the problems faced by social predators in establishing cognitive maps necessary for the successful navigation of the very large ranges that such species typically occupy. The olfactory–scent-marking system is especially well adapted for such mapping, and cortical systems, especially paleocortical structures like the hippocampus, are deeply implicated in such mapping (Olton, 1979). By the time true monkeys and apes appeared during the past 30 million years, there had been extreme reduction of the peripheral olfactory system in primate evolution. The early hominids were trying to make a wolflike living without adequate sensory machinery, I argued, and the auditory–vocal system was substituted for the normal olfactory–scent-marking machinery as a way to cope with the deficiency.

This kind of analysis is similar to other analyses that I have used to explain the evolution of unusual brain adaptations, including the early encephalization of mammals at least 150 million years ago. The next section reviews such analyses in more detail. The point on the evolution of language is that, according to my argument, a new kind of communication was an unexpected bonus that resulted from the evolution of the language system, primarily because of the design features inherent in the auditory–vocal channel. If vocal marks are used instead of scent marks to construct a map, conspecifics will share the auditory–vocal map with one another both in its construction ("naming") and in its reconstruction (repeating or remembering a name). Communication with this system would occur not as commands and forced responses but as sharing of a cognitive structure, sharing of consciousness. In communicating by means of this strange system, the reality of one individual becomes the reality of others that use the same language, at least to the extent that this channel contributes to the constructed reality of an individual.

In the operation of the sensorimotor system, there is continuous *motor* differentiation of sounds uttered by the self from those uttered by others; there is less differentiation of the auditory *sensory* information. The speech signal's uniqueness is partly its peculiar construction as a sensory and motor event, with major interaction between auditory feedback and the work of the sound-production apparatus (Liberman, 1974). Beyond this, the reality constructed by vocalizations of others must differ from the reality constructed by one's own vocalization. It is in this way that realities are distinguished and that a self is placed as a peculiar object in the constructed real world.

The story is about the *beginnings* of language, the source of its evolution. Had language evolved only under selection pressure for better communication, its neurological evolution could have been simpler and cheaper and based on less brain tissue. An adequate system for this predatory social primate would fit into the brain of a crow (Nottebohm, 1975; N. Thompson, 1976), a bird that communicates as elaborately as most primates. A wolf might be another model, and again there is no evidence for much brain to house its control system for communication. Even a system as elaborate as that discovered by Seyfarth and his associates (1980) in vervets could be handled by a small powerful neural control box. For these green monkeys, the communicated message might be "Run up a tree" – unambiguous, and easily followed. A message with human language, on the other hand, would have the form "I see a leopard." The listener would then have to share the image and act accordingly – make his own decision about what to do. Animal communications are typically commands. Action is directed and options are avoided. Language is quite different.

Scenarios for the evolution of language in which the auditory–vocal channel is fundamental (Hockett, 1960; cf. Sebeok, 1977) are consistent with the present analysis. Scenarios that emphasize gestures or facial expressions (which do "communicate," of course) are not (e.g., Dingwall, 1979; Hewes, 1976; Parker & Gibson, 1979). Had human language evolved from gestural systems, it would very likely not have evolved with as extensive a neocortical and hippocampal involvement as is present, nor would the language areas of the brain be as intimately associated with the neocortical fields for the localization of hearing and the motor control of mouth and tongue. Wernicke's area and Broca's area would be elsewhere relative to the "homunculus" that is mapped in the human brain, perhaps near the hand and thumb areas.

To conclude this section, two points: First, we note that the present human grade of intelligence, as characterized by uniquely human consciousness, is one in which the individuals of the species have a communication system in which there is sharing of elements of the constructed real world, sharing of consciousness. This is really what is unique about human language, not its logical structure or its infinite vocabulary (cf. Chomsky, 1972), and this is the unique feature of human intelligence. It is this feature that makes human intelligence so strange and social a phenomenon, one that led Eccles (1979) to insist that in describing the "human mystery," we should recognize a real world, his and Popper's (Popper & Eccles, 1977) World III, consisting of the accumulated cultural heritage stored in libraries and elsewhere. The relationship between language and constructed reality has been appreciated by Whorf (1956) and Sapir (1949). The relationship between language and mental maps was for Ludwig Wittgenstein one of the fundamental insights for his early *Tractatus* (Malcolm, 1958). This first point is that there is a fundamental role for language in human cognition, human awareness or consciousness, human intelligence, and the reality that is constructed by human brains.

The second point is less dramatic. For all its wonder and compellingness, consciousness is really a small if important element in the human (and presumably animal) experience. Almost all authors who have attacked this question, Jaynes (1977) most elegantly, make this point. In skilled action, in the process of learning, in fact in most ongoing behavior, consciousness seems to track the actual behavior. One speaks and then one hears oneself, and it is only in the hearing that there is acute awareness (D. A. Norman, personal communication). If there is awareness prior to or during speech, it may be accompanied by various failures of the act, just as skilled acts become impossible or at least very difficult if one tries to monitor or control them consciously. Most behavior is carried out without simultaneous conscious direction, though it is not "unconscious." It can easily be recalled or predicted and then examined and evaluated, but consciousness usually interferes with the action of the moment.

Human intelligence and various animal intelligences share many features, but all are unique for their niches. A difficulty to be faced by any human analyst is appreciation of the artifacts that inevitably arise in the analysis of one intelligence by another. The special role of language in human intelligence interferes with our picture of the intelligence of other species. One of my pleasures in reading *Lilly on Dolphins* (Lilly, 1975) was to discover Lilly's recognition of exactly this problem in his work with these small whales, a pleasure that was only slightly attenuated by his lively, mystical faith in the superiority of his subjects.

12.4.   ENCEPHALIZATION AND INTELLIGENCE

The evolutionary perspective of this chapter is based on an analysis of the history and nature of structural encephalization in vertebrates (Jerison, 1973, 1979b). The raw data are anatomical and paleontological on brain–body relations, and these data are translated into data on neural information-processing capacity evolving under the ecological and other environmental constraints of the past 400 million years.

There is hard evidence of structural encephalization in a number of vertebrate lineages. The earliest birds and the earliest mammals about which data on encephalization are available (*Archaeopteryx* and *Triconodon*) lived about 150 million years ago, and their brains were clearly larger than those of their contemporaries of similar body size among the reptiles (Hopson, 1977; Jerison, 1973). The earliest primate, the prosimian *Plesiadapis* of about 60 million years ago, was more encephalized than any of its contemporaries. And there are unique features in the history of encephalization in cetaceans and in the human lineage (the Hominidae), events of about 18 million years ago and of the past 3 million years or so, respectively (Herman, 1980; Kennedy, 1980).

Periods of rapid encephalization in certain lineages were probably interspersed among relatively long steady states, and evolution by "punctuated equilibria," as discussed earlier (cf. Stanley, 1979), could describe the history of encephalization. The reptiles, for example, appear to represent a large class of vertebrates in which, with few exceptions, the balance of encephalization among species has been the same for the past 200 million years. Among the mammals, the living Virginia opossum and many insectivores are at the same grade of encephalization as *Triconodon* of 150 million years ago.

The evidence for such generalizations about encephalization has been the subject of a certain amount of controversy (Hopson, 1977, 1979; Jerison, 1979a; Quiroga, 1980; Radinsky, 1978), but the broad outline is probably correct. The generalizations are important as the basis for conjectures on the course of evolution of intelligence and the place of intelligence among behavioral adaptations. It is, therefore, appropriate to review briefly the way encephalization is measured and the main results of its measurement. Because of the special place of within-species variation in the analysis of human intelligence, I will describe and try to explain the important differences between analyses based on diverse samples of species and those involving closely related species or several populations of a single species (cf. Jerison, 1977a, 1979b).

Encephalization represents an amount of brain size beyond that required by body size, and because total brain size is related to total information-processing capacity

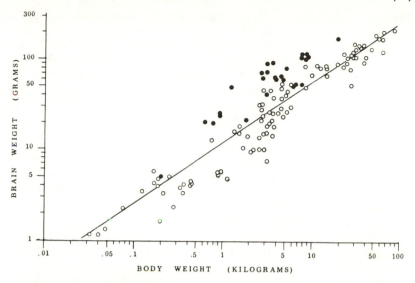

Figure 12.8. Brain and body size in 123 species of mammals. Filled points are primates. The line is Equation 2 with k = .12; that is, Equation 3 or 3a. (Data from "A Record of the Body Weight and Certain Organ and Gland Weights of 3690 Animals" by G. Crile and D. P. Quiring, *Ohio Journal of Science*, 1940, 40, 219–259.)

(see Figures 12.4 and 12.5 and the accompanying discussion), encephalization is a measure of processing capacity after an adjustment for body size. It is, thus, a measure of intelligence as defined here. There is some danger that this very simple syllogism will be interpreted as justifying a view of the brain as a homogeneous mass of tissue without specialized functions or meaningful localization of function. That is not the case, of course, and it is important to reconcile the analysis of encephalization with the implications of our knowledge of localization of function in the brain (Welker, 1976a, 1976b). This section is, therefore, devoted to a description of measured encephalization, an analysis of its meaning in relation to intelligence, and a review of the course of encephalization and its implication for the evolutionary history of intelligence.

MEASURING ENCEPHALIZATION

If the brain weights and body weights of a large number of species are plotted as points on double-logarithmic graph paper, the resulting cloud of points fits rather well about a line with a slope of about 2/3. An example of such a graph is presented in Figure 12.8. This graph shows how encephalization can be treated as a biometric problem in regression analysis. The line is Equation 2 (p. 730), with $k = .12$, the basic "allometric" equation for many numerical analyses of encephalization. In exponential rather than logarithmic form it is

$$E = .12P^{2/3} \tag{3}$$

with brain weight E and body weight P in grams. As a regression equation it is

$$\log E = 2/3 \log P + \log .12 \tag{3a}$$

The slope is 2/3, and a residual from the regression could be measured as a value of k_i for species i with brain and body weights E_i and P_i.

Dimensionally, k is a length in centimeters (Jerison, 1977a), and for this reason, a minor modification of this empirical numerical approach may be preferred, based on the dimensionless "encephalization quotient," EQ, a ratio of actual brain weight E_i to expected brain weight E for a given species. This is the same as the ratio k_i/k or $\log k_i - \log .12$, which is, of course, the residual with respect to the regression, Equation 3a.

The numerical computation of EQ is with Equation 4:

$$EQ = E_i/.12P_i{}^{2/3} \tag{4}$$

To illustrate, one of the smaller primates in the sample of Figure 12.8 is a squirrel monkey with $E = 24$ g and $P = 903$ g (Crile & Quiring, 1940, p. 240). A 903-g mammal, according to Equation 3, has an expected brain weight of 11.2 g, and this is the value of the denominator of Equation 4 for the squirrel monkey. The computed EQ for the squirrel monkey is, therefore, 24/11.2, or 2.1. The distance of the squirrel monkey datum from the "regression" line in Figure 12.8 is fairly typical for all the primates, and $EQ = 2.1$ means that primates are about twice as encephalized as average mammals.

This is the sort of generalization that can be made legitimately about encephalization. Convex polygons drawn about sets of brain–body data of the type in Figure 12.8 can yield the same information. In Figure 12.9, such polygons are drawn for prosimians (Figure 12.9A) and for higher primates (Figure 12.9B). Figure 12.9 provides information for many judgments about progressive encephalization of primates, including hominids. The living prosimians are seen to be "average mammals," for example, because their polygon falls on the regression line. In their evolution during the past 60 million years, the prosimians progressed from the grade of *Plesiadapis* (*P*), which was below that of living species, to that of *Tetonius* (*T*) and *Necrolemur* (*N*), tarsierlike species of about 55 and 45 million years ago. The later species are close to or lie within the polygon that describes living prosimians and average living mammals. This is an example of the evidence for rapid evolution of encephalization, followed by a long period of equilibrium. The prosimians as a group reached their present grade about 50 million years ago, having evolved to that grade during the previous 10 million years.

A comparable account can be derived for higher primates. The earliest of these on which there are data is the Paleogene (Oligocene) *Aegyptopithecus* (*Ae*) of about 30 million years ago, and we have here the interesting suggestion that, although the earliest higher primates may have been "higher" in some morphological traits, they apparently lagged in encephalization. Hominid history leading directly to man can also be read that way. The australopithecines (Hominid: *A*) of from about 4 million years to 1 million years ago were only slightly above the grade of other higher primates. But within about 1.5 million years of evolution, hominids rapidly became encephalized through the habiline (*h*) and pithecanthropine (*e*, for *Homo erectus*) grades. Like the earliest simians, the earliest hominids also lagged in encephalization compared to other traits (cf. Washburn & Harding, 1970). The story that can be read from Figure 12.9B is told more simply later in Figure 12.11.

It is possible to draw polygons like those of Figure 12.9 through many assemblages of data, grouped according to natural zoological categories. Most of the major vertebrate groups have been analyzed in this way with respect to encephalization (Hopson, 1979; Jerison, 1973; Northcutt, 1981; Platel, 1974; Quiroga, 1980).

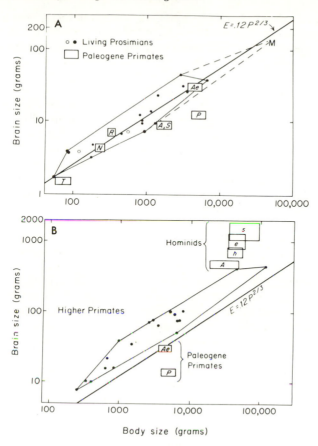

Figure 12.9. Convex polygons enclosing primate data, shown relative to Equation 3. *A*, the early anthropoid *Aegyptopithecus* (*Ae*), compared with the polygon of living prosimians. Fossil species: *Tetonius* (*T*), *Necrolemur* (*N*), *Rooneyia* (*R*), *Adapis* (*A*), *Smilodectes* (*S*), *Plesiadapis* (*P*), and *Megaladapis* (*M*). *B*, higher primates compared with one another, with the Paleogene fossils *Aegyptopithecus* and *Plesiadapis*, and with the hominids *Australopithecus* (*A*), *Homo habilis* (*h*), *H. erectus* (*e*), and *H. sapiens* (*s*). Rectangles about hominid data indicate range of variations according to present estimates. Paleogene includes Paleocene, Eocene, and Oligocene epochs, from about 63 million years ago to 22.5 million years ago. (Data from "Données nouvelles sur l'encéphalisation des Insectivores et des Prosimiens" by R. Bauchot and H. Stephan, *Mammalia*, 1966, 30, 160–196; "Encéphalisation et niveau evolutif chez les Simiens" by R. Bauchot and H. Stephan, *Mammalia*, 1969 33, 225–275; *Evolution of the Brain and Intelligence* by H. J. Jerison [New York: Academic Press, 1973]; "Brain, Body, and Encephalization in Early Primates" by H. J. Jerison, *Journal of Human Evolution*, 1979, 8, 615–635.)

There is a major advantage in this graphic way of characterizing encephalization in that the vertical displacement of the polygons (e.g., simians vs. prosimians in Figure 12.9) can be the measure. This method requires no empirical or theoretical equations. The results of numerical versions of analyses like these are summarized later, in Figure 12.11, as the history of vertebrate encephalization, to suggest a fundamental pattern in the evolution of intelligence. Before we turn to these, however, it is important to consider some limitations of the numerical analyses, which require additional assumptions about the allometric analysis of brain–body relations.

THE ALLOMETRIC COEFFICIENT

In the data of Figures 12.8 and 12.9, there is little question that the regression line has a slope of about 2/3. that is, the allometric exponent is approximately $\alpha = 2/3$ for Equation 1 (p. 730). The result is typical for large heterogeneous samples of species, but in a group of similar species, or within a species, the allometric coefficient is usually less than 2/3. The difference among allometric coefficients for different kinds of samples must signify that the computed value is determined by more fundamental aspects of the allometry of brain and body. Lande (1979) has discussed this issue in an analysis based on population genetics by determining the effect of selection exclusively for body size or exclusively for brain size within a species. It was possible for Lande to predict an allometric coefficient $\alpha = .36$ in mice when selection is only on body size, from a mathematical expression in which the terms are the coefficients of variation, heritabilities, and additive genetic correlation of brain and body weight. Lande's analysis also explains the unusual $\alpha = .77$ in mouse strains bred for brain size (Roderick, Wimer, & Wimer, 1976). The exponent 2/3 for diverse species is explained as a macroevolutionary effect of selection primarily for enlarged brains in mammalian evolution, in effect, of encephalization. This approach is consistent with other arguments that brain size and body size may be decoupled in evolution (Jerison, 1973).

Another kind of explanation, which is consistent with Lande's but emphasizes functional effects of encephalization, is concerned with geometric constraints on information-processing in nervous systems (Jerison, 1977a). The 2/3 exponent in equations like Equation 3 is fundamental for this view as a constraint of body surface on brain volume. According to the theory, the exponent reflects the two-dimensional mappings of sensory and motor surfaces in the organization of a three-dimensional vertebrate brain. The analysis leads to the fundamental brain–body relationship being reexpressed as:

$$E = .12mP^{2/3} + A \tag{5}$$

The dimensionless constant m is linearly related to the amount of amplification (multiplication) of a basal sensorimotor representation, or map, for the projection systems of the brain. In the cortical representation of the retina, for example, there are 12 replications in rhesus monkeys (Zeki, 1978) and presumably a smaller number in rats (Merzenich & Kaas, 1980) – a difference that could be associated with a computed $m = 1$ in monkeys and $m = .5$ in rats. The constant A is a fraction of brain weight in grams, which is not accounted for by the projection systems. A is a mnemonic for "added" tissue, or for association system of the brain, but it should not be conceived as a localized association system restricted to particular nonprojection regions. The theory is about amount, not about location, of tissue. Equation 5 could be exactly true even if there were no identifiable association areas, that is, even if the entire cortex could be accounted for by projection systems as discussed by Diamond (1979) and by Masterton & Berkley (1974). The added tissue could be interdigitated, or buried within projection systems, and would not be identifiable as "association" cortex by present methods.

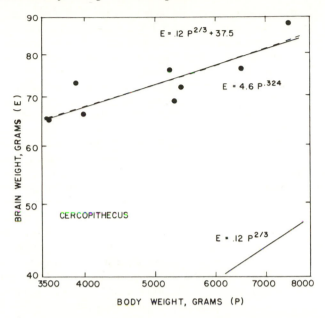

Figure 12.10. Brain–body relations in *Cercopithecus* monkeys. Equation 3, also shown in Figures 12.8 and 12.9, is the line at the lower right. The solid line fitting the data is a least squares fit with Equation 1, i.e., an empirical allometric equation. The dashed line is Equation 5 with $m = 1$, $A = 37.5$ g. Note that Equation 1 and Equation 5 are almost identical within this range of values. Equation 5 has a theoretical rationale (Jerison, 1977a; Lande, 1979). (Data from "Encéphalisation et niveau evolutif chez les Simiens" by R. Bauchot and H. Stephan, *Mammalia*, 1969, 33, 225–275.)

Lande's is a dynamic and mathematically sophisticated analysis of the course of allometric evolutionary change, based on genetics and population biology rather than neurobiology. My geometric theory, on the other hand, emphasizes the neurobiological constraints implied by allometry for the processing capacities of brains of different species. There are differences between the predictions of the theories for allometric relationships, but these are too small to provide critical tests of the views as alternatives, nor is it clear that the two views are inconsistent with one another.

It is instructive to compare the approaches with the help of the data presented in Figure 12.10, on eight species of *Cercopithecus* monkeys. Lande's approach uses the straight solid line fitted through the points, the allometric equation (Equation 1, section 12.1), and is concerned with the exponent $\alpha = .324$ in that equation. My approach implies the dashed line, which represents Equation 5, and which is also almost congruent with the allometric line. In my approach the values .12 and 2/3 are fixed constants, not determined by the data; the data are used to estimate the "free parameters" m and A, and the approach is as parsimonious as allometry in which the parameters k and α are estimated from the data. In any case, it is impossible to use these data to distinguish between Lande's approach and mine.

In Lande's approach the estimated $k = 4.6$ is not interpreted as being of biological interest. The important term is $\alpha = .324$, and its meaning (in conjunction with data on heritability and variability) is that during the evolution of the species of monkeys

of Figure 12.10, selection pressures were on body size. The difference among species in brain size is viewed as a kind of passive evolutionary response owing to the
genetic correlation between brain and body. This analysis is entirely consistent with
the approach presented here on the issue of the control for a body-size factor in brain
size: The species of *Cercopithecus* would be treated as equivalent in encephalization,
and the expected brain size for a given body size would be estimated allometrically
with $\alpha = .324$. It is not clear, however, that the value of $k = 4.6$ could be used in
some way to estimate the degree of encephalization (see Jerison, 1973, p. 59).

In my geometric approach, the parameter m has a value of 1.0 for *Cercopithecus* of
Figure 12.10, a number that can be interpreted only with the help of other data on
other species. It is clearly higher than in rats ($m = .5$), as noted earlier, indicating
more "amplification" in the monkey's central nervous system. Data on ungulates (A.
Filler, personal communication) indicate that $m = .7$ for a very diverse sample of
bovids, which are average mammals by other criteria ($EQ = 1$, approximately). Thus
monkeys would have more amplification in their mappings (projection systems) in
the brain than do other mammals. The value of m does not, of course, provide a true
measure of amplification; it is a relative measure. If amplification is defined as the
number of central neurons relative to the number of peripheral neurons in a projection system, data on the auditory and visual systems indicate much larger numbers
to represent true amplification, at least on the order of 10^3 or 10^4 (see Jerison, 1973,
p. 416).

The additive, or association, factor in my approach is evaluated as 37.5 g in
Cercopithecus. This does not mean that 37.5 g of brain are devoted to associative
functions. The *A* factor should be interpreted as accounting for 37.5 g of the brain
weight in each species. Much of the weight is unrelated to processing information. It
is the weight of connective tissue, blood and blood vessels, and so forth, as well as
nerve cells. The approach merely states that in a statistical partitioning of the brain
weight, a constant amount in each of the species in this group is encumbered by the
presence of associative systems in the brain. The implication is that there is a similar
amount of processing in all eight species that would be describable as associative
rather than related to maps.

Both Lande's theory and mine can be correct. Lande's theory shows us how things
could have happened to produce the present situation in animal brains and bodies,
and the geometric theory tells us what this could mean for the distribution of processing capacities among living vertebrates. My geometric theory enables us to
relate divergences from an allometric exponent of 2/3 to processing capacity.

A single measure of encephalization, such as *EQ*, is a heuristic composite of the
two factors m and *A*. In connecting this theory to Lande's, it should be noted that
factor m is an encephalization factor that remains functionally coupled to body size,
though responsive to selection pressures on brain size. Factor *A*, on the other hand,
is a decoupled encephalization factor both functionally and with respect to selection
pressures, based entirely on selection for enlarged brains.

SEX AND RACE

Within-species variation in the human species in brain size is explained by the
geometric theory as an effect of body size. Sex differences in brain size are approximately one standard deviation; adult male European brains average about 1350 g,
and female brains average about 1225 g (Jerison, 1979b). Taking body weights as 70

kg and 50 kg for the two sexes and fitting Equation 5 to these data, we can calculate $m = 3$; $A = 740$ g. The threefold increase in the amplification in humans over that in monkeys may reflect the enormous expansion in the human brain of sensorimotor control systems that control lips, tongue, and speech production, the hand–eye coordination system, and other systems that are related to a map of the real world as something experienced and acted upon. The A factor can be explained entirely by the size of the conventional speech and language areas and their contralateral homologues, though frontal and other association fields would also clearly be subsumed within this partitioning of the brain.

The important point is that relatively simple assumptions about the nature of encephalization explain the remarkable sex difference. The computation is based on the assumption that the sexes are exactly equal in their values of m and A, and this assumption leads to acceptable results in terms of our knowledge of brain–behavior relations.

There are also real race differences in brain size within the human species, which are smaller than the sex differences (Ashton & Spence, 1958; Tobias, 1970). These can probably be explained in the same way as sex differences. The data on race are confounded by nutritional effects, which are minor for brain size but severe for body size. The estimation of m and A in different racial populations is presently a futile exercise. It is enough to note that the available data are consistent with the idea that the human sexes and races are equal in encephalization.

PUNCTUATED HISTORY OF ENCEPHALIZATION

Despite the caveats developed about the index EQ, this single heuristic measure is extremely useful for summarizing encephalization. The distributions of EQ presented in Figure 12.2 illustrated graphically the way relative brain size changed, at least in the orders of mammals represented in those curves. The advance in encephalization, the comparability of carnivore and ungulate encephalization, and the increasing diversity in encephalization were all clearly shown. The history of encephalization can be described by changes in mean values of EQ, which are essentially the distance between centroids of minimum convex polygons, such as those illustrated in Figure 12.9, from the diagonals in those illustrations, Equation 3.

That history is summarized in Figure 12.11; data on primates in Figure 12.9 are the entire basis for the primate lines drawn in Figure 12.11, and this explanation should help identify some of the simplifications in the latter illustration. Broken lines indicate extrapolations. It is impossible to indicate the diversity of encephalization within any lineage; all lineages are represented by mean values. The rapid encephalization of prosimians between about 40 and 60 million years ago was already discussed; in Figure 12.11 it is shown as the steep prosimian solid line, which reached the steady state of "average" living mammals ($EQ = 1$) earlier than the other "average" mammalian groups presented here, the ungulates and carnivores. Simians (higher primates) are shown diverging from prosimians, with the earliest of their lineage remaining at a prosimian grade. Three of the hominid lineages are shown, with lines ending at about the time of their extinction.

The most important fact in Figure 12.11 is the extent to which the data can be represented by horizontal lines. These are the equilibria, the evidence of conservation – of conservative evolution. Living reptiles are at the same grade as the earliest fossils that are known. There are living mammals at the same grade as Mesozoic

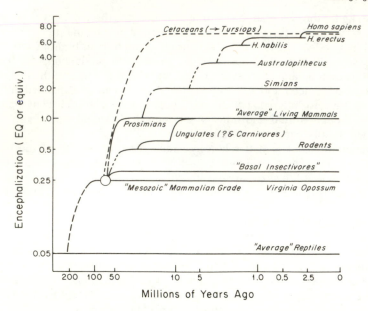

Figure 12.11.   The course of encephalization in various vertebrate lineages. Solid lines indicate fairly complete records; dashed lines show regions of extrapolations. The circle at about 60 million years ago on the mammalian line is the approximate beginning of the great adaptive radiation of mammals. Note that "time" is on a logarithmic scale.

species. Rodents are about half as encephalized as "average" mammals, and have been at that grade as long as data on their brains are known, as of the Oligocene about 30 million years ago. This means, of course, that big brains are not essential for survival. They are required for some niches, but a majority of vertebrates have evolved and diversified without notable encephalization. The line for "average" reptiles is also the line for average fish, and that lowest grade of encephalization is the grade for the majority of living vertebrate species.

A second feature of Figure 12.11 is the rapid evolution to higher grades in each lineage, the "punctuations" of the equilibria. These are more than pure conjecture. The evidence is generally about the equilibrium level, and advances across levels are not normally represented by fossil data, but this situation reflects only the prevalence of fossils. In several instances, most notably the beginning of the simian line and much of the prosimian line, there are records of the rapidly evolving intermediate grades, of missing links, as it were. To take another example, the earliest bird, *Archaeopteryx*, was a missing link in encephalization between a reptilian and avian grade (Jerison, 1973; cf. Hopson, 1977).

The cetacean line is shown as conjectural because of the limited data. There are a total of six fossil specimens from essentially two grades, one reached about 40 million years ago and comparable to that of the prosimians at that time (note the convergence of the curves) and a second achieved about 18 million years ago and comparable to the australopithecines. The essentially sapient grade of encephalization in the bottlenose dolphin, *Tursiops truncatus,* is a grade with unknown evolutionary history; the fossil history of the genus *Tursiops* covers about the same interval as and is less known than that of *Homo*. Living *Tursiops* could fall almost exactly on a human line as defined by $m = 3$, $A = 740$; there is a reported mean dolphin body weight of 233 kg (Gihr & Pilleri, 1969), and for the human m, A, this corresponds to a brain weight of 2,103 g. The reported mean brain weight in *Tursiops* associated with that body weight was 2,048 g. The difference between man and dolphin is about 2.5%, surely within our margin for error.

Those are the sorts of data on which Figure 12.11 is based. Now let us consider a few exceptions or unusual cases. The most interesting of these is in the evolution of cartilaginous fish, sharks and their relatives. There is unpublished evidence of a Permian shark, about 250 million years ago, which has an endocast comparable in size to that of the living horned shark, *Heterodontus*. These and several other living species of shark are at a mammalian (rodent) grade of encephalization. The lessons of traditional comparative anatomy that sharks are primitive animals are clearly not appropriate for their intelligence, as defined in this chapter. According to the available evidence, they are the first vertebrates to have experimented with significant encephalization. Their present successful adaptations should clearly be reevaluated and, perhaps, related to behavioral intelligence (Northcutt, 1981).

Another notable exception to the pattern revealed in Figure 12.11 occurred in the evolution of dinosaurs. Within one group, the ostrichlike dinosaurs, there has evidently been significant encephalization that approached and may have reached the avian and mammalian grade. This conclusion is based on the work of the Canadian paleontologist Dale Russell and is reviewed by Hopson (1977, 1979, 1980).

HUMAN ENCEPHALIZATION AND LATERALIZATION

The hominid data presented in Figure 12.11 are among the best documented (Holloway, 1974). The australopithecines, both skull and body of which are now known from about 4 million years ago, represent a rather stable brain–body system. There have been conjectures about allometric effects in hominids beginning with this genus (Pilbeam & Gould, 1974), based on limited data. Most of the work with this material has been by anthropologists: Holloway and Pilbeam, just cited, and also McHenry (1975) and Tobias (1971). These positions are reviewed in Jerison (1975) and Kennedy (1980), as well as elsewhere. The evolutionary consequences of these views have been incorporated in Lande's (1979) theory.

There is still uncertainty about the status of the habilines, *Homo habilis*. One specimen (KNM ER 1470) of about 2 million years ago has an endocast of about 775 cc, a volume that is close to the erectus grade, but in other respects the habilines seem to be a good australopithecine species (Kennedy, 1980). The detailed data on pithecanthropines (*Homo erectus*) are beginning to suggest some advance within the species during the interval between 1.6 million years and 0.5 million years ago, from which this group is known. The advent of *Homo sapiens* as Neandertals or pre-Neandertals has been recorded in the endocasts, and it is clear that the Neandertals had brains at or perhaps above the living human grade in encephalization (Jerison, 1973; Kennedy, 1980; Kochetkova, 1973/1978).

There has been a report of asymmetric lateralization of the endocast of the Chapelle-aux-Saints Neandertal, of about 40,000 years ago (LeMay, 1975). I have seen the endocast and am much less confident of the evidence of asymmetry. When Boule and Anthony (1911) prepared the endocast, they penciled their impressions of the probable placement of the Sylvian fissure onto the endocast, and it is from these penciled "data" that LeMay reached her conclusions. The difficulty may be appreciated in part from Connolly's (1950) discussion of this endocast in the context of many other endocasts of living and fossil hominids and other primates. The fissural pattern of the brain is *not* represented clearly on the lateral surfaces of primate endocasts in the size range of those of living humans. Connolly also points out that, in primate endocasts, there is occasionally a misrepresentation of the Sylvian fissures in the endocast. The fossil "evidence" from subjective markings on one endocast is too slight to be taken as at all conclusive. There may have been asymmetry, but it has not really been determined, nor is it easy to determine on endocasts by present methods.

The reason for LeMay's observation on Chapelle-aux-Saints is partly that genuine morphological asymmetry in the human brain has been discovered within the past decade or so. The most striking asymmetry is in temporal lobe cortex buried in the Sylvian fissure. The region is called the *planum temporale* behind auditory cortex (Heschl's gyrus), which is probably part of Wernicke's speech and language area. Geschwind and Levitsky (1968) found that in 65% of the 100 human brains that they examined the left hemisphere *planum* is more extensive than that of the right hemisphere. This finding has since been verified as an asymmetry that appears in the fetal brain (Witelson & Pallie, 1973) and is probably a genetically determined human trait. Asymmetries have since been discovered in the external morphology of the human brain, as well as in the brain of the chimpanzee, though not in rhesus monkeys (LeMay & Geschwind, 1975; Yeni-Komshian & Benson, 1976). These are in the pattern of the Sylvian fissure and are exactly the kind of asymmetry that LeMay found in pictures of the Chapelle-aux-Saints Neandertal. The Sylvian is slightly longer and placed lower in the left hemisphere than in the right.

The functional asymmetry of the living human brain (Sperry, 1974) is certainly unique in the human species, because it involves a uniquely human language system and its localization (Levy, 1974). Some authors (e.g., Levy, 1977) view this as an amplification of processing capacity, because most species appear to be functionally symmetric in the organization of their brains. There are some suggestions, as noted earlier, of functional asymmetries in nonhuman primates (Peterson, Beecher, Zoloth, Moody, & Stebbins, 1978), though it hardly seems likely that the asymmetry is as unusual as in humans. In effect, asymmetric organization of the brain may be equivalent to encephalization without increment in brain size. The total processing capacity may be the same in symmetrically and asymmetrically organized brains, but the latter might be able to process a greater variety of information, because there may be less duplication of the processed information.

ENCEPHALIZATION AND PROCESSING CAPACITY

The punctuations in Figure 12.11 are marks in the history of vertebrates that can be used as focuses for conjectures about the place of intelligence in the history of life. The punctuations were the times when there were major changes in the organization of the brain and increments in processing capacity. The most completely developed conjectures (Jerison, 1973) involve the evolution of mammals from a reptilian grade between 150 and 200 million years ago and the evolution of the hominids from a pongid grade. The analysis of the evolution of cognition and consciousness described in Section 12.3 is derived from these attempts to reconstruct the selection pressures and adaptations during those critical evolutionary periods.

The central issue is, why evolve more brain? Brain tissue is among the most metabolically costly in the body, and it is most efficient to solve behavioral problems with a minimum of neural tissue, to evolve adaptations and neural control systems that will keep the size of the control system small. Encephalization occurred often enough to make it clear that it was not accidental but a genuine adaptive response. There may be clues to the reasons for this heavy bioenergetic investment in the events of the first major encephalization of land vertebrates, the reptile–mammal transition. We can reconstruct these events as an exercise in imaginative evolutionary neurobiology and natural history.

The story begins about 220 million years ago, near the end of the Permian period, with the mammallike reptiles the dominant land vertebrates. These must have been "normal" reptiles, moderately large diurnal species relying on retinotectal vision for primary information about events at a distance, and they must have been at the top of the food chain as well as at other points in the chain – with herbivorous and carnivorous species (Olson, 1972). The next 50 million years were a period of a kind of competition between mammallike reptiles and ruling reptiles (dinosaurs, etc.).

As the story is reconstructed (cf. Crompton, Taylor, & Jagger, 1978) the ruling reptiles won the competition for the major reptilian niches, and the only route to survival for species of mammallike reptiles was to find and invade niches not typical for reptiles. They found those niches, nocturnal niches for life at twilight and at night. But to do well as nocturnal animals, the mammallike reptiles also evolved some specialized adaptations. They became small; they evolved internally regulated temperature to reduce reliance on sunlight, and they evolved sensory and behavioral systems that enabled them to be adequate "reptiles" without visual information about events at a distance. The new sensory information was scotopic visual, auditory, and olfactory, with tactile information from vibrissae. The mammallike reptile species that took this route became a true mammalian species. The other mammallike reptiles became extinct, about 150 million years ago.

If this narrative is correct, there must have been major reorganization of the brain in the transition from reptile to mammal. This follows from the way information processing in the several sensory systems is partitioned between processing near the sense organ and more central processing. In the visual system, an enormous amount of processing takes place in the neural retina, which contains millions of neurons. In reptiles, the region of the inner ear, or organ of corti, has only a few hundred neurons, and the auditory system is a small part of the brain. "Reptiles" that evolved into mammals with expanded auditory systems would have been able to do only some of the expansion at the sense organ. (The inner ear of typical mammals has about 35,000 neurons in the spiral ganglion.) Much of the processing analogous to that in the neural retina would have had to take place within the brain proper of mammals. Thinking in terms of synaptic chains, the retina contains neurons of at least Order I–III, with many internuncials involved in feedback loops and analysis. The peripheral auditory (and olfactory as a second potential distance-sense) system is entirely an afferent system, limited essentially to neurons of Order I. For higher-order analysis, the auditory system is represented in the brain proper, whereas the visual system does a significant amount of higher-order analysis in the retina.

The shift from vision to nonvisual distance senses is thus a sufficient explanation for the enlargement of the brain. Encephalization in the earliest mammals was probably an adaptation in response to a packing problem: where to put the neurons from nonvisual systems that had evolved to do the kind of processing that is done by retinal neurons in "normal" reptiles.

Although this analysis tells us why encephalization probably occurred, and how it successfully handled an adaptive dilemma, it does not provide any insight of any fundamental changes in the work of the brain. There are insights, if we consider how the additional processing would work.

The new processing would enter into the hierarchical work of the brain, which at certain levels amounts to the creation of reality, the world of awareness and experience. Certain "chunks" of neural information are the "pieces" of reality, and it has been one of our insights that hierarchical organization is the simple way for complex systems to be put together. Imagining an early mammal as little more than a modified reptile specialized to live at night, because it can use audition and olfaction and (probably a newly evolved) night vision based on a rod system in the retina, we recognize that there would have to be chunks in these animals' neural hierarchies to integrate information from other chunks. If they have chunks labeled "echoes" and others labeled "odor" and still others labeled "dimly seen things," it might be appropriate to have a superchunk labeled "object" that would integrate the information from the other chunks as having come from the same thing. There would be a need for still more superchunks called "space" and "time" to complete the map of events at a distance. All of these become part of the work of the brain when information accumulates from different sources about the same thing. The reality created by the brain must be more elaborate in order to be consistent with the varieties of information that must be integrated.

When I first wrote in this vein (Jerison, 1973), I suggested that the creation of models of possible realities, such as the real world of human experience, may have been limited to birds and mammals as large-brained vertebrates. Without any real new evidence, but with a better sense of the enormous size and complexity of the nonmammalian brain (Northcutt, 1981), I would no longer restrict this kind of model building, essentially the beginnings of consciousness, to "higher vertebrates." I would join Griffin (1976) and Humphrey (1978) in seeing this as a common adaptation of vertebrates. There may be no vertebrate brains that are small enough to be able to work in "machine language," and all may require an amount of chunking that reifies the information of the brain into a real world of experience.

Encephalization implies this kind of organization of the brain. The idea of consciousness as an aspect of an integration that results in the creation of a reality has important implications for the human situation, where encephalization has involved a novel neural system, the speech and language system. The point is in the question presented at the beginning of these paragraphs: Why so much nerve tissue? The answer appears to be that this is how to do the work of sensory analysis and integration of the mammalian (or vertebrate) kind.

Encephalization is not associated with other kinds of neural control. It is not associated with endothermy – the maintenance of body temperature by internal controls. In fact, the ectothermy of living reptiles probably encumbers more neural tissue than does endothermy, because ectothermy uses complex neural machinery of skeletal musculature for behavioral controls: physical movements into and out of sunlight or close to or away from the ground. Endothermy is essentially a reflex autonomic control of peripheral blood flow, shivering, sweating, and salivating.

The question Why so much neural tissue? remains even for the analysis of animal communication. Elaborate patterns of communication are known in wolves, for example, yet these are not unusually encephalized species. They are "average mammals" in Figure 12.11. The same thing is true in birds, as mentioned earlier. Human communication has involved enormous encephalization, but that should be understood as a biological oddity resulting from communication with a system that is essentially a cognitive one, and it is effected with certain disadvantages, in comparison to other mammalian systems. Animal communication should be reliable and unambiguous. It is dangerous to control it with learned, malleable behaviors. Communication should work best as part of the innately established ethogram of a species, and that is how it works in most species (Moynihan, 1970). Where learning is involved in establishing local dialects in birds or mammals, the learning is completed expeditiously, and the adult (or other communicator) rarely sends ambiguous messages. It is hard to imagine human verbal language, with its notorious ambiguities, evolving as a natural communication system. The ambiguities are often resolved by "body language," which is the human communication system that is the likely homologue for the "languages" of other species (cf. Myers, 1976).

ENCEPHALIZATION, LANGUAGE, AND HOMINID NICHES

The present consensus is that early hominids were social predators in a wolflike niche but limited by the neurobiological adaptations of higher primates (Washburn & Harding, 1970). As mentioned in the portion of Section 12.3 entitled "Self-consciousness and language," such a niche entails serious information-processing problems: Higher primates with much-reduced olfactory bulbs must use "novel" sensorimotor systems in place of the normal olfactory and scent-marking systems of proper carnivores. A useful analogy is to the early mammals and their discovery of "novel" systems to replace the normal vision of diurnal reptiles.

Human language evolved from the novel system that was ancestrally equivalent to the olfactory and scent-marking system that is used by wolves to map their range. That is the conjecture defended here. Our language is thus a peculiar sensory–cognitive system, deeply involved in the way we know (create) reality, which also serves as a major communication system. The peculiarity of that communication system, that we can share realities with others even to the extent of sharing an author's realities by living the lives and experiencing the worlds created in novels, is unique compared to "natural" communication. Instead of commanding, we tell stories. In an earlier example, the human "command" was in the form, "See the leopard," not "Climb the tree," a form that invites the listener to share an experience rather than ordering the listener to act.

Language, seen thus, explains self-consciousness as a peculiar kind of awareness. Human reality is a construction from conventional sensory information but also from language as a kind of supersensory system. In analysis of reality (a superchunk, as it were), its elements (chunks) are readily described and referred to things outside the skin. But linguistic elements do not have such referents. They were generated inside the skin and their referent was inside the skin. Names are different from the things that are named. This aspect of the self as an object is internal; it is an object that names names. We can build further, noting that it is possible to get inside the skin, dissect bodies and brains, and seek physical locations for this strange self. We can rediscover the mind–body problem, or the mind–brain problem . . . and this may be a good place to leave it (Rieber, 1980).

The special feature of human intelligence is surely the unique role of language. The neurobiology of language is only beginning to be analyzed. It is more than a left-hemisphere function, of course. From a biological perspective, furthermore, we anticipate that language will be a major source of variance in any effective human intelligence test. Because language and cognitive skills can only develop in a normal environment (just as auditory and visual functions require a normal environment for their normal development in infancy and childhood as sensory systems), it is something of a biological oddity to find psychologists seeking to test intelligence as independent of the environment (culture) within which it developed. Normal human intelligence as a trait of the species should be defined with respect to the environment in which it develops and the environment (e.g., the school) in which it is used.

VARIETIES OF INTELLIGENCES

Processing capacity can be used in many different ways, and in the various adaptations of encephalized species we see the necessary diversity of intelligence in animal life. Encephalization has evolved to similar grades in many different species, as indicated in Figures 12.3 and 12.11, and there may be common as well as unique features of these varieties of intelligence.

The previous discussion puts intelligence primarily within the domain of the creation of reality, of consciousness, and, broadly speaking, of cognition. But cognitive adaptations can be involved in many functional categories. The human cognitive system that we know as the language system is deeply involved in human communication, whereas in other species, cognition and communication are less closely intertwined.

When we think of human intelligence, we think of problem solving, of performance on tests, and of skill at intellectual games, or of Piagetian stages in reaching the adult condition. And we may be tempted to apply this human model to other species. That is a mistake, of course, but a reasonable mistake. At best, it is a point of departure, and at worst, it is a source of confusion in an analysis that begins with uncertainty and confusion about the trait in question. Intelligence is defined in human terms. It is only with some effort that we realize that the biological basis of human intelligence, in encephalization and the evolution of language, has probable analogues in the encephalization of other species. Species-typical behaviors that evolved in other highly encephalized species should be as dramatic as human language as adaptations. The challenge of comparative psychology is to discover those adaptations and tame them intellectually, that is, to learn to understand them by translating them into human terms.

There have been outstanding successes: the discovery of the "language" of bees and echolocation in bats by ethologists, the successful teaching of "language" to apes and dolphins, the discoveries of cognitive capacities in apes both in the laboratory and in the field, and the discoveries of "cultures" in Japanese macaques. All of these represent varieties of intelligences. Their evolutionary histories have been difficult to reconstruct. But it is possible to reconstruct the correlated encephalization, at least in vertebrates.

CONSERVATION AND PROPER MASS

There are two important principles that have not been mentioned in this chapter so far, which must be mentioned both for their importance and for their relevance to the varieties of intelligences correlated with encephalization. One of these is the principle of conservation, essentially that evolution is conservative: Old adaptations tend to be kept and new adaptations tend to be cheap, in energetic or informational terms. The question Why encephalization? is essentially a question about an evolutionary change that seems not to be conservative. Yet we have seen in Figure 12.11 that encephalization is indeed a stable phenomenon – long periods of equilibrium with only occasional periods of rapid change. The conservation principle asserts that adaptations are appropriate to niches. There is not much place in this framework for a generalized adaptive trait called intelligence that could fit any niche. We should expect intelligences in the plural, more or less tailored to various adaptive niches, not a single kind of animal intelligence.

The second principle is more strictly neurobiological. I have called it *proper mass,* because it needed a name as an important and well-known principle. When the functional areas of the brain are mapped, there are both interspecific and intraspecific variations and disproportionalities in the maps that reflect the importance of the functions in the life of the animal. Brain maps are distorted homunculi or animalculi, and the distortions reflect what is important (Welker, 1976a, 1976b). Bats as echolocators have a large fraction of their brains associated with acoustic processing: Much of their neocortex is auditory, and they have remarkably enlarged inferior colliculi – the midbrain auditory centers (Suga & Jen, 1976). Humans have large fractions of their brains associated directly with language in the "language areas" of the brain, and their sensory and motor systems show very large representations of eye, thumb, lips, and tongue, which are correlated with our elaborate hand–eye coordination and speech production, that are part of human language (Penfield & Roberts, 1959). Our specializations are reflected in our brains, at the species level.

In the analysis of encephalization, we have considered the brain as a whole, but the specialized functions of the brain are reflected in special enlargement of certain parts and occasional diminution of other parts. To an extent, brains and bodies of different species can be mapped onto one another (in the mathematical sense). This is probably the reason that the data on encephalization are as orderly as they are. This is the reason that the $P^{2/3}$ term, which is a measure that is proportional to body surface, can appear in the equations of encephalization and represent a common aspect of the projection areas, or maps, in the brain for different species. There is also a balancing of specializations. When species are equally encephalized but differently specialized, we anticipate that each will be emphasizing a different system. Welker and Campos (1963) illustrate this nicely in procyonids, with the raccoon specialized for tactile information from its forepaws and the coati mundi specialized for tactile information from its snout. Forepaw areas are much enlarged in the somatosensory cortex of the raccoon, and snout areas are enlarged in coati mundi. The proper masses of the several specializations balance one another (see also Welker, 1976a).

The great mystery of the whale brain is partly a problem of determining what all that tissue is doing. There is so much tissue that, even with reservations about its unusual organization (Bullock & Gurevich, 1979), we should be confident that there are unimagined cognitive capacities among whales that await discovery.

Human intelligence, which can reconstruct the intelligences of so many other species, is at one of the vertebrate maxima on this dimension. Its peculiar feature is human verbal intelligence. The asymmetric organization of the human brain is related to that behavioral adaptation and is part of our uniqueness. But human intelligence is, in principle, commensurate with intelligence in other species as measurable by encephalization, which is the measure of the processing capacity encumbered by this human adaptation.

12.5. CONCLUSION

A biological chapter on intelligence is inevitably an anomaly. The topic is defined in human terms, and the human species is too small a part of animal life to sustain the definition. But our concern is with the human trait of intelligence as it arose in the evolutionary process: Human intelligence in the context of hominid evolution and, further, in the context of primate, mammalian, and vertebrate evolution. The biology of intelligence has to be an analysis of the human trait in its broadest context. That was the goal of this chapter.

In this broad biological context, intelligence transcends its human manifestation. It is related to information-processing capacity, and it can appear in many different guises. In the human species it is very much related to language as we know it in everyday situations. Yet the same analyses that we perform, as humans, with language – logical operations, constructions of knowledge and of experience (as in the reading of a novel), constructions of the very reality that we know – may be performed in other ways by other species. This chapter has reviewed our present understanding of the differences among species on these dimensions, with special emphasis on mammals and primates and on the evolutionary history that led to the present diversity. There are also major problems in the concept of intelligence, and the approach to knowledge about it is a problem in the philosophy and sociology of science, and a problem in philosophy as well as in science. Many of these issues, which arise in the study of human intelligence, appear easier to resolve, or at least easier to state, when considered in relation to animal intelligence and its evolutionary history.

NOTE

I received many helpful criticisms and suggestions from L. M. Herman, I. L. Jerison, R. Lande, M. McGuire, and C. E. Taylor, as well as many other colleagues, about an earlier draft of this chapter. To the extent that these could be incorporated in the final draft, the present chapter is more accurate and easier to read. I appreciate the help of these people enormously and regret only that I could not make all the changes they suggested and thus must accept the onus for the inevitable errors in a review of this type.

REFERENCES

Aristotle. The parts of animals. 653a.28 (W. Ogle, Trans.). In *Great books of the Western world* (Vol. 9). Chicago: Encyclopedia Brittanica, 1952. (Originally published, ca. 335 B.C.)

Ashton, E. H., & Spence, T. F. Age changes in the cranial capacity and foramen magnum of hominoids. *Proceedings of the Zoological Society, London*, 1958, *130*, 169–181.

Bailey, R. E., & Bailey, M. B. 1980. A view from outside the Skinner box. *American Psychologist*, 1980, *35*, 942–946.

Baillarger, J. De l'étendue de la surface du cerveau et de ses rapports avec le developpement de l'intelligence. *Annales Medico-Psychologiques* (Series 2), 1853, *5*, 1–9.

Bateson, P. P. G., & Hinde, R. A. (Eds.). *Growing points in ethology*. Cambridge: Cambridge University Press, 1976.

Bauchot, R., & Stephan, H. Données nouvelles sur l'encéphalisation des Insectivores et des Prosimiens. *Mammalia*, 1966, *30*, 160–196.

Bauchot, R., & Stephan, H. Encéphalisation et niveau evolutif chez les Simiens. *Mammalia,* 1969, *33,* 225–275.

Bindra, D. *A theory of intelligent behavior.* New York: Wiley-Interscience, 1976.

Bitterman, M. E. The comparative analysis of learning. *Science,* 1975, *188,* 699–709.

Boule, M., & Anthony, R. L'encéphale de l'Homme fossile de la Chapelle-aux-Saints. *L'Anthropologie,* 1911, *22,* 129–196.

Brandt, A., Jr. Sur le rapport du poids du cerveau à celui du corps chez différents animaux. *Bulletin de la Société Impériale des Naturalistes de Moscou,* 1867, *40*(3–4), 525–543.

Bridgman, P. W. *Dimensional analysis* (Rev. ed.). New Haven: Yale University Press, 1931.

Bridgman, P. W. *The way things are.* New York: Viking Press, 1959.

Broca, P. P. Nouvelle observation d'aphemie produite par une lésion de la moitié postérieure des deuxième et troisième circonvolutions frontales gauches. *Bulletins de la Société Anatomique de Paris,* 1861, *36,* 398–407.

Brodmann, K. Neue Forschungsergebnisse der Grosshirnrindenanatomie mit besonderer Berücksichtung anthropologischer Fragen. *Verhandlungen des 85ste Versammlung Deutscher Naturforscher und Aerzte in Wien,* 1913, 200–240.

Brookshire, K. H. Vertebrate learning: evolutionary divergences. In R. B. Masterton, C. B. G. Campbell, M. E. Bitterman, & N. Hotton (Eds.), *Evolution of brain and behavior in vertebrates.* Hillsdale, N.J.: Erlbaum, 1976.

Buell, S. J., & Coleman, P. D. Dendritic growth in the aged human brain and failure of growth in senile dementia. *Science,* 1979, *206,* 854–856.

Bullock, T. H., & Gurevich, V. S. Soviet literature on the nervous system and psychobiology of cetacea. *International Review of Neurobiology,* 1979, *21,* 47–127.

Buss, A. R. *A dialectical psychology.* New York: Irvington/Halstead/Wiley, 1979.

Carroll, J. B. *Individual difference relations in psychometric and experimental cognitive tasks* (Report No. 163). Chapel Hill: University of North Carolina, L. L. Thurstone Psychometric Laboratory, 1980.

Carroll, J. B., & Maxwell, S. E. Individual differences in cognitive abilities. *Annual Review of Psychology,* 1979, *30,* 603–640.

Casseday, J. H., & Diamond, I. T. Symmetrical lateralization of function in the auditory system of the cat: Effects of unilateral ablation of the cortex. *Annals of the New York Academy of Sciences,* 1977, *299,* 255–263.

Chomsky, N. *Language and mind* (Enlarged ed.). New York: Harcourt Brace Jovanovich, 1972.

Connolly, C. J. *External morphology of the primate brain.* Springfield, Ill.: Thomas, 1950.

Craik, K. J. W. *The nature of explanation.* (Reprinted, 1967, with postscript.) Cambridge: Cambridge University Press, 1943.

Crile, G., & Quiring, D. P. A record of the body weight and certain organ and gland weights of 3690 animals. *Ohio Journal of Science,* 1940, *40,* 219–259.

Crompton, A. W., Taylor, C. R., & Jagger, J. A. Evolution of homeothermy in mammals. *Nature,* 1978, *272,* 333–336.

Cronbach, L. J. Review of *Cyril Burt, psychologist,* by L. S. Hearnshaw. *Science,* 1979, *206,* 1392–1394.

Dareste, G. M. C. Sur les rapports de la masse encéphalique avec le développement de l'intelligence. *Bulletins de la Société d'Anthropologie de Paris,* 1862, *3,* 26–55.

Darwin, C. *The origin of species* (6th ed.). London: Murray, 1872. (Originally published, 1859. Reprinted, New York: Modern Library, 1936.)

Darwin, C. *The descent of man and selection in relation to sex.* London: Murray, 1871. (Reprinted, New York: Modern Library, 1936.)

Dawkins, R. *The selfish gene.* London: Oxford University Press, 1976.

DeFries, J. C. Quantitative aspects of genetics and environment in the determination of behavior. In L. Ehrman, G. S. Omenn, & E. Caspari (Eds.), *Genetics, environment, and behavior.* New York: Academic Press, 1973.

DeFries, J. C., Vandenberg, S. G., & McClearn, G. E. Genetics of specific cognitive abilities. *Annual Review of Genetics,* 1976, 179–207.

Diamond, I. T. The subdivisions of neocortex: A proposal to revise the traditional view of sensory, motor, and association areas. *Progress in Psychobiology and Physiological Psychology,* 1979, *8,* 1–43.

Dimond, S. J. Symmetry and asymmetry in the vertebrate brain. In D. A. Oakley & H. C. Plotkin (Eds.), *Brain, behaviour and evolution*. London: Methuen, 1979.

Dimond, S. J., & Blizard, D. A. (Eds.). Evolution and lateralization of the brain. *Annals of the New York Academy of Sciences*, 1977, *299*, 1–501.

Dingwall, W. O. The evolution of human communication systems. In H. Whitaker & H. Whitaker (Eds.), *Studies in linguistics* (Vol. 4). New York: Academic Press, 1979.

Dobzhansky, T. *Genetics of the evolutionary process*. New York: Columbia University Press, 1970.

Dubois, E. Sur le rapport du poids de l'encéphale avec la grandeur du corps chez les mammifères. *Bulletins de la Société d'Anthropologie de Paris*, 1897, *8*(4), 337–376.

Dubois, E. The brain-cast of pithecanthropus erectus. *Proceedings of the Fourth International Congress of Zoology, Cambridge*, 1898, pp. 79–96.

Dubois, E. Die phylogenetische Groshirnzunahme autonome Vervollkommung der animalen Funktionen. *Biologia Generalis*, 1930, *6*, 247–292.

Eccles, J. C. *The human mystery (Gifford Lectures, 1977–1978)*. New York: Springer-Verlag, 1979.

Edinger, T. Anthropocentric misconceptions in paleoneurology. *Proceedings of the Rudolf Virchow Medical Society of the City of New York*, 1962, *19*, 56–107.

Edinger, T. Paleoneurology, 1804–1966: An annotated bibliography. *Advances in Embryology and Cell Biology*, 1975, *49*(1–6), 1–258.

Eisenberg, J. F., & Kleiman, D. Olfactory communication in mammals. *Annual Review of Ecology and Systematics*, 1972, *3*, 1–31.

Eldredge, N., & Cracraft, J. *Phylogenetic patterns and the evolutionary process*. New York: Columbia University Press, 1980.

Elias, H., & D. Schwartz, Cerebro-cortical surface areas, volumes, lengths of gyri and their interdependence in mammals, including man. *Zeitschrift fur Säugetierkunde*, 1971, *36*, 147–163.

Elliott, M. H. The effect of change of reward on the maze performance of rats. *University of California Publications in Psychology*, 1928, *4*, 19–30.

Engels, F. *Dialectics of nature*. London: Lawrence & Wishart, 1940.

Falconer, D. S. *Introduction to quantitative genetics*. New York: Ronald Press, 1960.

Farb, P. *Word play: What happens when people talk*. New York: Knopf, 1975.

Ferrier, D. *The functions of the brain*. London: Smith, Elder, 1876.

Fisher, R. A. *The genetical theory of natural selection*. Oxford: Clarendon Press, 1930. (Reprinted, with corrections, New York: Dover, 1958.)

Gallup, G. G., Jr. Self-recognition in primates: A comparative approach to the bidirectional properties of consciousness. *American Psychologist*, 1977, *32*, 329–338.

Gallup, G. G., Jr. Self-awareness in primates. *American Scientist*, 1979, *67*, 417–421.

Galton, F. Regression towards mediocrity in hereditary stature. *Journal of the Anthropological Institute*, 1885, *15*, 246–262.

Garcia, J. The futility of comparative IQ research. In N. A. Buchwald & M. A. B. Brazier (Eds.), *Brain mechanisms in mental retardation*. New York: Academic Press, 1975.

Garcia, J., Hankins, W. G., & Rusiniak, K. W. Behavioral regulation of the milieu interne in man and rat. *Science*, 1974, *185*, 824–831.

Gardner, B. T., & Gardner, R. A. Two-way communication with an infant chimpanzee. In A. M. Schrier and F. Stollnitz (Eds.), *Behavior of nonhuman primates* (Vol. 1). New York: Academic Press, 1971.

Geschwind, N., & Levitsky, W. Human brain: Left–right asymmetries in temporal speech region. *Science*, 1968, *161*, 186–187.

Gihr, M., & Pilleri, G. Hirn-Körpergewichts-Beziehungen bei Cetaceen. *Investigations on Cetacea*, 1969, *1*, 109–126.

Gingerich, P. D. Cranial anatomy and evolution of early Tertiary Plesiadapidae (Mammalia, Primates). *University of Michigan Papers on Paleontology*, 1976, *15*, 1–140.

Gould, S. J. Grades and clades revisited. In R. B. Masterton, W. Hodos, H. J. Jerison (Eds.), *Evolution, brain, and behavior: Persistent problems*. Hillsdale, N.J.: Erlbaum, 1976.

Gould, S. J. Morton's ranking of races by cranial capacity. *Science*, 1978, *200*, 503–509.

Gould, S. J. Is a new and general theory of evolution emerging? *Paleobiology*, 1980, *6*, 119–130.

Greenough, W. T., & Juraska, J. M. Experience-induced changes in brain fine structure. In M. E. Hahn, C. Jensen & B. C. Dudek (Eds.), *Development and evolution of brain size: Behavioral implications*. New York: Academic Press, 1979.

Griffin, D. R. *The question of animal awareness.* New York: Rockefeller University Press, 1976.

Hahn, M. E., Jensen, C., & Dudek, B. C. (Eds.). *Development and evolution of brain size: Behavioral implications.* New York: Academic Press, 1979.

Hall, K. R. L. Tool-using performances as indicators of behavioral adaptability. *Current Anthropology,* 1963, 4, 479–494.

Halstead, W. C. *Brain and intelligence.* Chicago: University of Chicago Press, 1947.

Hamilton, C. R. Investigation of perceptual and mnemonic lateralization in monkeys. In S. Harnad, R. W. Doty, L. Goldstein, J. Jaynes, & G. Krauthamer (Eds.), *Lateralization in the nervous system.* New York: Academic Press, 1977.

Harlow, H. F. The formation of learning sets. *Psychological Review,* 1949, 56, 51–65.

Harnad, S. R., Steklis, H. D., & Lancaster, J. (Eds.). Origins and evolution of language and speech. *Annals of the New York Academy of Sciences,* 1976, 280, 1–914.

Hearnshaw, L. S. *Cyril Burt, psychologist.* Ithaca, N.Y.: Cornell University Press, 1979.

Hebb, D. O. *The organization of behavior.* New York: Wiley, 1949.

Herman, L. M. Cognitive characteristics of dolphins. In L. M. Herman (Ed.), *Cetacean behavior: Mechanisms and functions.* New York: Wiley, 1980.

Herman, L. M., & Tavolga, W. N. The communication systems of cetaceans. In L. M. Herman (Ed.), *Cetacean behavior: Mechanisms and functions.* New York: Wiley, 1980.

Hewes, G. W. The current status of the gestural theory of language origin. *Annals of the New York Academy of Sciences,* 1976, 280, 482–504.

Hill, J. H. Apes and language. *Annual Review of Anthropology,* 1978, 7, 89–112.

Hinde, R. A. *Animal behavior* (2nd ed.). New York: McGraw-Hill, 1969.

Hinde, R. A., & Stevenson-Hinde, J. (Eds.). *Constraints on learning.* New York: Academic Press, 1973.

Hockett, C. F. The origin of speech. *Scientific American,* 1960, 203(3), 89–96.

Hodos, W., & Campbell, C. B. G. *Scala naturae:* Why there is no theory in comparative psychology. *Psychological Review,* 1969, 76, 337–350.

Holloway, R. L., Jr. Casts of fossil hominid brains. *Scientific American,* 1974, 231(1), 106–115.

Hopson, J. A. Relative brain size and behavior in archosaurian reptiles. *Annual Review of Ecology and Systematics,* 1977, 8, 429–448.

Hopson, J. A. Paleoneurology. In A. C. Gans, R. G. Northcutt, & P. Ulinski (Eds.), *Biology of the reptilia* (Vol. 9). London: Academic Press, 1979.

Hopson, J. A. Relative brain size in dinosaurs: Implications for dinosaurian endothermy. In D. K. Thomas & E. C. Olson (Eds.), *A cold look at warm blooded dinosaurs.* Washington, D.C.: American Association for the Advancement of Science, 1980.

Humphrey, N. K. Vision in a monkey without striate cortex: A case study. *Perception,* 1974, 3, 241–255.

Humphrey, N. K. The social function of intellect. In P. P. G. Bateson & R. A. Hinde (Eds.), *Growing points in ethology.* Cambridge: Cambridge University Press, 1976.

Humphrey, N. K. Nature's psychologists. *New Scientist,* 1978, 78, 900–903.

Hunt, E. Mechanics of verbal ability. *Psychological Review,* 1978, 85, 109–130.

Hunt, E., Lunneborg, C. E., & Lewis, J. What does it mean to be high verbal? *Cognitive Psychology,* 1975, 7, 194–227.

Hunter, W. S. The delayed reaction in animals and children. *Behavior Monographs,* 1913, 2, 1–86.

Huxley, J. S. *Problems of relative growth.* London: Allen & Unwin, 1932.

Huxley, J. S. Evolutionary processes and taxonomy with special reference to grades. *Uppsala Universitets Arsskrift,* 1958, pp. 21–39.

Huxley, T. H. *Man's place in nature (with other anthropological essays).* New York: D. Appleton, 1899. (Originally published, 1863.)

Isaac, G. L. Stages of cultural elaboration in the Pleistocene: Possible archaeological indicators of the development of language capabilities. *Annals of the New York Academy of Sciences,* 1976, 280, 275–288.

Itani, J., & Nishimura, A. The study of infrahuman culture in Japan. In W. Montagna (Ed.), *Symposia of the Fourth International Congress of Primatology* (Vol. 1). Basel: Karger, 1973.

James, W. *Principles of psychology* (2 vols.). New York: Holt, 1890.

Jaynes, J. *The origin of consciousness in the breakdown of the bicameral mind.* Boston: Houghton Mifflin, 1977.

Jensen, A. R. g: Outmoded theory or unconquered frontier. *Creative Science and Technology,* 1979, 2, 16–29.

Jensen-Jazbutis, G. T. Clinical-anatomical study of microcephalia vera: A microcephalic brother and sister with atrophy of the left mamillary body. *Journal für Hirnforschung,* 1970, *12,* 287–305.

Jerison, H. J. *Evolution of the brain and intelligence.* New York: Academic Press, 1973.

Jerison, H. J. Fossil evidence of the evolution of the human brain. *Annual Review of Anthropology,* 1975, *4,* 27–58.

Jerison, H. J. Paleoneurology and the evolution of mind. *Scientific American,* 1976, 234(1), 90–101. (a)

Jerison, H. J. Discussion paper: The paleoneurology of language. *Annals of the New York Academy of Sciences,* 1976, 280, 370–382. (b)

Jerison, H. J. The theory of encephalization. *Annals of the New York Academy of Sciences,* 1977, 299, 146–160. (a)

Jerison, H. J. Should phrenology be rediscovered? *Current Anthropology,* 1977, *18,* 744–746. (b)

Jerison, H. J. Brain, body, and encephalization in early primates. *Journal of Human Evolution,* 1979, 8, 615–635. (a)

Jerison, H. J. The evolution of diversity in brain size. In M. E. Hahn, C. Jensen, & B. C. Dudek (Eds.), *Development and evolution of brain size: Behavioral implications.* New York: Academic Press, 1979. (b)

Jerison, H. J. Allometry, brain size, cortical surface, and convolutedness. In E. Armstrong & D. Falk (Eds.), *Primate brain evolution: Methods and concepts.* New York, Plenum, 1982. (a)

Jerison, H. J. Problems with Piaget and pallia. *Behavioral and Brain Sciences,* 1982, 5, 284–287. (b)

Johnson, C. *Introduction to natural selection.* Baltimore: University Park Press, 1976.

Kawai, M. Newly acquired precultural behavior of the natural troop of Japanese monkeys on Koshima Islet. *Primates,* 1965, 6, 1–30.

Kennedy, G. E. *Paleoanthropology.* New York: McGraw-Hill, 1980.

King, M-C., & Wilson, A. C. Evolution at two levels in humans and chimpanzees. *Science,* 1975, *188,* 107–116.

Klüver, H. *Behavior mechanisms in monkeys.* Chicago: University of Chicago Press, 1933.

Kochetkova, V. I. *Paleoneurology* (H. J. Jerison & I. L. Jerison, Eds. and trans.). Washington, D.C.: Winston, 1978. (Originally published, Moscow: Moscow University Press, 1973.)

Konorski, J. *Integrative activity of the brain.* Chicago: University of Chicago Press, 1967.

Kosslyn, S. M. *Image and mind.* Cambridge, Mass.: Harvard University Press, 1980.

Kuhn, T. S. *The structure of scientific revolutions* (2nd ed.). Chicago: University of Chicago Press, 1970.

Lande, R. Natural selection and random genetic drift in phenotypic evolution. *Evolution,* 1976, 30, 314–334.

Lande, R. Quantitative genetic analysis of multivariate evolution, applied to brain:body size allometry. *Evolution,* 1979, 33, 402–416.

Lande, R. Microevolution in relation to macroevolution. (Review of *Macroevolution: Pattern and process* by S. S. Stanley.) *Paleobiology,* 1980, 6, 233–238. (a)

Lande, R. Genetic variation and phenotypic evolution during allopatric speciation. *American Naturalist,* 1980, *116,* 463–479. (b)

Lapique, L. Sur la relation du poids de l'encéphale au poids du corps. *Comptes Rendus des Séances de la Société de Biologie et de Ses Filiales,* 1898, 50, 62–63.

Lapique, L. Tableau générale des poids somatique et encéphalique dans les espèces animales. *Bulletins de la Société d'Anthropologie de Paris,* 1907, 8(5), 248–262.

Lartet, E. De quelques cas de progression organique verifiables dans la succession des temps géologiques sur des mammifères de même famille et de même genre. *Comptes Rendus de l'Academie des Sciences,* 1868, 66, 1119–1122.

Lashley, K. S. Persistent problems in the evolution of mind. *Quarterly Review of Biology,* 1949, 24, 28–42.

LeMay, M. The language capabilities of Neanderthal man. *American Journal of Physical Anthropology,* 1975, 42, 9–14.

LeMay, M., & Geschwind, N. Hemispheric differences in the brains of great apes. *Brain, Behavior and Evolution,* 1975, *11,* 48–52.

Lenneberg, E. H. *Biological foundations of language*. New York: Wiley, 1967.

Leuret, F., & Gratiolet, P. *Anatomie comparée du système nerveux considéré dans ses rapports avec l'intelligence* (2 vols.) Paris: J.-B. Bailliere, 1857.

Levy, J. Psychobiological implications of bilateral asymmetry. In S. Dimond & J. G. Beaumont (Eds.), *Hemisphere function in the human brain*. London: Paul Elek, 1974.

Levy, J. The mammalian brain and the adaptive advantage of cerebral asymmetry. *Annals of the New York Academy of Sciences*, 1977, *299*, 264–272.

Lewontin, R. C. *The genetic basis of evolutionary change*. New York: Columbia University Press, 1974.

Lewontin, R. C. Adaptation. *Scientific American*, 1978, *239*(3), 212–230.

Liberman, A. M. The specialization of the language hemisphere. In F. O. Schmitt & F. G. Worden (Eds.), *The neurosciences: Third study program*. Cambridge, Mass.: MIT Press, 1974.

Lilly, J. C. *Lilly on dolphins*. Garden City, N.Y.: Doubleday, Anchor Press, 1975.

Lilly, J. C. *Communication between man and dolphin*. New York: Crown, 1978.

Lorenz, K. *Evolution and modification of behavior*. Chicago: University of Chicago Press, 1965.

Lubbock, J. (Lord Avebury). *On the senses, instincts, and intelligence of animals with special reference to insects*. London: Kegan Paul, Trench, 1888.

Mackintosh, N. J. *The psychology of animal learning*. New York: Academic Press, 1974.

Malcolm, N. *Ludwig Wittgenstein: A memoir*. London: Oxford University Press, 1958.

Malcolm, N. *Problems of mind: Descartes to Wittgenstein*. New York: Harper & Row, 1971.

Manouvrier, L. Sur l'interprétation de la quantité dans l'encéphale et dans le cerveau en particulier. *Bulletins de la Société d'Anthropologie de Paris*, 1883, *3*, 137–323.

Marsh, O. C. Small size of the brain in Tertiary mammals. *American Journal of Science and the Arts*, 1874, *8*, 66–67.

Marsh, O. C. Dinocerata. *U.S. Geological Survey, Monograph*, 1886, *10* (Whole No.). 1–243.

Marshack, A. Some implications of the paleolithic symbolic evidence for the origin of language. *Annals of the New York Academy of Sciences*, 1976, *280*, 289–311.

Mason, W. A. Environmental models and mental modes: Representational processes in the great apes and man. *American Psychologist*, 1976, *31*, 284–294.

Masterton, R. B., & Berkley, M. A. Brain function: Changing ideas on the role of sensory, motor, and association cortex in behavior. *Annual Review of Psychology*, 1974, *25*, 277–312.

Masterton, R. B., & Skeen, L. C. Origins of anthropoid intelligence: Prefrontal system and delayed alternation in hedgehog, tree shrew, and bush baby. *Journal of Comparative Physiological Psychology*, 1972, *81*, 423–433.

Maynard Smith, J. *The evolution of sex*. Cambridge: Cambridge University Press, 1978. (a)

Maynard Smith, J. The evolution of behavior. *Scientific American*, 1978, *239*(3), 176–192. (b)

McClearn, G. E., & DeFries, J. C. *Introduction to behavior genetics*. San Francisco: W. H. Freeman, 1973.

McHenry, H. M. Fossils and the mosaic nature of human evolution. *Science*, 1975, *190*, 425–432.

Merzenich, M. M., & Kaas, J. H. Principles of organization of sensory-perceptual systems in mammals. *Progress in Psychobiology and Physiological Psychology*, 1980, *9*, 1–42.

Morgan, C.`L. *Animal life and intelligence* (2nd ed.). London: William Clowes, 1891. (Originally published, 1890.)

Morgan, C. L. *Introduction to comparative psychology*. London: Walter Scott, 1894.

Morgan, C. L. *Habit and instinct*. London: Arnold, 1896.

Mountcastle, V. B. An organizing principle for cerebral function: The unit module and the distributed system. In G. M. Edelman & V. B. Mountcastle (Eds.), *The mindful brain*. Cambridge, Mass.: MIT Press, 1978.

Moynihan, M. H. Control, suppression, decay, disappearance and replacement of displays. *Journal of Theoretical Biology*, 1970, *29*, 85–112.

Myers, R. E. Function of corpus callosum in interocular transfer. *Brain*, 1956, *79*, 358–363.

Myers, R. E. Comparative neurology of vocalization and speech: Proof of a dichotomy. *Annals of the New York Academy of Sciences*, 1976, *280*, 745–760.

Nissen, H. W. Phylogenetic comparison. In S. S. Stevens (Ed.), *Handbook of experimental psychology*. New York: Wiley, 1951.

Northcutt, G. L. Forebrain and midbrain organization in lizards and its phylogenetic significance. In N. Greenberg & P. D. MacLean (Eds.), *Behavior and neurology of lizards* (DHEW Publication No. [ADM]77-491). Washington, D.C.: National Institute of Mental Health, 1978.

Northcutt, R. G. Evolution of the telencephalon in nonmammals. *Annual Review of Neuroscience*, 1981, *4*, 301–350.

Nottebohm, F. A zoologist's view of some language phenomena with particular emphasis on vocal learning. In E. H. Lenneberg & E. Lenneberg (Eds.), *Foundations of language development: A multidisciplinary approach.* New York: Academic Press, 1975.

Olson, E. C. The habitat: Climatic change and its influence on life and habitat. In R. N. Fiennes (Ed.), *Biology of nutrition.* Oxford & New York: Pergamon, 1972.

Olton, D. S. Mazes, maps, and memory. *American Psychologist*, 1979, *34*, 583–596.

O'Sullivan, C., Fouts, R. S., Hannum, M. E., & Schneider, K. Chimpanzee conversations: Language cognition and theory. In S. A. Kuczaj II (Ed.), *Problems, theories and controversies in language development: Language, cognition and culture.* Hillsdale, N.J.: Erlbaum, in press.

Parker, S. T., & Gibson, K. R. A developmental model for the evolution of language and intelligence in early hominids. *Behavioral and Brain Sciences*, 1979, *2*, 367–408.

Passingham, R. E. Primate specialization in brain and intelligence. *Symposia of the Zoological Society, London*, 1981, *46*, 361–388.

Pavlov, I. P. Experimental psychology and psycho-pathology in animals. In I. P. Pavlov (Ed.), *Lectures on conditioned reflexes* New York: Liveright, 1928. (Originally published, 1903.)

Pearson, K. S. Mathematical contributions to the theory of evolution: III. Regression, heredity and panmixia. *Philosophical Transactions of the Royal Society of London*, 1896, *187A*, 187–318.

Pearson, K. S. *The grammar of science* (2nd ed., rev. and enlarged). London: Adam & Charles Black, 1900.

Penfield, W., & Roberts, L. *Speech and brain-mechanisms.* Princeton: Princeton University Press, 1959.

Peters, R. P., & Mech, L. D. Scent-marking in wolves. *American Scientist*, 1975, *63*, 628–637.

Peterson, M. R., Beecher, M. D., Zoloth, S. R., Moody, D. B., & Stebbins, W. C. Neural lateralization of species-specific vocalizations by Japanese macaques (*Macaca fuscata*). *Science*, 1978, *202*, 324–326.

Pilbeam, D., & Gould, S. J. Size and scaling in human evolution. *Science*, 1974, *186*, 892–901.

Platel, R. Poids encéphalique et indice d'encéphalisation chez les reptiles sauriens. *Zoologischer Anzeiger*, 1974, *192*, 332–382.

Popper, K. R., & Eccles, J. C. *The self and its brain.* New York: Springer-Verlag, 1977.

Posner, M. I. *Chronometric explorations of mind.* Hillsdale, N.J.: Erlbaum, 1978.

Premack, D. *Intelligence in ape and man.* Hillsdale, N.J.: Erlbaum, 1976.

Premack, D. Does the chimpanzee have a theory of mind? *Behavior and Brain Sciences*, 1978, *4*, 515–526.

Premack, D., Woodruff, G., & Kennel, K. Paper-marking test for chimpanzee: Simple control for social cues. *Science*, 1978, *202*, 903–905.

Quiroga, J. C. The brain of the mammal-like reptile *Probainognathus jenseni* (Therapsida, Cynodontia): A correlative paleo-neurological approach to the neocortex at the reptile-mammal transition. *Journal für Hirnforschung*, 1980, *21*, 299–336.

Radinsky, L. B. The fossil evidence of anthropoid brain evolution. *American Journal of Physical Anthropology*, 1974, *41*, 15–28.

Radinsky, L. Evolution of brain size in carnivores and ungulates. *American Naturalist*, 1978, *112*, 815–831.

Rensch, B. *Evolution above the species level.* London: Methuen, 1959.

Richards, D. G., Wolz, J. P., & Herman, L. M. *Generalized vocal mimicry of computer-generated sounds by the bottlenosed dolphin.* Unpublished manuscript, 1981.

Riddel, W. I. Cerebral indices and behavioral differences. In M. E. Hahn, C. Jensen, & B. C. Dudek (Eds.), *Development and evolution of brain size: Behavioral implications.* New York: Academic Press, 1979.

Rieber, R. W. (Ed.). *Body and mind: Past, present, and future.* New York: Academic Press, 1980.

Robinow, M. *The relationship of head circumference to height and weight in healthy and malnourished infants.* Paper presented to the child development section of the meeting of the American Academy of Pediatrics, Chicago, 1968.

Rockel, A. J., Hiorns, R. W., & Powell, T. P. S. The basic uniformity in structure of the neocortex. *Brain*, 1980, *103*, 221–224.

Roderick, T. H., Wimer, R. E., & Wimer, C. C. Genetic manipulation of neuroanatomical traits. In L. Petrinovich & J. L. McGaugh (Eds.), *Knowing, thinking and believing*. New York: Plenum, 1976.

Romanes, G. J. *Mental evolution in animals*. London: Kegan Paul, 1883.

Romero-Herrera, A. E., Lehmann, H., Joysey, K. A., & Friday, A. E. On the evolution of myoglobin. *Philosophical Transactions of the Royal Society of London*, 1978, *283B*, 61–163.

Rose, R. J., Harris, E. L., Christian, J. C., & Nance, W. E. Genetic variance in nonverbal intelligence: Data from the kinships of identical twins. *Science*, 1979, *205*, 1153–1155.

Rosenzweig, M. R. Responsiveness of brain size to individual experience: Behavioral and evolutionary implications. In M. E. Hahn, C. Jensen, & B. C. Dudek (Eds.), *Development and evolution of brain size: Behavioral implications*. New York: Academic Press, 1979.

Rozin, P. The evolution of intelligence and access to the cognitive unconscious. *Progress in Psychobiology and Physiological Psychology*, 1976, *6*, 245–280.

Russell, B. *The problems of philosophy*. London: Oxford University Press, 1912. (Reprinted, 1959.)

Russell, B. *Freedom and organization*. London: Allen & Unwin, 1934.

Russell, B. *A history of Western philosophy*. New York: Simon & Schuster, 1945.

Russell, B. Mind and matter. In B. Russell, *Portraits from memory and other essays*. New York: Simon & Schuster, 1956.

Ryle, G. *The concept of mind*. London: Hutchinson, 1949.

Sapir, E. *Selected writings of Edward Sapir in language, culture and personality* (D. G. Mandelbaum, Ed.). Berkeley and Los Angeles: University of California Press, 1949.

Savage-Rumbaugh, E. S., Rumbaugh, D. M., & Boysen, S. Do apes use language? *American Scientist*, 1980, *68*, 49–61.

Schaaffhausen, H. Sur le crâne de Néanderthal. *Bulletins de la Société d'Anthropologie de Paris*, 1863, *4*, 314–317.

Schiller, P. *Paul Broca*. Berkeley and Los Angeles: University of California Press, 1979.

Schneirla, T. C. The study of animal behavior: Its history and relation to the museum. *Curator*, 1958, *1*, 17–35. (Also in *Selected writings of T. C. Schneirla* [L. R. Aronson et al., Eds.]. San Francisco: W. H. Freeman, 1958.)

Sebeok, T. A. (Ed.). *How animals communicate*. Bloomington: Indiana University Press, 1977.

Seidenberg, M. S., & Petitto, L. A. Signing behavior in apes: A critical review. *Cognition*, 1979, *7*, 177–215.

Seligman, M. E. P. On the generality of the laws of learning. *Psychological Review*, 1970, *77*, 406–418.

Seligman, M. E. P., & Hager, L. (Eds.). *Biological boundaries on learning*. New York: Appleton-Century-Crofts, 1972.

Seyfarth, R. M., Cheney, D. L., & Marler, P. Monkey responses to three different alarm calls: Evidence of predator classification and semantic communication. *Science*, 1980, *210*, 801–803.

Sherrington, C. S. *The integrative action of the nervous system*. New Haven: Yale University Press, 1906.

Simon, H. A. How big is a chunk? *Science*, 1974, *183*, 482–488.

Simpson, G. G. *The major features of evolution*. New York: Columbia University Press, 1953.

Singer, D. W. *Giordano Bruno: His life and thought*. New York: Henry Schuman, 1950.

Skinner, B. F. The experimental analysis of behavior. *American Scientist*, 1957, *45*, 343–371.

Snell, O. Die Abhängigkeit des Hirngewichtes von dem Körpergewicht und den geistigen Fähigkeiten. *Archiv für Psychiatrie und Nervenkrankheiten*, 1891, *23*, 436–446.

Sperry, R. W. Lateral specialization in the surgically separated hemispheres. In F. O. Schmitt & F. G. Worden (Eds.), *The neurosciences: Third study program*. Cambridge, Mass.: MIT Press, 1974.

Sperry, R. W., Stamm, J. S., & Miner, N. Relearning tests for interocular transfer following division of optic chiasma and corpus callosum in cats. *Journal of Comparative and Physiological Psychology*, 1956, *49*, 529–533.

Stanley, S. M. *Macroevolution: Pattern and process*. San Francisco: W. H. Freeman, 1979.

Suga, N., & Jen, P. H.-S. Disproportionate tonotopic representation for processing CF-FM sonar signals in the mustache bat auditory cortex. *Science*, 1976, *194*, 542–544.

Szentágothai, J. The neuron network of the cerebral cortex: A functional interpretation (The Ferrier Lecture, 1977). *Proceedings of the Royal Society, London* (Series B), 1978, *201*, 219–248.

Teleki, G. Chimpanzee subsistence technology: Materials and skills. *Journal of Human Evolution*, 1974, *3*, 575–594.

Terrace, H. S., Petitto, L. A., Sanders, R. J., & Bever, T. G. Can an ape create a sentence? *Science*, 1979, *206*, 891–902.

Thompson, D'Arcy W. *On growth and form* (2nd ed.). Cambridge: Cambridge University Press, 1942.

Thompson, N. S. My descent from the monkey. In P. P. G. Bateson & P. H. Klopfer (Eds.), *Perspectives in ethology* (Vol. 2). New York: Plenum, 1976.

Thorndike, E. L. Animal intelligence: An experimental study of the associative processes in animals. *Psychological Monographs*, 1898, 2, (4, Whole No. 8).

Thorpe, W. H. *Animal nature and human nature*. London, Methuen, 1974.

Thouless, R. H. *Mind and consciousness in experimental psychology (the seventeenth Arthur Stanley Eddington Memorial Lecture)*. Cambridge: Cambridge University Press, 1963.

Tobias, P. V. Brain-size, grey matter and race – fact or fiction? *American Journal of Physical Anthropology*, 1970, *32*, 3–26.

Tobias, P. V. *The brain in hominid evolution*. New York: Columbia University Press, 1971.

Tolman, E. C. *Purposive behavior in animals and men*. New York: Appleton-Century-Crofts, 1932.

Tolman, E. C. Cognitive maps in rats and men. *Psychological Review*, 1948, *55*, 189–208.

Valentine, J. W., & Campbell, C. A. Genetic regulation and the fossil record. *American Scientist*, 1975, *63*, 673–680.

Van Lawick-Goodall, J. Tool using in primates and other vertebrates. In D. S. Lehrman, R. A. Hinde, & E. Shaw (Eds.), *Advances in the study of behavior* (Vol. 3). New York, Academic Press, 1970.

Van Valen, L. A new evolutionary law. *Evolutionary Theory*, 1973, *1*, 1–30.

Van Valen, L. Two modes of evolution. *Nature*, 1974, *252*, 298–300. (a)

Van Valen, L. Brain size and intelligence in man. *American Journal of Physical Anthropology*, 1974, *40*, 417–424. (b)

Van Valen, L. Taxonomic survivorship curves. *Evolutionary Theory*, 1979, *4*, 129–142.

von Bonin G. Brain weight and body weight in mammals. *Journal of General Psychology*, 1937, *16*, 379–389.

von Frisch, K. *The dancing bees*. London, Methuen, 1953.

von Haller, A. *Elementa Physiologiae corporis humanis* (Vol. 4). Lausanne, 1762.

von Uexküll, J. *Streifzüge durch die Umwelten von Tieren und Menschen*. Berlin: Springer-Verlag, 1934. Translated in C. H. Schiller (Ed.), *Instinctive behavior: The development of a modern concept*. New York: International Universities Press, 1957.

Warren, J. M. Possibly unique characteristics of learning by primates. *Journal of Human Evolution*, 1974, *3*, 445–454.

Warren, J. M. A phylogenetic approach to learning and intelligence. In A. Oliverio (Ed.), *Genetics, environment and intelligence*. New York: Elsevier/North Holland, 1977.

Washburn, S. L., & Harding, R. S. Evolution of primate behavior. In F. O. Schmitt (Ed.), *The neurosciences: Second study program*. New York: Rockefeller University Press, 1970.

Watson, J. B. *Animal education*. Chicago: University of Chicago Press, 1903.

Watson, J. B. Psychology as the behaviorist views it. *Psychological Review*, 1913, 20, 158–177.

Weiner, J. S. *The Piltdown forgery*. London: Oxford University Press, 1955.

Weiskrantz, L. Trying to bridge some neuropsychological gaps between monkey and man. *British Journal of Psychology*, 1977, *68*, 431–445.

Welker, W. I. Brain evolution in mammals. In R. B. Masterton, M. E. Bitterman, C. B. G. Campbell, & N. Hotton (Eds.), *Evolution of Brain and Behavior in Vertebrates*. Hillsdale, N.J.: Erlbaum, 1976. (a)

Welker, W. I. (Ed.). Neocortical mapping studies. *Brain, Behavior and Evolution*, 1976, *13*, 241–243. (b)

Welker, W. I., & Campos, G. B. Physiological significance of sulci in somatic sensory cerebral cortex in mammals of the family Procyonidae. *Journal of Comparative Neurology*, 1963, *120*, 19–36.

Westfall, R. S. Newton and the fudge factor. *Science*, 1973, *179*, 751–758.

Whitney, G. Genetic considerations in studies of the evolution of the nervous system and behavior. In R. B. Masterton, W. Hodos, & H. Jerison (Eds.), *Evolution, brain, and behavior: Persistent problems*. Hillsdale, N.J.: Erlbaum, 1976.

Whorf, B. L. *Language, thought and reality* (John B. Carroll, Ed.). Cambridge, Mass.: MIT Press, 1956.

Wilson, E. O. *Sociobiology*. Cambridge, Mass.: Harvard University Press, 1975.

Wilson, E. O. *On human nature*. Cambridge, Mass.: Harvard University Press, 1978.

Witelson, S. F., & Pallie, W. Left hemisphere specialization for language in the newborn: Neuroanatomical evidence of asymmetry. *Brain*, 1973, *96*, 641–647.

Woodruff, G., Premack, D., & Kennel, K. Conservation of liquid and solid quantity by the chimpanzee. *Science*, 1978, 202, 991–994.

Wright, R. V. S. Imitative learning of a flaked stone technology – the case of an orangutan. In S. L. Washburn & E. R. McCown (Eds.), *Human evolution: Biosocial perspectives*. Menlo Park, Calif.: Benjamin/Cummings, 1978.

Yeni-Komshian, G. H., & Benson, D. A. Anatomical study of cerebral asymmetry in the temporal lobe of humans, chimpanzees and rhesus monkeys. *Science*, 1976, *192*, 387–389.

Yerkes, R. M. *The dancing mouse: A study in animal behavior*. New York: Macmillan, 1907.

Young, R. M. *Mind, brain and adaptation in the nineteenth century*. Oxford: Oxford University Press, Clarendon Press, 1970.

Zeki, S. M. Functional specialization in the visual cortex of the rhesus monkey. *Nature*, 1978, *274*, 423–428.

13 *Genetics and intelligence*

SANDRA SCARR AND LOUISE CARTER-SALTZMAN

13.1. INTRODUCTION

The idea of genetic differences as a source of individual and group differences in intelligence is one of the most controversial in the history of psychology. Some experts believe that evidence to date is insufficient to confirm that genetic differences affect individual or group differences in anything we measure as intelligence (Kamin, 1974, 1981; Schwartz & Schwartz, 1974; Taylor, 1980). Other experts claim that the evidence indicates a very high degree of genetic determination of differences in intelligence (Eysenck, 1973, 1979, 1981; Jensen, 1973a, 1978a). Most investigators in behavior genetics conclude from the evidence that about half ($\pm .1$) of the current differences among individuals in U.S. and European white populations in measured intelligence result from genetic differences among them (Loehlin, Lindzey, & Spuhler, 1975; R. Nichols, 1978; Plomin & DeFries, 1980; Scarr, 1981b).

It is curious that so many experts examining the same evidence could reach such different conclusions. To understand the controversy and the differing views, we will examine some of the history of investigations of genetic differences in intelligence and will reconsider the major evidence. Further, we will describe the profoundly varied approaches in genetics to the study of human behavior, which are often confused by behavioral scientists. The chapter will review the older and the more recent evidence on genetic and environmental differences in general and specific abilities and will propose a future for research.

This chapter must seem to be redundant with the many reviews of genetics and intelligence that have appeared in the last 10 years. The psychological community has been informed by reviews of the literature (Bouchard, 1976; DeFries and Plomin, 1978; Jencks, 1972; Jensen, 1973a; Kamin, 1974; Lindzey et al., 1971; Loehlin, Lindzey, and Spuhler, 1975; McClearn, 1970; McGuire and Hirsch, 1977; Nichols, 1978; Scarr-Salapatek, 1975; Thiessen, 1970). The genetics community has been informed by reviews of genetics and intelligence literature (Anderson, 1974; Childs et al., 1976; Lewontin, 1975; Morton, 1972).

We identify three legitimate reasons for producing yet another review of the literature on genetics and intelligence: (a) readers of this volume do not have access to the reviews (we discount this reason); (b) startling new data or ideas have appeared since the last reviews (in part true); and (c) we have a new, beneficial perspective to bring to the review of the literature, a vanity we would indeed like to entertain.

WHAT WE USED TO KNOW

More than 40 years ago, the distinguished psychologist R. S. Woodworth was asked by the Social Science Research Council to review the research on heredity and environment (Woodworth, 1941) that had recently been obtained from several studies of twins and foster (adopted) children and of nursery schools. There was much dispute at the time between the Stanford (Terman, McNemar, & Burks), Minnesota (Leahy & Goodenough), and Iowa (Wellman, Skodak, & Skeels) groups concerning the interpretation of evidence favoring either heredity or environment as the predominant source of intellectual differences in the U.S. white population. Woodworth began his evaluative volume with the following statement, which serves as a suitable introduction for this chapter as well:

If the individual's hereditary potencies could somehow be annulled he would immediately lose all physiological and mental characteristics and would remain simply a mass of dead matter. If he were somehow deprived of all environment, his hereditary potencies would have no scope for their activity and, once more, he would cease to live. To ask whether heredity or environment is more important to life is like asking whether fuel or oxygen is more necessary for making a fire. But when we ask whether the *differences* obtaining between human individuals or groups are due to their differing heredity or to differences in their present and previous environments, we have a genuine question and one of great social importance. In a broad sense both heredity and environment must be concerned in causing individuals to be different in ability and personality, but it is a real question whether to attach more importance to the one or the other and whether to look to eugenics or euthenics for aid in maintaining and improving the quality of the population. [P. 1]

After a judicious review of the evidence from studies of twins reared together and apart, and from studies of foster children, orphanage children, and those with and without nursery-school experience, Woodworth wrote a conclusion that stands today as a fine summary of our knowledge about genetic and environmental differences in intelligence. We reprint it here in full to inform the reader that the research of the past 40 years has only firmed the conclusions and elaborated the theoretical and methodological bases for those judgments. We have had to rediscover these facts, because the intervening intellectual history largely buried them in an avalanche of naive environmentalism (Scarr & Weinberg, 1978). It is true that methods of analysis and the measurement of intelligence have both advanced since the 1920s and 1930s but, curiously, the conclusions have not changed.

As the preceding survey had found repeatedly, there are serious difficulties in the way of separating the factors of heredity and environment when our interest lies in such traits as human intelligence and personality. There are sampling difficulties, inadequacies in even the best available tests for mental abilities, and much vagueness as regards the proper measures of environment. Also we have no direct indication of the individual's hereditary constitution, of his particular combinations of genes. It is not to be wondered at if the results of elaborately planned investigations leave us unsatisfied and uncertain. A few findings do seem to be well assured.

Heredity and environment differ as between families, and also as between the children of the same parents growing up in the same home. By noticing how much siblings differ in comparison with children from the community at large we can estimate the total effect of intra-family variation in heredity and environment combined, as compared with the inter-family variation. We find the inter-family component in the total variance of the population to be smaller than the intra-family component. From the examination of foster children compared with own children in similar homes we gather that the inter-family differences are due partly to differences in heredity and partly to differences in home environment and about equally to the two factors. That is, own children from different homes differ in part because their families have somewhat distinctive heredity and in part because the home influences are different.

As to the intra-family differences, the fact that there are some even between identical twins reared together proves that such differences are due in part to environment. But the relatively small differences between these twins leave the major part of the intra-family differences still undissected. Since siblings in general differ in heredity, they differ correspondingly in the effective environment, dependent as that is on their own characteristics. The environmental factors that differ as between children in the same home are often too subtle to be easily controlled or measured, and no promising beginning has been made toward estimating their respective shares in the production of individual differences. Differences between own children in the same home are sometimes the result of prenatal and natal accidents. But for the rest they are due to the combination or interaction of heredity and environment, and that is about all we can say at present.

The most striking feature of these results is the small share that can be attributed to inter-family differences in environment. Not over a fifth, apparently, of the variance of intelligence in the general population can be attributed to differences in homes and neighborhoods acting as environmental factors. The reason is probably to be sought in the large degree of uniformity of environment produced by the schools and other public and semipublic agencies. It is still possible that raising the intellectual level of the environment would raise the general level of intelligence, while not by any means annulling the individual differences due to heredity.

The gains of foster children and of other children in changed and improved environments have been much less striking than might have been expected. About 5 or 10 points in IQ is all that can be claimed for the average gain, with much individual variation above and below this average. Even this amount of gain is not established beyond doubt – nor, to be sure, is it proved that still better environments would fail to register much larger gains. Somewhat larger gains and losses have indeed been indicated in some of the identical twin pairs who received very unequal educational opportunities.

An important result of several foster-child studies is the good showing made by many children whose own parents are rated very low in the socio-economic scale. Instead of saying that these children have made good in spite of poor heredity, we must conclude that their heredity was good or fair in spite of the low status and unsatisfactory behavior of their own parents. Their heredity was obviously good enough to permit them to do what they have actually done. By this test of accomplishment some children of feebleminded parents are proved to have average heredity. But to infer that all or even most children of inferior parents are possessed of average heredity would be going far beyond the present evidence, because of the elimination of especially unpromising children that has always occurred before the samples were made available to the investigators. To assure a gifted young couple that they could do as much for the next generation by adopting any "normal" infant as by having a child of their own would be a scandalous exaggeration of the known facts. [Pp. 84–86]

This compact summary of knowledge about genetic and environmental differences deserves several readings, for Woodworth makes virtually all the general points about intellectual differences that are salient today.

1.   Both heredity and environment contribute to differences among and within families.
2.   Intrafamily differences are subtle and undissected. Sibling differences depend in part on their own genetic differences and in part on their environments, with which we now know birth order differences are correlated.
3.   Interfamily environmental differences among U.S. whites are a very small part of the total individual variation in IQ, probably, as Woodworth says, because of the uniformity of environments produced by public schooling and other public agencies.
4.   It is still possible to raise the general level of intelligence by improving the environment, but that will not by any means annul individual differences due to heredity.

5.   The gains made by adopted children reared in improved environments are not dramatic (unless they are minority children, who were not studied at that time), and differences between separated monozygotic (MZ) twins are not large unless their educational differences have been large.
6.   Children from very disadvantaged backgrounds, however, often proved to be of normal intelligence when given the opportunities of foster homes.

The notions of the 1930s about fixed heredity were obviously wrong. On the other hand, Woodworth concludes, two intellectually gifted parents could not adopt any "normal" infant in the expectation that that child would intellectually match an offspring of their own. Heredity does play a substantial role in determining individual differences in intelligence.

A BRIEF POLITICAL HISTORY OF GENETIC DIFFERENCES IN IQ

There is a remarkably high ratio of cant to data in this field. Many people express opinions (and write polemics in reviews), and relatively few people do empirical research. Since the mid 1970s the ratio is improving as more investigators see the possibilities of important research questions and approaches, particularly through the study of adopted children (DeFries & Plomin, 1978; Scarr-Salapatek, 1975).

To understand the controversy about the very study of genetic variance in intelligence, one must assume a political frame of mind and believe that genetic differences have awful consequences. On the one hand, one may decide to suppress the evil consequences of such knowledge and its possible uses. On the other hand, one might appoint oneself the guardian of an awful truth: that genetic differences among human beings and among groups of people are so pervasive, so terrifyingly strong, that the knowledge is essential to bring before the public for their consideration in social policy issues. Now the stage is set for a confrontation, a noisy conflict that has persisted from the early 20th century to the present (see Block & Dworkin, 1976, for a good collection of articles).

Terman (1922), Yerkes (1923), and Brigham (1923) engaged in polemic debate with the great literary columnist Walter Lippmann (see Cronbach, 1975, for a reference list, 1922–1923). Lippmann argued for the malleability of intelligence and for the role of cultural differences in IQ test scores. Like any sensible liberal, Lippmann recognized that the tests sampled culturally bound knowledge and skills. Terman, Yerkes, and Brigham pigheadedly argued for the immutability of intelligence and for the cultural fairness of their testing programs. They lost (Block & Dworkin, 1976; Cronbach, 1975). Later another great columnist, Joseph Alsop, effectively tackled Jensen's views on racial differences in intelligence. As Cronbach said, psychologists who gain the limelight often lose their academic heads.

Within the academic community, Neff (1938) challenged the hereditarian views of the Stanford school and discounted the research of Terman and Burks. The Iowans (Skeels, 1938; Wellman, 1940) advocated the environmental effects of early interventions while McNemar (1940) wrote scathing commentaries on their statistics. On the race issue, Herskovits (1926) and Klineberg (1963) were especially forceful in their views against the idea of racial differences in intelligence. Their evidence was scanty, but their values were strong. Later "validation" of their hopes and beliefs was offered by the American Anthropological Association, which adopted a resolution declaring all races biologically identical. The resolution responded to

Jensen and to the furor caused by his 1969 article in the *Harvard Education Review* (see Jensen, 1973b).

> Discussion of the inheritance of human intelligence consists of two slippery slopes joined by a razor's edge. One slope descends to antiracism at any intellectual cost, the other to intellectual freedom at any social cost. The shabby misuse of IQ testing in the support of past American racist policies has created understandable anxiety over current research on the inheritance of human intelligence. But the resulting personal attacks on a few scientists with unpopular views has had a chilling effect on the entire field of human behavioral genetics and clouds public discussion of its implications. . . .
> The political capture of a discipline in the United States is highly unlikely, but feelings run high. No controversy within the academic world has been more cruelly divisive; none better illustrates the maxim that tragedy is a clash of rights. There appears to be only one solution to the dilemma: a return to an uncompromising ethic of objectivity, based on a careful decoupling of the collection and analysis of data from the discussion of their social and political implications.

A similar view was expressed by a prestigious group of geneticists:

> The application of the techniques of quantitative genetics to the analysis of human behavior is fraught with complications and potential biases, but well-designed research on the genetic and environmental components of human psychological traits may yield valid and socially useful results and should not be discouraged. [Statement adopted by the Genetics Society of America, 1975.]

Some doubt that well-designed research on genetic variation in human behavior is possible. Lewontin (1975), for example, sets forth requirements for the design of adoption studies that cannot be met in any population: We cannot randomize genotypes over environments, finding genotypes and environments that are representative of the entire range of the population to which inferences are to be made; still ". . . the failure to adhere to clean experimental design renders all work uninterpretable. It is simply not true that approximate designs give approximate results" (Lewontin, 1975, p. 403). Furthermore, Lewontin and other critics doubt that the study of genetic variation in human behavior is worth any effort. "Finally, from a scientific standpoint or from one of valid inferences about social policy, the problem of assaying genetic components of IQ test differences seems utterly trivial and hardly worth the immense effort that would be needed to carry out decent studies" (Lewontin, 1975, p. 403). Kamin (1981) echoes similar sentiments:

> The great merit of Scarr's plentiful empirical research lies, in my view, in the demonstration that no scientific gain is to be had from further "behavior genetic" research on the heritability of IQ. The same data set from which Scarr concludes that IQ is substantially heritable can also be used – since Scarr is willing to share her raw data – to show that IQ is not at all heritable. The data are not, after all, the product of clearly designed and well controlled experimentation. They are necessarily correlational data, collected in difficult and inevitably flawed field settings. The patterns discerned within such data are many, and complex. The interpretation of these complex patterns, I believe, must reflect the investigator's theoretical bias. [P. 468]

Layzer (1972, 1974) and Feldman and Lewontin (1975), for example, deny any legitimate use for the information about the "heritability" of behavioral phenotypes in human populations. They point to the possible existence of genotype–environment correlations and interactions as rendering any studies of genetic and environmental variances indeterminant. They further argue that studies of sources of variation in human populations are misleading and lack serious implications for any scientific or practical purpose.

We must distinguish those problems which are by their nature numerical and statistical from those in which numerical manipulation is a mere methodology. Thus, the breeding structure of human populations, the intensities of natural selection, the correlations between mates, the correlations between genotypes and environments, are all by their nature statistical constructs and can be described and studied, in the end, only by statistical techniques. It is the numbers themselves that are the proper objects of study. It is the numbers themselves that we need for understanding and prediction.

Conversely, relations between genotype, environment, and phenotype are at base mechanical questions of enzyme activity, protein synthesis, developmental movements, and paths of nerve conduction. We wish, both for the sake of understanding and prediction, to draw up the blueprints of this machinery and make tables of its operating characteristics with different inputs and in different milieus. For these problems, statistical descriptions, especially one-dimensional descriptions like heritability, can only be poor and, worse, misleading substitutes for pictures of the machinery. . . . At present, no statistical methodology exists that will enable us to predict the range of phenotypic possibilities that are inherent in any genotype, nor can any technique of statistical estimation provide a convincing argument for a genetic mechanism more complicated than one or two Mendelian loci with low and constant penetrance. Certainly the simple estimate of heritability, either in the broad or narrow sense, but most especially in the broad sense, is nearly equivalent to no information at all for any serious problem of human genetics. [Feldman & Lewontin, pp. 1167–1168]

WHAT ARE THE QUESTIONS?

One's evaluation of the answers that can be supplied by statistical and mechanistic models surely depends on one's question. Answers to questions about the current intellectual state of human populations, the distribution of intelligence, and the likely success of improving intellectual phenotypes through intervention with *known* environmental manipulations call for a statistical model of contemporary sources of variance in the population. Knowledge of evolutionary history, selection pressures, or enzyme activity at a few loci will not help. Nor will appealing to the unpredictable effects of yet-to-be-devised interventions help solve the problems of the here and now.

We can find a useful analogy by considering another population statistic, birth rate. Suppose that one proposed to study the birth rate of a developing country in order to devise a family planning program. The logic of Feldman and Lewontin's argument (see also Medawar, 1977) against studying sources of variance in populations would oppose such a study, because (a) statistical studies will not inform us about the mechanisms and physiology of reproduction; (b) the correlations between reproduction and social structure render the birth rate a meaningless statistic; and (c) knowledge of the birth rate will not permit us to advise the Joneses or the Smiths about their reproductive plans. We submit that each of these objections is based on questions not addressed by studies of population variability or reproductive rate; different questions require different studies.

It seems that some scientists fear that knowledge of the current sources of intellectual differences in a population will foreclose attempts to search for ways to improve the intellectual status or distribution of resources of the population. If current differences in intelligence are attributable half to genetic differences, about 10% to differences among family environments, and the rest to differences among individuals within families, should we abandon a commitment to improve children's lives? We, the authors, fail to see the connection.

As Anderson (1974) pointed out:

Genetics as a discipline cuts across the four levels of biological study – molecular, cellular, organismal, and populational. At each level testable hypotheses can be stated and the results at one level may lead to questions which may be investigated at other levels.

Genetic studies treat variability as the primary focus for investigation, not merely as noise to be eliminated or disregarded. This variation must be examined both within families and between families. If only one pair of genes is involved, the incidence among relatives will follow simple ratios, but with multigenic inheritance there is a more complex set of expectations. [Pp. 20–21].

Consider the following questions that one might ask about the role of genetic differences in intelligence:

1.   How do genes affect intelligence? (Which pathways of gene–protein–enzyme activity to physiology and brain function cause differences in intelligence?)
2.   What are the sources of individual (and group) differences in intelligence? (What are the sources of *variation* in a population at the present time?)
3.   Why and in what ways does human intelligence differ from that of other primates? (What is the evolutionary history of primate species?)
4.   Why is there a distribution of individual differences in intelligence within a population and perhaps between populations? (What is the evolutionary history and structure of human populations?)

DEVELOPMENTAL VERSUS INDIVIDUAL DIFFERENCES

Confusion about the different nature of each of these questions has led many critics of the study of genetics and intelligence to commit amazing feats of illogic. Most common is the confusion of questions (a) and (b) in the psychological literature. It is asserted that one cannot study the sources of individual differences in a population because both genes and environments determine individual development. Well, yes, we all assume that human development requires both genes and environments. Still, as Woodworth said, that statement does not answer question (b), about sources of variation. Many species-typical developments depend on the same or functionally equivalent genotypes and environments for development within bounds that are normal for the species. Individual differences depend on functional differences in genotypes and/or environments that cause noticeable variations in phenotypes (Scarr, 1978).

Populations can be described only in statistical terms, because they are *distributions* of individuals. Although one can reify some frequent "type" as representative of a population, it is quickly apparent that more is lost than is gained by typological thinking (Hirsch, 1967). As Dobzhansky (1950) and his students (e.g., McDonald & Ayala, 1974) have demonstrated, a naturally occurring population is most often genetically diverse, and the more environmental diversity its range of habitats contains, the more genotypically and phenotypically diverse the individuals within a population will be. An evolutionary history of selection pressure does not generally lead to the elimination of all variability, for a variety of reasons (see Kidd & Cavalli-Sforza, 1973). Thus, an understanding of the role of genetic differences in human intelligence necessitates questions about the *distribution* of intelligence in the population. There are many possible questions about the evolution of intelligence, genetic drift, local adaptations, adaptation to various niches within a population, developmental changes in the distribution of intelligence, and so forth, but one question surely is: Why do individuals within a population vary in intelligence at the present time?

USES AND ABUSES OF THE TERM *INTELLIGENCE*

It has become fashionable to adopt a nihilistic position regarding the nature and definition of intelligence. No one knows what intelligence is, it is often said, although *everyone* knows that the term is a "fuzzy" construct! We create confusion by using it at several levels that are not necessarily related to one another. The term can be applied or misapplied at four levels. In our view, *intelligence* should be reserved for the individual level of cognitive functioning.

At a cultural level, the prescribed and habitual solutions to problems make better or worse use of the available resources in relation to the demands of size and density of the population. The *adaptation* of a cultural group can be evaluated by the degree to which there is a balance between the needs of the population and the available resources that the group knows how to use (see M. Harris, 1975). "Intelligent" cultures are better described by their adaptation.

At the level of social organization, one can speak of the structures and functions of the organization as working more or less effectively to deal with the problems presented by the society. Effective social organizations have structured social roles and allocate those roles appropriately to individuals. Thus, intelligence at the societal level is better described as the *organization and allocation* of social roles.

In small groups, there are also social roles to be allocated, but the structure of such groups is often informal and shifting. Incumbents change roles over short periods of time. One can evaluate the effectiveness of such groups by criteria of problem solving, use of time, satisfactions of members, and so forth, as is frequently done in the literature on street gangs, boy scout troups, and other informal small groups. At the group level, "intelligent" groups solve everyday problems (which movie to see, when to rumble) in ways that satisfy most members and make better than worse use of time and resources.

Also in small groups, one can look at the adequacy of individuals' role performance. Intelligent behavior in small groups requires that one take into account the social and material resources in the setting. On the basketball court, playing intelligently does not mean that one takes every available shot oneself. Rather, one is most effective if one's shot-taking decisions take into account the positions and shooting prowess of one's teammates. Similarly, intelligent behavior in many other small group situations requires that one withhold some uses of one's individual cognitive skills so that the group may function most effectively. This means that small groups are not likely to be good settings in which to sample individual intelligence.

We should reserve the term *intelligence* for those *individual* attributes that center around reasoning skills, knowledge of one's culture, and ability to arrive at innovative solutions to problems. *Intelligence* should be reserved to describe cross-situational attributes in individuals that they carry with them into diverse situations.

INTELLIGENCE AND SOCIAL COMPETENCE

Social competence is most clearly defined as an individual's success in filling social roles. The most socially competent people are those who can fill many social roles well; less competent people are those who have few options in social roles and who fill them badly. This definition confounds breadth of role options with performance in roles, but some weighted combination is necessary to capture what is meant by social competence. Some people fill a few roles well but are quite limited in their options. Others have qualifications to fill many roles but do none of them well.

People who are intelligent by the individual definition are likely to have greater social competence, because breadth of role options is related to intelligence, as is goodness of role performance. Intelligence is, however, only one component in social competence, although perhaps a major one. The correlation between the two is probably middling. People who are considered socially competent need not have high intelligence. Depending upon the roles they choose or have thrust upon them, the performance of those with average or low-average intellectual levels may be quite adequate.

Looking unintelligent in social roles depends upon a *mismatch* of the role to the person; for example, a professor of psychology coaching a basketball team or most basketball coaches teaching psychology. Looking intelligent in social roles is not what we mean by *intelligence,* a term reserved for those mental processes already mentioned.

Any people but the more retarded should be able to find social roles in which they fit and behave competently. People of lesser intelligence will not have the breadth of options that more intelligent people have, nor are they as likely to fill the roles they do have as competently, on the average, as more intelligent people, but they can be socially competent at some level.

POLITICAL PROBLEMS WITH THE TERM *INTELLIGENCE*

As we all recognize, the term *intelligence* is surrounded with a halo of valuation that threatens to include all manner of virtues. Many avoid the term in writing and public speaking because of the unusual amount of surplus meaning. This is a case of bad money driving out good, because there is a perfectly good domain of behaviors to be described by *intelligence.* We use terms like *cognitive skills, intellectual skills,* and *abstract reasoning* because others may take offense at the possible exclusion of virtues that they value and that their friends and relatives seem to have.

Not all good things about people are "intelligence," nor is the relationship of measured intelligence to the allocation of resources as strong as it is to educational level, reading achievement, and mathematics skills. The allocation of social and economic resources seems to be tied more closely to educational landmarks and motivation to work hard than to intelligence per se.

Acknowledging the public problems with the use of the term *intelligence,* we propose that it be available to close friends and colleagues to apply to those individual, mental processes in the domain described earlier. In sum, the field of intelligence is not served well by blurred distinctions among levels of analysis nor among meanings of the term *intelligence.* We should find other words to apply to cultures, social organizations, small groups, and individual behaviors in social contexts. Although the term has an aura of virtue, its application to other contexts or behaviors will not improve anyone's functioning.

INTELLIGENCE AT A POPULATION LEVEL

A serious view of intelligence should include a consideration of the population level. The population that is best adapted to a typical human environment includes people with diverse skills. The benefits of their diverse talents are shared through their social interdependence. This is a far more realistic picture of human evolution and the role of intelligence than the Social Darwinian notion of a best-adapted phenotype. In a real human society, no one phenotype is adapted best. Intelligence as a population concept refers to the distribution of skills in a population of humans who work and live together in interdependent, socially organized ways.

The application of a population concept to intelligence in modern industrial societies is easy. If we had to do our own home building the result would indeed be primitive, because we do not have skills that are comparable to those of a specialized architect, builder, carpenter, or plumber. Neither do they know how to deliver human services or investigate educational and psychological problems, for which they depend on people like us. Not only are these differently developed skills, but they require different kinds of intelligence. A well-adapted society, then, is one that fosters diversity of intelligence.

Even in less industrial societies, division of labor makes the diversity of intelligence an adaptive advantage. In the most primitive form, there is at least a division of labor by sex. It seems to us not accidental that women all over the world are socialized to be nurturant, whereas men are socialized to be more independent. Although these particular forms of the division of labor are no longer fashionable in postindustrial societies such as the United States (and we agree they should not be, because child rearing and participation in the economy need no longer be related to gender), it is likely that until this century, an important division of labor was that by gender, each sex requiring a somewhat different set of intellectual and social skills.

In contemporary preindustrial societies, the division of labor is not only by gender. People who are good storytellers often have suitable roles, as do those who are particularly good builders, farmers, fishermen (rarely women), embroiderers, weavers, and so forth. It is interesting that one modern government program that was readily accepted by the Quechua women on the eastern slopes of the Andes in Ecuador was the sponsorship of especially good weavers to teach the young weavers in other villages. Women weavers who attained status in their own villages for their skill at devising and weaving intricate patterns were traditionally the teachers of young women in other villages, and thus the government program was compatible with a long-established recognition of this form of intelligence. Husbands and children of particularly good weavers suffer their absences with pride in their accomplishments (S. Scarr's personal knowledge from fieldwork).

A complex society requires variation in intelligence for optimal adaptation. Given that a distribution of skills is required, the next question concerns levels of skills. One would generally think that individuals are better adapted if they have the highest possible levels of intelligence. Certainly, to be seriously retarded and unable to take care of oneself is maladaptive. At an intellectual level of mild retardation, however, some individuals may make a population better adapted. It is easier to defend the idea that a population needs some people of high intelligence, who define and solve problems for the society as a whole. People of more average abilities carry out the major work of the society, but the mildly retarded, who complain less about tedium and who are willing to do jobs that few others want and to get satisfaction from them, may fulfill roles, too. We are speculating when we say that the continued presence of large numbers of mildly retarded persons in every society suggests that their fitness, as witnessed by their above-average reproductive rate, means that they have productive or at least adapted roles in most societies.

Whatever one concludes about the contribution of the mildly retarded to the overall adaptation of a population, we believe that populations require a range of intellectual levels and specific skills to be optimally adapted.

13.2.   MOLECULAR AND POPULATION GENETICS

MECHANISMS AND VARIANCE

When laypeople think of the term *genetic,* they are likely to think of the material segments of chromosomes that produce some mysterious products that govern our growth and development. The lay model is based on a linear, causal stream of determinism that flows from molecular to molar levels of analysis. This molecular model has been developed through the study of major aberrations in the genetic code that lead inexorably to noticeably different, abnormal phenotypes. The scientific success of molecular genetics is a sociological phenomenon, worthy of study in its own right. Our purpose here is to describe the phenomena in intelligence to which molecular models do and do not (yet?) apply and to propose the efficacy of the lesser known evolutionary population genetic models for complex phenotypes, such as intelligence.

More than 150 known gene defects are associated with mental retardation (Anderson, 1972). Development can go awry in many ways. At the minimum, we know that so many genes must perform properly in the chorus for the performance of normal intelligence to go on stage. Genes that fail to code for enzymes required for normal metabolism are inborn errors, many of which result in mental retardation, such as in phenylketonuria (PKU), galactosemia, and Lesch-Nyhan syndrome. Other single gene disorders code for incorrect enzymes, fail to code for proper proteins, or produce indigestible products somewhere in the gene action pathway. The literature in genetics is replete with examples of rare and specific gene defects that lead to mental retardation.

We believe, however, that models of gene-action-gone-awry tell us very little about the role of genetic differences in intelligence per se. Perhaps they serve to confirm the views that genetic variants are present in the human organism, that normal intellectual development is a complex feat of genetic programming, and that genetic variation "counts" in explaining normal variation in intelligence. If one begins with an evolutionary view of intelligence, however, all of those points are obvious from the start. One cannot fail to note, too, the extensive literature on chromosomal abnormalities. Still, is it surprising that having the species-typical amount of genetic material should make the development of intelligence in the normal range more likely or that having an abnormal amount of chromatin makes mental retardation more likely? Having too many or too few sex chromosomes is not as disastrous to intelligence as too many or too few other chromosomes (the last is evidently lethal as there are no living examples). Nevertheless, intellectual development is adversely affected by the wrong amount of genetic material. We will discuss briefly, however, the status of molecular and simple genetic research on behavior, particularly intelligence, following the outline and spirit of Reed (1975), who reviewed the role of genetic defects in intellectual development.

SIMPLE GENETICS MODELS

Only since 1956 has the correct number (46) of human chromosomes been known. As in all sexually reproducing organisms, these chromosomes come in pairs, one of each pair coming from the father via the sperm and the other one of the pair coming from the mother via the egg. The fertilized egg, then, unless something goes awry, has 46 chromosomes in its nucleus. These 46 packages of DNA contain the genetic code that will direct the development of the future person and will make him or her genetically different from everyone else except his or her identical twin. This DNA will provide the individual's *genotype,* the set of genes derived from his or her ancestors. This may or may not be expressed in visible or measurable traits as the individual's *phenotype.* The phenotype expression of the genotype depends on the genotype itself and on all the environmental influences that impinge upon the individual from the time of conception to death.

Autosomes and sex chromosomes. The genetic code that each individual carries is in the DNA arranged on the chromosomes. There are two kinds of chromosomes. One kind comprises the 22 pairs of *autosomes.* These chromosomes are in matched pairs and carry most of the genetic code for development. In addition, each person has one pair of *sex chromosomes.* This pair is alike in females, XX, and unlike in males, XY. The X chromosome is large and carries many genes, whereas the Y found in males is considerably smaller and appears to be primarily involved with initiating the development of the male sex glands or gonads. Thus, males are vulnerable to any deleterious genes carried on their single large X. Unlike females, they have no second X to supply the corresponding genes for normal processes that can overrule or mask the unfortunate effects of the deleterious genes. Hence, a number of X-linked disorders, including several forms of mental retardation, occur almost exclusively in males. The male needs only the one gene to exhibit symptoms of the disease, whereas the female needs two genes, one on each of her X chromosomes, to have a sex-linked disorder. This can happen only if her father has the disease and her mother either has the disease or is a carrier. In the more likely cases, in which the mother is a carrier, 50% of the time the daughter would get both X chromosomes carrying the gene. Because severely retarded males rarely reproduce, the chances are remote of finding such a retarded woman.

The pattern of inheritance in X-linked disorders is that of unaffected carrier women having half of their sons affected. This happens because each son gets one or the other of his mother's X chromosomes. Half of the time, on an average, the son will get the X chromosome that carries the gene for the disorder. Half the daughters of carrier women will be themselves carriers (because they, too, get one of their mother's X chromosomes) and will have a risk of having half their sons affected. The well-known historical example is that of Queen Victoria, who had hemophiliac sons and carrier daughters, who, in turn, affected their sons.

Autosomal recessive and dominant inheritance. There are two other simple patterns of genetic inheritance in addition to the X-linked type. These are related to the genes located on the 22 pairs of autosomes. Many disorders, in which the presence of the abnormal gene affects the production of an enzyme needed for a biochemical process, appear only when the abnormal gene is present in both members of the chromosome pair. This is called *autosomal recessive* inheritance. In the case of albinism, production of the pigment melanin is prevented, and albinism is the resulting phenotype. If, however, one defective gene is present but its mate on the other chromosome is not defective, then enough enzyme can be produced to supply sufficient melanin and the carrier appears to be normal. Parents who are related to each other have a greater chance of being carriers of the same recessives and thus run a greater chance of having affected children. When a child is diagnosed as having one of the many rare forms of mental retardation with autosomal, recessive inheritance, one of the best guesses about the parents is that they are genetically related.

On the other hand, when the presence of one deleterious gene is enough to cause the appearance of the anomaly, the inheritance is that of an *autosomal dominant,* and the trait appears in every generation, going from affected parent to affected child. The heterozygote almost always shows the trait phenotypically. (The double dose of the gene in the homozygote may have such a severe effect that the fetus is aborted spontaneously.) The chance of a child's being affected when one parent is affected is about 50%. One example is Huntington's chorea, which results in gross mental deterioration in middle age.

Most human traits are affected by several genes or have a *multigenic* inheritance. These traits show a continuous gradation in phenotype in contrast to those recessive or dominant ones in which there is an "all or none" discrete ratio. One example is intelligence, which has a range in the population from retarded to superior with most phenotypes clustering around an average or mean. *Genetic predictions in regard to multigenic traits have to be based on empirical data from population statistics.* Simple genetic models just do not apply, but more about that later.

Chromosomal anomalies.   Gross chromosomal abnormalities involve much more DNA than differences between single genes. Such abnormalities usually produce very serious disorders, which are generally manifest at birth and which present an array of seemingly unrelated symptoms. When the normal balance of the chromosome complement is upset by the absence of a chromosome, the presence of an extra one, or the lack of some parts of chromosomes, the total development of the individual is disrupted. Down's syndrome with its many congenital defects of the eye, heart, skeleton, and brain is one example. Many early spontaneous abortions are the result of such chromosomal abnormalities. Estimates go as high as 46% for the proportion of aborted fetuses that may have *monosomies* (one chromosome missing), *trisomies* (one extra chromosome present), or other chromosomal abnormalities (Witschi, 1971).

About 1 in 200 live births shows some sort of gross chromosomal abnormality. These mishaps appear to be due either to a failure in the separation of the chromosomes in the last meiotic division of the oocyte that forms the egg or to a similar occurrence in the first or very early mitotic divisions of the egg itself. If the failure occurs in the first few divisions of the fertilized egg, *mosaicism* usually results, with some cell lines in the body showing one chromosome complement and some showing another. The risk of recurrence here depends upon the type of chromosomal anomaly involved. Often the risk is related to the age of the mother.

This classification of autosomal recessives and dominants and X-linked, multigenic, and chromosomal aberrations may seem quite clear cut. Because each individual has many thousands of other genes acting upon his development, and each person, even an identical twin, has had a different environment from conception on, however, it follows that the phenotypic expression of a certain genotype will differ somewhat from person to person. In some cases the trait may not be expressed at all (reduced penetrance), whereas in other cases it may be made more severe by the action of other genes in the chromosome complement or by special environmental stresses. Some conditions resembling known genetic disorders are the result of special environmental influences, for example, the blindness, deafness, and retardation of infants born to mothers who had rubella during early pregnancy.

Methods of research on genetic anomalies. Because the expression of a trait can vary so greatly from person to person, the incidence of a given disorder in the population is difficult to ascertain with an acceptable degree of accuracy. The genetics of a particular trait, however, cannot be understood fully until the incidence of the trait in a particular population, for example, an extended kinship, can be contrasted with its incidence in the population as a whole. Does a particular family line show an unusually high incidence of mental retardation? Is mental retardation more frequent in certain socioeconomic levels? Does close proximity to nuclear power plants increase the incidence of such genetic defects?

The methods used to measure the phenotypes and to investigate the mode of inheritance vary widely with the trait. Phenotypes may be defined by biochemical analysis, by intelligence tests, by personality inventories, by neurological examination, and so forth. Suspected modes of inheritance can be investigated by chromosome counts, by pedigree analysis, by population studies, by the incidence of cousin marriages, by twin and family studies, and so forth.

Longitudinal studies of family *pedigrees* can reveal patterns of inheritance through several generations of persons related in different degrees to each other. The pedigree method is useful with simple Mendelian traits. A strong case can be made for the high *heritability* of a trait that increases in frequency with closer degrees of relationship. The study of population variances is the approach for multigenic traits.

Identical twins share the same DNA and therefore the closest genetic relationship; as a result they have been favorite subjects for research, because the differences between them can be ascribed to environmental influences. Often such studies include fraternal twins, who have only half their genes in common and are essentially siblings born at the same time. If the *concordance* of a trait in identical twins is greater than that in fraternal twins (that is, if the trait in one identical twin appears also in the other identical twin more often than the trait appears in both fraternal twins), an estimate of heritability can be made. Twin and family methods are used very frequently in studies of behavioral traits.

Rare recessive disorders are more often found in the offspring of first- or second-cousin marriages. The offspring of related parents have an increased risk of inheriting the same deleterious recessive gene from a common ancestor of the parents. Thus, a useful technique in defining the pattern of inheritance for a particularly rare trait is to look for an increased incidence of cousin marriages among the parents of affected children.

The range in the heritability of traits is large because the phenotypes of some traits are more susceptible to environmental differences than others. As far as anyone knows, blood groups have 100% genetic variance. No environmental differences have been found that can affect the ABO blood groups. At the other end of the range one might put starvation, an environmental factor that is 100%

effective in eliminating genetic differences. However, even in circumstances of starvation, some persons will survive longer than others, perhaps by virtue of their particular genotype (better utilization of food, lower metabolic rate, etc.), and epidemics of contagious disease rarely spare no one.

The importance of genetic differences is most clear in the cases of genetic anomalies in which the phenotypes can be divided into discrete classes of those affected and those not affected, but even here, genetic and environmental modifiers affect the development of the trait. In cases of multigenic inheritance, both genes and environment always play their part in affecting observable phenotypic differences.

GENE ACTION AND INTELLECTUAL DEVELOPMENT

If gene action pathways in human development were known, writing this chapter would involve no speculation. In fact, only bits and pieces of the genetics of developmental processes are known. The basic DNA–RNA protein-synthesis code is well established. Knowledge of fetal development at a morphological level is fairly complete, but how does morphological development through the fetal period, and indeed the life span, relate to protein synthesis at a cellular level? What causes some cells to differentiate and develop into the cortex and others into hemoglobin? How do gene action and morphological development relate to intellectual development from birth to senescence? How do cells, which all originate from the same fertilized ovum and which all carry the same genetic information, program the development of different organs and systems and in different behavioral stages?

Jacob and Monod (1961) have hypothesized that several different kinds of genes exist: structural genes to specify the proteins to be synthesized, operator genes to turn protein synthesis on and off in adjacent structural genes, and regulator genes to repress or activate the operator and structural genes in a larger system (Lerner, 1968; Martin & Ames, 1964). The instructions that a cell receives must be under regulatory control that differentiates the activity of that cell at several points in development.

Genes and chromosome segments are "turned on" at some but not other points in development. Enlargements of a chromosome section (called puffs) have been observed to coincide with RNA synthesis in the cell. Puffs occur on different portions of the chromosomes at different times in different cells, indicating the existence of regulatory mechanisms in development.

Regulatory genes are probably the ones responsible for species and individual differentiation through control of the expression of structural genes. Most of the structural genes, which are directly concerned with enzyme formation, are common to a wide array of species and function in approximately the same way. They provide the fundamental identity of life systems. The diversity of individuals and species is due in large part to the regulatory genes, which modify the expression of basic biochemical processes. "In other words, the greatest proportion of phenotypic variance, at least in mammalian species, is probably due to regulatory rather than structural genes – genes that activate, deactivate, or otherwise alter the expression of a finite number of structural genes" (Thiessen, 1972, p. 124).

Several cellular regulatory mechanisms have been suggested (Lerner, 1968).

First, the cytoplasms of different cells contain different amounts of material and may contain different materials. As cell division proceeds, daughter cells receive unequal amounts of cytoplasm, which may relate to their progressive differentiation. Second, the position of the developing cells may influence their course. Outer cells may have potentialities for development different from those surrounded by other cells. Third, the cell nuclei become increasingly differentiated in the developmental process. Progressively older nuclei have a more limited range of available functions; they become more specialized in the cell activities they can direct. Specialization of nuclei is related to the differentiation of organs and functions in different portions of the developing organism.

The regulation of developmental processes over the life span is accomplished through the gene-encoded production of hundreds of thousands of enzymes and hormones. During embryogenesis, changes in enzyme concentrations and development correlate precisely (Hsia, 1968).

For example, *cholinesterase* activity shows particularly close relationships with neural development. As early as the closure of the neural tube, high cholinesterase activity has been found in association with morphogenesis of the neuraxis. . . . Nachmansohn has shown that cholinesterase is synthesized in the developing nervous system of the chick embryo exactly at the time that synapses and nerve endings appear. [Pp. 96–97]

Any behavior represented phenotypically by the organism *must* have a genetic and organismic substrate. It does not appear without central nervous system (CNS) regulation, and such regulation does not occur without brain myelenization, synaptic transmission, and previous experience encoded chemically in the brain.

Enzymatic differentiation is specific to the state of development, the particular organ, particular regions within organs, and the type of enzyme. Development proceeds on a gene-regulated path by way of enzymatic activity. Generalizations are very risky from one point in time to another and from one organ part to another.

Several enzyme systems are active in the embryo but disappear with the cessation of growth. Other enzymes are absent in the embryo but appear later, and still others are present in low activity in the embryo and greatly increase in activity at the time an organ becomes functionally mature and remain active throughout life to regulate functional organ activity. A third class of enzymes is activated only with maturation and remain active the rest of adult life (Hsia, 1968, pp. 96–107).

Interference with regulatory mechanisms at a cellular or organ system level can result in a variety of phenotypic abnormalities. The result of interference is often related to the stage of development at which it occurs. For example, male rabbit fetuses castrated on the 19th day of gestation resemble a female at birth. Castration on any day up to the 24th results in a gradation of femininity, but if castration is performed on the 25th day or later, the development of male genitalia is not affected. Figure 13.1 is a schematic presentation of the biochemical development of the embryo and the influence of environment at all levels of development.

Hormonal activity is critically important to the stimulation of protein synthesis and to the differentiation of male embryos from the basic female form. Minute quantities of fetal testosterone at critical periods in development affect genital differentiation as well as CNS differences that seem to last a lifetime (Levine, 1967). Stimulation of protein synthesis is provided by growth hormones as well as

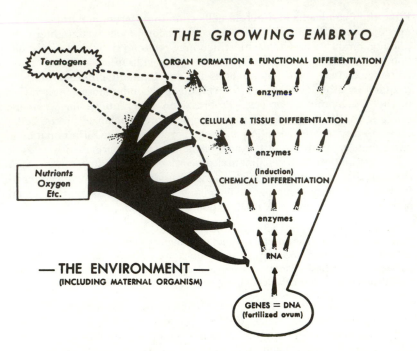

Figure 13.1.   Model of the biochemical development of the growing embryo and the influence of environment at all levels of development. (From "Experimental Studies on Congenital Malformations" by J. G. Wilson, *Journal of Chronic Diseases*, 1959, *10*, 111. Reprinted by permission.)

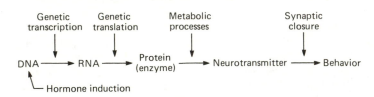

Figure 13.2.   Model of hormone-gene flow from cellular to behavioral levels. (From "A Move toward a Species-Specific Analysis in Behavior Genetics" by D. D. Thiessen, *Behavior Genetics*, 1972, *2*, 115. Reprinted by permission.)

sex hormones, cortisone, insulin, and thyroxine (Thiessen, 1972, p. 95). A model of hormone–gene flow is presented by Thiessen, as shown in Figure 13.2.

Normal development can be disrupted at a biochemical level in many ways. Defects in the biochemical pathways between gene action and normal cell metabolism number in the hundreds. In the glucose to glycogen pathway alone, seven independent genetic errors result in genetic anomalies (Hsia, 1968). Environmental pathogens can, of course, intervene in normal development. Radiation, infectious diseases, drugs, and other specific environmental factors are responsible for some congenital abnormalities in the developing fetus. The effect of ioniz-

Table 13.1. *Timetable of radiation malformations in mice and man*

Age (days)		Embryo (mm)	Nervous system	Other
Mouse	Man			
0–9	0–25		No damage	
9	$25\frac{1}{2}$	2.4	Anencephaly (extreme defect of forebrain)	Severe head defects
10	$28\frac{1}{2}$	4.2	Forebrain, brain stem, or cord defects	Skull, jaw, skeletal, visceral defects, anophthalmia
11	$33\frac{1}{2}$	7.0	Hydrocephalus, narrow aqueduct, encephalocele, cord, and brain stem defects	Retinal, skull, skeletal defects
12	$36\frac{1}{2}$	9.0	Decreasing encephalocele, microcephaly, porencephaly	Retinal, skull, skeletal defects
13	38	12.0	Microcephaly, bizarre defects of cortex, hippocampus, callosum, basal ganglia, decreasing toward term	Decreasing skeletal defects

Source: Hsia (1968), after Hicks.

ing radiation on CNS development is detailed in Table 13.1. Rubella, mumps, toxoplasmosis, and viral infections produce characteristic anomalies when contracted by the fetus in the first trimester of pregnancy. Mental retardation is a prominent feature of many genetic and environmental disturbances in the developmental process. Single genes currently account for more than 159 abnormalities of mental development (Anderson, 1972).

Another genetic pathway that has received considerable attention is that of phenylalanine. Although many behavioral scientists recognize that a block in this pathway can produce PKU, most are not aware that four other identifiable genetic syndromes result from additional blocks in the same pathway, as shown in Figure 13.3. Three of the genetic blocks result in other forms of mental retardation, but all are susceptible to dietary intervention in infancy.

THE VOID BETWEEN MOLECULAR MODELS AND NORMAL VARIATION

How can the extensive knowledge that has been accumulated about the molecular nature of gene action and the many forms of mental retardation associated with single gene and chromosome defects help in unraveling the mystery of normal intellectual variation? On this subject, those behavioral and human geneticists who prefer mechanistic models become understandably vague. They can offer only the hope that future knowledge will provide full accounts of the mechanisms underlying normal intelligence and hence variations in the normal range. One hope is that a few of the major genes might be found to account for a major portion of the variability in intelligence. Even though hundreds of gene loci may be involved in the program for normal intelligence, perhaps only two or three control half or more of the phenotypic variation. The normal distribution of quantitative traits need not depend on small contributions of many genes; in fact, three or four loci without complete dominance will generate a nicely Gaussian curve of

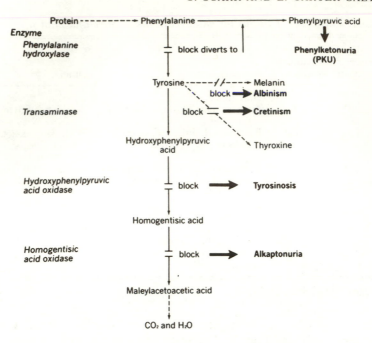

Figure 13.3.   Genetic blocks in the metabolism of phenylalanine. (From *Heredity, Evolution, and Society,* 2nd ed. by I. Michael Lerner and William J. Libby [San Francisco: W. H. Freeman and Co.] Copyright © 1976. Reprinted by permission.)

phenotypes, as shown in Figure 13.4. The search for major genes is an active area of research; with the development of linkage studies and pedigrees, it is hoped that specific gene loci can be located that make the largest contributions to intellectual variation. The next section will examine critically that line of research. We express strongly negative opinions about the mechanistic model; readers may well disagree.

ARGUMENTS FOR POPULATION GENETIC MODELS

Recently, Andrew Pakstis, a graduate student with Scarr at the University of Minnesota, discovered several important linkages between genetic blood group markers and skin color reflectance. The blood group markers are independently segregating, single genes, located on 3 of the 60 or so chromosome segments that make up the new combination of genetic material that children receive from their parents. Evidently, three of the four to six genes for skin color are located on the same chromosome segments as three of the blood group markers. We know this to be the case, because siblings who have the same blood group genes on these segments also have more similar skin color than do brothers and sisters who have different blood group markers. Our statistical procedures show that these results would occur by chance only one in several million trials.

What are we to make of these results? It seems probable that three of the genes that code for metabolic processes leading to the production of melanin in skin

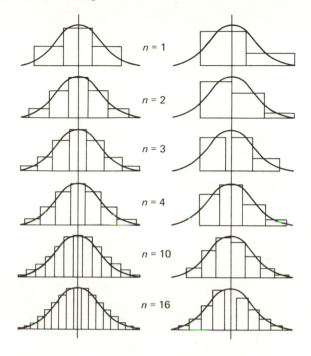

Figure 13.4. Gradual approximation to normal curve of phenotypes controlled by n pairs of genes: *left,* no dominance; *right,* complete dominance for all genes. (Adapted from *Animal breeding plans* by J. L. Lusk [Ames, Iowa: Iowa State College Press], 1945.)

cells have been found. Most geneticists, and indeed most other scientists, would mentally model the gene action from the DNA to the melanin in a linear, causal chain, with each step in the sequence permitting the occurrence of the subsequent steps, given the presence of appropriate enzymes at each step. In fact we already have a well-detailed metabolic pathway for one – perhaps, the major – pathway for the production of melanin, as shown in Figure 13.3. More important, the idea that specific genes can be identified does not strike us as outlandish.

In addition, our analysis has identified two major genes for abstract reasoning. A linear causal chain for the production of abstract reasoning abilities was hastily rejected, of course, because many environmental events have important effects on the development of abstract reasoning abilities from the earliest years to adolescence, when we measured them. Authorities in the field, however, have explicitly denounced the idea of genes directly influencing behavior. The accepted account for the relation between gene action and behavioral development was summarized by Delbert Thiessen (1972, p. 87).

The lengthy, often tortuous, path from DNA specificity to metabolic synchrony explains why behavior must be considered a pleiotropic reflection of physiological processes. Gene influence in behavior is always indirect. Hence the regulatory process of a behavior can be assigned to structural and physiological consequences of gene action and developmental canalization. The blueprint for behavior may be a heritable characteristic of DNA, but its ultimate architecture is a problem for biochemistry and physiology. Explaining gene-behavior relations entails knowing every aspect of the developmental pattern: its inception, its relation to the environment, its biochemical individuality, and its adaptiveness.

The advice of the experts is to apply a Mendelian, linear, causal model to the gene action that produces melanin (and single gene mental defects) and to reject that same model for normal abstract reasoning. Note, however, that Thiessen retains a commitment to explaining causally the genetic architecture of behavior, even if the causal sequence is fraught with developmental uncertainties.

Our argument is that in neither the case of skin color nor of abstract reasoning is a mechanistic model appropriate to account for the phenotypes we observe. Mechanistic models are hopelessly reductionist and will not "explain" human behavior or any other complex phenotype. Furthermore, they are misleading in their emphasis on efficient or proximal causes.

THE SCHIZOPHRENIA OF GENETICS

In genetics, as in other sciences, the natural-science model is the dominant force. Molecular models of gene action pathways is to genetics as mechanics is to physics. The gene action pathway illustrated in Figure 13.3 is an example of the mechanistic model in genetics. Parallel to mechanistic models, however, are the statistical models of evolutionary biology, with their manifestations in ethology, behavior genetics, and population genetics. Darwinian models are probabilistic and in that sense are indeterminant on the level of individual organisms. The level of analysis is a breeding population, whose members are more likely to mate, reproduce, live, or die within that population than within others. The essential evolutionary concepts, variation and selection, refer to differences among individuals, and selection is said by most authorities to act primarily at an individual level. Individuals are merely temporary receptacles for the gene pool; the level of interest is that aggregate of interbreeding individuals called the population.

The levels of analysis in molecular and population branches of genetics are entirely different, as are the methods. In addition, the emphases in their explanatory models are at variance, to say the least. It is not surprising that a sociological look at genetics as a field reveals that molecular geneticists talk to and publish with cell biologists and biochemists, whereas evolutionary biologists communicate with demographers and the few behavioral scientists who will listen. The Animal Behavior Society and the Society for the Study of Social Biology represent this nexus of population analysts. Developmental geneticists talk to pediatricians and physiologists but rarely to those concerned with human behavioral development.

Mather (1971) described in uncritical terms the contrast between Mendelian interest in deterministic genetic models and biometrical (or population) genetic concerns with probabilistic models of genetic variation in populations.

The Mendelian approach depends on the successful recognition of clearly distinguishable phenotypic classes from which the relevant genetical constitution can be inferred. It is at its most powerful when there is a one-to-one correspondence of phenotype and genotype, though some ambiguity of the relationship, as when complete dominance results in the heterozygote and one homozygote having the same phenotype, is acceptable [p. 351]. . . . The biometrical approach is from a different direction starting with the character rather than the individual determinant. It makes no requirement that the determinants be traceable individually in either transmission or action. It seeks to measure *variation* in a character and then, by comparing individuals and families of varying relationship, to *partition* the differences observed into fractions ascribable to the various genetical (or for that matter non-genetical) phenomena. [P. 352]

Mather does not warn us fully of the uncertainties in the pathways from genes to the characteristic of interest, even when there is "one-to-one correspondence of phenotype and genotype." Take, for example, the well-known case of mental retardation resulting, it is said, from the absence of the enzyme phenylalanine hydroxylase in the presence of the protein phenylalanine, ingested in many foods. This is the same pathway illustrated in Figure 13.3. Is there a one-to-one correspondence between genotype and phenotype for the recessive homozygote? Of course not; the distribution of intellectual attainment among children with PKU, treated or untreated, is considerable. Although untreated children are severely retarded, *on the average,* individuals vary from unmeasurably low IQ levels to dull normal, a range of 60 to 80 points! Yet, all have the same DNA sequence that fails to code for the enzyme to metabolize phenylalanine. Somewhere, at the cellular level, at the more general physiological levels, and at the level of organism–environmental transactions there are uncertainties in the development of the phenotype. The "expression" of PKU varies among individuals in a probability distribution.

Now, let us turn to the effects of diet on the "expression" of PKU. As popularly understood, the virtual elimination of phenylalanine from the diet of infants and young children without the enzyme phenylalanine hydroxylase prevents mental retardation. Does this mean that all treated children develop the same intellectual level? Of course not. There is, on the average, a beneficial effect of reduced phenylalanine on the intellectual development of PKU children, but individual IQs vary from moderately retarded to bright average, again a range of more than 60 IQ points. We are not referring here to the ontogenetic effects of diet administered at earlier and later periods of infancy – surely an earlier diet regimen is more beneficial than a later one – but to the variability among children who all received the diet from the first months of life.

Now, let us examine the notion of dominance and recessivity as Mather describes it. The heterozygotes, in the case of PKU, are the carrier parents, whose intellectual distribution is normal, varying from retarded to superior. The average IQ level is like that of the dominant homozygote, the normal population. In other words, there is what Mather calls complete dominance in PKU. (See Bessman, Williamson, & Koch, 1978, for a study of carriers whose IQ levels are 10 points lower than those of noncarrier siblings.)

Unfortunately, that satisfyingly simple, mechanistic view applies only at the behavioral level of analysis. An examination of the level of phenylalanine hydroxylase activity in the heterozygote shows that it is *midway* between the two homozygotes. When loaded with phenylalanine, the heterozygote metabolizes the protein at a rate about half of that of the normal homozygotes. This convenient difference between normals and carriers enables carriers to be detected and thus counseled if they want to be parents. What does this fact do to the notion of "complete dominance"? The idea of dominance and recessivity depends entirely on the level of analysis of the phenotype, and therefore it is impossible to speak of a one-to-one correspondence between genotype and phenotype. In addition, of course, heterozygote carriers vary in their enzyme activity, from nearly normal to nearly defective levels. So it is with all known genetic defects: The variability among those identically afflicted at the single locus is considerable.

There are very many other examples of the points illustrated by PKU. Down's syndrome children, with an extra Chromosome 21, are far more alert, function at much higher levels of personal care, and communicate far better with others when they are reared by affectionate caretakers, rather than impersonal custodians. Black Africans have lower rates of hypertension under the dietary and stress conditions of village than of urban life. To return to the example of skin color, sunlight, hormones associated with age and gender, and probably diet, all affect the degree to which melanin is produced in the skin cells. Women are paler than men on the average, and people darken after puberty. Clearly, some genotypes produce more melanin than others under the same exposure to sunlight. Vary the exposure to sunlight, however, and you will discover that some genotypes who were *paler* phenotypes than others under *lower* exposure to sunlight are now *darker* than others under higher levels of sunlight. They have a greater *responsiveness* to the sunlight and produce melanin at rates that vary more directly with exposure. Others produce little melanin regardless of exposure levels. This homely example points to a more profound objection to mechanistic models of gene action.

To wit, the mechanistic notion of a one-to-one correspondence between genotype and phenotype is largely a myth, fashioned from models for the blood and serum proteins, in which the relationship between genotype and phenotype seems *not* to be vulnerable to interventions from other genes or from environments at any level. As is often the case with perfect models, they have very limited applicability. For intellectual phenotypes in the normal range, the relationship between genotype and phenotype can be only very partially explained by mechanistic models of gene action.

FUDGE FACTORS

Molecular genetics, like all sciences, has "fudge factors" to account for phenotypic variability. "Penetrance," "expression," and "buffering" are concepts invoked to explain (?) why the same gene, coding for the same disorder, fails to produce identical phenotypes. All of these concepts attempt to account for the *probabilistic* relationship between genotype and phenotype. Such concepts are needed because the mechanistic model invoked to link gene action to phenotype is a reductionist one. By reducing the level of analysis, both methodological and explanatory, to gene action, such models assert a form of determinism that excludes so many possible, intervening events that they are largely indeterminant when applied to phenotypic variability in the real world.

The disadvantages of mechanistic models in psychology and behavior genetics may far outweigh their explanatory assets. Mechanistic models are not now, and never will be, in our view, preferable to probabilistic models to account for the genetic determination of abstract reasoning, skin color, or mental retardation associated with PKU. Such models "work" only under conditions in which all other possible effects on phenotypic development are held constant, as they never are in the real world. An explanation of the variation that exists in vivo in situ requires probabilistic models with greatly lessened generality. *Local conditions –*

the particular combinations of events that affect development – and the *time frame* of effects – the ontogenetic time during which the phenotype develops and is susceptible to change – both limit the applicability of mechanistic models to explain the relationship of genotype to phenotype.

Linear causal models that begin with the gene and proceed directly to the phenotype – whether physical or behavioral – explain *some* of the variance among people's observable traits. We do not deny the results of Pakstis's linkage study. Chromosomes have material reality, and on several of those tangible chromosome segments are located DNA sequences that affect the development of skin color and abstract reasoning (McKusick & Ruddle, 1977). Mechanistic models, however, do not emphasize the most important facts about the relationship of genotype to phenotype: *that developmental environments shape phenotypic development in such ways as to render that relationship entirely probabilistic and not determinant, within even our wildest dreams of specifying all of the events that shape (intellectual) development.* Even if one knows the genotype, as in simple Mendelian disorders, such as PKU, the genetic background of individuals and their particular developmental histories will so alter the expression of the single gene as to make population thinking preferable even here. In the case of normal intellectual variation, there is little hope that we will ever know the genotype in a mechanistic sense. Even if the gene action pathways for the hundreds of loci were known, and the systematic interactions among the loci known, the relationship between genotype and phenotype would still be rendered indeterminant for individuals by idiosyncratic genetic and environmental events.

Contrary to the claims of Feldman and Lewontin (1975), Monod (1971), and many others, the most fruitful questions about the nature of genetic and environmental differences in intelligence are asked and answered at a population level. The question To what extent are existing intellectual differences among individuals due to genetic and to what extent to current environmental differences in a specified population? is scientifically important and has many possible implications for the design of environmental programs to enhance people's lives (see DeFries, Vandenberg & McClearn, 1976; R. Nichols, 1978; Scarr & Weinberg, 1978; and Willerman, 1979, for a variety of opinions on this matter). Questions about individual variability in normal intelligence at a mechanistic level of determinism have not been fruitful and do not promise to become so.

GENETIC FIXITY

A great danger in the application of mechanistic linear models to the genetic study of behavior is that they lead to erroneous ideas about the *fixity* of genetic effects. They permit malleability in the development of the phenotype only incidentally, as residual, unexplained error.

As Paul Weiss (1969, pp. 33–34) so eloquently said about genetic determination:

The term "genetically determined" means three different things to three different groups of people: (1) the broad-gauged student of genetics, who is thoroughly familiar with the underlying facts and uses the term simply as a shorthand label to designate unequivocal relations between certain genes and certain "characters" of an organism; (2) scientists in various other branches who are not familiar with the actual content of the term and accept it literally in its verbal symbolism; and (3) the public at large, to whom the term frequently imparts a fatalistic outlook on life, frustrating in its hopelessness, of an inexorably pre-set existence and fixed course towards a pre-ordained destiny.

By contrast, probabilistic models of development and of population dynamics may include mechanistic parts, where applicable, in the larger theory of change. In most evolutionary accounts, however, little emphasis is put on efficient and proximal causes. Rather, evolutionary changes are interpreted in terms of reproductive fitness and adaptation, final causes. In Aristotelian logic, final causes are reasons or goals for a particular adaptation. Mechanistic models emphasize what Aristotle called efficient causes, which are the proximal, immediate antecedents for an event. This difference in emphasis between mechanistic and probabilistic models has been the source of a great deal of the anguish about sociobiology. The idea of human behavioral adaptations having evolved, genetic bases that limit variability and bias learning have been interpreted within the mechanistic model of efficient causes to mean that human behavior is on a "fixed course towards a pre-ordained destiny," to quote Paul Weiss.

"Environmentalists sometimes misunderstand the very implications of population genetics, thinking that heredity would imply 'like class begets like class.' Probably the opposite is true. Only very strong social and environmental forces can perpetuate an artificial class; heredity does not" (Li, 1971, p. 172). Li has presented a simple but comprehensive polygenic model for intelligence that explains parent–child regression, variability within families, and the other phenomena observed for phenotypic IQ. The most important single consequence of the genetic model is that the offspring of any given class of parents will be scattered in various classes; conversely, the parents of any given class of offspring will have come from various classes. This effect is shown in Figure 13.5. Parents at the high and low *extremes* of the distribution contribute offspring primarily to the upper or the lower *halves* of the distributions whereas parents in the middle of the distribution contribute children to all classes in the distribution. On the average, the children will have less extreme scores than their parents, but the total distribution of phenotypic IQ will remain relatively constant from one generation to another (unless selective forces or radical environmental changes intervene).

To the redistribution of offspring from parental to offspring classes in each generation, Li adds the Markov property of populations: "The properties of an individual depend upon the state (in this case, genotype) in which he finds himself and not upon the state from which he is derived. A state is a state; it has no memory" (p. 173). Thus, the distant descendants of Jean Bernoulli are distributed into the various classes of mathematical ability in exactly the same way as the distant descendants of one whose mathematical ability was subnormal. Family members who are as much as six to eight generations apart are practically unrelated even though they retain the same family name.

Whether present-day family groups and social classes are genetically artificial groups is debatable (Eckland, 1979; Herrnstein, 1971; Scarr & Weinberg, 1978), because one assumption of Li's model is random mating, which is violated by an IQ correlation of about .40 between parents. Even under conditions of high assortative mating, however, there is considerable regression of offspring scores toward the population mean and the majority of IQ variation is found among the offspring of the same parents. Fear not! The population may be relatively stable but individual determinism is not yet upon us.

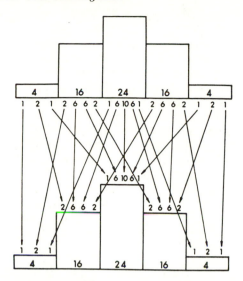

Figure 13.5. The distributions of offspring and parents in five phenotypic classes in a random mating population. (From "A Tale of Two Thermos Bottles: Properties of a Genetic Model for Human Intelligence" by C. C. Li, in R. Camcro [Ed.], *Intelligence: Genetics and Environmental Influences* [New York: Grune & Stratton, 1971]. Reprinted by permission.)

13.3.   ANALYSES OF VARIATION IN HUMAN INTELLIGENCE

To analyze variation at a population level, one must estimate the magnitude of genetic and environmental variances in a given interbreeding group. Both genetic and environmental variances may be analyzed into several components, although not without some difficult and questionable assumptions.

INDIVIDUAL VARIATION IN A POPULATION

The relative contributions of genetic and environmental differences to phenotypic diversity within a population depend upon six major parameters: (a) range of genotypes, (b) range of environments, (c) favorableness of genotypes, (d) favorableness of environments, (e) covariance of genotypes and environments, and (f) interactions of genotypes and environments. The range of genotypes and environments can independently and together affect the total variance of a behavioral, polygenic train in a population. The mean favorableness of genotypes and environments can independently and together affect the mean values of phenotypes.

Two separate problems are involved in understanding the effects of mean favorableness and ranges of genotypes in a population: first, the frequency of genes, and second, the distribution of genes among the genotypes. Gene frequencies are affected by two principal processes: differential reproduction, or *natural selection,* and *sampling errors.* Genotype frequencies are affected by *assortative mating.* Two populations (or two generations of the same population) may have equal gene frequencies but different genotype frequencies if assortative mating for a behavioral trait is greater in one population than in the other.

Natural selection.   Changing environmental conditions, such as the introduction of more complex technology, may affect the rate of reproduction in different segments of the IQ distribution in a generation. We know, for example, that severely mentally retarded persons in the contemporary white populations of Europe and the United States do not reproduce as frequently as those who can hold jobs and maintain independent adult lives (Bajema, 1968; Higgins, Reed, & Reed, 1962). Being severely retarded renders one less likely to be chosen as a mate and less likely to produce progeny for the next generation. If one segment of the phenotypic IQ range has been strongly and consistently selected against, as severely mentally retarded persons are in contemporary industrial populations, then the range and favorableness of the total gene distribution will be slowly changed. If, in another population, high phenotypic IQ were disadvantageous for mate selection and reproduction, then the genic distribution would be reduced at that end. It does not seem likely that high phenotypic IQ has ever been strongly selected against within a population.

Sampling.   Gene frequencies can also be affected by genetic drift, or random sampling error. Not every allele at every gene locus is equally sampled in every generation through reproduction. Rare genes, especially, may disappear through failure to be passed on to the next generation, and the frequencies of other alleles may be randomly increased or decreased from generation to generation.

   A special case of restriction in genic range is nonrandom sampling from a larger gene pool in the formation of a smaller breeding group. If, for example, an above-median sample from the IQ group migrated to a distant locale and bred primarily among themselves, the gene frequencies within the migrant group might eventually vary considerably from those of the nonmigrant group, all other things being equal.

Assortative mating.   The distribution of genes in genotypic classes within a population can vary because of assortative mating. To the extent that "likes" marry "likes," genetic variability is decreased within families and increased between families. Assortative mating for IQ also increases the standard deviation of IQ scores within the total (white) population by increasing the frequency of extremely high and extremely low genotypes for phenotypic IQ. On a random mating basis, the probability of producing extreme genotypes is greatly reduced because extreme parental genotypes are unlikely to find each other by chance. The sheer frequency of middle-range genotypes makes an average mate the most likely random choice of an extreme genotype for both high and low IQ. The offspring of such matings will tend to be closer to the population mean than will the offspring of extreme parental combinations because children's IQ values are distributed around the mean parental value (with some regression toward the population mean). The phenotypic distribution under conditions of random mating will tend to have a leptokurtic shape with a large modal class and low total variance.

The range of environments within a population can also affect phenotypic variability. Uniform environments can restrict phenotypic diversity by eliminating a major source of variation. Because environments can be observed and manipulated, many studies on infrahuman populations demonstrate the restriction of variability through uniform environments (Manosevitz, Lindzey, & Thiessen, 1969).

Far more important, however, for the present discussion is the favorableness of the environment. Environments that do not support the development of a trait can greatly alter the mean value of the trait. If unfavorable environments are common to all or most members of a population, then the phenotypic variance of the population can be slightly reduced and the mean value can be drastically lowered. The most likely effects of very suppressive environments are that they lower the mean of the population, decrease phenotypic variability, and consequently reduce the correlation between genotype and phenotype (Henderson, 1970; Scarr-Salapatek, 1971b). A contrast can be made between uniform environments that support the development of a particular behavior and uniform environments that are suppressive and not supportive of optimal development (P. L. Nichols, 1970). Uniform environments of a good quality may reduce total variability and raise the mean of the population.

The ranges of genotypes and environments and the favorableness of the environment control a large portion of the total phenotypic variance in IQ. The two additional factors, covariance and interaction, are probably less important (Jinks & Fulker, 1970), at least within the white North American and European populations.

COVARIATION

Covariation between genotypes and environments is expressed as a correlation between certain genotypic characteristics and certain environmental features that affect phenotypic outcome; for example, the covariance between the IQs of children of bright parents, which is likely to be higher than average, and the educationally advantaged environment offered by those same parents to their bright children. Retarded parents, on the other hand, may have less bright children under any environmental circumstances but also may supply those children with educationally deprived environments. Covariation between genotype and environment may also depend upon the genotype and the kind of response it evokes from the environment. If bright children receive continual reward for their educationally superior performance while duller children receive fewer rewards, environmental rewards can be said to covary with IQ. Finally, children build their own niches, selecting those aspects of the environment that are most compatible with their phenotypes, which include their genotypes (Plomin, DeFries, & Loehlin, 1977).

INTERACTION

Covariance is sometimes confused with *interaction*, but they are quite different terms. When psychologists speak of genetic–environment interaction, they are usually referring to the reciprocal relationship that exists between an organism and its surrounding. The organism brings to the situation a set of characteristics that affect the environment, which in turn affects the further development of the organism and vice versa. This is not what quantitative geneticists mean by interaction. The psychologists' term would better be *transaction* between organism and environment, because the statistical term *genetic–environment interaction* refers to the *differential* effects of various organism–environment transactions on development.

Behavioral geneticists, whose experimental work is primarily with mouse strains and drosophila, often find genotype–environmental interactions of considerable importance. The differential response of two or more genotypes to two or more environments is interaction. In studies of animal learning, where genotypes and environmental conditions can be manipulated, so-called maze-dull rats, who were bred for poor performance in Tryon's mazes, were shown to perform as well as so-called maze-bright rats when given enriched environments (Cooper & Zubek, 1958) and when given distributed rather than massed practice (McGaugh, Jennings, & Thompson, 1962).

Studies of genotype–environment interaction in human populations are quite limited. Biometrical methods that include an analysis for interaction have failed to show any substantial variance attributable to nonlinear effects on human intelligence (Erlenmeyer-Kimling, 1972; Jinks & Fulker, 1970). This is not to say that genotype–environment interaction may not account for some portion of the variance in IQ scores in other populations or in other segments of white populations (e.g., the disadvantaged).

HERITABILITY

Heritability is a summary statement of the proportion of the total phenotypic variance that is due to additive genetic variance (narrow heritability) or to total genetic variance (broad heritability). Heritability (h^2) is a *population statistic*, not a property of a trait (Fuller & Thompson, 1978). Estimates of h^2 differ from population to population as genetic and environmental variances change as proportions of the total variance. (For the calculation of differed kinds of heritability estimates, see Falconer, 1960.)

The six parameters of individual variation within a population (ranges and favorableness of genotypes and environments, covariation, and interactions) discussed here, are the major contributors to the total phenotypic variance in any population. The proportions of genetic variance and environmental variance may well vary from one population to another depending upon the ranges and favorableness of the two sets of variables, their covariances, and their interactions. The variance terms and heritability statistics are frequently used in twin and family studies to estimate the relative importance of genetic and environmental differences to account for phenotypic IQ differences.

METHODS OF ANALYSIS FOR TWIN AND FAMILY STUDIES

The simplest and most defensible method of analysis of twin and family studies is to calculate a statistical measure of resemblance between pairs of persons in two sets who differ in their degrees of genetic and/or environmental relatedness, and stop there. No one objects to the calculation of regressions coefficients for child IQ on parental IQ or the use of intraclass correlations for twins and siblings. These are basic measures of the degree to which pairs of individuals in various relationships resemble each other, compared with randomly paired people. One may even test for the significance of the difference between coefficients.

Comparisons of coefficients of resemblance between relatives of different degrees or persons of the same genetic relatedness reared in environments with greater or lesser similarity are based on some assumptions that legitimate the comparison. The major assumption in comparisons of identical (MZ) and fraternal (DZ) twins is that the environments of MZs do not create more similarities than those of DZs. This assumption has been tested in several ways and found to be satisfactory, as will be reviewed in a later section. In the case of comparisons of adopted and biologically related children, a similar objection can be raised to the lack of comparability of environmental variances are similar for the two kinds of relatives. Again this assumption has been tested and found satisfactory (Scarr, Scarf, & Weinberg, 1980).

From the comparison of coefficients of resemblance for persons of different degrees of relatedness, one can calculate a "heritability" coefficient. The assumptions at this stage are many and difficult to defend. Is there parental assortative mating, which decreases the genetic variance within families for DZ twins and siblings and increases their genetic resemblance? What can one assume about the role of gene–environment correlation and interaction (nonlinear type) in phenotypic resemblance? What about broad "heritability" versus narrow "heritability"; the former can be calculated, with certain assumptions, from a variety of family data, and the latter can be calculated from parent–child data, again with certain assumptions. Rather than detail here the many assumptions and objections to "heritability" analyses, we refer the reader to sources listed in the next section.

BIOMETRICAL ANALYSIS

The next, large step in complex analysis of kinship data is the application of models of several or many degrees of simultaneous relationship. We are not experts on biometrical methods. For mathematically sophisticated treatments of this extensive literature, the reader is referred to articles by the Birmingham group (Eaves, 1975, 1976; Eaves et al., 1977; Jinks & Fulker, 1970; Martin, 1975; Martin et al., 1978), the Hawaii group (Morton & Rao, 1977), the North Carolina group (Elson & Stewart, 1971; Haseman & Elston, 1970), and the Stanford group (Cavalli-Sforza & Feldman, 1973, 1977). One group of economists (Taubman, Behrman, & Wales, 1978) is also involved in similar analyses of twin data. Telling criticisms of the biometrical enterprise have been made by Goldberger (1975, 1978).

Jencks (1972) was the first, to our knowledge, to apply Sewell Wright's path models to the complement of family and twin data sets from U.S. studies. Since that time, there has been considerable interest in expanding the application of path models to the study of population variation. Although Jencks misspecified a parameter in his model (Loehlin, Lindzey, & Spuhler, 1975), the method is increasingly used. An example of a path model of parent–child resemblance is given in Figure 13.6.

The additive genotypes for two phenotypes of the parent (A_x and A_y) lead to those of the children (A_{x_o} and A_{y_o}). In this model, the parent phenotypes do not directly affect the child's phenotypes, nor do the environments of the parents directly affect the child's environments or phenotypes. Do you agree with these assumptions? If not, you may draw a different model, and so it goes. The authors

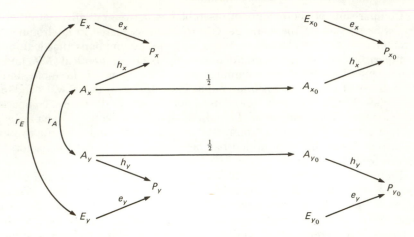

Figure 13.6.   Path diagram of bivariate resemblance between parental phenotypes (P_x and P_y) and offspring phenotypes (P_{x_0} and P_{y_0}). (From "Genetic correlations, Environmental Correlations, and Behavior" by J. C. DeFries, A. R. Kuse, & S. G. Vandenberg, in J. R. Royce [Ed.], *Theoretical Advances in Behavior Genetics* [Alphen aan den Rijn, The Netherlands: Sythoff and Woodhoff, 1979]. Reprinted by permission.)

suggest that this model is applicable to studies in which the parents do not provide the rearing environment. The objections that Goldberger raises with the biometrical approach are that the assumptions that must be made are largely indefensible and that the statistical manipulations of the data exaggerate the already large statistical errors in twin and family correlations. By relaxing any of the assumptions, or by making others, Goldberger has shown that quite different results can be obtained. We do not care to enter this fray.

In simple lay language, biometrical models attempt to estimate genetic and environmental parameters from sets of family and twin data, primarily intelligence tests, by making assumptions about the nature of the genetic and environmental effects (e.g., Is there gene–environment correlation that acts from parental phenotype to child phenotype or from parental genotype to child phenotype?). With simultaneous equations and matrix algebra, they solve for the best fits to the available data. Unfortunately, the data are not, as a group, robust enough to withstand extensive manipulations without yielding solutions that can be seriously challenged by doubters, nor are the models defensible without recourse to the data.

Lewontin (1974a) tackled Morton (1974) and his colleagues (Rao, Morton, & Yee, 1974), and by implication many other biometricians, for an alleged confusion of the analysis of variance and the analysis of causes. The latter, Lewontin says, is what we "really" want to know about genetic effects on human development, because only by a knowledge of the mechanisms underlying genetic effects can we arrive at "correct schemes for environmental modification and intervention" (p. 409). Analysis of the variation in a population cannot do this, because "its results are a unique function of the present distribution of environment and genotype" (p. 409). Only where there is perfect or nearly perfect additivity between genotypic and environmental effects, he says, can the analysis of variance estimate functional relationships between genotypes and environments. Lewontin doubts that linear combinations of gene and environmental effects are the rule and presents many examples of interactions, both hypothetical and from rates of survival for drosophila larvae.

One must ask how likely it is that genotype–environment interactions account for a major portion of the variance in human intelligence. Erlenmeyer-Kimling (1972) reviewed the scanty literature on possible interaction effects of genes and environments on human intelligence and found no evidence. Neither have there been good methods for testing for interaction effects. The issue is whether or not it is plausible that, with the exception of extreme deprivation or extreme over-stimulation (which could be defined in sensory and affective terms), some children develop better phenotypes under impoverished than under enriched environments, whereas others profit more from sensory and affectively rich than from poor environments?

In our view, those who propose that genotype–environment interactions are major determinants of intellectual variation in populations are more interested in putting roadblocks in the way of studies of normal human variation than in clarifying the scientific issues. It is not accidental that they call upon a mechanistic model for "real" understanding of human variation and deny the legitimacy of statistical models, which are feasible approaches to understanding the individual differences that exist in a population at the present time. In fact, Lewontin confuses the individual level of analysis, for which mechanistic studies are appropriate, with the population level of analysis, for which analysis of variation is the appropriate model. For social policy planning of intervention programs, the latter may, in fact, be more important in deciding whether and how to distribute *known* resources. We agree that knowledge of the mechanisms by which genetic effects are translated into phenotypic behaviors would be handy in designing intervention programs, but treatment of the mentally ill and the mentally retarded has proceeded with reasonably good effects without benefit of mechanistic knowledge in most cases. Life goes on even without complete information.

Many have argued that knowledge of sources of variation in a population is irrelevant to social policy (see Scarr-Salapatek, 1971a; Jensen, 1973b). The empirical, trial-and-error approach would be necessary in any case to test the effects of an intervention. Let us say here that we do not agree and will deal with this issue in the concluding section of the chapter.

13.4. TWIN AND FAMILY STUDIES

INTRODUCTION

In this section we will present the heart of the research on genetic differences in normal intelligence. Necessarily, the many studies will be condensed into fewer paragraphs, beginning with studies of familial mental retardation, followed by a review of twin and family studies of normal intelligence. Because of the recent surge in studies of adoptive families, particular attention will be given to these remarkable new data.

MENTAL RETARDATION: A POPULATION VIEW

Assuming that 2% of the general population is retarded, Reed and Anderson (1973) estimated that 17% of the retarded children have a retarded parent. If no

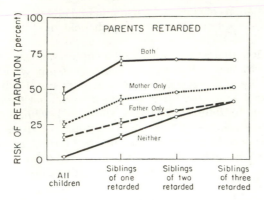

Figure 13.7.   Risk of mental retardation among offspring, by presence or absence of retardation in parents and siblings. The vertical bars for the first two points in each line indicate ±1 standard error. The standard errors for the remaining points are larger but are difficult to estimate. (From "Genetics and Intelligence" by V. E. Anderson, in J. Wortis [Ed.], *Mental Retardation and Developmental Disabilities: An Annual Review*, Vol. 6 [New York: Brunner/Mazel, 1974]. Reprinted by permission.)

retarded persons were to reproduce, the frequency of retardation in the next generation would drop to 1.7%. If the retarded were to reproduce at the same rate as the general population, retardation would rise to 2.2% and 26% of the retarded children would have a retarded parent.

The increased risk of retardation in families is graphically shown in Figure 13.7. The risk of familial mental retardation rises from 2% for all children without retarded parents or siblings to more than 70% when both parents are retarded and there is at least one retarded sibling. These data are drawn from the Reed and Reed (1965) study of some 80,000 individuals sampled in the state of Minnesota who were the descendants (mostly distant) or retardates institutionalized in the early years of this century.

It has not been possible to differentiate a major gene model from a polygenic one in the determination of familial mental retardation. Such a discrimination depends upon the rarity of the trait, and mental retardation is too common to make the choice among models possible (Anderson, 1974, p. 33). Pauls (1972) studied nearly 6,000 individuals, none of whose parents was retarded, and calculated a heritability estimate for retardation of .62, very close to contemporary estimates for intelligence in general. Analysis of the family data produced no evidence that major genes accounted for a major part of the retardation.

Quantitative genetic theory

As Anderson indicated in his review (1974), several features of the literature on mental retardation are relevant to a quantitative genetic theory: First, the frequency of retardation is higher among males; second, retarded females are more likely to reproduce than retarded males; third, the risk of retardation is higher among the offspring of female than male retardates. In summary, the risk of retardation is highest among the sons of affected mothers and lowest among the daughters of affected fathers. As Anderson indicates, these results are congruent with a hypothesis that familial mental retardation results from multigenes with a sex-modified threshold, which predicts that when a trait is more common among males, the least risk will be for the female relatives of retarded males. Because more severely affected females than males reproduce, the offspring of retarded mothers have a higher rate of retardation than the offspring of (less severely) retarded males. The females have, on the average, greater "genetic loading" for retardation, and therefore part of the maternal effect for retardation may be genetic. Another part may be the rearing environment, which is more related to the mother's mental status than the father's.

Familial versus clinical retardation

Although there are overlapping or indistinct boundaries between categories, most workers in the field of retardation hold that there are two broad categories of retarded individuals: the lower-grade mental defectives with major chromosome, genetic, or traumatic disabilities, and the higher grade, "familial" retardates, without histories of specific etiology or known defect, who just have much lower than average IQ and social competencies. Roberts (1952) found that the siblings of severely mentally retarded children are more likely to have normal IQ scores than are the siblings of familial mental retardates. If the causes of severe defects are rare chromosomal single gene and environmental events, then the sibs are unlikely to be affected; if the higher-grade mental retardates are the lower end of the normal curve of polygenic inheritance for intelligence, then their sibs are likely to have lower IQs as well.

Kamin (1974, pp. 136–141) questioned the methods of the Roberts study and ridiculed the results. To reexamine Roberts's hypotheses with new data, Johnson, Ahern, and Johnson (1976) looked at the siblings and parents of 289 retarded probands, reported by Reed and Reed (1965). Forty-seven of the probands had no IQ score or no sibling; data on the 242 remaining probands and their siblings are presented in Table 13.2.

It is clear from the table that higher-grade retardates ($X^2 = 26.22$, $p = .001$) have more retarded siblings than lower-grade retardates. Of the siblings of retardates with IQs lower than 40, 21.5% are retarded. Of the siblings of retardates with IQ scores above 40, 31.0% are retarded. Also in keeping with Roberts's results, the siblings of the higher-grade retardates were more likely to be of higher-grade retardation themselves. If severely retarded probands had affected sibs, the sibs were likely to be severely retarded themselves.

The authors suggested that the groups, clinical and familial retardates, were not as clearly divisible as is sometimes suggested, for the severely retarded had some higher-grade retarded sibs. Still, the parents of the retardates with IQ scores below 40 were far less likely to be described occupationally as indigent or unskilled than the parents of higher-grade retardates, thus supporting the notion of familial retardation. The percentage of parents who were themselves retarded also differed between the groups: of the severely retarded probands, 12.7% had two defective parents and 28.8% had one defective parent; of the probands with IQ scores > 40, 22.3% had both parents defective and 33.8% had one defective parent. Interestingly, the defective parents of the severely retarded probands were equally divided between mothers and fathers, whereas the mothers of the higher-grade retardates were more likely to be retarded than the fathers, in keeping with

Table 13.2. *Status of full siblings of Reed and Reed probands by IQ level of probands*

| IQ level of probands[a] | Number of probands[a] | Sibs | | | Total number of sibs | Percentage retarded of retarded normal, and unknown sibs | Number of probands with one or more retarded sibs | Percentage of probands with retarded sibs | Mean IQ of retarded sibs of probands[d] |
		Dead[b]	Retarded	Normal or of unknown ability[c]					
0–19	47	81	34	169	284	16.70	17	36.17	28.21 (N = 19)
20–29	32	57	41	104	202	28.28	14	43.75	34.21 (N = 19)
30–39	31	33	35	127	195	21.60	17	54.84	35.78 (N = 9)
40–49	54	65	77	195	337	28.31	35	64.85	47.56 (N = 18)
50–59	37	40	42	119	201	26.09	21	59.46	58.12 (N = 17)
60–79[e]	41	56	68	106	230	39.08	33	80.49	60.50 (N = 24)
Total	242	332	297	820	1449	26.59[f]	137	56.61[f]	45.32[g]

[a] Only probands with IQ scores and full siblings are included in this table.
[b] Includes recorded miscarriages, stillbirths, infant and neonatal deaths.
[c] Internal evidence (Reed & Reed, 1965, Table 27, p. 39) indicates that persons of unknown ability nearly always are of normal ability, despite the fact that too little is known about them to state that they are of normal ability.
[d] Only sibs with known IQ scores are included.
[e] Only one proband was above IQ 69.
[f] Percent of total population (N = 106).
[g] Mean for total population (N = 106).
Source: Johnson, Ahern, & Johnson (1976).

Table 13.3. *Mean intraclass correlations from twin studies of various traits*

Trait	N of (studies)	M intraclass correlation		Difference $r_{MZ} - r_{DZ}$	
		r_{MZ}	r_{DZ}	M	SD
Ability					
General intelligence	30	.82	.59	.22	.10
Verbal comprehension	27	.78	.59	.19	.14
Number and mathematics	27	.78	.59	.19	.12
Spacial visualization	31	.65	.41	.23	.16
Memory	16	.52	.36	.16	.16
Reasoning	16	.74	.50	.24	.17
Clerical speed and accuracy	15	.70	.47	.22	.15
Verbal fluency	12	.67	.52	.15	.14
Divergent thinking	10	.61	.50	.11	.15
Language achievement	28	.81	.58	.23	.11
Social studies achievement	7	.85	.61	.24	.10
Natural science achievement	14	.79	.64	.15	.13
All abilities	211	.74	.54	.21	.14

Source: R. Nichols (1978), Table 1.

the polygenic theory developed by Anderson (1974), which posits a greater genetic loading for retarded women than men.

TWIN STUDIES OF INTELLIGENCE

Robert Nichols (1978) compiled 211 studies of intelligence and abilities that compare the resemblance of MZ and DZ twins. His results for 1,100 to 4,500 pairs of MZs and a like number of DZs are given in Table 13.3. For general intelligence, the mean correlation for MZ twins, derived from a variety of tests, is .82; for DZ twins, .59. Although the MZ correlation exceeds the DZ coefficient by .22, it is clear that being genetically related and being reared as twins in the same family are potent determinants of individual differences in measured intelligence. From the comparison of MZ and DZ correlations in the 30 studies, one can estimate the broad heritability of IQ in the white U.S. population of adolescents (who made up most of the studies' subjects) as somewhere between .3 and .7, with a most likely value of about .5, given a correction for assortative mating of the parents but no correction for the reliability of the tests. Nichols corrected for the unreliability of measurement and estimated that genetic differences accounted for about .60 to .70 of the IQ variation.

As anyone fond of distributions and sampling theory would have smilingly predicted, the studies summarized by R. Nichols (1978) form a distribution of results. The population of studies of general intelligence and other abilities has means and variances of its own. In Figure 13.8 a dot indicates the results of each study and an arrow points to the weighted mean correlation coefficient for MZ and DZ twins for each measure. As expected, there are some outlying values, and more studies clustered nearer to the middle of the distribution. In these cases, however, there are some unusually low correlation values, outlying by them-

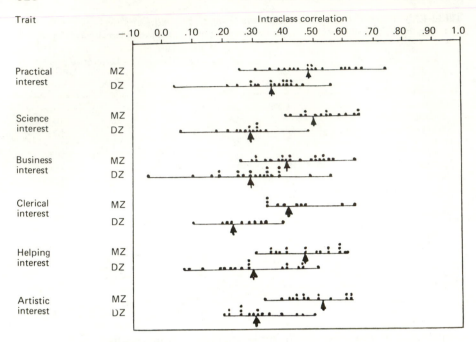

Figure 13.8.   Intraclass correlations from twin studies of various abilities. Correlations obtained in each study for MZ (identical) and DZ (fraternal) twins are indicated by dots; the mean correlation, weighted by the number of cases, is indicated by an arrow below the horizontal line representing the range of correlations for each trait. (From "Twin Studies of Ability, Personality, and Interests" by R. C. Nichols, *Homo*, 1978, *29*, 158–173. Reprinted by permission.)

selves, that raise suspicions about measurement, test administration, sampling restriction, and the like.

Critics of the twin-study method have seized upon the outliers in distributions of studies to raise questions about the overall pattern of results. Kamin (1974), in particular, has made much of equivocal findings from some twin and adoption studies (Kamin, 1981). McAskie and Clarke (1976) use the variance of parent–child study results for the same purpose. It seems to us that a more sophisticated, statistical look at the twin-study results is persuasive evidence for the greater average similarity of MZ than of DZ co-twins on measures of general and specific abilities. The greater similarity of MZ twins is usually interpreted as due to their greater genetic similarity, but that conclusion is based on a critically important assumption: that the environments of MZ twins do not bias their behavioral similarities by their more similar treatment.

Environmental similarity of MZ and DZ twins

Identical twins, it is said by critics of twin studies, are treated more similarly by their parents and others than are fraternal twins; therefore, the usually greater behavioral similarity of MZ twins is due not to their greater genetic relatedness but to the more similar environmental response to their identical appearance

(Kamin, 1974). Three approaches have been taken in testing the effects of greater environmental similarity of MZ than of DZ twins. First, Scarr (1968) and Scarr and Carter-Saltzman (1979) compared the actual intellectual, personality, and physical similarities of twins who were correctly and incorrectly classified as MZ and DZ by themselves, their parents, and others. There appeared to be little bias from the belief in zygocity, as the incorrectly classified MZs and DZs were as similar on most measurements as the correctly classified pairs. On intellectual measures, belief in zygocity had no significant effect on actual similarity. On personality and physical measures, both actual zygocity and belief in zygocity were related to measured similarities. It is hard to imagine that twins grow taller or shorter or have greater or lesser skeletal maturity because someone believes them to be identical or fraternal twins. Thus, we conclude that for personality and physical measures, actual similarity is a basis for the judgment of zygocity, rather than the reverse.

Lytton (1977) has taken a second approach to the issue of environmental similarity between identical and fraternal twins. With extensive observations of the parental response and initiation of interactions with very young twins, Lytton showed that the parents of MZs treat their children more similarly than do the parents of DZs, because the identicals give the parents more similar stimuli to respond to. He observed no difference in parental treatment of MZs and DZs that would create additional similarities or differences to bias comparisons between the types of twins. A third approach to the study of the role of more similar environment for identical than for fraternal twins was developed by Plomin, Willerman, and Loehlin (1976). Their reasoning was as follows: If identical twins are more similar *because* they are treated more similarly, then those identicals who experience more similar environments should be more similar than those identicals who experience less similar environments. Sharing the same room, friends, classrooms, and receiving similar parental treatment, for example, should increase the behavioral similarity of some MZs over that of others. In short, those aspects of environments that differ *between* identical and fraternal co-twins ought to affect the degree of similarity *among* identical twins as well. (Fraternal twins were not used, because some pairs are genetically more similar than others, a confounding factor in any analysis of greater and lesser environmental similarity. To some extent, greater genetic similarity may lead some DZ pairs to select and receive more similar environments than others.) The result of the analysis by Plomin and colleagues of the effect of greater similarities of the environmental factors on MZ and.DZ twins was clear: greater environmental similarity does not inflate actual intellectual or personality similarities among identical twins. Rather, it seems likely that more similar genotypes develop greater behavioral similarity and select more similar environments more often than less similar (e.g., DZ) genotypes. The greater environmental similarity of MZ than of DZ twins is, therefore, primarily a result and not a cause of behavioral similarity.

Results without Sir Cyril Burt

It seems appropriate to mention here the famous review of the literature on genetic differences on intelligence by Erlenmeyer-Kimling and Jarvik (1963). They presented a chart of 52 studies, clearly excluding some of the twin studies with low correlations that R. Nichols (1978) included in his summary and showing the

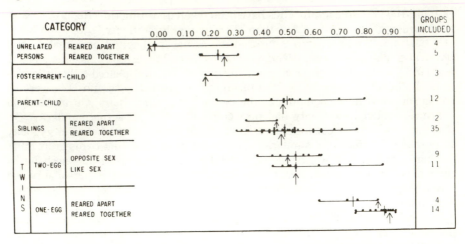

Figure 13.9.   IQ correlations of unrelated persons, first-degree relatives, and twins reared together and apart. Vertical lines indicate median value and arrows indicate values reported by Burt. (From "Burt's IQ Data" by B. Rimland and H. Munsinger, *Science,* 1977, *195,* 246–248. Copyright © 1977 by the American Association for the Advancement of Science. Reprinted by permission.)

median correlations for the various degrees of kinship and rearing closeness. Unfortunately, their chart included data from the "studies" of Sir Cyril Burt, now considered questionable at least, fraudulent at most (Hearnshaw, 1979).

The older, selected studies of genetic differences in measured intelligence supported a conclusion that about 70% of the variance among individuals in the white populations of the United States and Great Britain was due to genetic variation. The omission of Burt's data does little to change that picture, as Rimland and Munsinger (1977) showed in their annotated graph (here Figure 13.9) from Erlenmeyer-Kimling and Jarvik (1963). The regularity of these data and the magnitude of the differences among kinship groups, with some variance due to rearing together, supported a strong genetic hypothesis. More recent data, as will be shown, support a more moderate position on the heritability of general intelligence.

Rowe and Plomin (1978) compared Burt's data with those of Jencks (1972), which were based entirely on U.S. samples. Their data, given in Table 13.4, again support more moderate estimates of heritability than do Burt's data.

Twin family studies

A particularly interesting design for the estimation of genetic and environmental effects on intelligence is the study of the children of identical twins. Suppose that identical twin males marry two unrelated women and each has two children. The children of one are equally related genetically to the co-twin, with whom the children do not live, and are not related at all to the spouse of the co-twin. Thus, these families provide example of parent–child pairs together and in different households (albeit correlated environments). Furthermore, the children of the MZ twins are more than ordinary first cousins; they are half siblings, having

Table 13.4. *A comparison of data from Burt's studies and from other behavior genetic studies*

	Burt's studies[a]		Other behavior genetic studies	
	Correlation	N/pairs	Correlation	N/pairs
MZ together	0.930	95	0.857[b]	526
DZ together	0.537	127	0.534[c]	517
MZ apart	0.841	53	0.741[d]	69
Sibs together	0.525	264	0.545[e]	1671
Unrelated together	0.267	136	0.376[f]	259

Note: MZ = monozygotic twins; DZ = dizygotic twins.
[a]From Burt (1966). The correlations for the group tests, individual tests, and final assessments were converted to z scores, weighted by N, averaged, and converted back to correlations. Jensen (1974, p. 18) noted one misprint in Burt's (1966) Table 2 in which the final assessment correlation was 0.453 instead of 0.534 and the correction was noted in our calculations.
[b]From Jencks (1972), Table A-6, column headed Identical Twins. Correlations from studies on IQ (excluding Burt's data) were converted to Z scores and averaged within each study reported; then the weighted average for all studies was computed and the resultant z score was converted back to a correlation. The data included in this calculation were Holzinger, Otis IQ and Binet IQ; Newman, Freeman, & Holzinger, Stanford–Binet IQ and Otis IQ; Schoenfeldt, Project Talent IQ Composite; Blewett, Thurstone PMA; Eysenck & Prell, Wechsler–Bellevue; and Herman & Hogben, Otis Advanced Group Test.
[c]From Jencks (1972), Table A-6, column headed Fraternal Twins. Same studies as in b above.
[d]From Jencks (1972), Table A-12. Included were Juel–Nielsen, Raven's Progressive Matrices, Wechsler–Bellevue Verbal, and Wechsler–Bellevue Performance; Newman, Freeman, & Holzinger, Stanford–Binet IQ and Otis IQ; and Shields, Non-verbal Intelligence.
[e]From Jencks (1972), Table A-7. Included were Conrad & Jones; Hart; Madsen; McNemar; Outhit; and Hildreth.
[f]From Jencks (1972), Table A-8 (panel 1). Included from panels 1 and 2 were Stanford–Binet data from Freeman, Holzinger, & Mitchell; Leahy; and Skodak; and from panel 1, Burks's Stanford–Binet data.
Source: Rowe & Plomin (1978), Table 1.

genetically the same father and a different mother. The design also provided for the study of ordinary full sibs, spouse correlations, and maternal versus paternal effects, depending upon the gender of the MZ twin pair. Nance and Corey (1976) have proposed models for the analysis of such data, and Rose (1979) has reported initial data from 65 such family constellations for the Wechsler Block Design. The data for Block Design and fingerprint ridge count are given in Table 13.5.

One notable result is that the regression of genetic offspring on genetic parent (whether actual parent or twin uncle/aunt) is only slightly lower when they do not reside in the same household, whereas the regression of offspring on the genetically unrelated spouse of the twin is zero. The twin, sibling, and half-sibling data are all consistent with the parent–child results and heritability estimates in the .4 to .6 range. A comparison of the Block Design and fingerprint ridge count data shows a very similar pattern of family resemblance, with the physical measure being more heritable (an estimated range of .68 to .84). The study of twin families seems to be a very appealing one that will yield more defensible estimates of genetic variance than the study of twins alone.

Another study that incorporates both twins and siblings is the Louisville Twin

Table 13.5. *Regression and correlation analyses of Block Design test scores and fingerprint ridge counts*

	Block Design		Ridge count	
	Coefficient	N	Coefficient	N
Regressions				
Son/daughter on father/mother	.28 ± .04	572	.42 ± .05	564
Nephew/niece on twin uncle/aunt	.23 ± .06	318	.37 ± .05	310
Nephew/niece on spouse uncle/aunt	−.01 ± .06	241	−.06 ± .07	247
Offspring on midparent	.54 ± .07	254	.82 ± .07	254
Correlations				
Monozygotic twins	.68 ± .06	65	.96 ± .03	60
Full siblings	.24 ± .08	297	.36 ± .08	296
Half siblings	.10 ± .12	318	.17 ± .12	310
Father–mother	.06 ± .10	102	.05 ± .10	98

Study (R. S. Wilson, 1977). The twins and one of their siblings were tested at about the age of 8 years with the WISC. The data are shown in Table 13.6. The correlations for siblings are very close to those for DZ twins, with whom they are genetically related as sibs and who are genetically related to each other as ordinary sibs. (Twins were designated A and B, according to the alphabetical order of their legal first names.) Identical twins are far more similar in WISC scores than any of the sibling groups. Wilson concludes, and we agree, that

> The concordance for full-scale IQ and verbal IQ showed no significant change from dizygotic twins to sibling pairs to twin-sibling sets, so the unique experiences of being born and raised as twins did not promote significantly greater similarity in IQ. Nor did the differential experiences of twin versus singleton lead to greater disparities in school-age IQ among the twin-sibling sets. From this perspective, the concordance among age-matched zygotes from the same family was negligibly related to the experiences of being a twin or a singleton. The more potent determinants appeared to be the proportion of shared genes plus the common family environment. [P. 214]

Not only are the full-scale Verbal and Performance scores per se heritable in a range of .5 to .8, but the *pattern* of Verbal and Performance scores also shows evidence of moderate heritability. The fourth column in the table gives the correlations of the difference between the two subscores for the related pairs. The patterns of the first-degree relatives are correlated about .24, whereas those of the identical twins are correlated .49.

MZ twins reared apart

We, like DeFries, Vandenberg, and McClearn (1976), believe that adoption studies offer the best evidence for genetic differences in intelligence. Although most laypeople find the study of identical twins reared apart most compelling, reasons of nonrandom selection and nonrandom assignment to environments render the study of MZs apart less useful than research on adopted children. If there were a study of identical twins reared in uncorrelated environments, genetic differences would be controlled, whereas both within-family and between-families environments would vary. This would be an ideal study of genetic differences. Unfortu-

Table 13.6. *Within-pair correlations on the Wechsler scale for different sets of siblings and twins*

	Full-scale IQ	Verbal IQ	Performance IQ	Difference between Verbal and Performance IQs	No. of sets
Sibling–sibling pairs	.46	.42	.37	.21	56
Sibling and monozygotic twin A	.41	.46	.24	.24	65
Sibling and monozygotic twin B	.46	.48	.29	.26	65
Sibling and dizygotic twin A	.47	.35	.47	.17	53
Sibling and dizygotic twin B	.28	.39	.09	.24	53
Dizygotic twins (8 years)	.45	.41	.41	.27	71
Monozygotic twins (8 years)	.82	.79	.67	.49	86

Note: In those families where two siblings were available, the sibling closest to age 8 was used.
Source: Data from R. S. Wilson (1977), Tables 2 and 3.

nately for science, too few pairs of MZs are reared apart and thus are too peculiarly sampled to make these subjects useful to social science. The most notable studies of MZ twins reared in separate households for at least most of their growing years (but not entirely separated and not reared in uncorrelated environments) are those of Newman, Freeman, and Holzinger (1937) and Shields (1962). The average IQ correlation of MZs reared in correlated but not the same households is .76, considerably higher than that of DZ twins reared in the same household. Thus these studies provide some evidence of the importance of genetic differences in intelligence.

ADOPTIVE FAMILY STUDIES

Adopted children, on the other hand, provide almost as useful data as the rare identical twins reared apart, and they are far more available. Adopted children are not genetically descended from the family of rearing, and therefore environmental differences between families are not confounded with genetic differences in the children if the adopted children are randomly placed by adoption agencies. Theoretically, regressions of adopted child outcomes or adoptive family characteristics will provide genetically unbiased estimates of true environmental effects in the population. Unfortunately, adoptive families are selected by agencies for being above average in many virtues, including socioeconomic status. Thus, they are always an unrepresentative sample of the population. Although it is possible that the adoptive family coefficients are good background estimates of the population values, it is difficult to know without modeling the way in which the families were selected. An easier way to correct for the possible bias of selected adoptive families would be to have a comparison sample of biologically related children in the same adoptive families or a sample of biological families that are similarly selected.

A complete adoption-study design would include comparable information on the intelligence of the natural parents of the adopted children. No study to date has reported IQ data on both the natural mothers and the fathers of adopted children, but the adoption study currently being conducted by Robert Plomin and his colleagues at the University of Colorado will provide information on the IQs of both natural parents as well as the IQs of the adoptive parents and the adopted children. The studies of Skodak and Skeels (1949) and Horn, Loehlin, and Willerman (1979) reported IQ test scores on the natural mothers of the adopted children. Other studies have been forced to use educational level of the natural parents as indexes of intelligence, because no IQ tests were given to most of the natural parents.

Bias in the adoption-study methods?

Comparisons of adopted and biologically related children assume that the greater behavioral similarity usually found among biological relatives is due to their greater genetic similarity. Critics of behavior genetic methods assert, to the contrary, that important biases creep into comparisons of genetically related and unrelated families or members of families through parental and child expectations of greater similarity among biological relatives than among adoptive relatives. If biological parents see themselves in their offspring and expect them to develop greater similarity to the parents, then the children may develop more similarly in many ways. Adoptive parents, knowing that there is no genetic link between them and their children, may expect less similarity and thus not pressure their children to become like the parents. The greater expectation of similarity among biological than adoptive relatives could well bias the comparisons of genetically related and unrelated families, confounding genetic relatedness with environmental pressures.

To test the hypothesis that knowledge of biological or adoptive status influences actual similarity, Scarr, Scarf, and Weinberg (1980) correlated absolute differences in objective test scores with ratings of similarity by adolescents and their parents in adoptive and biological families. Although biological family members see themselves as more similar than adoptive family members, there are also important generational and gender differences in perceived similarity that cut across family type. Moderate agreement is shown among family members on the degree of perceived similarity, but no correlation exists between perceived and actual similarity in intelligence or temperament. Family members more accurately perceive shared social attitudes. Knowledge of adoptive or biological relatedness is related to the degree of perceived similarity, but perceptions of similarity are not related to measured similarities and thus do not constitute a bias in comparisons of measured differences in intelligence or temperament in adoptive and biological families.

Three famous adoption studies

As we indicated by the extensive quotations from Woodworth at the beginning of the chapter, the adoption studies of the 1920s and 1930s were crucial to his conclusions about the role of genetic and environmental differences in intelligence in the white, nonethnic population of the United States at that time. Despite their detractors (Kamin, 1974), the studies are remarkable and are unlikely to be appreciated by contemporary psychologists unless they have more intimate contact with them.

Barbara Burks (1928, 1938), Alice M. Leahy (1935), and Marie Skodak and Harold Skeels (Skeels, 1938; Skodak, 1938; Skodak & Skeels, 1949) contributed unique and valuable information to the nature–nurture debate. Their studies supported the following points: (a) the above-average intellectual level of adopted children reared in advantaged homes, and hence the malleability of IQ scores, and (b) the lesser resemblance of adopted than natural children to their adoptive parents, and hence the role of genetic resemblance in intellectual resemblance. It is worthwhile to look more closely at these three studies, particularly in light of Kamin's (1974) criticisms of them.

THE PIONEER, BARBARA BURKS.   Burks (1928) set out in her dissertation for Stanford University to answer the question, "To what extent are ordinary differences in mental level due to nature and to what extent are they due to nurture?" Even in 1928 she said, "Few scientific problems have been the subject of so much speculation and controversy. . . . This is probably attributable to two facts: the practical and theoretical significance of the problem itself, and the extreme difficulty of gathering data which cannot be applied with more or less plausibility to the support of either the nature or nurture hypothesis" (p. 219).

From her review of the literature of the time, such as Galton's *Hereditary Genius,* Burks notes the consistent decrease in correlations between relatives for "physical traits" as genetic relatedness decreases; the consistency in individual test scores over time; and the marked differences in average intelligence among racial and social class groups. All of these phenomena, she said, might conceivably be due either to hereditary or environmental differences or to both. What was (is) needed, Burks proposed, was one additional experimental step for the whole set of data "to become invested with definite meaning" – the isolation of the effects of heredity and environment.

To this end, she conducted her study of 214 adoptive (called foster) families and 105 control (biologically related) families in California, from San Francisco to San Diego. The foster families were selected through adoption agencies' records, to which Burks applied seven criteria, which included age at adoption, ethnic background, intactness of the family and accessibility. Control families were matched for intactness, the child's age, sex, and preschool experience, and the parents' ethnicity, locality, type of neighborhood, and father's occupational field. Burks and her two assistants traveled the state to visit each family and to spend 4 to 8 hours assessing the mental level of the child and both parents, the cultural and material level of the home, and parental ratings of the children's character and temperament. In her report of the study, Burks was meticulous in telling the reader of the problems of sample recruitment, assessment procedures, and the like. Her data analyses were brilliant and far more advanced than those of most behavioral scientists of the time. Her use of multiple correlations and path analysis, then being developed by the geneticist Sewell Wright at the University of Wisconsin, should amaze contemporary readers, for no electronic calculators or computers were available. More important, although grossly misrepresented in secondary sources, her conclusions were appropriate and balanced.

Reference should be made to the educational opportunities of the children examined, which were good. . . . If the children had varied considerably in educational opportunity, . . . and if, in addition, home environment and educational opportunity had been correlated, it would have

Table 13.7. *Intelligence distribution of children, in IQ*

	Foster	Control		Foster	Control
175–179	—	—	105–109	32	15
170–174	—	—	100–104	32	13
165–169	—	—	95–99	27	5
160–164	1	—	90–94	16	5
155–159	1	1	85–89	7	—
150–154	1	2	80–84	2	—
145–149	1	1	75–79	3	2
140–144	—	2	70–74	2	—
135–139	3	7	65–69	1	—
130–134	7	3	60–64	—	—
125–129	8	10	55–59	—	—
120–124	16	13	50–54	1	—
115–119	24	18	45–49	—	—
110–114	28	8	40–44	1	—
M				107.4	115.4
SD				15.09	15.13
N				214	105

Source: Burks (1928), Table 11.

been quite difficult to separate the effects of the two upon the mental variability of our children. . . .

Thus, the study is based upon children homogeneous as to race and educational opportunity; sufficiently homogeneous in health and physique to avoid confusion; and about as variable in hereditary endowment and in home environment (including kindred social mores) as white children of ordinary communities.

The study does not purport to demonstrate what proportions of the *total* mental development of an individual are due to heredity and to environment. Biologists have frequently pointed out the futility of attempting such a demonstration, since *any development whatever would be impossible without the contributions of both nature and nurture.* But if we direct our attention to the contributions of ordinary differences in heredity and ordinary differences in environment to *mental differences* (i.e., I.Q. variance), it is possible to draw some significant conclusions. The causes which affect human differences, rather than the causes which condition the absolute developmental level of the human species have, after all, the more vital bearing upon social and educational problems.

Given a group of school children such as our subjects (which surely are representative of the largest single element in the American juvenile population), it will later be seen that the data gathered in this investigation lead to the conclusion that *about 17 percent of the variability of intelligence is due to differences in home environment.* It will further appear that the best estimate the data afford of the extreme degree to which the most favorable home environment may enhance the I.Q., or the least favorable environment depress it, is about 20 I.Q. points. This amount is larger, no doubt, than some of the firmest believers in heredity would have anticipated, but smaller than the effects often attributed to nurture by holders of an extreme environmentalist's view. To the writer, these results constitute an important vindication of the potency of home environment. But even more significant appear to be the implications of these basic results, e.g., that *not far from 70 percent of ordinary white school children have intelligence that deviates less than 6 I.Q. points up or down from what they would have if all children were raised in a standard (average) home environment;* that, while home environment in rare, extreme cases may account for as much as 20 points of increment above the

Table 13.8. *Child's IQ correlated with environmental and hereditary factors*

Factor	Type of r	Foster			Control		
		r	PE	N	r	PE	N
Father's MA	PM	.07	.05	178	.45	.05	100
Mother's MA	PM	.19	.05	204	.46	.05	105
Mid-parent MA	PM	.20	.05	174	.52	.05	100
Father's vocabulary	PM	.13	.05	181	.47	.05	101
Mother's vocabulary	PM	.23	.04	202	.43	.05	104
Whittier index	PM	.21	.04	206	.42	.05	104
Whittier index (using 5-yr.-olds only)	PM	.29	.08	63	—	—	—
Culture index	PM	.25	.05	186	.44	.05	101
Culture index (using 5-yr.-olds only)	PM	.23	.08	60	—	—	—
Grade reached by father	PM	.01	.05	173	.27	.06	102
Grade reached by mother	PM	.17	.05	194	.27	.06	103
Parental supervision rating 3 or 4 *vs.* 5 or 6	B	.12	.05	206	.40	.09	104
Income	PM,K	.23	.05	181	.24	.06	99
No. of books in home library	PM,K	.16	.05	194	.34	.06	100
Owning or renting home	B	.25	.07	149	.32	.10	100
No. of books in child's library	PM,K	.32	.04	191	.32	.06	101
Private tutoring (in music, dancing, etc.)	B						
Boys		.06	.10	77	.43	.11	46
Girls		.31	.08	108	.52	.09	56
Five-year-girls only		.50	.12	31	—	—	—
Home instruction by members of household (hrs. weekly)	PM						
Ages 2 and 3		.34	.04	181	−.05	.07	101
Ages 4 and 5 (children over 5)		.15	.06	129	−.03	.08	71
Ages 6 and 7 (children over 7)		.03	.07	88	.24	.09	46
Ages 2 and 3 (5-yr.-olds only)		.18	.09	51	—	—	—
Ages 4 and 5 (5-yr.-olds only)		.13	.09	52	—	—	—
Father's rating of child's intelligence	PM	.49	.04	164	.32	.06	98
Mother's rating of child's intelligence	PM	.39	.04	181	.52	.05	101

Note: PE = probable error; MA = mental age; PM = product–moment correlation; B = biserial correlation; K = Professor Kelley's auxiliary score method.
Source: Burks (1928), Table 31.

expected, or congenital, level, heredity (in conjunction with environment) may account in some instances for increments above the level of the generality which are five times as large (100 points). [Pp. 222–223]

The major data that led Burks to these conclusions are shown in Tables 13.7 and 13.8. In the first table, the distribution of Stanford–Binet IQ scores of the foster and control children are given. The mean of the adopted children's scores was 8 points below that of the control children, but the adopted children's scores were half of a standard deviation (SD) above the population mean of California schoolchildren on whom this version of the Stanford–Binet was standardized. Burks noted that, based on the facts about the natural parents of the adopted children, their expected mental level was not more than 2 to 3 points above 100. "But the average IQ level actually found in this group was 107. Can this discrepancy be accounted for through superior environmental advantage? Probably it can be" (p. 304). She estimated that the total complex of environmental variables in the adoptive homes was between one-half and one standard deviation above the average. Because the multiple correlation of home environment with foster children's IQ scores was .42 (corrected for attenuation), a positive increment of one-half to one *SD* in home environment would predict a rise in child IQ of 3 to 6 points, or very close to what was actually found.

The second table shows the correlations between the major parental and home variables and child's IQ. Even a glance will reveal that the IQ scores of biological offspring bear closer resemblance to their parents' intelligence and to the home environment provided by the parents than do the scores of adopted children to their adoptive parents. From these correlations, Burks calculated the multiple correlations of home environment and child IQ.

In the same volume in which Barbara Burks published her research, Freeman, Holzinger, and Mitchell (1928) described their very large study of foster children adopted at any time between early infancy and late adolescence, at an average age of 4½ years. Newman et al. (1937), in contrast to Burks, found that foster children bore a remarkable intellectual resemblance to their adoptive parents. Although the authors concluded that home environments accounted for the high degree of resemblance for unrelated parents and children, the specter of the highly selective placement of older children haunted the study. Although it is difficult to predict the intellectual level of an infant, it is not difficult to estimate the IQ of a 5-year-old when he or she was in the care of the agency for an average of 11 months before placement in the adoptive home.

ALICE M. LEAHY'S STUDY.   Alice M. Leahy (1935), the author of the second important study of adopted children, summarized her predecessors' work as follows:

In contrast to the low coefficients of correlation between test intelligence of child and foster home found by Burks, Freeman secured coefficients that ranged from .32 to .52 when certain subclassifications were used, and .48 for his entire population. From this he concluded that environment is capable of exercising an influence on mental ability commensurate with that established for true parent and child in which both heredity and environment are operative. [P. 248]

Leahy concluded that selective placement in the Freeman and colleagues (1928) study raised serious and unanswerable questions about the results and planned her own study to avoid the problems of selective placement. She selected families whose adopted children were placed before 6 months of age and control (biologically related) families with identical environmental distribution. She, like Burks, limited her sample to white Northern European children, legally adopted by married couples who were still together at the time of the study. She matched the control group on the child's sex, age, parents' school attainments, father's occupation, and residence in towns where educational opportunities would be advantageous. Also like Burks, Leahy combed her state of Minnesota to find and interview the 193 adoptive and 193 control families. Three interviews and test sessions totaling 5 to 7 hours were held with each family. Both parents and children were given mental tests and interviews to assess the psychological status of the child and the qualities of the home environment. Like Burks's study, this work was Leahy's Ph.D. dissertation, an effort that shames most contemporary theses.

By limiting her sample to very early adoptions and by sampling in the state of Minnesota, Leahy's sample excluded all children who were for any reason suspected

Table 13.9. *Distribution of IQ of adopted and control children*

Stanford–Binet IQ	Adopted children	Control children
160–164	0	2
155–159	1	1
150–154	0	0
145–149	1	2
140–144	2	0
135–139	1	6
130–134	6	7
125–129	11	19
120–124	26	13
115–119	21	19
110–114	31	23
105–109	33	21
100–104	23	26
95–99	21	24
90–94	6	17
85–89	10	5
80–84	0	7
75–79	1	2
M	110.5	109.7
SD	12.5	15.4
N	194	194

Source: Leahy (1935), Table 3.

of possible mental abnormality, either because of parental problems or because of early suspicions about the child (pp. 273–274). The average Stanford–Binet IQ scores of her adopted and control children were nearly identical, as shown in Table 13.9. The IQ scores of both groups of children, reared in very similar, above-average families, were two-thirds of a standard deviation above average. It seems that both groups were environmentally advantaged and genetically select, because the children of feebleminded persons, the insane, and those suspected of immoral (lower-class) behavior would not have been permitted early adoption under the state laws of the 1920s.

Leahy analyzed her data with correlations for parent–child resemblance in the adoptive and biologically related families. Table 13.10 gives the results of her study which support Burks's conclusions about the predominant role of heredity for individual differences in measured intelligence. The greater resemblance of biologically related children to their parents led Leahy to the following conclusions.

1. Variation in IQ is accounted for by variation in home environment to the extent of not more than 4%; 96% of the variation is accounted for by other factors.

2. Measurable environment does not shift the IQ by more than 3 to 5 points above or below the value it would have had under normal environmental conditions.

3. The nature or hereditary component in intelligence causes greater variation than does environment. When nature and nurture are operative, shifts in IQ as great as 20 IQ points are observed with shifts in the cultural level of the home and neighborhood.

An additional feature of Leahy's analyses, which were in general less sophisticated than Burks's earlier work, was the comparison of IQ scores of the adopted and

Table 13.10. *Child's IQ correlated with other factors*

Correlated factor	Adopted children			Control children		
	r	PE[a]	N	r	PE[a]	N
Father's Otis score	.19	.06	178	.51	.04	175
Mother's Otis score	.24	.06	186	.51	.04	191
Midparent Otis score	.21	.06	177	.60	.03	173
Father's S–B[b] vocabulary	.26	.06	177	.47	.04	168
Mother's S–B vocabulary	.24	.06	185	.49	.04	190
Midparent S–B vocabulary	.29	.06	174	.56	.03	164
Environmental status score	.23	.06	194	.53	.03	194
Cultural index of home	.26	.06	194	.51	.04	194
Child training index	.22	.06	194	.52	.04	194
Economic index	.15	.06	194	.37	.04	194
Sociality index	.13	.06	194	.42	.04	194
Father's education	.19	.06	193	.48	.04	193
Mother's education	.25	.06	192	.50	.04	194
Midparent education	.24	.06	193	.54	.03	194
Father's occupational status	.14	.06	194	.45	.04	194

Note: r corrected for unequal range in child's IQ.
[a]PE = probable error.
[b]S–B = Stanford–Binet Intelligence Scale.
Source: Leahy (1935), Table 11.

control children by the occupational status of their fathers in the family of rearing. Her remarkable results led Burks (1938) to reanalyze her own data in similar fashion. Burks's tabulations of her own and Leahy's data are given in Table 13.11.

Leahy found that the average IQ scores of adopted children reared in professional families exceeded those of adopted children reared in slightly skilled and unskilled families by 5 IQ points. Children born and reared in families of the same social class groups differed on the average by 16.5 IQ points. Burks found the same 5 point difference for adopted children and a 12-point difference for genetic offspring of similar families. These data laid the groundwork for contemporary studies of the effects of family environments (Scarr & Weinberg, 1978; Scarr & Yee, 1980).

SKODAK AND SKEELS'S STUDY OF NATURAL MOTHERS AND ADOPTED CHILDREN. Perhaps the most widely cited of the early adoption studies in the contemporary literature is that of Skodak and Skeels (1949), a follow-up study on 100 children adopted from mothers whose IQ they had tested at the time of the child's delivery. Like Burks, they found a substantial gain in the children's IQ scores over what would have been expected had the children been reared by their mothers. Jensen (1973c) has estimated that the children would have averaged IQ 96 under natural-parent rearing, whereas at the average age of 13 years they actually scored IQ 107 on the same version (1916) of the Stanford–Binet on which their mothers had averaged IQ 86. On the 1937 version of the Binet they scored an average of IQ 117. Altogether their intellectual development in the adoptive families was prodigious and spoke well for the adoptive home environments. Table 13.12 gives the results.

The relative benefits of the home environments were, however, very much tem-

Table 13.11. *Means and dispersions of intelligence scores by occupational group*

	Stanford study, occupation of father (or foster father)				Minnesota study, occupation of father (or foster father)				
	Profess.	Semi-prof.[a]	Lower bus.	Skilled labor	Profess.	Bus. mgr.	Skilled trades[b]	Semi-skilled	Slightly skilled & day labor
Foster children									
M (IQ)	109.1	108.6	108.0	104.6	112.6	111.6	110.6	109.4	107.8
SD (IQ)	17.2	14.5	14.3	16.7	11.8	10.9	14.2	11.8	13.6
N	32.0	47.0	41.0	43.0	43.0	38.0	44.0	45.0	24.0
Control children									
M (IQ)	118.7	118.5	115.5	106.1	118.6	117.6	106.9	101.1	102.1
SD (IQ)	15.4	12.2	18.6	12.4	12.6	15.6	14.3	12.5	11.0
N	18.0	33.0	27.0	18.0	40.0	42.0	43.0	46.0	23.0
Foster parents[c]									
M	221.8	207.3	201.2	184.7	59.6	59.6	49.6	39.7	38.4
SD	22.6	30.8	29.7	30.3	8.0	6.7	11.9	12.3	11.2
N	24.0	40.0	34.0	34.0	—	—	—	—	—
Control parents[c]									
M	221.6	221.8	192.0	176.2	64.6	57.1	51.8	44.0	38.3
SD	24.4	30.4	33.4	31.6	5.4	10.0	11.5	11.5	9.0
N	18.0	32.0	27.0	18.0	—	—	—	—	—

[a]Includes higher business.
[b]Includes clerical.
[c]The Stanford study data are for Stanford–Binet mental age in months of foster fathers and control fathers. In the Minnesota study, data are for midfoster parent and midparent point score on the Otis Test of Mental Ability.
Source: Burks (1938), Table 1, p. 279.

Table 13.12. *IQ scores of adopted away children from 2 to 13 years of age*

Test	Age	MIQ	SD	Range	Mdn
I	2 yrs. 2 mo.	117	13.6	80–154	118
II	4 yrs. 3 mo.	112	13.8	85–149	111
III	7 yrs. 0 mo.	115	13.2	80–149	114
IV (1916)	13 yrs. 6 mo.	107	14.4	65–144	107
IV (1937)	13 yrs. 6 mo.	117	15.5	70–154	117

Source: Skodak & Skeels (1949), Table 4.

pered by the genetic endownment of the children. Not only did the children's IQ scores correlate more highly with the biological mothers' than with the educational levels of the adoptive families, but there was a definite association between the IQ levels of the children and the IQ levels of their natural mothers, regardless of the advantages of the home environment. Skodak and Skeels's table (Table 13.13) shows the results of comparisons between children of mothers of "inferior and of

Table 13.13. *Comparisons between children of mothers of inferior and of above average intelligence*

Case no.	True mother's IQ	True mother's educ.	Foster midpar. educ.	Foster father occup.[a]	Test I	Test II	Child's IQ Test III	Test IV	Test IV (1937)
Group A									
8B	64	8	16	I	126	125	114	96	106
10B	64	11	8	III	125	109	96	87	100
18B	65	8	9	VI	114	102	112	122	118
53G	63	8	13	III	127	121	119	101	111
54G	67	9	12	III	116	113	113	91	102
58G	54	8	13	III	117	114	119	98	113
60G	66	8	10	V	105	109	90	105	115
67G	65	6	12	IV	110	111	114	95	103
70G	63	1	10	II	110	113	107	101	118
76G	67	7	15	I	109	92	87	74	84
82G	53	3	12	IV	81	37	80	66	74
M	63	7	12	3.2	113	109	105	96	104
Mdn	64	8	12	III	114	111	96	96	106
Group B									
17B	128	12	12	III	120	128	148	127	145
22B	109	13	11	III	102	107	113	108	130
57G	109	13	16	III	99	126	139	132	130
61G	109	13	15	II	112	113	125	128	135
71G	113	12	19	II	128	112	114	114	122
72G	110	12	8	VI	116	92	105	103	104
73G	105	8	9	IV	125	111	129	110	131
87G	109	13	11	III	128	145	125	119	133
M	111	12	12.5	3.3	116	117	125	118	129
Mdn	109	12.5	11.5	III	117	112.5	125	117	130

[a] I = professional, managerial; II = business and managerial; III = skilled trades and clerical; III = semiskilled; IV = unskilled.
Source: Skodak & Skeels (1949), Table 15.

above average intelligence." By 4 years of age (Test 2), the children whose natural mothers had above-average IQ scores were performing on IQ tests well above the children whose mothers had low scores. Although the samples are small, the data are compelling.

Using the Skodak and Skeels data and scores from her own University of California Guidance Study, Marjorie Honzik (1957) published two of the most reprinted graphs in the history of psychology. Undeterred by our predecessors, we reproduce these graphs once again for their dramatic illustration of the effects of genetic resemblance on intellectual resemblance. Figures 13.10 and 13.11 show that with increasing age, biological offspring come to resemble their parents. Adoptive parents' educational levels (here a proxy for intelligence) bear little resemblance to the intelligence of their adopted children. These data are entirely consonant with our later studies of adoptive and biologically related families with young children and with adolescents.

Surely, the other moral from this story concerns the high average IQ scores of the children. If we assume that the natural mothers were an intellectually average

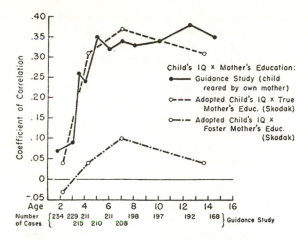

Figure 13.10. Education of mother in relation to child's IQ. (From "Developmental Studies of Parent–Child Resemblance in Intelligence" by M. P. Honzik, *Child Development,* 1957, 28(2), 215–228. Copyright © 1957 by the Society for Research in Child Development, Inc. Reprinted by permission.)

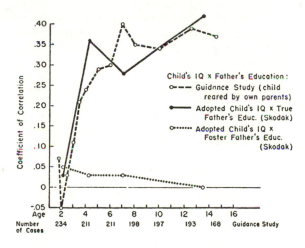

Figure 13.11. Education of father in relation to child's IQ. (From "Developmental Studies of Parent–Child Resemblance in Intelligence" by M. P. Honzik, *Child Development,* 1957, 28(2), 215–228. Copyright © 1957 by the Society for Research in Child Development, Inc. Reprinted by permission.)

sample of the general population, as was later found to be true of Pearson and Amacher's (1956) sample of unmarried mothers in Minnesota for 1948–1952, then the adopted children's IQ scores are not alarmingly high. The IQ scores of the mothers are, however, unwarrantedly low; the tests were given soon after the delivery of the child and its relinquishment, and the mothers subsequent depression might account for the low scores. In addition, one might venture the guess that the largely rural Iowa mothers were culturally disadvantaged on the Stanford–Binet;

their genetic value did not shine through on the test as much as it would have had they been reared in circumstances more congruent with the test samples of knowledge.

Kamin (1974) poses objections to each of the three studies chosen here for emphasis. Matching adoptive and control families on socioeconomic variables left other variables unmatched. Adoptive parents were several years older on the average than biological parents; income levels for older fathers were higher, even when occupational levels were matched; adopted children had fewer siblings than did children in biological families. Kamin implies that these sources of differences between biological and adoptive families contribute to, or indeed account for, the large differences in resemblance between the adoptive and biological families. More recent research will speak to many of his proposed explanations, but even within these older studies one can ask how reasonable it is to raise questions about the effective environments of adopted and biologically related families. Is there any evidence that parent–child resemblance depends on the number of siblings, when the family sizes varied from 1 to 4 or 5? Also, is it not just as likely that adopted children in smaller families would come to resemble their parents more, because of closer association with the adults in the household? Are not older parents supposed to spend more time with their children? Hence again, one would predict greater resemblance between the adopted children and their older, less frivolous parents. After all, adoptive parents chose to have the child, which certainly cannot be said for many biological parents.

Alas, it is useless to argue with ad hoc, environmentalist arguments that employ adventitious variables to discredit well-designed research. Peter Urbach (1974) summed up the plight of naive environmentalism in the face of the evidence for *some* genetic variance in intelligence:

The hereditarian programme has anticipated many novel facts. . . . When the environmentalist programme has attempted to account for the novel facts produced by the hereditarian programme, it has been unable to do so except in an ad hoc fashion. . . . In this part of my paper I have considered some of the predictions made by the environmentalist programme, especially in regard to social class and racial differences in average IQ. I have shown that almost none of these predictions has been confirmed and that when predictions have failed, environmentalists have rescued their theories in an ad hoc fashion. This patching-up process has left the environmentalist programme as little more than a collection of untestable theories which provide a passe partout which explains everything because it explains nothing. [Pp. 134–135, 253]

RECENT TWIN AND FAMILY STUDIES

In this section we will review several studies of twins and siblings from the past four years (1976–1980). After a brief overview of the findings, we will take closer looks at the Hawaii Family Study, the Texas Adoption Project, and the Minnesota Adoption Studies.

Plomin and DeFries (1980) compiled recent studies of twins and families and reported family correlations for seven groups, as shown in Table 13.14. Plomin's comparisons would imply that, unlike Wilson's (1977) results, the twin experience per se increases similarity, but unfortunately, the "intelligence" measures are diverse and the age groups of relatives vary, which makes comparisons difficult to interpret.

It is impressive that so many pairs of relatives have been studied in the past four years. In fact, the three family studies to be reviewed in more detail have contributed

Table 13.14. *Correlation coefficients for new "intelligence" data*

	Correlation	N (pairs)
Genetically identical		
Same individual tested twice	.87[a]	456
Identical twins reared together	.86[b]	1,300
Genetically related (first degree)		
Fraternal twins reared together	.62[b]	864
Nontwin siblings reared together	.31[c]	455
Parent–child living together	.35[d]	2,715
Parent–child separated by adoption	.29[e]	342
Genetically unrelated		
Unrelated children reared together	.25[f]	553
Adoptive parent–adopted child	.15[g]	1,578

[a] Obtained over an average period of 15 months for scores of 456 individuals on the first principal component derived from the 15 tests of specific cognitive abilities used in the Hawaii Family Study of Cognition (Kuse, 1977).

[b] From Loehlin & Nichols (1976), Table 4–10.

[c] From DeFries, Johnson, Kuse, McClearn, Polvina, Vandenberg, & Wilson (1979), Table 9. Average weighted correlation for 216 brother–sister pairs, and 125 sister–sister pairs in 830 families of European ancestry for the first principal component score derived from scores on the 15 tests of specific cognitive abilities in the Hawaii Family Study of Cognition.

[d] From DeFries, Johnson, Kuse, McClearn, Polvina, Vandenberg, & Wilson (1979), Table 8. Average weighted correlation for 672 father–son pairs, 692 mother–daughter pairs, 666 mother–son pairs, and 685 father–daughter pairs in 830 families of European ancestry for the first principal component score derived from scores on the 15 tests of specific cognitive abilities in the Hawaii Family Study of Cognition.

[e] From the Texas Adoption Study (DeFries & Plomin, 1978, Table 9).

[f] Average weighted correlation for three recent adoption studies: Texas Adoption Study, .28 for 282 pairs of unrelated children reared in the same family (DeFries & Plomin, 1978, Table 9); a transracial adoption study, .33 for 187 pairs (Scarr & Weinberg, 1977, Table 6); and an adoption study of adolescents, −.03 for 84 pairs (Scarr & Weinberg, 1978).

[g] Average weighted correlation for four recent adoption studies: Texas Adoption Study, .18 for 541 adoptive mother–adopted child pairs, .12 for 454 adoptive father–adopted child pairs (DeFries & Plomin, 1978, Table 9); a transracial adoption study, .23 for 109 adoptive mother–adopted child pairs, .15 for 111 adoptive father–adopted child pairs (Scarr & Weinberg, 1977, Table 4); an adoption study of adolescents, .09 for 184 adoptive mother–adopted child pairs, .16 for 175 adoptive father–adopted child pairs (Scarr & Weinberg, 1978); and a study by Fisch et al., .08 for 94 adoptive mother–adopted child pairs (1976).

all the nontwin data with the exception of 94 pairs of adoptive mothers and children (Fisch et al., 1976).

The Hawaii Family Study of Cognition

In the Hawaii Family Study, a battery of 15 tests of specific cognitive abilities was administered to 6,581 members of 1,816 intact families living on the island of Oahu.

The families, recruited through church groups, community groups, and various other means, consisted of biological parents and one or more children of 13 years or older. The scores for the cognitive battery were age corrected, and the resemblances of various biological family members were calculated. The study is reported most fully by DeFries, Johnson, Kuse, McClearn, Polvina, Vandenberg, and Wilson (1979). That report presents spouse correlations, single-parent–single-child correlations, regressions of midchild on midparent, and sibling correlations, for the two largest ethnic groups in Hawaii – Americans of European ancestry (AEA) and Americans of Japanese ancestry (AJA). The goal of the study was to ascertain the degree of "familiality" of specific cognitive abilities. There was no variation in the degree of familial relatedness or the degree of environmental similarity.

SPOUSE CORRELATIONS.   The resemblance between husbands and wives in this study was lower than has been reported in many other studies (Jensen, 1978b). Jensen reported a mean spouse correlation of .45 for 43 studies of intelligence. In the Hawaii study, the age-adjusted spouse correlations for the first principal component (the closest measure to IQ) were .23 and .15 for the AEA and AJA samples, respectively. The spouse correlations for the individual tests in the battery ranged from −.08 (Subtraction and Multiplication) to .29 (Pedigrees, a verbal reasoning task). The authors believe that their spouse correlations are lower than the reported literature because (a) the spouses are highly correlated for age and thus the age corrections lowered the correlations; (b) spouses may not be as highly correlated for specific abilities as for g and verbal intelligence, although their general factor correlates .73 with the Wechsler Adult Intelligence Scale (WAIS) full-scale IQ; (c) the families who participated may have been drawn from a restricted range of the intellectual population distribution. Volunteers for social science studies are always self-selected samples, and it is very likely that the volunteers for the Hawaii study also represented a biased sample.

PARENT–CHILD CORRELATIONS.   Table 13.15 gives the correlations of single parents and single children for the test battery, the composite factors, and the first principal component. As one can see, the correlations for vocabulary and the first principal component are fairly high (.3 to .4), whereas the family resemblance for many of the other tests is low. Because the samples are very large, the standard errors around the correlations are quite low. It seems from this study and from the Minnesota Adoption Study (Carter-Saltzman, 1978) of adolescents' and their parents' specific cognitive abilities that biological family correlations for specific abilities are dramatically lower than for measures of g.

The regression of midchild on midparent value was used as the principal index of parent–child resemblance. The authors point out, however, that between-families environmental influences may be an important source of variance for tests of mental ability. For this reason the regression coefficients presented here should be regarded only as measures of familiality and not as direct estimates of heritability.

The corrected coefficients in Table 13.16 may be compared across tests for evidence of differential familiality. The Spearman rank correlation between the AEA and AJA corrected coefficients across the 15 individual tests in the total AEA and AJA samples is 0.76. With regard to the four varimax rotated principal component scores, the regressions are moderately high for verbal and spatial measures and somewhat lower for visual memory and perceptual speed in both ethnic groups. In

Table 13.15. *Single-parent–single-child correlations for cognitive test and principal component scores in total Hawaiian AEA and AJA samples*

Tests and composites	AEA				AJA			
	Father–son	Mother–daughter	Mother–son	Father–daughter	Father–son	Mother–daughter	Mother–son	Father–daughter
Tests								
Vocabulary	.31	.30	.35	.32	.38	.36	.40	.31
Visual memory (immediate)	.03	.11	.08	.10	.01	.07	.08	.17
Things	.19	.27	.22	.19	.18	.19	.15	.23
Mental rotations	.20	.30	.13	.20	.20	.11	.17	.24
Subtraction and multiplication	.29	.24	.21	.14	.19	.22	.12	.09
Elithorn Mazes ("lines and dots")	.11	.17	.16	.07	.13	.09	.15	.19
Word beginnings and endings	.21	.25	.19	.27	.25	.22	.25	.17
Card Rotations	.26	.34	.21	.23	.24	.17	.10	.11
Visual memory (delayed)	.14	.10	.16	.22	.13	.10	.07	.07
Pedigrees	.27	.33	.28	.29	.18	.38	.27	.27
Hidden Patterns	.24	.32	.24	.27	.09	.19	.13	.22
Paper Form Board	.28	.33	.29	.35	.21	.29	.20	.27
Number comparisons	.25	.24	.21	.17	.25	.07	.20	.24
Social perception	.10	.17	.11	.14	.10	.22	.10	.16
Progressive Matrices	.23	.25	.32	.25	.09	.25	.24	.20
Composites								
Spatial	.33	.38	.29	.31	.26	.22	.20	.32
Verbal	.24	.26	.29	.32	.38	.36	.33	.31
Perceptual speed and accuracy	.30	.29	.22	.17	.25	.08	.13	.15
Visual memory	.11	.12	.15	.18	.06	.10	.11	.10
First principal component (unrotated)	.30	.40	.35	.35	.25	.34	.31	.27
N (pairs)	672	692	666	685	241	248	244	237

Note: AEA and AJA are Americans of European and Japanese ancestry, respectively. Correlations greater than .09 are significantly ($p \le .05$) different from zero for AEA subjects, whereas those greater than .14 are significant ($p \le .05$) for AJA subjects.
Source: DeFries, Johnson, Kuse, McClearn, Polvina, Vandenberg, & Wilson (1979).

Table 13.16. *Regressions of midchild on midparent for cognitive test and principal component scores in total Hawaiian AEA and AJA samples*

Tests and composites	Uncorrected		Corrected[a]	
	AEA	AJA	AEA	AJA
Tests				
Vocabulary	.64	.55	.67	.57
Visual memory (immediate)	.15	.12	.26	.21
Things	.41	.35	.55	.47
Mental rotations	.43	.40	.49	.45
Subtraction and multiplication	.38	.34	.40	.35
Elithorn Mazes ("lines and dots")	.24	.23	.27	.26
Word beginnings and endings	.39	.42	.55	.59
Card Rotations[b]	.46	.30	.52	.34
Visual memory (delayed)	.31	.18	.50	.29
Pedigrees	.52	.45	.72	.63
Hidden Patterns[b]	.45	.27	.49	.29
Paper Form Board	.51	.46	.61	.55
Number comparisons	.38	.29	.46	.36
Social perception	.26	.18	.38	.26
Progressive Matrices[b]	.52	.24	.60	.28
Composites				
Spatial[b]	.60	.42	.64	.45
Verbal	.54	.48	.61	.55
Perceptual speed and accuracy	.41	.34	.46	.38
Visual memory	.31	.18	.43	.25
First principal component (unrotated)[b]	.60	.42	.62	.43
N (families)	830	305	830	305

Note: AEA and AJA are Americans of European and Japanese ancestry, respectively. Standard errors for AEA and AJA coefficients range from .04 to .05 and from .06 to .08.
[a]Corrected for test reliability.
[b]AEA and AJA regression coefficients significantly ($p \leq .05$) different.
Source: DeFries, Johnson, Kuse, McClearn, Polvina, Vandenberg, & Wilson (1979), Table 5.

contrast to this finding of differential familiality, Loehlin and Nichols (1976) found no evidence of differential heritability among various mental ability tests when they analyzed extensive twin data. Such results suggest that it may be between-families environmental variance that differs in relative importance among various measures of mental ability.

The unrotated first principal component score may be used as a measure of general intelligence. Parent–offspring regressions (uncorrected) for this measure are .60 and .42 for the total AEA and AJA samples, respectively. These values are similar to the estimate of .46 obtained by Williams (1975) for WAIS/WISC full-scale IQ. Because the regression of offspring on midparent value provides an "upper-bound" estimate of heritability, assuming positive environmental covariance, these results indicate that the heritability of general intelligence in these populations is less than .6.

SIBLING RESEMBLANCE.   If between-families environmental influences contributed equally to parent–child and sibling resemblance, the difference between single-parent–single-child and sibling correlations could be used to obtain an estimate of dominance variance. However, since siblings share a rearing environment, whereas parents and children do not, it seems logical to assume that between-families environmental influences may contribute more to sibling than to parent–child resemblance. Sibling correlations for the total AEA and AJA samples are presented in Table 13.17. Because the AJA sibling correlations are based on relatively small sample sizes, they are less reliable. The AEA correlations are somewhat more reliable and correspond reasonably well to the single-parent–single-child correlations. Median AEA sibling correlations are .25 (brother–sister), .26 (brother–brother), and .16 (sister–sister); corresponding values for single-parent–single-child correlations are .23 (father–son), .25 (mother–daughter), .21 (mother–son), and .22 (father–daughter). This comparison suggests that between-families environmental influences on specific cognitive abilities are not more important for sibling resemblance and that dominance variance for such characters is not relatively large.

In addition, the Hawaii Family Study has reported on the nearly identical factor structures of cognitive abilities in the two major ethnic groups, AEA and AJA (De-Fries et al., 1974) and across the ages of the children and parents sampled in their study. The authors have also tried to estimate genetic and environmental parameters from their data on biological families, but we find the assumptions tenuous and the results questionable. For these results, see DeFries, Johnson, Kuse, McClearn, Polvina, Vandenberg, & Wilson (1979).

The Hawaii Family Study is the largest study of the specific cognitive abilities of families in two large ethnic groups in not notably disadvantaged environments. The lack of related persons who vary in genetic or environmental relatedness, however, limits the inferences that can be drawn from it.

The Texas Adoption Project

The Texas Adoption Project was begun in 1973 soon after the investigators discovered an adoption agency that had routinely administered IQ and personality tests to the unwed mothers in their care. The agency tested their clients in order to provide them with occupational and educational counseling and to provide adoptive parents with some general information concerning the background of their adoptive children.

The project's sample included only those mothers who had been tested between 1963 and 1971. Of the 1,381 eligible unwed mothers, 364 were included in the final sample. IQ tests were administered to the final sample of 300 adoptive families by 22 licensed psychologists across the state. The adopted children ranged from 2 to 20 years, with an average age of about 8 years. The adoptive families were well above average socioeconomically and intellectually. The biological mothers also came from advantaged families, because the private agency for unwed mothers from which the sample was drawn asked that the families of the unwed mothers contribute "significant amounts of money to offset the costs of caring for their daughters" (Horn, Loehlin, & Willerman, 1979, p. 182). The average IQ of the natural mothers of the adopted children in this sample was 108.7 on the Beta test. The average IQ scores of the adoptive parents on the same test was 113.8 and on the WAIS 113.9. The IQ scores of the adopted and biological offspring of the adoptive families are given in

Table 13.17. *Sibling intraclass correlation (± SE) for cognitive test and principal component scores in total Hawaiian AEA and AJA samples*

Tests and composites	AEA			AJA		
	Brother–sister	Brother–brother	Sister–sister	Brother–sister	Brother–brother	Sister–sister
Tests						
Vocabulary	.33 ± 0.06	.32 ± 0.09	.38 ± 0.09	.51 ± 0.11	.17 ± 0.15	.39 ± 0.16
Visual memory (immediate)	.21 ± 0.07	.04 ± 0.09	.02 ± 0.08	.06 ± 0.12	−.08 ± 0.12	−.08 ± 0.13
Things	.17 ± 0.07	.28 ± 0.10	.14 ± 0.08	.43 ± 0.11	.05 ± 0.14	.26 ± 0.17
Mental rotations	.25 ± 0.07	.35 ± 0.09	.16 ± 0.09	.18 ± 0.12	.16 ± 0.15	.24 ± 0.17
Subtractions and multiplication	.29 ± 0.07	.38 ± 0.09	.26 ± 0.09	.38 ± 0.12	.14 ± 0.15	.35 ± 0.17
Elithorn Mazes ("lines and dots")	.11 ± 0.07	.06 ± 0.09	.07 ± 0.08	.34 ± 0.12	.07 ± 0.14	.00 ± 0.14
Word beginnings and endings	.27 ± 0.07	.33 ± 0.09	.25 ± 0.09	.30 ± 0.12	.11 ± 0.15	.41 ± 0.16
Card Rotations	.33 ± 0.06	.17 ± 0.09	.25 ± 0.09	.27 ± 0.12	.33 ± 0.15	.26 ± 0.17
Visual memory (delayed)	.14 ± 0.07	.19 ± 0.09	.13 ± 0.08	.21 ± 0.12	.01 ± 0.13	−.05 ± 0.13
Pedigrees	.22 ± 0.07	.28 ± 0.10	.16 ± 0.09	.28 ± 0.12	.02 ± 0.14	.36 ± 0.17
Hidden Patterns	.30 ± 0.07	.28 ± 0.10	.18 ± 0.09	.43 ± 0.11	−.05 ± 0.12	.04 ± 0.15
Paper Form Board	.35 ± 0.06	.26 ± 0.10	.20 ± 0.09	.28 ± 0.12	.08 ± 0.14	.19 ± 0.17
Number comparisons	.27 ± 0.07	.19 ± 0.09	.23 ± 0.09	.38 ± 0.12	.08 ± 0.14	.14 ± 0.16
Social perception	.12 ± 0.07	.09 ± 0.09	.14 ± 0.09	.31 ± 0.12	.27 ± 0.15	.19 ± 0.17
Progressive Matrices	.20 ± 0.07	.19 ± 0.09	.16 ± 0.09	.33 ± 0.12	.12 ± 0.15	.41 ± 0.16
Composites						
Spatial	.36 ± 0.06	.29 ± 0.10	.25 ± 0.09	.39 ± 0.12	.17 ± 0.15	.29 ± 0.17
Verbal	.27 ± 0.07	.30 ± 0.10	.26 ± 0.09	.55 ± 0.10	.21 ± 0.15	.44 ± 0.16
Perceptual speed and accuracy	.33 ± 0.06	.29 ± 0.10	.28 ± 0.09	.34 ± 0.12	.19 ± 0.15	.32 ± 0.17
Visual memory	.22 ± 0.07	.19 ± 0.09	.10 ± 0.08	.16 ± 0.12	.01 ± 0.13	−.10 ± 0.12
First principal component (unrotated)	.31 ± 0.06	.36 ± 0.09	.25 ± 0.09	.53 ± 0.11	.01 ± 0.13	.44 ± 0.16
N (families)	216	114	125	66	44	37

Note: AEA and AJA are Americans of European and Japanese ancestry, respectively.
Source: DeFries, Johnson, Kuse, McClearn, Polvina, Vandenberg, & Wilson (1979), Table 9.

Table 13.18. *IQs of children, by test*

	Adopted children			Biological children		
	M	SD	N	M	SD	N
WAIS[a]	111.0	8.69	5	112.9	8.60	22
WISC[b]	111.9	11.39	405	111.2	11.55	123
S–B[c]	109.2	13.22	59	113.8	11.18	19

Note: WAIS given to children aged 16 or older, WISC to children aged 5–15, Stanford–Binet to children aged 3 and 4, with one or two exceptions at borderline ages. S–B IQs adjusted to 1970 norms.
[a]WAIS = Wechsler Adult Intelligence Scale.
[b]WISC = Wechsler Intelligence Scale for Children.
[c]S–B = Stanford–Binet Intelligence Scale.

Table 13.19. *Correlation of parent's Beta IQ with child's IQ tests*

	Child test			
Correlational pairing	r for Wechsler performance IQ	N for Wechsler performance IQ	r for Wechsler or Binet total IQ	N for Wechsler or Binet total IQ
Adoptive father				
Biological child	.29	144	.28	163
Adopted child	.12	405	.14	462
Adoptive mother				
Biological child	.21	143	.20	162
Adopted child	.15	401	.17	459
Unwed mother				
Her child	.28	297	.31	345
Other adopted child in same family	.15	202	.19	233
Biological child in same family	.06	143	.08	161

Note: NS refers to the number of pairings (= the number of children) – the same parent may enter more than one pairing. In the case of twins, the second twin was excluded from the unwed mother–other child comparisons.
Source: Horn, Loehlin, & Willerman (1979).

Table 13.18. Unlike the Burks (1928) study and the Minnesota Adoption Studies, but consonant with Leahy's (1935) results, the Texas Adoption Project found no average difference between the IQ scores of the adopted and biological children of the same families.

PARENT–CHILD CORRELATIONS. Table 13.19 gives the correlations for adoptive and biological parents with their children. Although the biological relatives tend to have higher correlations with their offspring than the adoptive relatives, all of the correlations are quite low. The magnitude of the IQ correlation of the biological mother with her child is as high as the correlations of the adoptive parents with their own offspring. There is evidence for considerable selective placement in these families;

Table 13.20. *IQ correlations among biological and adoptive siblings*

Correlational pairing	Verbal IQ		Performance IQ		Wechsler or Binet IQ	
	r	df/df w b	r	df/df w b	r	df/df w b
Among biological children	.14	40/35	.33	40/35	.35	46/39
Among adopted children	.19	132/121	.05	132/121	.22	167/150
Between biological and adopted	.21	159/97	.24	159/97	.29	197/116
All unrelated children	.21	266/195	.18	266/195	.26	330/235

Note: r = intraclass or interclass correlations. df_w = degrees of freedom within families = $\Sigma(n_i - 1)$, where n_i is the number of children in family i entering into the correlations. df^b = degrees of freedom between families = number of families entering into the correlation -1. For twins, only the first member of the pair was included.
Source: Horn, Loehlin, & Willerman (1979).

for example, the IQ score of the biological mother of one adopted child is correlated .19 with the IQ score of another (unrelated) adopted child being reared in the same family and .08 with the biological child of that family.

SIBLING CORRELATIONS. The overall IQ correlation of biological offspring of the adoptive parents was .35. Genetically unrelated children reared together had IQ scores that correlated .26, a statistically lower coefficient but still quite high. Table 13.20 gives the sibling data. The parent–child data from this study suggest moderate heritability for IQ. The means of the groups of unwed mothers, adoptive parents, and biological and adopted children of the adoptive families do not agree. The authors speculate about the reasons for the higher-than-expected IQ levels of the adopted children and suggest several reasons for the lack of mean differences between the adopted and biological children of the adoptive families.

A path model is presented for the parent–child data. As the authors point out, their initial path model may not be the most appropriate analysis of the data, but it implies a narrow heritability (additive genetic variance only) of .45 to .53; because there is very little estimated dominance variance, the same estimates are appropriate for broad h^2, as well.

ENVIRONMENTAL AND GENETIC EFFECTS ON IQ SCORES OF ADOPTED CHILDREN. Willerman (1979) divided the Texas adoptees into two extreme groups by the IQ scores of their natural mothers. For the low-IQ group he selected natural mothers with IQ scores below 95, and for the high-IQ group, mothers with IQ scores of 120 or above. Table 13.21 shows the adoptive midparent IQ, the mean IQ scores of the offspring of the high-IQ and low-IQ natural mothers, and the percentage of the adopted children with IQ scores below 95 or equal to or above 120.

Although there is some evidence of selective placement for the adopted children, because the adoptive parent groups differ by 4 points in IQ, the 13-point IQ difference between the offspring of high-IQ and low-IQ mothers shows that individuals of different genetic backgrounds differ in their responsiveness to the generally good environments of adoptive homes. Although the offspring of the low-IQ mothers score

Table 13.21. *IQs of adoptees as a function of biological mother's IQ*

Biological mother (Beta)	Adoptive midparent (Beta)	Adoptee (WISC/Binet)	Adoptees ≥ 120 IQ	Adoptees ≤ 95 IQ
Low IQ				
(N = 27; M = 89.4)	110.8	102.6	0%	15%
High IQ				
(N = 34; M = 121.6)	114.8	118.3	44%	0%

Note: WISC = Wechsler Intelligence Scale for Children; Binet = Stanford–Binet Intelligence Scale.
Source: Willerman (1979).

above the population mean, they are not as bright as the offspring of high-IQ mothers in similar environments.

The Minnesota Adoption Studies: transracial adoption

Two large adoption studies were launched in 1974 for two quite different purposes. The transracial adoption study was carried out from 1974 to 1976 in Minnesota to test the hypothesis that black and interracial children reared by white families (in the culture of the tests and of the schools) would perform on IQ tests as well as other adopted children (Scarr & Weinberg, 1976).

In the transracial families were 143 biological children, 111 children adopted in the first year of life (called the early adoptees) and 65 children adopted from 12 months of age to 10 years. Most of the later adoptees were in fact placed with adoptive families before 4 years of age, but they were not the usually studied adopted children who have spent all of their lives after their first few months with one adoptive family, and they had checkered preadoptive histories.

The 101 participating families included 176 adopted children, of whom 130 were socially classified as Black (29 with two Black natural parents and 101 with one Black natural parent and one natural parent of other or unknown racial background), and 25 as White. The remaining 21 included Asian, North American Indian, and Latin American Indian children. All of the adopted children were unrelated to the adoptive parents. Adopted children reared in the same home were unrelated, with the exception of four sibling pairs and one triad adopted by the same families, who were excluded from the analyses of family similarity.

IQ LEVELS OF FAMILY MEMBERS. Both the parents and the natural children of the families were found to score in the bright average to superior range on age-appropriate IQ tests. The black and interracial adopted children were also found to score above the average of the white population of Minnesota, regardless of when they were adopted. The black children adopted in the first 12 months of life scored on the average at IQ 110 (Scarr & Weinberg, 1976). This remarkable result was interpreted to mean that adopted children were scoring at least 20 points above comparable children being reared in the black community. The dramatic change in the IQ scores and the higher school performance of the black and interracial children seemed to mean that (a) genetic racial differences do not account for a major portion of the IQ

Table 13.22. *Comparisons of biological and unrelated parent–child IQ correlations in 101 transracial adoptive families*

	N (pairs)	r
Parents–biological children		
Adoptive mother–own child	141	.34
Natural mother–adopted child[a]	135	.33
Adoptive father–own child	142	.39
Natural father–adopted child[a]	46	.43
Parents–unrelated children		
Adoptive mother–adopted child	174	.21[b]
Natural mother–own child of adoptive family[a]	217	.15
Adoptive father–adopted child	170	.27[b]
Natural father–own child of adoptive family[a]	86	.19

[a]Educational level, not IQ scores.
[b]Among early adopted only ($N = 111$), $r = .23$ for adoptive mother–adopted child, and $r = .15$ for adoptive father–adopted child.

or academic test performance difference between racial groups, and (b) black and interracial children reared in the culture of the tests and the schools perform as well as white adopted children in similar families (Burks, 1928; Horn, Loehlin, & Willerman, 1979; Leahy, 1935; Scarr & Weinberg, 1978). The adopted children scored 6 points below the natural children of the same families, however, as Burks (1928) had discovered and a second adoption study by Scarr and Weinberg also found.

PARENT–CHILD CORRELATIONS.   The adoptive families had adopted at least one black child, but these same families also included other adopted children and many biological offspring. The children ranged in age from 4 to about 18. Because of the age range, children from 4 to 7 years were given the Stanford–Binet, children from 8 to 16 the WISC, and older children and all parents the WAIS. The adopted children averaged age 7 and the natural children about 10. Table 13.22 shows the parent–child IQ correlations for all of the adopted children in the transracial adoptive families, regardless of when they were adopted. It is worth noting that the total sample of adopted children is just as similar to the adoptive parents as the early adopted group. The midparent–child correlation for all adoptees is .29 and for the early adoptees, .30. Mothers and all adopted children are equally similar, and fathers are more similar to all adoptees than they are to the early adopted children.

Table 13.22 also shows the correlations between all adopted children's IQ scores and their natural parents' educational levels (used as a proxy for IQ). These correlations are as high as the IQ correlations of biological parent–child pairs and exceed those of the adoptive parent–child IQ scores. The natural midparent–child correlation of .43 is significantly greater than the adoptive midparent–child correlation of .29.

Because the adoptive parents are quite bright, the variance in their scores was considerably restricted. In Table 13.22 the correlations between parents and their natural and adopted children are not corrected for restriction of range in the parents' IQ scores. When corrected, the correlations of biological offspring with their parents rise to .49 and .54, and the midparent–child correlation is .66. Adopted-child–adoptive-midparent IQ resemblance rises to .37 (Scarr & Weinberg, 1977).

Table 13.23. *Sibling IQ correlations among natural and adopted children of adoptive families*

	N (pairs)	r
Natural sibs		
All IQ scores	107	.42
Stanford–Binet	10	.50
WISC and WAIS	63	.54
Natural sib–adopted sib		
All IQ scores	230	.25
Stanford–Binet	57	.23
WISC and WAIS	63	.20
Natural sib–early adopted sib		
All IQ scores	34	.30
All adopted sibs		
All IQ scores	140	.44
Stanford–Binet	36	.31
WISC and WAIS	50	.64
Early adopted sibs		
All IQ scores	53	.39

Note: Stanford–Binet = Stanford–Binet Intelligence Scale; WISC = Wechsler Intelligence Scale for Children; WAIS = Wechsler Adult Intelligence Scale.

When the IQ scores of the parents are corrected for restriction of range, the magnitude of the resemblance between biological parents and their nonadopted children exceed that of the natural parents' educational level and the IQ scores of their adopted offspring, but the latter are still higher than the correlations of corrected IQ score correlations for the adoptive parents and adopted children.

The correlations between natural parents and adopted children and the biological children of the adoptive parents are estimates of the effects of selective placement. If agencies match educational and social class characteristics of the natural mothers with similar adoptive parents, then the resemblance between adoptive parents and children is enhanced by the genetic, intellectual resemblance of natural and adoptive parents. Selective placement also enhances the correlation between natural parents and their adopted offspring, because the adoptive parents carry out the genotype–environment correlation that would have characterized the natural parent–child pairs, had the children been retained by their natural parents. Thus, neither the adoptive parent–child correlations nor the natural parent–adopted child correlations deserve to be as high as they are. In another paper, Scarr and Weinberg (1977) subtracted half of the selective placement coefficient of .17 from both the natural parent–adopted child correlation, a solution proposed by Willerman (1977). Other corrections could be justified by the data set, but the "ultimate" solution(s) must be left to biometricians. Scarr and Weinberg's simple figuring of these data yields heritabilities of .4 to .7.

SIBLING CORRELATIONS. In Table 13.23, the sibling correlations reveal a strikingly different picture. Young siblings are quite similar to each other, whether genetically related or not. The IQ correlations of the adopted sibs, genetically unrelated to each other, are as high as those of the biological sibs reared together. Children reared in

Table 13.24. *Means, standard deviations, and correlations of adoptive and biological family characteristics*

	1	2	3	4	5	6	7	8	9	10	11	M	SD
												Biological children	
Adopted children													
1. Child's IQ		.26	.24	.10	.22	−.19	−.21	.39	.39			112.82	10.36
2. Father's education	.10		.51	.61	.44	.01	−.36	.56	.24			15.63	2.83
3. Mother's education	.10	.51		.36	.39	.02	−.36	.43	.46			14.68	2.24
4. Father's occupation	.12	.57	.25		.47	.01	−.30	.37	.13			62.47	24.73
5. Family income	.06	.50	.40	.46		.00	−.25	.38	.19			24,987.34	8,770.43
6. Birth rank	−.19	.05	.03	.06	.15		.08	−.00	.03			1.62	.63
7. Family size	−.05	.04	.11	−.00	.21	.10		−.30	−.10			3.85	1.48
8. Father's IQ	.15	.53	.30	.40	.45	.08	.14		.20			118.02	11.66
9. Mother's IQ	.04	.29	.44	.19	.21	.07	.12	.30				113.41	10.46
10. Natural mother's age	−.10	.04	.03	.12	−.02	−.11	−.04	−.10	.03				
11. Natural mother's education	.21	.33	.24	.29	.43	.09	.14	.20	.10	.07			
12. Natural mother's occupation	.12	−.00	.13	.11	.06	−.06	.11	.11	.15	.28	.33		
M	106.19	14.90	13.95	60.30	25,935.00	1.43	2.87	116.53	112.43	22.46	11.97		
SD	8.95	3.03	2.06	24.14	10,196.78	.57	1.20	11.36	10.18	5.80	1.66		

Note: Adopted children $N = 150$, biological children $N = 23\%$. $r \geq .16$, $p < .05$.
Source: Scarr & Weinberg (1978).

the same family environments who are still under the major influence of their parents score at similar levels on IQ tests. The IQ correlations of the adopted sibs result in small part from their correlations in background, such as their natural mothers' educational levels (.16) and age at placement in the adoptive home (.37), which is in turn related to the present intellectual functioning of the children – the earlier the placement the higher the IQ score. Age of placement is itself correlated with many other background characteristics of the child and is a complex variable (Scarr & Weinberg, 1976). It seems that some families accepted older adoptees and others did not and that the families differed on the average in the rearing environments. The correlation among the early adopted siblings is fully .39. Even among the families who had early adoptees, differences in family environments and selective placement accounted for an unexpectedly large resemblance between unrelated children.

The major point is that the heritabilities calculated from young sibling data are drastically different from those calculated from the parent–child data. As Christopher Jencks pointed out in his earlier book (1972), the correlations of unrelated young siblings reared together do not fit any biometrical model, because they are too high. This study only makes the picture worse.

The Adolescent Adoption Study

This study was conceived to assess the cumulative impact of differences in family environments on children's development at the end of the child-rearing period (Scarr & Weinberg, 1978; Scarr & Yee, 1980). All of the adoptees were placed in their families in the first year of life, the median age being 2 months. At the time of the study they were 16 to 22 years of age. The short form of the WAIS was given to both parents and to two adolescents in most of the 115 adoptive families. A comparison group of 120 biological families had children of the same ages. Both samples of families were of similar socioeconomic status (working class to upper-middle class) and of similar IQ levels, except that the adopted children scored about 6 points lower than the biological children of similar parents. Table 13.24 gives these results.

PARENT–CHILD AND SIBLING CORRELATIONS.   Table 13.25 gives the parent–child and sibling correlations for the WAIS IQ and the four subtests on which it is based. The parent–child IQ correlations in the biological families were about .4 when uncorrected for the restriction of range in the parents' scores. The adoptive parent–child correlations, however, were lower than those of the younger adopted children and their parents, and the IQ correlation of adopted adolescents reared together is zero. Unlike the younger siblings (who, after all, are also of different races), these white adolescents reared together from infancy do not resemble their genetically unrelated siblings at all.

The IQ "heritabilities" from the adolescent study vary from .38 to .61, much like the parent–child data in the study of younger adoptees, but very unlike those data on younger sibs. The interpretation of these results (Scarr & Weinberg, 1978) is that older adolescents are largely liberated from their families' influences and have made choices and pursued courses that are in keeping with their own talents and interests. Thus, the unrelated sibs have grown less and less alike. This hypothesis cannot be tested fully without longitudinal data on adopted siblings; to date all of the other adoption studies sampled much younger children, at the average age of 7 or 8. We

Table 13.25. *Correlations among family members in adoptive and biologically related families (Pearson coefficients on standardized scores by family member and family type) for intelligence test scales*

Child score	Reliability[a]	Biological[b]				Adoptive[c]			
		MO	FA	CH	MP	MO	FA	CH	MP
Total WAIS IQ	(.97)	.41	.40	.35	.52	.09	.16	−.03	.14
Subtests									
Arithmetic	(.79)	.24	.30	.24	.36	−.03	.07	−.03	−.01
Vocabulary	(.94)	.33	.39	.22	.43	.23	.24	.11	.26
Block Design	(.86)	.29	.32	.25	.40	.13	.02	.09	.14
Picture Arrangement	(.66)	*.19*	*.06*	.16	*.11*	−.01	−.04	.04	−.03
n		270	270	168	268	184	175	84	168

Note: MO = mother–child; FA = father–child; CH = child–child; MP = midparent–child; WAIS = Wechsler Adult Intelligence Scale. Italicized numbers = biological > adoptive correlation, $p < .05$.
[a]Reliability reported in the WAIS manual for late adolescents.
[b]120 families.
[c]104 families.
Source: Scarr & Weinberg (1978), Table 5.

can think of no other explanation for the markedly low correlations between the adopted sibs at the end of the child-rearing period, in contrast to the several studies of younger adopted sibs, who are embarrassingly similar.

EFFECTS OF FAMILY BACKGROUND ON IQ, APTITUDE, AND ACHIEVEMENT SCORES.   For contrast with the material that is forthcoming, let us look first at the effects of family environments on young adoptees' IQ scores. Table 13.26 shows two regression equations, one for the biological children and one for the early adopted children of the transracial adoptive families. The predictive variables are more substantially related to the IQ scores of the biological children, with an R^2 of .30, compared with an R^2 of .156 for the young adoptees. The major difference in the two equations is the predictive value of the parents' IQ scores for the biological children's IQ scores. The IQ scores are correlated, of course, with parental demographic characteristics, whose coefficients are pulled in a negative direction when they coexist in the equation.

Now let us look at similar data for the adolescent adoptees and their biological, comparison families. The nonadopted adolescents' IQ, school aptitude, and achievement test scores were regressed on family demographic characteristics, sibling order, and parental IQ. The adopted adolescents' scores were regressed on those variables plus the natural mothers' age, education, and occupational status. The goal of these analyses was to estimate how much the indexed differences in family environments contributed to individual differences in IQ and school test scores. The contribution of genetic differences to test-score differences is grossly underestimated by this procedure, because the only parental scores available are from the WAIS IQ for the biological parents. There are no comparable data on the natural parents of the adopted children nor are there school test scores on any of the parents. Nonetheless, it is interesting to examine the pattern of R^2s obtained from the regres-

Table 13.26. *Regressions of child IQ on family
demographic characteristics and parental IQ in
transracial adoptive families with their own children*

	Biological children[a]		Early adopted children[b]	
	B[c]	Beta	B[c]	Beta
Mother's IQ	.474	.32	.141	.13
Father's IQ	.513	.40	−.028	−.02
Father's education	.682	.14	.389	.09
Mother's education	−.943	−.15	1.501	.25
Father's occupation	−.174	−.23	.008	—[d]
Family income	.445	.06	−.371	−.06
Total R^2	.301		.156	
Adjusted R^2	.269		.116	

[a]$N = 143$.
[b]$N = 111$.
[c]B = unstandardized regression coefficient.
[d]$F < .01$; variable did not enter the equation.

sion of the IQ, aptitude, and achievement scores on social and genetic background. Table 13.27 summarizes the regression analyses. (Detailed versions of the regressions are given in Scarr & Yee, 1980.)

Let us concentrate on the adoptive families first. Because the parents in this case provide only the social environment, it is possible to estimate the effects of differences in these environments, which range socioeconomically from working class to upper-middle class. The R^2 values, shrunken for each equation, give the estimated percentages of variance in test scores accounted for by socioeconomic differences *between* families – that is, those social environmental features that siblings share – and by environmental differences between siblings *within* the same families, which are indexed here by sibling order (in biological families this would be called birth order).

Between-families effects. The most striking result is that differences in adoptive families' income, parents' education, fathers' occupation, and parents' IQ scores account for none of the variance in their adolescents' IQ scores. In fact, the uncorrected R^2 for the regression of adopted adolescents' IQ scores on their adoptive parents' characteristics is only .02, which shrinks to −.01 with correction. This means that differences in social class and intellectual *environment* of the families have virtually no effect on IQ differences among their children at the end of the child-rearing period. By comparison, the same variables accounted for 11.6% of the IQ variance among the younger adopted children.

The same analysis for the biologically related adolescents is given at the bottom of Table 13.27. In contrast to .01, their corrected R^2 is .26 for the same measures of between-families differences in social class and parental IQ. This value is identical to the shrunken R^2 for the younger sample of biological children in the transracial adoptive families. In the case of biological children, of course, these differences between families are due to both environmental and genetic differences, the latter

Table 13.27. R^2 *estimates of the effects of social environmental and genetic differences on IQ, aptitude, and achievement test scores in adopted and biologically related adolescents, stepwise regressions*

	\multicolumn{7}{c}{Adjusted R^2s}						
	WAIS IQ	Verbal aptitude	Num. aptitude	Total	Read achiev.	Math	Total
Adopted adolescents, social environmental indexes							
Between families[a]	−.01	.05	.03	.04	.09	.08	.10
Within families[b]	.02	.02	.00	.01	.01	.05	.03
Total environment	.02	.07	.03	.05	.10	.13	.13
Genetic indexes[c]	.06	.08	.02	.05	.07	.07	.09
Total R^2	.08	.15	.05	.10	.17	.20	.22
n	150	147	128	128	140	128	128
Biologically related adolescents, social environmental indexes, and genetic indexes							
Between families[a]	.26	.19	.13	.18	.14	.14	.18
Within families[b]	.03	.04	.04	.07	.01	.02	.02
Total R^2	.29	.23	.17	.25	.15	.16	.20
n	237	231	158	158	195	187	181

[a]Parental education, father's occupation, family income, parental WAIS IQs.
[b]Sibling order.
[c]Natural mother's education, occupation, and age (to correct for young mothers).

being of overwhelming importance in explaining the IQ differences both among younger children and adolescents in these families.

As we move from IQ to school test scores, there are three important trends to notice: First, the effect of differences in social environments *between* families increases as the tests sample more recently taught material; second, natural mothers' genetic contribution to test-score differences is similar and moderate across the various tests; and third, the contribution of biological parents' IQ scores to their offsprings' test-score differences is far less for school aptitude and achievement tests than for IQ tests.

The first point is that the major difference in explained variance between IQ and school achievement test scores is that social class differences – that is, differences *among* families – account for the majority of the explained variability in achievement scores and for virtually none of the IQ differences. In one sense, then, school achievement tests are more biased against working-class environments than are IQ tests.

Natural mothers' effects. The index of genetic differences is admittedly very weak. Information was available on only one of the natural parents and was limited to educational and occupational level at the time of the child's birth, and age, which was entered into the regression equations to correct for any underestimation of younger mothers' educational and occupational levels. Regardless of the limitations of those variables, one can see from Table 13.27 that natural mothers' characteristics are substantially related to their offsprings' intellectual achievements, even though any variance due to selective placement has been removed by entering social environmental variables into the equations first.

Biological parents' IQ effects. The detailed tables of regression analyses (available in Scarr & Yee, 1980) show that parental IQs decline from 15% of the variance in adolescents' IQ scores (holding everything else in the equation constant) to less than 2% of the variance in aptitude and achievement test scores (again holding constant education, income, and other variables). Parental IQ is by far the best predictor of IQ differences among biologically related children, but parental education and family income are as good predictors of school aptitude score differences and better predictors of school achievement scores. This does not mean that the genetic differences are less important for aptitude and achievement scores, as will be seen from both the natural mothers' data and from sibling correlations of test scores, to be discussed. It does mean, however, that parental IQ differences are more closely related to their offsprings' differences in IQ than in school achievements. If we had obtained reading and mathematics achievement scores for the parents, however, it may well be that the between-families genetic differences would remain relatively constant across the various tests, whereas the impact of social environments would rise, giving a higher total between-families R^2 for achievement than IQ test scores. From the adopted family results, it is clear that environmental differences among families are a trivial source of IQ differences and a substantial source of differences in school test scores.

Sibling correlations. Another method for checking on the effects of family environment on test scores is to calculate the correlations between pairs of siblings who are genetically unrelated but who have been reared together from early infancy, as are the adopted children in the adolescent study. Their sibling correlations are given in Table 13.28, with the corresponding biological sibling correlations for comparison.

As one can see, the effects of being reared in the same household, neighborhood, and schools are negligible unless one is genetically related to one's brother or sister. The correlations on the biological siblings are modest but statistically different from zero.

With the most simpleminded version of the heritability coefficient and an assumption that parental assortative mating is the same for aptitude and achievement as it is for IQ, we multiply the difference between the biological and adopted siblings' correlations by 1.6. The heritability estimates vary from .22 to .61, with a median of .37. Although these values are not .8, as some would claim, neither are they zero. There seems to be no consistent difference in heritability by the kind of test.

The negligible differences in heritability for IQ, aptitude, and achievement scores in this study of late adolescents is congruent with Lloyd Humphreys's findings of equal heritabilities for all cognitive measures in the Project Talent data (Humphreys, 1981) and with those of the Texas Adoption Study, which showed equal sibling resemblances in IQ and school achievement measures in a sample of younger children (Willerman, Horn, & Loehlin, 1977). In other words, there seems to be no

Table 13.28. *Sibling correlations of IQ, aptitude, and achievement test scores of adopted and biologically related adolescents*

| | Biological | | Adopted | | $h^2 = 1.6$ |
	N (pairs)	r	N (pairs)	r	$(r_{bio} - r_{adopt})$
WAIS					
Verbal	168	.23	84	.07	.26
Performance	168	.21	84	.07	.22
IQ	168	.35	84	−.03	.61
Aptitude					
Verbal	141	.29	68	.13	.26
Numerical	61	.32	49	.07	.40
Total	61	.32	49	.09	.37
Achievement					
Reading	106	.27	73	.11	.26
Math	104	.35	58	−.11	.53
Total	104	.33	58	−.03	.58

Source: Scarr & Yee (1980).

greater sibling resemblance for one or another kind of intellectual achievement, when they are all *g* loaded. Humphreys and we agree, however, that some specific skills may have different heritabilities.

It seems that the effects of family environments vary with the age of the child and the material sampled on the test. Younger children appear to be far more influenced by differences among families. Children reared in working-class families are more disadvantaged in comparison with upper-middle-class children when the tests sample specifically and recently taught material, that is, by school achievement tests rather than IQ tests. Finally, the evidence from these studies argues from a heritability of intellectual measures in the .4 to .7 range, and not .8.

Other adoption studies

One of the most interesting and novel adoption studies was done of working-class families in France who had relinquished one child for adoption but retained others to rear themselves (Schiff et al., 1978). The authors found a small sample of children of working-class families who had been adopted into upper-middle-class families. The average IQ of the adoptees was 110.6, whereas that of their nonadopted siblings was only 94.7. Similarly, in school the adoptees seldom failed grades (13%), whereas 55% of the nonadopted sibs had failed. The authors' conclusion that there are no important genetic differences between social groups that are relevant to school failure directly contradicts the findings of the Texas and Minnesota adoption studies. Willerman (1979) suggested that the range of environments in the U.S. studies may be too narrow to provide a test of such social class environmental effects. One is reminded that population statistics are highly sensitive to the ranges and variances of the genetic and environmental sources of variation, which may well differ from population to population.

From the Netherlands, Claeys (1973) reported on the Primary Mental Abilities and field independence of 84 adopted children. The average level of performance of the adopted children was about 10 points above the levels that are average for the social class from which they came and was equal to or better than the performance level of biological offspring of the families of the same social class as the adoptive families. Like Schiff and colleagues in France, Claeys found no evidence for genetic differences between social class groups. One wonders if social mobility by ability has been so restrained in Europe that there is no association between intelligence and social class, as there seems to be in U.S. studies.

Fisch and colleagues (1976) used another version of an adoption-study design, comparing 94 children adopted by nonrelatives with 50 children kept by their biological mothers, who eventually married men who adopted the children. The children in both groups were matched by gestational age, birth weight, sex, and socioeconomic status of the mother at the time of the birth. Although the authors collected data on physical growth and health as well, we include here only the information on IQ and school achievement. The adopted children did not have higher Stanford–Binet IQ scores at 4 years or WISC IQs at 7 than their controls; in addition, their IQ scores were not as high as those of the biological offspring of families of the same socioeconomic status as their adoptive families. The adopted children did perform better than controls on two WISC subtests and on measures of reading and spelling, indicating the effects of adoptive homes on school achievement.

Racial differences in intelligence

In view of all the most relevant evidence which I have examined, the most tenable hypothesis, in my judgment, is that genetic, as well as environmental, differences are involved in the average disparity between American Negroes and whites in intelligence and educability, as here defined. All the major facts would seem to be comprehended quite well by the hypothesis that something between one-half and three-fourths of the average IQ difference between American Negroes and whites is attributable to genetic factors, and the remainder to environmental factors and their interaction with the genetic differences. [Jensen, 1973, p. 363]

The evidence to which Jensen refers is (a) the unbiased nature of cognitive tests (see also, Jensen, 1980), (b) the heritability of individual differences within each racial group studied, (c) the inability of environmental factors that account for individual variation within racial groups to account for differences between racial groups, and (d) the poor performance of U.S. black groups in comparison with that of Indians and Mexican-Americans, whose social conditions are even worse than those of blacks. Jensen admits that none of these arguments addresses directly the issue of genetic racial differences between blacks and whites in the United States.

In 1975, Loehlin, Lindzey, and Spuhler published their review of the literature on racial differences in intelligence (sponsored by the Social Science Research Council). Their equivocal conclusion led many social scientists to take the position that the possibility of genetic differences between the races was an open issue. Since that time, three investigations of the possible genetic origins of racial differences in performance on school and IQ tests have rejected the hypothesis of genetic differences as the major source of intellectual differences between the races. First, a study of transracial adoption (Scarr & Weinberg, 1976) showed that black and interracial children reared by socioeconomically advantaged white families score very well on standard IQ tests and on school achievement tests. Being reared in the culture of the test and the school resulted in intellectual achievement levels for black children that were comparable to those for adopted white children in similar families. Therefore, it is highly unlikely that genetic differences between the races could account for the major portion of the usually observed differences in the performance levels of the two groups.

A second study, on the relation of black ancestry to intellectual skills within the black population (Scarr et al., 1977), showed that having more or less African ancestry bore no relation to how well one scored on cognitive tests. In other words, holding social identity and cultural background factors constant, socially classified blacks with more African ancestry scored as highly on the tests as blacks with less African ancestry. A strong genetic difference hypothesis cannot account for this result.

Briefly, blood groups were used to estimate the proportion of each person's African and European ancestry. This is roughly possible because the parent populations differ in the average frequencies of many alleles at many loci and differ substantially at a few loci. Therefore, particular alleles could be assigned probabilities as to their origins in one of the two populations. Although there is undoubtedly a large error term in these estimates, they had several satisfactory characteristics, such as appropriately large sibling and skin color correlations. What is most important here is that the estimates of ancestry did not correlate with any measures of intellectual performance in the black sample. Thus, we concluded that degree of white ancestry had little or no effect on individual levels of performance within the black group. We must look to other explanations.

The third study was of black and white twins in Philadelphia (Scarr & Barker, 1981). Briefly, the black 10- to 16-year-olds scored one-half to one standard deviation below the whites on every cognitive measure. The social class differences between the races were not sufficiently large, as Jensen has reminded us, to account solely for the magnitude of this performance difference between the racial groups. The major hypothesis was that black children have less overall familiarity with the information and the skills being sampled by the tests and the schools. The use of twins in this study enabled a comparison of three major predictions of the cultural difference hypothesis with those of a genetic difference hypothesis. The cultural difference hypothesis predicts:

1. Black children will score relatively worse on these tests that are more culturally loaded than on more "culture-fair" tests when the instructions for all tasks are equally understood.
2. The cultural differences of the blacks constitute a "suppressive environment" with respect to the development of the intellectual skills sampled by typical tests, and therefore black children will show less genetic variability in their scores and more environmental variability (Scarr-Salapatek, 1971a).
3. Differences among black children will be more dependent on differences among their family environments in the extent to which they aid children in the development of test-relevant skills, and therefore (a) the twin correlations will be higher for black twins, and (b) there will be less difference between MZ and DZ coefficients in the black groups than in the white groups.

A genetic difference hypothesis predicts:

1. Black children will score relatively worse on those tests that are loaded more highly on a g factor than on more verbal, culturally loaded tests.
2. The proportions of genetic and environmental variability will be the same in both racial groups.
3. Family environments will be no more important in black than in white racial groups in determining individual variation.

We believe that the pattern of results supports a general cultural difference hypothesis far better than a genetic difference view. The major intellectual results are:

1.   Black children have lower scores on all of the cognitive tests, but they score relatively worse on the more culturally loaded of the conceptual tests.
2.   The cognitive differences among the black children are less well explained by genetic individual differences, by age, and by social class differences than are those of the white children.
3.   The similarity of the black co-twins, particularly the DZs, suggests that differences in families determine more of the cognitive differences among black than white children but that those between-families differences are not usually the socioeconomic variables that are measured in the white community.

The results of the Scarr and Barker study support the view that black children are being reared in circumstances that give them only marginal acquaintance with the skills and the knowledge being sampled by the tests that were administered. Some families in the black community encourage the development of these skills and knowledge, whereas others do not. The hypothesis that most of the differences among the cognitive scores of black children and white children are due to genetic differences between the races cannot, in our view, account for this pattern of results. Therefore, in three studies, the hypothesis of genetic differences between the races fails to account for the IQ performance differences.

13.5.   SEPARATE COGNITIVE ABILITIES

INTRODUCTION

Discussions about the behavior genetics of separate cognitive abilities often focus on data from multivariate studies indicating that some abilities that correlate highly with one another are more heritable than other clusters of abilities. There is considerable dispute about the strength of such a claim and about its implications for a theory of intelligence. Many behavior geneticists continue to doubt that different kinds of intellectual functioning are differentially heritable (Loehlin & Nichols, 1976; R. Nichols, 1978). Despite the general finding of moderate to high correlations among tests of specific cognitive abilities, the existence of sharp discontinuities of intellectual performance have kept alive the hope that there may be discrete and uncorrelated components of information processing that contribute to what we loosely construe as intelligence. The existence of idiots savants, individuals with subnormal psychometric IQ scores who excel in specific areas such as music, art, or numerical abilities, has been cited as testimony to the separate abilities approach to intelligence (Anastasi & Levee, 1959; Minton & Schneider, 1980). Additional support for this position has come from evidence of differential rates of decline with age for verbal and spatial abilities (Botwinick, 1977; Wechsler, 1950).

There would be no good rationale for asking questions about genetic and environmental mechanisms for separate cognitive abilities if we believed that all cognitive abilities developed in the same way and responded identically to differences in genetic constitution, biological factors, and environmental circumstances. We know, however, that this is not the case. There is good evidence for discontinuities in cognitive development, not only from the factor analytic studies that are commonly cited but from studies of cognitive dysfunction. We know, for example, that women with Turner's syndrome, a chromosomal anomaly involving the X chromosome, although normal or above normal in verbal functioning, often show deficits in spatial thinking. If this genetic anomaly had deleterious effects on intellectual functioning in general, we would expect to see an overall decrement in cognitive skills. Similarly, if the physical consequences of Turner's syndrome (short stature, webbed neck, absence of secondary sexual characteristics, infertility, and others) led to treatment by parents, siblings, and teachers that depressed cognitive performance, we would not expect the performance depression to be restricted to spatial thinking.

Attempts to specify and elaborate the routes from genes to behaviors have not met with great success when general level of intellectual functioning has been the object of study. It is possible, however, that the mechanistic approach will have greater utility with respect to specific cognitive abilities. In certain clinical syndromes with known or suspected genetic etiologies (Turner's syndrome, autism, dyslexia), only certain kinds of cognitive functions are disrupted while others are quite intact. Other conditions have known genetic antecedents, but the precise nature of the cognitive impairment has not been fully explored (PKU, Down's syndrome, Klinefelter's syndrome, and Huntington's chorea, for example). Carrying out the necessarily detailed biochemical analyses on probands and their families may seem arduous and painstaking, but only by doing such studies can we hope to understand the biological substrates of abnormal cognitive development and discover effective treatments for affected individuals.

The bulk of recent behavior genetic research on IQ and general intellectual ability has focused on normal development rather than on clinical populations. The same has not been true in studies of specific cognitive abilities. Researchers seem here to fall into two camps: those who take a population approach and administer cognitive tests to large numbers of individuals who differ in the extent to which they share common genes and common rearing environments; and those who sample from populations with a specific deficit and either study those individuals intensively or study those individuals *and* their relatives, in an attempt to explore the possible biological and sociocultural mechanisms underlying the condition. In the first approach, the goal is to determine what proportion of total variance can be attributed to genetic and nongenetic factors. Although the second approach may also attempt to explain some variance in the population, the major focus seems to be one of developing explanatory, mechanistic models that might lead to effective interventions, at whatever level.

MULTIVARIATE STUDIES OF SPECIFIC COGNITIVE ABILITIES

No convincing evidence exists that any one kind of cognitive ability is substantially more heritable than any other. Although some studies have reported greater familiality for verbal abilities, others have found no significant differences. The most comprehensive and largest twin studies to date have come up with mixed results and have led us to conclude that such studies cannot be used to support the notion of genetically mediated differences in the relative degree of familial resemblance across different cognitive abilities (Bruun, Markkanen, & Partanen, 1966; Loehlin & Nichols, 1976; Schoenfeldt, 1968). Although the heritability estimates for specific and general cognitive abilities from twin studies do not differ significantly (.42 for specific abilities, and .48 for general IQ), an examination of the magnitudes of the MZ and DZ correlations suggests that within-family environmental influences may affect specific cognitive abilities more than they affect general cognitive functioning (Plomin, DeFries, & McClearn, 1980).

Family studies have also come up with inconsistent findings. Williams (1975)

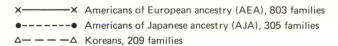

x———————x Americans of European ancestry (AEA), 803 families
●- - - - - -● Americans of Japanese ancestry (AJA), 305 families
△— — — —△ Koreans, 209 families

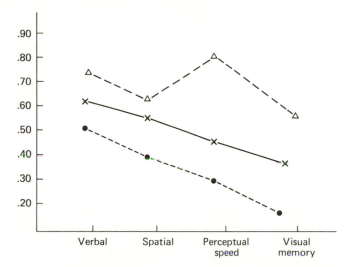

Figure 13.12.   Regressions of midchild on midparent for four factor scores in three ethnic groups. (From "Parent–Offspring Resemblance for Specific Cognitive Abilities in Korea" by J. Park et al., *Behavior Genetics*, 1978, 8(1), 43–52. Reprinted by permission.)

reported that family resemblance was greater for Verbal than for Performance subscales on Wechsler tests in a study of 55 10-year-old boys and their parents. Verbal test correlations were not consistently higher than correlations for other tests, however, in Loehlin, Sharan, & Jacoby's (1978) study of cognitive performance in 192 Israeli families with two children aged 13 or older.

Data from the largest family study to date, the Hawaii Family Study, have been combined with data from a study of 209 Korean families (Park et al., 1978) in Figure 13.12 in an attempt to present comparable information (the same measures were used in both studies) for three different ethnic groups. After age corrections had been made, midchild scores were regressed on midparent scores for individual cognitive tests and for factor scores. Both the Americans of European ancestry and the Americans of Japanese ancestry had somewhat higher familial similarity on verbal and spatial factors than on perceptual speed and visual memory (see Figure 13.13). This pattern is not evident for the Korean sample, however, in which, although the value for visual memory is the lowest of the four factors, all factors reflect substantial familiality. Park and colleagues (1978) have suggested two explanations for the discrepancy in results. First, the Korean families were tested in nuclear family groups rather than in large groups of several families as in the Hawaii study. This would tend to increase between-families differences. Second, assortative mating coefficients for the Korean sample were higher than for the Hawaiian sample. This may be the result of the cultural practice of matchmaking in Korea and could result in greater genetic variance in that population.

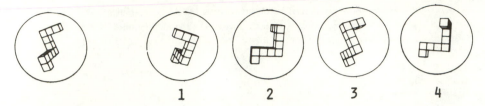

Figure 13.13.   Sample item from Vandenberg and Kuse's Mental Rotations Test. (From "Mental Rotations: A Group Test of Three-dimensional Spatial Visualization" by S. G. Vandenberg and A. R. Kuse, *Perceptual and Motor Skills*, 1978, 47, 599–604. Reprinted by permission.)

Table 13.29. *Assortative mating for intelligence test scales*

	Biological	Adoptive
Child score	Father-mother	Father-mother
Total WAIS IQ	.24	.31
Subtests		
Arithmetic	.19	−.04
Vocabulary	.32	.42
Block Design	.19	.15
Picture Arrangement	.12	.22
n	120	103

Note: WAIS = Wechsler Adult Intelligence Scale.
Source: Scarr & Weinberg (1978), Table 5.

Few adoption studies have examined specific cognitive abilities, but those that have are consistent with the twin and family studies in that they report significantly higher correlations for biological relatives than for adoptive relatives but do not present convincing evidence that one kind of cognitive process is more heritable than another (Carter-Saltzman, 1978; Claeys, 1973; Scarr & Weinberg, 1978). Tables 13.25 and 13.29 will make it clear that although biological relatives are more similar than adoptive relatives on WAIS subtests, the patterns of correlations (especially when assortative mating coefficients are taken into account) do not allow us to make any strong statements about differential heritability of specific abilities.

SPATIAL THINKING

It is probably fair to say that spatial abilities have received more attention from behavior geneticists than any other kind of cognitive processes, and there are several reasons why this is so. First, there are substantial individual and group differences in some kinds of spatial thinking. In particular, strong and consistent sex differences in "spatial visualization" have been replicated many times and have led to the formulation and testing of specific genetic models to account for the distributional and family correlational patterns obtained. Second, psychologists have been somewhat more precise in their definitions of spatial ability than in definitions of other cognitive abilities, so the phenotype under consideration can be clearly differentiated from other cognitive phenotypes. Factor-analytic studies have greatly facilitated this differentiation and have even enabled us to distinguish among various kinds of spatial thinking (not all of which show the aforementioned sex differences). Finally, some clinical subgroups have shown striking patterns of deficits and advantages in spatial thinking. Women who have Turner's syndrome, a known genetic disorder, show a definite disturbance of spatial thinking. The knowledge that these women differ from other women by the absence of sex chromatin in their cells (they are missing the second X chromosome) has led investigators to focus attention on possible X-chromosome involvement in spatial thinking. Autistic children, on the other hand, often are exceptionally good at spatial tasks but do poorly on measures requiring verbal skills. Autism appears to be a disorder with multiple causes, but a genetic etiology seems probable for some children.

Definition of spatial thinking

Since the 1930s, factor-analytic studies have provided strong support for the existence of two separate kinds of spatial abilities, visualization and orientation (McGee, 1979). In a recent review of human spatial abilities, McGee (1979) defines *visualization* as involving

the ability to mentally manipulate, rotate, twist, or invert a pictorially presented stimulus object. The underlying ability seems to involve a process of recognition, retention, and recall of a configuration in which there is movement among the internal parts of the configuration . . . or the recognition, retention, and recall of an object manipulated in three-dimensional space . . . or the folding or unfolding of flat patterns. [P. 893]

Orientation is said to involve "the comprehension of the arrangement of elements within a visual stimulus pattern and the aptitude to remain unconfused by the changing orientation in which spatial configuration may be presented" (McGee, 1979, p. 893). Whether or not either of these abilities bears any relationship to the ability to navigate through three-dimensional space in everyday life has not been investigated.

Several questions still remain unanswered about the specificity of the two spatial factors. Many of the studies from which claims of such distinct abilities were drawn involved subjects limited in age range (usually age 10 to 20), and few studies included female subjects or analyzed the results separately by sex. Several investigators have reported positive and significant correlations between the visualization and orientation factors (Borich & Bauman, 1972; Goldberg & Meredith, 1975; Karlins, Schuerkoff & Kaplan, 1969; Yen, 1975).

Sex differences

Differences between the sexes favoring males have been found across a wide range of spatial tasks by many different investigators. The strongest and most consistent differences have been discerned on tasks that have a visualization component, and this difference is rarely detected before puberty. Although some early sex differences in spatial abilities have been reported (see Vandenberg &

Kuse, 1979, for review), the most discriminating tests that tap visualization have proved too difficult for both young boys and young girls. An example of such a task is illustrated in Figure 13.13. A subject is presented with a two-dimensional representation of a three-dimensional figure and is then asked to choose from an array of similar representations those that are rotations of the original prototype. The rotations can be either in the picture plane, perpendicular to the picture plane, or, conceivably, diagonal to the picture plane. This particular measure is Vandenberg and Kuse's (1978) pencil and paper adaptation of Shepard and Metzler's (1971) task that was designed to address questions about information processing time as a function of degrees of rotation. The most striking sex differences emerge in adolescence, when males move well ahead of their female peers, most of whom never manage to catch up (L. J. Harris, 1979a, 1979b; Maccoby & Jacklin, 1974). It should be noted, of course, that not all females lack spatial visualization ability, although there are more males than females in whom this talent is expressed.

Questions about the nature of the mechanisms underlying this sex difference still remain unresolved, despite the considerable vigilance of several investigators. Hypotheses about the effects of sociocultural, physiological, endocrinological, and genetic mechanisms have been tested. We will review the genetic models that have been proposed and will assess the state of the field in the light of family studies that have been conducted to date. It is sometimes forgotten that behavior genetic methodologies allow us to test environmental models as well as genetic models. Some of the data obtained from family studies have indeed been used to explore the power and specificity of environmental effects on the development of spatial thinking.

X-linkage model of inheritance

Results from twin studies and studies of biological and adoptive families have indicated that spatial abilities are as heritable as other kinds of cognitive abilities (Claeys, 1973; DeFries, Vandenberg & McClearn, 1976; McGee, 1979; Osborne & Gregor, 1968; Vandenberg, 1962; Williams, 1975). Due to the difficulties inherent both in accurate assessment of the phenotype – there is, for instance, no absolute cut-off level on a particular test above which one can reliably diagnose the presence of spatial visualizing ability – and in correct designation of genotype, speculations about the genetic mechanisms influencing sex differences have been somewhat vague. A hypothesis involving X-linkage was most clearly articulated by Bock and Kolakowski (1973), who proposed that spatial visualization ability, although probably influenced by multiple autosomal alleles, was "enhanced" by a recessive gene located on the X chromosome. The frequency of this gene was calculated to be about .50 in North American white populations. It would therefore be expected that about 50% of all males and about 25% of all females in these populations would express the trait of enhanced ability, because males express whatever is on their single X chromosome whether it is dominant or recessive, whereas females would be required to have two of the recessive Xs.

The distribution of scores in a large number of studies involving spatial tests supported the hypothesis (Bock & Kolakowski, 1973; Bouchard & McGee, 1977; Corah, 1965; Guttman, 1974; Hartlage, 1970; Loehlin, Sharan, & Jacoby, 1978; O'Connor, 1943; Stafford, 1961; Yen, 1975): generally about one-quarter of the females scored above the median score for males. Family correlations also followed the expected patterns. Equally high mother–son and father–daughter correlations would be expected because a son receives his only X chromosome from his mother, and a father passes on his only X chromosome to his daughter; the correlation between fathers and sons should be very close to zero because sons receive no X chromosomes from their fathers; and the correlation between mothers and daughters should be intermediate because neither mothers nor daughters necessarily express what is coded on a single X chromosome. Therefore, the order of correlations for an X-linked trait should be as follows: mother–son = father–daughter > mother–daughter > father–son. For sibling correlations, sisters are expected to be most similar because they share the paternally derived X and have a 50% chance of sharing an X chromosome from the mother; brothers would have a 50% chance of having the same maternal X chromosome; and brother–sister pairs would be the least similar because their 50% chance of sharing the maternally derived X is offset by the certainty that the sister will receive an X from the father, whereas the brother will not. The expected order of sibling correlations, then, is: sister–sister > brother–brother > sister–brother.

Since 1973, however, several studies have tested the X-linkage hypothesis, usually with quite large samples of families and often with the same measures across studies. For more detailed treatments of these investigations, the reader is referred to recent reviews by McGee (1979) and Vandenberg and Kuse (1979). The overwhelming conclusion that has been drawn from the more recent studies is that the X-linkage hypothesis cannot be supported on the basis of the rank order of intrafamilial correlations. Comparisons across investigations have been difficult in the past, in part because each researcher used a different test to measure spatial ability. This has not been true in recent behavior genetic research, and the correlations from family studies that used the same three tests – mental rotations (Vandenberg & Kuse, 1978), Card Rotations (French, Ekstrom, & Price, 1963; Ekstrom, French, & Harman, 1976), and Hidden Patterns (Thurstone & Thurstone, 1941) – are presented in Tables 13.30 and 13.31. Mental Rotations is a test of spatial visualization; Card Rotations measures orientation ability, and Hidden Patterns measures the ability to pick out a simple line figure from a more complex drawing.

Although the recent family correlational results clearly cannot be used to support an X-linkage hypothesis, nongenetic factors could be invoked to explain the poorness of fit. It is probable that only linkage analysis will be widely accepted as a critical test of the hypothesis. The X-linkage model would seem quite viable if it could be demonstrated that relatives who were identical for some marker known to be located on the X chromosome were also more similar in spatial skills than relatives who differed on the critical marker. Only one such experiment has been done to date, and the results gave tentative support to the involvement of the X chromosome in field dependence but found no evidence for X-linkage of visualization abilities. Goodenough and colleagues (1977) administered a battery of seven spatial ability tests to sons in 67 Italian families with at least three sons. All of the sons were also tested for red–green color blindness and typed on the XG(a) blood group, both phenotypes known to be located at different parts of the X chromosome. For each marker phenotype the spatial test correlations of sons who were identical for the marker were compared with correlations of sons who differed from one another. No evidence of linkage was found in the analyses of color

Table 13.30. *Parent–offspring correlations of spatial scores*

	Father–son	Mother–daughter	Mother–son	Father–daughter
Mental Rotations Test (spatial visualization)				
AEA, Hawaii[a]	.20 (672)	.30 (692)	.13 (666)	.20 (685)
Colorado[b]	.25 (81)	.04 (81)	.10 (81)	.32 (81)
Minnesota[c]	.04 (94)	.23 (119)	.04 (94)	.17 (119)
Minnesota[d]	.23 (185)	.16 (196)	.20 (204)	.17 (172)
Israel[e]	.32 (153)	.21 (182)	.12 (168)	.08 (157)
AJA, Hawaii[a]	.20 (241)	.11 (248)	.17 (244)	.24 (237)
Korean[f]	.22 (99–103)	.46 (113–121)	.26 (100–105)	.41 (107–117)
Card Rotations Test (spatial orientation)				
Colorado[b]	.25 (81)	.03 (81)	.16 (81)	.15 (81)
AEA, Hawaii[a]	.26 (672)	.34 (692)	.21 (666)	.23 (685)
AJA, Hawaii[a]	.24 (241)	.17 (248)	.10 (244)	.11 (237)
Korean[f]	.12 (99–103)	.61 (113–121)	.36 (100–105)	.54 (107–117)
Israel[g]	.27 (183)	.40 (201)	.27 (183)	.32 (201)
Hidden Patterns Test (disembedding figures)				
AEA, Hawaii[a]	.24 (672)	.32 (692)	.24 (666)	.27 (685)
AJA, Hawaii[a]	.09 (241)	.19 (248)	.13 (244)	.22 (237)
Korean[f]	.51 (99–103)	.65 (113–121)	.58 (100–105)	.56 (107–117)
Israel[g]	.40 (183)	.22 (201)	.44 (183)	.38 (201)
Israel[e]	.24 (153)	.18 (182)	.17 (168)	.19 (157)

Note: Numbers in parentheses = *n*; AEA and AJA are Americans of European and Japanese ancestry, respectively.
[a]DeFries, Johnson, Kuse, McClearn, Polvina, Vandenberg, & Wilson, 1979.
[b]Spuhler, 1976.
[c]Carter-Saltzman, 1977.
[d]McGee, 1978.
[e]Guttman & Shoham, 1979.
[f]Park et al., 1978.
[g]Loehlin et al., 1978.

blindness, but sons who shared the same XG(a) typing were more similar on the two tests of field dependence (rod-and-frame test and Embedded Figures Test) than sons who differed in blood type. It should be noted that the one test included to measure the visualization factor, Stafford's (1961) Identical Blocks Test, provided no support whatever for the X-linkage model. The absence of positive results, however, does not disprove the hypothesis, because a gene influencing spatial thinking could be located on the X chromosome but be quite far from both of the markers tested. Only positive results can be interpreted with certainty. Clearly this kind of study needs to be done with new and larger samples. It could prove most informative.

Turner's syndrome and spatial performance

Studies of the cognitive performance patterns of women with Turner's syndrome are of particular interest for several reasons. First, Turner's syndrome has a known genetic antecedent involving the X chromosome. In the classic Turner's syndrome, there is a total absence of sex chromatin; that is, the entire second X chromosome is missing, leaving the patient with a total of only 45 chromosomes (45,X). Some Turner's women are mosaics, with some of their cells showing the classic 45,X patterns and others having the normal chromosome complement.

Table 13.31. *Sibling correlations of spatial scores*

	Sister–sister	Brother–brother	Sister–brother
Mental Rotations Test (spatial visualization)			
California[a]	.41 (103)	.32 (84)	.27 (191)
Minnesota[b]	.21 (112)	.50 (132)	.33 (249)
AEA, Hawaii[c]	.16 (125)	.35 (114)	.25 (216)
AJA, Hawaii[c]	.24 (37)	.16 (44)	.18 (66)
Card Rotations Test (spatial orientation)			
AEA, Hawaii[c]	.25 (125)	.17 (114)	.33 (216)
AJA, Hawaii[c]	.26 (37)	.33 (44)	.27 (66)
Israel[d]	.52 (51)	.44 (42)	.24 (99)
Hidden Patterns Test (disembedding figures)			
Israel[d]	.55 (51)	.76 (42)	.39 (99)
AEA, Hawaii[c]	.18 (125)	.28 (114)	.30 (216)
AJA, Hawaii[c]	.04 (37)	−.05 (44)	.43 (66)

Note: AEA and AJA are Americans of European and Japanese ancestry, respectively.
[a]Yen, 1975.
[b]Bouchard & McGee, 1977.
[c]DeFries, Johnson, Kuse, McClearn, Polvina, Vandenberg, & Wilson, 1979.
[d]Loehlin et al., 1978.

Still others show variations of the short arm of the second X chromosome: deletions, translocations, or complete absence of the arm (Serra et al., 1978; Stern, 1973). The X-linkage hypothesis about the transmission of spatial abilities has evoked considerable interest in studying possible X-chromosome involvement in spatial thinking. If spatial visualization were X-linked, one would expect the spatial performance of Turner's syndrome women to resemble that of normal males, because any information coded on the X-chromosome should be expressed. In contrast to that expectation, Turner's women perform exceptionally poorly, on the average, on tests of spatial thinking. In addition, this deficit seems to be quite specific to spatial thinking; performance on tests of verbal ability is at or above normal levels.

Garron (1977) reported on a sample of 67 Turner's syndrome women, aged 6 to 31 years, and 67 control subjects, who were matched for age, race, education, residence, social class, marital status, and ethnic and religious backgrounds. All subjects were administered the version of the Wechsler Intelligence Scale that was appropriate to their ages (WAIS or WISC), and Turner's subjects were classified according to karyotype and presence or absence of a variety of physical stigmata. Garron's general conclusions from the study were as follows (p. 125):

1. There is no increased incidence of either severe or moderate general mental retardation, as such is usually understood, among persons with Turner's syndrome.
2. The distribution of intelligence, and the presence of specific cognitive deficits, is similar in all groups of persons with Turner's syndrome, regardless of karyotype and/or somatic stigmata.
3. The cognitive deficits are equally characteristic of children and adults with Turner's syndrome, although the expression of these deficits may be influenced by particular stages of intellectual development.
4. The nature of these deficits may be understood better by an emphasis on the cognitive processes involved, rather than simply by an emphasis on the stimulus attributes.

Table 13.32. *Performance profiles of Turner's females and controls*

	Verbal IQ	Performance IQ	Verbal–Performance IQ
WISC			
Probands	95.6	89.1	6.5
Controls	99.4	105.5	−6.1
WAIS			
Probands	104.1	88.4	15.7
Controls	109.5	104.0	5.5

Note: WISC = Wechsler Intelligence Scale for Children; WAIS = Wechsler Adult Intelligence Scale.
Source: Garron (1977).

Although direct comparisons of WAIS Verbal IQ, Performance IQ, and full-scale IQ revealed significant differences between adult proband and control groups (see Table 13.32), comparisons of cognitive factors showed significant differences in favor of controls of numerical ability and perceptual organization factors but not for the verbal comprehension factor. Analyses of WISC factors yielded the same results.

When one examines the patterns of Verbal and Performance IQ scores for Garron's older (age 16 and up) and younger subjects the most striking finding is the large discrepancy between Verbal and Performance scales in the adult probands. It is at puberty that large differences between males and females begin to appear on spatial tests (Maccoby & Jacklin, 1974), and female enrollment in mathematics courses begins to decline (Fennema & Sherman, 1977). Indeed, in Garron's sample the control subjects showed a reversal of pattern from the younger to the older group, although the size of the Verbal–Performance gap remained constant.

In a study of 13 Turner's probands aged 12 to 22 years and 13 controls matched on full-scale IQ, age, race, education, parents' marital status, and SES, Silbert, Wolff, and Lilienthal (1977) also found that Wechsler Performance IQs were significantly depressed relative to Verbal IQs in the Turner's sample. In addition to age-appropriate Wechsler IQ tests, subjects were given six tests of spatial perception and organization, three tests of sensorimotor sequencing, three automatization measures, and three auditory tests. Across all the spatial tests administered, Silbert and colleagues (1977) reported deficits in Turner's patients only for "tasks requiring the integration of spatial elements into synthetic wholes or the remembering of total spatial configurations" (p. 19). They did not find differences on tests that required that spatial arrays be analyzed and broken down into component parts. There were no differences between groups on the automatization measures, but the Turner's patients again did more poorly than controls on all three auditory measures (Seashore Rhythm Test, Seashore Tonal Memory Test, and Auditor Figure-Ground Test).

The authors concluded that Turner's patients may have a selective deficit of right-hemisphere functioning that affects synthetic spatial thinking and configurational auditory processing. The idea is intriguing and surely bears further investigation. It seems the next step would be to assess Turner's subjects with some of the standard measures of differential hemispheric processing: verbal and nonverbal dichotic listening tests; tachistoscopic presentation of verbal and nonverbal information to the right and left visual fields; electroencephalograph (EEG) measurements of cortical activity while carrying out different cognitive operations.

As Serra and colleagues (1978) suggested, it is possible that the expression of spatial cognitive abilities is dependent on a normal gonadal hormonal environment, and that, in turn, may depend on sex heterochromatin in the prenatal period.

Hormonal models for differences in spatial ability

Models linking spatial performance to hormonal events – prenatally, at puberty, and in adulthood – have made a respectable showing over the past fifteen years, and most are still viable today. These models have tried to account for cognitive differences as a function of maturation rate (Waber, 1976, 1977), physical androgyny (Klaiber, Broverman, & Kobayashi, 1967; Mackenberg, et al., 1974; Petersen, 1976), and hormonal fluctuations during the menstrual cycle (Englander-Golden, Willis, & Deinstbier, 1976; Klaiber, et al., 1974). Although research in this area is of great importance and will surely enhance our eventual understanding of the biological mechanisms underlying cognitive performance patterns, no studies to date have employed behavior genetic methods. For recent reviews and critiques of these models the reader is referred to Dan (1979), McGee (1979), Petersen (1979), and Waber (1979).

For the present we will briefly discuss a condition of known genetic origin that results in abnormal hormonal concentrations, and we will synthesize some of the hypotheses about the relationships among sex chromosomes, hormones, and cognitive performance.

Adrenogenital syndrome (AGS). The adrenogenital syndrome, caused by an autosomal recessive gene, is a metabolic dysfunction involving an enzyme insufficiency that causes the adrenal gland to secrete excessive amounts of adrenal androgens throughout the lifetime. Since 1950, cortisone treatment has been available to patients with this disorder, and the treatment leads to a reduction of androgen secretions. Therefore, most current cases have suffered only prenatal exposure to abnormally high androgen levels (Reinisch, Gandelman, & Spiegel, 1979). The existence of both genotypic males and females who have been exposed to elevated androgen levels at a specific phase of development allows us to examine the specific effects of prenatal androgen on cognitive performance patterns.

In studies with appropriate controls, no significant differences in specific cognitive abilities have been found between AGS subjects and controls (Baker & Ehrhardt, 1974). Females with AGS do not provide evidence that prenatal exposure to excessive androgen specifically enhances spatial ability. Baker and Ehrhardt (1974) used parents and siblings of AGS patients as controls and found no significant differences between any groups on Verbal or Performance IQ. They did, however, find that the AGS subjects, their parents, and their siblings, all performed above the population norms for IQ. This finding raises the intriguing possibility that both unaffected heterozygotes and homozygotes for AGS share some genetically mediated characteristic that is related to high IQ.

Sex chromosomes, hormones, and cognitive performance.   It has been suggested that the Y chromosome retards maturation rate, permitting fuller expression of the genome in males than in females (Ounsted & Taylor, 1972). This would presumably be reflected in more complete penetrance in males (already proposed in some of the genetic models reviewed above), as well as in greater male variance for a wide array of phenotypes. Wilson and Vandenberg (1978) have reported that in the Hawaii study, variance was greater for males than for females on 11 of 15 cognitive tests (the difference was significant for mental rotations, Subtraction and Multiplication, and Word Beginnings and Endings). Existing data sets can be examined for sex differences in variances, and the question can partially be addressed in that manner. In addition, it should be possible to look at the rates of physical maturation and cognitive development in individuals with Y-chromosome anomalies.

McGee (1979) has proposed that there may be an X-linked gene that controls the timing of androgen release at puberty and has related his suggestion to the work of Petersen (1976) and Broverman and colleagues (1968), who found that high spatial performance was associated with late maturation and low androgenization (determined by physical characteristics) in males, and with highly androgenized body types in females. This notion is consistent with Waber's (1976, 1977, 1979) reports that for both males and females, late-maturers performed at higher levels than early-maturers on tests of spatial ability. These formulations would be strengthened considerably by data indicating a strong positive relationship between the timing of puberty and ratings of physical androgeny. One would also want to look at familial patterns in the timing of the onset of puberty to see if there was any evidence of X-linked inheritance. To our knowledge such studies have not yet been undertaken.

Studies of the relationship between cognitive performance profiles and hormonal status have not been numerous, but we do not know of a single one in which affected subjects showed higher spatial than verbal performance. Dawson (1972) has reported higher Verbal than Performance scores on Wechsler tests for four different groups of subjects with sex hormone anomalies: genetic males with testicular feminization (Masica, Money, & Ehrhardt, 1969); males with Klinefelter's syndrome; females with Turner's syndrome; and West African males with gynaecomastia (breast-enlargement) due to kwashiorkor (Dawson, 1967a; 1967b). As discussed above, even AGS subjects had higher Verbal than Performance scores in those instances where differences were found. It may be that an optimal balance of steroid hormones at one or more periods during development is a prerequisite for the development of high spatial ability. Levine (1971) has suggested that early hormones are crucial during some critical periods of neurological differentiation. He proposed that "the function of gonadal hormones in infancy is to organize the central nervous system with regard to neuroendocrine control of behavior" (p. 15), and he suggested that the differential responsiveness of males and females to externally administered hormones might be dependent upon hormonal events occurring in the prenatal and neonatal periods (Levine, 1971).

Visual perception and cognition

The existence of individual differences in visual perception is well established (Berry, 1971; Pick & Pick, 1970; Segall, Campbell, & Herskovits, 1966). Strangely enough, no one seems to have tried to relate those differences – for example, in visual acuity, lens pigmentation, illusion susceptibility, persistence of a visual image, brightness judgment, and many other basic aspects of visual processing – to performance on cognitive tests of visuospatial performance. Instead, the very limited literature on individual differences in vision has concentrated on linking such variation to differences in age (see Pick & Pick, 1970, for review), culture (Deregowski, 1973; Segall et al., 1966) or sex (McGuinness, 1976a; 1976b; McGuinness & Lewis, 1976). Although individual differences in visual perception do exist, we do not know how such differences might relate to differences in more cognitive processes.

A few studies have investigated the possibility that visual-perceptual mechanisms might be affected by genetic variability. Fuller and Thompson (1978) have reviewed a set of older twin studies (published between 1939 and 1953) and have concluded that amid a host of methodological flaws and outdated techniques, the studies suggest that genetic factors do influence the determination of some aspects of visual perception. To our knowledge almost all of the behavior genetic research published on this topic since 1953 has concerned susceptibility to visual illusions.

Genetic factors have been found to contribute to susceptibility to both primary illusions (those that show a decrease in errors with age) and secondary illusions (those that show an increase in errors with age) and to an illusion that shows a quite complex relationship to age changes. Twin-studies data supporting this general conclusion have been reported for the Müller–Lyer Illusion (Smith, 1949) and the double trapezium illusion (Matheny, 1971), a secondary illusion.

In a family study including 203 mother–father–offspring triads and 303 sibling pairs, Coren and Porac (1979) found evidence of significant family resemblance for the Müller–Lyer Illusion and for the underestimated segment of the Ebbinghaus Illusion. In their very informative review of the possible cognitive and sensory processes underlying illusion susceptibility, the authors concluded that several heritable optical and neural mechanisms might be responsible for both the Müller–Lyer Illusion and the underestimated part of the Ebbinghaus Illusion but that no such mechanisms could be invoked to explain Ebbinghaus overestimation. The reader is referred to Coren and Porac (1979) for a brief review of the studies on heritable variation of visual sensory and neural processes. In an earlier paper, the same authors (1978) reported that the magnitude of the Ebbinghaus Illusion increases with age for the underestimation portion and decreases with age for the overestimation portion. It is not unreasonable to suspect that age differences are also responsive to genetic factors.

One of the most interesting investigations into the relationship of illusion susceptibility to cognitive processes was a co-twin control study done by Matheny (1972a) as a follow-up to his 1971 paper on the Ponzo Illusion. In the earlier paper, Matheny (1971) found that MZ twins had significantly smaller intrapair differences on the Ponzo Illusion than did DZ twins. He later selected 34 pairs of 9- to 11-year-old MZ twins who were discordant on the magnitude of their susceptibility to the Ponzo Illusion; he examined their differences on WISC subtests in order to test Pollack's (1969) hypothesis that high illusion susceptibility was related to high performance on tests of numerical sequencing and analogical reasoning. The WISC subtests of interest were Digit Span and Similarities. Pollack's hypothesis was confirmed for the female twins (21 pairs) but not for the males (13 pairs). It is a nice demonstration of the relationship between visual perception and cognition, holding genetic factors constant.

Patterns of visual exploration were investigated in a study of 70 MZ and 50 DZ twin pairs between the ages of 5 and 11 years (Matheny, 1972b). The children were given cards with multiple pictures of common objects arranged in various patterns, and they were asked to name each picture. Ratings of twin similarity were based on whether the twins started at or near the same place in the visual array and whether they named the pictures according to similar or different spatial patterns. Both older and younger MZ twins were significantly more similar than the DZs in their visual exploratory strategies. Matheny interpreted the greater similarity of the MZ pairs as a reflection of similarities in genetically mediated cognitive strategies related to memory and intelligence.

Although there has been relatively little work by behavior geneticists on visual perception, the existing data suggest that both genetic and nongenetic factors are important in the development of perceptual processes and that such processes are related to cognitive functioning. The field is wide open for a more programmatic approach to the problem.

Sex differences

The robust sex difference in spatial visualization leads to questions about sex differences in visual perception. Are there any? If so, do we know anything about how such differences develop? It will perhaps be surprising to some students of perception and cognition that there is considerable evidence for the existence of sex differences in visual perception (see McGuinness, 1976a, 1976b, for reviews). A few of the differences are male superiority in both dynamic and static visual acuity (Burg, 1966; J. Roberts, 1964); longer persistence of visual sensation (as measured by the Ganzfeld and the afterimage) in males than females (McGuinness & Lewis, 1976); female superiority in some perceptual learning and visual discrimination tasks (Laughlin & McGlynn, 1967; Pishkin, Wolfgang, & Rasmussen, 1967; Stevenson et al., 1968); greater amount of lens pigmentation in males (Girgus, Coren, & Porac, 1977).

Investigations of susceptibility to visual illusions have found no sex differences for two-dimensional, static illusions (Fraisse & Vautrey, 1956; Pressey & Wilson, 1978; Porac et al., 1979), but they have discovered sex differences for Necker cube reversals (Immergluck & Mearini, 1969), an illusion that involves reorganization of a three-dimensional array. This finding is not at all inconsistent with what has been reported for the spatial cognitive tasks. Although sex differences are sometimes found for two-dimensional spatial tests, those findings are less robust and less consistent across studies. The only family studies on visual illusions to date have been limited to two-dimensional illusions.

This brief review of the literature on processes of visual perception and cognition has made one thing abundantly clear: Much work remains to be done. We know that there are individual differences in some aspects of visual perception, but we know little about the relationship between visual perception and spatial cognition. We also know that genetic differences contribute to differences in perceptual processes, but again, we do not have the data necessary for determining if the same genetic differences affect both perceptual and cognitive processes.

Conclusions: spatial thinking

Clearly, individuals differ greatly in spatial thinking. The results of numerous behavior genetic studies have led us to conclude that genetic factors do contribute to the observed differences, although it is difficult to estimate precisely the magnitude of that contribution. Of all cognitive abilities that have been psychometrically assessed, none has shown greater sex differences, at least in North American Caucasian populations, than spatial visualization. To date, the mechanisms mediating those differences have not been specifically delineated, although several genetic models have been proposed and tested. Some of these models have involved differential penetrance in males and females and have most recently been subjected to complex statistical analyses.

Perhaps the most intriguing (and most widely tested) hypothesis has been the one invoking X-linkage, and that question is as yet unresolved. The most recent family correlational data do not favor the hypothesis of a recessive gene on the X-chromosome that enhances spatial visualization, but distributional data and the results of recent linkage study still do not allow us completely to discard the idea. Although the pattern of cognitive abilities of women with Turner's syndrome seems in direct opposition to the X-linkage hypothesis, it is possible that early (possibly prenatal) hormonal events set the stage for the subsequent unfolding of a pattern of spatial thinking. Turner's syndrome women may differ in such hormonal events both from men and from other women with a normal chromosome complement.

Because hormonal status and spatial thinking may in some way be related, it is also possible that the timing of androgen release at puberty and/or the rate of sexual maturation may be related to level of spatial ability. The extent to which genetic factors are important to such a relationship has not yet been addressed with behavior genetic methods. It is only through a longitudinal behavior genetic study that one would be able to demonstrate a clear relationship between hormonal events, spatial performance (at a later point in time), and genetic constitution.

Studies of Turner's syndrome women have allowed us to isolate and test a variety of factors that might relate to spatial thinking. We should do more cognitive testing of subjects with genetic anomalies, particularly those that influence hormonal status. Such experiments may provide us with our best opportunities to find out how genotypes are translated into behavioral phenotypes.

The importance of nongenetic factors in the development of spatial thought should not be slighted and can be addressed through classic behavior genetic studies, cross-cultural studies, and training studies. A combination of these techniques may even lead to new insights about the selection pressures to which subpopulations of our species were subjected in their evolutionary histories.

13.6. THE IMPLICATIONS OF INTELLECTUAL DIVERSITY AND GENETIC DIFFERENCES FOR IMPROVING INTELLIGENCE

One implication of evolutionary theories of intelligence, with their emphasis on adaptation and diversity, is that intelligence will not be randomly distributed in the population. Related persons are more likely to share similar talents, whether high g, musical talent, or spatial skills. Two corollaries of this proposition are (a) more intelligent children tend to be reared by more intelligent parents, and (b) the effects of attempts to improve intelligence are very difficult to predict because apparent environmental differences are often confounded with genetic differences.

As the justifiably maligned Professor Sir Cyril Burt noted a half-century ago, more highly intelligent children come from the working class than the middle class; although proportionally more highly intelligent children come from middle-class families, the smaller numbers of such families mean that in absolute numbers working-class parents contribute more talented children to the next generation than do middle-class parents. Nonetheless, high intelligence in children is associated with high intelligence in parents, by genetic and perhaps environmental transmission.

The correlation of parent and child intelligence means that more intelligent children also tend to have more intellectually advantaged rearing environments. In some psychological circles this may be called the "double-whammy" effect. In behavior genetic circles, it is called a genotype–environment correlation of the passive kind. This means that parental behaviors such as reading to children, discussing topics of intellectual interest with them, and listening to children's opinions are not an arbitrary set of parenting skills applied willy-nilly to any child. Rather they are a set of skills used by intelligent parents with their usually more intelligent children. One is tempted to hypothesize that if parents read to, discussed topics with, and listened to only less intelligent children, the less intelligent would be like the more intelligent children. The adoptive studies discussed earlier suggest that the effects of parental child-rearing practices per se may be substantial in the early years and wane with the children's advancing independence of familial influences. Early intervention studies do *not* suggest that children of parents who are taught how to stimulate them intellectually approach the level of intelligence of children of bright parents who rear their genetically bright children.

In fact, there may be a trade-off between teaching the child apart from the (relatively dull) parents, when the teachers are bright, university-trained people, and training the less bright parents to teach their children, when the effects of the training will be realized after hours and may even be applied by the parent to other children. The quality and intensity of *nonparental* programs may be equivalent to the quantity and extensiveness of *parental* programs.

The natural correlation between parental child rearing and child IQ depends on genotypic correlations of the parent with the child and also on the child's genotype for intelligence. Bright children evoke more intelligent environments from others by selecting more intellectual stimulation. Even if an intervention program provides a stimulating environment, the child may not make full use of it. A bright child automatically gains extra stimulation from that environment by asking smart questions, following complex arguments and presentations, and evoking intellectual interactions from other people.

Thus, it is hard to predict what effects deliberate attempts to improve the intellectual development of children will have. Before discussing the role of environmental interventions on intellectual development, let us consider the family-based intervention.

QUANTITATIVE PREDICTION

Suppose that we find, as Scarr and her colleagues at Yale have in research in Bermuda, that some rough measures of particular mothers' teaching skills are strongly related to children's conceptual development, degree of cooperation with adults in learning tasks, and social competencies. Does this mean that teaching other mothers to be better teachers will enhance their children's intelligence, cooperation, and social competencies? The answer is probably yes, but the question of interest is, How much?

Measured in standard deviation units, the prediction of improvement in children's scores is a direct function of the unstandardized coefficient from the regression of children's scores on mothers' teaching skills. That is, if, as Scarr and her colleagues found, the regression of children's cognitive and social competencies on their mothers' teaching skills is about .67, then every standard deviation improvement in mothers' teaching skills ought to pay off in two-thirds of a standard deviation in children's skills. Let us be concrete with a familiar scale, that of IQ. The regression equation reported predicts that a one *SD* improvement in mothers' teaching skills yields 10 IQ points in the children, a practically important payoff.

Many studies of family situation in the developmental literature stop right there with the implication hanging and untested. For example, the Caldwell HOME Scale (Caldwell, 1978), based on such research, takes naturally occurring correlations of the sort reported and implies that huge gains are to be found in the improvement of the mother's interaction or teaching of the child whose family scores are below average on such scales.

Something must be wrong with the predicted payoff of 10 IQ points for every SD improvement in mothers' teaching skills. No study of intervention has shown such striking effects. What is wrong, of course, is that the mother's teaching skills are related to many other facts about her: her home, her whole environment, and most likely her genetic background. Her genotype is correlated with the environment she provides for herself and the child, whose genotype is correlated with both the mother's genotype and the rearing environment. For example, the mother's IQ is correlated with her 24- to 30-month-old's intellectual or social characteristics; although she may be more irritable than before the child was born, she has probably not lost many skills and certainly has not learned any from her offspring. The child's IQ, on the other hand, is more likely to be affected directly by the mother's IQ, both genetically and environmentally. Let us also assume that the mother's IQ is not directly affected by her skills in teaching a 2-year-old but rather that her teaching skills are another manifestation of her developed intellect. These reasonable assumptions give us the model shown in Figure 13.14.

Given the correlation between the mother's teaching skills and her own IQ and the full impact of the mother's transmission of her IQ to the child by genetic means only (the most conservative assumptions from an intervention point of view), it is still the case that the mother's teaching skills have a partial coefficient of .35 for the child's IQ score; in fact, this figure is obtained after removing the variance in child IQ and teaching skills due to the ethnicity–social class of the family. Thus, an improvement of the mother's teaching skills by one *SD* may well improve the child's IQ score by .35 *SD* or 5 to 6 IQ points, on the average.

Now let us consider another model where mothers' teaching skills are to some extent a function of their child's responsiveness and cooperation in learning. We know from the mothers' ratings of their child's personality and from our own ratings of the children's personalities that young children who are seen by their mothers and by us as cooperative, responsive, and not overly active actually receive better teaching in our experimental situation than children who are seen by their mothers and by us as less cooperative, less responsive, and overly active. The child plays a role in how well he or she is taught.

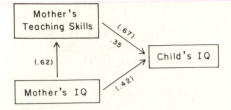

() = zero order correlation coefficients

Figure 13.14.   Correlations among child's IQ, mother's teaching skills, and mother's IQ (in parentheses); the partial regression coefficient of child IQ on mother's teaching skills with mother's IQ is partialed out. (Reprinted from *Facilitating Infant and Early Childhood Development,* by Lynne A. Bond and Justin M. Joffe [Eds.]. By permission of University Press of New England. Copyright 1982 by the Vermont Conference on the Primary Prevention of Psychopathology.)

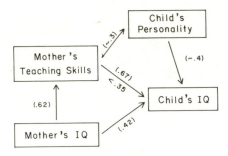

() = zero order correlation coefficients

Figure 13.15.   Correlations and regressions of mother and child variables. (Reprinted from *Facilitating Infant and Early Childhood Development,* by Lynne A. Bond and Justin M. Joffe [Eds.]. By permission of University Press of New England. Copyright 1982 by the Vermont Conference on the Primary Prevention of Psychopathology.)

Now we have a mediating variable, child personality, between the mother's teaching skills and the child's IQ. Actually, the child's personality affects not just how the mother teaches him or her but how able we are to assess his or her IQ. David Wechsler's view of functioning intelligence as part of general personality and not just cognitive skills is valuable here, because in the real world one has to be able to use effectively what one has cognitively. One's theoretical view of this matter is important in creating the intervention model to predict the payoff. Consider Figure 13.15. The payoff from improving mothers' teaching skills is complicated by the degree to which the program addresses and "improves" the children's cooperation, attention, and responsiveness and lowers their activity in learning situations. If the intervention has no effect on a child's personality then the payoff from raising the mother's teaching skills will be considerably less than the .35 SD cited before. (We have not done this calculation.) If, on the other hand, mothers who teach better gain more attentive, cooperative learners, who will

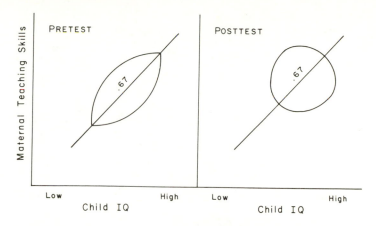

Figure 13.16. Hypothetical distributions of scores on pre- and posttests if mothers with the lowest initial scores gained the most from intervention. (Reprinted from *Facilitating Infant and Early Childhood Development,* by Lynne A. Bond and Justin M. Joffe [Eds.]. By permission of University Press of New England. Copyright 1982 by the Vermont Conference on the Primary Prevention of Psychopathology.)

further reinforce their mothers' teaching skills, and so forth, the effect of child personality on payoff from the intervention may be minimal or even salutary.

Now let us consider three other possibilities: (a) The mother's improvements in teaching skills are a function (positive or negative) or her initial intellectual level; (b) the child's gain in IQ is a function of his or her initial intellectual level (positive or negative correlation); and (c) both maternal and child interactions of intellectual level occur with gain from the program. These modifications of the prediction models can be fitted on the average results predicted by the former models, but they may be important for policy reasons. If, as rarely happens, those who need the intervention most benefit the most from it, one could rejoice, especially at the result shown in Figure 13.16. Although the best slope might be much the same in the posttest as in the pretest, the R^2 of the child's IQ regressed on maternal teaching skills would be greatly reduced by the restriction in variance caused by the negatively correlated gains of both mother and child with their initial scores.

The more usual and opposite result, although everyone benefits from the intervention to some extent, is that those who are more intelligent gain more from the program, as studies of "Sesame Street" watchers have shown. See Figure 13.17. The only way to keep the bright from getting more from absolutely everything is to lock them in closets while the rest are being taught. Otherwise, they will use their time to learn more, and more efficiently, than others.

On the other hand, Richard Snow and Elanna Yalow (chapter 9, this volume) have shown that certain forms of teaching are actually better geared to slow learners and impede the learning efficiency of faster learners subjected to the treatment. Making instructional programs highly *explicit* and *redundant* enhances the learning of those who do not ordinarily make connections and generalizations and impedes the learning of those who do. If an intervention program is particularly geared to mothers who do not teach well because they do not know

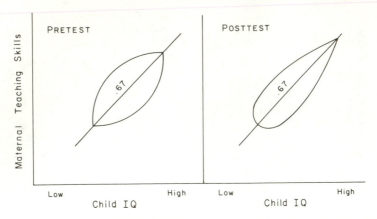

Figure 13.17.   Hypothetical distributions of scores on pre- and posttests if mothers with the highest initial scores gained the most from intervention. (Reprinted from *Facilitating Infant and Early Childhood Development,* by Lynne A. Bond and Justin M. Joffe [Eds.]. By permission of University Press of New England. Copyright 1982 by the Vermont Conference on the Primary Prevention of Psychopathology.)

how to make teaching sufficiently explicit for young children and because they do not spontaneously analyze the tasks that they want to teach, then such programs may bore brighter mothers into not gaining while enhancing the learning of less bright mothers. Given the social goals of most intervention programs, we ought to gear them to people who need them most, taking into account the functional relationships between the mother's and the child's characteristics and the functional level of the mother's intelligence.

IMPLICATIONS

The major implications of this loose thinking about the effects of interventions on the amelioration of intelligence are that we must take into account the genetic nature of differences in intelligence and we must recognize that genotype–environment correlations are of major importance in understanding the efficacy of interventions. People are different and they process information from their environments differently. Predictions and expectations from attempts to ameliorate intelligence must take realistic account of these facts.

As Jencks (1980) and Axelrod and Scarr (in press) have noted, the correct statistic for predicting the effects of environmental interventions is not heritability but, according to the latter authors, the reaction range. What one wants to know about the probable effects of changes in the social environment is the probable improvement in the intelligence of the persons receiving the treatment. Even if the heritability of intelligence were very high, changing the environments of those persons who are forecast to have low intelligence would have indeterminant effects, as long as genotypes of that sort were not regularly exposed to such environments in the populations studied. Poor genotypes for intelligence are rarely exposed to very stimulating environments, and exceptionally good genotypes are rarely exposed to really poor environments. The correlation between genotypes of parents and children guarantee that few gross mismatches will occur. Of course, some bright parents have retarded children, and some retarded parents have bright children. Most parents' and children's intellectual levels fall in the middle of the range, but it is rare that parents with midparent IQ scores of, say, 140 have a child who scores below IQ 110. Similarly, it is rare for parents whose average IQ score is 70 to have a child who scores above IQ 110.

NEEDED: MODELS OF HOW GENES AND ENVIRONMENTS WORK
TOGETHER

Certainly, one of the major emotional objections to ideas about genetic differences in behavior is that the term *genetic* implies immutability. Interventions, except dietary and biochemical, seem less likely to improve the lot of the less fortunate if the cause of their misfortune is genetic.

It is true, of course, that if the sole reason for differences, let us say between the college entrance rate of lower-class and middle-class youngsters, is the economic disadvantage of the former, then providing free tuition and scholarships will equalize their rates of college attendance. For many economically disadvantaged youth, low-interest loans, free tuition, and scholarships do, in fact, provide the environmental remedy to their problem.

In most cases, however, genetic differences cause and are correlated with environmental differences among people. On the average, lower-class youngsters are less qualified by several criteria to gain entrance into higher education; for example, their reading and writing skills are often not as well developed as those of middle-class children, and their work habits in academic settings are less pleasing to school authorities. Although much of the difference in skills and motivation between middle- and lower-class youngsters may arise from differences in their rearing environments, the research on class differences reported earlier in this chapter suggests that genetic differences are implicated as well. In addition, there is a correlation between genetic differences and differences in the rearing histories of middle- and lower-class youth. Although there are many academically able children in lower-SES homes, the proportion is smaller than in the middle class, and the environments provided by lower-SES families are less conducive, on the average, to the development of academic skills.

Jencks (1980) has provided an interesting scheme for understanding the ways in which genetic and environmental differences can be correlated and the ways in which genetic differences can cause environmental differences. Jencks argues that instead of implicitly equating genetic differences with physical causes and environmental differences with social causes, we should recognize that the two dimensions are independent of one another. Table 13.33 presents a fourfold classification of phenomena affecting IQ test performance.

Cell I includes traditional "genetic" causes of variation, most often defects. Genetic differences are invoked to explain the exogenous cause of the disorder, and physical factors are the endogenous forces to explain the genetic effects. Jencks points out that with earlier screening, diet therapy can minimize the effects of the PKU disorder; thus, children born in places where screening is routine will be minimally impaired, whereas those born in places where screening is not done will be mentally retarded. Therefore, the effects of the genetic difference between PKU and normal children interacts with socially determined variations in medical care. Similar examples could be drawn from other genetic

Table 13.33. *Sources of variation in test performance*

Proximate endogenous cause	Exogenous cause	
	Genetic	Nongenetic
Physical	(I) PKU	(II) Lead poisoning
Social	(III) Sexism	(IV) Language spoken at home

Source: Jencks (1981).

disorders that can be minimized by early diagnosis and effective treatment, such as galactosemia. Many genetic disorders for which no effective treatment has yet been devised also illustrate this category.

Cell II includes lead poisoning, a condition that has little or no important genetic variation, as far as we know. Exposure to lead poisoning is a physical environmental source of variation. Malnutrition and living near the Love Canal also fit into this category. The physical environment can be detrimental to one's health and intellectual development. Although there may well be individual genetic differences in susceptibility to damage from lead and other toxic chemicals and from protein–calorie malnutrition, the major source of variation here is the physical environment. Note, however, that all of the cited examples are socially correlated. As Jencks said, virtually all physical determinants of test-score differences are themselves socially determined.

In Cell III, Jencks includes test-score variation that is caused endogenously by social environmental differences but whose exogenous cause is genetic. Sex and race are two prime examples of genetic differences whose relation to IQ test scores may be more due to differences in socialization than to genetic differences in intelligence between groups.

Cell IV contains sources of variation that are causally independent of both genetic differences and physical variations. Jencks's example is the language an individual learns to speak at home. Note that one's native language is sure to be correlated with many social and physical factors, for example, that Arabic speakers tend to be darker skinned and poorer than most Swedish speakers. Other examples might include the political party of one's choice, one's religion, and preferences of certain foods.

The point of Jencks's presentation is that what we commonly label *genetic* is spuriously limited to physical modes of effect, thereby disguising the nongenetic physical causes of intellectual variation, and what we label *environmental* is confused with social causation, which may well have a genetic basis, as in the examples of sex and race.

What we need to know is *how* genes and environments combine to affect intellectual development. It is important to know whether or not a social change will ameliorate a condition, whether its exogenous cause is genetic or not. It is important to know if a genetic difference among people has its effect through physical or social routes. Pellagra and scurvy are fundamentally different from genetically caused vitamin insufficient metabolisms. Sex differences in spatial abilities are probably different from those of assertiveness or shoulder width. We do not know the extent to which socialization affects spatial skills, but we have a pretty good idea that it affects assertiveness. Hormones at puberty have differential effects on the two sexes' shoulder development and may have some effect on spatial abilities. It is important to know.

Axelrod and Scarr (in press) agree with Jencks that the extent of heritability is not the information one needs for effective interventions. Rather we need to know how, by which routes, genetic differences have their effects. Knowing the degree to which a characteristic in a population differs among individuals for genetic reasons, however, is a starting point – helpful but not sufficient information to plan interventions.

REFERENCES

Alexander, D., & Money, J. Turner's syndrome and Gerstmann's syndrome: Neuropsychologic comparisons. *Neuropsychology, 1966, 4,* 265–273.

Anastasi, A., & Levee, R. F. Intellectual defect and musical talent. *American Journal of Mental Deficiency,* 1959, *64,* 695–703.

Anderson, V. E. Discussion. In L. Ehrman, G. S. Omenn, & E. Caspari (Eds.), *Genetics, environment, and behavior*. New York: Academic Press, 1972.

Anderson, V. E. Genetics and intelligence. In Joseph Wortis (Ed.), *Mental retardation (and developmental disabilities): An annual review* (Vol. 6). New York: Brunner/Maze, 1974.

Axelrod, R., & Scarr, S. Human intelligence and public policy. *Scientific American,* in press.

Baker, S. W., & Ehrhardt, A. A. Prenatal androgen, intelligence and cognitive sex differences. In R. C. Friedman, R. N. Richart, & R. L. Van de Wiele (Eds.), *Sex differences in behavior*. New York: Wiley, 1974.

Bajema, C. J. Relation of fertility of occupational status, IQ, educational attainments, and size of family origin: A follow-up study of male Kalamazoo public school population. *Eugenics Quarterly,* 1968, *15,* 198–203.

Bekker, F. F., & Van Gemund, J. J. Mental retardation and cognitive deficits in Xo Turner's Syndrome. *Maandschr. Kindergeneesk,* 1968, *36,* 148–156.

Berry, J. W. Muller-Lyer susceptibility: Culture, ecology, race? *International Journal of Psychology,* 1971, *6,* 193–197.

Bessman, S. P., Williamson, M. L., & Koch, R. Diet, genetics, and mental retardation interaction between phenylketonuric heterosygous mother and fetus to produce nonspecific diminution in IQ: Evidence in support of the justification hypothesis. *Proceedings of the National Academy of Sciences* (U.S.A.), 1978, *75,* 1562–1566.

Bishop, P. M. F., Lessof, M. H., & Polani, P. E. Turner's syndrome and allied conditions. In C. R. A Alstin (Ed.), *Sex differentiation and development*. Cambridge: Cambridge University Press, 1960.

Block, N. J., & Dworkin, G. (Eds.). *The IQ controversy: Critical readings*. New York: Pantheon Books, 1976.

Bock, R. D., & Kolakowski, D. Further evidence of sex-linked major-gene influence on human spatial ability. *American Journal of Human Genetics,* 1973, *25,* 1–14.

Borich, G. D., & Bauman, P. M. Convergent and discriminant validation of the French and Guilford–Zimmerman spatial orientation and spatial visualization factors. *Educational and Psychological Measurement,* 1972, *32,* 1029–1033.

Botwinick, J. Intellectual abilities. In J. C. Birren & K. W. Schaie (Eds.), *Handbook of the psychology of aging*. New York: Van Nostrand Reinhold, 1977.

Bouchard, T. J. Genetic factors in intelligence. In A. R. Kaplan (Ed.), *Human behavior genetics*. Springfield: Charles C. Thomas, 1976.

Bouchard, T. J., Jr., & McGee, M. G. Sex differences in human spatial ability: Not an X-linked recessive gene effect. *Social Biology,* 1977, *24,* 332–335.

Brigham, C. C. *A study of American intelligence*. Princeton, N.J.: Princeton University Press, 1923.

Brigham, C. C. Intelligence tests of immigrant groups. *Psychological Review,* 1930, *37,* 158–165.

Broverman, D. M., Klaiber, E. L., Kobayashi, Y., & Vegel, W. Roles of activation in inhibition in sex differences in cognitive abilities. *Psychological Review,* 1968, 75, 23–50.

Bruun, K., Markkanen, T., & Partanen, J. Inheritance of drinking behavior: A study of adult twins. Helsinki: Finnish Foundation for Alcohol Research, 1966.

Burg, A. Visual acuity as measured by dynamic and static tests: A comparative evaluation. *Journal of Applied Psychology,* 1966, 50, 460–466.

Burks, B. S. The relative influence of nature and nurture upon mental development: A comparative study of foster parent–foster child resemblance and true parent–true child resemblance. *27th Yearbook of the National Society for the Study of Education,* 1928, 27(1), 219–316.

Burks, B. On the relative contributions of nature and nurture to average group differences in intelligence. *Proceedings of the National Academy of Sciences,* 1938, 24, 276–282.

Caldwell, B. M. Home observation for measurement of the environment. Unpublished manuscript, University of Arkansas, 1978.

Carter-Saltzman, L. Patterns of cognitive abilities in relation to handedness and sex. In M. Wittig & A. Petersen (Eds.), *Determinants of sex-related differences in cognitive functioning.* New York: Academic Press, 1978.

Cavalli-Sforza, L. L., & Feldman, M. Cultural versus biological inheritance: Phenotypic transmission from parents to children: A theory of the effect of parental phenotypes on children's phenotypes. *American Journal of Human Genetics,* 1973, 25, 618–637.

Cavalli-Sforza, L. L., & Feldman, M. The evolution of continuous variation III: Joint transmission of genotype, phenotype, and environment. Unpublished manuscript, Stanford University, 1977.

Childs, B., Finucci, J. M., Preston, M. S., & Pulver, A. E. Human behavior genetics. In H. Harris & K. Hirschhorn (Eds.), *Advances in human genetics* (Vol. 7). New York: Plenum, 1976.

Claeys, W. Primary abilities and field-dependence of adopted children. *Behavior Genetics,* 1973, 3, 323–338.

Cohen, L. B., & Salapatek, P. *Perception, space, and sound:* Vol. 2. *Infant perception: From sensation to cognition.* New York: Academic Press, 1975.

Cooper, R., & Zubek, J. Effects of enriched and restricted early environments on the learning ability of bright and dull rats. *Canadian Journal of Psychology,* 1958, 12, 159–164.

Corah, N. L. Differentiation of children and their parents. *Journal of Personality,* 1965, 33, 300–308.

Coren, S., & Porac, C. A new analysis of life-span age trends in visual illusion. *Developmental Psychology,* 1978, 14 (2), 193–194.

Coren, S., & Porac, C. Heritability in visual–geometric illusions: A family study. *Perception,* 1979, 8,

Cronbach, L. J. Five decades of public controversy over mental testing. *American Psychologist,* 1975, 30 (1), 1–14.

Dan, A. J. The menstrual cycle and sex-related differences in cognitive variability. In M. A. Wittig & A. C. Petersen (Eds.), *Sex-related differences in cognitive functioning.* New York: Academic Press, 1979.

Dawson, J. L. M. Cultural and psychological influences upon spatial–perceptual processes in West Africa: Part 1. *International Journal of Psychology,* 1967, 2, 115–128. (a)

Dawson, J. L. M. Cultural and psychological influences upon spatial–perceptual processes in West Africa: Part 2. *International Journal of Psychology,* 1967, 2, 171–185. (b)

Dawson, J. L. M. Effects of sex hormones on cognitive style in rats and man. *Behavior Genetics,* 1972, 2, 21–42.

DeFries, J. C., Ashton, G. C., Johnson, R. C., Kuse, A. R., McClearn, G. E., Mi, M. P., Rashad, M. N., Vandenberg, S. G., & Wilson, J. R. Parent–offspring resemblance for specific cognitive abilities in two ethnic groups. *Nature,* 1976, 261, 131–133.

DeFries, J., Johnson, R. C., Kuse, A. R., McClearn, G. E., Polvina, J., Vandenberg, S. G., & Wilson, J. R. Familial resemblance for specific cognitive abilities. *Behavior Genetics,* 1979, 9, 23–43.

DeFries, J. C., Kuse, A. R., Vandenberg, S. G. Genetic correlations, environmental correlations, and behavior. In J. R. Royce (Ed.), *Theoretical advances in behavior genetics.* Alphen aan den Rijn, The Netherlands: Sythoff and Woordhoff, 1979.

DeFries, J. C., & Plomin, R. Behavioral genetics. *Annual Review of Psychology,* 1978, 29, 473–515.

DeFries, J. C., Vandenberg, S. G., & McClearn, G. E. Genetics of specific cognitive abilities. *Annual Review of Genetics,* 1976, *10,* 179–207.

DeFries, J. C., Vandenberg, S. G., McClearn, G. E., Kuse, A. R., Wilson, J. R., Ashton, G. C., & Johnson, R. Near identity of cognitive structure in two ethnic groups. *Science,* 1974, *183,* 338–339.

Deregowski, J. B. Illusion and culture. In R. L. Gregory & G. M. Gombrich (Eds.), *Illusion in nature and art.* New York: Scribner's, 1973.

Dobzhansky, T. The genetic nature of differences among man. In S. Persons (Ed.), *Evolutionary thought in America.* New Haven: Yale University Press, 1950.

Eaves, L. J. Testing models for variation in intelligence. *Heredity,* 1975, *34,* 132–136.

Eaves, L. J. The effects of cultural transmission on continuous variation. *Heredity,* 1976, *37,* 51–57.

Eaves, L. J., Last, D., Martin, N. G., & Jinks, J. L. A progressive approach to non-additivity and genotype–environmental covariance in the analysis of human differences. *British Journal of Mathematical and Statistical Psychology,* 1977, *30,* 1–42.

Eckland, B. K. Genetic variance in the SES–IQ correlation. *Sociology of Education,* 1979, *52,* 191–196.

Ekstrom, R. B., French, J. W., & Harman, H. H. *Kit of factor-referenced cognitive tests.* Princeton, N.J.: Educational Testing Service, 1976.

Elston, R. C., & Stewart, J. A general model for the genetic analysis of pedigree data. *Human Heredity,* 1971, *21,* 523–542.

Englander-Golden, P., Willis, K. A., & Deinstbier, R. A. *Intellectual performance as a function of repression and menstrual cycle.* Paper presented at the meeting of the American Psychological Association, September, 1976.

Erlenmeyer-Kimling, L. Gene–environment interactions and the variability of behavior. In L. Ehrman, G. S. Omenn, & E. Caspari (Eds.), *Genetics, environment and behavior.* New York: Academic Press, 1972.

Erlenmeyer-Kimling, L., & Jarvik, L. F. Genetics and intelligence: A review. *Science,* 1963, *142,* 1477–1479.

Eysenck, H. J. *The inequality of man.* London: Temple Smith, 1973.

Eysenck, H. J. *The structure and measurement of intelligence.* New York: Springer Verlag, 1979.

Eysenck, H. J. The nature of intelligence. In M. Friedman, J. P. Das, & N. O'Connor (Eds.), *Intelligence and learning,* pp. 67–85. New York: Plenum, 1981,

Falconer, D. S. *Introduction to quantitative genetics.* New York: Ronald Press, 1960.

Feldman, M. C., & Lewontin, R. The heritability "hang-up." *Science,* 1975, *190,* 1163–1168.

Fennema, E., & Sherman, J. Sex-related differences in mathematics achievement, spatial visualization, and affective factors. *American Educational Research Journal,* 1977, *14,* 51–71.

Ferguson-Smith, M. A. Karyotype–phenotype correlations in gonadal dysgenesis and their bearing on the pathogenesis of malformations. *Journal of Medical Genetics,* 1965, *2,* 142–155.

Fisch, R. O., Bilek, M. K., Deinard, A. S., & Chang, P. N. Growth, behavioral and psychologic measurements of adopted children: The influences of genetic and socioeconomic factors in a prospective study. *Behavioral Pediatrics,* 1976, *89,* 494–500.

Fraisse, P., & Vautrey, P. The influence of age, sex, and specialized training on the vertical–horizontal illusion. *Quarterly Journal of Experimental Psychology,* 1956, *8,* 114–120.

Freeman, F. N. Holzinger, H. J., & Mitchell, B. C. The influence of environment on the intelligence, school achievement and conduct of foster children. *The 27th Yearbook for the National Society for the Study of Education,* 1928, *27*(1), 103–217.

French, J. W., Ekstrom, R. B., & Price, L. A. *Kit of Reference Tests for Cognitive Factors.* Princeton, N.J.: Educational Testing Service, 1963.

Fuller, J. L., & Thompson, W. R. *Behavior genetics.* (2nd ed.) New York: Wiley, 1978.

Garron, D. C. Intelligence among persons with Turner's syndrome. *Behavior Genetics,* 1977, *7,* 105–127.

Garron, D. C., & Vander Stoep, L. Personality and intelligence in Turner's syndrome. *Archives of General Psychiatry,* 1969, *21,* 339–346.

Girgus, J. S., Coren, S., & Porac, C. Independence in in vivo human lens pigmentation from U.V. light exposure. *Vision Research,* 1977, *17,* 749–750.

Goldberg, M. B., & Meridith, W. A longitudinal study of spatial ability. *Behavior Genetics*, 1975, 5, 127–135.

Goldberg, M. B., Scully, A. L., Solomon, I. L., & Stenibach, H. L. Gonadal dysgenesis in phenotypic female subjects. *American Journal of Medicine*, 1968, 45, 529–543.

Goldberger, A. S. Statistical inference in the great IQ debate. *Institute for Research on Poverty Discussion Papers*, 1975, 301–375.

Goldberger, A. S. *Models and methods in the IQ debate: Part 1* (Rev). Paper No. 7801, University of Wisconsin—Madison, 1977.

Goldberger, A. S. Pitfalls in the resolution of IQ inheritance. In N. E. Morton & C. S. Chung (Eds.), *Genetic epidemiology*. New York: Academic Press, 1978.

Goodenough, D. R., Gandini, E., Olkin, I., Pizzamiglio, L., Thayer, D., & Witkin, H. A. A study of X chromosome linkage with field dependence and spatial visualization. *Behavior Genetics*, 1977, 7, 373–387.

Guttman, R. Genetic analysis of analytical spatial ability: Raven's Progressive Matrices. *Behavior Genetics*, 1974, 4, 273–284.

Hammerton, J. L. *Human cytogenetics* (Vol. 2). New York: Academic Press, 1971.

Harris, L. J. Sex differences in spatial ability: Possible environmental, genetic and neurological factors. In M. Kinsbourne (Ed.), *Asymmetrical function of the brain*. Cambridge, England: Cambridge University Press, 1979. (a)

Harris, L. J. Sex related differences in spatial ability: A developmental psychological view. In C. B. Kopp (Ed.), *Becoming female: Perspectives on development*. New York: Plenum, 1979. (b)

Harris, M. *Cows, pigs, wars, & witches: The riddles of culture*. New York: Vintage Books, 1975.

Hartlage, L. C. Sex-linked inheritance of spatial ability. *Perceptual and Motor Skills*, 1970, 31, 610.

Haseman, J. K., & Elston, R. C. The estimation of genetic variance from twin data. *Behavior Genetics*, 1970, 1, 11–19.

Hearnshaw, L. Structuralism and intelligence. *International Review of Applied Psychology*, 1975, 24, 85–92.

Hearnshaw, L. *Cyril Burt, psychologist*. Ithaca, N.Y.: Cornell University Press, 1979.

Henderson, N. D. Genetic influences on the behavior of mice as can be obscured by laboratory rearing. *Journal of Comparative and Physiological Psychology*, 1970, 3, 505–511.

Herrnstein, R. IQ. *Atlantic*, September 1971, 43–64.

Herskowits, M. J. On the relation between Negro–white mixture and standing in intelligence tests. *Pedagogical Seminary*, 1926, 33, 30–42.

Higgins, J. V., Reed, E. W., & Reed, S. C. Intelligence and family size: A paradox resolved. *Eugenics Quarterly*, 1962, 9, 84–90.

Hirsch, J. *Behavior–genetic analysis*. New York: McGraw-Hill, 1967.

Hirsch, J. Behavior–genetic analysis and its biosocial consequences. In R. Cancro (Ed.), *Intelligence: Genetic and environmental influences*. New York: Grune & Stratton, 1971.

Honzik, M. P. Developmental studies of parent–child resemblance in intelligence. *Child Development*, 1957, 28, 215–228.

Horn, J. M., Loehlin, J. C., & Willerman, L. Intellectual resemblance among adoptive and biological relatives: The Texas Adoption Project. *Behavior Genetics*, 1979, 9, 177–207.

Hsia, D. Y. Y. *Human developmental genetics*. Chicago: Yearbook Medical, 1968.

Humphreys, L. The primary mental ability. In M. Friedman, J. P. Das, & N. O'Connor (Eds.), *Intelligence and learning*. New York: Plenum, 1981, 87–102.

Immergluck, L., & Mearini, M. C. Age and sex difference in response to embedded figures and reversible figures. *Journal of Experimental Child Psychology*, 1969, 8, 210–221.

Jacob, F., & Monod, J. Genetic regulatory mechanisms in the synthesis of proteins. *Journal of Molecular Biology*, 1961, 3, 318–356.

Jencks, C. *Inequality: A reassessment of the effect of family and schooling in America*. New York: Basic Books, 1972.

Jencks, C. Heredity, environment, and public policy reconsidered. *American Sociological Review*, 1980, 45, 723–736.

Jensen, A. R. How much can we boost IQ and scholastic achievement? *Harvard Educational Review*, 1969, 39, 1–123.

Jensen, A. R. *Educability and group differences*. New York: Harper & Row, 1973. (a)

Jensen, A. R. *Genetics and education*. New York: Harper & Row, 1973. (b)

Jensen, A. R. Let's understand Skodak and Skeels, finally. *Educational Psychologist*, 1973, *10*, 30–35. (c)

Jensen, A. R. The current status of the IQ controversy. *Australian Psychologist*, 1973, *13*, 7–27. (a)

Jensen, A. R. Genetic and behavioral effects of nonrandom mating. In R. T. Osborne, C. E. Noble, & N. Weyl (Eds.), *Human variation: Biopsychology of age, race and sex.* New York: Academic Press, 1978. (b)

Jensen, A. R. *Bias in mental testing.* New York: Basic Books, 1980.

Jinks, J. L., & Fulker, D. W. Comparison of the biometrical, genetical, MAVA, and classical approaches to the analysis of human behavior. *Psychological Bulletin*, 1970, *73*, 311–349.

Johnson, C. A., Ahern, F. M., & Johnson, R. C. Level of functioning of siblings and parents of probands of varying degrees of retardation. *Behavior Genetics*, 1976, *6*, 473–477.

Kamin, L. J. *The science and politics of IQ.* Potomac, Md.: Erlbaum, 1974.

Kamin, L. J. Commentary. In S. Scarr, *IQ: Race, social class, and individual differences: New studies of old issues*, pp. 467–482. Hillsdale, N.J.: Erlbaum, 1981.

Karlins, M. Schuerkoff, C., & Kaplan, M. Some factors related to architectural creativity in graduating architecture students. *Journal of General Psychology*, 1969, *81*, 203–215.

Kidd, K. K., & Cavalli-Sforza, L. L. An analysis of the genetics of schizophrenia. *Social Biology*, 1973, *20*, 254–265.

Klaiber, E. L., Broverman, D. M., & Kobayashi, Y. The automatization of cognitive style, androgens, and monoamine oxidase (MAO). *Psychopharmacologia*, 1967, *11*, 320–336.

Klaiber, E. L., Broverman, D. M., Vogel, W., & Kobayashi, Y. Rhythms in plasma MAO activity, EEG, and behavior during the menstrual cycle. In M. Ferin, F. Halberg, R. M. Richart, & R. L. Van de Wiele (Eds.), *Biorhythms and human reproduction.* New York: Wiley, 1974.

Klineberg, O. Negro–white differences in intelligence test performance: A new look at an old problem. *American Psychologist*, 1963, *18*, 198–203.

Kuse, A. R. *Familial resemblance for cognitive abilities estimated from two test batteries in Hawaii.* Unpublished doctoral dissertation, University of Colorado, 1977.

Laughlin, P. R., & McGlynn, R. P. Cooperative versus competitive concept attainment as a function of sex and stimulus display. *Journal of Personality and Social Psychology*, 1967, *7*, 398–402.

Layzer, D. Science or superstition: A physical scientist looks at the IQ controversy. *Cognition*, 1972, *7*, 265–269.

Layzer, D. Heritability analyses of IQ scores: Science or numerology. *Science*, 1974, *183*, 1259–1266.

Leahy, A. M. Nature–nurture and intelligence. Genetic Psychological Monographs, 1935, *17*, 237–308.

Leao, J. C., Vorhess, M. L., Schlegel, R. J., & Gardner, L. I. XX/Xo mosaicism in nine preadolescent girls: Short stature as presenting complaint. *Pediatrics*, 1966, *38*, 972–981.

Lerner, I. M. *Heredity, Evolution, and Society.* San Francisco: Freeman, 1968.

Levine, S. Sex differences in the brain. In J. L. McGaugh, N. M. Weinberger, & R. E. Whalen (Eds.), *Psychobiology.* San Francisco: Freeman, 1967.

Levine, S. Sexual differentiation: The development of maleness and femaleness. *California Medicine*, 1971, *114*, 12–17.

Lewontin, R. C. The analysis of causes and the analysis of variance. *American Journal of Human Genetics*, 1974, *26*, 400–411. (a)

Lewontin, R. C. *The genetic basis of evolutionary change.* New York: Columbia University Press, 1974. (b)

Lewontin, R. C. Genetic aspects of intelligence. *Annual Review of Genetics*, 1975, 387–405.

Li, C. C. A tale of two thermos bottles: Properties of a genetic model of human intelligence. In R. Cancro (Ed.), *Intelligence: Genetic and environmental influences*, pp. 162–181. New York: Grune & Stratton, 1971.

Lindsten, J. *The nature and origin of X chromosome aberrations in Turner's syndrome.* Stockholm: Almqvist and Wiksell, 1963.

Lindzey, G., Loehlin, J., Monosevitz, M., Thiessen, D. Behavioral genetics. *Annual Review of Psychology*, 1971, *22*, 39–94.

Loehlin, J. C., Lindzey, G., & Spuhler, J. N. *Raw differences in intelligence.* San Francisco: Freeman, 1975.

Loehlin, J. C., & Nichols, R. *Heredity, environment, and personality: A study of 850 sets of twins.* Austin, Tex.: University of Texas Press, 1976.

Loehlin, J. C., Sharan, S., & Jacoby, R. In pursuit of the "spatial gene": A family study. *Behavior Genetics,* 1978, *8,* 27–41.

Lusk, J. L. *Animal breeding plans.* Ames, Iowa: Iowa State College Press, 1945.

Lytton, H. Do parents create, or respond to, differences in twins? *Developmental Psychology,* 1977, *13* (5), 456–459.

Maccoby, E. E., & Jacklin, C. N. *The psychology of sex differences.* Stanford, Calif.: Stanford University Press, 1974.

Mackenberg, E. J., Broverman, D. M., Vogel, W., & Klaiber, E. L. Morning-to-afternoon changes in cognitive performances and in the electroencephalogram. *Journal of Educational Psychology,* 1974, *66,* 238–246.

Manosevitz, M., Lindzey, G., & Thiessen, D. (Eds.). *Behavioral genetics.* New York: Appleton-Century-Crofts, 1969.

Martin, N. G. The inheritance of scholastic abilities in samples of twins: 2. Genetic analysis of examination results. *Annals of Human Genetics,* 1975, *39,* 219–229.

Martin, N. G., Eaves, L. J., Kearsey, M. J., & Davies, P. The power of the classical twin study. *Heredity,* 1978, *40,* 97–116.

Martin, R. G., & Ames, B. N. Biochemical aspects of genetics. *Annual Review of Biochemistry,* 1964, *33,* 235–256.

Masica, D. N., Money, J., & Ehrhardt, A. A. Fetal sex hormones and cognitive patterns: Styles in the testicular feminizing syndrome and androgen insensitivity. *Johns Hopkins Medical Journal,* 1969, *124,* 34–43.

Matheny, A. P. Genetic determinants of the Ponzo illusion. *Psychonomic Science,* 1971, *24,* 155–156.

Matheny, A. P. Cognitive factors associated with the Ponzo illusion: A study using the Coturn method. *Psychonomic Science,* 1972, *29,* 91–93. (a)

Matheny, A. P. Hereditary components of the response to the double trapezium illusion. *Perceptual and Motor Skills,* 1973, *36,* 511–513.

Mather, K. On biometrical genetics. *Heredity,* 1971, *26,* 349–364.

McAskie, M., & Clarke, A. M. Parent–offspring resemblances in intelligence: Theories and evidence. *British Journal of Psychology,* 1976, *67*(2), 243–273.

McCall, R. B. *Intelligence and heredity.* Homewood, Ill.: Learning Systems, 1975.

McClearn, G. E. Behavioral genetics. *Annual Review of Genetics,* 1970, *4,* 437–468.

McClearn, G. E., & DeFries, J. C. *Introduction to behavioral genetics.* San Francisco: Freeman, 1973.

McDonald, J. F., & Ayala, F. J. Genetic response to environmental heterogeneity. *Nature,* 1974, *250,* 572–574.

McGaugh, J. L., Jennings, R. D., & Thompson, C. W. Effect of distribution of practice on the maze learning of descendents of Tryon maze bright and maze dull strains. *Psychological Reports,* 1962, *10,* 147–150.

McGee, M. G. Human spatial abilities: Psychometric studies and environmental, genetic, hormonal, and neurological influences. *Psychological Bulletin,* 1979, *86,* 889–918.

McGuinness, D. Away from a unisex psychology: Individual differences in visual sensory and perceptual processes. *Perception,* 1976, *5,* 279–294. (a)

McGuinness, D. Sex differences in the organization of perception. In B. Lloyd & J. Archer (Eds.), *Exploration of sex differences.* London: Academic Press, 1976. (b)

McGuinness, D., & Lewis, I. Sex differences in visual persistence: Experiments on the Ganzfeld and afterimages. *Perception,* 1976, *5,* 295–301.

McGuire, T. R., & Hirsch, J. *General Intelligence* (g) *and Heritability* (H^2h^2). New York: Plenum, 1977.

McKusick, V. A., & Ruddle, F. H. The status of the gene map of the human chromosomes. *Science,* 1977, *196,* 390–406.

McNemar, Q. E. A critical examination of the University of Iowa studies of environmental influences upon the IQ. *Psychological Bulletin,* 1940, *37,* 63–92.

Medawar, P. B. Unnatural science. *New York Review of Books,* 1977.

Minton, H. L., & Schneider, F. W. *Differential psychology.* Monterey, Calif.: Brooks/Cole, 1980.

Mittwoch, U. *Genetics of sex differentiation.* New York: Academic Press, 1973.

Money, J. Two cytogenetic syndromes: Psychologic comparisons and specific-factor quotients. *Journal of Psychiatric Research,* 1964, *2,* 223–231.

Money, J., & Alexander, D. Turner's syndrome: Further demonstration of the presences of specific cognitional deficiencies. *Journal of Medical Genetics,* 1966, *3,* 47–48.

Monod, J. [*Chance and necessity: An essay on the natural philosophy of modern biology*] (Austryn Wainhouse, Trans.). New York: Knopf, 1971.

Morton, N. E. Human behavioral genetics. In L. Ehrman, G. S. Omenn, & E. Caspari (Eds.), *Genetics, environment, and behavior.* New York: Academic Press, 1972.

Morton, N. E. Analysis of family resemblance: 1. Introduction. *American Journal of Human Genetics,* 1974, *26,* 318–330.

Morton, N. E., & Rao, D. C. Genetic epidemiology of IQ and socio-familial mental defect. Unpublished manuscript, University of Hawaii, 1977.

Nance, W. E., & Corey, L. A. Genetic models for the analysis of data from families of identical twins. *Genetics,* 1976, *83,* 811–826.

Neff, W. S. Socioeconomic status and intelligence: A critical survey. *Psychological Bulletin,* 1938, *35,* 727–757.

Newman, H. G., Freeman, F. N., Holzinger, K. J. *Twins: A study of heredity and environment.* Chicago: University of Chicago Press, 1937.

Nichols, P. L. *The effects of heredity and environment on intelligence test performance in 4 and 7 year old white and Negro sibling pairs.* Unpublished doctoral dissertation, University of Minnesota, 1970.

Nichols, R. Twin studies of ability, personality, and interests. *Homo,* 1978, *29,* 158–173.

Nichols, R. C. Policy implications of the IQ controversy. In L. S. Shulman (Ed.), *Review of research in education.* Itasca, Ill.: Peacock, 1979.

O'Connor, J. *Structural visualization.* Boston: Human Engineering Laboratory, 1943.

Ohno, S. *Sex chromosomes and sex-linked genes.* Berlin: Springer Verlag, 1967.

Osborne, R. T., & Gregor, A. J. Racial differences in heritability estimates for tests of spatial abilities. *Perceptual and Motor Skills,* 1968, *27,* 735–739.

Ounsted, C., & Taylor, D. (Eds.). *Gender differences: Their ontogeny and significance.* London: Churchill Livingston, 1972.

Park, J., Johnson, R. C., DeFries, J. C., McClearn, G. E., Mi, M. P., Rashad, M. N., Vandenberg, S. G., & Wilson, J. R. Parent–offspring resemblance for specific cognitive abilities in Korea. *Behavior Genetics,* 1978, *8,* 43–52.

Pauls, D. *A genetic analysis of mental retardation and high intelligence.* Unpublished doctoral dissertation, University of Minnesota, 1972.

Pearson, J. S., & Amacher, P. L. Intelligence test results and observations of personality disorder among 3,594 unwed mothers in Minnesota. *Journal of Clinical Psychology,* 1956, *12,* 16–21.

Petersen, A. C. Physical androgyny and cognitive functioning in adolescence. *Developmental Psychology,* 1976, *12,* 524–533.

Petersen, A. C. Hormones and cognitive functioning in normal development. In M. A. Wittig & A. C. Petersen (Eds.), *Sex-related differences in cognitive functioning.* New York: Academic Press, 1979.

Pick, H. L., Jr., & Pick, A. D. Sensory and perceptual development. In P. H. Mussen (Ed.), *Carmichael's manual of child psychology* (34d ed.) New York: Wiley, 1970.

Pishkin, V., Wolfgang, A., & Rasmussen, E. Age, sex, amount and type of memory information in concept learning. *Journal of Experimental Psychology,* 1967, *73,* 121–124.

Plomin, R., & DeFries, J. C. Genetics and intelligence: Recent data. *Intelligence,* 1980, *4,* 15–24.

Plomin, R., DeFries, J. C., & Loehlin, J. C. Genotype–environment interaction and correlation in the analysis of human behavior. *Psychological Bulletin,* 1977, *34,* 309–322.

Plomin, R., DeFries, J. C., & McClearn, G. E. *Behavioral genetics: A primer.* San Francisco: Freeman, 1980.

Plomin, R., Willerman, L., & Loehlin, J. C. Resemblance in appearance and the equal environments assumption in twin studies of personality. *Behavior Genetics,* 1976, *6,* 43–52.

Polani, P. E. Chromosomal factors in certain types of educational sub-normality. In P. W. Bowman & H. V. Mautner (Eds.), *Mental retardation: Proceedings of the First International Congress.* New York: Grune & Stratton, 1960.

Pollack, R. H. Some implications of ontogenetic changes in perception. In J. Flavell & D.

Elkind (Eds.), *Studies in cognitive development: Essays in honor of Jean Piaget*. New York: Oxford University Press, 1969.

Porac, C., Coren, S., Girgus, J. S., & Verde, M. Visual–geometric illusions: Unisex phenomena. *Perception*, 1979, 8, 401–412.

Pressey, A. W., & Wilson, A. E. Another look at age changes in geometric illusion. *Bulletin of the Psychonomic Society*, 1978, 12, 333–336.

Rao, D. C., Morton, N. E., & Yee, S. Analysis of family resemblance: II-A linear model for familial correlation. *American Journal of Human Genetics*, 1974, 26, 331–359.

Reed, E. W. Genetic anomalies in development. In Frances D. Horowitz, E. M. Hetherington, S. Scarr-Salapatek, & G. M. Siegal (Eds.), *Review of child development research*. Chicago: University of Chicago Press, 1975.

Reed, E. W., & Reed, S. C. *Mental retardation: A family study*. Philadelphia: Saunders, 1965.

Reed, S. C., & Anderson, V. E. Effects of changing sexuality on the gene pool. In F. F. La Cruz & G. D.LaVeck (Eds.), *Human sexuality and the mentally retarded*. New York: Brunner/ Mazel, 1973.

Reinisch, J. M., Gandelman, R., & Spiegel, F. S. Prenatal influences on cognitive abilities: Data from experimental animals and human endocrine syndromes. In M. A. Wittig & A. C. Peterson (Eds.), *Sex-related differences in cognitive functioning*. New York: Academic Press, 1979.

Rimland, B., & Munsinger, H. Burt's IQ data. *Science*, 1977, 195, 248.

Roberts, J. *Binocular visual acuity of adults*. Washington, D.C.: U.S. Department of Health, Education and Welfare, 1964.

Roberts, J. A. F. The genetics of mental deficiency. *Eugenics Review*, 1952, 44, 71–83.

Rose, R. J. Genetic variance in non-verbal intelligence: Data from the kinship of identical twins. *Science*, 1979, 205, 1153–1155.

Rowe, D. C., & Plomin, R. The Burt controversy: A comparison of Burt's data on IQ with data from other studies. *Behavior Genetics*, 1978, 8, 81–84.

Scarr, S. Environmental bias in twin studies. *Eugenics Quarterly*, 1968, 15, 34–40.

Scarr, S. Comments on psychology, behavior genetics, and social policy from an anti-reductionist. In R. A. Kasschau & C. Cofer (Eds.), *Psychology's Second Century – Enduring Issues*. New York: Praeger, 1981a, 147–175.

Scarr, S. Genetic differences in "g" and real life. In M. Friedman, J. P. Das, & N. O'Connor, *Intelligence and learning*. New York: Plenum, 1981b, 103–120.

Scarr, S. On quantifying the intended effects of interventions: A proposed theory of the environment. In L. A. Bond & J. M. Joffe (Eds.), *Facilitating infant and early childhood development*. Hanover, N.H.: University Press of New England, 1982.

Scarr, S., & Barker, W. The effects of family background: A study of cognitive differences among black and white twins. In S. Scarr, *IQ: Social class and individual differences*, pp. 261–315. Hillsdale, N.J.: Erlbaum, 1981.

Scarr, S., & Carter-Saltzman, L. Twin method: Defense of a critical assumption. *Behavior Genetics*, 1979, 9, 527–542.

Scarr, S., Pakstis, A. J., Katz, S. H., & Barker, W. B. The absence of a relationship between degree of white ancestry and intellectual skills within a black population. *Human Genetics*, 1977, 39, 69–86.

Scarr, S., Scarf, E., & Weinberg, R. A. Perceived and actual similarities in biological and adoptive families: Does perceived similarity bias genetic inferences? *Behavior Genetics*, 1980, 10, 145–158.

Scarr, S., & Weinberg, R. A. IQ test performance of black children adopted by white families. *American Psychologist*, 1976, 31, 726–739.

Scarr, S., & Weinberg, R. A. Intellectual similarities within families of both adopted and biological children. *Intelligence*, 1977, 1(2), 170–191.

Scarr, S., & Weinberg, R. A. The influence of "family background" on intellectual attainment. *American Sociological Review*, 1978, 43, 764–692.

Scarr, S., & Yee, D. Heritability and educational policy: Genetic and environmental effects on IQ, aptitude, and achievement. *Educational Psychologist*, 1980, 15, 1–22.

Scarr-Salapatek, S. Race, social class, and IQ. *Science*, 1971, 174, 1285–1295. (a)

Scarr-Salapatek, S. Unknowns in the IQ equation. *Science*, 1971, 174, 1223–1228.

Scarr-Salapatek, S. Genetics and intelligence. In F. D. Horowitz (Ed.), *Review of child development research* (Vol. 4). Chicago: University of Chicago Press, 1975.

Schiff, M., Duyme, M., Dumaret, A., Stewart, J., Tomkiewicz, S., & Feingold, J. Intellectual status of working-class children adopted early into upper-middle-class families. *Science,* 1978, 200, 1503–1504.

Schoenfeldt, L. F. The hereditary components of the Project TALENT two-day test battery. *Measurement and Evaluation in Guidance,* 1968, *1,* 130–140.

Schwartz, M., & Schwartz, J. Evidence against a genetical component to performance on IQ tests. *Nature,* 1974, 248, 84–85.

Segall, M. H., Campbell, D. T., & Herskovits, M. J. *The influence of culture on visual perception.* Indianapolis: Bobbs-Merrill, 1966.

Serra, A., Pizzamiglio, L., Boari, A., & Spera, S. A comparative study of cognitive traits in human sex chromosome aneuploids and sterile and fertile euploids. *Behavior Genetics,* 1978, 8, 143–154.

Shaffer, J. W. A specific cognitive deficit observed in gonadal aplasia: Turner's syndrome. *Journal of Clinical Psychology,* 1962, 18, 403–406.

Shepard, R. N., & Metzler, J. Mental rotation of three-dimensional objects. *Science,* 1971, *171,* 701–703.

Shields, J. *Monozygotic twins brought up apart and brought up together.* London: Oxford University Press, 1962.

Silbert, A., Wolff, P. H., & Lilienthal, J. Spatial and temporal processing in patients with Turner's syndrome. *Behavior Genetics,* 1977, 7, 11–21.

Skeels, H. M. Mental development in children in foster homes. *Journal of Consulting Psychology,* 1938, 2, 33–43.

Skodak, M. Children in foster homes. *University of Iowa Child Welfare,* 1938, 15 (4), 191.

Skodak, M., & Skeels, H. M. A final follow-up study of one hundred adopted children. *Journal of Genetic Psychology,* 1949, 75, 85–125.

Smith, G. *Psychological studies in twin differences.* Lund, Sweden: Gleerup, 1949.

Stafford, R. E. Sex differences in spatial visualization as evidence of sex-linked inheritance. *Perceptual and Motor Skills,* 1961, *13,* 428.

Stempfel, R. S., Jr. Abnormalities of sexual development. In L. E. Gradner (Ed.), *Endocrine and genetic diseases of childhood.* Philadelphia: Saunders, 1969.

Stern, C. *Principles of human genetics* (2nd ed). San Francisco: Freeman, 1960.

Stevenson, H. W., Hale, G. A., Klein, R. E., & Miller, L. K. Interrelations and correlates in children's learning and problem solving. *Monographs of the Society for Research in Child Development,* 1968, 33.

Taubman, P., Behrman, J., & Wales, T. The roles of genetics and environment in the distribution of earnings. In Z. Griliches, W. Krelle, H. J. Krupp, & O. Eyne (Eds.), *Income distribution and economic inequality.* New York: Halstead Press, 1978.

Taylor, H. J. *The IQ game: A methodological inquiry into the heredity–environment controversy.* New Brunswick, N.J.: Rutgers University Press, 1980.

Terman, L. M. The great conspiracy. *New Republic,* 1922, 33, 116–120.

Theissen, D. D. Philosophy and method in behavior genetics. In A. R. Gilgen, (Ed.), *Scientific psychology: Some perspectives.* New York: Academic Press, 1970.

Theissen, D. D. *Gene organization and behavior.* New York: Random House, 1972.

Thurstone, L. L., & Thurstone, T. C. *Factorial studies of intelligence.* Chicago: University of Chicago Press, 1941.

Urbach, P. Progress and degeneration in the "IQ debate": 1 and 2. *British Journal of Philosophical Science,* 1974, 25, 99–135, 235–259.

Vandenberg, S. G. The hereditary abilities study: Hereditary components in a psychological test battery. *American Journal of Human Genetics,* 1962, *14,* 220–237.

Vandenberg, S. G. & Kuse, A. R. Spatial ability: A critical review of the sex-linked major-gene hypothesis. In M. A. Wittig, & A. C. Petersen (Eds.), *Sex-related differences in cognitive functioning.* New York: Academic Press, 1979.

Vandenberg, S. G., & Kuse, A. R. Mental Rotations: A group test of three-dimensional spatial visualization. *Perceptual and Motor Skills,* 1978, 47, 599–604.

Waber, D. P. Sex differences in cognition: A function of maturation rate? *Science,* 1976, *192,* 572–574.

Waber, D. P. Sex differences in mental abilities, hemispheric lateralization and rate of physical growth at adolescence. *Developmental Psychology,* 1977, 13, 29–38.

Waber, D. P. Cognitive abilities and sex-related variations in the maturation of cerebral cortical functions. In M. A. Wittig & A. C. Petersen (Eds.), *Sex-related differences in cognitive functioning.* New York: Academic Press, 1979.

Wechsler, D. *The measurement of adult intelligence* (3rd ed.). Baltimore: Williams & Williams, 1950.

Weiss, P. The living system: Determinism stratified. In A. Koestler & J. R. Smythies (Eds.), *Beyond reductionism.* Boston: Beacon Press, 1969.

Wellman, B. L. Iowa studies on the effects of schooling. *Thirty-ninth Yearbook of the National Society for the Study of Education,* 1940, 2, 377–399.

Willerman, L. Personal communication, 1977.

Willerman, L. Effects of families on intellectual development. *American Psychologist,* 1979, 34, 923–929.

Willerman, L., Horn, J. M., & Loehlin, J. C. The aptitude–achievement test distinction: A study of unrelated children reared together. *Behavior Genetics,* 1977, 7, 465–470.

Williams, T. Family resemblance in abilities: The Wechsler scales. *Behavior Genetics,* 1975, 5, 405–409.

Wilson, E. O. Unpublished manuscript, Harvard University, 1977.

Wilson, J. R., & Vandenberg, S. G. Sex differences in cognition: Evidence from the Hawaii family study. In T. E. McGill, D. A. Dewsbury, & B. D. Sachs (Eds.), *Sex and behavior: Status and prospectus.* New York: Plenum, 1978.

Wilson, R. S. Twins and siblings: Concordance for school-age mental development. *Child Development,* 1977, 48, 211–216.

Witschi, E. Overripeness of the egg as a possible cause in mental and physical disorders. In I. I. Gottesman & L. Erlenmeyer-Kimling (Eds.), *Differential reproduction in individuals with mental and physical disorders. Social Biology Supplement,* 1971, 18, S9–S15.

Woodworth, R. S. *Heredity and environment: A critical survey of recently published material on twins and foster children.* A report prepared for the Committee on Social Adjustment. New York: Social Science Research Council, 1941.

Yen, W. M. Sex-linked major-gene influences on selected types of spatial performance. *Behavior Genetics,* 1975, 5, 281–298.

Yerkes, R. M. Testing the human mind. *Atlantic Monthly,* 1923, 131, 358–370.

14 *The development of intelligence*

ROBERT S. SIEGLER AND D. DEAN RICHARDS

In this chapter, we examine three approaches to intellectual development: psychometric, Piagetian, and information processing. The psychometric approach provides a quantitative perspective on the nature of intellectual growth. The Piagetian approach provides a qualitative perspective on the same phenomenon. The information-processing approach provides numerous analyses of specific thought processes that are components of intelligence: memorial strategies, transitive inference, analogical reasoning, counting, and a variety of other memorial and problem-solving processes.

The reasons that we chose to examine both general theories of intellectual growth and the development of specific thought processes stem in large part from our views about the nature of intelligence. These views are quite similar to those expressed by Neisser (1979). Neisser proposed that intelligence be viewed as a family-resemblance concept, that is, as a concept with no defining attributes but with prototypical instances, a hierarchical organization, and a stable correlational structure. To Neisser's thesis we add a developmental dimension; intelligence at different points in life may be viewed in terms of different prototypes, different hierarchical organizations, and different correlational structures. To evaluate this hypothesis, it will be necessary to discuss briefly the idea of family-resemblance concepts and then to consider how the idea might apply to the development of intelligence.

Wittgenstein's (e.g., 1953) analysis of the nature of concepts is central in this approach to studying intelligence. His key insight was that not all concepts could be defined in terms of a single shared feature or even in terms of combinations of shared features. Instead, many concepts seem to be organized more in terms of family resemblances. Much as members of a biological family may not share any one physical feature yet may look alike, so exemplars of concepts may fail to contain any common conceptual feature yet may still recognizably fall within the category. Wittgenstein's classic example for illustrating this point is the concept of *games*. Chess, solitaire, baseball, and golf share few obvious similarities but are nonetheless all considered games. Games frequently involve competition among two or more participants but do not always do so. They often but not always require physical activity. Winning is usually defined in absolute terms, but not always (e.g., when a person plays golf by himself). There does not seem to be any sharp demarcation between games and nongames; some cases may strike us as more and less gamelike, but no formal definition seems possible that would include all exemplars and would exclude all nonexemplars.

Rosch (1974, 1978; Rosch et al., 1976) has elaborated Wittgenstein's ideas, provided a large amount of psychological evidence supporting them, and extended them to many concepts. Recently, Neisser (1979) noted that the ideas also seemed to

897

apply to the concept of intelligence. Neisser suggested that intelligence has many facets but no defining attributes. He further argued that these facets correlate fairly highly but far from perfectly. Thus, two people may be classified as intelligent yet may share almost no traits.

If we do not possess even an implicit formal definition of intelligence, how do we judge a new acquaintance as intelligent or unintelligent? Neisser contended that we do so by comparing our observations with a prototype – the quintessentially intelligent person. Although no one has ever met such a person, we are able to use the correlational structure embodied in the term *intelligent* to imagine what he or she might be like.

What might a prototypic intelligent person look like? In order to find out, we asked students in an introductory psychology class at Carnegie-Mellon University (before the course began) to list five traits that they thought best characterized an intelligent adult and to weight them according to their relative importance. Whether viewed in terms of frequency of mention as one of the five most important traits or in terms of citations as the most important trait, the same five characteristics emerged as the most important (in order): reasoning, verbal ability, problem solving, learning, and creativity.

We asked the students to do the same task for 6-month-olds, 2-year-olds, and 10-year-olds. As illustrated in Table 14.1, the prototypes of intelligent people of other ages were quite different from the prototypes of adults. In the extreme case, at age 6 months, recognition ability, motoric coordination, and alertness were the three most frequently mentioned attributes. None of these were mentioned at all in characterizing intelligent adults or 10-year-olds. Problem solving and reasoning became increasingly important with age, whereas perceptual and motor abilities became less so. Verbal ability and the ability to learn were considered important at all ages from 2 years on.

We also asked the students to estimate the average correlation between the traits, with 1.00 indicating a perfect relationship, 0 indicating no relationship, and .50 indicating a moderate relationship. The pattern of correlations revealed some close relationships among the traits but also considerable distinctiveness. For example, the average estimate of the correlation between problem solving and verbal ability was .65, between problem solving and learning it was .66, and between verbal ability and learning .58. By contrast, the average estimated correlation between motor coordination and verbal ability was .28, and that between verbal ability and reasoning was .31. All of these correlations were computed on data produced by students who thought that both of the traits characterized intelligence at a given age; thus the rankings indicate that the students thought that important characteristics of intelligence need not be closely related, though they also thought that there was a common core of related characteristics.

The three major approaches to intellectual development – psychometric, Piagetian, and information processing – mirror this same tension between conceptualizing intelligence as a consistent trait and as a collection of loosely related skills. As we mentioned above, the psychometric and Piagetian approaches have emphasized unities among intellectual skills, whereas the information-processing approach has tended to emphasize individual skills in isolation. As might have been predicted from the view of intelligence as a family-resemblance concept, neither emphasis alone has proved adequate. To briefly foreshadow points that we will make later in greater detail, many of the types of commonalities among intellectual skills that are postu-

Table 14.1. *Five traits most frequently mentioned as characterizing intelligence at different ages*

6-month-olds	2-year-olds	10-year-olds	Adults
Recognition of people and objects	verbal ability	verbal ability	reasoning
Motor coordination	learning ability	learning ability; problem solving; reasoning (all three tied)	verbal ability
Alertness	awareness of people and environment		problem solving
Awareness of environment	motor coordination		learning ability
Verbalization	curiosity	creativity	creativity

Source: Siegler & Richards (1980).

lated by Piagetian and psychometric approaches have not been found. Consider Flavell's (1982) evaluation of research on Piagetian stages:

There is also the well known fact that empirical studies have generally not found as much chronological synchrony or concurrence among same-stage acquisitions as Piaget's stage theory would predict. Diverse abilities and concepts that one would expect the child to acquire at the same time, because they are assumed in the theory to reflect the emergence of the same cognitive structure, often do not appear to develop concurrently.

Now consider Sternberg's (1977) critique of the efforts of psychometricians to use factor analysis to induce the common basis of intelligence in diverse domains:

Factor analysis is not an appropriate method for discovering the components underlying intelligence. . . . [There] are four intrinsic limitations that restrict the kinds of interpretations that should be drawn from factor analytic results. Two of these are statistical and two are psychological. Because of the statistical limitations, factor analysis lacks inferential power for distinguishing among theories. Because of the psychological limitations, factors cannot be components of intelligence. [Pp. 29, 36]

These critiques should not be taken as unqualified support for the information-processing approach, which does not postulate strong commonalities among intellectual skills. As Keating (1980) commented:

Although one- or two-factor theories are not adequate to describe the nature of intelligence, the existence of a certain amount of empirical "g" cannot be ignored. . . . That is, there is at least something common to success on a wide variety of tasks. If developmental theories are entirely content-constrained, this empirical fact is difficult to account for.

One conclusion that might be drawn from these comments is that the strengths of each approach should be combined into one coherent and powerful approach to studying intellectual development. Indeed, some attempts to utilize the strengths of each possible pair of the three approaches have been made. Keating and Bobbitt (1978) have attempted to integrate psychometric and information-processing approaches; Uzgiris and Hunt (1966), Green, Ford, and Flamer (1971), and Goldschmid and Bentler (1968) have attempted to integrate psychometric and Piagetian approaches; and Klahr and Wallace (1976), Case (1978a), and Siegler (1976) have attempted to combine Piagetian and information-processing approaches.

Each of these efforts has yielded useful findings, but no one of them has proved to be a panacea. It is possible that the optimal integration of approaches simply has not yet been found, but another possibility is that the relative fragmentation of current approaches to intellectual development is not undesirable. Just as in many cases there is no single definition that fits very well all exemplars of a concept, there may be no single approach that is well suited to studying all aspects of intellectual development. Each major approach has evolved procedures for selecting which aspects of intellect to focus upon, which types of issues to raise, which methodological procedures to apply to analyzing findings, and which representational languages to use to characterize them. There may be no overall maximally effective approach but rather several local maximums: approaches that are optimal given constraints on other features.

This point can be made more explicitly when we consider what some of the constraining features might be for each of the three approaches. First, consider some of the questions that are central to each. The psychometric approach poses such questions as: How can intellectual development be quantified? How can such quantifications be used to predict later intellectual achievements? How can the intelligence of individual children be meaningfully compared? What factors make up intelligence, and do the factors change with age? The Piagetian approach poses a quite different set of questions. How do children come to understand the basic categories of space, time, and causality around which man organizes the universe? What stages of thought give rise to children's distinctive understandings of these phenomena? How similar is children's reasoning across different types of phenomena? How is incoming information assimilated into the child's existing mental organization, and how does the mental organization accommodate to incoming information? The information-processing approach poses a third set of questions. How are symbols manipulated so as to give rise to observable performance? Are differences in children's and adults' cognition due to differences in capacity limits (size of echoic memory, rate of symbol manipulation in visual short-term memory) or to differences in memory strategies and the knowledge base? Do children and adults represent information in the same format? How does the information-processing system adjust to the demands of particular task environments?

The three approaches also differ in the procedures by which they identify tasks as being of interest. Psychometricians emphasize discrimination between age groups, moderately high correlations with items on existing intelligence tests, and predictive validity as the crucial standards for selecting new items to study. Piagetians look to Kantian philosophy and to the physical sciences as prime sources of tasks that correspond to important psychological processes. Information-processing psychologists reanalyze tasks studied by psychometricians and Piagetians, analyze educationally relevant problems such as reading and mathematics, and design new tasks that are analogous to structures and functions of computers (e.g., sensory buffers, retrieval from long-term memory). A third way in which the approaches differ is in their preferred methodologies. Psychometric approaches rely heavily on complex correlational methods such as factor analysis. Piagetian approaches emphasize clinical interviews and children's verbal explanations of their reasoning. Information-processing approaches focus on reaction-time patterns, eye movement patterns, and error patterns. Finally, the different approaches are associated with different representational languages for modeling intellect. Psychometricians' models are phrased in terms of factor structures; Piagetians' models are phrased in terms of algebraic structures; and information processors' models are phrased in terms of computer simulations and flow diagrams.

As we mentioned above, we do not think that the associations among these basic issues, task selection procedures, methodologies, and representational languages are accidental. Analyses of eye movement patterns can be extremely revealing of how an individual reads, but it is difficult to imagine a general model of intellect based on eye movement patterns. Factor analyses can indicate commonalities among diverse skills but do not seem at all promising for showing how individuals execute each of the skills. Piagetian clinical interviews can isolate qualitative differences among modes of reasoning but provide little guide as to how to quantify individual differences. The appropriateness of real-time analyses is obvious if tasks are designed to examine the human equivalents of computer processes, but the application of real-time analyses to children's understanding of Kantian categories is far less direct. Thus, to paraphrase Rosch, the groupings of issues, task selection procedures, methodologies, and representational languages into separate research approaches may not be arbitrary but rather highly determined.

We have argued that there is a match between the family-resemblance nature of the intelligence concept and the diverse approaches that have evolved for studying it. Each approach seems well suited for investigating certain aspects of intellectual development, but no one of them seems well suited for investigating every aspect. The approaches also fit well together, subsuming as a group most of the issues we would want a theory of intellectual development to cover. Thus, despite the inadequacies of each approach considered individually, the combination of psychometric, Piagetian, and information-processing perspectives has resulted in a relatively clear and comprehensive picture of intellectual development.

In the remainder of this chapter, we attempt to support this viewpoint in the following way. First, we examine each of the three major approaches, ending each discussion with a list of the substantive conclusions that the approach has contributed. It is our contention that no single approach would have allowed all of these conclusions, yet also that all of them are valid. Even if the reader totally rejects our view of intelligence and decides that a single all-encompassing approach to intellectual development is both feasible and desirable, these conclusions provide a set of constraints within which any such theory would need to operate. Next, we examine a topic that has been given too little attention by all three approaches but that is beginning to receive more attention: learning. Finally, we conclude the chapter by briefly raising several issues that as yet no one has dealt with very well but that we feel will and should be important foci of future research.

14.1.   THE PSYCHOMETRIC APPROACH TO INTELLECTUAL DEVELOPMENT

One way to study intelligence is to treat it as a set of quantifiable dimensions along which people can be ordered. There are numerous variants of this psychometric approach, ranging from Spearman's emphasis on a single general intellectual capacity to Guilford's arsenal of 120 distinct factors. Psychometricians also differ in their characterizations of intelligence: they range from Spearman's (1904) "education of correlates," to Binet's (1911) "judgment," to Woodrow's (1921) "the capacity to acquire capacity." Nonetheless, psychometric approaches to intelligence form a recognizable group in their emphasis on quantifying and rank ordering people's intellectual skills, in their reliance on general tests of intelligence for their data base, and in their use of factor analysis to analyze the data.

It is impossible to discuss psychometric approaches to intellectual growth without considering the test instruments on which they are based. In this section, we will first describe in some detail the contents of several prominent intelligence tests. The focus will be on how items are selected and on whether the tests measure the same qualities at different ages. Next, the stability of intelligence test scores over both short and long time intervals will be examined. Finally, we will consider what intelligence test scores predict and what factors predict intelligence test scores; here, the objective is to determine the relationship of the type of intelligence measured by intelligence tests to other intellectual skills and other life status indicators that might be expected to be relevant to intellectual development.

PSYCHOMETRICALLY BASED DESCRIPTIONS OF INTELLECTUAL GROWTH

Item selection criteria. In order to evaluate the characterizations of intellectual development that emerge from intelligence tests, it is first necessary to consider how items are chosen for inclusion in them. This issue will be examined with reference to two of the most prominent measures of children's intelligence: the Stanford–Binet Intelligence Test and the Wechsler scales.

Stanford–Binet items are selected by two criteria (Anastasi, 1976). The primary criterion is how well items differentiate between children of different ages. The secondary one is how well performance on new items correlates with performance on items already on the test. The former criterion is consonant with Binet's view that the performance of a child of above-average intelligence resembles the performance of an older child and that the performance of a child of below-average intelligence resembles the performance of a younger child. This criterion considerably constrains the content of test questions, however – no questions on the test tap intellectual skills that do not vary appreciably with age. For example, recognition memory is relatively constant over age, reaching impressive levels by age 5 (Brown & Scott, 1971); therefore measures of recognition memory on the Stanford–Binet are limited to very young ages. The second criterion also constrains the content of test questions, because it limits new items to ones that correlate with existing items. For example, by many measures, mechanical ability improves with age; however, because tests of mechanical ability do not correlate highly with existing Stanford–Binet items, they are systematically excluded from the intelligence test.

The selection criteria also have led to the inclusion of items that do not appear intuitively to be major components of intelligence, even though they differentiate between age groups. For example, in the Level 3 test (corresponding to age 3 years), stringing beads and drawing a vertical line do not have the face validity of picture vocabulary and picture memory, but all are included in the assessment.

Items for the Wechsler tests (Wechsler Preschool and Primary Scale of Intelligence, or WPPSI; Wechsler Intelligence Scale for Children, or WISC; Wechsler Adult Intelligence Scale, or WAIS) are selected in a slightly different manner. Differentiation among age groups is not emphasized; rather, the primary selection criterion is the items' correlation with other accepted measures of intelligence. Like the Stanford–Binet criteria, this standard excludes some intuitively important aspects of intelligence. For example, as on the Stanford–Binet, no assessments of mechanical ability appear on the Wechsler tests, because such tests correlate moderately to poorly with other measures of intelligence.

What intelligence tests measure.   Now that we have discussed how intelligence test items are selected, we can examine the items that have been chosen. We will begin by considering the content of the Stanford–Binet for Levels 2, 4, and 10, corresponding to ages 2, 4, and 10, respectively.

On the Stanford–Binet Level 2 test, children are asked to place 3 shapes in the appropriate holes on a board, to recognize 7 body parts on a paper doll, to construct a tower of blocks, and to recognize 18 objects from line drawings. They also see an object hidden and are asked to find it after a time delay. In addition, the examiner observes whether children spontaneously use words in combination. On the Level 4 test, children are asked to recognize the same 18 line drawings as at Level 2, but this time they must succeed on 14 rather than on 3 of them. They are also asked to identify the missing object from a set of 3 and to complete a series of analogies involving opposites. Additional tests involve pointing to pictures of named objects, finding the form identical to an example from within a group of 10, and explaining the need for certain everyday items. The Level 10 test requires children to define a series of concrete words, to define a series of abstract words, and to count the blocks in a picture where the presence of some of the blocks must be inferred. They are also asked to supply reasons why certain situations exist in the world, to say as many words as they can in a specified time period, and to repeat a series of digits.

These test contents reveal a considerable amount about developmental changes in the nature of intelligence, that is, what an intelligent child of 2, 4, or 10 might be able to do that an unintelligent one could not. Probably the most striking change is quantitative; even an unintelligent 10-year-old can do all of the tasks at Levels 2 and 4. There are also changes, however, in the types of tasks that constitute developing aspects of intelligence at each age (i.e., the tasks that discriminate between intelligent and unintelligent children of each age). One dimension of change is in the role of motor coordination. Motor coordination plays a large role in several Level 2 tasks, such as building a tower of blocks and placing shapes in holes, but little role in Level 4 and 10 tasks. Another type of change, as mentioned above, is in the decreasing role of recognition memory. Yet a third change is the presence of tests of real-world knowledge and inferential ability on the Level 10 assessment; these are not examined on the earlier measures.

Comparing the contents at different ages of the WISC and WPPSI tests is more difficult: their subtests have virtually the same names at all ages. Thus we might expect the types of test items on the two scales to be very similar. Upon closer analysis, however, it becomes apparent that the use of a single title can mask large differences in test items. For example, the arithmetic test initially examines children's judgments as to which pile has more objects, then their ability to count out n objects, then their performance on arithmetic problems, and later their performance on simple algebra problems. Although all of these items call on mathematical skills, it is difficult to know whether the abilities they demand are closely related.

Perhaps the most dramatic age-related changes in item content occur on infant intelligence tests. To illustrate this point, we will focus on the Bayley Scales of Infant Development. This test is designed to test children ranging in age from 1 to 30 months. The 1- and 2-month tests examine gross head and body movements and eye

coordination. By ages 7 to 12 months, items assessing responses to verbal instructions, ability to find hidden objects, and standing and walking are included. By 18 to
30 months, the items concentrate on verbal communications skills and precise
motor movements, such as walking a straight line and jumping some minimum
distance.

Analyses of face validity, such as those above, can be revealing but are limited in
certain ways. Skills that seem inherently related may in fact be unrelated in people's
performance; skills that seem to have nothing in common may correlate substantially. The technique of factor analysis was developed specifically to deal with this
problem. We turn to studies using this technique in the next section.

Factor-analytic studies of intelligence test performance. Factor analysis subsumes
a number of procedures for extracting common sources of variance from different
measures. Sources of variance are determined on the basis of intercorrelation patterns. Scores on tests measuring a particular underlying variable (a factor) should
intercorrelate more highly than scores on tests measuring different factors. From a
developmental perspective, if a test taps the same construct at various age levels, it
should show the same underlying factors at each of them. Before considering
whether this criterion is met on intelligence tests, however, several limitations of
factor-analytic techniques must be noted. Results of factor analyses can depend
heavily upon seemingly arbitrary methodological assumptions, the particular items
chosen, and the particular subject population tested. In addition, there is no objective method for construing the content of a factor after it has been isolated by factor
analysis; the intercorrelation pattern is objectively present, but the interpretation of
the underlying factor is inevitably subjective to a large degree (Sternberg, 1977).
With these limitations in mind, we will examine the results of factor analyses of
some commonly used intelligence tests.

McNemar (1942) factor-analyzed 2- to 18-year-olds' performance on the Stanford–Binet. He found that performance at all ages reflected a large general factor,
and also that more specific "group" factors appeared at ages 2 and 2½, 5 and 6, and
18. This is not to say that the general factor was identical for all age groups. Although it appeared to be very similar at adjacent age levels, there was evidence that
it varied more over larger intervals. In particular, it became increasingly purely
verbal at older ages. McNemar concluded, "Some differences do exist in the common factor called for at various age levels" (1942, p. 122).

Factor analyses of the WISC suggest a more consistent factor structure over age
than that found for the Stanford–Binet. Kaufman (1975) factor-analyzed the WISC
for 11 age levels (6–17 years) and found two factors at 6 of the age levels and three
factors at the other 5. For all age levels, the first two factors closely corresponded to
the Verbal and Performance scales of the test. The third factor usually related to
"freedom from distractibility" and was found primarily in late childhood and in early
adolescence.

The factor structure of intelligence seems to change most often and most substantially in the first few years of life. McCall, Eichorn, and Hogarty (1977) examined
age-related changes in the factor structure of two commonly used intelligence tests
for very young children, the California First Year Test and the California Preschool
Test. Using a factor-analytic method termed *principal component analysis,* they
found differences in the nature of the general factor at 2, 8, 13, 21, and 36 months of
age. McCall and associates suggested that these differences reflect fundamental

alterations in the nature of intelligence. They characterized intelligence at each level as follows:

> Stage 1: The period of the newborn (0–2 months). The principal component of intelligence is responsiveness to the environment. Intelligence at this stage does not correlate with that at any other age.
>
> Stage 2: Complete subjectivity (2–7 months). The principal component is active interaction with the environment.
>
> Stage 3: Separation of means from ends (7–13 months). Imitation and elementary vocal behavior become important components of intelligence.
>
> Stage 4: Objectification of environmental entities (13–21 months). Labeling and verbal recognition become important components.
>
> Stage 5: Symbolic relations (21–36 months). Verbal behavior increases dramatically in importance. Correlations with later IQ scores begin to strengthen.

Factor analyses thus reveal changes in the nature of intelligence at early ages and slowly occurring changes at later ages as well. Verbal and other symbolic abilities become more important, and motor skills become less important dimensions of variation. This picture is strikingly similar to the Carnegie-Mellon students' stereotypes of intelligence at different ages. We now examine another set of issues relevant to the nature of intelligence at different ages: the stability of intelligence test scores over short and long time periods.

STABILITY OF INTELLIGENCE TEST PERFORMANCE

Reliability. Perhaps the basic prerequisite for a psychometric test is that it be reliable. Intelligence tests generally do very well on this criterion. For example, in the standardization sample, split-half reliabilities for the WISC-R were .94 for the Verbal Scale, .90 for the Performance Scale, and .96 for the Full Scale (Wechsler, 1974). Retest reliabilities over a 1-month period for the same test were .93, .90, and .95 for the Verbal, Performance, and Full scales, respectively. Split-half reliabilities were computed at ages 4 to 6 for all the WPPSI subscales but one (which required the retest method for technical reasons). The reliability of the Verbal Scale averaged .94, that of the Performance Scale .93, and that of the Full Scale .96 (Wechsler, 1967).

Stanford–Binet reliabilities are based upon the two forms (L and M) of the 1937 test. Alternate form reliabilities ranged from .83 for high-IQ 2½- to 5-year-olds to .98 for low-IQ 14- to 18-year-olds (Terman & Merrill, 1960). In general, the Stanford–Binet was found to be more reliable for older children than for younger and also more reliable for lower-IQ children than for higher. Anastasi (1976) noted that the increase in reliability with age is characteristic of psychometric tests. One reason is that testing conditions are better controlled for older children. In addition, development seems to proceed more rapidly at younger ages, and more variability between tests occurs in periods of rapid change. Overall, though, the reliabilities of both the Stanford–Binet and Wechsler tests are very high.

Stability over longer time periods. Long-term patterns of intellectual growth have been of great interest to psychometrically oriented investigators. Because of the inherent expense of collecting data on such long-term patterns, the tendency has been for numerous investigators to use the data from a relatively few longitudinal studies. Among the most commonly used data sources are the Fels Longitudinal

Study, the Berkeley Growth Study, and the California Guidance Study. These data bases yield a consistent picture of intellectual growth.

Honzik, Macfarlane, and Allen (1948) used the California Guidance Study data to examine the stability of intelligence test performance from age 2 through adulthood. They found relatively low correlations at early ages; for example, IQ test performance at ages 2 and 5 correlated only slightly ($r = .32$). By contrast, over a similar age span in later childhood (ages 9 to 12), the correlation was much higher ($r = .85$). Scores at relatively early ages correlated quite highly with adjacent scores but much less highly with scores at later ages. For example, scores at age 3 correlated .71 and .73 with scores at age 2½ and 3½, respectively, but only .43 with scores at age 9.

Sontag, Baker, and Nelson (1958) reported similar findings with the Fels data. Correlations at adjacent ages were quite high, even in early childhood: For example, intelligence at age 3 correlated $r = .83$ with intelligence at age 4. The relationship decreased as the time between testings increased; for example, the correlation between IQ at ages 3 and 12 was .46. There were also decrements in the magnitude of the correlation over time at older ages, but these were more gradual; test scores at ages 11 and 12 correlated very highly ($r = .90$), whereas those between ages 9 and 12 correlated somewhat less highly ($r = .81$).

Thus, two patterns seem to emerge from the temporal stability data: (a) The less time between testings, the more closely related the IQ test scores; and (b) the older the children, the more closely related the test scores within any given time interval.

A number of explanations have been advanced for the relative instability of very young children's intelligence test scores. Anderson (1940) suggested the "overlap hypothesis." This view starts with the assumption that young children possess a smaller body of knowledge than older ones. It follows that any variability attributable to other factors, such as an illness causing a child to miss two weeks of school, would exert a larger relative influence on the younger children's performance than on the older ones'. To the degree that extraneous factors affect different children on different test occasions, younger children's performance would be more variable than older children's.

Another explanation emphasizes that intelligence tests measure different skills in early childhood and late childhood. Items testing sensorimotor skills, which make up a large portion of infant intelligence tests, are quite different from the abstract verbal items used to assess later intelligence. Whether these changes in test contents reflect changes in the nature of intelligence or simply differences in the test instruments is not known. Some relevant evidence has been derived from presenting to young children items with more intuitive correspondence to abstract verbal intelligence. Such items, intended to measure vocabulary, syntax, and various perceptual skills, have if anything proved less predictive of later intelligence test scores than the conventional items (Bayley, 1970; Jones, 1954). This lack of predictive validity may be attributable to the particular items used, but another possibility is that it is due to a difference between younger and older cohorts in the nature and determinants of intelligence.

Our discussion of the stability of intelligence scores has centered on the strength of correlations between earlier and later performance. It is also possible to view stability in absolute terms. Most people's intelligence test scores vary within a fairly small range in middle and late childhood, adolescence, and adulthood, but greater variability is not uncommon. For example, in the study by Honzik and associates discussed above, 80% of the participants' IQ scores varied less than .5 standard deviations on the two test occasions. Among the remaining 20%, however, were several children whose scores increased or decreased by as much as 4.5 standard deviations. Other investigators have reported similar shifts. Moore (1967) reported one case in which a boy whose IQ was 78 at age 3 scored 151 at age 8. Such dramatic shifts in IQ are often associated with large-scale alterations of the environment: loss of a parent, removal to a foster home, onset of serious illness, and so forth.

To summarize, intelligence test scores are for most though not all children reasonably accurate predictors of later intelligence test scores. Let us now consider the utility of such test scores for predicting academic success.

PREDICTING ACADEMIC SUCCESS

Intelligence test scores often correlate highly with academic success. For example, McNemar (1942) reported that Stanford–Binet scores were related to age and grade placement; the IQ scores of children who were one grade ahead of their age group averaged 11 points higher than those of children in their normal age and grade location, whereas those who were behind one grade averaged 11 points lower than the normal group. Symmetrically, children two grades ahead were found to average 22 points more than children in their normal age and grade location, whereas those who were two grades behind averaged 22 points less than their age peers.

Numerous studies report moderate to high correlations between intelligence test scores and academic achievement. The correlations are generally highest for verbally oriented courses. For example, Bond (1940) reported that correlations between Stanford–Binet IQ scores and success in various high school studies ranged from .48 (geometry) to .73 (reading comprehension). Frandsen and Higginson (1951) reported correlations between WISC scores and performance on the Stanford Achievement Test that ranged between .45 (science) and .73 (literature). The Stanford–Binet and Wechsler tests appear to be equally accurate predictors of academic performance. Mussen, Dean, and Rosenberg (1952) reported correlations ranging from .44 to .81 between the WISC and tests of academic achievement and correlations from .45 to .76 between the Stanford–Binet and tests of academic achievement. The correlations between teacher ratings and these tests were .68 and .76 for the WISC and the Stanford–Binet, respectively. Thus, commonly used intelligence tests predict academic success in elementary and high schools quite well. Pushing the causal chain back one step, we may probe the reasons for differences in scores on these tests.

PREDICTORS OF INTELLIGENCE TEST SCORES

What variables influence intelligence test scores? The answer differs considerably for younger and older children, as a brief review of some of the extensive literature on this subject will show.

Predictors of infants' and preschoolers' intelligence. Broman, Nichols, and Kennedy (1975) conducted the most thorough study to date of the predictors of early intelligence test scores. They examined the relationship between Stanford–Binet test scores and 169 prenatal and postnatal predictor variables for more than 26,000 4-year-olds. Included among the predictors were the child's race, sex, and weight at birth, the mother's educational status, the father's presence or absence, and the family's socioeconomic status.

Race, socioeconomic status, and mother's SRA score (a nonverbal intelligence test) proved to be the best predictors of intelligence test scores at age 4. None of these accounted for as much as 20% of the variance, however. Even stepwise multiple regressions, combining a subset of the most effective predictors, could account for only 25% of the variance in the children's IQ scores. Thus, despite the huge number of potential predictors, no way was found to forecast which 4-year-olds would have high IQ scores and which would have low ones.

Bayley (1970; Bayley & Schaefer, 1964; Schaefer & Bayley, 1963) conducted a similar longitudinal study of predictors of early intelligence test scores. She found that a variety of maternal behaviors correlated little if at all with the test scores. For example, maternal intrusiveness was positively correlated with intelligence for girls of 1 to 3 months, virtually uncorrelated with it at 7 to 9 and 18 to 24 months, and negatively correlated with it at 42 to 54 months. Maternal irritability showed a positive correlation with intelligence among boys at 4 to 6 months, virtually no correlation at 18 to 24 months, and a negative correlation at 42–54 months. Also for boys, mother's punitiveness and child's intelligence were positively correlated at 4 to 9 months, uncorrelated at 13 to 15 months, and negatively correlated at 42 to 54 months.

Bayley reported that socioeconomic predictors showed a similarly inconsistent pattern. For example, parent's education was only slightly and sometimes negatively correlated with intelligence in infancy but was positively correlated with it for children of more than 24 months. Even then, it, like other indexes of socioeconomic status, rarely accounted for as much as 20% of the variance in intelligence test scores of children below age 5.

Predicting the intelligence of older children and adolescents. A different picture emerges when we examine the predictors of intelligence in later childhood and adolescence. Here the polarities of the predictors and even their magnitudes are quite stable. For example, in Bayley's data, the degree to which mothers perceived their children as a burden was negatively related to boys' IQ test scores, with the magnitude of the correlation nearly constant from ages 5 to 18 ($r = -.46$ to $-.52$). Mother's irritability was also negatively related to 5- to 18-year-old boys' IQ scores ($r = -.44$ to $-.51$). Maternal intrusiveness was consistently correlated with girls' intelligence test scores ($r = -.36$ to $-.47$), as was mother's intelligence ($r = .46$ to $.55$). Honzik (1957) reported correlations between mother's IQ and that of 7- to 15-year-old children ($r = .51$ to $.59$). She also reported correlations between mother's education and 7- to 15-year-olds' intelligence test scores of between .30 and .39 over the 8-year period.

Two basic interpretations might be advanced to account for the differences in the identity and stability of the predictors of younger and older children's intelligence test scores. One possibility is that existing test instruments are ineffective in tapping very young children's intelligence; if so, improvements in the test instruments might well yield consistent and stable predictors at early as well as later ages. The other interpretation is that the variable patterns stem not from faulty tests but from differences in the nature of intelligence at different ages. What it means to be an intelligent 6-month-old or 2-year-old may be very different from what it means to be an intelligent 10-year-old. In addition, different variables may influence the attainment of different types of intelligence. Seen from this perspective, the existing test data may be conveying an accurate picture; there may simply be little continuity between early and later intelligence to be found.

The psychometric approach has thus led to a number of conclusions about intellectual growth.

CONCLUSIONS

1. Reliable quantitative measurements of children's general intelligence can be obtained from at least age 4 or 5 years onward.

2. For children of these ages, measures of general intelligence possess considerable stability over a period of several years. The stability increases with children's ages and decreases with the length of the interest interval.

3. These quantitative measurements of intelligence quite accurately predict children's future performance in school. Again, predictive accuracy increases with children's ages and decreases with the interval between the test and the outcome measure.

4. Both parental personality and demographic variables predict the intelligence of older children, though the same cannot be said for children below 4 years of age.

5. The factor structure of intelligence, as obtained from IQ tests, is quite stable from 4 or 5 years onward, with the first two factors corresponding to verbal and performance components. Much greater changes in factor structure are seen in the first few years of life. Perceptual, motor, and recognitory skills occupy prominent places in early assessments of intelligence but lesser roles later on.

14.2.   THE PIAGETIAN APPROACH TO INTELLECTUAL DEVELOPMENT

Jean Piaget's theory of intellectual development stands in marked contrast with the psychometric approaches just reviewed. Psychometric approaches aim to quantify intellectual skills and to identify individual differences in them. Piaget's approach is more concerned with qualitative aspects of intelligence and with establishing universal patterns such as invariant orders of acquisition. The differences can be seen in the types of data that are collected: Psychometricians focus on the number of correct answers, whereas Piagetians place at least as much emphasis on the particular errors that children make. The large gulf between the approaches is ironic: Piaget acquired his first experience in psychology as an intelligence tester working for Binet. In administering Binet's test items Piaget noticed that children's errors were very informative, a realization that contributed much to the distinctive flavor of his work.

Piaget's theory covers the entire range of ages from infancy through adolescence. In examining his work, it is possible to observe many concepts evolving from rudimentary forms in infancy to more complex forms in childhood to even more complex forms in adolescence. One of Piaget's central assumptions was that age-related regularities in the types of reasoning are seen across these concepts and that these regularities reflect qualitatively distinct stages of development. Piaget argued for the existence of four developmental stages: the sensorimotor stage, the preoperational stage, the concrete-operational stage, and the formal-operational stage. We discuss essentials of each stage in the next section. Thereafter we examine Piaget's proposed mechanisms of stage transition. Finally, we evaluate subsequent research about

Piaget's theory in a number of areas: whether children do in fact use the qualitatively discrete reasoning forms described by Piaget, whether their reasoning is consistent over many tasks, as implied by the stage model, whether skills associated with a stage can be taught before the child reaches that stage, and whether the child's existing level of knowledge influences his or her reaction to new information. First we describe the four stages.

THE SENSORIMOTOR STAGE

The sensorimotor stage spans the first 2 years of life. During this period, reflexes, which Piaget believed to be the basic units of more complex activities, are elaborated in a number of ways. They come to be systematically repeated, are generalized to a wider range of objects and situations and are coordinated with each other into increasingly lengthy chains of behaviors. Consider the sucking reflex. Even before birth, neonates reflexively suck on any object that touches their mouths. A few months after birth, infants become able to bring their fingers to their mouths to suck. Soon after, they become able to grasp objects and to convey them to their mouths so they can suck on them. By the age of 6 months, an infant can spot an interesting object, raise it to his or her mouth, and suck on it. This represents the coordination of several previously reflexive behaviors: looking, reaching, grasping, bringing to the mouth, and sucking. The topography of the sucking response also changes during the sensorimotor period. Infants become able to accommodate their sucking reflexes to the requirements imposed by the shape, size, and consistencies of objects. Both the coordination and the generalization of sucking represent impressive improvements on the initial reflex.

One advantage of Piaget's method is that the development of individual concepts can be charted from early to advanced understanding. We will use the concepts of conservation and causation to illustrate the picture of development that emerges. Possessing the conservation concept means understanding that certain attributes of objects remain constant over certain transformations. During the sensorimotor stage, a seemingly simple but very important conservation concept is acquired – a concept that might be called *conservation of existence*, which Piaget called the *object permanence* concept. Although it is obvious even to young children that objects that move behind a barrier continue to exist, infants may not have the same understanding. The basic task that is used to study this phenomenon was formulated by Piaget (1954). The infant is playing with a toy. Suddenly the experimenter takes the toy and places it behind a screen a few inches in front of the infant. Piaget reported that infants below 6 months of age behaved as if the toy had simply ceased to exist. They seemed motorically capable of retrieving it but made no apparent efforts to do so and showed no signs of distress. It was as if they were governed by the strongest possible version of the adage "out of sight, out of mind." (We will present a more detailed analysis of this early form of conservation later in the chapter.)

The concept of causation also begins its development during the sensorimotor stage. Michotte (1962) showed infants films containing physically impossible events. For example, in one film a ball approached another ball and the second ball started moving before the first ball made contact. This event did not seem to surprise infants under 10 months of age but did surprise older ones. Michotte also showed a film of a train entering a tunnel engine first but emerging caboose first; again, children older than 10 months showed surprise at the odd chain of events, but younger ones did not. Michotte concluded that until age 10 months, infants lack firm notions of causation.

Piaget attributed infants' limited notions of conservation and causation to their lack of representational ability. In his view, sensorimotor-stage children deal exclusively with ongoing perceptions and actions. Language is impossible for them because they lack the ability to represent objects and actions in memory. These representational skills, however, develop substantially toward the end of the sensorimotor stage. At this point, the child enters the preoperational stage.

THE PREOPERATIONAL STAGE

Preoperational-stage children range from 2 to 7 years of age. As the primary development of the sensorimotor stage was the acquisition of representational skills, so the preoperational stage has as its primary development the growth and utilization of these skills. The most dramatic growth takes place in the area of language use. Vocabulary increases 100-fold between 18 and 60 months (McCarthy, 1954), and grammatical and sentence construction patterns become increasingly complex. There is also increasing diversity in the uses to which language is put. Very young children use language primarily for naming objects, for greeting and other social functions, and to obtain desired goals (Bloom, Rocissano, & Hood, 1976; Nelson, 1973). By 60 months of age, the range of functions has increased considerably, even encompassing playful usages such as puns, jokes, and riddles.

Piaget suggested a parallel growth in mental imagery. Within his theory, imagery is viewed as a representational system similar to language. As children become able to describe situations verbally, they are also believed to become able to represent them imaginally. Piaget viewed improvements in drawing ability and memory for static situations as reflecting this improved imaginal capacity.

An unfortunate aspect of research on preoperational-stage children is that Piaget and many subsequent investigators have dwelt upon children's inadequacies rather than on what they can do. Such children are described as being unable to solve conservation problems, transitivity problems, class-inclusion problems, and so on. This heavy emphasis on the preoperational child's failings often overshadows the phenomenal increases in all types of intellectual activities that do occur.

Piaget's emphasis on preoperational children's deficiencies is evident in his descriptions of their understanding of conservation and causation. Although they consistently answer correctly on the simplest conservation problem, object permanence, they rarely solve conservation problems dealing with specific attributes of the material (quantity, weight, number). These conservation tasks are usually presented in three phases. Children are first shown two or more identical objects (glasses of water, clay cylinders, etc.). After the children agree that the objects are equal on the crucial dimension (quantity of water, weight, etc.), the second phase of the procedure begins. The experimenter transforms one of the objects in a way that changes its appearance but leaves the crucial dimension constant – the water is poured into a taller but thinner glass or the clay cylinder is molded from a ball into a sausage. In the third phase, the experimenter asks if the objects remained equal on the crucial dimension (amount of material or weight). Although the correct answer to this question is yes, preoperational children almost always say no. Piaget believed that this was because they base their judgments on appearances rather than on logical considerations.

Piaget also devoted considerable attention to preoperational children's concept of causation. He asked children questions about the causes of complex physical phe-nomena such as "what causes the tides?" Preoperational-stage children gave such answers as "God wants there to be tides," "you need them for swimming," and "my Daddy makes them." Piaget (1969) argued that these answers reflect a number of characteristics of preoperational children's thinking: finalism (every event has a purpose), artificialism (all things conform to some grand pattern), animism (inani-mate objects have human qualities), and phenomenalism (events that occur to-gether in time and space are always causally connected). Conversely, such children were said not to appreciate the importance of the physical mechanisms that causally connect events.

Piaget generally characterized preoperational-stage children's reasoning as focus-ing on states rather than transformations. He attributed this to their lacking under-standing of reversibility (the notion that an operation can be reversed), identity (the notion that superficial changes leave essential qualities unchanged), and compensa-tion (the notion that changes in one dimension can be compensated for by changes in another). By contrast, he claimed that concrete-operational children possessed all of these operations.

THE CONCRETE-OPERATIONAL STAGE

Between ages 7 and 11, children master conservation, causality, transitivity, class inclusion, multiple classification, and seriation tasks. They come to understand reversibility, identity, compensation, and numerous other logical concepts. This understanding, however, is limited to concrete tasks. Abstract reasoning, long chains of deduction, and the realization that insufficient evidence is available to reach any conclusion are not yet possible, according to Piaget.

Although 7- to 11-year-olds can solve many conservation problems, some such problems are still said to be beyond their capabilities. One of these is conservation of volume. The child is shown a container of water and two balls of clay. The experi-menter demonstrates that the water level rises to the same height when each of the balls is placed in the container. Then, the experimenter remolds one of the balls into a different shape and asks if the water would still rise to the same height if the remolded ball were placed in it. Although Archimedes demonstrated that a given substance will displace the same amount of water regardless of its shape, even college students often fail to solve this problem.

Causality problems requiring the separation of variables were also said to be beyond the capabilities of concrete-operations-stage children. Inhelder and Piaget's (1958) pendulum problem is a good example of such a problem. Children are shown a frame from which a number of metal balls are hung by strings. Weight of the balls and length of the strings vary. The task is to determine what factor or factors influence the period of the pendulum. Length of the string is the only factor that actually influences it, but concrete-operations-stage children almost always con-clude either that weight is the only important factor or that weight and length of the string are both important factors. They reach this conclusion because they fail to vary the values of one dimension systematically while holding the other dimension's values constant.

Concrete-operations-stage children also have difficulty understanding the concept of proportionality. One task that has been used to study the development of this concept is Piaget and Inhelder's (1951) probability task. Children are presented with two piles of marbles each of which includes some red and some blue marbles. The children's task is to select the pile from which they would have the best chance of obtaining a red marble. Rather than comparing the proportions of red marbles in the two piles, concrete-operations-stage children either simply choose the pile containing more red marbles or subtract the number of blue marbles from the number of red marbles and choose the pile with the larger remainder.

Thus, despite the obvious cognitive progress that occurs during the concrete-operations stage, children within it are still limited in certain thought processes. Inhelder and Piaget (1958) characterized these limitations in the following ways. Hypothetical reasoning divorced from or contrary to experience is said to be beyond children at this stage. In addition, they lack understanding of how changes in one variable can be exactly compensated for by changes in another. They are also said to be unable to plan systematic experiments that will result in useful data regardless of the outcome. Inhelder and Piaget suggested that all of these limitations arise from one cause: Concrete-operational children concentrate on the here and now rather than on how the here and now relates to the total matrix of logical possibilities. In Piagetian terms, they lack a complete combinatorial thought system.

THE FORMAL-OPERATIONAL STAGE

Formal operations represent the apex of cognitive development. Children who attain this stage are said to solve all of the problems mentioned in the preceding section and many others. They can reason both concretely and abstractly, they can disentangle the influence of different variables, and they can generate all possible combinations of variables and events. In short, they possess the reasoning abilities of educated adults.

Although Inhelder and Piaget (1958) suggested that this stage is usually attained by age 12 or 13, they also reported that some people may never reach it. Also, even though the formal-operations stage is the norm in Western cultures, some primitive cultures may be entirely without it. The formal-operations stage is thus the only one of the four stages said not to be universal for individuals and cultures.

An interesting characteristic of formal-operational thinkers is their tendency to apply their new abstract reasoning abilities to all areas of life. Inhelder and Piaget attributed adolescent idealism in the realms of politics, religion, and ethics to this newfound ability to think in terms of logical possibilities rather than in terms of that which exists. The focus on logical possibilities is at first untempered by practical considerations, thus leading to the frequently noted intolerance of the young (e.g., Cowan, 1978).

Another interesting characteristic of the formal-operations stage is that in examining different-aged children's approaches to its tasks, one can see the full range of reasoning characteristic of the different stages. Consider children's knowledge about balance scales, one of the tasks used to measure understanding of proportionality. Sensorimotor-stage children have little idea of how balance scales work; they are unable to separate their own activities from those of the balance scale. Preoperational-stage children focus solely on the amounts of weight on the two sides of the fulcrum and base all judgments on the values on this dimension; they consistently predict that the side that has more weight will go down. Concrete-operations-stage children recognize the importance of both the amount of weight and the distance of the weights from the fulcrum, but they do not understand the proportional relationship between weight and distance; therefore they do not know which side will go down when one has more weight and the other has its weight farther from the fulcrum. Finally, formal-operational-stage children recognize the importance of both distance and weight and understand the proportional relationship between them; they therefore can solve any problem involving the balance scale.

MECHANISMS OF STAGE TRANSITION

Any comprehensive theory of cognitive development must specify not only what children know at different points but also how they progress from one knowledge state to another. Piaget defined three mechanisms that he believed important in such transitions: assimilation, accommodation, and equilibration. Assimilation and accommodation are reciprocal processes – children transform incoming information to conform to their present mental structures (assimilation), whereas the mental structures are transformed by the new information (accommodation). For example, upon seeing a new object, infants might try to grasp it as they have other objects (thus assimilating the new object to an existing scheme), but they must adjust their grasps to conform to the shape of the object (thus accommodating their schemes as well). The extreme case of assimilation is fantasy play, in which the physical characteristics of an object are ignored and the object is treated as if it were something else. The extreme case of accommodation is imitation, in which interpretation of the other person's actions is minimized and the child simply adjusts his or her behavior to that of the other. Assimilation is never present without accommodation and vice versa – children engaged in fantasy play must accommodate to the shape of the object if they intend to grasp or control it (elephants are virtually never assimilated as teacups in fantasy play), and gestures and actions that are imitated must be assimilated to conform to the child's smaller stature and generally poorer coordination.

Assimilation and accommodation take place continuously throughout life. In contrast, Piaget believed equilibration occurs only during large-scale transitions. The equilibration process occurs in three phases. At first, children are satisfied with their mode of thought and are in a state of equilibrium. Then they become aware of shortcomings in their preferred mode of thinking but are unable to replace it with anything better, resulting in a state of disequilibrium. Finally, a more suitable and sophisticated mode of thought is adopted that eliminates the shortcomings of the old mode; thus a new equilibrium is reached. For example, on the conservation-of-liquid-quantity task, the child might initially believe that taller liquid columns always contain more water; this initial equilibrium would serve the child well, as in most cases taller liquid columns do contain more water. The child might then come to realize that this formula does not always work and would enter a state of disequilibrium. He or she would consider alternatives, such as that wider glasses have more water, but these would be rejected also. Finally, the child would discover that pouring water does not affect quantity, despite perceptual appearances; thus he or she would reach a new equilibrium.

Although Piaget mentioned other factors involved in the process of stage transition, such as maturation, direct experience with materials, and socially transmitted information, he claimed that the involvement of these factors was limited to their influence on the equilibration process. In other words, these factors operate by helping to create a state of disequilibrium. Piaget believed such cognitive conflict is necessary for large-scale cognitive growth.

CURRENT STATUS OF PIAGET'S THEORY

As is probably evident from our description, Piaget's theory makes a number of controversial predictions. These include predictions about the typical developmental sequence, the consistency of children's performance across tasks and over time, and the possibility of teaching relatively young children to understand complex concepts. A huge body of research has been collected relevant to these issues. We will now review the basic findings that emerge from this research.

The developmental-sequence issue. Piagetian theory makes three predictions about the typical developmental sequence. First, it predicts the knowledge states through which children will progress on their way to mastery of each concept. Second, it predicts the order in which the knowledge states will emerge. Third, it predicts the approximate ages at which the knowledge states will be attained, at least for children in technologically advanced Western societies.

Probably the most basic issue raised by these predictions concerns how well Piaget's theory describes the contents of children's knowledge: Do children really know what Piaget says they do at different points in development? A number of early experiments that were aimed at evaluating Piaget's theory focused on this issue. These experiments seemed to provide considerable supportive evidence for all four of Piaget's stage descriptions (Corman & Escalona, 1969; Dodwell, 1960; Elkind, 1961a, b; Jackson, 1965; Lovell, 1961; Uzgiris, 1964). Strong methodological criticisms have been raised, however, about these studies' reliance on verbal explanation data. Such data can lead investigators either to underestimate what children know (because they lack the verbal facility to explain their reasoning) or to overestimate it (by allowing children to parrot explanations they have heard from parents or peers but do not fully understand).

On the other hand, recent work, using essentially nonverbal methodologies, has tended to support the conclusions of investigators who relied on the verbal explanation data. We have been involved in one such series of experiments in which we used a rule-assessment methodology to examine 10 cognitive developmental tasks: the balance scale, projection of shadows, probability, fullness, conservation of liquid quantity, conservation of solid quantity, conservation of number, speed, time, and distance problems (Siegler, 1976, 1978, 1981; Siegler & Richards, 1979; Siegler & Vago, 1978). On all 10 of these tasks, the types of discrete knowledge states described by Piaget emerged. The specific contents of the knowledge states also were similar to those he described, though often not identical to them. The way in which the rule-assessment approach works, and the way in which it can be applied to several particular tasks, will be described in a later section of this chapter.

The second prominent developmental-sequence issue concerns the order in which different levels of understanding are achieved. Much of the prominence of this issue stems from Piagetian statements such as the following:

The minimum programme for establishment of stages is the recognition of a distinct chronology in the sense of a constant order of succession. The average age for the appearance of a stage may vary greatly from one physical or social environment to another . . . but one could not speak of stage in this connection, unless (for example) in all environments the Euclidean structures were established after and not before the topological structures. [1960, p. 13]

Most studies of the ordering of knowledge states within specific concepts have supported Piaget's predictions, leading some investigators to conclude that the theory must be correct (Pinard & Laurendeau, 1969; Tanner, 1956). Other investigators, however, have questioned whether such findings are a test of the theory at all (Brainerd, 1978; Flavell & Wohlwill, 1969). These critics raise a provocative point. Given that both Knowledge State A and Knowledge State B occur on the Piagetian tasks, it may often be logically impossible to obtain anything but the predicted ordering. Consider the balance scale task. The expected developmental sequence is that children first base predictions solely on the amount of weight, then they consider both weight and distance from the fulcrum but do not understand the proportional relationship between them, and finally they consider both dimensions and understand that they are related proportionally. Given that all three knowledge states occur, however, how could the ordering be otherwise? That the different knowledge states occur is an important discovery, but their ordering may be a matter more of logic than of psychology and certainly does not confirm or disconfirm any particular theory.

This criticism is not the whole story, however. Some cases of invariant sequences cannot be attributed to the more advanced rule, including the less advanced one. For example, Siegler (1981) found that on conservation problems children first relied on perceptual cues (always choosing the glass with the taller liquid column) and later based judgments on the type of transformation that had been performed (e.g., if the experimenter added some water, there is more than before; if he or she did not add or subtract any, there is the same amount as before, etc.). There is no obvious way in which the earlier perceptual rule is included within the later transformation rule. The invariant order of this and all Piagetian examples that we know of can be predicted, however, on the basis of the inherent correlation between the predictions of the rules and the predictions of the correct formula. Given two partially correct rules, or a partially and a completely correct rule, children always progress toward the rule that more often has predicted the correct answer in the environments they have encountered. Basing conservation judgments on the relative heights of the liquid column will usually yield the correct answer, but basing them on the type of transformation will always do so. Basing balance scale judgments on the amounts of weight on each side will often yield correct predictions, but considering distance in those cases where weight is equal must more often do so. Thus the ordering of two rules may be predicted from the relative frequency with which they predict the correct answer in the environments that the children encounter.

The third developmental-sequence issue, the ages at which various tasks are mastered, has also been the source of considerable controversy. As long as researchers have used Piaget's basic assessment techniques, they usually have obtained age norms similar to his original ones, at least on sensorimotor, preoperational, and concrete-operational stages (e.g., Elkind, 1961a, b; Gratch, 1977). On modified versions of Piagetian tasks, however, children sometimes display understanding at much younger ages than they are supposed to. Children as young as 3 and 4 have been found able to solve some versions of the number-conservation task (Bryant, 1972; Gelman, 1972), the class-inclusion task (Markman, 1973; Markman & Siebert, 1976), the transitivity task (Bryant & Trabasso, 1971; Trabasso, Riley, & Wilson, 1975), and the seriation task (Greenfield, Nelson, & Salzman, 1972). This would seem to be a very surprising finding if children indeed fail these tasks because they lack the relevant logical structures, as Piaget hypothesized.

A difficulty of the opposite type has risen in connection with the age norms of Inhelder and Piaget's (1958) formal-operations tasks. Here the problem is that even college students often cannot solve the problems correctly, although 12- and 13-year-olds should theoretically be able to do so. On the balance scale and projection-of-shadows tasks, for example, no more than one-half of high school and college students generally demonstrate a formal-operations-level understanding (Jackson, 1965; Lee, 1971; Lovell, 1961; Martorano, 1977). In response to these findings, Piaget (1972a) modified his description of the stage. He indicated that the formal-operations stage represents an ideal that may be reached only in the child's area of greatest interest or knowledge, and he also conceded that the protocols in the Inhelder and Piaget (1958) book were chosen because they were illustrative of formal-operations thought rather than because they were representative of the way that most adolescents think.

Where does such research leave Piaget's theory as a description of the developmental sequence? On one dimension the theory fares very well: It seems that the discrete states of knowledge predicted by the theory really do appear. On the other hand, the accuracy of the predictions concerning the ordering of the knowledge states seems due more to the inherent correlations between the rules and the correct answers than to the validity of the theory. In addition, the age norms associated with the knowledge states seem increasingly tenuous: 3- and 4-year-olds display conceptual understanding on some tasks that they should not possess until age 7 or 8, and 19- and 20-year-olds fail to display conceptual understanding that they should have acquired by age 12 or 13. Thus it seems that the description of the developmental sequence is generally in the right direction but is wrong in some important particulars.

Consistency over tasks and time. One of the basic predictions of Piaget's theory is that children's performance will be consistent across a wide range of tasks. For example, Piaget and Inhelder (1941) stated that concrete-operational abilities "appear at the same time without our being able to seriate (them) into stages" (p. 246). An 8-year-old should be able to pass all concrete-operations-level tasks (conservation, class inclusion, seriation, transitivity, etc.) but should fail all formal-operations-level tasks (balance scale, projection of shadows, probability, pendulum, etc.). Flavell (1971b) termed this the concurrence assumption.

It has become increasingly apparent that the concurrence assumption is at best overstated. Consider three concrete-operations-level conservation tasks: conservation of number, conservation of solid quantity, and conservation of weight. Theoretically, all of these should be mastered simultaneously; a child should understand either all or none of them. Empirically, however, number conservation seems to be mastered at around age 5 or 6, solid quantity conservation at around age 7 or 8, and weight conservation at around age 9 or 10 (Elkind, 1961a; Katz & Beilin, 1976; Miller, 1976). Some investigators contend that number conservation may be understood even earlier, perhaps as early as age 3 or 4 (Bryant, 1974; Gelman, 1972; Mehler & Bever, 1967). These data do not support the idea of synchronous development, even within the concept of conservation.

Because of the prevalence of these asynchronies, the research question has shifted to whether concepts within a particular stage emerge in a consistent order. Research on this issue has produced a remarkably confusing picture. Consider the situation of one investigator (Brainerd, 1973) who attempted to determine the order of emergence of three concepts: conservation, transitivity, and class inclusion. From the reports of Piaget, Inhelder, and Szeminska (1960), Inhelder and Piaget (1964), and Piaget and Inhelder (1941), he inferred that the ordering would be class inclusion first, and transitivity and conservation second and synchronous. When he considered a different set of Genevan articles (Inhelder & Piaget, 1964; Piaget, 1952; Piaget et al., 1960), however, he derived a different expected ordering: conservation, then class inclusion, then transitivity. From the neo-Piagetian literature (Murray & Youniss, 1968; Smedslund, 1963, 1964), he derived yet a third expectation: Acquisition of both conservation and class inclusion would precede acquisition of transitivity. Brainerd's own findings corresponded to none of the above predictions; he found that transitivity developed first, conservation second, and class inclusion third.

What might give rise to such inconsistency? Flavell (1971b) pointed out that one problem is a fundamental ambiguity in the definition of the problem. When we say that Concept A precedes Concept B, do we mean that the earliest sign of competence on Concept A is achieved before the earliest sign of competence on Concept B, that final competence on A is achieved before final competence on B, or that on the average, competence on A is greater than competence on B? The importance of this definitional issue is underscored by a careful study performed by Keller and Hunter (1973). They examined the acquisition of three concepts – conservation of length, conservation of quantity, and transitivity of length. Each concept was measured by three tasks, all of which seemed to be appropriate measures. Keller and Hunter found that on the average, 7- and 8-year-olds most often solved the transitivity tasks, next most often the conservation-of-length tasks, and least often the conservation-of-quantity tasks. This is one possible developmental sequence. However, if only the most frequently passed task measuring each concept had been considered (as the most sensitive index of understanding), a different ordering would have been derived: first conservation of length, then transitivity, then conservation of quantity. The quantity-conservation concept emerged last in both of these analyses; it should be noted, though, that the most frequently passed quantity-conservation task was passed more often than two of the three conservation-of-length tasks.

These complexities stem from the fact that any concept can be measured in many ways and that no one of them has any special claim to being the "correct" one. The alternative measures often differ greatly in difficulty, thus making problematic the assertion that one concept is mastered later than another. The more frequently justifiable (but less exciting) statement seems to be that by most but not all measures, Concept A is understood before, after, or concurrently with Concept B.

The data on stability of performance over time are both clearer and more favorable to Piaget's theory. For example, Neimark (1975) performed a large-scale longitudinal study in which she examined intellectual development over a 4-year period, from third to sixth grade. She focused on children's understanding of the concepts of combinations and permutations. In terms of the Piagetian stage ratings, considerable stability was apparent. Most children either stayed at the same stage or progressed by one stage from 1 year to the next. Regressions and large jumps in skill were rare. This finding fits the basic prediction of Piagetian theory that cognitive development occurs one stage at a time, does not ordinarily skip stages, and proceeds in an invariant direction.

Training studies. Piaget's statements concerning the possibility of accelerating cognitive development through training are among his most controversial. Some of the statements appear to rule out the possibility that any training can be successful. Others suggest that training might at times be effective, but only if the child already possesses some understanding of the concept, if the training procedure involves active interaction with materials, and if it creates cognitive conflict. Both types of statements indicate that many young children will not be able to benefit from any training technique and that many training techniques will not benefit any children.

Not surprisingly, these claims have spurred a huge body of empirical research. Beilin (1977) reviewed cognitive-developmental training studies and found that more than 100 investigations had been conducted on conservation alone. Many attempts also have been made to teach other concrete-operational concepts such as transitivity, class inclusion, seriation, and multiple classification as well as formal-operational concepts such as the separation of variables, proportionality, and combinatorial reasoning.

The conclusion to be drawn from these studies seems clear. Concrete- and formal-operational skills can be taught to children long before they master these skills spontaneously. A huge variety of training methods have proved effective. Among the most successful are task-analytic approaches, which seek to inculcate specific skills that younger children may lack (Kingsley & Hall, 1967; Rothenberg & Orost, 1969); modeling approaches, in which effective conservation strategies are illustrated (Rosenthal & Zimmerman, 1972; Zimmerman & Rosenthal, 1974); social interaction approaches, in which children are shown that peers believe in conservation (Murray, 1972); and approaches relying on feedback and verbal rules, demonstrating that nonconservation responses are incorrect and that conservation responses are correct (Beilin, 1965; Field, 1977; Gelman, 1969). One or more of these approaches has been successfully applied to virtually all of Piaget's concrete- and formal-operational problems. In addition, the trained knowledge has been demonstrated to constitute "genuine understanding" by a variety of criteria: durability over time, generalizability to new tasks and materials, generation of appropriate rationales as well as correct answers, and at least some resistance to counterexamples.

Piaget has said on more than one occasion that he is the leading revisionist of Piagetian theory. Thus it is not terribly surprising that his Genevan group has modified its stance on training in response to the data cited above. The change is most apparent in a book by Inhelder, Sinclair, and Bovet (1974) entitled *Learning and the Development of Cognition*. This book includes training experiments on class inclusion and on conservation of number, liquid, and solid quantity; in all cases, the Genevans find it possible to teach children the concepts at relatively young ages. Their main emphasis, though, centers on the different benefits that children of different ages and different initial knowledge derive from training. Older and more knowledgeable children are invariably found to learn more efficiently and more completely. Thus Inhelder, Sinclair, and Bovet commented, "The nature and extent of a subject's progress depends on the assimilatory instruments the subject already has at his disposal" (p. 244).

We suspect that this emphasis on developmental differences in learning will prove far more tenable than the previous contention that certain types of training would never work and that children at certain ages could never learn. Indeed, the basic relation between age and knowledge on the one hand and learning on the other has already been amply demonstrated in non-Genevan work on such concepts as conservation of number, liquid quantity, and weight (Christie & Smothergill, 1970; Kingsley & Hall, 1967; Siegler & Liebert, 1972), separation of variables (Case, 1974), proportionality (Brainerd & Allen, 1971), and combinatorial reasoning (Siegler &

Liebert, 1975). We will explore the phenomenon in greater depth in a later section of this chapter.

Thus to the conclusions drawn earlier from psychometric studies, research within the Piagetian approach adds several more.

CONCLUSIONS

6. On many concepts, children progress through a sequence of qualitatively discrete, partially correct knowledge states prior to full understanding.

7. The sequence of partial understandings occurs in an invariant order. Given that two rules appear some time in development, children progress toward the rule that more often predicts the correct answer in the environments that they encounter.

8. It is possible to teach conceptual understanding at considerably younger ages than those at which the concepts are usually mastered. Still, there are developmental differences in the benefits that children derive from the instruction.

9. Tasks that can be analyzed as being formally similar are often mastered at very different ages. Relative to the Piagetian norms, some tasks are mastered earlier than they should be, whereas others are mastered later. In addition, a wide range of tasks corresponding to a given concept can be devised, and the ages at which these tasks are mastered vary greatly.

14.3.   INFORMATION-PROCESSING APPROACHES TO DEVELOPMENT

Perhaps the greatest weakness of the psychometric and Piagetian approaches is that they say little about the specific processes involved in intelligent performance. They may tell us that knowing the capital of Thailand predicts high-school grade-point average or that children do not understand from birth that objects have a permanent existence, but they fail to indicate how people retrieve "Bangkok" from their long-term memories or what symbol manipulations are involved in knowing that the ball still exists. Here the information-processing approach comes in.

The information-processing approach starts from a view of man as a manipulator of symbols. Its most basic goals are to describe the symbols that are manipulated (the representation) and to identify the ways in which they are manipulated (the processing). In trying to accomplish these goals, researchers must answer numerous questions about the nature of the information-processing system. Is information represented in a linguistic form, in an imaginal form, or in some type of amodal propositional form? Is most processing conducted in parallel or serially? Is the overall system best conceived in terms of separate memory storage units such as immediate, short-term, and long-term memories or in terms of a single system whose parts undergo varying degrees of activation at any one time?

Information-processing psychologists interested in development have concentrated their efforts in two areas: memory and problem solving. Those interested in the growth of memory have focused on changes in quantitative and qualitative characteristics of the overall memory system. In particular, they have attempted to explain developmental differences in terms of changes in four aspects of the memory system: memorial capacity, memorial strategies, metamemory, and the knowledge base. Developmentalists interested in problem solving, on the other hand, have focused more on the interface between the problem solver and the task environment. They have examined the demands imposed by different tasks in order to discover the strategies that children might bring to them. The different task-analytic techniques that they have used – computer simulations, flow chart analyses, and analyses of underlying principles – have emphasized psychological processes of different levels of specificity and have led to distinctive types of research.

Our discussion of information-processing approaches is organized in terms of this dichotomy between research on memory development and that on problem solving. The section on memory development is structured by the four alternative explanations of development: changes in basic memorial processes, in the use of memorial strategies, in metamnemonic knowledge, and in the extensiveness of the knowledge base. The section on problem solving centers on five arbitrarily chosen task environments that have been of interest to Piagetians and psychometricians as well as to information-processing psychologists: transitive inference, analogical reasoning, conservation, counting, and object permanence. Research programs in these areas have been chosen because they illustrate alternative task-analytic techniques as well as because they are of exemplary quality.

MEMORY DEVELOPMENT

Capacity approaches

One of the most striking features of human cognition is the limited amount of processing that can be done at one time. Lyndon Johnson is said to have characterized the intelligence of a political foe with the phrase "He can't walk and chew gum at the same time." Although most of us can perform these tasks simultaneously, there are many others that we cannot, for example, reading novels and performing mental arithmetic.

Capacity limitations can be conceived of in several ways. One of the first formulations was Miller's (1956) 7 ± 2 approach. Miller suggested that humans can store between five and nine chunks of information in short-term memory. The amount of information within a chunk varies, but the number of chunks is said to be constant and limited. A second approach is that of Kahneman (1973). Kahneman suggested that the bottleneck could be viewed in terms of a limited resource of attention; each task claims a certain amount of processing resources, and when the resources are entirely allocated, the addition of a new task is either impossible or forces inferior performance on the original tasks. A third view identifies information-processing speed as the limiting factor. Only a certain number of operations can be executed in a given unit of time; this time constraint may limit the tasks that can be performed simultaneously.

Developmental claims based on each of these conceptualizations have been advanced. Pascual-Leone (1970) formulated an M-space approach, in which the number of slots in working memory increased with age. Manis, Keating, and Morrison (1981) derived an approach based on Kahneman's work in which the ability to allocate attention efficiently improved with age. Wickens (1974) and Miller (1969) emphasized speed of information processing as a variable changing with age.

These models of age-related increases in capacity have led to several distinct types of research. One approach, associated with the slot models of short-term memory, has been to assess the number of slots in a child's memory and then to relate the measured capacity to performance on other tasks. The backward digit-span task is often used as a measure of capacity (cf. Case, 1974; Pascual-Leone, 1970). Children are presented with a series of digits in a slow even cadence (7 4 8 9 4 2) and then are asked to recite them backward (2 4 9 8 4 7). The reason that these researchers have cited for relying on backward rather than on forward span is that the backward format limits the types of strategies that children can use to augment their recall, a desirable quality in a measure of capacity (Pascual-Leone, 1970).

Backward digit span has been found to increase from two digits at age 5 or 6 to six digits during adolescence. These values are taken to represent the child's short-term memory capacity, or M-space, at the given age. M-space has been found to be related to performance on a wide variety of measures of problem-solving ability and memory (Case, 1974, 1978b; Pascual-Leone, 1970; Scardemalia, 1977). The explanation advanced is that young children, with limited short-term memory capacity, are not able to keep in mind simultaneously all of the information necessary to perform the most demanding components of various tasks.

Different procedures have been used to measure the speed of information processing. In one study, Miller (1969) examined the time it took 8-year-olds and adults to shift their gaze from an initial position on a screen to a new target elsewhere in their field of vision. Adults shifted more quickly, despite the fact that the 8-year-olds and the adults would both have had very substantial experience with the visual skill in question. Miller concluded that the difference was due to adults' greater capacity for rapid information processing.

These capacity models of development encounter two types of difficulty. First, they are difficult to distinguish operationally from each other. Excepting physiological evidence, it is unclear how we could ever determine whether central processing capacity was best defined in terms of discontinuous slots, in terms of a continuous resource that could be allocated, or in terms of differential speed of symbol manipulation. It would seem that any behavioral data that could be explained in terms of one model could be explained equally easily in terms of the others (cf. Anderson, 1978; Townsend, 1974).

The second difficulty lies in distinguishing any of the capacity models from models that explain developmental changes in terms of increased knowledge or improved strategies. Strategies often enter into performance on tasks intended as direct measures of capacity (Baron, 1978; Brown, 1978; Chi, 1978). Performance on tasks that minimize the potential use of strategies tends to be invariant or close to invariant over a broad age range (Brown, 1974; Frank & Rabinovitch, 1974; Hoving, Spencer, Robb, & Schulte, 1978; Morrison, Holmes, & Haith, 1974). In addition, estimated capacity proves to depend heavily on theoretically irrelevant task parameters such as the number of objects to be remembered (Trabasso & Foellinger, 1978).

The fact that we cannot presently demonstrate developmental changes in capacity does not mean that no such changes occur or that they are unimportant. There clearly are physiological limits on the intellectual activities that people can perform, and these may change with age. The problem is that it is extremely difficult to interpret any particular set of data as demonstrating age-related changes in memorial capacity. Thus the most reasonable reaction to claims concerning such changes may be akin to the Scottish legal verdict "case unproven."

Strategies

Within psychology, the term *strategies* has been used in many different ways; some definition of what we mean by *strategies* therefore seems desirable. A strategy may be thought of as a qualitative algorithm, with the variables corresponding to cognitive processes. Such an algorithm may include both the conditions under which it is to be used and the processes involved in its execution. For example, an algorithm for the rehearsal strategy might read: If there is material that needs to be recalled serially, repeat the first N chunks in order, next repeat the first N chunks and N more after that, redefine all of the already repeated material as the first N chunks, and continue the process recursively until the material is exhausted. Such a strategy could be made arbitrarily complex as expertise in its use grew. For example, to the "bare bones" rehearsal strategy might be added additional strictures concerning optimal rates of rehearsal, what to do if a previously rehearsed item cannot be remembered, how to allocate attention differentially to difficult items, and so on.

The mastery of increasingly sophisticated mnemonic strategies seems to play a large role in intellectual development. One investigator recently went so far as to state, "The major reviews of the literature in this area are in essential agreement that differences in memory abilities can so far be ascribed entirely to differences in strategies" (Baron, 1978, pp. 411–412). Investigators have shown that these strategies are employed in all phases of the memorization process: when the material is initially encoded, when it is stored, and when it is finally retrieved. In addition to a plethora of task-specific strategies, several more general strategies can be utilized across many tasks. These include rehearsal, organization, elaboration, and allocation of study time.

Rehearsal. Rehearsal involves the cumulative repetition of material that a person is trying to memorize. An everyday example of the strategy is the usual approach to memorizing telephone numbers; when we look up a number, we simply repeat to ourselves the seven or ten digits until we have completed dialing. Young children rarely rehearse spontaneously; some researchers have questioned whether rehearsal would help them if they did use it (Reese, 1962).

Some of the first studies on the development of rehearsal strategies were conducted by Flavell and his students. In one study (Keeney, Canizzo, & Flavell, 1967) each child was presented with seven pictures of objects to be remembered. Then a space helmet was placed on the child's head; this helmet hid the child's eyes but allowed the experimenter to watch for lip movements. It was found that very few 5-year-olds but almost all 10-year-olds moved their lips or said the words aloud in the 15-sec period between when the pictures were presented and when the children were asked to recall them. Children who rehearsed recalled more than those who did not. When original nonrehearsers were later taught to rehearse the words, their recall improved to the level of peers who rehearsed spontaneously.

In addition to these developmental differences in the probability of rehearsal, the quality of older and younger children's rehearsal also differs. Ornstein, Naus, and Liberty (1975) asked 8-, 11-, and 13-year-olds to rehearse aloud after the presentation of each of 18 unrelated words. Their reason for this request was to allow them to observe the ways in which each child rehearsed. Ornstein and colleagues found that the rehearsal approaches of the youngest and oldest children differed greatly. The 8-year-olds typically rehearsed items in isolation – after the item "cat," they would say "cat, cat, cat." The 13-year-olds, by contrast, would combine the past few words with the newly presented one – after the word "cat," they would say "desk, lawn, sky, shirt, cat." The younger children's approach did not yield the primacy effect characteristic of successful use of rehearsal, whereas that of the older ones did; the older children also recalled more words. In a second experiment, Naus, Ornstein, and

Aivano (1977) instructed both 8- and 11-year-olds to use three different items in their rehearsal sets. This produced characteristic serial position effects and greatly reduced but did not eliminate the age differences in recall. On yet closer examination of the children's rehearsal, Naus and colleagues found that the older children continually changed the members of the rehearsal set, whereas the younger ones regularly included the first two items from the entire set along with the newly presented item. In a subsequent experiment, these variations in rehearsal-set membership were found to be tied to the amount recalled (Ornstein, Naus, & Stone, 1977).

Instructing young children to use rehearsal strategies in one situation often is insufficient to persuade them to use it in others, even if the strategy proved effective in the first case. Keeney, Canizzo, and Flavell found that the children they had taught to rehearse abandoned the strategy when they were later given a similar memorization task but no explicit instructions to rehearse. Similarly, Hagen, Hargrove, & Ross (1973) found that when the experimenter stopped prompting children to rehearse, their recall declined to the level of children who had never been taught the rehearsal strategy, and they no longer appeared to rehearse. Thus, although the evidence is now overwhelming that young children can be taught to use rehearsal strategies effectively, it is less clear that they can be taught to transfer the strategies to new tasks and to maintain them over time.

Organization.   Organizing material to be memorized into taxonomic categories has been found to aid recall substantially. In the typical task, people are presented with a list containing between 12 and 40 words that they will later be asked to recall. For example, a list might include 4 types of furniture, 4 animals, and 4 professions. The words within the list are presented in random order; of primary interest is whether in recall children group together words that share a common taxonomic category. The paradigm can also be used to study subjective organization. Rather than examining the degree to which items within a taxonomic category are recalled in succession, the investigator focuses on the degree to which people recall the same words in succession across trials, regardless of their taxonomic relatedness.

Even very young children's recall is influenced by the semantic relatedness of terms. For example, Goldberg and associates (1974) reported that 2-year-olds' interresponse times for recalling two-item lists are faster for semantically related than for semantically unrelated items. It is also the case, however, that the degree of utilization of semantic relationships steadily increases from early childhood through college. Young children often use phonemic features, such as rhyming patterns, to link words; older children and adults concentrate more exclusively on semantic connections (Bach & Underwood, 1970; Hasher & Clifton, 1974).

There are also age-related changes in the quality of those semantic organizations that are used. Young children tend to use similarity or associative strength as the basis for their semantic organizations; older children and adults more often rely on taxonomic relatedness (Flavell, 1970). Young children also tend to divide lists into a greater number of categories each having fewer members (Worden, 1975). Finally, their categories and categorization schemes are less stable, with considerable reorganization often occurring from one trial to the next (Moely, 1977).

Efforts to teach children to use organizational strategies have yielded results similar to those of efforts to teach them rehearsal strategies. Children as young as 4 or 5 years clearly can be taught to use organizational strategies (Moely et al., 1969).

On the other hand, such instruction results in less transfer, less durability over time, and less effective implementation than the same instruction given to older children (Liberty & Ornstein, 1973; Rosner, 1971; Williams & Goulet, 1975). Thus, the ability to execute the strategies does not seem to guarantee their use.

Elaboration.   Elaboration refers to activities that link together in some meaningful way two or more items that are to be memorized. For example, a child who needed to remember schoolbooks, lunch, and an arithmetic assignment might form an image of a peanut butter and jelly sandwich placed between two pages of a book, with the assignment placed between the peanut butter and the jelly. Such imagery has been found to facilitate recall in a variety of circumstances (Delin, 1968).

One of the crucial features governing the effectiveness of elaboration is the degree of activity involved in the interaction. Sentences involving a highly active interaction between two words (e.g., the LADY flew on a BROOM on Halloween) facilitate children's recall to a much higher degree than sentences describing more static interactions (e.g., the LADY had a BROOM; Buckhalt, Mahoney, & Paris, 1976). Similarly, interactive images are more effective than images lacking such interactions (Reese, 1977).

Older and younger children's uses of the elaboration strategy differ in a number of ways. Older children are more likely than younger ones to use the strategy spontaneously (Paris & Lindauer, 1976). When they do use it, their sentences and images are more likely to involve active interactions. Finally, older and younger children seem to be differentially influenced by self-generated and experimenter-generated elaborations. Older children seem to benefit more from elaborations that they make up themselves (Reese, 1977), whereas younger ones seem to benefit more from those of the experimenter (Turnure, Buium, & Thurlow, 1976). This finding may reflect differences in the quality of the elaborations. Older children's elaborations may be particularly meaningful to them, thus leading to superior recall, whereas the elaborations of younger children may be obscure or unmemorable, thus producing inferior recall.

Allocation of study time.   Perhaps the most frequent use that children make of memory strategies is in deciding how much time to spend studying and how to allocate the time among different parts of the material. Flavell, Friedrichs, and Hoyt (1970) examined 4- to 10-year-olds' study strategies. The task involved memorizing the pictures that appeared in each of 10 windows. In order to see the picture in a given window, the child needed to press a button that would reveal it; this requirement provided an objective index of the time each child spent on each picture. In general, older children spent more time studying than younger ones. They engaged in a greater variety of subsidiary strategies, such as naming the pictures, rehearsing them cumulatively, and testing themselves. Each of these activities was associated with greater recall.

Masur, McIntyre, and Flavell (1973) used an identical procedure to examine the items upon which 7-year-olds, 9-year-olds, and adults focused in their study period. Both 9-year-olds and adults were more likely than 7-year-olds to focus upon those items that they failed to recall previously. This strategy helped only the adults, however; the 9-year-olds did as well when they studied items that they previously answered correctly as when they studied items that they previously missed. Brown (1978) suggested a possible explanation. In order to succeed on the study task, she argued, children needed to identify the missed items, select those items for further study, and maintain the memories of the previously recalled items. She hypothesized that the maintenance process may have been difficult for the 9-year-olds, thus negating the potential effectiveness of focusing on previously missed items.

Another study skill that has received some attention is notetaking. Danner (1976) examined 8-, 10-, and 12-year-olds' ability to take good notes on a prose passage. The task involved 12 sentences, 4 on each of three topics. A good note taker was defined as one who, when restricted to noting 3 sentences, would choose 1 representing each of the three topics. Only 20% of the youngest children used this strategy, but almost 90% of the oldest ones did.

In general, there is a developmental trend toward increasingly precise shaping of study strategies to task demands. Even preschoolers take some strategic steps when they know they will later be asked to recall material. In particular, they make use of external objects as retrieval cues (Wellman, Ritter, & Flavell, 1975). Older children have available a much greater range of strategies and adapt them to much finer differentiations in the task demands, however. For example, Rogoff, Newcombe, and Kagan (1974) told 4-, 6-, and 8-year-olds that their recognition of 40 pictures would be tested after a few minutes, 1 day, or 7 days. Only the oldest children studied for a longer time when anticipating the longer delays. Similarly, Horowitz and Horowitz (1975) reported that 11-year-olds but not 5-year-olds adopted different strategies when anticipating a test of recall than when anticipating a test of recognition.

Several trends emerge in this review of our knowledge of memory strategies. First, the use of such strategies increases with age, particularly between the ages of 5 and 10. Second, the strategies are increasingly finely adjusted to meeting task demands. Third, the strategies can be taught to children younger than those who generally use them spontaneously, but such instruction often fails to generalize over time and to new tasks. Some investigators (Brown, 1978; Flavell & Wellman, 1977) have suggested that understanding of one's own memory processes – metamemory – might be a crucial determinant of such generalization. We now turn to research on this topic.

Metacognition

Why do people use memory strategies in some situations but not in others? One frequently cited possibility is that they do so in response to their knowledge concerning their own memorial capabilities, the nature of the task demands, and the potential effectiveness of the strategies in augmenting their memorial capabilities. For example, they may use the rehearsal strategy because of what they know about serial lists, their ability to remember serial lists without rehearsing, and their ability to remember serial lists with rehearsing.

Metacognitive research has been controversial from its inception. Part of the reason is that its relationship to consciousness has not been defined; measures of metacognitive knowledge have usually been based on interview data, and psychologists have a long tradition of distrusting the validity of such introspections. Another reason is that for some people, the metacognitive metaphor summons an image of a homunculus directing the operations of the information-processing system; how metacognition influences cognitive operations has rarely been specified. A third objection is that the metacognitive construct is superfluous; in this view, knowledge about when to use a strategy is embedded in the strategy itself, and there is no need to distinguish between metacognition and strategies.

Such arguments seem to us quite compelling, but counterarguments have been raised. Some recent metacognitive research has used measures that do not demand conscious introspection (e.g., Markman, 1979). Entirely mechanistic formalisms, such as production systems, can use metacognitive knowledge to direct cognitive activities (Greeno, Riley, & Gelman, 1979; Sacerdoti, 1977). Finally, although metacognitive knowledge may initially be embedded within strategies, it may come to play an autonomous role, for example, by motivating a search for new strategies if the original ones do not seem adequate. With these objections and counterarguments in mind, we may consider recent metacognitive research.

Knowledge of memory limitations. One focus of metamnemonic research has been on children's knowledge of their own and other people's memorial limitations. Kreutzer, Leonard, and Flavell (1975) posed children perhaps the most basic question in this domain: "Do you forget?" Almost all children beyond first grade indicated that they did forget at times, but a fairly substantial minority of kindergarteners (30%) denied that they ever encountered such memorial difficulties.

The number of objects that children think they can remember has also been of interest. Flavell, Friedrichs, and Hoyt (1970) presented nursery schoolers, kindergarteners, second graders, and fourth graders with groups of 10 pictures. They then asked the children how many of the pictures they thought they could remember. They found that more than half of the nursery schoolers and kindergarteners thought they could remember all 10 pictures, whereas very few older children thought they could. (In fact, none of the children could remember so many pictures.) The two younger groups' predictions of the number of pictures they would remember were higher than the predictions of the two older groups, but the children in the two older groups actually remembered more. Thus the older children appeared to be more aware of their memorial abilities and limitations.

How does knowledge of memory limitations improve? One plausible explanation is that experience with tasks requiring accurate assessments is essential. The evidence is equivocal, however. Typically, in studies addressing this issue, children are presented with alternating trials in which they first estimate how many items they will remember and then see how many items they actually do remember. To such experience 4- and 5-year-olds have proven surprisingly unresponsive; many continue to make the same unrealistic estimates after a number of feedback trials (Markman, 1973; Moynahan, 1973; Yussen & Levy, 1975), though in some experiments fairly substantial gains have been noted (Salatas & Flavell, 1976). Thus the means by which children develop more accurate estimates of their memorial capabilities remain unclear.

Knowledge about strategies. Investigators of metamemory have also been interested in the strategies that young children think would be effective in augmenting their mnemonic performance. Kreutzer, Leonard, and Flavell (1975) asked kindergarteners and first, third, and fifth graders what they would do to try to remember a telephone number. Almost all of the third and fifth graders indicated that they would write down the number, rehearse, or take some other step to maintain it in memory; only 60% of the kindergarteners indicated that they would use any such strategy. In addition, 95% of the third and fifth graders but only 40% of the kindergarteners indicated either that they knew it was wisest to phone quickly before getting a drink of water or that they might encounter difficulty remembering if they got the drink first.

Moynahan (1973) examined children's knowledge of organizational strategies. She asked 7-, 9-, and 10-year-olds to assess the relative difficulty of learning lists of unrelated and taxonomically related items. The 9- and 10-year-olds were more likely than the 7-year-olds to predict that the taxonomically related items would be easier to recall. A study by Tenney (1975) suggests that this result was not attributable to the younger children's not knowing the taxonomic relationships. Tenney provided 5-, 8-, and 11-year-olds with a first word and asked them to provide three associates of the word, three other words within the same category, or three other words that would be easy to remember if the first word was given. For example, they might initially be presented with the word *green* and might be asked for three other words that they thought of along with *green*, three other colors, or three other words that they thought would be easy to remember if *green* was provided as a cue. All age groups were able to provide three other color words upon request, and clustered them together in recall when they did so. When asked to provide other words that would be easy to remember along with *green*, however, the 5-year-olds did not usually choose other colors and had considerable difficulty remembering the words that they did select. Older children chose colors when asked for easy-to-remember words and had little difficulty remembering them.

One of the most consistent findings of metamnemonic research concerns children's knowledge of the usefulness of external memory aids. The finding of Kreutzer and associates that some 5-year-olds and almost all 8- and 10-year-olds would write down a telephone number if they were asked to remember it provides one example. Another example, provided by the same investigators, involved a question concerning what children would do to be sure to remember their ice skates the next day. The kindergarteners and first, third, and fifth graders suggested a variety of ideas, almost all of them relying on external aids: Put the skates someplace where they would easily be seen, write oneself a note, tie a string around one's finger, or attach the skates to one's body. No more than 10% of the children at any age suggested relying on one's memory as the best strategy. Reliance on external memory aids is forbidden in standard psychological experiments but likely plays a large role in children's everyday mnemonic activities.

Knowledge about ongoing performance. Monitoring one's comprehension of and performance on tasks is another aspect of metamemory. Markman (1977) examined 6-, 7-, and 8-year-olds' ability to recognize their failure to comprehend instructions. Children were enrolled as consultants helping an experimenter develop instructions for a new card game to be taught to other children. The experimenter presented to children the existing instructions, which were grossly incomplete; the intent was to examine the point at which the children would ask clarifying questions. If children did not ask such questions spontaneously, a series of 10 probes was given, with each probe more explicit than the last in indicating the need for the child to question the instructions. Not surprisingly, older children realized that the instructions were incomplete earlier than younger children did. It took children of all three ages a large number of probes before they reached this awareness, though. The youngest children rarely did so until they had been asked to play the largely undefined card game. Markman suggested that young children may need to enact instructions in order to know that they do not comprehend.

As anyone who has ever tried to assemble model airplanes or to learn new games from written instructions can attest, comprehension monitoring can be a difficult task for people well beyond age 8. Markman (1979) demonstrated this finding experimentally. She presented prose passages containing self-contradictory information to 8-, 10-, and 11-year-olds. For example, in a passage on making baked alaskas, the children read: "To make it they put the ice cream in a very hot oven. The ice cream in Baked Alaska melts when it gets that hot. Then they take the ice cream out of the oven and serve it right away. When they make Baked Alaska, the ice cream stays firm and does not melt" (p. 646). Again the crucial measure was when in a series of probes the child asked a question.

Markman found that almost half of the children who heard such directly contradictory information did not note the fact, even after such probes as "did everything make sense?" The children's lack of comprehension was not due to failure to remember the stories; when asked to repeat them, the children were quite accurate. The difficulty persisted when the contradictory information was presented in two successive sentences. Even when warned that the stories might be flawed, many 8-year-olds did not detect the contradictions; 10- and 11-year-olds, however, usually did detect the inconsistencies after such warnings.

Markman's explanation of these findings emphasized the flexibility of children's processing skills. She suggested that children might concentrate on the empirical truthfulness of statements rather than on their logical compatibility. Thus, monitoring one's comprehension may be far from an automatic process; it may require attentiveness to one's own knowledge state as well as to the material.

Metamnemonic knowledge and memorial performance. Early investigations of metamemory were fueled by the hope that there would be a simple, direct relationship between metamnemonic knowledge and memorial performance. This hope has been dashed; some investigators have found no links at all, whereas others have found only relatively weak ones (Markman, 1973; Moynahan, 1973; Salatas & Flavell, 1976).

Flavell and Wellman (1977) described several factors that probably contribute to the relatively small relationship that has emerged. Consider some factors that might lead a child who knows about a strategy not to use it. The child might know about the strategy but might think that some other strategy was superior in the particular situation. He or she might know about the strategy but judge the task sufficiently simple to perform without it. The child might know abstractly about the strategy but not be very good in executing it: Under such circumstances, he or she might not even try to use it. Finally, the child might be familiar with the strategy, recognize its utility for the situation, and be skilled in using it but simply decide that it was not worth the bother; Flavell and Wellman termed this the "original sin" hypothesis.

Although the relationship between metamemory and memorial performance has emerged as more complex than "improved metamemorial performance leads to improved memorial performance," this does not mean that the two are unrelated. Particularly suggestive is a study by Wellman, Drozdal, Flavell, Salatas, & Ritter (1975). These investigators found two types of links between metamemorial knowledge and memory performance. On some tasks, the two correlated positively from the earliest ages examined. On other tasks, they were uncorrelated at early ages but correlated positively at later ages. This finding is concordant with the Piagetian notion that part of advanced thinking is the ability to view one's own behavior abstractly, as an object to be analyzed and improved (e.g., Inhelder & Piaget, 1958).

Thus, although the early findings concerning the relationship between meta-mnemonic knowledge and memorial performance are not encouraging, stronger relationships may yet emerge with more focused assessments.

The knowledge base

For the same reasons that fish will be the last to discover water, developmental psychologists until recently devoted almost no attention to changes in children's knowledge of specific content. Such changes are so omnipresent that they seemed uninviting as targets for study. Instead of being investigated, improved content knowledge was implicitly dismissed as a by-product of more basic changes in capacities and strategies. (For purpose of illustration, consider the historic emphasis on learning principles and the lack of emphasis on the material being learned in such areas as concept formation, discrimination learning, and the various mediation paradigms.) Recently, however, researchers have suggested that knowledge of specific content domains is a crucial dimension of development in its own right and that changes in such knowledge may underlie other changes previously attributed to the growth of capacities and strategies.

Work on children's knowledge of specific content has attempted to establish several points. First, content knowledge enters into recall in a great many situations; such findings are often lumped under the heading of constructive recall. Second, knowledge of content domains influences the ease with which mnemonic strategies can be acquired. Third, memorial performance improves during periods of development in which there is little improvement in strategies but substantial improvements in content knowledge. Fourth, and most dramatic, under some circumstances differences in content knowledge can outweigh all other age-related differences; more knowledgeable younger children can recall more material in their area of expertise than less knowledgeable adults. We will discuss each of these topics.

Constructive memory. When people are given a prose passage and then are asked to recall it, they rarely produce exactly the same story. Some parts are left out, others are embellished, yet others that were only implied are recalled as if they were explicit. In many cases, even adults are unable to distinguish sentences that they have heard from sentences whose meaning was implicit in the story (e.g., Bransford & McCarrell, 1974).

One implication of such findings is that as children's knowledge bases grow more elaborated and rich, their memories for incoming information should also. Support for this viewpoint can be found in analyses of children's intrusion errors. Brown, Smiley, Day, Townsend, and Lawton (1977) presented second, fourth, and sixth graders with a brief story and then asked them to recall it. They found that although the number of intrusion errors was similar for the three age groups, the older children's intrusions were more often relevant to the theme of the story: 79% of the sixth graders' intrusions were theme relevant, whereas only 51% of the second graders' were so. Brown and associates explained this difference in terms of preexisting knowledge. The older children knew more about the topic of the stories (life among Eskimos or desert Indians) and therefore were more likely to make plausible additions to what they were told. In everyday learning situations, such theme-relevant intrusions, rather than representing errors, would be an encouraging sign that existing information and new information were being integrated.

A related consequence of growing knowledge bases may be an increased likelihood of drawing appropriate inferences. These can be helpful in recall, as a study by Paris and Lindauer (1976) illustrates. The experimenter presented 7-, 9-, and 11-year-olds with sentences in which the instrument of action was either made explicit (e.g., "The girl swept the floor with a broom") or left implicit (e.g., "The girl swept the floor"). Later, the children were provided with the instrument as a retrieval cue for the sentence. The performance of 11-year-olds was similar regardless of whether the instrument was explicitly identified in the original sentence. By contrast, 7- and 9-year-olds recalled more of the sentences in which the instrument was explicitly mentioned. Paris and Lindauer interpreted this finding as indicating that the older children were more likely to infer the instrument in the absence of its naming.

In perhaps the most controversial experiment on reconstructive memory, Piaget and Inhelder (1973) reported that with appropriate changes in the knowledge base, memory of an event can become more accurate with the passage of time. They showed 3- to 8-year-olds a row of sticks, ordered from shortest to longest, and told the children to study the row in preparation for a later recall test. A week later, the children were asked to draw the row of sticks that they had seen. Six to eight months later, the test was repeated. The most interesting finding of the study concerned changes in the drawings between the first and second testing. The reproductions of the 5- to 8-year-olds actually became more accurate; the children were more likely to draw a seriated row on the second than on the first testing. Piaget and Inhelder interpreted this change in terms of improved knowledge of seriation leading to a more accurate memorial representation of the sticks.

Liben (1975) suggested that the locus of Piaget and Inhelder's effect might lie in the children's decoding of their mnemonic representation. To test this hypothesis, she presented kindergarteners and first, second, and third graders with a task in which they were asked to imagine and to draw a row of 10 sticks standing up straight in a row. Although the children were not asked to reproduce any particular seriated row, their drawings nevertheless became seriated increasingly with age, from 19% seriated drawings among the kindergarteners to 82% among the third graders.

The Piaget and Inhelder findings may be most interesting for the questions that they raise about the nature of memory. By most definitions, it is logically impossible for a child to remember material that has not been presented. From this viewpoint, the Liben findings would be interpreted as suggesting that Piaget and Inhelder's phenomenon did not involve episodic memory at all. On the other hand, Piaget and Inhelder distinguished between two types of memory: memory in the strict sense, which they defined as memory for the sensory attributes of the stimuli shown in a particular situation, and memory in the wider sense, defined as inseparable from intelligence and knowledge. They argued that memory in the wider sense inevitably influences memory in the strict sense, that old and new memories are inextricably intertwined, and that distinctions between them are largely artificial. Liben (1977) largely agreed with this view and presented evidence that the drawings of children who have and have not seen the original configuration differ in some ways. (A third view is also possible, that the entire phenomenon of memory improvement over time is artifactual. For research supporting this position, see Maurer, Siegel, Lewis, Kristofferson, Barnes, and Levy, 1979.)

Content knowledge and the acquisition of strategies. Differences in strategic knowledge are often used to explain differences in older and younger children's ability to acquire information about specific content. This equation can be reversed, however; knowledge of specific content may influence the acquisition of strategies. Several observations are consistent with this view. Training younger children to use strategies rarely brings their performance to the level of older children's (Belmont & Butterfield, 1971). Training retardates to use strategies rarely improves their performance to the point where it equals that of "normals" (Brown, 1978). Preventing adults from using any apparent strategy reduces their performance, but it still remains higher than that of children (Chi, 1977). Several investigators have suggested that these remaining differences are caused by different content knowledge among members of the different groups (Chi, 1978; Myers & Perlmutter, 1978; Ornstein, 1978).

Chi (in press) presented somewhat more direct evidence that knowledge of the content to be remembered can play a role in the acquisition of strategies. She examined how well a 5-year-old could learn an alphabetic retrieval strategy for her classmates' names. Although the strategy was novel, the child learned it rather easily. By contrast, the same child encountered much difficulty applying the alphabetic strategy to a set of names of people she did not know. Chi (in press) concluded that powerful strategies may be acquired only after content knowledge is well understood.

Memorial growth in the absence of improved strategies.   As mentioned above, children do not often rehearse, organize, elaborate or use other easily detectable strategies before age 5. Nevertheless, their memorial performance improves substantially between birth and that age. Myers and Perlmutter (1978) argued that growth of content knowledge likely contributes to this improvement. They found that differences between 2- and 4-year-olds' recall were greater for related than for unrelated words. Blocking items from the same conceptual category produced similarly greater benefits for 4- than for 2-year-olds. Myers and Perlmutter found little evidence of deliberately invoked strategies such as rehearsal, organization, or elaboration among either the younger or the older children. Instead, they concluded that the older children's superior performance was due to their superior knowledge about the material being learned.

Age versus knowledge.   Chi (1978) provided the most dramatic demonstration to date of the potential impact of the knowledge base. She compared the memorial and metamemorial performance of 10-year-olds and adults on two tasks: a standard digit-span task and a chess task. The 10-year-olds were skilled chess players, whereas the adults were novices at the game. The primary chess memory task involved displaying an organized arrangement of pieces on a board for 10 sec, then covering the arrangement and asking the child or adult to reproduce it on a second chess board. The primary metamemorial task involved asking the children and adults to predict how many trials it would take them to reproduce correctly all of the pieces on the board.

On both of the chess tasks, the children outperformed the adults (Figure 14.1). Their reproductions of the chess boards were more accurate, and they were better able to anticipate how many trials they would take to memorize the entire arrangement. These findings were not attributable to the children's being generally smarter or possessing better memories. On the standard digit-span task, adults showed the

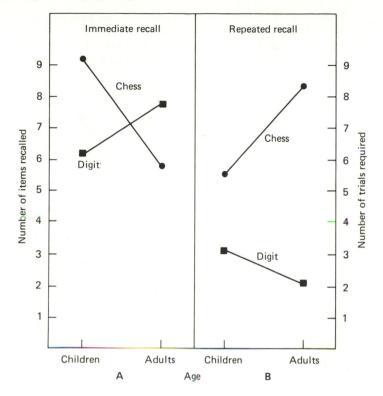

Figure 14.1. Recall of chess and digit stimuli by children and adults. (From "Knowledge Structures and Memory Development" by M. T. Chi, in R. S. Siegler, Ed., *Children's Thinking: What Develops?* [Hillsdale, N.J.: Erlbaum, 1978]. Reprinted by permission.)

usual superiority of recall. Thus differences in knowledge can outweigh whatever other memorial differences exist between children and adults.

Wagner (1978) made a similar point in a cross-cultural investigation conducted in Morocco. The groups that he studied included two of particular interest in the present context: Koranic scholars and rug sellers. The Koranic scholars were generally well schooled and their schooling involved a great deal of memorization; thus, their general mnemonic skills were presumably developed to a high degree. The rug sellers had little formal education but a high degree of knowledge about the experimental stimuli: rugs. The task involved a continuous recognition procedure, in which subjects were asked to identify stimuli as previously presented or new (cf. Shepard & Teeghtsoonian, 1961). The rug sellers proved to be more proficient than the Koranic scholars in recognizing which rugs they had seen and which they had not. Wagner hypothesized that the rug sellers' greater knowledge of the stimuli aided them in identifying distinctive features, thus enhancing their recall. By contrast, the Koranic scholars' highly developed general mnemonic skills appeared to be limited to meaningful verbal material in which serial strategies could be used (e.g., the Koran).

Before ending this discussion of the effects of the knowledge base, a word of caution is in order. Research on the topic is still in an extremely preliminary phase. Many of the effects being attributed to differential content knowledge receive this explanation as a sort of default option; the investigator does not know what else to attribute the effects to. Similarly, demonstrating that differential content knowledge can outweigh the influence of other capabilities that are acquired with age and education does not mean that knowledge generally overshadows the other factors, only that it may do so. In addition, at present we have only vague notions of the mechanisms by which content knowledge influences memory. With these caveats in mind, we remain optimistic about this area of research. We now know that content knowledge can substantially influence memory for new information, and we may soon know more about the mechanisms by which this occurs.

DEVELOPMENT OF PROBLEM-SOLVING SKILLS

In this section we examine information-processing approaches to five problem-solving tasks: transitive inference, analogical reasoning, conservation, counting, and object permanence. The focus of this research, as of most information-processing research on problem solving, is on the interaction between the problem solver and the task environment. In order to understand the research, it is necessary to have some understanding of the general idea of task analysis and of the particular forms that task analyses can take.

Task analysis encompasses a set of quite diverse research strategies, but it is possible to discern several common characteristics. As the terms *task* and *analysis* imply, the approach involves the breaking down of a complex problem into smaller, more precisely specifiable components. These components are then combined into one or more models of overall performance. Such models may be derived either from a priori consideration of the structure of the task or from empirical data on how people actually perform it (cf. Resnick, 1976). Often but not always, the models are intended as real-time depictions of people's activities; first they do this, then they do that, and so on. Again, often but not always, the models are stated as flow diagrams or as computer simulations; the purpose is to increase the precision of the description beyond that allowed by standard written language.

Several variants of the task-analytic approach have been developed. These differ in their level of specificity, in whether they attempt to depict real-time processing, and in their characteristic types of evidence. The most common approach is to analyze tasks at the level of flow charts. Such models usually, though not always, contain assumptions about the temporal order of processing; thus they are real-time models. Experimental methods using reaction times and patterns of correct answers and errors are the typical means of testing the models. The models are usually specific at the level of the behavior that they predict, though unanalyzed components often reside within the boxes of the diagrams.

The computer simulation approach is somewhat less common. As in the flow chart strategy, the goal is to develop real-time models. The level of analysis of computer simulation models is more specific, though. Where a flow diagram might contain 10 or 15 boxes, a computer simulation might include 100 separate statements. The standards of evidence also differ. The first goal of a computer simulation is that it should run. This provides a sufficiency proof by demonstrating that the model is sufficiently complete and well specified to produce the desired behavior. Another goal is that the simulation is consistent with the known general properties of human information processors. For example, short-term memory capacity is limited, as is the speed with which processes can be performed. A third goal is that the simulation demonstrate how different systems, such as semantic memory and immediate perceptions, might interact to produce behavior. Less emphasis is placed on experimental means of verification than in the flow diagram approach, and what verification is done is typically performed for a single person rather than for a broader population. Empirical testing is difficult because many parts of simulation models have no obvious behavioral implications and because simulations typically are designed at the level of individuals rather than groups.

The newest and thus far least common task-analytic approach is to elucidate principles involved in conceptual understanding. The principles approach does not aim at producing real-time models. Instead, the emphasis is on knowledge implicit in the production of behavior. Patterns of correct answers and errors are the main evidence used to indicate children's understanding of principles. Analyses of principles are typically less specific than either flow chart or computer simulation models. Principles do not completely specify what behavior is expected, because a child may understand a principle and still not produce the corresponding behavior because of extrinsic difficulties (not understanding the task, short-term memory limitations, insufficient appreciation of the domain of applicability of the principles, and so on). The broader level of aggregation of the principles approach is not altogether a weakness, however; it sometimes allows investigators to discover types of understanding that they might otherwise miss. Below we describe several analyses of task environments of interest, in which the flow diagram, computer simulation, and principle approaches have been used.

Transitive inference.   Transitive inference has been studied by psychometricians, Piagetians, and information-processing psychologists alike (Burt, 1919; Piaget, 1921; Sternberg, 1980). The problems usually take the form

$$A > B$$
$$B < C$$
$$\therefore A > C$$

and the subject's possible responses are "true," "false," and "can't tell." Investigators have generally found that children below age 7 rarely solve these problems. Until recently, the most influential explanation for this finding was that advanced by Piaget (1970). Piaget attributed the young children's failure to their not possessing the logical structures necessary to understand the reversible nature of transitive relationships (i.e., that $A > B$ implies that $B < A$) and to their not being able to seriate an extended list of asymmetric relations.

Trabasso and his coworkers (e.g., Bryant & Trabasso, 1971; Riley & Trabasso, 1974; Trabasso, 1975) challenged this interpretation. Within their task analysis, children are seen as needing to memorize the pair-wise relations (e.g., $A > B$), to integrate the pair-wise relationships into some overall form, and then to make the inference from this integrated representation. This analysis suggested that young children's difficulty might lie in remembering the original premises rather than in the logical inference process as such. If this was the case, then ensuring that children remembered the premises would be expected to lead to appropriate inferences as well.

Bryant and Trabasso (1971) tested this prediction. They presented preschoolers with five different-colored sticks that varied in length. First they taught the children the relation between each adjacent pair (e.g., Stick 1 is longer than Stick 2). Then, after the children mastered each relation, the experimenter presented in random order all four pairs (1 and 2, 2 and 3, 3 and 4, 4 and 5); this procedure continued until the children were correct on 24 consecutive questions. Finally, the crucial third phase was administered. Here, children were asked not only about the original pairs but also about other pairs whose relation could only be inferred (e.g., Sticks 2 and 4). Bryant and Trabasso's basic expectation was that once children memorized all of the premises (the original pairs) they would also do well on the untrained inference problems. This expectation was strongly supported. When children memorized the original pairs, they also drew the appropriate inferences. For example, 13 of 17 4-year-olds in the study performed without error in the test phase.

Since this initial experiment Trabasso and his associates have expanded their investigation in a number of directions. Perhaps the greatest attention has been given to specifying the representation within which children and adults maintain the premises in memory. The basic model that has emerged is a linear array in which all of the sticks are lined up from shortest to longest. Given such a representation, it is a relatively simple matter to draw the proper inference; simply locate within the array the two sticks asked about and choose the one closer to the tall end.

One type of evidence used to support this model involves the order in which the premises are memorized when all are presented together (cf. Trabasso et al., 1975). Adults and 6- and 9-year-olds seem to build their representations from the outside in; that is, they first master the extreme relationships (Stick 1 is longer than Stick 2; Stick 5 is longer than Stick 6), then the next most extreme ones (Stick 2 is longer than Stick 3; Stick 4 is longer than Stick 5), and last the middle one (Stick 3 is longer than Stick 4). Exactly this pattern of memorization has been observed in studies of linear orders outside of the transitive inference context (e.g., Potts, 1972). In representing a wide variety of spatial information, people master the extreme (and anchor) relations first and build inward from there.

A second type of evidence used to support the model involved a comparison of subjects' performance in the transitive inference situation with their performance in a visible display condition. In the display condition, children saw six different-colored sticks, ordered from shortest to longest, and were asked the usual inference questions (e.g., whether the red stick was longer than the blue stick). Performance under the display and the standard conditions was indistinguishable, both in terms of the pattern of errors and in terms of reaction times (Trabasso et al., 1975). It seemed to make little difference whether the linear array was in the subject's head or in the visible environment.

A third type of evidence was derived from studying inferences more than one step removed from the original premises. Trabasso, Riley, and Wilson (1975) presented 6-year-olds, 9-year-olds, and adults with six-stick arrays; this allowed the investigators to contrast zero-step inferences (Stick 2 vs. Stick 3; Stick 3 vs. Stick 4) with one-step inferences (Stick 2 vs. Stick 4; Stick 3 vs. Stick 5) and with two-step inferences (Stick 2 vs. Stick 5). If information were represented in terms of the original premises, the zero-step inferences would presumably be most quickly and accurately recalled, as these were the originally memorized premises. On the other hand, if information was represented in terms of an integrated linear array, the relationship involving the most discrepant elements (the two-step inferences) would be recalled most quickly and accurately (cf. Potts, 1972). The latter situation proved clearly to be the case. The two-step inferences were made more rapidly and more often correctly than the zero-step ones. Again, this pattern has emerged in numerous other studies of linear orderings.

The story until now has had little developmental content; in terms of the basic representations and processes, young children closely resemble adults. People of different ages differ substantially, however, in the range of situations under which they form these representations and in the efficiency with which they do so. One differentiating factor involves the linguistic form in which questions are presented during the training period. Bryant and Trabasso trained children using both marked terms (which stick is shorter) and unmarked ones (which stick is longer). Riley and Trabasso (1974) noted that this was a departure from the usual transitivity format in which only one linguistic form is used and suggested that it might have been important in helping the children succeed in the Bryant and Trabasso experiment. Therefore they contrasted the previous training procedure with one that was identical except for use of only the marked or only the unmarked form in training.

The effectiveness of the two training conditions differed considerably; 87% of the 4-year-olds instructed with both linguistic forms met the training criterion for mastery; 35% of those given only one or the other linguistic form did so. Riley and Trabasso suggested that this difference resulted because young children who were instructed with a single form encoded the relations absolutely (Stick 1 is long; Stick 2 is short) rather than relatively (Stick 1 is longer than Stick 2). Such absolute encoding would produce contradictions and confusion as Stick 2 was eventually found to be both long and short. One difference between young children and older ones may thus be that older children are more apt to code the original premises in relative terms.

A second difference between younger and older children involves the rapidity with which they memorize adjacent pairs. Eventually, young children memorize all of the pairs, but they are much slower than adults in doing so. The reason may be that they take longer to decide on the integrated linear array as the appropriate representation (Falmagne, 1975). The question of which representations young children generate before arriving at the linear array has not yet been addressed by Trabasso and colleagues.

Trabasso's analysis thus implicates at least three factors in the development of transitive inference: memorial skills, linguistic understanding, and ability to choose appropriate representations. Intellectual development on the task seems to involve improvement in the range of conditions under which appropriate representations are formed more than improvement in the inference process as such. The series of experiments elegantly illustrates the advantages of breaking tasks into their components and examining the components separately rather than assuming that children's difficulty must be with the logic of the task.

Analogical reasoning. Sternberg and Rifkin (1979) applied componential analysis, a sophisticated form of task analysis, to studying the development of analogical reasoning. The type of analogy problem that they used is shown in Figure 14.2. In these problems, Elements A, B, and C are given; the task is to select Element D so that the relation between C and D is the same as that between A and B. Thus, the basic form of the analogies is A:B :: C:?.

Sternberg and Rifkin first analyzed this task in terms of the attributes and values of its stimuli. The stimuli (the men in the Figure 14.2 example) can differ in four

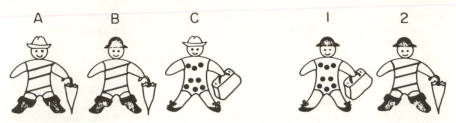

Figure 14.2. Representative analogy item. (From "The Development of Analogical Reasoning Processes" by R. J. Sternberg and B. Rifkin, *Journal of Experimental Child Psychology*, 1979, 27, 195–232. Copyright © 1979 by Academic Press. Reprinted by permission.)

attributes: their hats, their jerseys, their footwear, and the objects in their hands. Each of these attributes can take on two values: hats can be light or dark, jerseys can be striped or polka dotted, footwear can be shoes or boots, and the objects carried can be umbrellas or lunch boxes. The child's task is to choose a fourth man who is identical to and different from the third exactly as the second man is identical to and different from the first. That is, since Man B differs from Man A in hat color and is similar in jersey, umbrella, and footwear, Man D must be different from Man C in hat color and similar in jersey, umbrella, and footwear. This formula is fit by Alternative 1, making it the correct answer.

Sternberg and Rifkin further analyzed the task in terms of the required processing of these attributes and values. They hypothesized that people execute four mandatory components and perhaps also two optional ones. Encoding, inference, application, and response are the mandatory components, mapping and justification the optional ones. Encoding involves noting the attributes and their values for each figure. Inference involves establishing the similarities and differences between Choices A and B on each attribute. Mapping involves finding the relationship between A and C; this step is not formally necessary to solve analogy problems but may at times be undertaken. Application involves discovering a relationship between C and D that parallels that between A and B. If neither possibility allows a precise analogy, a next step of justification is taken, involving the formulation of an explanation of why one answer is superior to the other. Finally a response is made.

The Figure 14.2 example can be used to illustrate how this componential analysis works. To simplify the explanatory task, we will assume that all processes are executed exhaustively. In the encoding stage, the child would note the attributes and values of each element: that the first man had a light hat, a striped jersey, boots, and an umbrella, that the second man had a dark hat, a striped jersey, boots, and an umbrella, and so on for each of the five men. In the inference stage, the child would determine the relationship between Men A and B: that they were different in their hat colors and similar in their jerseys, boots, and umbrellas. If the child executed the mapping component, he or she would determine the relationship between C and A: that they were different in all values except for hat colors. In the application stage, the child would seek an alternative that bore the same relationship to C that B did to A – that is, an alternative that was different in hat color but similar in the other attributes. Possibility 1 meets this specification exactly, so that no justification stage would be undertaken. Finally, the response "1" would be made.

Using this componential analysis, Sternberg and Rifkin formulated four models of analogical reasoning. The models include the same components but differ in whether the components are executed exhaustively or in a self-terminating fashion. Exhaustive operations involve comparing values on all attributes for a given pair of stimuli before moving on to the next step. For example, exhaustive execution of the inference process in our example would involve noting all four of the relationships between A and B: that jersey colors, footwear, and materials in hand are the same and that hat colors are different. Self-terminating inferencing would involve noting only one relationship before going on to see if the problem could be solved on that basis. Many problems can be; in our example, if the subject focused on jersey color, B has the same jersey color as A, and only Choice 1 has the same color as C, therefore Choice 1 must be correct.

As we have mentioned, Sternberg and Rifkin's models differ primarily in which operations are exhaustive and which are self-terminating. In Model 1, all components are executed exhaustively. In Model 2, all are executed exhaustively save application. As soon as one possible answer matches the predicted values for D, the search is terminated. In Model 3, both mapping and application are self-terminating. Once all relationships between A and B have been noted, C is compared to A on a particular attribute and the two response alternatives are compared on their attribute to see if one but not the other has the proper relation to C. If so, the process is terminated and the answer is given; if not, the mapping is made on a second attribute, the application performed on that attribute, and so on. Finally, Model 4 involves self-terminating processing on inference, mapping, and application processes: A single relationship between A and B is noted, the relationship of A to C on that attribute is determined, and the response alternatives are checked to see if one but not both has the predicted value on the attribute. If so, that choice is the answer; if not, the cycle starts over with a second attribute.

A large number of the Figure 14.2 type of analogy problems were presented to 8-year-olds, 10-year-olds, 12-year-olds, and adults. The primary measure of performance was solution latencies on correctly solved items. The main standard used to compare the fit of the alternative models was percentage of variance accounted for, although other criteria such as the total number of parameters (the fewer the better), and the number of parameters accounting for significant variance (the more the better) were also employed when competing models accounted for similar percentages of variance (see Sternberg & Rifkin, 1979, for details).

Results proved to differ substantially, depending on whether the stimuli in the analogy problems involved separable or integral attributes (cf. Garner, 1974). With the separable attributes, a modified version of Model 4 (one involving self-terminating encoding, inferencing, and application) proved to be the best supported for all age groups. With the integral attributes, the pattern was more complex. Eight-year-olds used the version of Model 4 with self-terminating encoding, inferencing, and application. Ten-year-olds used the originally hypothesized version of Model 4, with self-terminating inferencing, mapping, and application. Twelve-year-olds and adults used Model 3, in which only mapping and application are self-terminating.

How could these developmental changes be interpreted? With respect to the component operations used, children and adults were very similar. Differences existed, however, in whether the operations were executed in exhaustive or self-terminating fashion. Older children and adults tended increasingly toward exhaustive processing, at least on the integral stimuli. This was especially the case with regard to encoding. On all other parameters, adults were considerably faster than 10-year-olds, a result that is hardly surprising. What is surprising is that adults took more time than children (in absolute as well as relative terms) to encode the initial stimuli.

Sternberg and Rifkin suggested that the differences in encoding might be due to memory limitations among the younger children. Exhaustive encoding requires the encoder to memorize the values of all attributes for a given term. Self-terminating encoding requires memorization of only one attribute at a time. The substantial memory burden entailed by exhaustive encoding seems to pay off in lower error rates and reduced need to return to the operation, but the immediate cost of the memorization effort may be too great for the younger children.

Conservation.   Klahr and Wallace (1973, 1976) presented a computer simulation of the development of conservation concepts. Although we will not discuss the simulation itself here, our description of the theory should indicate the specificity of thinking that the simulation approach encourages.

We have already described the standard conservation procedure. One of two identical objects (or sets of objects) is transformed in a way that leaves the dimension in question unchanged but alters some more perceptually salient dimension; the child needs to indicate that the two alternatives remain the same on the dimension of interest even though they no longer look the same.

Many variants of this basic conservation procedure have been developed. Rather than the usual *equivalence* procedure with two rows of objects, children may be presented with an *identity* procedure in which a single object or row of objects is transformed. The question in such identity procedures is whether the object or row of objects is the same or different on the relevant dimension as it was before – for example, whether the number of objects remains the same. A second variant is called conservation of inequality. Rather than making the object or rows of objects initially identical on the dimension of interest, the researcher can make them initially unequal on it. For example, one row could have four checkers and the other three. Finally, quantity-altering transformations (addition and subtraction) as well as quantity-preserving ones can be performed. Instead of simply spreading a row of checkers, the experimenter could add a checker.

Klahr and Wallace hypothesized that conservation understanding develops from empirical experience with transformations, materials, and quantitative operators. They assigned a special role to conservation of number, believing that understanding of the other types of conservation grows from knowledge in this domain. Finally, within conservation-of-number tasks, they contended that experience with problems involving very small numbers of elements is central. Their hypothesized developmental progression leading to conservation is sufficiently complex that it is not surprising that children take several years to master all of its steps.

The first step in the developmental sequence is learning to apply quantitative operators to a set in order to obtain a quantitative representation. That is, the child must have some way of representing three objects as "three." Klahr and Wallace believe that at least initially this is done by subitizing, a very rapid process applicable to sets of between one and four objects. A child who can subitize can note the numerousness of small sets both before and after a transformation is applied. This allows the child to make observations of the form "spreading apart three checkers leaves three checkers," "spreading apart two dimes leaves two dimes," "spreading apart three marbles leaves three marbles," and so on. Klahr and Wallace label such observations *specific sequence detections.* After some number of specific sequence

Table 14.2. *Possible number-conservation outcomes, given two initially identical rows of objects*

Transformation	Relation between x and y' on length dimension	Relation between x and y' on width dimension	Quantitative relation between x and y'
No addition/no subtraction	=	=	=
No addition/no subtraction	>	<	=
No addition/no subtraction	<	>	=
Addition	<	<	<
Addition	<	=	<
Addition	=	<	<
Addition	<	>	<
Addition	>	<	<
Subtraction	>	>	>
Subtraction	>	=	>
Subtraction	=	>	>
Subtraction	>	<	>
Subtraction	<	>	>

Note: x refers to the untransformed row. y' refers to the transformed row after the transformation.
Source: Klahr & Wallace (1976, Table 5.2).

detections, the child might draw the more general inference that "spreading objects apart (at least within the range of two to four objects) leaves the number of objects unchanged." This higher level of abstraction is termed *common sequence detection*. Once it is accomplished, there is no longer a need to requantify after the transformation; the result is already known.

This initial conservation knowledge spreads in several directions. Of special importance within Klahr and Wallace's analysis are the extensions to addition and subtraction transformations and to situations of initial inequality between rows. Learning the effects of all of the possible transformations (adding, subtracting, and neither adding nor subtracting) on all of the possible initial relationships between the two rows ($x > y$, $x = y$, $x < y$) yields the knowledge represented in Table 14.2. This knowledge, when extended to sets of arbitrary numerousness, represents mature understanding of number conservation.

Before children can use this knowledge in its widest application, however, they must learn to apply it to large as well as small arrays. This application necessitates a quantification operator usable on sets of all sizes. For conservation of number, counting provides such an operator. Through its use, children can establish that the pattern for large sets is identical to that for small; spreading and contracting leave the numerosity of sets of all sizes unchanged, and addition and subtraction change all of them. Once this identity of the effects of transformations is realized at the level of common sequences, counting of the transformed set can be eliminated.

Additional steps are necessary to generalize the knowledge to other types of conservation. Here estimation becomes the important quantitative operator. Only a process of estimation can indicate the initial equality of the quantity of liquid in the two containers, or the amount of clay in two clay balls, and only a process of estimation can be used to judge whether the quantities remain equal following the pouring transformation. The development of these types of conservation is more protracted than the development of number conservation for two reasons. First, estimates yield less precise results than counting or subitizing and thus are less easy to rely upon. Second, children's initial estimates are usually based upon values of a single dimension, such as the heights of the water in the two containers. It is only when this unidimensional approach is shown to be untrustworthy that it is abandoned. This process takes a long time, as the unidimensional strategy usually works quite well (relative heights are highly correlated with relative quantities in most situations). When the strategy is finally disconfirmed, and the correct approach adopted, conservation development is complete.

Klahr and Wallace presented relatively little empirical evidence to support their theory. Subsequent work, however, has provided considerable supportive data. For example, Siegler (1981) found that on the number-conservation task, addition and subtraction transformations are mastered prior to the quantity-preserving transformation. This result supports Klahr and Wallace's emphasis on the distinctiveness of the three arithmetic operations. Siegler (1981) also found that in the process of mastering number conservation, children first justify their correct responses in terms of counting and pairing and then shift to justifying them in terms of the type of transformation. Only when this latter type of justification is used are the children likely to solve liquid and solid quantity problems. This finding supports Klahr and Wallace's position that understanding of number conservation is functionally related to understanding of other types of conservation. The converging evidence provided by counting and pairing may make it easier for children to discover the role of transformations on number problems; once this discovery has been made, it may in turn facilitate children's learning about the transformations' roles in other conservation contexts.

Although we do not have the space to discuss the details of Klahr and Wallace's computer simulation, a few points about it should be made. First, it demonstrates that their theory is sufficient to account for performance on the task; computers do only what they are told and refuse to fill in unspecified details. Second, the simulation is closely related to other models that Klahr and Wallace have developed for transitive inference and class inclusion; inspection of the three simulations reveals the points of overlap as well as the features distinct to each task. Third, the simulation reveals the complexity of even a "simple" task such as number conservation; more than 60 separate "productions" are required to perform the task, and the productions often require the child to hold a considerable amount of information in memory. Fourth, the models reveal a difficulty that the simulation approach shares with the Piagetian approach and other approaches to studying intellectual development. Change processes are not simulated – Klahr and Wallace's models describe the knowledge states through which children progress but fail to address the processes through which change occurs. Some recent self-modifying production system simulations of adult performance (e.g., Anderson, Kline, & Beasley, 1979; Anzai & Simon, 1980) have begun to address this issue, but as yet these simulations have not been extended to modeling development.

Counting.   Gelman and Gallistel (1978) analyzed children's counting in terms of the principles underlying performance. They described five principles that they believe guide preschoolers' counting. The one–one principle corresponds to the knowledge that each object in an array must be assigned one and only one number word. The stable-order principle concerns the need to recite the number words in a constant order. The cardinal principle indicates that the last number in a counting sequence corresponds to the cardinal value of the set. The abstraction principle defines the objects or events that can be counted. The order-irrelevance principle states that the pairing between a particular item and a particular number word is arbitrary, that any item in an array can be counted first, second, or last.

Gelman and Gallistel examined a variety of aspects of children's counting to determine whether they understood these principles. The types of performance that were said to indicate understanding of each principle tell us much about the principles' meaning. Therefore we will examine these criteria in some detail.

A child who, for a five-item array, said "one-two-three-four-five" would be said to understand the one–one principle. Understanding would also be indicated by the response "one-three-seven-eight-nine" or "A-B-C-D-E," because these sequences contain one count term for each item, though not the conventional ones. Instances in which the child produced one count term more or less than required were also accepted, at least provisionally, as showing understanding of the one–one principle; the problem in such cases was thought to be lack of skill in execution or counting rather than lack of understanding.

Understanding of the stable-order principle was indicated when the child repeated either the standard list of numbers or some nonstandard list in a consistent order. A child who counted a five-item array "one-two-three" would qualify, as would a child who counted it "one-four-eight," as long as the child consistently followed the sequence.

Understanding of the cardinal principle could be demonstrated in several ways. The child could indicate understanding of the importance of the last term in the count series by repeating it ("one-two-three-*three*"), by verbally stressing it ("one-two-*three*"), or by simply saying the correct number of objects in the set without going through the count sequence. This last criterion was included because older children often do not count small sets aloud in response to the question "How many are there?" By saying only the last number, they indicate their understanding of its special importance.

The abstraction principle was measured in terms of the range of objects children would count. Children who understood this principle would count abstract as well as concrete sets (the set of minds in the room) and heterogeneous as well as homogeneous sets (a single set including all of the pencils and minds in the room as well as a single set including only the pencils).

Finally, the order-irrelevance principle was in a sense a composite of all of the other rules. It was assessed in an experiment of its own. On one trial within this procedure, children were presented with a row of five objects: from left to right, a pencil, a doll, a house, a book, and a ladder. They were asked to count the objects so that the pencil would be the fourth object. One way to do this would be to start at the position farthest left except for the pencil and to return to it when appropriate. That is, the child might count the doll as 1, the house as 2, the book as 3, the pencil as 4, and the ladder as 5. Alternatively, the child might view the arrangement circularly rather than linearly and count the objects in the order: house, book, ladder, pencil, doll. A child who could count under these circumstances would be demonstrating understanding of all of the principles and skill in manipulating them as well.

Gelman and Gallistel found that even very young children perform in accordance with these standards when they count small arrays. More than 70% of 3-year-olds produced the same number of tags as objects to be counted for Set Sizes 2, 3, 4, and 5. More than 80% of them used the number tags in a stable order for arrays of these sizes. Roughly half indicated in one way or another understanding of the cardinal principle. Essentially all of the children conformed to the criteria for understanding of the abstraction principle; all objects were treated as countable. Only on the order-irrelevance principle did the majority of 3-year-olds show little evidence of understanding with the small sets.

The data concerning children's counting of larger arrays were different. Here young children demonstrated little understanding. Although more than 70% of 3-year-olds used the correct number tags in counting 2-to-5-item sets, fewer than 40% did so in counting 7-, 9-, or 11-item ones. Understanding of the cardinality principle ranged from 50% to 75% on 2-to-5-item sets, but from 20% to 35% on 7-, 9-, and 11-item ones. This difference suggested a question for Gelman and Gallistel's approach: If a child cannot state a principle, and acts in accord with it in only a few of the situations to which it applies, in what sense can he or she be said to understand it? That is, what differentiates understanding of a principle from skill in executing a procedure of limited generality?

Gelman and Gallistel's data indicated that the development of counting after age 3 mostly involves changes in the range of situations in which children give evidence of understanding. Skill in applying the principles fell off much less steeply with set size for 5-year-olds than for 3-year-olds. There was also a dramatic change in ability to integrate the principles, as evidenced by performance in the order-irrelevance experiment. Whereas only 6% of 3-year-olds showed consistent mastery of this task, 81% of 5-year-olds did. Thus, although impressive understanding of counting may be attained early, considerable development also occurs beyond this initial period.

Object permanence.   We know far less about infant intellectual development than about such development in later childhood. A few acquisitions, however, have been carefully investigated. One of the most interesting of these is the object-permanence concept, the notion that objects continue to exist when they move beyond the visual field.

No investigator of object permanence seems to have formulated an explicit task analysis of the problem. In surveying experiments in the area, however, we detected an implicit task analysis carried out by the field as a whole. This task analysis can be formulated in terms of principles similar to Gelman's counting principles. A child who understands object permanence should understand the following.

1.   Objects continue to exist in some form when they are outside the visual field as well as when they are within it.
2.   An object will remain where it was last placed unless someone or something moves it.
3.   An object's identity will remain the same when it is hidden.
4.   If no object is hidden in a previously empty space, no object will be found there.
5.   Objects can be regained by reaching behind barriers.
6.   Objects can be regained by reaching under covers.

Experiments on object permanence have examined the development of each of these principles.

Piaget's (1954) original experiment, described above, would appear to have demonstrated that very young infants do not understand the first principle, that objects continue to exist outside the visual field. An alternative explanation, however, is that the infants understand the principle but lack the motoric coordination to retrieve the object. Bower and Wishart (1972) tested this interpretation. Five-month-olds first saw a toy hidden under a transparent cup; the large majority of infants retrieved it. Then the infants saw the same toy hidden under an opaque cup. Only 2 of 16 retrieved it. This experiment allows rejection of the motoric coordination interpretation and also of the interpretation that the failure to retrieve the toy was due to a lack of motivation. Neither of these interpretations explain why the infants would retrieve the toy in the first situation but not in the second.

Even when infants know that an object can be retrieved when hidden, they may not realize that it must reappear where it was last placed. Several investigators (Evans, 1973; Evans & Gratch, 1972; Gratch & Landers, 1971; Landers, 1971) have reported that when 9-month-olds see a toy hidden under an opaque cup, they retrieve it. When the toy is then hidden under a second opaque cup, however, the infants look under the first one. Frequently, they do not seem to look at the second hiding cup when the object is being placed there; they continue to focus on the initial location (Gratch, 1977). They look under the first cup even when a different toy is placed under the second cup. Not until 11 or 12 months do infants seem to know that a toy will be found where it was last hidden.

The third principle involves the notion that an object's identity remains unchanged, that is, that the same toy that was hidden must reappear. LeCompte and Gratch (1972) and Saal (1974) found that 18-month-olds reacted with deep puzzlement when the toy found differed from the one that had been hidden. In contrast, 6- and 9-month-olds showed mild initial surprise or no initial reaction at all. Subsequent reactions of the young infants involved simple inspection of the toy by the 6-month-olds and the beginnings of puzzlement by the 9-month-olds. Thus the principle of a constant identity of objects, as opposed to their continued existence, seems to emerge relatively late in infancy.

Appel (1971) investigated the development of the notion "nothing hidden, nothing to be found." Nine- and 12-month-old infants were presented with a situation in which the experimenter either hid a toy on five trials or simply rapped on the hiding place with an empty hand on the trials. Neither age group searched in the no-toy-hidden condition. Then the infants who had previously seen a toy being hidden were presented with the no-toy-hidden procedure. The majority of infants continued searching for at least one trial, and many persevered over two or three trials. Appel concluded that the infants had only a diffuse understanding of the notion that a toy must be hidden in order to be found.

The type of obstruction used to hide the toy exerts an effect on whether infants will retrieve it. Brown and Bower (1978) found that infants of ages 5 to 8 months would often reach behind a screen to retrieve a toy but would not reach under a cloth to get it. They attributed this difference to differential understanding of the relations *behind* and *under*. In order to solve the retrieval task, infants must motorically understand the nature of these relationships, at least that objects can be retrieved behind and under objects. Brown and Bower's data suggest that such understanding may be acquired somewhat independently for the two relations.

These studies demonstrate how complex even a simple concept such as object permanence can be. Principles that to adults seem not only to be obvious but almost identical emerge one by one over a fairly protracted period of infancy. Real-time models, in which we are able to trace what occurs in the infants' minds from the time the object disappears to the time they retrieve or forget about it, seem an exciting if difficult next extension.

To the conclusions about intellectual development drawn from the psychometric and Piagetian approaches, research within the information-processing approach has thus contributed several more.

CONCLUSIONS

10. At present there is little evidence for developmental changes in the capacity of short-term memory that cannot also be explained in terms of changes in strategies or the knowledge base. Basic capacities may change, but it is exceptionally difficult to provide unambiguous evidence of their existence.

11. Between ages 5 and 10 years, children increasingly use general mnemonic strategies, including rehearsal, elaboration, and organization. The quality of children's implementation of the strategies also improves during this period. Use of such strategies can be taught to children younger than would ordinarily use them, but frequently the children revert to their original approaches when tested later in time or with different material.

12. Children possess considerable knowledge of their own memory limitations and of procedures that can be used to overcome the limitations. As yet, however, this knowledge has not been linked to memorial performance.

13. Children's knowledge of specific content undergoes enormous development. This growth may account for changes in measures of basic capacities, strategies, and metamemory, rather than the other way around, as psychologists have traditionally believed. Under some circumstances, differences in content knowledge can overwhelm all other age-related differences in memory: More knowledgeable children can remember more than less knowledgeable adults.

14. Children's use of logical reasoning skills is influenced by a variety of factors other than understanding of the logic itself, including memorial skills, linguistic understanding, and ability to select the appropriate representation for the problem.

15. Developmental differences in problem solving may at times be due less to the component operations that are performed than to the resources that are allocated to each component. Comprehensive encoding may be especially important for efficient problem solving.

16. Concepts that to adults seem to constitute single entities may to children represent separate concepts. For example, the notion of number conservation may be differentiated by young children according to the particular objects involved, the number of objects, the type of linear transformation, and the type of quantitative operator.

17. Understanding of higher-order principles may guide even very young children's performance in areas with which they have much experience, such as counting.

14.4.   THE DEVELOPMENT OF LEARNING SKILLS

At the outset of this paper, learning was given considerable emphasis as one of the intuitively important aspects of intelligence. Superior ability to learn was rated by the Carnegie-Mellon undergraduates as one of the most important characteristics of intelligent 2-year-olds, 10-year-olds, and adults. Historically also, learning and intelligence have been viewed as being closely related: In a 1921 symposium on the nature of intelligence, for example, a number of investigators identified intelligence with rapid and complete learning and explicitly stated that the usefulness of IQ tests depended upon the assumption that children who knew more now had been better at learning earlier (e.g., Colvin, 1921, p. 136; Haggerty, 1921, p. 213; Henman, 1921, p. 145).

Despite its intuitive importance for a comprehensive theory of intellectual growth, learning has scarcely been mentioned thus far in this chapter. This fact reflects the state of the discipline rather than our own preference. Scholars taking the three major approaches have devoted little attention to it. Psychometric tests examine what children already know and what problems they can already solve rather than their ability to acquire new information. Piagetian approaches predict limits on children's ability to learn within a given stage, but until recently no experiments had been performed to test this assumption. Information-processing researchers have noted within their own literature the same paucity of research on the topic. For example, Anderson (1976) commented that "interest in the mechanisms of procedural learning seems to have died in cognitive psychology with the demise of stimulus–response theories" (p. 20). Voss (1978) noted, "The study of learning indeed exists within cognitive psychology . . . [but] it must be conceded that the cognitive view of learning is vague, is abstract, and most important is lacking a substantive data base" (p. 13).

Why this disparity between the obvious importance of learning and the lack of recent attention to it? One answer is that it is much easier to study systems in steady states than systems undergoing transitions. All of the data produced by a system in a steady state can be predicted by a single description of that state, whereas the data produced by a system undergoing transition will have been produced by several different states, thereby necessitating several descriptions. In addition, in unsteady states it is usually far from obvious which data were produced by which state. Thus, the tactic of studying steady states prior to studying learning, adopted by researchers within all three approaches, seems justifiable in the short run. The study of learning cannot be put off forever, though, and the time seems ripe for examining the role of learning in intellectual development.

For the past few years, our own research has dealt with the question of how existing knowledge influences learning. Two of the concepts upon which we have focused in pursuing this question are proportionality and time. The rule-assessment approach that we have used to study these concepts has been strongly influenced by the Piagetian and information-processing approaches and slightly influenced by the psychometric approach as well. We now describe this rule-assessment approach and the research on learning that has flowed from it.

THE RULE-ASSESSMENT APPROACH

The rule-assessment approach focuses upon conceptual development. It can be summarized in terms of five core assumptions.

1. Children's conceptual understanding progresses through a regular sequence of qualitatively discrete rules.

2. These rules are ordered in terms of increasing correlation with the correct rule in environments that the children encounter. Children will not adopt a new rule that is less highly correlated with the correct rule than the rule that they are already using.

3. The effectiveness of a learning experience is largely determined by whether the learning experience distinguishes the child's existing rule from the correct rule. If

the learning experience does not discriminate between the two rules, the child will continue to use the original rule. If the learning experience does discriminate between the two rules, the child will either adopt a more advanced rule or will enter into a "rule search" state characterized by uncertainty as to which rule is correct.

4. A major reason why children do not immediately adopt the correct rule for all concepts and why they have difficulty in learning it consists in the limited encoding of the correct rules' component dimensions. Understanding of concepts frequently requires integration of several component dimensions. Failure to encode one or more of them can restrict children's ability to learn the concept (as can lack of knowledge of the appropriate method for combining the dimensions).

5. Failure to encode a dimension may be caused by lack of knowledge of the dimension's importance or lack of perceptual salience relative to other dimensions in the situation in which the concept is to be applied. Increasing a child's knowledge of the dimension's importance or increasing the dimension's perceptual salience can lead to improved ability to learn, which in turn can lead to improved knowledge.

The research that we have done to test this model of conceptual development has a cyclical flavor. First, we develop means for determining what children already know about a concept; we will shortly describe the rule-assessment method that we have used for this purpose. Next, we use these assessments of existing knowledge to predict children's ability to learn new information about the concept. If the assessments of existing knowledge fail to predict adequately the learning that occurs, this failure is taken as indicating a need to develop more comprehensive assessments of the children's initial knowledge. These more comprehensive assessments typically include direct measures of the children's encoding. We then examine the usefulness of the new assessments in predicting when learning will occur and what form it will take.

Central to this approach is a methodology for determining which rule an individual child is using. The basic strategy that has been used involves the formulation of problem types that yield distinct patterns of correct answers and errors for children using different rules. To date, this error-analysis methodology has been applied to studying children's rules on 11 tasks: the balance scale, projection of shadows, probability, fullness, conservation of liquid quantity, conservation of solid quantity, conservation of number, speed, time, distance, and the Tower of Hanoi (Klahr & Robinson, 1981; Siegler, 1976, 1978, 1981; Siegler & Richards, 1979; Siegler & Vago, 1978). Two examples may help illustrate how the approach works and how it can be used to study the relationship between existing knowledge and learning.

EXISTING KNOWLEDGE OF THE BALANCE SCALE

Consider the balance scale task shown in Figure 14.3. On each side of the fulcrum were four pegs on which metal weights could be placed. The arm of the balance could tip left or right or could remain level, depending on how the weights were arranged. A lever (not shown in Figure 14.3) could be set to hold the arm motionless. The child's task was to predict which (if either) side would go down if the lever were released.

Siegler (1976) suggested that children's knowledge about this task could be represented in terms of the four decision trees shown in Figure 14.4. A child using Rule I considers only the number of weights on each side of the fulcrum. If they are the

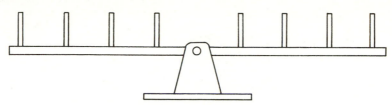

Figure 14.3. The balance scale. (From "Three aspects of cognitive thought" by R. S. Siegler, *Cognitive Psychology*, 1976, 8, 481–520. Copyright © 1976 by Academic Press. Reprinted by permission.)

same, the child predicts "balance"; otherwise, the child predicts that the side with the greater weight will go down. Someone using Rule II relies exclusively on weights if the two sides have different amounts of weight, but if their weights are equal, he or she also considers the distances of the weights from the fulcrum. A person using Rule III always considers both weight and distance and solves problems consistently correctly if one or both are equal; however, if one side has more weight and the other side has its weight farther from the fulcrum, the Rule III user does not know what to do and therefore muddles through, or guesses. Rule IV represents mature knowledge of the task. Because it includes the torque calculation, children using it always make the correct prediction.

It seemed possible to determine which, if any, of these four rule models accurately characterized a child's knowledge about the balance scale by examining that child's pattern of predictions on the six types of problems shown in Figure 14.5. Children who used the different rules would produce dramatically different response patterns on these problems. Those using Rule I would always predict correctly on balance, weight, and conflict–weight (i.e., cases in which distance and weight are both unequal and the side with the greater weight goes down) problems and would never predict correctly on the other three problem types. Children using Rule II would behave similarly except that they would also solve distance problems. Those adopting Rule III would invariably be correct on all three nonconflict problem types and would perform at a chance level on the three types of conflict problems. Those using Rule IV would solve all problems of all types.

Siegler (1976, Experiment 1) used these problem types to examine 5-, 9-, 13-, and 17-year-olds' existing knowledge about balance scales. In the experimental condition of interest here (the existing knowledge condition), children were simply asked to predict which side of the balance scale would go down if the lever were released. In order to be classified as using a rule, the child's predictions needed to conform to those of the rule on at least 26 of the 30 items. The rule models fit the predictions of 90% of children of all ages: 5-year-olds most often used Rule I, 9-year-olds most often Rule II or III, and 13- and 17-year-olds most often Rule III. Few children of any age used Rule IV. Children's explanations of how they made their choices closely paralleled their predictions; more than 80% of children were classified as using the same rule on the two measures by "blind" raters. Thus the results supported both the particular rule models as characterizations of children's knowledge about the balance scale and the rule-assessment methodology as a psychometric technique for determining what children know.

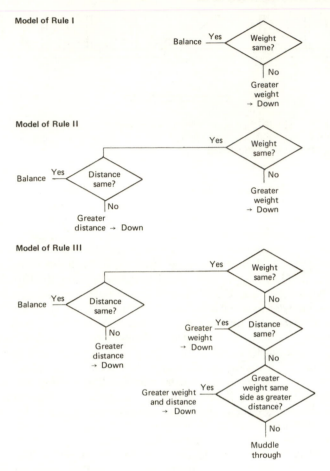

LEARNING ABOUT BALANCE SCALES

The ability to assess children's existing knowledge allowed investigation of the relationship between initial knowledge and learning. In particular, it allowed us to address the following hypothetical question: "If two children of different ages but with identical task-specific initial knowledge were presented with the same learning experiences, would they emerge with the same final knowledge about the task?"

The experimental strategy that was used to study this issue involved a pretest–training–posttest design. First, 5- and 8-year-olds were pretested to create groups of different-aged children who used the same initial rule (Rule I). Then the children were provided a series of feedback trials on conflict–weight, conflict–distance, and conflict–balance items in which they saw a balance scale configuration of weights on pegs, predicted which way the arm would tilt when the lever was released, and then observed as the lever was released and their prediction confirmed or disconfirmed. One or two days later, they were given a no-feedback posttest to determine the effects of the experience.

The results were quite different for older and younger children. Younger children

Model of Rule IV

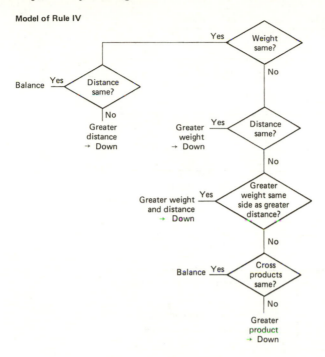

Figure 14.4. Decision tree models of rules for performing the balance scale task. (From "Three Aspects of Cognitive Development," by R. S. Siegler, *Cognitive Psychology,* 1976, *8,* 481–520. Copyright © 1976 by Academic Press. Reprinted by permission.)

made no progress; none of them adopted rules beyond Rule I. Older children, however, derived great benefits from exposure to the conflict problems; 70% of them advanced to Rule II or Rule III. This finding suggested that there were age differences relevant to learning above and beyond the initial rules that the children used.

The encoding hypothesis. Why might these differing reactions to conflict problems have occurred? Detailed examination of a few children suggested the encoding hypothesis: that children may fail to learn because they are not encoding all of the relevant dimensions. In the case of the balance scale, the 5-year-olds seemed to see the configurations solely in terms of two piles of weights, one on the left and one on the right, rather than as two piles of weights each a particular distance from the fulcrum. The specific number of pegs separating the weights from the fulcrum on each side did not seem to be represented. If such limited encoding was occurring, it might well explain why 5-year-olds in the conflict problem condition had difficulty learning that a difference in distance could more than compensate for an opposing difference in weight.

In order to determine the validity of this encoding explanation, it was necessary to measure encoding independent of the predictive knowledge tapped by the rule assessments. To do this, 5- and 8-year-olds were briefly presented with balance scale configurations of weights on pegs. Then the scale was hidden from sight and a

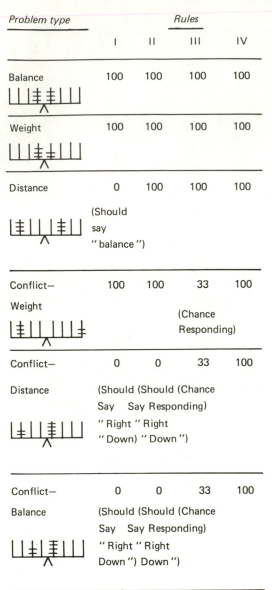

Problem type	Rules			
	I	II	III	IV
Balance	100	100	100	100
Weight	100	100	100	100
Distance	0 (Should say "balance")	100	100	100
Conflict— Weight	100	100	33 (Chance Responding)	100
Conflict— Distance	0 (Should Say "Right "Down)	0 (Should Say Responding) "Right "Down")	33 (Chance	100
Conflict— Balance	0 (Should Say "Right Down")	0 (Should Say Responding) "Right Down")	33 (Chance	100

Figure 14.5. Problem types used for assessing rules on balance scale task. (From "Three Aspects of Cognitive Development" by R. S. Siegler, *Cognitive Psychology*, 1976, 8, 481–520. Copyright © 1976 by Academic Press. Reprinted by permission.)

second identical scale was presented. The task was to reproduce on the second scale the arrangement of weights on pegs that had been observed on the first.

An advantage of this approach was that it allowed independent assessment of encoding on the weight and distance dimensions. A child could place the correct number of weights on each side of the fulcrum, could place the weights the correct distance from the fulcrum, could do both, or could do neither. If the encoding explanation was correct, it would be expected that the 8-year-olds, who had bene-fited from the conflict problems, would be shown to encode both weight and distance dimensions, whereas 5-year-olds, who had not benefited, would be shown to encode weight but not distance.

In Experiment 3A of Siegler (1976), the encoding task was presented to 5- and 8-year-olds. The children were shown balance scale problems for 10 sec apiece; then the initial arrangement was hidden and the children were asked to "make the same problem" by placing weights on the pegs of a second, identical, balance scale. After the encoding task, children were presented with the usual predictions test to assess their rule for judging which side of the balance scale would go down. The pattern of results was entirely consistent with the encoding hypothesis. Five-year-olds were much more accurate in encoding weight than distance, whereas 8-year-olds were similarly accurate on the two dimensions. These differing patterns of encoding contrasted with the very similar predictions performance of the older and younger children; both groups consistently used Rule I.

Next, children were provided with encoding instruction. They were first told to count the disks on the one side of the fulcrum, then to count the number of pegs separating those disks from the fulcrum, then to rehearse the result (e.g., "three weights on the fourth peg"), and then to do the same for the other side. After the instruction, the child was given the encoding test, followed by the predictions posttest.

This instructional procedure substantially changed 5-year-olds' encoding. They now encoded accurately both weight and distance. The improved encoding perfor-mance of the 5-year-olds was not accompanied by improvements in their predictions performance; the majority of both older and younger children continued to use Rule I. This finding set the stage for a direct test of the encoding hypothesis. If (a) the reason that 5-year-olds had not earlier benefited from the conflict problem feedback experience was that they did not encode distance, and if (b) they now encoded distance, then (c) they should now benefit from experience with the conflict prob-lems. The children who had been taught to encode were therefore brought back 2 or 3 days later and were given the feedback on conflict problems that we described above. Then they were given the standard predictions test to determine the feedback problem's effects.

Experience with conflict problems now improved the performance of 5-year-olds as well as 8-year-olds. Virtually all children adopted a rule more advanced than Rule I. The majority adopted Rule III. The older children showed somewhat more im-provement than the younger ones, but at the minimum, reducing the differences in encoding substantially reduced the differential responsiveness to experience pre-viously observed. Thus assessment of two aspects of children's existing knowledge – their performance rules on the predictions task and their encoding – proved useful in predicting and improving their ability to learn.

EXISTING KNOWLEDGE OF TIME

Another concept on which we have studied the interaction between children's exist-ing knowledge and their ability to learn is the concept of time. Our first experiment in the area (Siegler & Richards, 1979) was intended to assess existing knowledge of

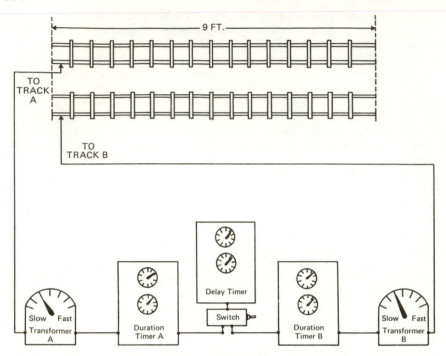

Figure 14.6.   Schematic diagram of train apparatus on time, speed, and distance tasks. (From "Three Aspects of Cognitive Development" by R. S. Siegler, *Cognitive Psychology*, 1976, *8*, 481–520. Copyright © 1976 by Academic Press. Reprinted by permission.)

time. The task was quite similar to Piaget's (1969) cars problem. Children were shown two parallel tracks for an electric train (see Figure 14.6), each with a locomotive on it. The two locomotives could start at the same or at different points, could stop at the same or at different points, and could travel the same or different distances. They could start at the same or at different times, could stop at the same or at different times, and could travel the same or different total times. Finally, they could travel at the same or at different speeds.

On the basis of Piaget's (1969) descriptions, we expected children to use one of three rules on this task (see Figure 14.7). Rule I children would base their judgments on where the cars stop; whichever car stopped farther ahead would be said to have traveled for the longer time. Rule II children would judge similarly if the two trains stopped at different points but would choose the train that started farther back if the trains stopped at the same point. Rule III children would judge in terms of starting and stopping times; in other words, they would use the correct approach.

In order to test these hypothesized rules, we needed to formulate problem types that would yield discriminative patterns. The six problem types that were chosen are shown in Table 14.3. These yielded distinct patterns for the rules corresponding to each of the seven physical dimensions along which the trains' activity could vary: time of travel, distance traveled, speed, end point, end time, beginning point, and beginning time. A child responding consistently on the basis of any one of the seven

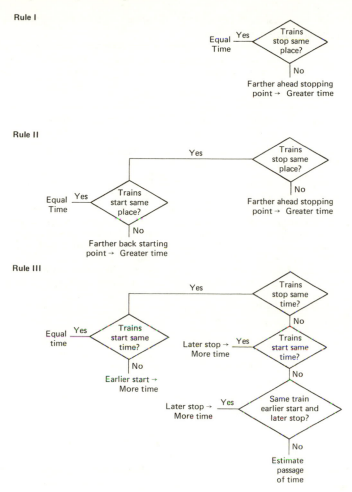

Figure 14.7. Rule models for time task. (From "When do children learn: the relationships between existing knowledge and the acquisition of new knowledge" by R. S. Siegler and D. Klahr, in R. Glaser, Ed., *Advances in Instructional Psychology*, Vol. 2. [Hillsdale, N.J.: Erlbaum, 1982]. Reprinted by permission.)

dimensions would answer differently on at least two of the six problem types from a child responding on the basis of any other dimension. Note that in order to limit the problems' difficulty, the two trains always either started simultaneously or stopped simultaneously. The procedure followed in the experiment was quite simple. Participants of four ages – 5-year-olds, 8-year-olds, 11-year-olds, and adults – were each presented with problems of the types shown in Table 14.3. No feedback was given at any time.

The data were essentially consistent with expectation. Five-year-olds most often chose the train that ended at the point farthest down the track, 8- and 11-year-olds tended to choose the train that traveled the greater distance, and adults chose the train that traveled the greater total time.

Table 14.3. *Specific response and percentage of correct answers predicted by each rule for each problem type on time concept*

	Problem type 1	Problem type 2	Problem type 3	Problem type 4	Problem type 5	Problem type 6
Train A.	0____6	0____9	0___9	0____6	0____6	0____5
Train B.	2____6	0____5	4½___9	0____5	0__4	2_5
Rule I	A longer 100	Equal 0	A longer 100	B longer 0	A longer 100	B longer 0
Rule II	A longer 100	A longer 100	A longer 100	B longer 0	A longer 100	B longer 0
Rule III	A longer 100	A longer 100	A longer 100	A longer 100	A longer 100	A longer 100

Note: Numbers in the column heads, under problem type, correspond to the number of seconds since the beginning of the trial. Lengths and relative positions of lines correspond to distances traveled and spatial positions. Thus in the example in problem type 1, one train (A) would start at the beginning of the trial and would travel for 6 sec, whereas the other (B) would start 2 sec after the trial began and would also stop at 6 sec. The two trains would start from parallel points, but Train A would finish farther up the track. The numbers in the table's cells represent the predicted percentage of correct answers.
Source: Siegler & Richards (1979).

ACQUIRING NEW KNOWLEDGE ABOUT TIME

The next question was whether we could use these assessments of children's existing knowledge about time to predict their ability to acquire new information about it. In particular, would our findings that young children relied on end-point cues and older children on distance cues allow us to predict the type of feedback problems that would advance their understanding?

First, we selected 5- and 11-year-olds with the desired initial knowledge states. Then we presented the children with feedback problems. These problems differed in whether they distinguished time from end point and/or distance. In a problem that discriminated between dimensions, answers based on each dimension would differ (e.g., the problem would discriminate between distance and time if the train that traveled the shorter distance also traveled the longer time, because reliance on the time cue would lead to choosing one train and reliance on the distance cue would lead to choosing the other). In a problem that did not discriminate between dimensions, judgments based on the two dimensions would be identical (e.g., distance would not be distinguished from time if the train that traveled the longer distance also traveled the longer time; reliance on either cue would lead to choosing the same train).

Thus, in Siegler and Richards (in preparation), some children received feedback problems that discriminated between time and both distance and end-point cues (e.g., Problem Type 4 in Table 14.3); some received problems that discriminated between time and distance but not end point (e.g., Problem Type 3 in Table 14.3); some received problems that discriminated between time and end point but not distance (e.g., Problem Type 2 in Table 14.3); and some received problems that did not discriminate between time and distance or end point (e.g., Problem Type 1 in Table 14.3).

As in the balance scale experiments, the results on the time concept demonstrated that the effectiveness of learning experiences is a joint function of children's initial knowledge and the particular dimension(s) among which the learning experience discriminates. Five-year-olds who were given problems that did not discriminate between end point and time continued to use the end-point rule; 14 of the 20 children who were given such feedback problems used the rule on the posttest. Five-year-olds who were given feedback problems that discriminated between end point and time shifted away from Rule I; only 3 of the 20 continued to use it. Whether or not the problems discriminated between time and distance had no effect on the 5-year-olds' performance. Among the 11-year-olds, the greatest effects of feedback were seen in the number of children adopting Rule III. Of those who saw distance distinguished from time, 10 of 20 adopted this most advanced rule. Of those who did not see distance distinguished from time, only 4 of 20 shifted to it. Whether or not the problems distinguished end point from time had no effect on the 11-year-olds' performance. Thus, knowing the child's initial rule allowed us to predict which types of learning experiences would be effective and which types of learning experiences would not be.

Encoding and inference processes on the time concept. We were quite surprised to find that even among the 11-year-olds who were given distance-distinguishing feedback problems, only one-half learned the time rule. This result led us (Siegler & Richards, in preparation) to consider exactly how children might solve the task. Recall that the problems involved either both trains starting at the same time or both trains stopping at the same time, so that all items could be solved by reliance on two rules: (a) if two events start at the same time and one ends later than the other, then the event that ended later lasted for more time; and (b) if one event starts before another and they end at the same time, then the event that started first lasted for more time.

What would children need to do to use these rules? Our task analysis indicated that they could determine which train traveled for the longer time by (a) encoding which train started first; (b) encoding which train stopped last; and (c) drawing the appropriate inference based on the encoded information. This approach suggested that children's difficulty might lie either in not encoding the appropriate information or in not drawing the appropriate inference.

In order to examine these possibilities, we needed to develop means of assessing encoding and inference processes independent of children's judgments of time. To assess encoding, we presented children with problems in which the trains' activities were as previously described. Instead of invariably asking which train traveled for the longer time, however, we only asked this question on 9 of the 27 trials. On the other 18, we asked either which train started first (or whether they started at the same time) or which train stopped last (or whether they stopped at the same time). The order of questions was randomized so that children could not anticipate which type of information to focus upon; they would need to take in all three, just as they had needed to on the original task. It was found that children frequently erred on the encoding as well as on the total time questions. Error rates were 24% on beginning time, 16% on ending time, and 31% on total time questions.

We next attempted to assess children's understanding of the inference rules. The same children whose encoding had been tested were brought back the next day and were presented with two written questions: "If the red and blue trains started at the same time and the blue train stopped last, which one would have gone for the greater amount of time (or would they have gone for the same amount of time)?" "If the red train started first, and the red and blue trains stopped at the same time, which train would have gone the greater amount of time (or would they have gone for the same amount of time)?" This procedure eliminated all encoding problems, because the questions as written included the desired encodings.

Such abstract inference questions proved more difficult to answer than might have been anticipated. The 11-year-olds erred on 25% of the inference items, suggesting that lack of knowledge of the correct inference rules as well as inadequate encoding may have contributed to children's difficulty in solving the time problems. We further probed these possible sources of difficulty by examining the effects of teaching children more sophisticated encoding and inference skills. Our experiment utilized a 2 (Encoding Instruction: Present or Absent) × 2 (Inference Instruction: Present or Absent) factorial design. Encoding instruction involved telling the 11-year-old subjects to identify aloud at the beginning of each trial the train that started first (or to say that the trains started at the same time) and to identify aloud at the end of each trial the train that stopped last (or to say that they stopped at the same time). Inference training involved telling children the solutions to the abstract inference problems previously used to test knowledge of the inference rules. After the manipulation(s), children in each group were presented with the items testing encoding of beginning time, encoding of ending time, and judgments of total time.

The results of this experiment provided additional evidence that encoding and inference processes constitute important sources of difficulty in solving these problems. The encoding manipulation by itself improved children's encoding of both beginning and ending time relationships but did not improve their performance on the total time problems. Inference training by itself had little effect on encoding but moderately aided performance on the total time problems. Encoding and inference training together greatly improved children's encoding and their performance on the total time problems. In this last condition the overall error rates were below 5% on total time, beginning time, and ending time problems. Among the 16 children, 15 met the criterion for using the time rule.

Like the balance scale results, these findings on the time concept indicate that instruction in encoding, together with other types of instructions, can aid children's learning. Superficially, the balance scale and time findings differ in the type of instruction that was found to be useful in combination with encoding; however, this difference may mask a deeper similarity. Inference training involved directly teaching children an algorithm for solving the time task; feedback training consisted of problems that allowed induction of such an algorithm for the balance scale. The overarching principle may be that one effective way to promote intelligent behavior is to call attention to the important dimensions of problems and then either explicitly or implicitly to indicate the algorithm by which the dimensions are to be combined. At this very general level, the present conclusion resembles past analyses of such classic psychological tasks as discrimination learning (e.g., Zeaman & House, 1963) and concept learning (e.g., Haygood & Bourne, 1965). The present approach goes beyond these previous ones, however, in using assessments of existing knowledge to predict the usefulness of alternative instructional approaches. This research allows us to add two final conclusions to our list.

CONCLUSIONS

18. There is a strong relationship between children's initial knowledge and the lessons that they induce from learning experiences. If the learning experience does

Table 14.4. *Conclusions about the development of intelligence*

1. Reliable quantitative measurements of children's general intelligence can be obtained from at least age 4 or 5 years onward.
2. For children of these ages, measures of general intelligence possess considerable stability over a period of several years. The stability increases with the children's ages and decreases with the length of the interval between the tests.
3. These quantitative measurements of intelligence quite accurately predict children's future performance in school. Again, predictive accuracy increases with the children's ages and decreases with the length of the interval between the initial test and the eventual outcome measure.
4. Both parental personality and demographic variables predict the intelligence of older children, though the same cannot be said for children below 4 years of age.
5. The factor structure of intelligence, as obtained from IQ tests, is quite stable from 4 or 5 years onward, with the first two factors corresponding to verbal and performance components of the tests. Much greater changes in factor structure are seen in the first few years of life. Perceptual, motor, and recognitory skills occupy prominent places in early assessments of intelligence but much lesser roles later on.
6. On many concepts, children progress through a sequence of qualitatively discrete, partially correct knowledge states prior to full understanding.
7. The sequence of partial understandings occurs in an invariant order. Given that two rules appear at some time in development, children progress toward the rule that more often predicts the correct answer in the environments that they encounter.
8. It is possible to teach conceptual understanding at considerably younger ages than those at which the concepts are usually mastered. However, there are also developmental differences in the benefits that children derive from the instruction.
9. Tasks that can be analyzed as being formally similar are often mastered at very different ages. Relative to the Piagetian norms, some tasks are mastered earlier than they should be, whereas others are mastered later. In addition, a wide range of tasks corresponding to a given concept can be devised, and the ages at which these tasks are mastered varies greatly.
10. At present there is little evidence for developmental changes in the capacity of short-term memory that cannot also be explained in terms of changes in strategies or the knowledge base. This statement means not that there are no changes in basic capacities but just that it is exceptionally difficult to provide unambiguous evidence of their existence.
11. There is a large increase between ages 5 and 10 years in the use of general mnemonic strategies, rehearsal, elaboration, and organization among them. The quality of children's implementation of the strategies also improves during this period. Use of such strategies can be taught to children younger than would ordinarily use them, but frequently the children revert to their original approaches when tested later in time or with different material.
12. Children possess considerable knowledge of their own memory limitations and of procedures that can be used to overcome the limitations. As yet, however, no simple links between this knowledge and memorial performance have been demonstrated.
13. Children's knowledge of specific content undergoes enormous development. This growth may account for changes in measures of basic capacities, strategies, and metamemory, rather than the other way around, as has traditionally been believed. Under some circumstances, differences in content knowledge can overwhelm all other age-related differences in memory: more knowledgeable children can remember more than less knowledgeable adults.
14. Children's use of logical reasoning skills is influenced by a variety of factors other than understanding of the logic itself: memorial skills, linguistic understanding, and ability to select the appropriate representation for the problem, among them.
15. Developmental differences in problem solving may at times be due less to the particular component operations that are performed than to the resources that are allocated to each component that is performed. Comprehensive encoding may be especially important for efficient problem solving.

(*continued*)

Table 14.4. (*cont.*)

16. Concepts that to adults seem to constitute single entities may to children represent many separate concepts. For example, the notion of number conservation may be differentiated by young children according to the particular objects involved, the number of objects, the type of linear transformation, and the type of quantitative operator.
17. Understanding of higher-order principles may guide even very young children's performance in areas with which they have much experience, such as counting.
18. There is a strong relationship between children's initial knowledge and the lessons that they induce from learning experiences. If the learning experience does not discriminate between their existing rule and the correct solution, they continue to use their existing rule. If the learning experience does indicate that their existing rule is incorrect, they will most often move toward the next higher rule in the typical developmental sequence if this rule is consistent with the learning experience.
19. A younger and an older child with the same initial rule for performing a task may derive quite different lessons from the identical learning experience. One reason for this variation can be differential encoding; more comprehensive encoding is associated with greater ability to learn.

not discriminate between their existing rule and the correct solution, they continue to use their existing rule. If the learning experience does indicate that their existing rule is incorrect, they will most often move toward the next higher rule in the typical developmental sequence if this rule is consistent with the learning experience.

19. A younger and an older child with the same initial rule for performing a task may derive quite different lessons from the identical learning experience. One reason for this different learning may be differential encoding; more comprehensive encoding is associated with greater ability to learn.

We have now presented 19 conclusions about intellectual development (see Table 14.4). Obviously, our list is to some degree arbitrary; more, fewer, or different conclusions could have been included. Notwithstanding, we believe that all 19 conclusions are valid and that all represent important characteristics of intellectual growth. We are also convinced that no single approach to studying the development of intelligence could have produced all of them. Thus the existence of several alternative approaches to studying intellectual development seems justified.

14.5.   SOME LARGE, UNRESOLVED ISSUES

What continuities exist between infant and childhood intelligence? How much consistency is there in children's reasoning across different tasks? In what ways are more intelligent younger children similar to less intelligent older ones, and in what ways are they different? Does the nature of intelligence change in the course of development? At present, we are not very close to answering any of these questions. On the logic that the best predictor of future behavior is past behavior, we might conclude that we probably will not come much closer to answering them in the next 5 or 10 years, either. An alternative position, however, is that some of the conceptual and methodological advances that we have reviewed here make substantial progress likely. We will argue the optimistic case.

To date, little evidence has been reported to suggest the continuity of early and later intelligence. Perhaps there is little continuity to be found, or perhaps we simply have not developed appropriate ways of measuring the continuity that does exist. If the latter possibility obtains, the recent trend toward identifying young children's intellectual competencies may prove to be an important advance. This recent trend has taken two distinct forms. Some researchers have devised versions of complex cognitive tasks on which young children can succeed; the concepts and cognitive skills involved include conservation (Bryant, 1974), seriation (Greenfield, Nelson, & Salzman, 1972), use of mnemonic strategies (Wellman, Ritter, & Flavell, 1975), and counting (Gelman & Gallistel, 1978). Studies of this type might lead future researchers to ask (for example) whether the 2- and 3-year-olds who are the first to master Gelman and Gallistel's counting principles are also the first later to master the types of counting-based arithmetic strategies described by Groen and Resnick (1977).

The other form of the approach is to devise tasks that young children may not be able to solve but on which they can display partial knowledge of complex concepts. Examples of this strategy include studies applying the information integration approach to such concepts as conservation, velocity, area, and equity (Anderson, 1980; Anderson & Butzin, 1978; Anderson & Cuneo, 1978; Wilkening, 1979); studies applying the rule-assessment approach to such concepts as proportionality, conservation, velocity, time, and distance (Siegler, 1976, 1978, 1981; Siegler & Richards, 1979); and studies applying the componential approach to such concepts as analogical reasoning, transitive inference, and linear syllogisms (Sternberg, 1979, 1980; Sternberg & Rifkin, 1979). Within this approach, continuities in intellectual development could be examined by determining whether those children who are first to gain early forms of understanding of a concept are also the first to gain more advanced forms of understanding later. For example, are the children who at early ages first adopt the additive rule on Wilkening's (1979) area estimation task the same ones who later first adopt the (correct) multiplicative rule? Thus analyses that stress the cognitive skills that young children do possess may reveal considerably more continuity in intellectual development than has been evident.

Research on the second issue, the degree of similarity in reasoning across tasks, has to date yielded a paradoxical picture. On the one hand, virtually every assessment of intellectual skills, starting with Binet's intelligence tests, has demonstrated substantial positive correlations among measures of reasoning. On the other, attempts to specify the basis of the correlations have met with very limited success. In particular, the types of consistent reasoning patterns that seemed to be promised by Piaget's theory have not emerged.

The task-analytic approaches that we have described may prove useful in attacking this problem. To date, these approaches have most often been applied to analyzing particular tasks. Still, recent efforts to analyze several tasks within a common framework have yielded encouraging results. Keating and Bobbitt (1978) analyzed children's performance on four widely used information-processing tasks in terms of shared components; they found that the same processing variables predicted performance on all of them. Sternberg (1979) extended the analysis of analogical reasoning that we have described to performance on linear syllogism and metaphoric understanding tasks and reported similarly encouraging findings. Siegler (1981) applied his analysis of the balance scale task to six proportionality and conservation problems and reported substantial intertask consistency in young children's approaches, though less in those of older children. Thus, analyzing individual tasks into components and searching for similarities across the analyses may prove useful in suggesting where to look for intertask consistency.

Improved methods for studying the relationship between existing knowledge and learning may make possible progress on the third issue, the relationship between more intelligent younger children's and less intelligent older ones' thinking. This issue has been of interest since the early days of psychometrics. Binet proposed that young children were intelligent to the degree that their performance approximated that of older peers. His hypothesis was embodied in the long-time Stanford–Binet equation for calculating intelligence quotients ($IQ = MA/CA$).

Binet's hypothesis has been tested to some extent in comparisons of mentally retarded and normal children of the same mental ages; to date, more similarities than differences have appeared. Disparities may be due, however, to the fact that most studies focused on the children's spontaneous performance rather than on their ability to learn. It seems at least plausible that the major difference between more and less intelligent children lies in the rapidity and completeness with which they acquire new information. Improvements in our ability to assess children's existing knowledge may prove useful in testing this notion. If we can demonstrate that children of differing intelligence are initially similar in their knowledge about a particular topic, we can then test whether they are similar or different in their ability to learn about it. If learning differs, we can search for the source of the differential learning ability. This research strategy has already proved useful in comparing the acquisition processes of children of different ages (Siegler, 1976, 1978); it may prove similarly useful in comparing those of children of differing intelligence.

The final question is the one with which we began this chapter: Is intelligence the same or a different quality at different ages? In addressing this question, we might first ask what considerations would lead an observer to conclude that intelligence might be different in different developmental periods. The standard that is most often cited is "qualitative change" in reasoning. For example, Piaget argued that concrete and formal operational intelligence are separated by a qualitative change in the underlying logical structures (cf. Flavell, 1971b, pp. 423–425). Unfortunately, the term *qualitative* has proven exceptionally elusive of definition; no one has devised a clear way of deciding whether or not a change is qualitative.

Regardless of whether we define age-related changes as qualitative, however, our impression of what is changing most rapidly seems to be a major component in our judgments of what constitutes intelligence at different ages. Stage theorists such as Piaget, Kohlberg, and Bruner all named their stages for the child's most recent achievement, the type of reasoning that they believed constitutes the largest departure from past modes. A similar tendency is apparent among laymen. When the Carnegie-Mellon undergraduates whose characterizations of intelligence at different ages we described earlier, were asked 3 months later what qualities of intelligence changed most at those ages, their answers were very similar. For example, when they were asked to name the largest change in cognitive functioning that occurred at any age, the majority choice was the acquisition of language at about age 2. Earlier, when the students had been asked to characterize intelligence at the four ages, this age–trait pairing also was the most often cited (87% of the students cited language as an important part of intelligence at around age 2). Thus there seems to be a close link between impressions of what is changing most rapidly at particular ages and characterizations of intelligence at those ages.

Given the importance of impressions of change, we might wish to know just how accurate our impressions are. The type of dramatic, clear-cut changes that Piaget's stage theory envisioned do not seem consistent with the data reviewed in this chapter. Some forms of conceptual understanding are manifested much earlier than they should be, and others are not manifested until much later. On the other hand, the empirical research is consistent with the hypothesis that especially great progress is made in particular domains at particular times. Perceptual and motor growth seems especially striking in the first few years of life; slithering, crawling, walking, grasping, enunciating, localizing sounds, and discriminating among patterns all develop substantially between birth and age 2. Language seems to grow especially rapidly between ages 2 and 5; vocabulary, for example, increases 100-fold between 18 months and 5 years. A variety of memorial strategies, including rehearsal, elaboration, and reorganization, seem first to be generally utilized between ages 5 and 8 or 9. Metamnemonic development also seems to be particularly great in this last age period.

It is entirely possible that our impression of especially rapid growth in these domains at these ages is primarily a function of the particular perceptual, motor, linguistic, and mnemonic tasks that we have chosen to study. Alternatively, the impressions may be valid for our culture but may have nothing to do with mental or chronological age per se; instead, they may simply reflect the demands that the culture places on children at various ages. These issues are probably irresolvable. Still, the difficulty of ever knowing just how valid our impressions are should not deter us from at least keeping the issue in mind. Binet started with an impressionistic analysis of intelligence 80 years ago; his work includes some of the most profound achievements of all psychological research. We can hope that continuing consideration of the nature of intelligence at different ages will at least lead to increasingly informed impressions of when and how large-scale intellectual development occurs. Such notions may constitute more than a trivial achievement.

REFERENCES

Anastasi, A. *Psychological testing* (4th ed.). New York: Macmillan, 1976.

Anderson, J. E. The prediction of terminal intelligence from infant and preschool tests. *Thirty-Ninth Yearbook of the National Society for the Study of Education*, 1940, Part 1, 385–403.

Anderson, J. R. *Language, memory and thought*. Hillsdale, N.J.: Erlbaum, 1976.

Anderson, J. R. Arguments concerning representations for mental imagery. *Psychological Review*, 1978, *85*, 249–277.

Anderson, J. R., Kline, P. J., & Beasley, Jr., C. M. A general learning theory and its application to schema abstraction. In G. Bower (Ed.), *The psychology of learning and motivation* (Vol. 13). New York: Academic Press, 1979.

Anderson, N. H. *Information integration theory: A case history in experimental science*. New York: Academic Press, 1980.

Anderson, N. H., & Butzin, C. A. Integration theory applied to children's judgments of equity. *Developmental Psychology*, 1978, *14*, 593–606.

Anderson, N. H., & Cuneo, D. O. The height + width rule in children's judgments of quantity. *Journal of Experimental Psychology: General*, 1978, *107*, 335–378.

Anzai, Y., & Simon, H. A. The theory of learning by doing. *Psychological Review*, 1979, *86*, 124–140.

Appel, K. J. *Three studies in object conceptualization: Piaget's sensorimotor stages four and five*. Unpublished doctoral dissertation, University of Houston, 1971.

Bach, M. J., & Underwood, B. J. Developmental changes in memory attributes. *Journal of Educational Psychology*, 1970, *61*, 292–296.

Baron, J. Intelligence and general strategies. In G. Underwood (Ed.), *Strategies in information processing*. New York: Academic Press, 1978.

Bayley, N. Development of Mental Abilities. In P. H. Mussen (Ed.), *Carmichael's manual of child psychology* (Vol. 1, 3rd ed.). New York: Wiley, 1970.

Bayley, N., & Schaefer, E. S. Correlations of material and child behaviors with the development of mental abilities: Data from the Berkeley Growth Study. *Monographs of the Society for Research in Child Development,* 1964, (6, Serial No. 97).

Beilin, H. Learning and operational convergence in logical thought development. *Journal of Experimental Child Psychology,* 1965, 2, 317–339.

Beilin, H. Inducing conservation through training. In G. Steiner (Ed.), *Psychology of the 20th century,* Vol. 7: *Piaget and Beyond.* Zurich, Switzerland: Kindler, 1977.

Belmont, J. M., & Butterfield, E. C. Learning strategies as determinants of memory deficiencies. *Cognitive Psychology,* 1971, 2, 411–420. (a)

Binet, A. *Les idees modernes sur les enfants.* Paris: Flammarion, 1911.

Bloom, L., Rocissano, L., & Hood, L. Adult–child discourse: Developmental interaction between information processing and linguistic knowledge. *Cognitive Psychology,* 1976, 8, 521–552.

Bond, E. A. *Tenth grade abilities and achievements.* Contributions to Education No. 813 New York: Teachers College, 1940.

Bower, T. G. R., & Wishart, J. G. The effects of motor skill on object permanence. *Cognition,* 1972, 1, 165–172.

Brainerd, C. J. Order of acquisition of transitivity, conservation, and class inclusion of length and weight. *Developmental Psychology,* 1973, 8, 105–116.

Brainerd, C. J. The stage question in cognitive-developmental theory. *Behavioral and Brain Sciences,* 1978, 1, 173–181.

Brainerd, C. J., & Allen, T. W. Experimental induction of the conservation of "first order" quantitative invariants. *Psychological Bulletin,* 1971, 75, 128–144.

Bransford, J. D., & McCarrell, N. S. A sketch of a cognitive approach to comprehension: Some thoughts about what it means to comprehend. In W. B. Weimer & D. S. Palermo (Eds.), *Cognition and symbolic processes.* Hillsdale, N.J.: Erlbaum, 1974.

Broman, S. H., Nichols, P. L., & Kennedy, W. A. *Preschool IQ: Prenatal and early developmental correlates.* Hillsdale, N.J.: Erlbaum, 1975.

Brown, A. L. The role of strategic behavior in retardate memory. In N. R. Ellis (Ed.), *International review of research in mental retardation* (Vol. 1). New York: Academic Press, 1974.

Brown, A. L. Knowing when, where, and how to remember: A problem of metacognition. In R. Glaser (Ed.), *Advances in instructional psychology.* Hillsdale, N.J.: Erlbaum, 1978.

Brown, A. L., & Scott, M. S. Recognition memory for pictures in preschool children. *Journal of Experimental Child Psychology,* 1971, 11, 401–412.

Brown, A. L., Smiley, S. S., Day, J. D., Townsend, M. A. R., & Lawton, S. C. Intrusion of a thematic idea in children's comprehension and retention of stories. *Child Development,* 1977, 48, 1454–1466.

Brown, E. E., & Bower, T. G. R. The problem of object permanence. *Cognition,* in press.

Bryant, P. E. The understanding of invariance by very young children. *Canadian Journal of Psychology,* 1972, 26, 78–96.

Bryant, P. E. *Perception and understanding in young children.* New York: Basic Books, 1974.

Bryant, P. E., & Trabasso, T. Transitive inferences and memory in young children. *Nature,* 1971, 232, 456–458.

Buckhalt, J. A., Mahoney, G. J., & Paris, S. G. Efficiency of self-generated elaborations by EMR and nonretarded children. *American Journal of Mental Deficiency,* 1976, 81, 93–96.

Burt, C. The development of reasoning in school children. *Journal of Experimental Pedagogy,* 1919, 5, 68–77.

Case, R. Structures and strictures: Some functional limitations on the course of cognitive growth. *Cognitive Psychology,* 1974, 6, 544–574.

Case, R. Intellectual development from birth to adulthood: A neo-Piagetian approach. In R. Siegler (Ed.), *Children's thinking: What develops?* Hillsdale, N.J.: Erlbaum, 1978. (a)

Case, R. Piaget and beyond: Toward a developmentally based theory and technology of instruction. In R. Glaser (Ed.), *Advances in instructional psychology.* Hillsdale, N.J.: Erlbaum, 1978. (b)

Chi, M. T. Age differences in memory span. *Journal of Experimental Child Psychology,* 1977, 23, 266–281.

Chi, M. T. Knowledge structures and memory development. In R. S. Siegler (Ed.), *Children's thinking: What develops?* Hillsdale, N.J.: Erlbaum, 1978.

Chi, M. T. Knowledge development and memory performance. In M. Friedman, J. P. Dos, and N. O'Connor (Eds.), *Intelligence and learning*. New York: Plenum Press, in press.

Christie, J. F., & Smothergill, D. W. Discrimination and conservation of length. *Psychonomic Science*, 1970, *21*, 336–337.

Colvin, S. What I conceive intelligence to be. *Journal of Educational Psychology*, 1921, *12*, 136–139.

Corman, H. H., & Escalona, S. K. Stages of sensorimotor development: A replication study. *Merrill-Palmer Quarterly*, 1969, *15*, 351–361.

Cowan, P. A. *Piaget with feeling*. New York: Holt, Rinehart & Winston, 1978.

Danner, F. W. Children's understanding of intersentence organization in the recall of short descriptive passages. *Journal of Educational Psychology*, 1976, *68*, 174–183.

Delin, P. S. Success in recall as a function of success in implementation of mnemonic instructions. *Psychonomic Science*, 1968, *12*, 153–154.

Dodwell, P. E. Children's understanding of number and related concepts. *Canadian Journal of Psychology*, 1960, *14*, 191–205.

Elkind, D. Children's discovery of the conservation of mass, weight, and volume: Piaget replications, Study 2. *Journal of Genetic Psychology*, 1961, *98*, 219–227. (a)

Elkind, D. The development of quantitative thinking: A systematic replication of Piaget's studies. *Journal of Genetic Psychology*, 1961, *98*, 37–46. (b)

Evans, W. F. *The Stage IV error in Piaget's theory of object concept development: An investigation of the role of activity*. Unpublished doctoral dissertation, University of Houston, 1973.

Evans, W. F., & Gratch, G. The Stage IV error in Piaget's theory of object concept development: Difficulties in object conceptualization or spatial localization? *Child Development*, 1972, *43*, 682–688.

Falmagne, R. J. *Reasoning: Representation and process*. Hillsdale, N.J.: Erlbaum, 1975.

Field, D. The importance of the verbal content in the training of Piagetian conservation skills. *Child Development*, 1977, *48*, 1583–1592.

Flavell, H. H. Structures, stages, and sequences in cognitive development. *Minnesota Symposium on Child Psychology* (Vol. 13). Hillsdale, N.J.: Erlbaum, 1982.

Flavell, J. H. Developmental studies of mediated memory. In H. W. Reese & L. P. Lipsitt (Eds.), *Advances in child development and behavior* (Vol. 5). New York: Academic Press, 1970

Flavell, J. H. First discussant's comments: What is memory development the development of? *Human Development*, 1971, *14*, 272–278. (a)

Flavell, J. H. Stage-related properties of cognitive development. *Cognitive Psychology*, 1971, 2, 421–453. (b)

Flavell, J. H., Friedrichs, A. G., & Hoyt, J. D. Developmental changes in memorization processes. *Cognitive Psychology*, 1970, *1*, 324–340.

Flavell, J. H., & Wellman, H. M. Metamemory. In R. V. Kail, Jr., & J. W. Hagen (Eds.), *Perspectives on the development of memory and cognition*. Hillsdale, N.J.: Erlbaum, 1977.

Flavell, J. H., & Wohlwill, J. F. Formal and functional aspects of cognitive development. In D. Elkind & J. H. Flavell (Eds.), *Studies in cognitive development: Essays in honor of Jean Piaget*. New York: Oxford University Press, 1969.

Frandsen, A. N., & Higginson, J. B. The Stanford–Binet and the Wechsler Intelligence Scale for Children. *Journal of Consulting Psychology*, 1951, *15*, 236–238.

Frank, H. S., & Rabinovitch, M. S. Auditory short-term memory: Developmental changes in rehearsal. *Child Development*, 1974, *45*, 397–407.

Garner, W. R. *The processing of information and structure*. Potomac, Md.: Erlbaum, 1974.

Gelman, R. Conservation acquisition: A problem of learning to attend to relevant attributes. *Journal of Experimental Child Psychology*, 1969, 7, 167–187.

Gelman, R. The nature and development of early number concepts. In H. W. Reese (Ed.), *Advances in child development and behavior* (Vol. 7). New York: Academic Press, 1972.

Gelman, R., & Gallistel, C. R. *The child's understanding of number*. Cambridge, Mass.: Harvard University Press, 1978.

Goldberg, S., Perlmutter, M., & Myers, N. Recall of related and unrelated lists by two-year-olds. *Journal of Experimental Child Psychology*, 1974, *18*, 1–8.

Goldschmid, M. L., & Bentler, P. M. The dimensions and measurement of conservation. *Child Development*, 1968, *39*, 787–802.

Goodnow, J. J. A test of milieu differences with some of Piaget's tasks. *Psychological Monographs,* 1962, 76(36, Whole No. 555).

Gratch, G. Review of Piagetian infancy research: Object concept development. In W. F. Overton & J. M. Gallagher (Eds.), *Knowledge and development* (Vol. 1). New York: Plenum Press, 1977.

Gratch, G., & Landers, W. F. Stage IV of Piaget's theory of infants' object concepts. *Child Development,* 1971, 42, 359–372.

Green, D. R., Ford, M. P., & Flamer, G. B. (Eds.). *Measurement and Piaget.* New York: McGraw-Hill, 1971.

Greenfield, P. M., Nelson, K., & Salzman, E. The development of rule-bound strategies for manipulating seriated cups: A parallel between action and grammar. *Cognitive Psychology,* 1972, 3, 291–310.

Greeno, J. G., Riley, M. S., & Gelman, R. Young children's counting and understanding of principles. Unpublished manuscript, University of Pittsburgh, 1979.

Groen, G. J., & Resnick, L. B. Can preschool children invent addition algorithms? *Journal of Educational Psychology,* 1977, 69, 645–652.

Hagen, J. W., Hargrave, S., & Ross, W. Prompting and rehearsal in short-term memory. *Child Development,* 1973, 44, 201–204.

Haggerty, M. A. Intelligence and its measurements: A symposium. *Journal of Educational Psychology,* 1921, 12, 212–216.

Hasher, L., & Clifton, D. A developmental study of attribute encoding in free recall. *Journal of Experimental Child Psychology,* 1974, 7, 332–346.

Haygood, R. C., & Bourne, Jr., L. E. Attribute- and rule-learning aspects of conceptual behavior. *Psychological Review,* 1965, 72, 175–195.

Henman, V. A. C. Intelligence and its measurement: A symposium. *Journal of Educational Psychology,* 1921, 12, 195–198.

Honzik, M. P. Developmental studies of parent–child resemblance in intelligence. *Child Development,* 1957, 28, 215–228.

Honzik, M. P., Macfarlane, J., & Allen, L. The stability of mental test performance between 2 and 18 years. *Journal of Experimental Education,* 1948, 4, 309–324.

Horowitz, A. B., & Horowitz, V. A. The effects of task-specific instructions on the encoding activities of children in recall and recognition tasks. Paper presented at the biennial meeting of the Society for Research in Child Development, Denver, April 1975.

Hoving, K. L., Spencer, T., Robb, K., & Schulte, D. Developmental changes in visual information processing. In P. A. Ornstein (Ed.), *Memory development in children.* Hillsdale, N.J.: Erlbaum, 1978.

Inhelder, B., & Piaget, J. *The growth of logical thinking from childhood to adolescence.* New York: Basic Books, 1958.

Inhelder, B., & Piaget, J. *The early growth of logic in the child.* London: Routledge & Kegan Paul, 1964.

Inhelder, B., Sinclair, H., & Bovet, M. *Learning and the development of cognition.* Cambridge, Mass.: Harvard University Press, 1974.

Jackson, S. The growth of logical thinking in normal and subnormal children. *British Journal of Educational Psychology,* 1965, 35, 255–258.

Jones, H. E. The environment and mental development. In L. Carmichael (Ed.), *Manual of child psychology* (2nd ed.). New York: Wiley, 1954.

Kahneman, D. *Attention and effort.* Englewood Cliffs, N.J.: Prentice-Hall, 1973.

Katz, H., & Beilin, H. A test of Bryant's claims concerning the young child's understanding of quantitative invariance. *Child Development,* 1976, 47, 877–880.

Kaufman, A. S. Factor analysis of the WISC-R at eleven age levels between 6½ and 16½ years. *Journal of Consulting and Clinical Psychology,* 1975, 43, 135–147.

Keating, D. P. Toward a multivariate developmental theory of intelligence. In D. Kuhn (Ed.), *Intellectual development beyond childhood.* San Francisco: Jossey-Bass, 1980.

Keating, D. P., & Bobbitt, B. L. Individual and developmental differences in cognitive processing components of ability. *Child Development,* 1978, 49, 155–167.

Keeney, T. J., Cannizzo, S. R., & Flavell, J. H. Spontaneous and induced verbal rehearsal in a recall task. *Child Development,* 1967, 38, 935–966.

Keller, H. R., & Hunter, M. L. Task differences on conservation and transitivity problems. *Journal of Experimental Child Psychology,* 1973, 15, 287–301.

Kingsley, R. C., & Hall, V. C. Training conservation through the use of learning sets. *Child Development*, 1967, *38*, 1111–1126.

Klahr, D., & Robinson, M. Formal assessment of problem-solving and planning processes in pre-school children. *Cognitive Psychology*, 1981, *13*, 113–148.

Klahr, D., & Wallace, J. G. The role of quantification operators in the development of conservation of quantity. *Cognitive Psychology*, 1973, *4*, 301–327.

Klahr, D., & Wallace, J. G. *Cognitive development: An information processing view.* Hillsdale, N.J.: Erlbaum, 1976.

Kreutzer, M. A., Leonard, C., & Flavell, J. H. An interview study of children's knowledge about memory. *Monographs of the Society for Research in Child Development*, 1975, 40(1, Serial No. 159).

Landers, W. F. The effect of differential experience on infants' performance in a Piagetian Stage IV object-concept task. *Developmental Psychology*, 1971, *5*, 48–54.

LeCompte, G. K., & Gratch, G. Violation of a rule as a method of diagnosing infants' level of object concept. *Child Development*, 1972, *43*, 385–396.

Lee, L. C. The concomitant development of cognitive and moral modes of thought: A test of selected deductions from Piaget's theory. *Genetic Psychology Monographs*, 1971, *85*, 93–146.

Liben, L. Evidence for developmental differences in spontaneous seriation and its implications for past research on long-term memory improvement. *Developmental Psychology*, 1975, *11*, 121–125.

Liben, L. Memory for a cognitive-development perspective: A theoretical and empirical review. In W. F. Overton & J. M. Gallagher (Eds.), *Knowledge and development*, Vol. 1: *Advances in research and theory*. New York: Plenum Press, 1977.

Liberty, C., & Ornstein, P. A. Age differences in organization and recall. The effects of training in categorization. *Journal of Experimental Child Psychology*, 1973, *15*, 169–186.

Lovell, K. A follow-up study of Inhelder and Piaget's "The growth of logical thinking." *British Journal of Psychology*, 1961, *52*, 143–153.

Manis, F. R., Keating, D. P., & Morrison, F. J. Developmental differences in the allocation of processing capacity. *Journal of Experimental Psychology*, in press.

Markman, E. M. Facilitation of part–whole comparisons by use of the collective noun "family." *Child Development*, 1973, *44*, 837–840.

Markman, E. M. Realizing that you don't understand: A preliminary investigation. *Child Development*, 1977, *48*, 986–992.

Markman, E. M. Realizing that you don't understand: Elementary school children's awareness of inconsistencies. *Child Development*, 1979, *50*, 643–655.

Markman, E. M., & Siebert, J. Classes and collections: Internal organization and resulting holistic properties. *Cognitive Psychology*, 1976, *8*, 561–577.

Martorano, S. C. A developmental analysis of performance on Piaget's formal operations tasks. *Developmental Psychology*, 1977, *13*, 666–672.

Masur, E. F., McIntyre, C. W., & Flavell, J. H. Developmental changes in appointment of a study time among items in a multitrial free recall task. *Journal of Experimental Child Psychology*, 1973, *15*, 237–246.

Maurer, D., Siegel, L. S., Lewis, Terri, L., Kristofferson, M. W., Barnes, R. A., & Levy, B. A. Long-term memory improvement? *Child Development*, 1979, *50*, 106–118.

McCall, R. B., Eichorn, D. J., & Hogarty, P. S. Transitions in early mental development. *Monographs of the Society for Research in Child Development*, 1977, *42* (Serial No. 171).

McCarthy, D. Language development in children. In L. Carmichael (Ed.), *Manual of child psychology*. New York: Wiley, 1954.

McNemar, Q. *The revision of the Stanford–Binet Scale.* Boston: Houghton Mifflin, 1942.

Mehler, J., & Bever, T. G. Cognitive capacity of very young children. *Science*, 1967, *158*, 141–142.

Michotte, A. *Causalité permanence et réalité phénoménales.* Louvain, Belgium: Publications Universitaires Belgium, 1962.

Miller, F. Effects of different amounts of stimulus familiarity on choice reaction time performance in children. *Journal of Experimental Child Psychology*, 1969, *8*, 106–117.

Miller, G. A. The magical number seven, plus or minus two: Some limits on our capacity for processing information. *Psychological Review*, 1956, *63*, 81–96.

Miller, S. A. Nonverbal assessment of conservation of number. *Child Development*, 1976, 47, 722–728.

Moely, B. E. Organizational factors in the development of memory. In R. V. Kail, Sr., & J. W. Hagen (Eds.), *Perspectives on the development of memory and cognition*. Hillsdale, N.J.: Erlbaum, 1977.

Moely, B. E., Olson, F. A., Halwes, T. G., & Flavell, J. H. Production deficiency in young children's clustered recall. *Developmental Psychology*, 1969, *1*, 26–34.

Moore, T. Language and intelligence: A longitudinal study of the first eight years, 1: Patterns of development in boys and girls. *Human Development*, 1967, *10*, 88–106.

Morrison, F. J., Holmes, D. L., & Haith, M. M. A developmental study of the effects of familiarity on short-term visual memory. *Journal of Experimental Child Psychology*, 1974, *18*, 412–425.

Moynahan, E. D. The development of knowledge concerning the effect of categorization upon free recall. *Child Development*, 1973, *44*, 238–246.

Murray, F. B. Acquisition of conservation through social interaction. *Developmental Psychology*, 1972, 6, 1–6.

Murray, J. P., & Youniss, J. Achievement of inferential transitivity and its relation to serial ordering. *Child Development*, 1968, *39*, 1259–1268.

Mussen, P., Dean, S., & Rosenberg, M. Some further evidence on the validity of the WISC. *Journal of Consulting Psychology*, 1952, *16*, 410–412.

Myers, N. A., & Perlmutter, M. Memory in the years from two to five. In P. A. Ornstein (Ed.), *Memory development in children*. Hillsdale, N.J.: Erlbaum, 1978, 191–218.

Naus, M. J., Ornstein, P. A., & Aivano, S. Developmental changes in memory: The effects of processing time and rehearsal instructions. *Journal of Experimental Child Psychology*, 1977, 23, 237–251. (a)

Neimark, E. D. Intellectual development in adolescence. In F. D. Horowitz (Ed.), *Review of child development research* (Vol. 4). Chicago: University of Chicago Press, 1975.

Neisser, V. The concept of intelligence. *Intelligence*, 1979, 3, 217–227.

Nelson, K. Structure and strategy in learning to talk. *Monographs of the Society for Research in Child Development*, 1973, 38(Serial No. 149).

Ornstein, P. A. Introduction: The study of children's memory. In P. A. Ornstein (Ed.), *Memory development in children*. Hillsdale, N.J.: Erlbaum, 1978.

Ornstein, P. A., Naus, M. J., & Liberty, C. Rehearsal and organizational processes in children's memory. *Child Development*, 1975, 26, 818–830.

Ornstein, P. A., Naus, M. J., & Stone, B. P. Rehearsal training and developmental differences in memory. *Developmental Psychology*, 1977, *13*, 15–24. (b)

Paris, S. G., & Lindauer, B. K. The role of inference in children's comprehension and memory for sentences. *Cognitive Psychology*, 1976, *8*, 217–227.

Pascual-Leone, J. A mathematical model for transition in Piaget's developmental stages. *Acta Psychologica*, 1970, *32*, 301–345.

Peluffo, N. Culture and cognitive problems. *International Journal of Psychology*, 1967, 2, 187–198.

Piaget, J. Une forme verbale de la comparaison chez l'enfant. *Archives de Psychologie*, 1921, *141–172*.

Piaget, J. *The child's concept of number*. New York: Norton, 1952.

Piaget, J. *The construction of reality in the child*. New York: Basic Books, 1954.

Piaget, J. The general problems of the psychobiological development of the child. In J. M. Tanner & B. Inhelder (Eds.), *Discussion on child development* (Vol. 4). London: Tavistock, 1960.

Piaget, J. [*The child's conception of time*] (A. J. Pomerans, trans.). New York: Ballantine, 1969.

Piaget, J. Piaget's theory. In P. H. Mussen (Ed.), *Carmichael's manual of child psychology* (Vol. 1, 3rd ed.). New York: Wiley, 1970.

Piaget, J. *Science of education and the psychology of the child*. New York: Viking, 1972. (a)

Piaget, J. Intellectual evolution from adolescence to adulthood. *Human Development*, 1972, *15*, 1–12. (b)

Piaget, J., & Inhelder, B. *Développement des quantités chez l'enfant*. Neuchâtel, Switzerland: Delachaux et Niestlé, 1941.

Piaget, J., & Inhelder, B. *La genèse de l'idée de hazard chez l'enfant*. Paris: Presses Universitaires de France, 1951.

Piaget, J., & Inhelder, B. *Memory and intelligence.* New York: Basic Books, 1973.

Piaget, J., Inhelder, B., & Szeminska, A. *The child's concept of geometry.* New York: Basic Books, 1960.

Pinard, A., & Laurendeau, M. "Stage" in Piaget's cognitive developmental theory: Exegesis of a concept. In D. Elkind & J. H. Flavell (Eds.), *Studies in cognitive development.* New York: Oxford University Press, 1969.

Potts, G. R. Information processing strategies used in the encoding of linear orderings. *Journal of Verbal Learning and Verbal Behavior,* 1972, *11,* 727–740.

Reese, H. W. Verbal mediation as a function of age level. *Psychological Bulletin,* 1962, *59,* 502–509.

Reese, H. W. Imagery and associative memory. In Robert V. Kail, Jr., & John W. Hagen (Eds.), *Perspectives on the development of memory and cognition.* Hillsdale, N.J.: Erlbaum, 1977.

Resnick, L. B. Task analysis in instructional design: Some cases from mathematics. In D. Klahr (Ed.), *Cognition and instruction.* Hillsdale, N.J.: Erlbaum, 1976.

Riley, C. A., & Trabasso, T. Comparatives, logical structures, and encoding in a transitive inference task. *Journal of Experimental Child Psychology,* 1974, *17,* 187–203.

Rogoff, B., Newcombe, N., & Kagan, J. Planfulness and recognition memory. *Child Development,* 1974, *45,* 972–977.

Rosch, E. R. Linguistic relativity. In A. Silverstein (Ed.), *Human communication: Theoretical perspectives.* New York: Halsted Press, 1974.

Rosch, E. R. Human categorization. In N. Warren (Ed.), *Studies in the internal structure of categories.* London: Academic Press, 1978.

Rosch, E. R., Mervis, C. B., Gray, W., Johnson, D. M., & Boyes-Braem, P. Basic objects in natural categories. *Cognitive Psychology,* 1976, *8,* 382–439.

Rosenthal, T. A., & Zimmerman, B. J. Modelling by exemplification and instruction in training conservation. *Developmental Psychology,* 1972, *6,* 392–401.

Rosner, S. The effects of rehearsal and chunking instructions on children's multitrial free recall. *Journal of Experimental Child Psychology,* 1971, *11,* 93–105.

Rothenberg, B. B., & Orost, J. H. Training of conservation of number in young children. *Child Development,* 1969, *40,* 707–726.

Saal, D. *A study of the development of object concept in infancy by varying the degree of discrepancy between the disappearing and reappearing object.* Unpublished doctoral dissertation, University of Houston, 1974.

Sacerdoti, E. D. *A structure for plans and behavior.* New York: Elsevier, 1977.

Salatas, H., & Flavell, J. H. Behavioral and metamnemonic indicators of strategic behaviors under remember instructions in first grade. *Child Development,* 1976, *47,* 81–89.

Scardamalia, M. Information processing capacity and the problem of horizontal décalage: A demonstration using combinatorial reasoning tasks. *Child Development,* 1977, *48,* 28–37.

Schaefer, F. S., & Bayley, N. Maternal behavior, child behavior, and their intercorrelations from infancy through adolescence. *Monographs of the Society for Research in Child Development,* 1963, *28*(3, Serial No. 97).

Shepard, R. N., & Teeghtsoonian, M. Retention of information under conditions approaching a steady state. *Journal of Experimental Psychology,* 1961, *62,* 55–59.

Siegler, R. S. Three aspects of cognitive development. *Cognitive Psychology,* 1976, *8,* 481–520.

Siegler, R. S. The origins of scientific reasoning. In R. S. Siegler (Ed.), *Children's thinking: What develops?* Hillsdale, N.J.: Erlbaum, 1978.

Siegler, R. S. Developmental sequences within and between concepts. *Monographs of the Society for Research in Child Development,* 1981, 46 (Serial No. 189).

Siegler, R. S., & Liebert, R. M. Learning of liquid quantity relationships as a function of rules and feedback, number of training problems, and age of subject. In *Proceedings of the 80th Annual Convention of the American Psychological Association,* 1972, 80, 117–118. (Summary) (b)

Siegler, R. S., & Liebert, R. M. Acquisition of formal scientific reasoning by 10- and 13-year-olds: Designing a factorial experiment. *Developmental Psychology,* 1975, *10,* 401–402.

Siegler, R. S., & Richards, D. D. Development of time, speed, and distance concepts. *Developmental Psychology,* 1979, *15,* 288–298.

Siegler, R. S., & Richards, D. D. College students' prototypes of children's intelligence. In *Processing of the 85th Conference of the American Psychological Association,* New York, 1980.

Siegler, R. S., & Richards, D. D. Using assessments of existing knowledge to predict learning. Article in preparation.

Siegler, R. S., & Vago, S. The development of a proportionality concept: Judging relative fullness. *Journal of Experimental Child Psychology*, 1978, 25, 371–395.

Smedslund, J. Development of a concrete transitivity of length in children. *Child Development*, 1963, 34, 389–405.

Smedslund, J. Concrete reasoning: A study of intellectual development. *Monographs of the Society for Research in Child Development*, 1964, 29(Serial No. 93).

Sontag, C. W., Baker, C. T., & Nelson, V. L. Mental growth and personality development: A longitudinal study. *Monographs of the Society for Research in Child Development*, 1958, 23(Serial No. 68).

Spearman, C. General intelligence objectively determined and measured. *American Journal of Psychology*, 1904, 15, 201–293.

Sternberg, R. J. *Intelligence, information processing, and analogical reasoning: The componential analysis of human abilities*. Hillsdale, N.J.: Erlbaum, 1977.

Sternberg, R. J. The development of human intelligence (Technical Report). New Haven: Yale University, 1979.

Sternberg, R. J. The development of linear syllogistic reasoning. *Journal of Experimental Child Psychology*, 1980, 29, 340–356.

Sternberg, R. J., & Rifkin, B. The development of analogical reasoning processes. *Journal of Experimental Child Psychology*, 1979, 27, 195–232.

Tanner, J. M. Criteria of the stages of mental development. In J. M. Tanner & B. Inhelder (Eds.), *Discussion on child development* (Vol. 1). London: Tavistock, 1956.

Tenney, Y. J. The child's conception of organization and recall. *Journal of Experimental Child Psychology*, 1975, 19, 100–114.

Terman, L. M., & Merrill, M. A. *Stanford–Binet Intelligence Scale*. Cambridge, Mass.: Riverside, 1960.

Townsend, J. T. Issues and models concerning the processing of a finite number of inputs. In H. B. Kantowitz (Ed.), *Human information processing: Tutorial in performance and cognition*. Hillsdale, N.J.: Erlbaum, 1974.

Trabasso, T. Representation, memory and reasoning: How do we make transitive inferences? In A. D. Pick (Ed.), *Minnesota Symposia on Child Psychology* (Vol. 9). Minneapolis: University of Minnesota Press, 1975.

Trabasso, T., & Foellinger, D. B. Information processing capacity in children: A test of Pascual-Leone's model. *Journal of Experimental Child Psychology*, 1978, 26, 1–17.

Trabasso, T., Riley, C. A., & Wilson, E. G. The representation of linear order and spatial strategies in reasoning: A developmental study. In R. J. Falmagne (Ed.), *Reasoning: Representation and process*. Hillsdale, N.J.: Erlbaum, 1975.

Turnure, J., Buium, N., & Thurlow, M. The effectiveness of interrogatives for prompting verbal elaboration productivity in young children. *Child Development*, 1976, 47, 851–855.

Turiel, E. An experimental test of the sequentiality of developmental stages in the child's moral judgment. *Journal of Personality and Social Psychology*, 1966, 3, 611–618.

Uzgiris, I. C. Situational generality of conservation. *Child Development*, 1964, 35, 831–841.

Uzgiris, I. C., & Hunt, J. M. An instrument for assessing infant psychological development. Unpublished manuscript, University of Illinois, 1966.

Voss, J. F. Cognition and instruction: Toward a cognitive theory of learning. In A. M. Lesgold, J. W. Pellegrino, S. D. Fokkema, & R. Glaser (Eds.), *Cognitive psychology and instruction*. New York: Plenum Press, 1978.

Wagner, D. A. Memories of Morocco: The influence of age, schooling, and environment on memory. *Cognitive Psychology*, 1978, 10, 1–28.

Wechsler, D. *Wechsler Intelligence Scale for Children*. New York: Psychological Corporation, 1967.

Wechsler, D. *Manual: Wechsler Intelligence Scale for Children* (Rev ed.). New York: Psychological Corporation, 1974.

Wellman, H. M., Drozdal, J. G., Jr., Flavell, J. H., Salatas, H., & Ritter, K. Metamemory development and its possible role in the selection of behavior. In G. A. Hale (Chair), Development of selective processes in cognition. Symposium presented at the Society for Research in Child Development, Denver, 1975.

Wellman, H. M., Ritter, K., & Flavell, J. H. Deliberate memory behavior in the delayed reactions of very young children. *Developmental Psychology*, 1975, 11, 780–787.

Wickens, C. D. Temporal limits of human information processing: A developmental study. *Psychological Bulletin,* 1974, *81,* 739–755.

Wilkening, F. Combining of stimulus dimensions in children's and adults' judgments of area: An information integration analysis. *Developmental Psychology,* 1979, *15,* 25–33.

Williams, K. G., & Goulet, L. R. The effects of cueing and constraint instructions on children's free recall performance. *Journal of Experimental Child Psychology,* 1975, *19,* 464–475.

Wittgenstein, L. *Philosophical investigations.* Oxford: Basil Blackwell, 1953.

Woodrow, H. What I conceive intelligence to be. *Journal of Educational Psychology,* 1921, *12,* 205–210.

Worden, P. E. Effects of sorting on subsequent recall of unrelated items: A developmental study. *Child Development,* 1975, *46,* 687–695.

Yussen, S. R., & Levy, Jr., V. M. Developmental changes in predicting one's own span of short-term memory. *Journal of Experimental Psychology,* 1975, *19,* 502–508.

Zeaman, D., & House, B. J. The role of attention in retardate discrimination learning. In N. R. Ellis (Ed.), *Handbook of mental deficiency: Psychological theory and research.* New York: McGraw-Hill, 1963.

Zimmerman, B. J., & Rosenthal, T. L. Conserving and retaining equalities and inequalities through observation and correction. *Developmental Psychology,* 1974, *10,* 260–268.

PART V

Metatheory of intelligence

ROBERT J. STERNBERG AND JANET S. POWELL

A major goal of science is reduction of complex phenomena to manageable and understandable terms. Scientists attempt to isolate a piece of a phenomenon and to specify all the characteristics of that piece and the factors affecting it. Later, the disparate pieces are reconnected in the hope that one will then understand the whole phenomenon. A tension arises, however, between the desire to break the phenomenon into small enough pieces so that it can be understood and the need to keep track of how the pieces relate to each other and how they relate to the whole phenomenon.

Intelligence research has, in general, concentrated on breaking "intelligence" into specifiable pieces; the result has been a rich diversity of theories of different aspects of intelligent performance. Theorists of intelligence, however, have not often enough stepped back from their individual theories to ascertain the relationships between various theories of intelligence and between each specific theory and intelligence as a whole.

Our goal in this chapter is to present a conceptual overview of theories of intelligence. We attempt to delineate (a) the aspects of intelligence that various theorists have succeeded in isolating, (b) the relations of these aspects of intelligence to each other, and (c) the relations of these aspects of intelligence to the construct as a whole. The underlying theme will be that theories and classes of theories differ largely in their restrictions. Our overview is divided into four main sections; each of the first three presents a single main thesis. First, we deal with some of the variation that exists in kinds of theories of intelligence, discussing in particular the problem of deciding on the type of data that should serve as the basis for the formulation of a theory of intelligence. Second, we describe the evolution of theories of intelligence and discuss the current state of theorizing about the nature of intelligence. Third, we discuss restrictions of scope on past theories of intelligence; we also suggest ways in which these theories are interrelated via the kinds of questions they successfully address. In the fourth and last section we summarize our main points and discuss the implications of our analysis for future theorizing about intelligence.

15.1.   FORMS OF THEORIES OF INTELLIGENCE

Theories of intelligence take two principal forms, explicit and implicit. We deal with each of these forms in turn.

EXPLICIT THEORIES OF INTELLIGENCE

Explicit theories of intelligence are based, or at least tested, on data collected from people performing tasks presumed to measure intelligent functioning. For example,

975

a battery of mental ability tests might be administered to a large group of people and the data from these tests analyzed in order to isolate the proposed sources of intelligent behavior in test performance. Although investigators proposing explicit theories might disagree as to the nature of these sources of intelligence – which might be proposed to be factors, components, schemata, or some other kind of psychological construct – they would agree that the data base from which the proposed constructs should be isolated should consist (directly or indirectly) of performance on tasks requiring intelligent functioning.

Internal validation of explicit theories. Internal validation involves determining how well a theory accounts for the data from the task domain to which a theory is addressed. For example, a differential theorist might address the question of what proportion of the individual-difference variance in a set of test scores is accounted for by a particular set of structural factors postulated in his or her theory; or an information-processing theorist might address the question of what proportion of the stimulus variance in a set of item means is accounted for by the particular set of process parameters postulated in his or her theory.

The theorist using internal validation to test a theory of intelligence usually defines the scope of intelligence in terms of that which is accounted for by the theory. The theorist may claim that the theory specifies the whole domain of behaviors to be labeled intelligent but is more likely to claim that the theory specifies an interesting subset of this domain (e.g., Anderson, 1976; Newell & Simon, 1972; R. J. Sternberg, 1981g). Although the theory determines the choice of tasks to be studied, in practice the theory has often been derived from prior analysis of the tasks whose selection it now specifies.

This approach to defining the scope of a theory of intelligence has the advantage of being theoretically based: One chooses tasks to study on the basis of a prior theory of what tasks matter and of what is involved in the performance of these tasks. (See Sternberg, Chapter 5, this volume, for further discussion of task selection.) Acceptance of the specified domain of tasks, however, depends upon acceptance of the theory. Although a successful demonstration of internal validity is certainly a necessary condition for acceptance of a theory of intelligence, it is not a sufficient condition; others may argue that whether or not the theory gives a good account of task performance, the tests or tasks under consideration form either an incomplete or incorrect basis for the formation of a theory of intelligence.

External validation of explicit theories. The theorist using external validation to test a theory of intelligence usually defines the scope of intelligence in terms of whatever correlates with external measures of intelligent functioning. The researcher thereby hopes to isolate critical aspects of intelligence – ones that are important in central measures or in many measures of intelligence. External validation involves determining the extent to which parameters (of whatever kind) of a theory account for data from a performance domain external to that encompassed by the theory but in which performance should be predictable from the parameters of the theory. For example, a differential theorist might correlate scores on factors such as "reasoning" and "verbal comprehension" with grades in school; or an information-processing theorist might correlate scores on process parameters such as "lexical access time" or "inference time" with scores on psychometric tests.

Reliance on external validation in the absence or near-absence of internal validation is probably what gave research on intelligence a reputation for being atheoretical. Items for some psychometric tests of intelligence have been chosen primarily on the basis of their correlations with each other or with external criteria (such as grades in school), without reference to an internally validated theory of intelligent performance. A better procedure is to supplement external validation with internal validation.

Internal plus external validation of explicit theories. The theorist using internal plus external validation to define the scope of a theory shows that parameters of a given theory not only account for performance on tasks in the domain encompassed by the theory, but that individual differences in these parameters are related to individual differences in other tasks that are indicative of intelligent functioning. Often, an attempt is made to choose "other" tasks that are more ecologically valid than those falling within the scope of the theory, even if this means that these other tasks involve aspects of performance other than intelligence.

This approach to defining the scope of a theory of intelligence has the advantage not only of being theoretically based but of demonstrating sensitivity to performance beyond the range of any single theory, which almost certainly will not include within its scope all tasks that might involve intelligent performance. A successful demonstration of external validity, like a successful demonstration of internal validity, would seem to be a necessary condition for an adequate theory of intelligence, in that probably no one would want to claim that intelligent behaviors are limited to those studied in the task domain under investigation. A demonstration of external validity, however, eventually encounters the same problem as a demonstration of internal validity – the need to accept some theoretically prespecified criterion of what intelligence is; and many people would argue that neither grades in school, performance on psychometric tests, nor any of the external criteria commonly used in investigations of intelligence are adequate standards against which to test the parameters of a theory. It is often not clear that the external criteria are any better than, or qualitatively different from, the internal ones (see, e.g., the studies of Hunt, Lunneborg, & Lewis, 1975, and R. J. Sternberg, 1977, where standard psychometric ability tests are used for external validation). In addition, in using external criteria as a basis for justifying the scope of the theory, one still runs the risk of eventual circularity – that is, that one will justify the theory on the basis of correlations with external criteria, only later to justify the choice of external criteria on the basis of the theory.

IMPLICIT THEORIES OF INTELLIGENCE

Implicit theories of intelligence are based, or at least tested, on people's conceptions of what intelligence is: Implicit theories need to be "discovered" rather than "invented" because they already exist, in some form, in people's heads. The goal in research on such theories is to find out the form and content of people's informal theories. Thus, one attempts to reconstruct already existing theories, rather than to construct new ones. The data of interest are people's communications (in whatever form) regarding their notions as to the nature of intelligence. For example, a survey of questions might be administered to a large group of people and the data from this survey analyzed in order to reconstruct people's belief systems about intelligence. Although investigators working with implicit theories of intelligence might disagree as to the structure and possibly even the content of people's beliefs, they would agree that the data base from which the proposed constructs should be isolated should consist of people's stated or implemented beliefs regarding intelligent functioning (Sternberg et al., 1981).

The theorist who uses implicit theories defines the scope of a theory of intelligence in terms of what people say intelligence is. Intelligence is viewed as a stipulative concept, one that achieves its meaning as a result of people positing it to mean a certain thing. A major proponent of this view, Neisser (1979), believes that intelligence does not exist except as a resemblance to a prototype, that is, as a degree of similarity between actual persons and some ideally intelligent person. Neisser notes that this view can be traced back at least to Thorndike (1924), who suggested that

for a first approximation, let intellect be defined as that quality of mind (or brain or behavior if one prefers) in respect to which Aristotle, Plato, Thucydides, and the like, differed most from Athenian idiots of their day, or in respect to which the lawyers, physicians, scientists, scholars, and editors of reputed greatest ability at constant age, say a dozen of each, differ most from idiots of that age in asylums. [P. 241]

Neisser believes that the task domain considered by standard intelligence tests, although too limited, does make sense as far as it goes, because these tests measure a person's resemblance to a prototypical intelligence test "smartie" who would get all the items right.

One question that arises in the implicit-theory approach is that of whose conceptions of intelligence should be used in determining the scope of theories of intelligence. The two most common answers are experts in the field of intelligence and laypersons in our culture, although some investigators have studied as well the conceptions of intelligence held by people in other cultures (e.g., Wober, 1974).

Implicit theories of experts.   The most famous study of experts' conceptions of the scope of intelligent behavior is that done by the editors of the *Journal of Educational Psychology* ("Intelligence and Its Measurement," 1921) 60 years ago. Fourteen experts gave their views on the nature of intelligence, with definitions such as the following:

1. the power of good responses from the point of view of truth or fact (E. L. Thorndike);
2. the ability to carry on abstract thinking (L. M. Terman);
3. having learned or ability to learn to adjust oneself to the environment (S. S. Colvin);
4. ability to adapt oneself adequately to relatively new situations in life (R. Pintner);
5. the capacity for knowledge and knowledge possessed (V. A. C. Henmon);
6. a biological mechanism by which the effects of a complexity of stimuli are brought together and given a somewhat unified effect in behavior (J. Peterson);
7. the capacity to inhibit an instinctive adjustment, the capacity to redefine the inhibited instinctive adjustment in the light of imaginally experienced trial and error, and the volitional capacity to realize the modified instinctive adjustment into overt behavior to the advantage of the individual as a social animal (L. L. Thurstone);
8. the capacity to acquire capacity (H. Woodrow);
9. the capacity to learn or to profit by experience (W. F. Dearborn).

There have been many, many definitions of intelligence since these were presented in the journal symposium, and an essay has even been written on the nature of definitions of intelligence (Miles, 1957). A problem with using these various definitions as a basis for specifying the scope of theories of intelligence is that it is not clear whether the scope one should set should be the disjunction of the various definitions, the conjunction of the various definitions, or some other function of them; nor is it clear how one would compute any of these functions, even if one could be decided upon. Certain themes do seem to run through subsets of the definitions, such as the capacity to learn from experience and adaptation to one's environment, but the perception of common themes is probably as much in the eye of the perceivers as in the minds of the experts. Clearly, one would like a nonarbitrary means of combining the perceptions of the various experts.

A contemporary version of this kind of study that does provide a means of combining the conceptions of various experts was conducted by Sternberg, Conway, Ketron, and Bernstein (1981). These investigators compiled a list of behaviors that were described as "intelligent," "academically intelligent," or "everyday intelligent" by laypeople filling out a brief open-ended questionnaire at a train station, a supermarket, or a college library. The complete list of behaviors was sent to "experts" in the field of intelligence (faculty members in psychology departments of major universities whose research interests were in the field of intelligence, broadly defined). These experts were asked to rate either how characteristic each behavior is of an ideally "intelligent," "academically intelligent," and "everyday intelligent" person, or how important each behavior is in defining their conception of an ideally "intelligent," "academically intelligent," and "everyday intelligent" person. Ratings for the 65 experts who responded to the "characteristicness" questionnaire were factor-analyzed; only items that were classified as high in importance by the experts (a mean rating of 6.3 or above on a 1–9 scale) were retained in the factor analysis.

Three major factors were obtained for the ratings of "intelligence," and thus these factors might be seen as an implicit-theory specification of the potential scope for explicit theories of intelligence. The first factor, Verbal Intelligence, showed high loadings for behaviors such as "displays a good vocabulary," "reads with high comprehension," "is verbally fluent," and "converses easily on a variety of subjects." The second factor, Problem Solving, showed high loadings for behaviors such as "able to apply knowledge to problems at hand," "makes good decisions," "poses problems in an optimal way," and "plans ahead." The third factor, Practical Intelligence, showed high loadings for behaviors such as "sizes up situations well," "determines how to achieve goals," "displays awareness to world around him or her," and "displays interest in the world at large." Factors for academic and everyday intelligence were somewhat similar to those for intelligence, although slanted, as one might expect, toward the academic and everyday sides of intelligence, respectively.

This approach to defining the scope of a theory of intelligence has the advantage of not just being based upon one particular expert's definition or theory of intelligence but rather of being based upon some kind of consensus of experts. The factor analysis of the rated views of the experts essentially distills out the common elements in their conceptions and thus provides a level of consensual validation that no one explicit theory can attain (as a means for defining the scope of theories of intelligence). In many respects, however, this approach is no less problematical than any other. For one thing, views held in common by experts are not necessarily essential or even peripheral elements of intelligence. When all is said and done, it has been the often idiosyncratic opinions of small numbers of geniuses, such as Freud, Piaget, or Skinner, that have most shaped people's views of the nature of many psychological phenomena. Scientific truth is not necessarily reached by majority rule. For another thing, the experts may not be on the right track at all.

Consider as an illustration a rather extreme case. Suppose the experts in a particular culture believe that intelligence is a function of the balance of fire, air, water, and earth in a person's body: The more nearly balanced these elements are, the higher is a person's intelligence. Experts in our culture would almost certainly ridicule this notion, or at least feel some degree of pity for misguided souls who harbor these beliefs. Still, it is quite conceivable that the experts of 100 years from now may ridicule our beliefs or have a great deal of pity for us as mere primitives in the study of intelligence. Indeed, scientific revolutions like those attributed to Newton, Copernicus, and Einstein have, in fact, resulted in rather thorough reconceptualizations of the nature of particular kinds of phenomena. Experts' views are not guaranteed to be either complete or correct.

Implicit theories of laypersons.   If one views intelligence as a cultural concept, then one may use laypersons' views as a basis for specifying the scope of a theory of intelligence. Neisser (1979) has collected informal data from Cornell undergraduates, and more formal studies have been conducted by Bruner, Shapiro, and Tagiuri (1958), Cantor and Mischel (1979), and Sternberg, Conway, Ketron, and Bernstein (1981). The data of Sternberg and his colleagues suggest that laypersons' conceptions of intelligence are remarkably similar to those of experts. Characteristicness ratings of experts and laypersons were correlated .96, and importance ratings were correlated .85. Thus, the two groups of individuals seem largely to agree in what behaviors are characteristic of and important in defining the ideally intelligent person. Differences in views among populations can be found, however. The behaviors that people in a college library described as "intelligent" were very similar to the ones they described as "academically intelligent;" those that people at a train station (largely business commuters) and in a supermarket (largely housewives) described as "intelligent" were very similar to the ones they described as "everyday intelligent." Self-ratings displayed similar patterns: the students' self-ratings correlated more highly with "academic intelligence" than with "everyday intelligence." The commuters showed the reverse pattern, and the supermarket patrons showed a pattern in-between the other two.

The use of laypersons' views of intelligence as a basis for defining the scope of explicit theories has many of the same advantages and disadvantages as the use of experts' views. On the one hand, laypeople are less likely to be biased by current scientific paradigms, which are not likely to remain in favor indefinitely. On the other hand, one might well argue that if experts in the field of intelligence do not know what intelligence is, no one else is likely to know, and certainly not people whose knowledge about the nature of intelligence is probably minimal or at least considerably less than that of experts.

CONCLUSIONS

There is no single optimal way to determine the ideal scope of theories of intelligence. The combined use of internal and external validation of explicit theories and of discovery of the implicit theories of experts and laypersons can give one a reasonable starting point for specifying scope. This view may seem as circular to some as any of the single views: Theories (whether implicit or explicit) are used to specify scope, and the scope decided upon is then used to justify the coverage of the theories. We prefer to characterize the relationship between statements of scope and theories as a spiral rather than as a circle. The use of scope to inform theory and of theory to inform scope does not really keep us coming back to where we started, as in a circle. Rather, specifications of scope result in successive modifications in theories, which in turn result in successive modifications in scope, as in a spiral. One goes around and around but does not end up in the same place as one started; rather, one progresses in some direction that one hopes (but cannot know) is bringing one closer to some kind of scientific truth.

The various approaches we have considered suggest that the kinds of tasks theorists of intelligence have tended to study – inductive reasoning, verbal comprehension, spatial visualization, and complex problem solving, to name a few – are probably on a (if not *the*) right track. It is possible to validate internally quite good models of performance on tasks such as these, using as the basis for modeling either task or subject variance; performance on these kinds of tasks is moderately correlated with performance on external criteria, such as school grades; and these are, in fact, skills that appear in both experts' and laypersons' implicit conceptions of intelligence. Thus, given our limited bases for knowledge, we have good reason to believe that much, if not most, of what we have been studying as "intelligent performance" is, in some sense at least, intelligent performance.

The various approaches also make it clear that the behaviors we are studying under the rubric of "intelligence research" probably form only a narrow subset of the total set of behaviors that should be of interest to us. Experts and laypersons alike seem to believe that some kind of real-world adaptive intelligence not measured by current tests is an important aspect of intelligence, but little theoretical work has been done on the nature of adaptive intelligence and, at present, we have little in the way of measurement operations to test such theories. Some work, of course, has been done (see, e.g., Archer, 1980; N. Frederiksen, 1962, 1966; Frederiksen, Saunders, & Wand, 1957; Guilford, 1967; Mehrabian, 1972; Rosenthal et al., 1979; Skemp, 1979), but we suggest that more and better theorizing in this area is necessary. We know that the external validity of the parameters of most extant theories of intelligence is at best moderate, and it seems to be a reasonable bet that at least part of the unexplained variance in interesting real-world performances might be accounted for by theory-based measurement of some kind of practical-intelligence facility. We predict that as new theories of intelligence evolve, they will increasingly deal with more ecologically valid, or real-world aspects of intelligence than have the theories we have seen to date. More abstractly, we believe that there will be an evolution in the *contents* that theories of intelligence address. We also believe that there is an evolution in progress with respect to the *structures* posited by theories of intelligence. We discuss this evolution in the next section.

15.2. THE EVOLUTION OF THEORIES OF INTELLIGENCE

Theories of intelligence, like theories of any other psychological construct, undergo an evolutionary process that theorists believe, or at least hope, brings us to successively deeper levels of understanding of the psychological construct under investigation.[1] Although it is not clear that there is any even potentially definitive end-state toward which this evolution is proceeding, it is likely that newer theories represent advancements in definable ways (see Kuhn, 1970). Basically, we believe that theories of intelligence within a given world view for understanding intelligence follow a certain course of evolutionary development and that this course is closely

parallel across approaches or world views, at least across the two that we believe
have been most influential in intelligence research in the recent past. In particular,
we believe that the evolution of theories of intelligence can be conceptualized in
terms of a three-stage model that seems to capture certain aspects of theory development in the correlational and experimental approaches to the study of intelligence
(Sternberg, 1981a; for an alternative view of evolution of psychometric theories in
particular, see Eysenck, 1967).

OVERVIEW OF THE EVOLUTIONARY MODEL

The three stages of our model of theory development represent successive degrees of
complexity (see Figure 15.1). The first two stages include two alternative instantiations of a given level of complexity. The two instantiations essentially compete with
each other, generating a tension that is responsible for theory development within a
given stage and for the eventual passage of theorizing about intelligence from one
stage to the next. Each new stage helps to diffuse tensions created by the preexisting
stage, and at the same time it generates new tension of its own. Tension in Stages 1
and 2 is generated by the two competing instantiations and by competing theories
within each instantiation. Tension in Stage 3 is generated by the lack of competing
instantiations; this tension creates a feeling that no qualitatively new level of advancement in understanding the nature of intelligence is possible within a given
approach.

Figure 15.1 shows the two competing views that characterize Stages 1 and 2 and
the single view that characterizes Stage 3. The model depicts a given unit of analysis
in the study of intelligence as a circle of the kind found in Euler diagrams. The
identity of the particular unit depends upon the world view being considered. This
unit might, for example, be a factor, an elementary information process, a schema,
or some other kind of entity. The model specifies only the existence of units and the
nature of their interrelations. It should be emphasized that the model also makes no
claims about how long theorizing remains within a given stage: It claims only that
the order of the stages of evolutionary development is fixed. Moreover, the model
applies to the spirit rather than to the letter of a given theory, which sometimes differ
in the approach taken to understanding intelligent behavior. Discussion of the model
will be accompanied by examples of its application to the correlational approach,
which studies primarily person variation, and the experimental approach, which
studies primarily stimulus variation.

STAGES OF THE MODEL

Stage 1. In Stage 1, two competing kinds of theories characterize thinking about
the nature of intelligence. One kind of theory (labeled 1a in the figure) is essentially
monistic: A single instantiation of the given unit of analysis dominates thinking
about intelligence. Other instantiations may exist, but they are of little or no consequence. The other kind of theory (1b) is essentially pluralistic: Many independent
instantiations of the given unit dominate thinking about intelligence. The fundamental tension in this stage is between monism and pluralism – between the one
and the many. Tension may exist within as well as between these general views; that
is, there may be alternative monistic and pluralistic theories. The fundamental ten-

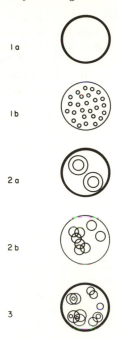

Figure 15.1. Schematic representation of the three stages of theory evolution. The unit of analysis within a given approach to intelligence is represented by a circle. Circles with heavy outer borders show emphasis upon a highest-order unit. Diagrams show alternative principles of organization for units in theories. The number of circles and placement of circles is meant to be illustrative only.

sion to be resolved, however, is between the notion of intelligence as emanating from a single latent source of task and person differences in intelligent performance and the notion of intelligence as emanating from multiple independent sources. The conflict between these two viewpoints is never resolved in favor of either of the original conceptualizations. Rather, the two points of view are eventually merged in Stage 2, but in two ways that again compete with each other.

Consider the application of Stage 1 to the development of correlationally based theories of intelligence. Two very early theories seem to be especially appropriate examples: those of Spearman (1904, 1923, 1927) and of Thomson (Brown & Thomson, 1921; Thomson, 1939). Spearman's theory of general intelligence, or *g*, is prototypical of monistic theories and is certainly the most famous one. In this theory, a single structural factor, referred to as the "general" factor, permeates performance on all of the various tests and tasks used to assess intelligent behavior. Spearman (1927) defined *g* primarily as an individual's level of mental energy. His theory of *g* is a good example of one in which the letter and the spirit of the theory may be seen as differing. Spearman explicitly contrasted his "two-factor" theory of intelligence, which allowed for both a general factor and for specific factors, with a monarchic theory, which allowed for only a single controlling entity. Our characterization of the theory as largely monistic derives from the fact that in both the bulk of Spearman's own work and of that which followed, the general factor received the lion's share of attention and was viewed as critical to an understanding of the nature of intelligence. Specific factors were perceived as necessary to account for statistical patterns of correlation; but because these factors applied only to single tests, they were never perceived as being of much interest (even to Spearman). Indeed, Spearman postulated as many specific factors as there are tests, and it is thus difficult to see how such factors could be of any great interest from a scientific point of view, which seeks at least some reduction of data.

Thomson's theory of general intelligence is prototypical of the pluralistic theories that characterize Stage 1. Thomson proposed that general intelligence can be conceived as comprising a very large number of independent structural "bonds," including reflexes, habits, learned associations, and the like. Performance on any one task would activate a large number of these bonds. Related tasks, such as those used in mental tests, would sample overlapping subsets of independent bonds. A factor analysis of a set of tests might give the appearance of a unitary general factor, but in Thomson's view, the communality among tests is attributable not to a unitary source of individual differences, such as mental energy, but rather to a multiplicity of sources, namely, those bonds that overlap across all tests. Thomson thus did not quibble with the validity of Spearman's mathematical discovery of a general factor but rather with Spearman's psychological interpretation of that discovery.

Stage 1 can also be applied to the development of experimentally based theories of intelligence, such as Gestalt theories (Koffka, 1935; Köhler, 1927, 1947; Wertheimer, 1945) and stimulus–response (S–R) theories (Guthrie, 1935; Thorndike, 1931; Watson, 1930). We believe that the Gestalt concept of *insight*, introduced in Köhler's (1927) work on the "mentality of apes," is the key to an understanding of the Gestalt conception of intelligence. According to Köhler,

We can, in our experience, distinguish sharply between the kind of behavior which from the very beginning arises out of a consideration of the structure of a situation, and one that does not. Only in the former case do we speak of insight, and only that behavior of animals definitely appears to us intelligence which takes account from the beginning of the lay of the land, and proceeds to deal with it in a single, continuous, and definite course. [P. 190]

In Köhler's view, then, insight is very closely linked to intellectual performance; indeed, only insightful behavior appears to us to be intelligent. In Wertheimer's (1945) terms, intelligent behavior is characterized primarily by productive (insightful) thinking rather than by reproductive (memorial) thinking. Thus, "insight" seems, in Gestalt psychology, to correspond to g in correlational psychology: It is the one primary source of intelligent behavior. Gestalt psychology, therefore, represents experimental psychology's monistic Stage 1a. Note that whereas in the psychometric conception of Stage 1a the unit for understanding intelligence is a cognitive structure, in the experimental conception the unit is a cognitive process. This difference between the two approaches continues to manifest itself throughout the stages.

The stimulus–response view of intelligence is particularly well stated by the noted associationist Thorndike and his colleagues (1926):

The hypothesis which we present and shall defend – asserts that in their deeper nature the higher forms of intellectual operation are identical with mere association or connection forming, depending upon the same sort of physiological connections but requiring *many more of them*. By the same argument the person whose intellect is greater or higher or better than that of another person differs from him in the last analysis in having, not a new sort of physiological process, but simply a large number of connections of the ordinary sort. [P. 415]

In Thorndike's view, therefore, intelligence is a function of the number of S–R connections one has formed. In the terminology of our evolutionary model, we view this conception as an example of Stage 1b. The S–R connections of Thorndike are closely analogous to the bonds of Thomson. In each case, intelligence is viewed as a function of the number of independent units (bonds or connections) that a person has formed and brings to bear upon the problems that confront him or her. Again, as in the correlational stream of research, Stage 1b theorizing stresses the pluralistic nature of the sources of intelligent behavior.

Stage 2. Stage 2 of the model posits that a resolution of the struggle between proponents of monistic and pluralistic theories is achieved by accommodating both conceptions of the nature of intelligence. Yet, two forms of this resolution appear, which are again represented by two competing kinds of theories. One kind of theory (2a in the figure) is essentially hierarchical: A single instantiation of the given unit of intelligence dominates others, but in fact, other instantiations of the unit are nested within each other. In general, instantiations of successively lower orders are nested within instantiations of successively higher orders. This view represents an integration of the two views of Stage 1 in that one instantiation of the unit of analysis clearly dominates all others, but there is at least one lower-order (and hence less important) instantiation of the unit as well. At each level, a higher-order instantiation dominates a lower-order one. This integration of Stages 1a and 1b emphasizes the "one" rather than the "many." The other kind of theory (2b) is essentially overlapping but non-hierarchical in nature: Multiple instantiations of the given unit are nonindependent of each other. They may overlap each other in any number of ways (functionally, structurally, causally, etc.), but they are always somehow interdependent in their functioning within a given theory. To the extent that any degree of overlap is common to all instantiations of the unit, the instantiations may be seen as giving rise to a higher-order instantiation that represents this overlap; but this higher-order instantiation of the unit is seen as secondary to the nature of the system and may even be viewed as epiphenomenal. This view represents an integration of the two views of Stage 1 in that there are multiple instantiations of a given unit, but these multiple interdependent instantiations may give rise to a less important second-order unit. This integration of Stages 1a and 1b emphasizes the "many" rather than the "one."

On the whole, Stage 2a is a closer descendant of Stage 1a than it is of Stage 1b in that Stage 2a theories emphasize the "one;" contrarily, Stage 2b is a closer descendant of Stage 1b than it is of Stage 1a in that Stage 2b theories emphasize the "many." Both Stages 2a and 2b may be viewed as more complicated and at the same time more sophisticated developments emanating out of the conflict that arose between the two views characterizing Stage 1. The conflict between Stages 2a and 2b, like that between Stages 1a and 1b, is never resolved in favor of either of the original conceptualizations. Rather, the two points of view are merged in Stage 3.

We will use two classes of correlationally based theories of intelligence – the hierarchical theories and the theories of primary mental abilities – to illustrate the application of Stage 2.

In our view, the hierarchical theories of intelligence (e.g., Burt, 1940; Cattell, 1971; Holzinger, 1938; Horn, 1968; Jensen, 1970; Royce, 1973; Vernon, 1971) represent one kind of resolution of the Stage 1 conflict. In each of these theories, Spearmanian g, or a close relative of it, dominates all other factors of intelligence, which are hierarchically nested under g. Usually, the general factor dominates group factors (which may themselves be of several orders), which in turn dominate specific factors (Burt, 1940; Holzinger, 1938; Vernon, 1971). The identities of these factors differ across theories. For example, in the Cattell–Horn theory, g is divided into subfactors, g_f (fluid ability) and g_c (crystallized ability); in the Vernon theory, g is divided into two major group factors, practical–mechanical ability (which is close in its conception to fluid ability) and verbal–educational ability (which is close in its conception to crystallized ability). Despite their differences, however, all of these theories are hierarchical, as specified by Stage 2a of the evolutionary model.

Competing with the hierarchical theories are the theories of primary mental abilities. In these theories, overlap is derived from correlations between individual differences in patterns of the various mental abilities. Correlation is not attributed to a higher-order factor, as in the hierarchical theories, but to direct relationships between abilities. Historically, the first such theory was Thurstone's (1938) theory of primary mental abilities. According to Thurstone, intelligence can be understood as comprising seven primary mental abilities: verbal comprehension, word fluency, reasoning, number, spatial visualization, memory, and perceptual speed. Thurstone believed these abilities to be primary and fundamental but correlated. Although Thurstone eventually admitted that a higher-order general factor could be extracted by factor-analyzing the correlated factors representing the primary mental abilities, he retained the view that the primaries were of fundamental interest and that any second-order general factor was of secondary interest, at best. Thurstone did not view his model as a hierarchical one, nor have his followers. A second theory of overlapping abilities, which is often viewed as an extension of Thurstone's theory, is the structure-of-intellect theory of Guilford (1967; Guilford & Hoepfner, 1971). In this theory, intelligence is viewed as comprising operations, contents, and products. There are 5 kinds of operations, 6 kinds of products, and 4 kinds of contents. Because the subcategories are independently defined, they are multiplicative ($5 \times 6 \times 4$), yielding 120 different factors of mental ability. An example of such a factor, generated by combining an operation, a content, and a product, would be cognition of figural relations. Guilford has represented his model as a large cube composed of 120 small cubes, each representing a factor. Although this form of representation might lead one to believe that Guilford intended his factors to be independent (in which case Guilford's model would be a Stage 1b model), Guilford (1980) has made clear in his recent writings that he never explicitly stated or intended his factors to be construed as uncorrelated. In fact, he has himself attempted some higher-order factor analyses. Thus, in his theory, as in Thurstone's, intelligence is seen as primarily consisting of a series of overlapping mental abilities, with the recognition that it might be possible to extract a general factor, or at least higher-order factors, from the lower-order ones. Such higher-order factors, however, are seen as of distinctly subsidiary interest in comparison with the primary abilities that constitute the main content of the theory.

Stage 2 can be applied also to the development of experimentally based theories of intelligence. Two classes of theories especially exemplify this stage: hierarchical, executive-based theories and nonhierarchical theories that do not specify executive processes that differ in kind from other processes. Note that as in Stage 1, the existence or nonexistence of a hierarchy pertains to kinds of processes, rather than to kinds of structures.

Hierarchical theories of intelligent behavior present a plausible strategy for information processing in task performance: An executive directs a sequence of elementary information processes. Sometimes the existence of the executive is implicit, although as Carroll (1976, p. 31) has noted, "the assumption of an executive process . . . seems an intuitive necessity if one is going to get the system in operation" (see also Carroll, 1981). At other times, the existence of the executive is explicit, as in the theory of Sternberg (1979, 1980c), which distinguishes metacomponents (executive processes) from other kinds of components; similarly, Brown (1978) distinguishes between metacognitive processes, such as predicting, checking, monitoring, and reality testing, and cognitive processes, such as those used in visual scanning or memory retrieval. Indeed, explicitly "metacognitive" theorists, such as Brown, are those most likely to propose the existence of executive processes that differ in kind from nonexecutive processes. In some theories, however, the distinction between the two kinds of processes, although not explicit, nevertheless seems to be there. For example, Atkinson and Shiffrin (1968) discuss only one kind of process – the control process – at any length in their article on human memory. Yet, they seem to make the same kind of distinction as that made by Brown, Sternberg, and others when they say, "we believe that the overall memory system is best described in terms of the flow of information into and out of short-term storage and the subject's control of that flow" (p. 83). Similarly, Newell, Shaw, and Simon (1958) discuss only one kind of process, the primitive information process, which operates on information in memory; but they present as a separate element of their theory "a perfectly definite set of rules for combining these processes into whole *programs* of processing" (p. 151). The formation of these rules and of the program that comprises them would seem, in their theory, to require some kind of executive processing. In some cases, kinds of processes are further differentiated within the hierarchy. For example, Hunt (1978) follows the lead of Schneider and Shiffrin (1977) in dividing mechanistic (nonexecutive) processes into automated and controlled ones. All of these theories, in our view, exemplify Stage 2a in that there are different orders of processes: executive ones that control nonexecutive ones and, in some theories, various kinds of nonexecutive ones.

An alternative conception of information processing does not distinguish between executive and nonexecutive processing (see, e.g., Chi, Glaser, & Rees, 1982). A well-known class of examples involves the notion of a production system (see Newell, 1973; Newell & Simon, 1972). A production is a condition–action sequence: If a certain condition is met, then a certain action is performed. Sequences of ordered productions are called production systems. Flow of control in a production system passes down an ordered list of productions until one of the conditions is met; the action corresponding to that condition is then executed, and control is returned to the top of the production list. Flow of control then passes down through the list again, trying to satisfy a condition. This sequence is repeated until a termination point is reached or until it is found that none of the conditions in a system of productions is satisfied. Production systems and other nonhierarchical systems differ from hierarchical systems in at least one key way: There is no executive or need for an executive. A separate, qualitatively distinct level of control is not seen as necessary. It is possible, for example, for production systems to create other production systems, to control other production systems, and to modify themselves (see Anderson, 1976; Klahr, 1979). Thus, a single unit of analysis is sufficient for understanding information processing: Production systems can handle in a unitary way what is handled in a dual way – by executive and nonexecutive processes – in a hierarchical theory. The productions in such a system are directly interdependent on each other: The one that is executed in a given pass through a list of productions depends in part upon its precedence in the list, and the ordering of the list is determined by those productions that created the given system. These generating productions do not differ in kind, however, from the productions they generate, and indeed, the generating productions may themselves be modified by the ones they create. The nonhierarchical nature of production systems combined with the direct interdependence of productions on each other lead us to classify production-system theories of intellectual functioning as Stage 2b theories.

Stage 3.   In Stage 3, the two views of Stage 2 are essentially merged into a single, all-encompassing view. The notion of different orders of units (hierarchy) is combined with the notion of overlap in units (nonhierarchy), as shown in panel 3 of Figure 15.1: Instantiations of a given unit may overlap other instantiations of the unit and at the same time nest within higher-order instantiations of the unit. The tensions between the one and the many, and between the hierarchical and the overlapping, are at least partly resolved by merging elements of all of these views into a single, integrated view. Subsequent tension, however, arises from the simultaneous realizations that (a) the questions that the approach was supposed to answer have still not fully been answered, although they have been addressed in a not totally unsatisfying way, and (b) there is nowhere qualitatively new to go with the chosen approach. The investigator is left with three basic options. The first is stagnation: Research continues within the third stage but seems not to go very far or very fast. Inevitably, people begin to lose interest in the approach to the problem and perhaps in the problem as well. The second option is a new subapproach (i.e., interpretation of the current world view): A new way of thinking within the approach is conceived, and thus the original problems and any new ones that have arisen since the original problems were posed can be investigated from a relatively new point of view. In essence, this option involves cycling backward to either Stage 1 or Stage 2. The third option is a new approach: A new way of studying intelligence is adopted that either deals with the old problems in a wholly new way or deals with new problems in a new way. In this case, theorizing starts again at Stage 1.

Stage 3 thus presents not so much a dead end as a challenge to the investigator to reconceptualize his or her approach to the study of intelligence. The view presented here should not be interpreted as suggesting that research on intelligence is futile or hopeless because it eventually ends up "stalling" in Stage 3. To the contrary, the evolution of theoretical accounts of intelligence shows that progress *is* being made, although it is always more clear from whence theories have come than to where they will go.

Consider the application of the Stage 3 notion to the development of correlationally based theories of intelligence. We find only one such theory that fits in this stage: Guttman's (1954, 1965) radex theory.

A *radex*, or "radial expansion of complexity," unites two distinct notions in a single theory. One notion is that of a difference in kind between tests; the other notion is that of a difference in degree. A radex is thus a doubly ordered system in that each of these notions generates a separate concept of structural order within a battery of tests. The double ordering corresponds to the union of the two kinds of ordering represented in Stage 2 of our model through the integrated theoretical development of Stage 3. The application of Guttman's various notions to test data is clearly stated in his own words:

Within all tests of the same kind, say of numerical ability, differences will be in degree. We shall see that addition, subtraction, multiplication, and division differ among themselves largely in the degree of their complexity. Such a set of variables will be called a *simplex*. It possesses a simple order of complexity. The tests can be arranged in a simple rank order from least complex to most complex. [Guttman, 1954, p. 260]

In other words, simplicially ordered tests are tests that are strictly hierarchically ordered from most to least complex, or vice versa (as in Stage 2a).

Correspondingly, all tests of the same degree of complexity will differ among themselves only in the kind of ability they define. We shall postulate a law of order here too, but one which is not from "least" to "most" in any sense. It is an order which has no beginning and no end, namely, a circular order. A set of variables obeying such a law will be called a *circumplex*, to designate a "circular order of complexity." Our empirical data will testify that different abilities such as verbal, numerical, reasoning, etc. do tend to have such an order among themselves. [Guttman, 1954, p. 260]

Circumplicially related abilities are not hierarchically ordered but rather are arranged circularly, with adjacent abilities essentially shading off into each other. Thus, adjacent abilities may be seen as overlapping each other, so that, for example, numerical ability shades off into reasoning ability (as in Stage 2b).

In the more general case, tests can differ among themselves simultaneously both in degree and in kind of complexity, and the general structure here is the radex. Thus, within a radex, one can usually isolate simplexes by keeping the content of the abilities constant and by varying the degree of complexity; and one can also usually isolate circumplexes by keeping degree of complexity constant and then varying the content. [Guttman, 1954, p. 261]

The radex, then, combining as it does the simplex and the circumplex, represents the combination of Stages 2a and 2b shown as Stage 3 in our evolutionary model.

We view Guttman's type of theory as a kind of culmination of correlationally based theorizing about the nature of intelligence. We do not believe Guttman's theory to be the only possible Stage 3 theory, although we have not actually found any others. We simply contend that this level of theorizing represents an end of the line for the evolution of correlationally based theories within the traditional factorial interpretation of correlational analysis. (Of course, future correlational theorizing may prove us wrong.) At this point, the choices open to investigators of individual differences are stagnation, a new subapproach, or a new approach. We have seen evidence of all three outcomes operating in parallel. First, during the 1960s and 1970s, some stagnation occurred in traditional factor-analytic studies of intelligence. Second, at the same time, some exciting new subapproaches of the individual-differences approach emerged, for example, latent-trait analysis (Whitely, 1980a) and confirmatory maximum-likelihood analysis (J. R. Frederiksen, 1980; Geiselman, Woodward, & Beatty, 1982; Whitely, 1980b). Third and finally, some investigators switched their allegiance to methods of analysis that were more experimentally based, as considered in this chapter.

We turn now to a discussion of how Stage 3 applies to the development of experimentally based theories of intelligence. A Stage 3 theory of intelligence would in some way combine aspects of theories with, and theories without, qualitatively distinct executive processes. Our evaluation of current experimental theories of intelligence does not lead us to believe that any of them are clearly Stage 3 theories. However, the evolutionary framework we have proposed leads to a rough sketch of what such a theory might look like. This sketch, provided in some detail in Sternberg

(1981a), involves two kinds of processing systems, a global one and local ones. The global one is drawn upon heavily in situations in which one is unfamiliar with procedures for coping with the task at hand. The global processing system is hierarchical, with executive processes controlling the selection, sequencing, and duration of nonexecutive processes. Each local system is specific to a task domain with which the individual is highly familiar and in which performance is largely automatized. Once a local processing system is activated by the global processing system, information processing becomes nonhierarchical; performance follows an automated sequence of actions. If the local processing system cannot handle a particular problem presented to it within a given task context, then control passes back to the global processing system, and hierarchical control is reinstated.

Thus, in processing information from old domains or domains in which one has acquired considerable expertise, the individual relies primarily upon automatic, local processing. A central executive initially activates a system consisting of locally applicable processes and a locally applicable knowledge base. Multiple local systems can operate in parallel. Performance in this system is both automatic and of almost unlimited capacity; attention is not focused upon the task at hand. Only knowledge that has been transferred to the local knowledge base is available for access by the storage and retrieval components utilized in a given task situation. An important detail to note is that the local system is activated by metacomponents from the global system. The metacomponents can, however, instantiate themselves as part of this local system; when used in this instantiation, they become automatic and do not differ functionally from components of any other kind.

In contrast, in domains in which one has little expertise, processing is largely focused in the global processing and knowledge system. As expertise develops, greater and greater proportions of processing are transferred to (i.e., packed into) a given local processing system. The advantage of the local system is that activation is of the system as a whole, rather than of individual components within the system, and thus its use requires much less attention than does the global system. Indeed, attention allocation for a whole local system is comparable to that for a single lower-order component activated by the global system. The disadvantages of the local system are that its knowledge base is limited and that only those processes that have been packed in a particular production-system sequence are available. Experts can use the local system to handle a wide variety of situations, because they have packed tremendous amounts of information into it and are able to process this information expeditiously. Novices can use local systems almost not at all, because these systems have as yet acquired relatively few processes and relatively little knowledge.

To summarize this sketchily proposed Stage 3 theory, the present view combines hierarchical and nonhierarchical viewpoints by suggesting that in the global mode information processing is hierarchical and controlled, and in the local mode it is nonhierarchical and automatic. Expertise develops largely from the successively greater assumption of information processing by local resources. When these local resources are engaged, parallel processing of multiple kinds of tasks becomes possible. Global resources, however, are serial in their problem-solving capabilities and are costly to use because of the conscious attention their use demands.

CONCLUSION

We have proposed a three-stage model of the evolution of theories of intelligence. We believe that the model applies to the evolution of two of the major approaches to studying intelligence – the correlationally based and the experimentally based – and possibly to other approaches as well. The model is characterized by competition between two conceptions of intelligence in each of Stages 1 and 2 .The competition is resolved in Stages 2 and 3 by combining the competing elements from the earlier stages. The third stage does not involve internal competition between alternative conceptions (although, as in earlier stages, there may be alternative theories within a given conception); rather, it involves the developing realization that for theorizing to progress, it will have somehow to change course.

The present view suggests that different questions are paramount in theorists' minds at different stages of the evolutionary process. At a general level, one might characterize the differences as follows. In Stage 1, the primary question is whether a theory of intelligence should be monistic or pluralistic; in Stage 2, the primary question is whether these two views should be, in some sense, integrated in a hierarchical or a nonhierarchical way; in Stage 3, the primary question is how hierarchical and nonhierarchical views can themselves be integrated in some sense. When Stage 3 comes to an end, the questions of just what intelligence is and how it should be studied are reconsidered, and possible new answers are considered (see Sternberg, 1981a). These answers, like the ones before them, will prove to be limited in various respects. We now turn to a consideration of these limitations.

15.3. LIMITS OF THEORIES OF INTELLIGENCE

All existing theories of intelligence, and probably any theories yet to be proposed, are limited in scope. In this section, we discuss the limitations on the range of phenomena to which theories of intelligence can apply and exemplify them from the correlational and experimental approaches to intelligence. We shall discuss limitations in the task, person, and situation domains.

TASK DOMAIN

Theories of intelligence can be limited in the range of tasks to which they apply. Various investigators may disagree as to just what the full range of tasks should be, because they may disagree as to just what tasks require "intelligent" behavior. We believe that the main restrictive elements in the task domain are ecological validity, diversity, difficulty, and aspects studied. The first three restrictions involve selection of tasks; the last restriction involves selection of particular aspects of task performance for psychological investigation.

Ecological validity. An ecologically valid task, as opposed to a highly artificial one, may be defined as one whose performance is required in adaptation to real-world environments. Restriction in ecological validity can occur both in the proximal domain in which the theory is internally validated – that is, in which the theory is immediately applied – and in the distal domain in which the theory is externally validated – that is, in the domain that serves as the basis for an outside comparison of task performance (see first section of this chapter).

An issue related to the task's ecological validity is the level of processing required by the task (Cermak & Craik, 1979; Craik & Lockhart, 1972; Craik & Tulving, 1975). The level of processing required to perform a task refers to the depth of meaning that must be accessed in order to complete the task. For example, a lexical decision task requires only a very low level of semantic involvement to complete, but a task requiring a person to judge the meaningfulness of a sentence entails a high degree of semantic involvement. The researcher's choice of tasks from this levels-of-processing continuum will greatly influence his or her view of intelligence. It is unclear at present what continuities in cognitive functioning exist across levels of processing. Some cognitive-correlates researchers, such as Hunt (1978) and Goldberg, Schwartz, and Stewart (1977), have studied a series of tasks postulated to require successively greater degrees of semantic processing and have found only moderate correlations of speed and accuracy measures for low-level tasks and tasks requiring a greater degree of semantic processing.

Both correlationally and experimentally derived and tested theories of intelligence have been subject to considerable restriction in their internal ecological validity. Most of the correlational theories have been based upon tasks of the kinds found on IQ tests, for example, vocabulary, analogies, mental rotations, arithmetic reasoning problems, and the like (Guilford, 1967; Thurstone, 1938; Vernon, 1971). Experimental theories have sometimes been based upon tasks of these kinds (Sternberg, 1977, 1979) and sometimes upon tasks of the kind studied in experimental psychologists' laboratories, for example, memory scanning, letter comparison, sentence-picture comparison, and the like (Hunt, 1978). Although these tasks may be the best proxies we now have for the kinds of performances we would ultimately like to predict, for example, a potential lawyer's ability to argue a case successfully or a future scientist's ability to conduct significant experiments, they are at best weak proxies (Olneck & Crouse, 1979). Attempts have been made in both the correlational and experimental domains to generate ecologically valid tasks and theories to serve as a basis for theorizing about intelligence in the real world (e.g., Cole, 1980; N. Frederiksen, 1962; Neisser, 1976; Thorndike, 1920), and these attempts continue into the present (Sternberg & Wagner, 1982). Still, any developments that provided a conceptual link between the proxies and the distal criteria would be of tremendous significance, especially if they also linked measurements of performance in real-world and testlike tasks. Perhaps what is needed most now are tasks at some middle level of ecological validity – ones that are susceptible to experimental analysis but closer to real-world performance than IQ test tasks. Real-world decision making, as in buying a house or deciding whether to undergo surgery, might provide models for such tasks.

Both correlational and experimental theories have also been subject to considerable restriction in the domains to which they have been externally validated. The external tests are usually well-established ones, such as the Stanford–Binet or the Wechsler, but such tests serve as modest bases for external validation, because these tests are usually no more ecologically valid than the tests that they are validating. Sometimes, school performance has been used as a criterion, which is at least one step up in the continuum of ecological validity. Experimental psychologists have been even more culpable: They have tended to use either criteria from the same domain of experimental tasks as the ones about which they are theorizing (e.g., Rose, 1978), or at best, intelligence test scores that are themselves of dubious ecological validity (e.g., Hunt, Frost, & Lunneborg, 1973; R. J. Sternberg, 1977, 1980c). We are aware of literally *no* experimental research that has tested parameters of information processing theories even against modestly ecologically valid criteria such as school grades.

Task diversity.   The derivation and testing of both correlational and experimental theories of intelligence have been subject to task restriction, but the level of restriction has been more severe in experimental theories than in correlational ones. The difference can probably be traced at least in part to differences inherent in the methodologies. Correlational methods force the theorist to deal with the problem of task diversity; experimental methods generally do not. Correlational theories based on or tested by factor analysis need correlations from a large number and variety of mental tasks as input. Restriction in the range of tests will result in biasing of the kinds of factors that can be obtained. Experimental theories based on or tested by stimulus-item manipulations can use scores from just a single kind of task as input, so long as the items of that task are varied, for example, the number of digits in the target set in the S. Sternberg (1969) memory-scanning task. The parameters of the theory are not biased by the choice of tasks, although their range may be limited. Experimental theorists are becoming more sensitive to the limitations of theories based upon small numbers of tasks (see Carroll, 1981; R. J. Sternberg, 1980c, 1981d), but the experimental theories still lack the breadth of data base that has characterized psychometric theories, especially the most ambitious ones (e.g., Guilford, 1967).

Task diversity has been a problem in the criterion domain as well as in the domain in which the theory is originally tested. The external tests against which correlational theories are validated are usually from the same domain of tests that served for internal validation, although occasionally achievement test scores and school grades have served as the basis for validation, which adds at least some range to the external measures. Tasks similar to the ones serving as the basis for internal validation of experimental theories, too, usually are used for external validation. For theories based on fairly low-level experimental tasks the use of IQ test types of tasks probably provides as much diversity in tasks as is found in any of the current efforts toward external validation. From a practical point of view, the unavailability or inaccessibility of interesting criterial data is usually the cause of restriction in the criterion domain. More effort seems to be needed to collect such data whenever the possibility exists.

Task difficulty. Because correlationally based theories need a fairly wide range in task difficulty in order to generate the individual differences necessary for doing factor analysis or other kinds of correlational analysis, correlational theories of intelligence have generally been tested on items varying widely in difficulty. The same cannot be said for experimental theories. They have generally been formed from and tested on laboratory tasks that are strikingly uniform in difficulty. Researchers who have used standard laboratory tasks, such as Hunt (1978), have generally worked with tasks on which error rates are on the order of 1–2% and almost always less than 5%. Researchers who have used tasks adopted from IQ tests, such as R. J. Sternberg (1979), have generally worked with tasks having higher error rates, say, on the order of 5–15%, but performance even on these tasks has been notable for its accuracy. The reason that performance on these tasks is so much more accurate than on the IQ tests is that the problems are usually simplified in being adapted to the reaction-time testing format. At the other extreme, problem-solving researchers, such as Newell and Simon (1972), have tended to use very difficult tasks, each taking many minutes to solve. An extension in the range of difficulty of experimental tasks both in the predictor and criterion domains is distinctly needed, and that need just now seems to be in the process of being recognized and acted upon (e.g., Whitely & Schneider, 1981).

Performance index.   Psychometric theories of intelligence have been derived from and tested on psychometric test data that are almost exclusively based on accuracy. For the most part, a battery of tests is administered, and each item on each test is scored as either right or wrong. Other response variables, such as latency, are usually ignored in psychometric assessments, even though research indicates that these response variables measure abilities that have scarcely been tapped by psychometric tests (Egan, 1976; R. J. Sternberg, 1980b). Although speeded administration of tests yields a combined measurement of speed and accuracy from which factors of intelligence are then derived, the relative contributions of speed and accuracy are usually unknown. Experimental theories have been more eclectic in their measurement of response variables, often considering speed and accuracy both separately and jointly (e.g., R. J. Sternberg, 1977, 1980b) and sometimes considering probabilities of various kinds of responses as well (e.g., Guyote & Sternberg, 1981). The greater eclecticism of the experimental theories applies to external as well as internal validation: Whereas the same response variable (accuracy) is usually used to validate psychometric tests against other psychometric tests, often different response variables (such as reaction time and accuracy) are used to validate information processing components (see, e.g., Hunt et al., 1973; Hunt, et al., 1975; R. J. Sternberg, 1977). We believe that it will be important for future theories to take into account multiple response variables, such as reaction time, response accuracy, and probability of a given response, if only because it now appears so evident that different variables can measure different aspects of psychological functioning. Indeed, the way in which a person trades off one aspect against another, for example, speed versus accuracy, may be an important feature of intelligent behavior.

Summary.   Restriction in task domain is a serious problem for all extant theories of intelligence. Restriction in ecological validity, in task diversity, and in task difficulty is probably more of a problem for existing experimental theories than for existing correlational ones, although when task selection is limited in correlational analyses, its effects are probably more invidious than when it is limited in experimental analyses. Probably restriction in indexes used to measure performance is more of a problem for correlational than for experimental theories. We believe that restriction in ecological validity is the most significant problem facing current tasks and theories, because ultimately, theories of intelligence are of interest only to the extent that they apply to situations in the real world. Current work on practical intelligence (e.g., Sternberg & Wagner, 1982) and on social intelligence (e.g., Archer, 1980; Sternberg & Smith, 1982) seems to represent steps toward what is needed to render theories of intelligence ecologically valid (see Chapter 11, this volume).

PERSON DOMAIN

Theories of intelligence can be limited in the range of persons to which they apply as well as in the attributes of those persons. The four main kinds of restrictions, we believe, are age, level of intelligence, range of sociocultural backgrounds, and aspects of abilities accounted for by a given theory. The first three restrictions involve selection of persons; the last restriction involves selection of particular aspects of their performance for psychological investigation.

Age.   All existing theories of intelligence are age-restricted to some extent, although recent findings on novelty-seeking and novelty-finding behavior in infants, children, and adults (Fagan & McGrath, 1981; Lewis & Brooks-Gunn, 1981; R. J. Sternberg, 1981b, 1981e) suggest the outline of a theory that may be broadly applicable across age levels, and Piaget's (1976) theory, of course, attempts to account in some detail for intelligent behavior from infancy through adulthood.

Correlational theories have usually been first generated and tested on the basis of adult performance and later extended to children's performance. Developmental investigations have shown the importance of actually testing theories based on adult performance on children of different ages, because aspects of the theories may not, in fact, hold up across age levels. Various developmental theories suggest changes in the factorial structure of intelligence with age. These changes may take a variety of forms, for example, changes in number of factors with age (Garrett, 1938, 1946), changes in the relevance or weights of factors with age (Hofstaetter, 1954), changes in the content (names) of factors within a given factor structure (McCall, Eichorn, & Hogarty, 1977; McCall, Hogarty, & Hulburt, 1972; McNemar, 1942), and changes in relative levels of abilities as represented by factors with age (Horn, 1968; Jarvik, Eisdorfer, & Blum, 1973). Because of these age-related differences in factorial structure or level, a theory of intelligence based on only one age group may have very limited generalizability to other age groups. Because of discontinuities in intellectual development, it is difficult even to hazard a guess as to how far generalization is obtained. (For further discussion of these and other developmental issues, see Sternberg & Powell, in press.)

Experimental theories, like correlational ones, have usually been first generated and tested on the basis of adult performance and only later extended to children's performance. In some cases, fits of theoretical predictions to data obtained for children have been comparable to those obtained for adults (e.g., Keating & Bobbitt, 1978; R. J. Sternberg, 1979, 1980a, 1982); in other cases, fits for children have been noticeably poorer than those obtained for adults (e.g., Keating et al., 1980). None of the experimentally based theories of intelligence has yet been widely tested on children's performance, and hence, their validity for children is still, to some extent, unknown.

Level of intelligence.   Correlational theories of intelligence require substantial individual differences in ability levels of tested subjects in order to be tested properly by correlational techniques such as factor analysis. Hence, investigators of these theories have often gone to great lengths to ensure wide ranges of ability levels in their samples. Because at least some of the theory testing has been done indirectly in the context of standardizations of nationally distributed IQ tests, resources for testing individuals of widely disparate ability levels have been particularly good. The same cannot be said for the resources available to many experimental psychologists. Although some theories, such as that of Hunt (1978), have been tested by various psychologists on a wide range of subject ability levels, other theories, such as that of R. J. Sternberg (1980c), have been tested almost exclusively on individuals of above-average and usually superior ability. Investigators who have restricted themselves to high-ability subjects have generally implied that their theories apply to low-ability subjects as well (see, e.g., R. J. Sternberg, 1981f), but these claims must be met with skepticism. In some cases, it is not even clear that the tasks on which the theories are based could be solved by individuals of distinctly below-average ability (e.g., R. J. Sternberg, 1981b), and even if they could be, there is no reason to assume that subjects of differing ability levels will use the same processes and strategies in performing intellectual tasks. Thus, there seems to be no substitute for testing a theory on subjects of widely ranging ability levels.

Range of sociocultural backgrounds.   The one theory of intelligence that has been tested in a wide variety of cultural settings is that of Piaget (see, e.g., Dasen, 1972, 1977). Psychometric theories have received some cross-cultural investigation (e.g., Vernon, 1969, 1979) but to a much lesser extent. Insofar as data are available, cross-cultural support for the Piagetian and correlational theories is fairly good, and there is even some tentative support for aspects of experimental theories (Cole & Scribner, 1974). The larger question, however, is whether what we in our culture measure as intelligence can reasonably be called intelligence in other cultures (Berry, 1980; Cole & Scribner, 1974; Laboratory of Comparative Human Cognition, Chapter 11, this volume; Wober, 1974), or whether we are merely imposing our own notions of intelligence upon other cultures. This question is largely unresolved, as are the methods by which it might be answered.

Aspects of performance accounted for.   The range of cognitive competencies that generate cognitive performances is so broad that it is unlikely that any one theory, or perhaps even any class of theories, could account for it. Carroll (1976, 1980, 1981) has proposed one taxonomy of these competencies, and we would propose another, recognizing that our taxonomy is very incomplete. In presenting this taxonomy (Table 15.1), we would note that it can be applied either to availability of functions, which might be dealt with in a competence model of human intelligence, or to accessibility of functions, which might be dealt with in a performance model.

Correlational theories generally have little to say about processes (with a few notable exceptions, e.g., Guilford, 1967; Guilford & Hoepfner, 1971), representations, and contents of representations. The theories do specify, in factorial terms, the forms taken by processing space and power, and occasionally, speed. Thus, in Thurstone's theory, one might view processing space as subdivided (at least functionally) into regions for verbal, spatial, numerical, perceptual, and other kinds of performance, with degree of speed and power a function of amount of space or of how efficiently this space is allocated in task performance. Only a handful of these theories specify motivational variables (e.g., Royce, 1973) and possible modes of interaction of these variables with cognitive ones.

Experimental theories are probably strongest in their specifications of processes, with a major source of disagreement among these theories being the kinds of processes and identities of processes into which performance should be parsed. Some of the theories specify representations (e.g., R. J. Sternberg, 1977), although it is not at all clear how alternative representations can be distinguished from one another (Anderson, 1976, 1978). None of the theories claims to specify the full knowledge base available to performing individuals, although recent theorizing has emphasized the importance of the knowledge base (e.g., Chi, Glaser, & Rees, 1982) and has shown how task performance can be influenced by it. Most of the theories have little to say about processing space (but see Case, 1974; Osherson, 1974) but quite a lot to say about processing power and processing speed (see, e.g., R. J. Sternberg, 1980c). The theories have almost nothing to say about motivation; at best, they acknowledge its importance (R. J. Sternberg, 1981c) without specifying how it can be parsed or just how it interacts with cognitive processing.

Table 15.1. *Taxonomy of cognitive competencies*

I. Processes
   A. Executive processes
      1. Ability to recognize the nature of problems
      2. Selection of nonexecutive processes
      3. Selection of strategies for combining nonexecutive processes
      4. Selection of representations upon which processes and strategies can act
      5. Allocation of processing resources across tasks and aspects of tasks
      6. Monitoring of solution progress
      7. Selection of relevant information from the total stream of incoming information
      8. Sensitivity to feedback
      9. Ability to translate feedback into an action plan
      10. Ability to act on one's action plan, actually implementing it
   B. Nonexecutive processes
      1. Components of task performance (e.g., encoding, inferring, mapping, applying, comparing, justifying, etc.)
      2. Components of information storage
      3. Components of information retrieval
II. Representations of information
   A. Digital representations (including propositions)
   B. Analogue representations (including images)
III. Contents of representations
   A. Amount of knowledge represented
   B. Real-world utility of knowledge represented
   C. Accuracy of knowledge represented
   D. Quality of organization(s) of knowledge represented (including accessibility of information when needed)
IV. Information processing capacities
   A. Processing space
   B. Processing power
   C. Processing speed
V. Motivations driving performance

Summary. Restriction in person domains is a problem in all theories of intelligence, but the problem differs in different classes of theories. Correlational theories tend to be strong in the range of levels of intelligence for which they are applicable, moderately strong in their range of applicability across ages, of unknown strength in their cross-cultural applicability, and relatively weak in the range of aspects of performance they can account for. Experimental theories tend to be strong where correlational theories are weak, and vice versa: Their applicability across levels of intelligence, age, and culture is very much in need of verification; but the range of aspects of performance they can account for in some detail has been quite impressive. In sum, both kinds of theories need extension in the person domain, but the restrictions with which they have to deal differ.

SITUATION DOMAIN

Situational variables have been all but totally ignored in theories and testing of intelligence. Tests are usually administered under conditions purposefully made as quiet, nondistracting, and generally sterile as possible. Intelligent performance in the real world, however, rarely takes place under these kinds of conditions, and therefore the attempt to provide an optimal working environment may actually detract from the predictive and ecological validity of the tests and tasks used to assess intelligent performance. We need to know more about people's abilities to work with the interruptions, distractions, upsets, and tensions that confront people in their real-world task performance.

We believe there are at least four main situational variables in the expression of intelligence. We propose that an examination of these variables can provide some degree of insight into situational constraints on behavior, but we make no claim that the variables are either orthogonal or exhaustive; to the contrary, the variables overlap and are certainly incomplete. The variables are internal versus external constraints on performance, usual versus unusual circumstances of performance, supportive versus adverse circumstances of performance, and maximal versus typical situational demands. The first variable is the broadest type of restriction and the one most likely to be mentioned in explaining differences between an individual's competence to perform and his or her actual performance. The other three continua are a more detailed exploration of the nature of the interaction between the internal and the external constraints on intelligent performance.

Internal versus external constraints.   Internal-state restrictions refer to potential limitations in performance deriving from transient emotional and motivational states, such as depression or elation, learned helplessness or feelings of control, inability to concentrate or particular ability to concentrate, and so on. Although such variables are usually written off as "noise" in psychometric testing, they are so much a part of everyday living that they seem worthy of investigation in their own right as systematic rather than chance influences upon performance. Recent work on state-specific retention (e.g., Bower, 1981) is an encouraging development, and we would like to see this genre of research carried over into the study of intelligent performance more generally.

External-state restrictions include sources of influence upon performance emanating from the environment, such as loud noises, frequent interruptions, insufficient illumination, inadequate resources for accomplishing the task at hand, and so on. Such restrictions are an integral part of the everyday task environment, of course. These sources of influence are not necessarily detrimental to performance (for example, distractions may be minimized, illumination may be optimized, ideal resources may be provided, and so on). Again, no body of literature systematizes the effects, either positive or negative, of variables such as these on different classes of intelligent performance. Indeed, the large majority of investigations have made serious efforts to hold these variables constant. They are not constant in everyday situations, however, and the standard policy may thus be self-defeating if one's goal is to understand intelligence as it operates in the real world. One of the reasons for the only moderate validities of most batteries of intelligence tests may well be that the conditions under which the tests are administered result in measurement of performance in situations that almost never simulate real-world situations. A person may perform well (or poorly) in a sterilized environment but fall apart (or come together) with the bombardment of distractions that accompany real-world performance.

Usual versus unusual circumstances of performance.   Almost everyone knows someone (perhaps oneself) who performs well when confronted with tasks in a familiar milieu but who falls apart when presented with perhaps very similar tasks in an unfamiliar milieu. For example, a person who performs well in his or her every-day environment may find it difficult to function effectively in a foreign country, even one that is similar in many respects to the home environment; or a person who plays good chess (or baseball) on his or her home turf may find it difficult to play in the opponent's home turf. It is known that test–retest reliability tends to be max-imized when the circumstances of administration are very similar on both occasions and that recall of stimulus material tends to be best when it occurs in the same setting as that in which the material was learned. Still, we do not have any good sense of what systematic effects situations have – of the extent to which individual differences in intelligent performance in the real world derive from people's differen-tial abilities to apply their knowledge and skills in a variety of situations, including both familiar and unfamiliar ones. Because, for many people, testing situations are relatively unfamiliar, some idea of what these situational effects are would seem to be essential: They are built into intellectual measurements to an extent that is presently unknown.

Supportive versus adverse circumstances of performance. When one has a series of tasks to perform over a prolonged period of time, it is almost inevitable that some-times the circumstances of performance will favor task performance and that other times the circumstances will disfavor it. For example, when writing a chapter for a book over a period of days, one finds no interruptions or sources of distraction on some days, and on other days one finds a new distraction every few minutes. A person who can continue to work reasonably effectively under sometimes adverse circumstances will have a considerable advantage over someone who always needs favorable circumstances. Again, we know little about people's flexibility in adapting to various amounts of stress in their environments, despite the fact that this flexibil-ity would seem to be an individual-difference variable that would have considerable impact upon people's abilities to function effectively in real-world situations.

Maximal versus typical situational demands. Intelligence tests are almost always administered under maximal-performance demands: One is encouraged to put forth one's best effort, and the pressure to do so is clear and present. Such tests may actually be more predictive of performance for people who are often under maximal-performance demands than for people who are usually under typical-performance demands, where there are no clear and present signals that one's best is required. We have found, for example, that people who perform well in the relatively struc-tured, obviously demanding environments of undergraduate school and of standard-ized testing often find themselves at a loss in graduate school, where much of the time one is left to produce at a rate and level that suits oneself. Obversely, some people may perform well when left to themselves but suffer overwhelming anxiety when they have to work under pressure. We believe that there is more involved here than a "test anxiety" trait: People seem to respond differentially well to differing levels of external demands for top performance, but we know little about how these differences affect intelligent performance either in test situations or in real-world ones.

Summary. Situational variables have been little studied in intelligence research, and there is virtually no systematic body of knowledge on the effects of such vari-ables on intelligent performance. Theories of intelligence in the correlational domain gave special attention to person variation; theories of intelligence in the experimental domain gave special attention to task variation. Still, neither type of theory has looked specifically at variance in the situational domain. The importance of situations is becoming widely recognized in the literature on personality (see, e.g., Bem & Allen, 1974; Bem & Funder, 1978; Cantor & Mischel, 1979; Mischel, 1971), if only out of necessity: Measurements based on theories of personality simply proved to be inadequate until situations were paid due respect (Mischel, 1971). Intelligence researchers have been blessed with better-looking statistics and hence have not been driven as hard to study situational effects, but we believe that the construct, predictive, and ecological validities of theories and measurements of intelligence will be as frozen as they have remained over the past few decades until situational variables are taken seriously.

CONCLUSION

A survey of the wide variety of restrictions confronting theories of intelligence makes one wonder how the theories are as successful as they are. Although we believe that theories of intelligence have succeeded well in many respects and have come a long way from, say, the earliest theorizing of Galton (1883), we also believe that at least some of the apparent success of theories of intelligence is illusory. The main reason for this is that there has been almost as much restriction in the criteria used to assess the success of our theories as there has been in the immediate person, task, and situation domains to which the theories have been applied. If one removes from the realm of potential criteria the restrictions that have characterized our actual criteria, then one begins to realize what a long way theories of intelligence have to go before they can account for anything except a data base that is highly restricted in terms of the persons, tasks, and situations from which it is derived. We hope that this section, by clarifying the restrictions that the theories face, will help point out the kinds of investigations that need to be conducted to remove these restrictions.

15.4.   SUMMARY AND CONCLUSIONS

One principal general theme runs through the three rather disparate preceding sections of this chapter: the restrictions to which theories of intelligence are subject. In each of the three sections, we have dealt with what we view as a different class of restrictions.

In the first section, we attempted to show that theories of intelligence can be restricted in terms of the class of phenomena to which they apply. Explicit theories apply to observable behaviors requiring the exercise of intelligence; implicit theories apply to people's conceptions of what these behaviors are and of how they are organized. An auspicious sign for theorizing about intelligence is that there seems to be some convergence between the two kinds of theories. For example, Sternberg, Conway, Ketron, and Bernstein (1981) found in people's conceptions of intelligence factors that seemed to correspond quite closely to Cattell and Horn's notions of fluid and crystallized abilities (e.g., Cattell, 1971), as well as to notions of Thorndike (1920), Guilford (1967), Sternberg and Wagner (1982), and others of some kind of practical intelligence or common sense that is distinct from academic intelligence (see also Neisser, 1976). We believe that although explicit and implicit theories need not converge in their conceptualizations, the extent to which they do lends credence to people's everyday beliefs and ecological validity to psychologists' theories. It appears that at least to some extent, what psychologists have been studying under the rubric of intelligence is a subset of the phenomena that ordinary people (as well as experts) have been referring to as "intelligence;" it is not merely some arcane construction bearing little or no resemblance to the ordinary language concept. The convergence in the two kinds of theories leads us to believe that despite the mystique of the concept of intelligence, it is a researchable entity that is susceptible to psychological understanding.

In the second section, we attempted to show how theories of intelligence evolve. We proposed a three-stage model of evolutionary development and showed how the model applies to the development of correlational and experimental theories. The first stage involves a dynamic tension between monistic and pluralistic theories; the second stage involves a dynamic tension that grows out of two possible resolutions of the Stage 1 conflict, the resolutions being those of hierarchical and nonhierarchical models. The third stage involves some kind of integration between these two kinds of models. Each successive stage can be viewed as a successive weakening of theoretical restrictions. The first stage includes just one entity of interest or multiple but essentially unrelated entities. The second stage includes multiple entities that are now allowed to interact, either by being hierarchically related to each other or by being essentially heterarchically related to each other. In the third stage, both hierarchical and heterarchical relations are allowed. This third stage, then, represents the least restrictive view in terms of the ways elements can interact with each other; the first stage represents the most restrictive view, in that elements are not allowed to interact at all.

The third section reviews the kinds of restrictions that theories can encounter in terms of their application to a range of tasks, persons, and situations. We suggested that tasks can be restricted in terms of their ecological validity, diversity, difficulty, and indexes of measured performance; that persons can be restricted in terms of their age, level of intelligence, range of sociocultural backgrounds, and the aspects of their performance that are accounted for; and that situations can be restricted in terms of internal versus external constraints on performance, usual versus unusual circumstances of performance, supportive versus adverse circumstances of performance, and maximal versus typical situational demands. Various theories and classes of theories of intelligence differ in terms of their freedom from these restrictions, although the domain of situational restrictions has been relatively uncharted in theories of any class. We believe that theories of intelligence will evolve toward greater freedom from the various kinds of restrictions to which current theories are subject, and we believe that such less restricted theories will soon become a part of psychological theorizing about the nature of intelligence.

NOTES

Preparation of this chapter was supported by Contract N0001478C0025 from the Office of Naval Research to Robert J. Sternberg. It was written while Janet S. Powell was supported by a National Science Foundation Graduate Fellowship.
1 This section is based on R. J. Sternberg (1981a).

REFERENCES

Anderson, J. R. *Language, memory, and thought.* Hillsdale, N.J.: Erlbaum, 1976.
Anderson, J. R. Arguments concerning representations for mental imagery. *Psychological Review,* 1978, *85,* 249–277.

Archer, D. *How to expand your social intelligence quotient.* New York: M. Evans, 1980

Atkinson, R. C., & Shiffrin, R. M. Human memory: A proposed system and its control processes. In K. Spence & J. Spence (Eds.), *The psychology of learning and motivation* (Vol. 2). New York: Academic Press, 1968.

Bem, D. J., & Allen, A. On predicting some of the people some of the time: The search for cross-situational consistencies in behavior. *Psychological Review,* 1974, *81,* 506–520.

Bem, D. J., & Funder, D. C. Predicting more of the people more of the time: Assessing the personality of situations. *Psychological Review,* 1978, *85,* 485–501.

Berry, J. W. Cultural universality of any theory of human intelligence remains an open question. *Behavioral and Brain Sciences,* 1980, *3,* 584–585.

Bower, G. H. Mood and memory. *American Psychologist,* 1981, *36,* 129–148.

Brown, A. L. Knowing when, where, and how to remember: A problem of metacognition. In R. Glaser (Ed.), *Advances in instructional psychology* (Vol. 1). Hillsdale, N.J.: Erlbaum, 1978.

Brown, W., & Thomson, G. H. *The essentials of mental measurement.* Cambridge, England: Cambridge University Press, 1921.

Bruner, J. S., Shapiro, D., & Tagiuri, R. The meaning of traits in isolation and in combination. In R. Taguiri & L. Petrollo (Eds.), *Person perception and interpersonal behavior.* Stanford, Calif.: Stanford University Press, 1958.

Burt, C. *The factors of the mind.* London, England: University of London Press, 1940.

Cantor, N., & Mischel, W. Prototypes in person perception. In L. Berkowitz (Ed.), *Advances in experimental social psychology.* New York: Academic Press, 1979.

Carroll, J. B. Psychometric tests as cognitive tasks: A new "structure of intellect." In L. B. Resnick (Ed.), *The nature of intelligence.* Hillsdale, N.J.: Erlbaum, 1976.

Carroll, J. B. *Individual difference relations in psychometric and experimental cognitive tasks* (NR 150–406 ONR Final Report). Chapel Hill, N.C.: L. L. Thurstone Psychometric Laboratory, University of North Carolina, 1980.

Carroll, J. B. Ability and task difficulty in cognitive psychology. *Educational Researcher,* 1981, *10,* 11–21.

Case, R. Structures and strictures: Some functional limitations on the course of cognitive growth. *Cognitive Psychology,* 1974, *6,* 544–573.

Cattell, R. B. *Abilities: Their structure, growth, and action.* Boston: Houghton Mifflin, 1971.

Cermak, L. S., & Craik, F. I. (Eds.), *Levels of processing in human memory.* Hillsdale, N.J.: Erlbaum, 1979.

Chi, M. T. H. Representing knowledge and metaknowledge: Implications for interpreting metamemory research. In F. E. Weinert & R. Kluwe (Eds.), *Learning by thinking.* Stuttgart, West Germany: Kuhlhammer, in press.

Chi, M. T. H., Glaser, R., & Rees, E. Expertise in problem solving. In R. J. Sternberg (Ed.), *Advances in the psychology of human intelligence* (Vol. 1). Hillsdale, N.J.: Erlbaum, 1982.

Cole, M. Niche-picking. Unpublished manuscript, University of California, San Diego, 1980.

Cole, M., & Scribner, S. *Culture and thought: A psychological introduction.* New York: Wiley, 1974.

Craik, F. I., & Lockhart, R. S. Levels of processing: A framework for memory research. *Journal of Verbal Learning and Verbal Behavior,* 1972, *11,* 671–684.

Craik, F. I., & Tulving, E. Depth of processing and the retention of words in episodic memory. *Journal of Experimental Psychology: General,* 1975, *104,* 268–294.

Dasen, P. R. Cross-cultural Piagetian research: A summary. *Journal of Cross-Cultural Psychology,* 1972, *3,* 23–40.

Dasen, P. R. *Piagetian psychology: Cross-cultural contributions.* New York: Gardner Press, 1977.

Egan, D. E. *Accuracy and latency scores as measures of spatial information processing* (Research Report No. 1224). Pensacola, Fla.: Naval Aerospace Medical Research Laboratories, 1976.

Eysenck, H. J. Intelligence assessment: A theoretical and experimental approach. *British Journal of Educational Psychology,* 1967, *37,* 81–98.

Fagan, J. F., & McGrath, S. K. Infant recognition memory and later intelligence. *Intelligence,* 1981, *5,* 121–130.

Frederiksen, J. R. Component skills in reading: Measurement of individual differences through chronometric analysis. In R. E. Snow, P.-A. Federico, & W. E. Montague (Eds.), *Aptitude, learning, and instruction: Cognitive process analyses of aptitude* (Vol. 1). Hillsdale, N.J.: Erlbaum, 1980.

Frederiksen, N. Factors in in-basket performance. *Psychological Monographs: General and Applied,* 1962, *76*(22, Whole No. 541).

Frederiksen, N. Validation of a simulation technique. *Organizational Behavior and Human Performance,* 1966, *1,* 87–109.

Frederiksen, N., Saunders, D. R., & Wand, B. The in-basket test. *Psychological Monographs,* 1957, *71* (9, Whole No. 438).

Galton, F. *Inquiry into human faculty and its development.* London: Macmillan, 1883.

Garrett, H. E. Differentiable mental traits. *Psychological Record,* 1938, *2,* 259–298.

Garrett, H. E. A developmental theory of intelligence. *American Psychologist,* 1946, *1,* 372–378.

Geiselman, R. E., Woodward, J. A., & Beatty, J. Individual differences in verbal memory performance: A test of alternative information-processing models. *Journal of Experimental Psychology: General,* 1982, *111,* 109–134.

Goldberg, R. A., Schwartz, S., & Stewart, M. Individual differences in cognitive processes. *Journal of Educational Psychology,* 1977, *69,* 9–14.

Guilford, J. P. *The nature of human intelligence.* New York: McGraw-Hill, 1967.

Guilford, J. P. Components versus factors. *Behavioral and Brain Sciences,* 1980, *3,* 591–592.

Guilford, J. P., & Hoepfner, R. *The analysis of intelligence.* New York: McGraw-Hill, 1971.

Guthrie, E. R. *The psychology of learning.* New York: Harper & Row, 1935.

Guttman, L. A new approach to factor analysis: The radex. In P. F. Lazarsfeld (Ed.), *Mathematical thinking in the social sciences.* Glencoe, Ill.: Free Press, 1954.

Guttman, L. A faceted definition of intelligence. In R. R. Eiferman (Ed.), *Scripta Hierosolymitana* (Vol. 14). Jerusalem, Israel: Magnes Press, 1965.

Guyote, M. J., & Sternberg, R. J. A transitive-chain theory of syllogistic reasoning. *Cognitive Psychology,* 1981, *13,* 461–525.

Hofstaetter, P. R. The changing composition of intelligence: A study of the *t*-technique. *Journal of Genetic Psychology,* 1954, *85,* 159–164.

Holzinger, K. J. Relationships between three multiple orthogonal factors and four bifactors. *Journal of Educational Psychology,* 1938, *29,* 513–519.

Horn, J. L. Organization of abilities and the development of intelligence. *Psychological Review,* 1968, *75,* 242–259.

Hunt, E. B. Mechanics of verbal ability. *Psychological Review,* 1978, *85,* 109–130.

Hunt, E. B., Frost, N., & Lunneborg, C. Individual differences in cognition. In G. Bower (Ed.), *The psychology of learning and motivation: Advances in research and theory* (Vol. 7). New York: Academic Press, 1973.

Hunt, E. B., Lunneborg, C., & Lewis, J. What does it mean to be high verbal? *Cognitive Psychology,* 1975, *7,* 194–227.

Intelligence and its measurement: A symposium. *Journal of Educational Psychology,* 1921, *12,* 123–147, 195–216, 271–275.

Jarvik, L. F., Eisdorfer, C., & Blum, J. E. *Intellectual functioning in adults.* New York: Springer, 1973.

Jensen, A. R. Hierarchical theories of mental ability. In W. B. Dockrell (Ed.), *On intelligence.* Toronto, Canada: Ontario Institute for Studies in Education, 1970.

Keating, D. P., & Bobbitt, B. L. Individual and developmental differences in cognitive-processing components of mental ability. *Child Development,* 1978, *49,* 155–167.

Keating, D. P., Keniston, A. H., Manis, F. R., & Bobbitt, B. L. Development of the search-processing parameter. *Child Development,* 1980, *51,* 39–44.

Klahr, D. *Self-modifying production systems as models of cognitive development.* Unpublished manuscript, Carnegie-Mellon University, 1979.

Koffka, K. *Principles of Gestalt psychology.* New York: Harcourt, Brace, 1935.

Köhler, W. *The mentality of apes.* New York: Harcourt, Brace, 1927.

Köhler, W. *Gestalt psychology: An introduction to the new concepts in modern psychology.* New York: Liveright, 1947.

Kuhn, T. S. *The structure of scientific revolutions* (2nd ed.). Chicago: University of Chicago Press, 1970.

Lewis, M., & Brooks-Gunn, J. Visual attention at three months as a predictor of cognitive functioning at two years of age. *Intelligence,* 1981, *5,* 131–140.

McCall, R. B., Eichorn, D. J., & Hogarty, P. S. Transitions in early mental development. *Monograph of the Society for Research in Child Development*, 1977, No. 171.

McCall, R. B., Hogarty, P. S., & Hurlburt, N. Transitions in infant sensorimotor development and the prediction of childhood IQ. *American Psychologist*, 1972, 27, 728–748.

McNemar, Q. *The revision of the Stanford–Binet Scale: An analysis of the standardization data*. Boston: Houghton Mifflin, 1942.

Mehrabian, A. *Nonverbal communication*. Chicago: Aldine, 1972.

Miles, T. R. On defining intelligence. *British Journal of Educational Psychology*, 1957, 27, 153–165.

Mischel, W. *Introduction to personality*. New York: Holt, Rinehart & Winston, 1971.

Neisser, V. *Cognition and reality: Principles and implications of cognitive psychology*. San Francisco: Freeman, 1976.

Neisser, V. The concept of intelligence. *Intelligence*, 1979, 3, 217–227.

Newell, A. Production systems: Models of control structures. In W. Chase (Ed.), *Visual information processing*. New York: Academic Press, 1973.

Newell, A., Shaw, J. C., & Simon, H. A. Elements of a theory of human problem solving. *Psychological Review*, 1958, 65, 151–166.

Newell, A., & Simon, H. A. *Human problem solving*. Englewood Cliffs, N.J.: Prentice-Hall, 1972.

Olneck, M. R., & Crouse, J. The IQ meritocracy reconsidered: Cognitive skill and adult success in the United States. *American Journal of Education*, 1979, 88, 1–31.

Osherson, D. N. *Logical abilities in children*: Vol. 2. *Logical inference: Underlying operations*. Hillsdale, N.J.: Erlbaum, 1974.

Piaget, J. *The psychology of intelligence*. Totowa, N.J.: Littlefield, Adams, 1976.

Rose, A. M. *An information processing approach to performance assessment* (NR 150-391 ONR Final Report). Washington, D.C.: American Institutes for Research, 1978.

Rosenthal, R., Hall, J. A., DiMatteo, M. R., Rogers, P. L., & Archer, D. *Sensitivity to nonverbal communication*. Baltimore: Johns Hopkins University Press, 1979.

Royce, J. R. The conceptual framework for a multi-factor theory of individuality. In J. R. Royce (Ed.), *Multivariate analysis and psychological theory*. New York: Academic Press, 1973.

Schneider, W., & Shiffrin, R. M. Controlled and automatic human information processing: I. Detection, search, and attention. *Psychological Review*, 1977, 84, 1–66.

Skemp, R. R. *Intelligence, learning, and action*. New York: Wiley, 1979.

Spearman, C. "General intelligence," objectively determined and measured. *American Journal of Psychology*, 1904, 15, 201–293.

Spearman, C. *The nature of "intelligence" and the principles of cognition*. London, England: Macmillan, 1923.

Spearman, C. *The abilities of man*. New York: Macmillan, 1927.

Sternberg, R. J. *Intelligence, information processing, and analogical reasoning: The componential analysis of human abilities*. Hillsdale, N.J.: Erlbaum, 1977.

Sternberg, R. J. The nature of mental abilities. *American Psychologist*, 1979, 34, 214–230.

Sternberg, R. J. The development of linear syllogistic reasoning. *Journal of Experimental Child Psychology*, 1980, 29, 340–356. (a)

Sternberg, R. J. A proposed resolution of curious conflicts in the literature on linear syllogisms. In R. Nickerson (Ed.), *Attention and performance VIII*. Hillsdale, N.J.: Erlbaum, 1980. (b)

Sternberg, R. J. Sketch of a componential subtheory of human intelligence. *Behavioral and Brain Sciences*, 1980, 3, 573–584. (c)

Sternberg, R. J. The evolution of theories of intelligence. *Intelligence*, 1981, 5, 209–230. (a)

Sternberg, R. J. Intelligence and nonentrenchment. *Journal of Educational Psychology*, 1981, 73, 1–16. (b)

Sternberg, R. J. The nature of intelligence. *New York University Education Quarterly*, 1981, 12, 3, 10–17. (c)

Sternberg, R. J. Nothing fails like success: The search for an intelligent paradigm for studying intelligence. *Journal of Educational Psychology*, 1981, 73, 142–155. (d)

Sternberg, R. J. Novelty-seeking, novelty-finding, and the developmental continuity of intelligence. *Intelligence*, 1981, 5, 149–155. (e)

Sternberg, R. J. Testing and cognitive psychology. *American Psychologist*, 1981, 36, 1181–1189. (f)

Sternberg, R. J. Toward a unified componential subtheory of human intelligence: I. Fluid abilities. In M. Friedman, J. Das, & N. O'Connor (Eds.), *Intelligence and learning*. New York: Plenum, 1981. (g)

Sternberg, R. J. A componential approach to intellectual development. In R. J. Sternberg (Ed.), *Advances in the psychology of human intelligence* (Vol. 1). Hillsdale, N.J.: Erlbaum, 1982.

Sternberg, R. J., Conway, B. E., Ketron, J. L., & Bernstein, M. People's conceptions of intelligence. *Journal of Personality and Social Psychology: Attitudes and Social Cognition*, 1981, *41*, 37–55.

Sternberg, R. J., & Powell, J. S. The development of intelligence. In P. Mussen (Ed.), *Carmichael's manual of child psychology* (3rd ed.). New York: Wiley, in press.

Sternberg, R. J., & Smith, C. Components of social intelligence. Unpublished manuscript, Yale University, 1982.

Sternberg, R. J., & Wagner, R. The nature and measurement of practical intelligence. Unpublished manuscript, Yale University, 1982.

Sternberg, S. The discovery of processing stages: Extensions of Donders' method. *Acta Psychologica*, 1969, *30*, 276–315.

Thomson, G. H. *The factorial analysis of human ability*. London, England: University of London Press, 1939.

Thorndike, E. L. Intelligence and its uses. *Harper's Magazine*, 1920, *140*, 227–235.

Thorndike, E. L. The measurement of intelligence: Present status. *Psychological Review*, 1924, *31*, 219–252.

Thorndike, E. L. *Human learning*. New York: Century, 1931.

Thorndike, E. L., Bregman, E. O., Cobb, M. V., & Woodyard, E. I. *The measurement of intelligence*. New York: Teachers College, 1926.

Thurstone, L. L. *Primary mental abilities*. Chicago: University of Chicago Press, 1938.

Vernon, P. E. *Intelligence and cultural environment*. London, England: Methuen, 1969.

Vernon, P. E. *The structure of human abilities*. London, England: Methuen, 1971.

Vernon, P. E. *Intelligence: Heredity and environment*. San Francisco: Freeman, 1979.

Watson, J. B. *Behaviorism* (rev. ed.). New York: Norton, 1930.

Wertheimer, M. *Productive thinking*. New York: Harper & Row, 1945.

Whitely, S. E. Latent trait models in the study of intelligence. *Intelligence*, 1980, *4*, 97–132. (a)

Whitely, S. E. Modeling aptitude test validity from cognitive components. *Journal of Educational Psychology*, 1980, *72*, 750–769. (b)

Whitely, S. E., & Schneider, L. M. *Generalizing componential theory to psychometric analogies* (NIE Technical Report NIE-81-2). Lawrence, Kansas: Department of Psychology, University of Kansas, 1981.

Wober, M. Towards an understanding of the Kiganda concept of intelligence. In J. W. Berry & P. R. Dasen (Eds.), *Culture and cognition: Readings in cross-cultural psychology*. London, England: Methuen, 1974.

Name index

Locke, J., 500, 502, 516
Locke, W. N., 366
Lockhart, R., 991
Lockhart, R. S., 6, 195
Loda, R. A., 597
Loehlin, J. C., 104, 565, 610, 792, 819, 821, 829, 834, 848, 849, 854, 861, 863, 865, 866, 867, 870
Loevinger, J., 42, 66, 67, 68, 320, 326, 327
Loftus, E. F., 208, 211, 214, 518–19
Loftus, G. R., 145, 518–19
Lohman, D. F., 6, 10, 78, 139, 141, 165n1, 543, 550
Lohnes, P. R., 79
London, M., 254
Lonner, W. J., 645
Lord, F. M., 65, 66, 67, 68, 79, 102, 453
Lord, F. W., 63, 332
Lorenz, K. Z., 174, 750
Loretan, J. O., 92
Lotan, M., 159
Lovell, K., 915, 917
Lubbock, Sir John, 736
Lubovsky, V. I., 440, 442, 449
Luce, R. D., 77
Luchins, A. S., 272, 312, 313
Luchins, E. H., 312, 313
Lumsdaine, A. A., 497
Lumsden, J., 68
Lund, N. J., 236
Lunneborg, C. L., 4, 9, 76, 79, 124, 125, 404, 550, 724, 977, 992
Lunzer, E. A., 236, 245, 248–9
Luria, A. R., 655, 695, 704
Luther, Martin, 500, 502
Lutkus, A. D.,, 254, 261
Lynn, R., 475
Lyon, D. R., 158, 196, 199, 206, 237, 409
Lytton, H., 829

McAlpine, W., 609
MacArthur, R. S., 661
McAskie, M., 828
McCall, R. B., 174, 904–5, 995
McCarrell, N. S., 930
McCarthy, D., 911
McCauley, C., 317, 410, 421
McClearn, G. E., 104, 744, 792, 815, 832, 846, 849, 866, 870
McClelland, D. C., 338, 343, 599, 601
McClelland, J. L., 9, 132–5, 136, 138, 146, 147, 149–50, 162, 399, 405, 406
McClure, W. E., 55
Maccoby, E. E., 870, 874
McCormick, E. J., 101
McCormick, W., 596
McCullough, C. M., 102–3
McDermott, R. P., 471, 693, 701
McDonald, J. F., 506, 798

McDonald, R. P., 70, 73
McElwain, D. W., 685
Macfarlane, J., 906
MacFarlane, J. W., 333
McFie, J., 678, 679
McGarvey, B., 78
McGaugh, J. L., 820
McGee, M. G., 139, 141, 542, 869, 870, 871, 875, 876
McGeogh, J. A., 209, 468, 469, 515,
McGlynn, R. P., 878
McGrath, S. K., 995
McGuinness, D., 877, 878
McGuire, M., 782n
McGuire, R., 376, 380
McGuire, T. R., 792
McGuire, W. J., 255
Machado, L. A., 538
McHenry, H. M., 775
Machover, S., 680
McIntyre, C. W., 925
McKay, H., 536–7, 538, 547
McKeachie, W. J., 497
Mackenberg, E. G., 875
Mackintosh, N. J., 182, 748, 752
Mackler, B., 596
McKusick, V. A., 815
Mackworth, N. H., 402
McLaughlin, D. H., 683
MacLeod, C. M., 12, 14, 129, 146, 149, 151, 152, 153, 163, 550
McLuhan, M., 689
MacMillan, D. L., 408
McNeil, J. T., 538
McNemar, Q., 83, 84, 172, 194, 506, 514, 518, 793, 795, 904, 907, 995
McPartland, J., 603
Madden, J., 623
Magnusson, D., 531
Mahoney, G. J., 925
Maier, N. R. F., 4, 7, 285, 287, 288, 291, 292, 293, 294–5
Malcolm, N., 726, 765
Malinowski, B., 649
Maltzman, I., 270, 544–5
Mandler, G., 210, 691
Mandler, J. M., 402, 694
Manis, F. R., 921
Manosevitz, M., 819
Manouvrier, Léonce-Pierre, 728, 729, 730
Mansfield, R. S., 545
Manuilenko, Z. V., 712n16
Marcus, S., 255
Marjoribanks, K., 103
Markey, P. R., 757
Markkanen, T., 866
Markham, E. M., 450, 462, 916, 927, 928, 929
Markova, A. K., 712n16

Subject index